# SURGICAL PATHOLOGY OF THE NERVOUS SYSTEM AND ITS COVERINGS

# SURGICAL PATHOLOGY OF THE NERVOUS SYSTEM AND ITS COVERINGS

**Fourth Edition**

## Peter C. Burger, MD

Professor, Department of Pathology
Johns Hopkins University School of Medicine
Baltimore, Maryland

## Bernd W. Scheithauer, MD

Professor, Department of Pathology and
Laboratory Medicine
Mayo Medical School
Consultant in Surgical Pathology
Mayo Clinic
Rochester, Minnesota

## F. Stephen Vogel, MD

Professor Emeritus, Department of Pathology
Duke University School of Medicine
Durham, North Carolina

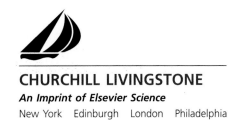

**CHURCHILL LIVINGSTONE**
*An Imprint of Elsevier Science*
New York   Edinburgh   London   Philadelphia

CHURCHILL LIVINGSTONE
*An Imprint of Elsevier Science*

The Curtis Center
Independence Square West
Philadelphia, Pennsylvania 19106

| | |
|---|---|
| Acquisitions Editor: | Natasha Andjelkovic |
| Developmental Editor: | Jennifer Shreiner |
| Project Manager: | Agnes Hunt Byrne |
| Production Manager: | Peter Faber |
| Illustration Specialist: | Robert Quinn |
| Book Designer: | Ellen Zanolle |

SURGICAL PATHOLOGY OF THE NERVOUS SYSTEM AND ITS COVERINGS

ISBN 0–443–06506–3

Printed in China

Last digit is the print number: 9 8 7 6 5 4 3 2 1

*To those patients*
*whose unfortunate illnesses*
*have provided us with information*
*we hope*
*will be beneficial to others*

# PREFACE

The breadth and depth of surgical neuropathology continues to expand as "new" entities are described, "old" lesions are subcategorized, intricate new grading systems are developed, and histopathologic evaluations are supplemented by molecular analysis. All of these advances are addressed in this extensively revised and enlarged edition of *Surgical Pathology of the Nervous System and Its Coverings*. The perennial problems of interpreting needle biopsy specimens and the analysis of specimens removed for seizure control are the subjects of new chapters. Discussions of many entities now include specific subsections covering tumor definition as well as clinical, radiologic, and pathologic features. To ensure that critical differential diagnostic lesions are not overlooked, a Diagnostic Checklist is attached to the discussion section of all major lesions. Many neuroradiologic images, both CT and MR, illustrate topographic and anatomic features relevant to pathologists and clinicians alike. To add both interest and utility to this book, nearly all macroscopic and microscopic illustrations are now in color. For similar reasons, multiple summary tables appear throughout the text. We have tried to make this a practical, user-friendly book, and hope that we have succeeded.

Peter C. Burger
Bernd W. Scheithauer
F. Stephen Vogel

# ACKNOWLEDGMENTS

One of the pleasures in completing this edition of *Surgical Pathology of the Nervous System and Its Coverings* is the opportunity to recognize the efforts of individuals who provided material or advice. We are therefore pleased to acknowledge the contributions of the photographic staff at Johns Hopkins University School of Medicine and Mayo Clinic. In Baltimore, Norman Barker has our deepest appreciation for his attention to detail in the preparation of photomicrographs and digital images of whole mount histologic sections. Ellen Winslow and Zuhair Kareem were similarly devoted to detail. In Rochester, Randy Ziegler and the late Louis Nichols fulfilled comparable roles; each took a personal interest in the project.

Patricia Goldthwaite's assistance in retrieving clinical histories, slides, and radiologic images was invaluable. Drs. Thomas Montine and Orest Boyko volunteered for the unglamorous task of reviewing proofs. Drs. Elias Melhem and Martin Pomper contributed radiographs and helpful suggestions. Drs. Henry Brem, William E. Krauss, and John C. D. Atkinson graciously opened their extensive files of operative photographs.

At Johns Hopkins, Rosemary Rogers readily offered help in preparing the manuscript. At Mayo Clinic, Carrie Sharp and Charice Mehring contributed greatly to this effort. Our thanks must also go to Mark Strauss for his advice and his patience and to Jennifer Shreiner who was always helpful as an interface between authors and the production staff at W.B. Saunders.

More generally, we are grateful for the culture of academic excellence at Johns Hopkins Medical Institutions and Mayo Foundation that encourages projects such as the preparation of this text.

Finally, we acknowledge the tolerance of our families for the unusual work schedules that let us accomplish much of this project in hours that otherwise would have been happily dedicated to vacations or domestic pursuits.

Peter C. Burger
Bernd W. Scheithauer
F. Stephen Vogel

# CONTENTS

# SKULL AND RELATED SOFT TISSUES

1

The diversity of anatomic structures in the head region and their juxtaposition to the central nervous system challenge both the clinician and pathologist with a heterogeneous array of neurologic signs and pathologic lesions. Despite the non-neural character of most of these, they do fall within the bailiwick of neuropathology, un-derscoring the catholic scope of the discipline and its intimate relation to general anatomic pathology.

## NON-NEOPLASTIC MASSES

### Fibrous Dysplasia

**Definition.** A benign, generally self-limiting fibro-osseous lesion.

**Clinical Features.** Fibrous dysplasia is a skeletal disorder of unknown etiology characterized by monostotic or polyostotic foci wherein normal bone is altered by abnormal fibro-osseous proliferation. Usually detected during the first three decades of life, it favors such sites as the long bones of the extremities, the ribs, and the skull (Figs. 1–1 to 1–7).[3] Spinal involvement is discussed in Chapter 10 on page 507. Fibrous dysplasia is sometimes associated with accelerated, but eventually stunted, skeletal growth as well as with extraskeletal abnormalities such as pigmented skin lesions and rarely sexual precocity. The last usually occurs in females and constitutes McCune-Albright syndrome when associated with cutaneous lesions and polyostotic fibrous dysplasia (Figs. 1–2 and 1–3).[4]

In the skull, fibrous dysplasia affects the facial, frontal, ethmoid, and sphenoid bones followed in incidence by the temporal, parietal, and occipital bones.[14] Signs and symptoms reflect the typical unilaterality of the monostotic form: facial involvement results in asymmetry, an orbital lesion produces proptosis,[6, 14] narrowing of an optic foramen compromises vision (see Fig. 1–8),[5, 6, 12–14] impingement on other foramina produces cranial nerve deficits,[8, 9, 11, 14] and a lesion of the vault causes a scalp mass.

The term "fibro-osseous dysplasia" can be used to describe skull base and gnathic lesions with an abundance of osseous trabeculae.

**Radiologic Features.** The lesions are usually focal, well-defined zones of rarefaction surrounded by a narrow rim of relatively sclerotic bone. The radiographic

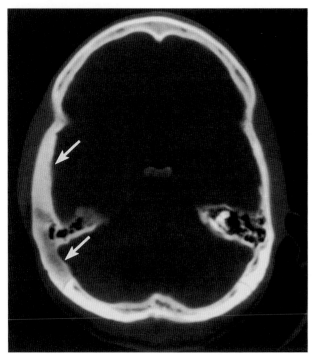

**FIGURE 1–1** FIBROUS DYSPLASIA

The thickened right temporal bone lesion in a 31-year-old man shows both "sclerotic" (anterior arrow) and "ground glass" (posterior arrow) appearances of fibrous dysplasia. (Courtesy of Dr. Elias Melhem, Baltimore, MD.)

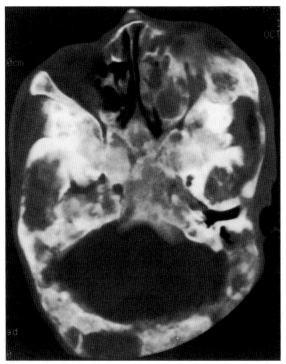

**FIGURE 1–2** FIBROUS DYSPLASIA IN McCUNE-ALBRIGHT SYNDROME

The thickening and variable lytic and sclerotic areas are apparent in this CT scan of the skull of a patient with long-standing McCune-Albright syndrome.

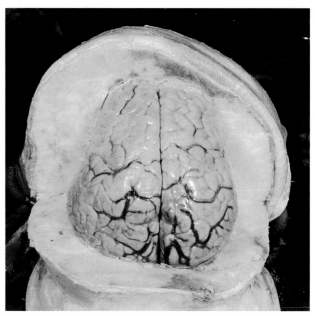

**FIGURE 1–3** FIBROUS DYSPLASIA IN McCUNE-ALBRIGHT SYNDROME

Fibrous dysplasia in its most exuberant form is illustrated in this 22-year-old woman with McCune-Albright syndrome. The massively thickened skull dwarfs the brain and encases it with the same intimate, yet separable, relationship that the fleshy fruit of an avocado has to its seed.

appearance varies somewhat depending on their content of trabecular bone or even focally calcified cartilage. Thus, mixed, sclerotic, and pagetoid patterns are encountered, as are cystic foci (Figs. 1–1, 1–2, and 1–5).[1] An occasional lesion bulges into surrounding soft tissue.

**Macroscopic Features.** Focal fibrous dysplasia of the cranial vault is typically a well-defined process, but the disease can be extensive and not present as a focal lesion. Such diffuse involvement with massive calvarial thickening is seen in McCune-Albright syndrome (Fig. 1–3). Some focal examples of fibrous dysplasia are composed predominantly of dense fibrous tissue, whereas others are granular and gritty because of spicules of bone (Fig. 1–6). Only a rare lesion is markedly sclerotic and requires decalcification. The presence of rich vascularity superimposes redness on their basic tan or gray color.

**Microscopic Features.** The soft lesions consist of dense fibrous tissue composed of plump spindle cells without cytologic atypia. Such cells may be disposed in a storiform pattern. Occasional tumors are somewhat myxoid in appearance. Mitoses are rare. Gritty ones contain spicules of "metaplastic" or "woven" bone. Such spicules are born as eosinophilic condensations of the osteoid and grow into short, curved or arcuate segments wherein the matrix is coarse and unaligned and osteocytes are large and undisciplined in arrangement. The spicules create letter forms jumbled as those in alphabet soup (Figs. 1–7 to 1–9). The borders of the spicules merge with the surrounding stroma without a conspicuous rim of osteoblasts (Figs. 1–9 and 1–10). Termed fibro-osseous metaplasia, such bone formation is in itself not abnormal. To some observers, its exclusive

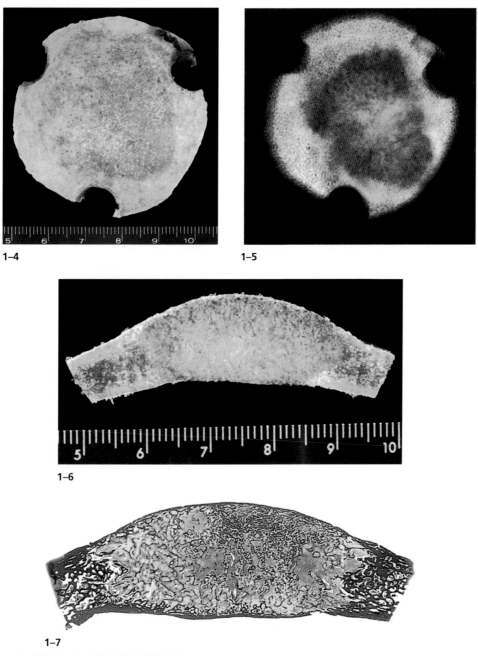

1–4

1–5

1–6

1–7

**FIGURES 1–4, 1–5, 1–6, AND 1–7**   FIBROUS DYSPLASIA

This sector of skull was excised from the frontal bone of an 18-year-old student who noted a painless enlargement over a 2-year period. An external view of the specimen (Fig. 1–4) and a radiograph (Fig. 1–5) emphasize the flocculent radiolucency of fibrous dysplasia. A cross section (Fig. 1–6) and its companion histologic section (Fig. 1–7, Masson) illustrate the expansile nature of fibrous dysplasia and its composition of fibrous tissue and irregular bony spicules.

presence is the hallmark of fibrous dysplasia, the manifestation of a basic defect wherein spicules are unable to complete their wonted maturation to lamellar bone. Occasional lesions form round, ossicle-like structures resembling the psammoma bodies of meningiomas.

As the fibrous dysplasia matures, the spicules broaden irregularly and their boundaries become more clearly demarcated in the now mature fibrous stroma. Over time, this appearance stabilizes, although even after many years no conversion to lamellar bone takes place. The irregularly thickened trabeculae with their jumbled configura-

tion of the cement lines may produce a pagetoid appearance. Also common are collections of foam cells or of giant cells. Chondroid metaplasia may be extensive.

**Differential Diagnosis.** Given variation in its sites of occurrence and radiographic appearance, the differential diagnosis of fibrous dysplasia can theoretically include a host of other lesions. However, the deforming nature of the process, especially when involving orbital and facial bones; the youth of the patients; and the distinctive histologic appearance of the lesion, when unaltered by pre-

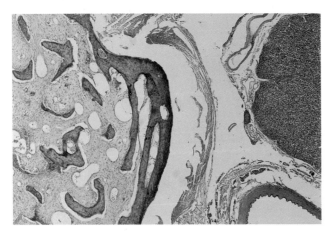

**FIGURE 1–8**   FIBROUS DYSPLASIA

Involvement of the orbit and the skull base may encroach on the optic nerve seen at the right of the illustration (H&E–Luxol fast blue).

vious treatment or superimposed fracture, point to the correct diagnosis.

   *Osteoma* is distinguished by the presence of osteoblasts around spicules of lamellar bone. Furthermore, in contrast to the predominant diploic involvement of fibrous dysplasia, osteomas grow from the cortex. The *hyperostosis associated with meningioma* is customarily seen at a more advanced age and is noted for spicules of new bone arrayed in a radial, "hair-on-end" fashion relative to the cortical surface (see Figs. 1–46 and 1–47).

**Treatment and Prognosis.** The lesions of fibrous dysplasia usually stabilize at or shortly after puberty. Nonetheless, surgery may be necessary for diagnosis, decompression of nearby structures, or correction of a deformity.[2] Sarcomatous degeneration, an uncommon complication, occurs more often after radiotherapy than as an event de novo.[7, 10, 17] Cranial examples are rare.[15–17]

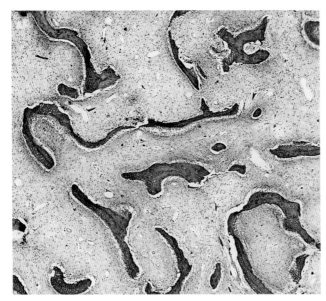

**FIGURE 1–9**   FIBROUS DYSPLASIA

As is characteristic of fibrous dysplasia, atolls of woven bone emerge from a sea of fibrous tissue.

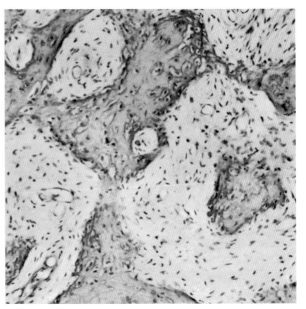

**FIGURE 1–10**   FIBROUS DYSPLASIA

Microscopically, fibrous dysplasia is characterized by irregular trabeculae of bone in a dense fibrous matrix. Note that cement lines are not oriented along lines of stress. As a rule, there is a paucity of osteocytes and only scant osteoblastic activity.

# Langerhans Cell Histiocytosis (Histiocytosis X, Eosinophilic Granuloma)

**Definition.** A proliferation of Langerhans cells usually associated with a mixed inflammatory infiltrate in which eosinophils are prominent.

**General Comments.** The disorder encompasses a group of histiocytic disorders that range from an innocuous solitary focus to multiple lesions of bone ("eosinophilic granuloma") and to an often lethal,

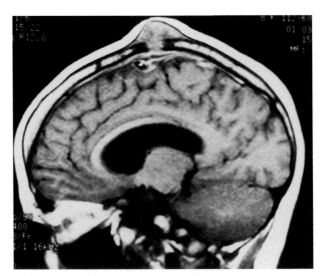

**FIGURE 1–11**   EOSINOPHILIC GRANULOMA

This 8-year-old girl presented with a bump on the bregma. There were no other osseous or soft tissue lesions.

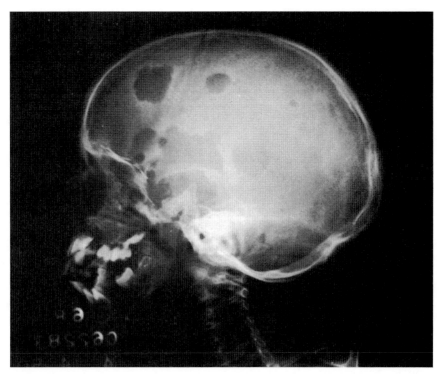

**1–12**

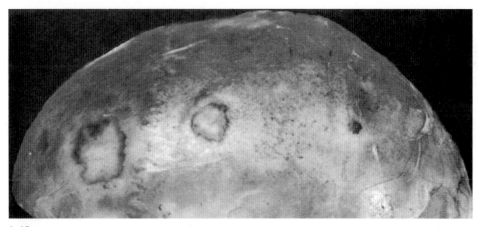

**1–13**

**FIGURES 1–12 AND 1–13**   MULTIFOCAL EOSINOPHILIC GRANULOMA

A $3\frac{1}{2}$-year-old girl expired 2 years after presentation with bleeding gums. During this interval, she had developed lymphadenopathy, hepatosplenomegaly, cutaneous foci, and multiple lytic skull lesions. The skull radiograph obtained shortly before death shows the discrete lesions within the vault, base of the skull, and jaws (Fig. 1–12). Three of these lesions can be seen in the skull cap obtained at autopsy (Fig. 1–13).

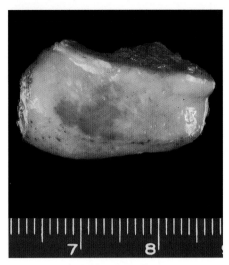

**FIGURE 1–14    EOSINOPHILIC GRANULOMA**

Discrete and expansile, this tender, lytic lesion was excised from the left parietal bone of a 2-year-old girl. The lesion is fleshy and mottled with yellow.

disseminated disorder with visceral involvement (Letterer-Siwe disease). Whether the latter is part of the disease spectrum is unsettled. The present discussion is limited to the far more common lesion of eosinophilic granuloma in both its solitary and multifocal variants. The rare lesions that arise in the brain are discussed on pages 146 to 148.

The benign course of eosinophilic granuloma in its solitary form suggests that it is an inflammatory rather than a neoplastic disorder. Nonetheless, clonality has been reported and with it the suggestion that the

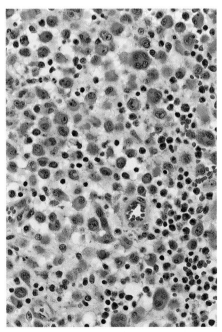

**FIGURE 1–15    EOSINOPHILIC GRANULOMA**

Pathognomonic of eosinophilic granuloma is the admixture of Langerhans cells and inflammatory cells, among which eosinophils are prominent. Note the typical convoluted, cleft nuclei of the Langerhans cells.

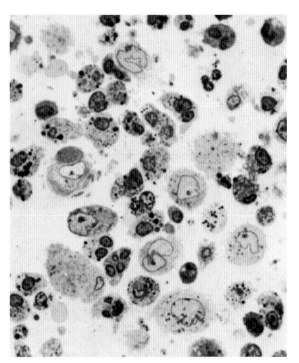

**FIGURE 1–16    EOSINOPHILIC GRANULOMA**

Langerhans cells, the principal cell type in eosinophilic granuloma, are well seen in a 1-µm Epon-embedded section. The densely granulated eosinophils contrast with the large pale histiocytes with their complex nuclear contours (toluidine blue–azure B).

process is neoplastic.[6] An additional study, however, failed to find evidence of T-cell receptor gene rearrangements.[7] In any case, the solitary lesion is a biologically benign process in almost all instances.

**Clinical Features.** Solitary eosinophilic granuloma of bone is the most common expression of Langerhans histiocytosis. Most lesions appear before age 30 and are especially frequent between 2 and 20 years. The process usually affects the cranial vault (Fig. 1–11). Tenderness and a palpable mass usually bring it to medical attention.

Multifocal eosinophilic granuloma generally makes its appearance in younger patients. With respect to the

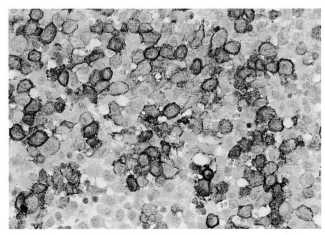

**FIGURE 1–17    EOSINOPHILIC GRANULOMA**

The Langerhans cells are immunoreactive for CD1A.

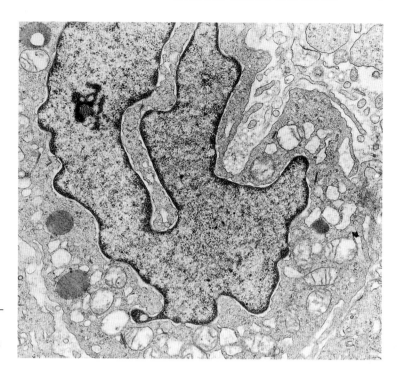

**FIGURE 1-18** EOSINOPHILIC GRANULOMA

The nuclear membranes of the histiocytes are sinuously redundant. The numerous and diagnostically important Langerhans granules are inconspicuous at this magnification (×11,000).

skull, the lesions usually affect both the vault and base (Figs. 1–12 and 1–13). Proptosis, growth retardation, and diabetes insipidus are predictable consequences. Otitis media may complicate mastoid involvement. When associated with skull base and sellar involvement as well as diabetes insipidus, the condition is referred to as Hand-Schüller-Christian disease.

**Radiologic Features.** Absolute osteolysis with a "justified" margin lacking in sclerosis is a characteristic feature. Occasional skull lesions show a "hole in a hole" appearance because of differential involvement of the inner and outer tables. A retained central nidus of radiodensity is also common. Some lesions become confluent and destructive in appearance. Periosteal new bone formation may be seen.

**Macroscopic Features.** At surgery, the soft, gray-tan to yellow lesions span several centimeters, elevate the galea, and extend through the full thickness of the skull (Fig. 1–14). Although they often adhere to the dura, the latter remains intact and unpenetrated.

**Microscopic Features.** The lesion is a mixture of large, pleomorphic histiocytes with ill-defined cytoplasmic boundaries and smaller inflammatory cells, among which eosinophils are often conspicuous (Figs. 1–15 and 1–16). The histiocytes may be dispersed or clustered, lending an epithelioid quality, but do not form truly cohesive sheets. Langerhans cells have folded and indented the nuclei, whose complex contours are best seen at high magnification, particularly in plastic-embedded semithin sections (see Fig. 1–16). Their nucleoli are small to

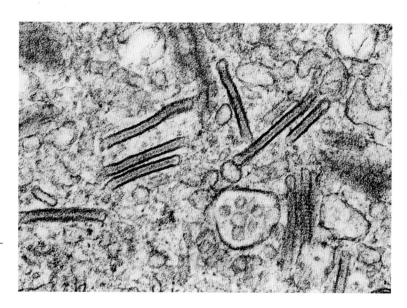

**FIGURE 1-19** EOSINOPHILIC GRANULOMA

The fine structure of the Langerhans granule is apparent when a cell is viewed under higher magnification. These enigmatic structures consist of an outer membrane ensheathing a striated, electron-dense core (×130,000).

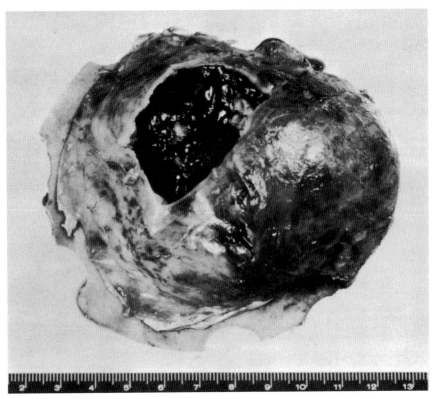

1–20

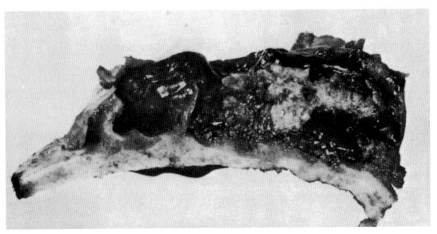

1–21

**FIGURES 1–20 AND 1–21**    ANEURYSMAL BONE CYST

A 77-year-old woman had noted a protrusion on her forehead for more than 20 years. During the 6 months before excision, the mass had rapidly enlarged and become tender. As is characteristic, the hemorrhagic cyst had expanded through the outer bony table and elevated the galea (Fig. 1–20). The inner table is only minimally involved (Fig. 1–21).

moderate in size. Mitoses in variable numbers show no relation to the subsequent course of the disease. Sometimes numerous scattered bi- or multinucleated histiocytes as well as foam cells embellish the lesion. Foam cells predominate in some examples and seemingly reflect the chronicity of the process.

Inflammatory cells vary in number and include mainly eosinophils, lymphocytes, and occasional plasma cells. The eosinophils may be dispersed or densely aggregated. Necrosis may be seen and is sometimes exten-

sive. In some instances, polymorphonuclear leukocytes are numerous and prompt consideration of osteomyelitis.

**Immunohistochemical Features.** Langerhans cells are immunoreactive for CD1A (Fig. 1–17) and S-100 protein.[2]

**Ultrastructural Features.** At the fine structural level, Langerhans, histiocytes bristle with small processes. Their cytoplasm contains both lysosomes and a

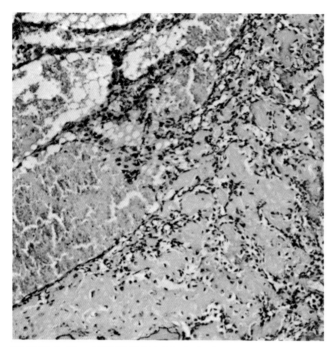

**FIGURE 1–22**    ANEURYSMAL BONE CYST

Prominent histologic features of aneurysmal bone cyst include multiple thin-walled vascular channels associated with considerable osteoid and fibrous tissue.

distinctive organelle known as the Birbeck granule (Figs. 1–18 and 1–19).[2] Formed of two parallel unit membranes sandwiching a striated electron-dense core, this pentalaminar structure often originates from fusion of cell surface membranes and ends in a bulbous terminal expansion.

**Treatment and Prognosis.** Solitary eosinophilic granuloma of the skull, especially in a teenager, is nearly always a self-limiting process cured by excision alone. An occasional lesion even regresses spontaneously. Small doses of irradiation may be of use in the presence of a recurrence.[1, 3] It is uncommon for additional lesions to appear and is even more unusual for the disease to extend into extraosseous tissue.

The prognosis of multifocal eosinophilic granuloma is variable. Lesions restricted to bone carry a favorable prognosis, although significant morbidity and mortality are associated with Hand-Schüller-Christian disease. Factors associated with significant morbidity, or an occasional fatal outcome, include an onset before 2 years and predominantly visceral or extraosseous involvement.[5] Splenomegaly, hepatomegaly with liver dysfunction, anemia, and thrombocytopenia are also unfavorable prognostic signs.[4]

## Aneurysmal Bone Cyst

**Definition.** A non-neoplastic, hemorrhagic, multicystic, and expansile lesion of bone.

**Clinical Features.** Aneurysmal bone cysts are lesions of uncertain genesis that occur in almost any bone, even the skull.[2–8] Most arise de novo, unaccompanied by a preexisting lesion. An association with prior fracture has been noted only occasionally. Areas similar to aneurysmal bone cyst are found in a variety of usually benign bone lesions, including giant cell tumor, chondroblastoma, chondromyxoid fibroma, and fibrous dysplasia, all of which can affect the skull. At this location, a tender, palpable scalp mass is usually responsible for its discovery (Figs. 1–20 and 1–21). Less often, the process expands inwardly to compress brain or cranial nerves. Like their extracalvarial counterpart, most aneurysmal bone cysts evolve over the first two decades.

**Radiologic Features.** Aneurysmal bone cysts appear to arise in the medullary cavity. The generation of new bone in the cyst wall does not offset the overall osteolytic nature of the lesion. Nonetheless, a thin rim of residual subperiosteal bone may be present. Cortical destruction may be complete. A "bubbly" appearance is seen in the expanded region body of the cyst, and blood-fluid levels can be noted.[7] Accordingly, computed tomographic (CT) and magnetic resonance (MR) scans may reveal internal septations.[8]

**Macroscopic Features.** Aneurysmal bone cysts are characterized by prominent vascular channels that impart a sponge-like appearance and are responsible for the effusion of blood during resection (see Fig. 1–21). Compact bone is inserted as delicate trabeculae between the vascular channels. Such intact specimens are uncommon. Instead, the typical specimen consists of fragments of red-brown, granular material.

**Microscopic Features.** Cavernous, pseudovascular channels are the hallmark of aneurysmal bone cyst. These consist of connective tissue septa of variable thickness and composition, some being merely strands of fibrous tissue and others consisting of granulation tissue and proliferating fibroblasts, which, although mitotically active, lack atypia. Osteoid, bone, and giant cells may also contribute to the lesion. These elements may also form solid tissue near the periphery of the lesion (Fig. 1–22). Occasional lesions are entirely solid ("solid ABC"). Leakage of blood, recent and/or remote, is evidenced by extravasated erythrocytes or hemosiderin-laden macrophages, respectively.

**Immunohistochemical Features.** The absence of endothelial cells is confirmed by lack of immunoreactivity for factor VIII–related antigen.[1]

**Differential Diagnosis.** The diagnosis of aneurysmal bone cyst is suggested generally by radiographic studies or on gross examination, especially when the specimen is intact. On the other hand, vigorous application of curettage often mutilates the lesion and obscures its vascular nature. In such fragments the giant cell component may be misinterpreted as *giant cell tumor*, and osteoid and proliferating spindle cells can be misinterpreted as *osteosarcoma*, particularly of the telangiectatic type. *Hemangioma* with its abundance of vascular spaces also enters into the differential, but its radiating bone spicules

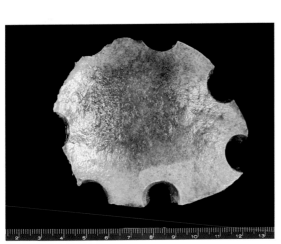

1–23

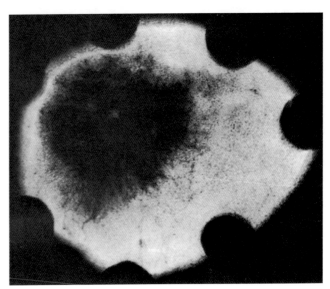

1–24

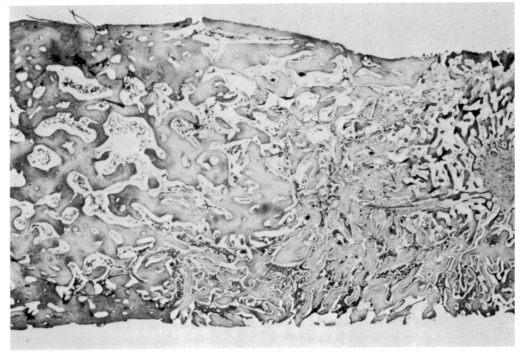

1–25

**FIGURES 1–23, 1–24, AND 1–25** PAGET'S DISEASE (OSTEOPOROSIS CIRCUMSCRIPTA)

This tender, lytic lesion was discovered incidentally in the occipital bone of a 65-year-old woman during a work-up for chronic brain syndrome. Typical of Paget's disease, the red-brown lesion contrasts with the surrounding white calvarium (Fig. 1–23). Although predominantly radiolucent, the lesion is mottled by radiodense foci (Fig. 1–24). A histologic section shows the characteristic resorption of the cortices and the abundance of trabeculae that are irregular in size and distribution (Fig. 1–25).

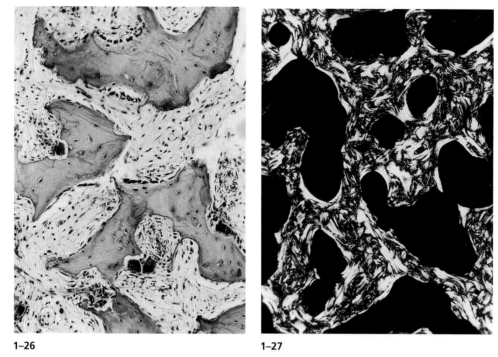

1–26                                    1–27

**FIGURES 1–26 AND 1–27    PAGET'S DISEASE**

As seen in Figure 1–26, the characteristic feature of Paget's disease is the energetic, but uncoordinated, activity of osteoblasts and osteoclasts. The jumbled pattern of bony spicules stands out when the mature lesion is viewed under polarized light (Fig. 1–27).

and lack of an exuberant fibroblast, giant cell, and osteoblastic response are impartial distinguishing features.

**Treatment and Prognosis.** The aneurysmal bone cyst is a benign lesion cured by total excision and often by simple curettage. Recurrence rarely follows even a subtotal resection.[6] Nonetheless, the prognosis is excellent.

## Paget's Disease

**Definition.** A skeletal disorder of unknown etiology affecting such diverse bones as the pelvis, femur, skull, tibia, and vertebrae.

**Clinical Features.** Although its consummate form includes obvious bone deformities related to osseous thickening and distortion, a more common manifestation is the clinically silent, monostotic lesion. Paget's disease usually becomes evident after the fourth decade and is somewhat more common in men.

The signs and symptoms of advanced cranial Paget's disease of the skull are usually referable to deformity of the skull base. The thickened bone impinges on canals and foramina to produce cranial nerve deficits, particularly deafness. The massive but weakened skull may settle, causing basilar impression and neurologic signs referable to pressure on the cranial nerves and medulla as well as the cervical spinal cord and nerves.[2, 3] Advanced disease may be associated with hydrocephalus and dementia.[5, 6, 9, 10] The osteoporosis circumscripta

stage is usually asymptomatic and is discovered radiologically in the presence or absence of known Paget's disease elsewhere.

**Macroscopic and Microscopic Features.** In the skull, the disorder is especially fascinating, not only because of the remarkable deformation that results but also because of the well-documented pathologic stages through which the bones are remodeled. The earliest phase is localized resorption of bone ("osteoporosis circumscripta") with resultant areas of radiolucency (Fig. 1–23 and 1–24).[1, 4, 8, 11] At this stage, the skull is not appreciably thickened but has a spongy, pitted appearance most apparent in cortex. Both increased vascularity and exposure of the marrow space impart a red to purple color. The destructive osteoclastic activity leaves a residue of widely spaced, narrow trabeculae separated by fibrovascular tissue devoid of marrow elements.

Coincident with the final stages of bone resorption, osteoblasts assert themselves and multiple trabeculae of new bone are formed (Figs. 1–25 to 1–27). Radiolucency may persist unless the spicules are sufficiently compacted or thickened to produce dense islands. Continued osteoblastic activity results in the formation of supernumerary and irregularly thickened trabeculae. The aberrant manner in which this remodeling occurs is apparent in their abnormal organization as well as in the jumbled, angular cement lines that are the hallmark of this disease (Fig. 1–28). This appearance results from the simultaneous, vigorous, and uncoordinated activity of both osteoblasts and osteoclasts—one undoing what the other has just completed. In its final form, the

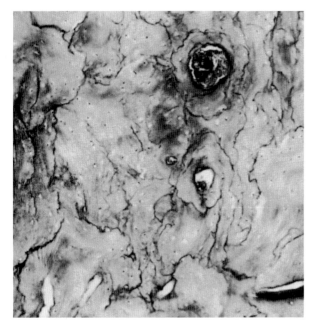

**FIGURE 1–28**   PAGET'S DISEASE

The mature lesion of Paget's disease exhibits the classic, mosaic pattern of cement lines.

medullary cavity and cortex of the skull are markedly thickened. Qualitatively, the abnormal bone has been likened to pumice stone (Fig. 1–29). Unlike that in fibrous dysplasia, the radiographic density of pagetoid bone is less than that of normal bone, from which it is sharply demarcated.

Very uncommonly, the appearance of a mass in a patient with known Paget's disease indicates "sarcomatous degeneration" to osteosarcoma or, less often, to fibrosarcoma. Its occurrence is suggested by radiographic lysis or the appearance of a palpable calvarial mass in a patient with established Paget's disease (Figs. 1–29 and 1–30).

**Differential Diagnosis.** Paget's disease of the skull is usually encountered in surgical material in the lytic stage, where it must be differentiated from a malignant neoplasm. Indeed, pagetoid bone may be seen in *osteosarcoma* and as a reaction to *metastatic carcinoma*. Furthermore, in florid disease the process may, to a limited extent, involve adjacent soft tissue.

**Treatment and Prognosis.** The development of sarcoma is a dreaded complication.[7, 12–18] Osteosarcoma, the most common type (see Fig. 1–29), may appear in pure form or in combination with fibrosarcoma or chondrosarcoma, either of which may occur alone. The high degree of malignancy of these sarcomas is reflected in the less than 2% 5-year survival reported in one study.[12] Giant cell tumors arising in the setting of Paget's disease are discussed on page 23.

## Mucocele

**Definition.** A non-neoplastic epithelial cyst originating within paranasal sinuses.

**General Comments.** Although their occasional association with other pathologic lesions suggests that occlusion

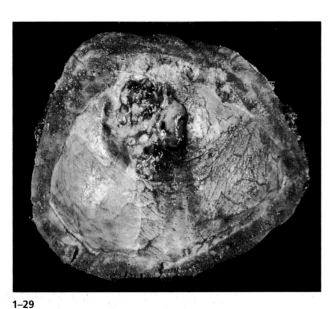

1–29

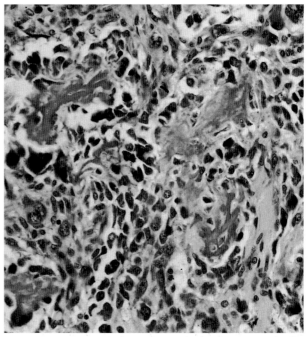

1–30

**FIGURES 1–29 AND 1–30**   OSTEOSARCOMA IN PAGET'S DISEASE

Sarcomatous degeneration of Paget's disease has produced a focal exophytic mass on the otherwise diffusely thickened calvarium (Fig. 1–29). As seen in Figure 1–30, such tumors are typically osteosarcomas.

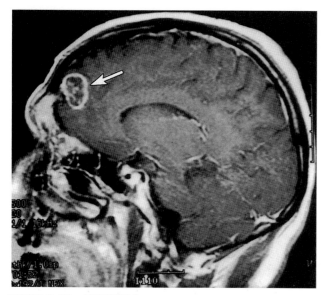

**FIGURE 1–31**   MUCOCELE

Mucoceles are discrete, sinus-based masses that may displace intracranial structures, in this case a frontal lobe. This lesion produced headaches in a 42-year-old man. Mucoceles are typically bright on T2-weighted MR scans because of their protein-rich, mucinous content. This lesion is contrast enchancing.

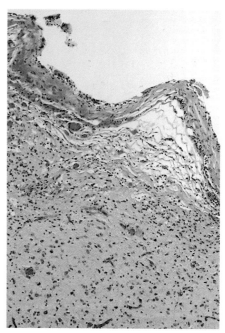

**FIGURE 1–32**   MUCOCELE

Mucoceles can compress and become secondarily attached to the brain.

of sinus ostia is the initiating factor, mucoceles are not an inevitable or even common result of such obstruction.

**Clinical Features.** Mucoceles may occur in any sinus, but the frontal is most frequently affected and is also the sinus most often affected by osteomas.[7, 8, 11, 12] Though benign and non-neoplastic, the lesion may expand slowly at the expense of adjacent bone, the latter yielding to the continual pressure. The fibrous walled cyst is then free to expand beyond the confines of its sinus and impinges on regional structures, such as orbital contents, cranial nerves, the pituitary, or even the brain (Fig. 1–31).[1-6, 8-13]

**Macroscopic Features.** The thin-walled lesion is filled with viscid material.

**Microscopic Features.** The lining is ciliated, columnar, mucus-producing epithelium (Fig. 1–32) but may be altered by squamous metaplasia and pressure atrophy. Fibrous wall mucoceles often contains foci of inflammatory cells, usually chronic. Long-standing examples may become denuded and are then lined only by histiocytes and occasional giant cells.

**Treatment and Prognosis.** Total resection is curative. Like certain other cystic lesions, such as colloid cyst of the third ventricle and craniopharyngioma, mucoceles can, albeit rarely, rupture into the cerebrospinal space, resulting in severe chemical meningitis.

## Cholesterol Granuloma

This inflammatory response to accumulated cholesterol produces an erosive mass at the petrous apex. Symptoms include dizziness, tinnitus, and hearing loss.[1] The process has a distinctive MR profile, being hyperintense (bright) on both T1- and T2-weighted images. Hemosiderin deposits at the edge of the lesion generate a rim of hypointense or dark T2 signal.[1-3] The destructive effect on the bone is well seen by CT (Fig. 1–33).

Histologically, cholesterol granulomas consist of an admixture of old hemorrhage, chronic inflammation, cholesterol clefts, and foreign body giant cells (Fig. 1–34). The lesions are effectively treated by simple excision alone.[1]

## BENIGN NEOPLASMS

### Hemangioma

**Definition.** A cavernous angioma or less often capillary hemangioma occurring in the skull.

**General Comments.** The majority of hemangiomas of bone involve the cranial vault, particularly the parietal and frontal bones,[2] or vertebrae. Most are solitary, but multiple lesions do occur.

**Clinical Features.** The lesion is usually seen as an outward expansion in the form of a painful scalp mass (Fig. 1–35). Less often, by inward extension, the mass compresses the brain.[5] Calvarial hemangiomas usually appear during midlife. The significant (3:2) female predilection is unexplained.

**Radiologic Features.** By MR, the expansile lesion is recognized by its hyperintense signal on both precontrast T1-weighted and T2-weighted images (Fig. 1–35).[1]

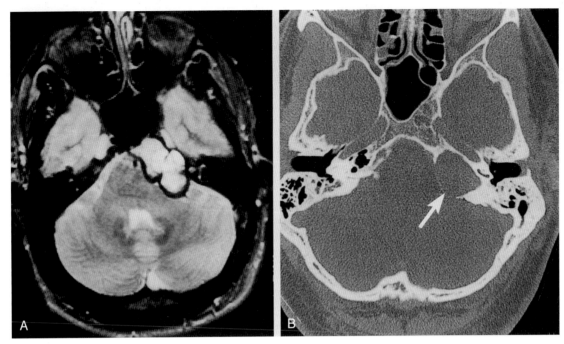

**FIGURE 1–33**    CHOLESTEROL GRANULOMA

A 35-year-old man presented with headaches, dysequilibrium, and hearing loss. Characteristically bright on T2-weighted MR images, the lesion is surrounded by a dark rim corresponding to hemosiderin-stained tissue (*A*). The erosive effects of the lesion on the petrous bone are seen in a CT scan (*B*).

In radiographs of the skull or the specimen, hemangiomas are lytic, sharply defined masses with a sclerotic border and often expansion of the bony profile with a distinctive, honeycomb trabecular pattern and radiating, sunburst-like spicules.[4]

**Macroscopic Features.** At surgery the lesion is often blue, with an obvious honeycombed architecture. Even in resected or fragmented specimens, hemangiomas appear as multiple blood-filled channels interposed between spicules of bone (Figs. 1–36 to 1–38). New bone is generally added to the convexity of the skull but does not overshadow the lesion's overall lytic effect.

**Microscopic Features.** In most cases, the vascular channels are those of a conventional cavernous angioma; that is, they are unaccompanied by muscle or elastic tissue and contain a variably thick layer of collagen. Hemangiomas of the capillary type are far less common. Bone, fat, and hematopoietic elements garnish the lesion (Figs. 1–38 and 1–39).

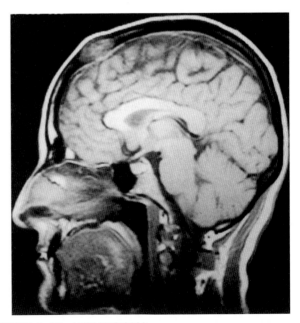

**FIGURE 1–35**    HEMANGIOMA

This 50-year-old woman noticed a bump on the head. In this precontrast T1-weighted MR image, the frontal lesion appears as a hyperintense mass because of blood and/or blood products.

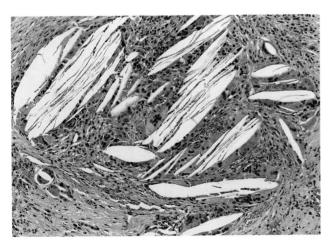

**FIGURE 1–34**    CHOLESTEROL GRANULOMA

Cholesterol clefts, foreign body giant cell reaction, and hemosiderin deposits are characteristics of this non-neoplastic lesion.

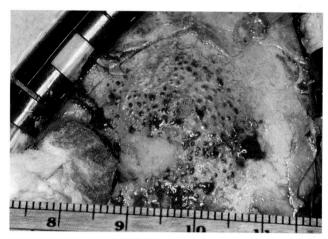

**FIGURE 1–36**   HEMANGIOMA

Exposed at surgery, the lesion is distinctive for the multiple vascular channels that reach its surface. The radiologic features of this lesion are illustrated in Figure 1–35. (Courtesy of Dr. Henry Brem, Baltimore, MD.)

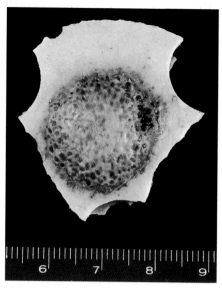

**FIGURE 1–37**   HEMANGIOMA

The excised hemangioma is a well-circumscribed, elevated mass. Collapsed vascular channels crater the surface.

**Differential Diagnosis.** When uninformed about the radiographic appearance of the lesion, the surgical pathologist might consider other vascular lesions of bone, including *aneurysmal bone cyst.* The latter, however, lacks endothelial lining cells; contains considerable osteoid, granulation tissue, and giant cells; and does not form radiating spicules.

**Treatment and Prognosis.** The hemangioma is benign, but it has a malignant counterpart in the skull, the angiosarcoma.[3] Hemangiomas respond well to conservative treatment, although radiation therapy has its place for nonresectable lesions at inaccessible sites.

# Glomus Tumor (Jugulotympanic Paraganglioma)

**Definition.** A benign localized or invasive neuroendocrine neoplasm originating from paraganglionic tissue in the region of the middle ear.

**General Comments.** Diminutive nests of paraganglionic tissue histologically resembling the normal carotid body have been identified in the adventitia of the jugular vein (glomus jugulare), along peripheral portions of the tympanic branch of the glossopharyngeal nerve (Jacobson's nerve), and in juxtaposition to the

**FIGURE 1–38**   HEMANGIOMA

The radiating spicules that characterize hemangioma are apparent in this surgical specimen of frontal bone of a 21-year-old woman. (From Dorfman HD, Steiner GC, Jaffe HL. Vascular tumors of bone. Hum Pathol 1971;2:349–376.)

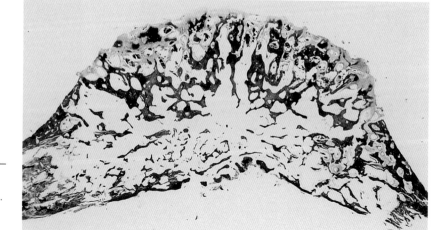

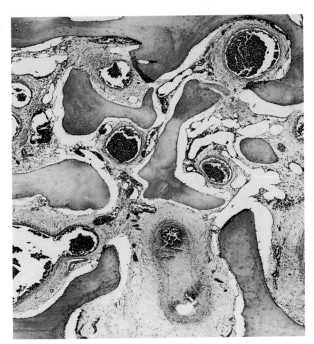

**FIGURE 1–39**   HEMANGIOMA

The anomalous vessels of this cranial hemangioma are variable in caliber and in their content of fibrous tissue.

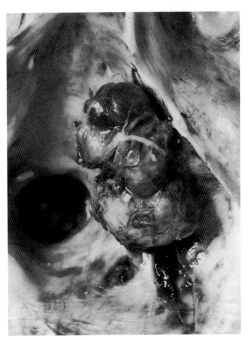

**FIGURE 1–41**   GLOMUS JUGULARE TUMOR

This bilobed neoplasm grew through the temporal bone into the right cerebellopontine angle of a 43-year-old man who had had a radical resection and radiotherapy of a glomus tumor of the middle ear 11 years prior to death.

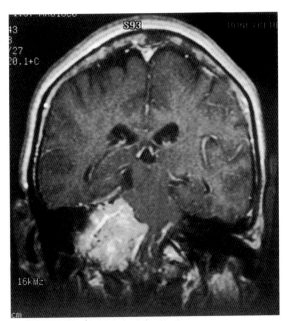

**FIGURE 1–40**   GLOMUS JUGULARE TUMOR

This contrast-enhancing cerebellopontine angle tumor produced multiple cranial nerve palsies in a 65-year-old woman.

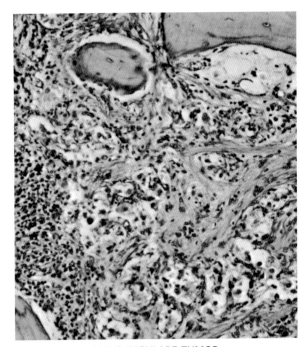

**FIGURE 1–42**   GLOMUS JUGULARE TUMOR

The neoplastic cells are characteristically assembled into nests, even as they infiltrate temporal bone.

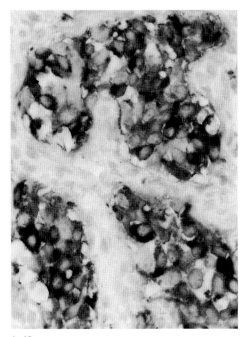 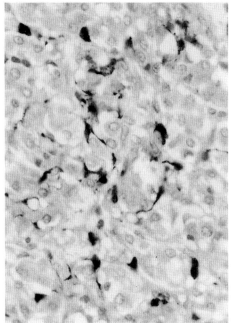

1–43                                    1–44

**FIGURES 1–43 AND 1–44**    GLOMUS JUGULARE TUMOR

Immunopositivity of glomus tumors for chromogranin (Fig. 1–43) confirms the cells' neurosecretory nature and readily excludes most other entities. Elongated sustentacular cells are immunoreactive for S-100 protein (Fig. 1–44).

postauricular branch of the vagus nerve (Arnold's nerve).[5, 15] Whereas glomus tumors arising in the latter two sites are sometimes termed "glomus tympanicum tumors," all three are customarily included under the umbrella term "jugulotympanic" paraganglioma in that they occur in a limited region and have identical histopathologic features. The once popular terms "chromaffin" and "nonchromaffin" paraganglioma are no longer in vogue. Instead, the paragangliomas are now termed "functional" and "nonfunctional" with respect to endocrine effects of catecholamine production.

An informative historical account reviews our understanding of the lesion.[5]

**Clinical Features.** Most paragangliomas in this region occur in women.[9, 14, 15, 16] Most glomus tumors are so positioned as to involve the middle ear, producing hearing loss, tinnitus, otic fullness or pounding, vertigo, and facial weakness.[5, 13, 15, 18] Passing through bony canals, the expanding lesions can compress the extracranial portions of other cranial nerves (Fig. 1–40). The tumors can emerge in the cerebellopontine angle as a discrete, lobulated mass compressing cranial nerves, brain stem, or cerebellum (Fig. 1–41).[1, 16] Approximately 40% of jugulotympanic paragangliomas show such intracranial extension.

Only a few glomus jugulare tumors produce clinically detectable amounts of catecholamines.[10, 15] Thus, signs of endocrine function (hypertension, palpitation, and sweating) are infrequent. They can, however, be induced by intraoperative tumor manipulation.

**Radiologic Features.** Their high vascularity is particularly evident on T2-weighted MR scans as a classical "salt-and-pepper" pattern resulting from the presence of "flow voids," the dark signal that emanates from flowing blood.[12, 18] On CT one may see infiltration along nerves as well as a ragged tumor outline related to bone invasion.

**Microscopic Features.** The round to polygonal cells of glomus tumors typically congregate in small nests (Zellballen) (Fig. 1–42) but may also lie dispersed between dilated vascular channels. Their spherical to ovoid nuclei with inconspicuous nucleoli frequently exhibit the salt-and-pepper pattern of neuroendocrine cells. Variation in cell size and chromatin content is evident in some tumors, but neither feature is of prognostic significance. Low-level mitotic activity may also be present. Ganglion cells are rarely seen. Most tumors exhibit a characteristic network of reticulin that defines small blood vessels and encircles small nests of cells. Stromal connective tissue varies in quantity and distribution, sometimes appearing as densely hyalinized masses.

**Immunohistochemical Features.** Chief cells, the principal constituent, are chromogranin and neuron-specific enolase (NSE) immunopositive (Fig. 1–43). The elongated sustentacular cells that surround Zellballen, and may lie among chief cells, are strongly S-100 protein, and occasionally glial fibrillary acidic protein (GFAP), reactive (Fig. 1–44).[6] Neuropeptide expression (somatostatin, serotonin, leu- and met-enkephalin) may also be seen. An enzyme active in catecholamine synthesis, tyrosine hydroxylase, can also be demonstrated.[17] Norepinephrine has been identified by histochemical methods.[3]

**Ultrastructural Features.** The ultrastructural features of glomus tumors are distinctive.[2, 7] Chief cells exhibit dense core granules measuring 100 to 400 nm (mean, 150 nm). Because of variations in cytoplasmic density, both "light" and "dark" chief cells are recognized. Both feature interdigitating cell processes and rudimentary junctions. A layer of basal lamina is present at the interface of Zellballen and stroma. In addition to well-developed Golgi, endoplasmic reticulum, and lysosomes, chief cells may contain numerous mitochondria and paranuclear intermediate filament whorls. Sustentacular cells are characterized by elongated nuclei with marginal chromatin, increased cytoplasmic electron density, and the presence of intermediate filaments. These "supporting" cells lack dense core granules.

**Differential Diagnosis.** Because of the position of the tumor and its characteristic histologic appearance, the surgeon usually directs the pathologist to the diagnosis. Nonetheless, other infiltrative tumors occur in this area. *Metastatic carcinoma* is more destructive of bone and is usually recognized by its anaplasia. Sharing features with glomus tumor, *meningiomas* may involve the petrous ridge and infiltrate bone and present a lobular pattern in histologic sections. Distinguishing features of the meningioma include the usual osteoblastic response it engenders, the tumor's whorled architecture, and the presence of psammoma bodies. The immunohistochemical demonstration of chromogranin reactivity and the absence of epithelial membrane antigen (EMA) staining remove any doubt regarding the nature of the lesion.

**Treatment and Prognosis.** Glomus tumors are potentially curable by excision,[13, 15, 18] but symptomatic recurrences, often late, and metastases can occur.[4, 8] In one study, one half of jugulotympanic examples recurred after surgical resection.[7] Radiation therapy is used in some centers.[7, 11]

# Meningioma

**Clinical Features.** Although meningiomas hesitate to invade the brain on their inner aspects, the opposite is true over their outer surfaces, where their dural attachment places them in broad and intimate contact with the skull. Bone invasion is frequent here but is not indicative per se of malignancy (Figs. 1–45 to 1–47).

Some pericranial "meningiomas" are thought to be hamartomatous and perhaps related to acoelous meningoceles.[15] Primary meningiomas in the lung,[6, 11] finger,[3] and mediastinum[26] are medical curiosities.

In addition to meningiomas that secondarily involve the cranial bones and soft tissues, rare examples appear truly ectopic in the skull (Figs. 1–48 to 1–50)[14, 18] or in extracranial soft tissues. Among the latter, favored sites include parotid gland,[2, 5, 10, 27] nose and paranasal region,[7, 12, 13, 20–24] neck,[7, 8] and scalp (Fig. 1–51).[1, 15, 17]

Meningiomas in bone are discovered most often during radiologic evaluation of unrelated neurologic dysfunction or are entirely fortuitous radiographic findings. In some instances, a meningioma occurs as a scalp mass and is detected by the patient, the physician, or, as he momentarily recaptures his historic role in medicine, the barber.

The presence of meningioma cells in the bone typically provokes an osteoblastic response with hyperostosis (see Figs. 1–45 to 1–47).[16, 19, 25] A lytic reaction is far less common.[9, 16] Although hyperostotic reactions can be observed anywhere in the skull, most occur either along the greater wing of the sphenoid bone and underlie an en plaque meningioma or in the frontal or parietal regions overlying a bregmatic or parasagittal tumor. In most instances, this osteoblastic activity is associated with the invasion of the bone, but infiltration is not a prerequisite; proximity alone may be adequate.[4]

**Radiologic Features.** The hyperostotic reaction of the skull is visualized first as irregular deposition of bone on the inner and only later on the outer table (see Fig. 1–46). Radiographs or CT scans show that much of this new bone, particularly that applied to the outer table, consists of radiating spicules that burst perpendicularly from the skull surface. Despite considerable deposition of new bone, the outlines of the inner and outer tables are generally preserved.

**Macroscopic Features.** In the case of primary intraosseous meningiomas, the skull is expanded to form a rock-hard mass. In cases in which meningeal meningiomas traverse the periosteum, a cap of soft tissue overlies the hyperostosis (see Fig. 1–45).

**Microscopic Features.** Although reactive bone formation is usually accompanied by infiltration of meningioma cells, osteoblastic activity may precede the advancing neoplasm. Ordinarily, the invading tumor resembles the parent neoplasm. In some instances, however, whorl and psammoma body formations are relinquished as the cells proceed through bone. Pleomorphism and mitotic activity are no more notable here than in the remainder of the tumor. As periosteum is breached, the cells often continue their centrifugal spread into soft tissues. Osteoblastic activity may be prominent.

Primary meningiomas in the subcutaneum are small masses of meningothelial cells embedded in a connective tissue stroma (see Fig. 1–51)

**Differential Diagnosis.** Bone involvement by meningioma must be distinguished from *metastatic carcinoma.* The latter usually produces a lytic lesion and exhibits the full histologic spectrum of anaplasia. Metastases of *neuroblastoma* produce radiating spicules of bone (see Fig. 1–89), but such tumors occur at a younger age and have an obviously distinguishing composition of primitive cells. Hemangiomas also feature radiating spicules and occur in adults, but they lack a meningothelial component. In the rare situation in which meningothelial cells are not present in the hyperostotic bone, the possibility of other osteoblastic skull lesions must be entertained; the most common is *osteoma.* This lesion, more fully discussed later, obscures the parallel arcs of the inner and outer tables and does not produce radiating spicules.

**Treatment and Prognosis.** Because intracranial meningiomas are prone to recur if not completely excised, bone invasion is of prognostic significance at locations that preclude a gross total excision. Extracranial

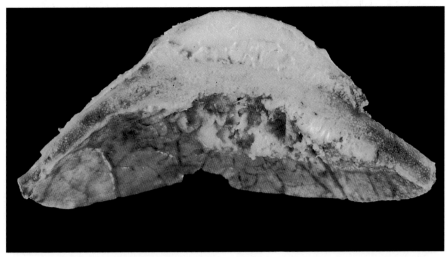

**1–45**

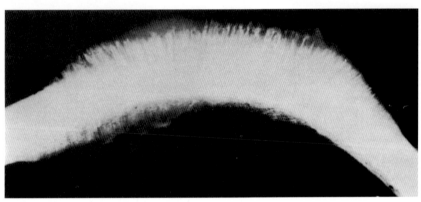

**1–46**

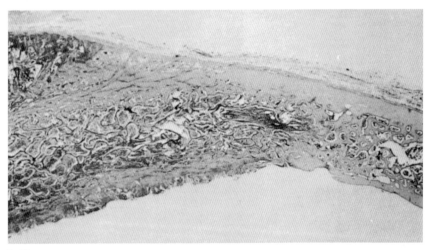

**1–47**

**FIGURES 1–45, 1–46, AND 1–47    MENINGIOMA WITH INVASION OF BONE**

During refraction, a lump was noted on the back of the head of a 44-year-old man who, on questioning, related a 4-week history of episodic right-sided numbness. Surgery disclosed a left parietal, parasagittal meningioma adherent to the falx and diffusely infiltrating the bone. Proximity of the lesion to the patent superior sagittal sinus precluded its total excision. Three years later, when the tumor had occluded this venous channel, it was again approached surgically. The portion of the calvarium removed at the first operation shows spicules that extend from the outer table (Fig. 1–45). A radiograph of the specimen demonstrates the characteristic radiating spicules of new bone as well as the general preservation of the calvarial silhouette (Fig. 1–46). Diffuse infiltration of the bone was seen microscopically (Fig. 1–47).

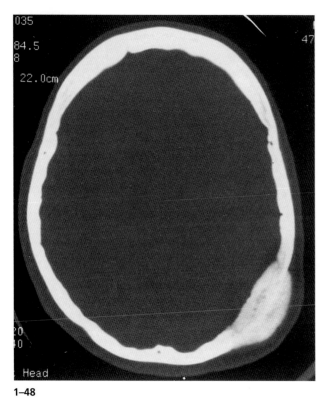

**1–48**

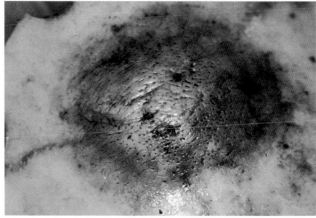

**1–49**

**FIGURES 1–48 AND 1–49**   PRIMARY INTRAOSSEOUS MENINGIOMA

Some meningiomas arise primarily in bone, as in this 27-year-old woman who presented with a bump on the head. As seen in a CT scan (Fig. 1–48), the lesion is markedly osteoblastic. No intracranial component was apparent by either neuroimaging or direct inspection at surgery; only a hard, smooth-surfaced, bony mass was seen (Fig. 1–49).

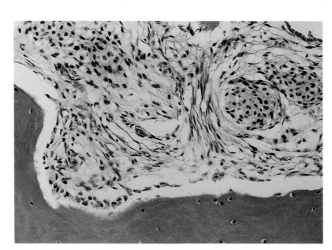

**FIGURE 1–50**   PRIMARY INTRAOSSEOUS MENINGIOMA

Meningothelial cells occupy lacunae of bone and induce osteoblastic activity. The radiologic and macroscopic features of the lesion are shown in Figures 1–48 and 1–49, respectively.

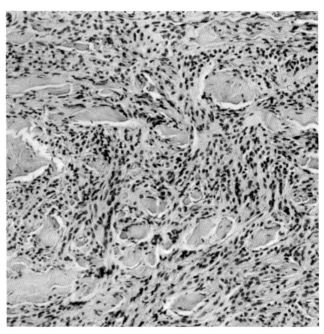

**FIGURE 1–51**   SUBCUTANEOUS MENINGIOMA

A mass had been present for 20 years in the scalp of a 41-year-old man before tenderness prompted its surgical excision. The meningioma appeared primary in subcutaneum; it was not attached to the skull and there was no intracranial component.

meningiomas, particularly those appearing in the scalp at birth, enlarge slowly and are usually cured by simple excision alone.[15]

## Osteoma

**Definition.** A benign local overgrowth of dense cortical bone.

**General Comments.** The osteoma is the quintessential benign tumor. Usually solitary, it consists of a localized proliferation of dense cortical bone. The relationship between osteoma and other "fibro-osseous lesions" is unclear. Its association with mucoceles is discussed on page 12.

**Clinical Features.** Most affect accessory nasal sinuses,[2, 5, 6] the outer and inner tables of the calvarium,[2] the skull base, or a paranasal sinus.[2] No bone of the cranial vault is immune, but the frontal bone is favored. Unquestionably, many skull osteomas remain occult for prolonged periods. When they surface symptomatically, they do so usually during the second through the fourth decades. The triad of Gardner's syndrome includes multiple osteomas as well as colonic polyposis and skin soft tissue tumors, most often epidermal inclusion cysts and fibromatosis.[3, 4, 7]

When symptomatic, osteomas come to medical attention because of their mechanical or cosmetic effects: a nasal sinus is obstructed, orbital contents are displaced, or the cranial contour is disfigured by a protuberance. The lesion enlarges primarily in an outward direction; only a few compress the brain.[2]

**Macroscopic Features.** Typically, the calvarial tumor presents as a nodular elevation that, on cross section, is an expansion of the cortex (Figs. 1–52 to 1–55). The

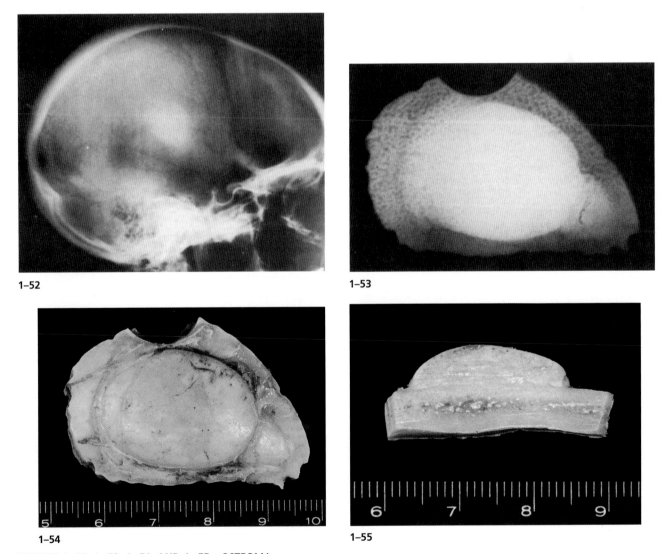

1–52

1–53

1–54

1–55

**FIGURES 1–52, 1–53, 1–54, AND 1–55    OSTEOMA**

A tender mass appeared beneath the right frontoparietal scalp of a 31-year-old woman and enlarged over a period of 8 months prior to excision. Radiographs of the skull (Fig. 1–52) and the excised specimen (Fig. 1–53) emphasize the lesion's discrete, smooth contours and extreme density. Osteomas grow predominantly from the outer table and remain inseparable from the calvarium (Fig. 1–54). The shape of the osteoma is variable; the present lesion forms an ivory button (Fig. 1–55).

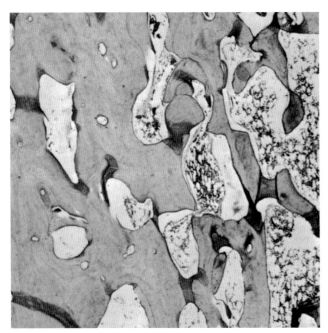

**FIGURE 1–56   OSTEOMA**

This mature osteoma consists of broad, compact trabeculae of lamellar bone.

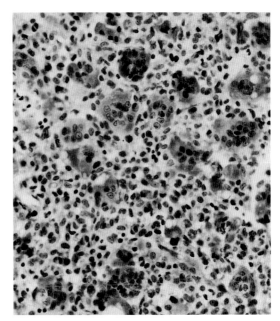

**FIGURE 1–57   GIANT CELL TUMOR**

The lesion has a densely cellular background of mononucleate cells in which some appear to coalesce to form multinucleate cells.

bone is petrous and eburnated, terms that accurately describe its extraordinary compactness.

**Microscopic Features.** Microscopically, the mature lesion consists of dense, sclerotic, lamellar bone similar to that of cortex (Fig. 1–56). Osteoblasts, present in young lesions, diminish with time and dwindle to the point of extinction in mature lesions. The varying ratios of bone to fibrous tissue are emphasized in the qualifying terms fibrous, mature, and ivory osteomas.[1]

**Treatment and Prognosis.** The prognosis after total surgical removal is excellent.[2]

## Giant Cell Tumor

Giant cell tumors are neoplasms of bone with variable degrees of aggressiveness. The vast majority arise in long bones. Most occur in adults, with a peak incidence in the third decade. Of 350 cases of giant cell tumor encountered at the Mayo Clinic, only 3 affected the skull.[5] In this location, they may arise de novo, predominantly during the third to fifth decades and usually involving the sphenoid bone (Fig. 1–57).[1, 4–6] They may rarely arise in other sites, such as the vault[2] or temporal bone.[3] Some appear at a later age in the setting of Paget's disease. Radiologically, they appear as an expanding, destructive lesion.[2, 3] Like their counterparts elsewhere in the body, some giant cell tumors of the skull continue to grow despite surgery and radiotherapy.

## Other Benign Neoplasms

Melanotic progonoma, also termed "retinal anlage tumor" or "pigmented neuroectodermal tumor of infancy," is a rare neoplasm usually encountered in the maxilla of young patients.[16, 21] Several have occurred in the cranial vault[5, 6, 12, 16, 28] and rare examples have been reported in the brain.[21, 37] The neoplasm contains epithelial-like arrangements of melanotic cells intermingled with a small cell component that resembles neuroblasts. Most progonomas are cured by excision alone, although recurrence and metastasis have occurred.

The plasmacytoma is an uncommon cranial lesion that always brings up the issue of the ultimate outcome, that is, does it evolve into multiple myeloma? According to one study, if myeloma is not discovered shortly after surgery for a plasmacytoma, it is unlikely to occur later.[4] Other studies have also suggested a nonrecurrent nature of solitary plasmacytoma.[7, 33] Nonetheless, we are cautious, particularly with reference to a lesion of the skull base, because these, we believe, are more likely to eventuate in myeloma.

Neuroradiologically, plasmacytomas are isointense to gray matter on T2-weighted MR images and show diffuse enhancement.[30] The distinction from chronic osteomyelitis, the main differential diagnosis, is easily achieved with immunostains for immunoglobulin light chains.

Angiofibroma,[8] chondroma,[1, 13, 26, 38] chondroblastoma,[3, 9, 23] chondromyxoid fibroma,[8, 10, 18, 22, 42] chondromyxoma,[31] hemangioendothelioma,[20, 24] desmoplastic fibroma,[35] ossifying fibroma,[11, 14, 25, 40, 41] ceruminoma,[32] lipoma,[39] osteoblastoma,[19, 27] osteochondroma,[2, 15, 17, 34] schwannoma,[36] and teratoma[29] have all occurred in the skull.

# MALIGNANT NEOPLASMS

## Chordoma

**Definition.** A neoplasm of notochordal tissue.

**General Comments.** During development, small nodules of notochordal tissue occasionally embed themselves within the dorsum sellae, project as polypoid masses from the clivus (ecchondrosis physaliphora), or become deeply ensconced in the roof of the nasopharynx. The coincident location of these embryonic structures and of cranial chordomas suggests that the "rests" are precursor lesions of chordomas. The notochordal origin of chordomas leaves unexplained why chordomas rarely occur along most of the vertebral column, a structure in which notochordal derivatives are abundant in the form of intervertebral disks. Aside from their shared axial location, an origin of chordoma from notochordal remnants is also implied by their common light microscopic and ultrastructural features.[5, 7, 8, 11, 31]

Rarely, an intracranial ecchordosis becomes sufficiently large to become symptomatic.[28] In such instances, one faces the semantic distinction between a "giant ecchordosis" and chordoma. The former's circumscribed nature and lack of bone involvement suggest a distinction.[30]

**Clinical Features.** This slowly growing, destructive neoplasm occurs with greatest frequency at the extremities of the axial skeleton. Most are commonly seen during the third through seventh decades and show a sex preference for men (ratio 1.5:1). Children are rarely affected.[1, 10] Spinal examples are discussed in Chapter 10 on pages 508 to 509.

Approximately 40% of chordomas arise at the base of the skull, where they arise in the clivus, that is, the region of the spheno-occipital synchondrosis (see Figs. 1–62 and 1–63). Growth of a clival tumor and destruction of bone result in (1) rostral extension to involve the sella and the cavernous as well as sphenoid sinuses, (2) dorsal displacement of the pons, and (3) posterolateral growth with emergence in the cerebellopontine angle. Only rare tumors are limited to the sella.[27] Recurrent chordomas can be massive.

Common symptoms include headache, cranial nerve palsies (especially of lateral gaze), visual field defects, and long tract signs.[1, 3, 4] Anteroinferior extension may produce a nasopharyngeal mass. Although notochordal rests are midline, the chordoma's growth is often asymmetric, and cranial nerve signs are therefore sometimes unilateral.

**Radiologic Features.** The destructive lesions are irregularly contrast enhancing and hyperintense on T2-weighted MR imaging (Fig. 1–58). The tumor's destructive effect on bone is well seen by CT, as is the frequent calcification. The small localized "ecchordoses" are nonenhancing.[28]

**Macroscopic Features.** Chordomas are lobulated, translucent, and gray and appear encapsulated in all areas but those of bone invasion. Their texture is typically soft or mucinous, but some are firm and

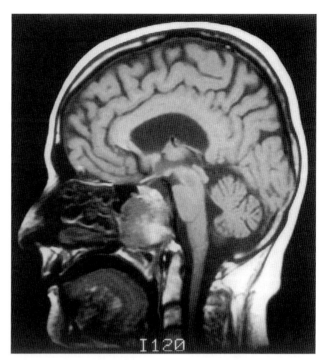

**FIGURE 1–58**   CHORDOMA

As visualized here on MR imaging, intracranial chordomas arise in the clivus, destroy bone, and produce a basilar mass.

resemble chondrosarcomas. Intraoperative hemorrhage may be profuse. Recurrences often produce multiple nodules in the original tumor bed.

**Microscopic Features.** The neoplastic cells are usually disposed in lobules of variable size separated by fibrous septa (Fig. 1–59). Tumor cells differ considerably in cy-

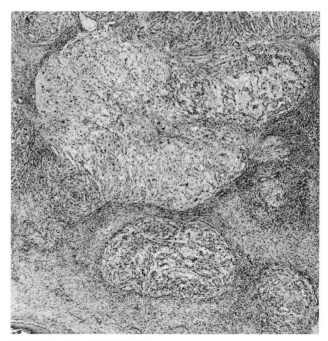

**FIGURE 1–59**   CHORDOMA

The characteristic lobularity of chordomas is readily evident at low magnification.

tologic appearance, configuration, and alignment. Some have well-defined, homogeneous, eosinophilic cytoplasm distinct from surrounding mucoid matrix. Such cells are variously arranged in sheets, clusters, cords, or narrow strands that resemble cords of the liver (Figs. 1–60 to 1–62). Most chordomas contain a spectrum of cells featuring varying amounts of mucin. When abundant, the distinction between intra- and extracellular mucinous material may be obscured (Fig. 1–63). Large cells markedly engorged with mucus vacuoles are termed "physaliphorous cells" (Greek, bubble-bearing) and are the hallmark of chordoma (Fig. 1–64). The frequent presence of transitional forms suggests that, by analogy with the developing notochord, the vacuolated cells evolve from those with solid cytoplasm.[7, 11] On occasion, chordoma cells show considerable nuclear pleomorphism and random mitotic figures.

In addition to their typical components, chordomas may contain areas of cartilaginous (Fig. 1–65) or less often osseous differentiation. Cartilaginous differentiation, the key feature of "chondroid chordoma," may be focal or so extensive as to dominate the histologic picture. Of disputed prognostic significance, this variant of chordoma is discussed later.[3, 6, 16, 21] Accompanying bone formation and fibroplasia are more often reactive than neoplastic in nature.

An uncommon complication of chordoma is malignant transformation, which adds an overtly sarcomatous element to the baseline lesion. In such tumors, the epithelioid component becomes markedly atypical and mitotically active, and a malignant spindle cell component appears.[14, 29]

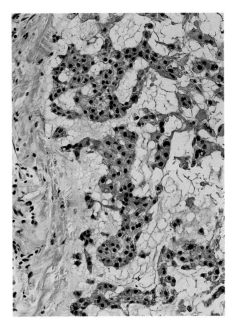

**FIGURE 1–60**   CHORDOMA

Cords of neoplastic cells somewhat resembling those of liver are a common feature of chordomas.

**Cytologic Features.** The cells with distinct cytoplasmic borders are strung out in a mucinous background. Variable vacuolation of cytoplasm is common (Fig. 1–66).

**Immunohistochemical Features.** Both chordoma and notochordal remnants are reactive for cytokeratins, EMA

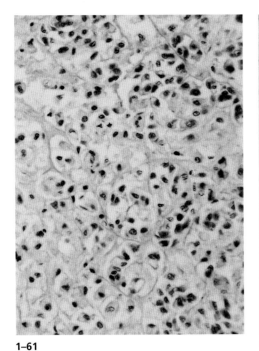

1–61

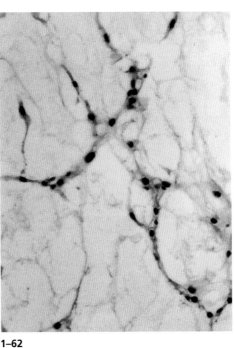

1–62

**FIGURES 1–61 AND 1–62**   CHORDOMA

Other histologic patterns of chordoma include irregular clusters of epithelial cells (Fig. 1–61) and interlacing strands of cells in a mucoid matrix (Fig. 1–62).

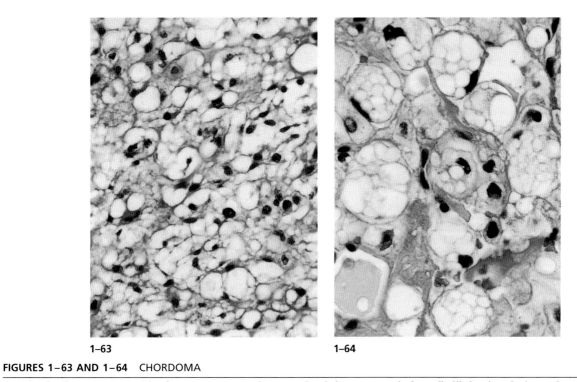

1–63                                    1–64

**FIGURES 1–63 AND 1–64**   CHORDOMA

Vacuolated cells are common in chordomas (Fig. 1–63). The term "physaliphorous" is applied to cells filled with multiple vesicles (Fig. 1–64).

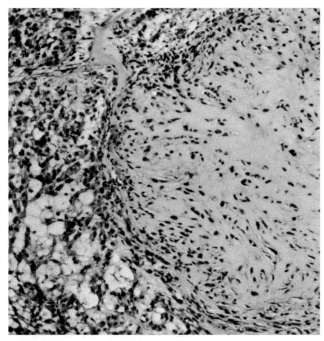

**FIGURE 1–65**   CHONDROID CHORDOMA

Foci of cartilaginous metaplasia may be encountered in the chordoma.

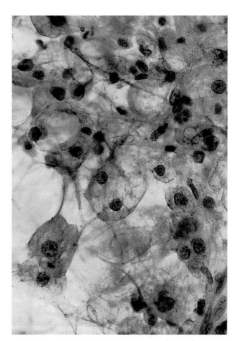

**FIGURE 1–66**   CHORDOMA

As seen in smear preparation, the cells of chordomas are often bland and epithelial in appearance. Note the cytoplasmic vacuoles.

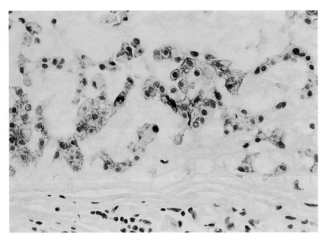

**FIGURE 1–67** CHORDOMA

The epithelial nature of chordoma and its progenitor cells is apparent in its strong staining for epithelial membrane antigen. This, and reactivity for cytokeratins, distinguishes chordoma from such mesenchymal neoplasms as chondrosarcoma.

(Fig. 1–67), and, in approximately 5% of cases, S-100 protein.[12, 14–17, 23, 25]

**Ultrastructural Features.** The presence of a mucinous substance, either within dilated cisternae or as extracellular cytoplasmic invaginations, imparts the vacuolar appearance seen by light microscopy.[5, 7, 11] As in the normal notochord, the cells of a chordoma are connected by well-formed desmosomes.[12, 14, 17, 24]

**Differential Diagnosis.** When the tumor occurs in the skull, the differential diagnosis of chordoma is simplified by the tumor's location, imaging characteristics, and distinctive macroscopic and microscopic features. However, its histologic appearance may be obscured by the cartilaginous differentiation, and the possibility of *chondrosarcoma* must be considered. In such cases, immunohistochemistry aids in this distinction. Unlike chondrosarcoma, chordomas have a decidedly epithelial immunotype that includes immunoreactivity for EMA and cytokeratins.[12, 13, 15, 22]

The lobular deposition of chordoma cells, and their production of mucin, invites confusion with *adenocarcinoma.* In contrast to chordoma, however, carcinoma is unlikely to produce a large, slow-growing, exophytic mass or one that at low magnification forms lobules lacking central necrosis. Although nuclear pleomorphism may be seen in either neoplasm, mitotic figures are much less common in the chordoma than the adenocarcinoma. Both tumors share immunoreactivity for EMA and cytokeratins, but S-100 protein reactivity is far more common in chordoma.[12, 13, 15, 26] Carcinoembryonic antigen is not encountered in chordoma.[13] Two other tumors with a conspicuous chordoid pattern, *chordoid meningioma* and *chordoid glioma of the third ventricle,* are discussed on pages 59 to 61 and 256 to 258, respectively.

**Treatment and Prognosis.** Its central location and the extent to which chordoma permeates bone preclude its total resection. Nonetheless, radiation therapy may extend life but is not curative. Just the same, in one series of patients treated between 1960 and 1984, the 5-year recurrence-free survival was 65%.[4] In yet another, the overall 5- and 10-year survival rates were 51% and 35%, respectively.[2, 3] Rather than conventional radiotherapy, the focused potential of proton beam therapy is increasingly being used in order to spare nearby vital structures.[9]

Although the cranial chordomas do not often metastasize, dissemination to skin, viscera (liver, lung), and spinal meninges has been recorded.[3] It has been proposed that chordomas exhibiting cartilaginous differentiation, so-called chondroid chordomas, have a more favorable prognosis.[6, 19, 20] This was not confirmed in two large studies in which this variant was of no prognostic significance.[3, 18] Instead, any beneficial effect could be attributed to the younger age of most patients with chondroid chordomas.

# Olfactory Neuroblastoma (Esthesioneuroblastoma, Esthesioneuroepithelioma)

**Definition.** A malignant, histologically varied neuroectodermal tumor that arises from specialized olfactory epithelium high in the nasal cavity.

**Clinical Features.** Occurring in almost any decade of life, the tumors produce nasal obstruction, epistaxis, and less often headache, anosmia, excess lacrimation, or ocular disturbances.[3, 13]

**Radiologic Features.** The intranasal mass frequently involves the cribriform plate and is well seen on either CT or MR scan (Fig. 1–68). Although initially in-

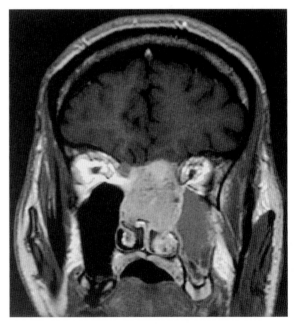

**FIGURE 1–68** OLFACTORY NEUROBLASTOMA

These distinctive tumors arise high in the nasal cavity, as in this 57-year-old woman who complained of nasal fullness. As seen in a contrast-enhanced image, the lesion penetrates the cribriform bone and elevates the left frontal lobe.

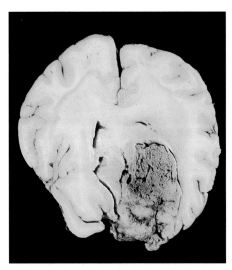

**FIGURE 1–69**   OLFACTORY NEUROBLASTOMA

A 29-year-old man presented with unilateral nasal obstruction, frontal headaches, and intermittent epistaxis. He refused further treatment and succumbed after 4 months as a consequence of intracranial extension. (Courtesy of Dr. Americo A. Gonzalvo, Tampa, FL.)

tranasal, with enlargement the tumors can penetrate the cribriform plate, mushroom into the intracranial compartment, and elevate the frontal lobes (Fig. 1–69).[11, 19, 21] The lesions are variably contrast enhancing.[9] Some lesions are calcified.

**Macroscopic Features.** Most olfactory neuroblastomas form polypoid, soft to friable but occasionally gritty tumors that are gray-red, highly vascular, and often hemorrhagic.

**Microscopic Features.** The histologic appearances of olfactory neuroblastoma are diverse, and mixed features are often represented in an individual case.[7, 13] Although there are overlaps in histologic features in high-grade olfactory neuroblastomas and epithelial intranasal tumors,

described later, most of the tumors fall into one of three readily recognizable categories, including somewhat paraganglioma-like lesions, tumors closely resembling conventional neuroblastoma, and neuroblastomas also featuring gland-like "olfactory rosettes" (esthesioneuroepithelioma). Many tumors show intermediate features.[13, 14]

The most common lesion, that somewhat resembling paraganglioma, is noted for its smooth-contoured, crisply defined lobules of considerably varying size (Figs. 1–70 and 1–71). In some cases, more diffuse, sheet-like growth predominates. These are composed of small, monomorphous, neurocyte-like cells with little cytoplasm and round nuclei featuring stippled (salt-and-pepper) chromatin and inconspicuous nucleoli. Although typically crowded in a patternless fashion, occasional tumors show a scant intercellular, fibrillary background or even patches of aligned "neuroblastic" processes. If present, Homer Wright rosettes are ill defined. Mitotic activity is variable but is often sparse. The stroma is quite vascular and, on occasion, even obscures the neoplastic element.

Although so delicate as to be inconspicuous in hematoxylin and eosin (H&E)–stained sections, a well-defined monolayer of S-100–positive cells circumscribes the lobules (see Fig. 1–76). Such cells and their processes may also be found within and partitioning the lobules. It is due to the presence of these cells that the lobules crudely mimic the Zellballen pattern of paragangliomas. In contrast to the latter, the lobules of olfactory neuroblastoma are generally larger and "bluer" given the scant cytoplasm of their cells. Exceptional lesions, while not as epithelioid as classic paraganglioma, feature more abundant cytoplasm.

Olfactory neuroblastomas more closely resembling conventional neuroblastoma are characterized by well-formed Homer Wright rosettes (Fig. 1–72) and process-rich neuropil (Fig. 1–73). Rosettes somewhat resembling the Flexner type, that is, ones with a lumen, may appear but are rarely seen in abundance. Differentiation toward ganglion cells or a ganglioneuroblastoma pattern is rare.

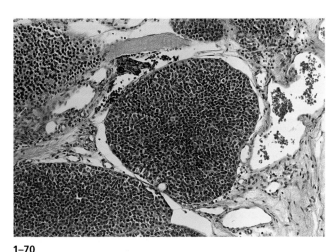

1–70

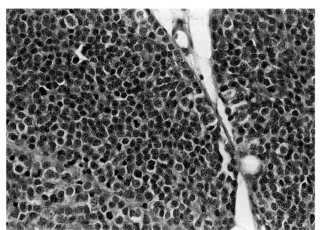

1–71

**FIGURES 1–70 AND 1–71**   OLFACTORY NEUROBLASTOMA

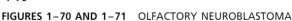

Lobulation and monomorphism typify olfactory neuroblastoma (Fig. 1–70). Note the paucity of cytologic atypia (Fig. 1–71).

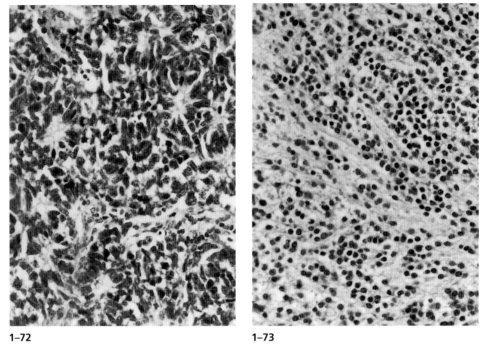

1–72                                          1–73

**FIGURES 1–72 AND 1–73**    OLFACTORY NEUROBLASTOMA

The neuroblastic nature of some olfactory neoplasms is expressed in the form of Homer Wright rosettes (Fig. 1–72) or the streaming of cells in a delicate fibrillary background (Fig. 1–73).

Complex patterns of neuroepithelium, including glands, tubules, and surfaces (Fig. 1–74), may be intimately admixed with more conventional, obviously paragangliomatous or neuroblastic tissue. In part, it is such a tumor that blurs the distinction of olfactory neuroblastoma from "neuroendocrine carcinoma" and creates definitional problems as to what is meant by the term olfactory neuroblastoma. The confusion is increased by (1) the finding of keratin and EMA staining in paraganglioma-like lesions and in tumors exhibiting Flexner or olfactory rosettes and (2) the occasional occurrence of

markedly epithelial-appearing tumors showing neuroblastic features only at the ultrastructural level.[7] Unlike olfactory neuroblastoma, neuroendocrine carcinomas are more obviously epithelial at the light microscopic level and show far stronger, more uniform immunostaining for EMA and keratin. Although the desire to separate these two tumor groups is understandable and it is possible in most instances, the occurrence of some lesions with intermediate features may make it difficult.[7, 16]

**Histologic Grading.** The best known histologic grading scheme, that of Hyams,[8] is based on degree of lobularity, differentiation (fibrillary matrix), nuclear pleomorphism, mitotic activity, necrosis, rosette and gland (olfactory rosette) formation, and calcification. This four-tiered system can be simplified into low grade (Hyams grades I and II) and high grade (Hyams grades III and IV). Although significant differences in outcome are said to correlate with these designations, we find that not all tumors are easily graded by this method. Suffice it to say that numerous mitoses, pleomorphism, and necrosis are limited to high-grade lesions. In our experience, however, the majority of olfactory neuroblastomas are of low grade. Indeed, without thorough immunohistochemical and selective ultrastructural study, it is likely that many so-called high-grade olfactory neuroblastomas are in fact other high-grade lesions, such as sinonasal undifferentiated carcinoma.

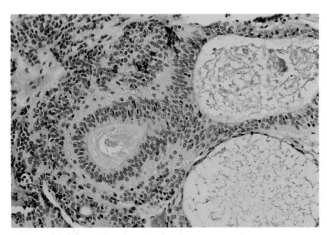

**FIGURE 1–74**    OLFACTORY NEUROBLASTOMA

This rare olfactory neuroblastoma has an overtly epithelial feature, olfactory rosettes. Such structures are both cytokeratin and EMA immunoreactive.

**Immunohistochemical Features.** All forms of olfactory neuroblastoma stain for one or several neuronal markers, including synaptophysin, NSE, microtubule-

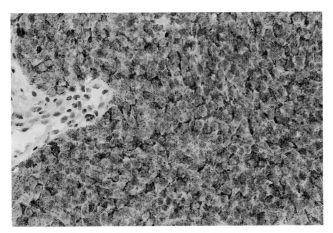

**FIGURE 1–75    OLFACTORY NEUROBLASTOMA**

Olfactory neuroblastomas are reliably synaptophysin positive.

associated protein, class III beta-tubulin, or neurofilament protein.[5, 6] Overall, synaptophysin is the most reliable marker (Fig. 1–75). Chromogranin staining is particularly strong in paraganglioma-like tumors, whereas neurofilament protein, microtubule-associated protein, and class III beta-tubulin reactivity are more often expressed in tumors with neuroblastoma-like features.[7] In a minority of cases, immunohistochemistry has also shown the presence of met-enkephalin, vasoactive intestinal polypeptide, and substance P.[7] Patchy or punctate paranuclear cytokeratin staining is occasionally seen in the lobular, paraganglioma-like variant.

Stains for S-100 protein, and to a lesser extent GFAP, stain sustentacular cells surrounding and within the lobules (Fig. 1–76).[2, 7] Whereas epithelial markers, such as cytokeratin and EMA, are absent in obviously neuroblastic tumors featuring Homer Wright rosettes, staining for both is often seen in Flexner or "olfactory" rosettes. In contrast to the limited staining for epithelial markers seen in olfactory neuroblastoma variants, they are strongly and uniformly expressed in neuroendocrine carcinomas.

**Proliferation Markers.** Several studies of Ki-67 and MIB-1 staining in olfactory neuroblastoma have reported variable indices, ranging from 0 to 43%.[7, 21, 23] MIB-1 labeling has been shown to correlate with frequency of tumor recurrence and metastatic spread as well as with survival.

**Ultrastructural Features.** The ultrastructural features of olfactory neuroblastoma are varied.[22, 23] Cells of the "paraganglioma-like" lesion are polygonal, rather cohesive, and contain scattered 80- to 230-nm dense core granules. Microtubule-containing processes vary in number. Accompanying sustentacular cells are relatively electron dense, contain intermediate filaments, lack granules, and possess long, narrow processes that often surround cell clusters (Fig. 1–77). These cells are covered on their outer or "stromal" aspect by a basal lamina.

Cells of the neuroblastic variant show their lush neuropil to consist of abundant neuritic processes containing neurofilaments and microtubules. Their terminations in particular often contain 100- to 170-nm dense core granules and, in some instances, clear vesicles. Synapses are less common. The apices of cells making up olfactory rosettes show bulbous cytoplasmic expansions, tufts of cilia with a 9+2 microtubule pattern, microvilli, and junctional complexes.[20]

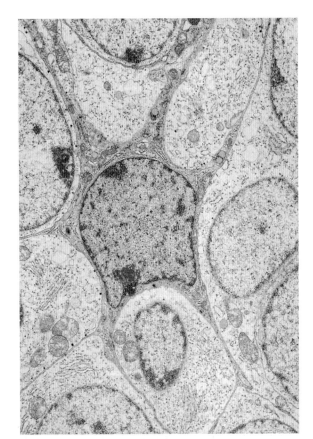

**FIGURE 1–77    OLFACTORY NEUROBLASTOMA**

An electron dense sustentacular cell grasps adjacent chief cells. Neurosecretory granules underlie the cell membrane of the latter (×12,000).

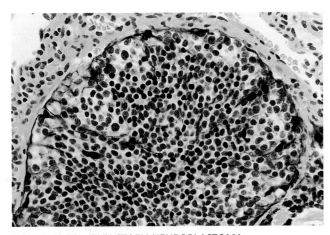

**FIGURE 1–76    OLFACTORY NEUROBLASTOMA**

S-100–positive sustentacular cells surround the lobules of neuronal cells but may also be present within lobules.

**Differential Diagnosis.** As a rule, olfactory neuroblastoma variants are so distinctive that there is little in the differential if classic histologic, immunohistochemical, or ultrastructural features are present. Nevertheless, the scope of tumors arising in the superior nasal cavity is broad and includes a variety of high-grade lesions that overlap, both practically and in some cases conceptually, with olfactory neuroblastomas. These include sinonasal undifferentiated carcinoma, malignant melanoma of small cell type, primitive neuroectodermal tumor (PNET) or Ewing's sarcoma, and malignant lymphoma.[12, 14] At the light microscopic levels, pituitary adenomas may be of concern but are easily excluded on anatomic grounds, as discussed in the following.

Unlike olfactory neuroblastoma, *sinonasal undifferentiated carcinoma* (SNUC) is a large cell, anaplastic tumor often featuring necrosis and immunoreactivity for both cytokeratin and EMA. Synaptophysin staining is seen in occasional examples showing neuroendocrine differentiation.[5, 12] Although there is potential overlap with rare examples of high-grade olfactory neuroblastomas, the SNUC is more obviously epithelial in nature.

*Melanoma* of the nasal cavity generally poses no problem in differential diagnosis with olfactory neuroblastoma. Some, however, are relatively small cell in appearance. Once the possibility of malignant melanoma is entertained, appropriate immunohistochemical studies easily resolve the issue.

Unlike *Ewing's sarcoma,* olfactory neuroblastoma is negative with the 013 antibody to the MIC2 antigen.[1] Malignant lymphomas are readily excluded with appropriate lymphoid markers.

Although *pituitary adenoma* may come to mind, particularly in the occasional olfactory neuroblastoma involving the subfrontal region or the sphenoid sinus, the sella is unaffected. Thus, simple attention to neuroimaging resolves this differential. Distinguishing features include the lobules of olfactory neuroblastoma, their circumscription by S-100–positive sustentacular cells, and the absence of immunoreactivity for any pituitary hormone.

**Treatment and Prognosis.** It has been repeatedly shown that completeness of resection is the single factor most affecting prognosis.[15] One large, long-term study concluded that surgery alone was effective for low-grade examples if the surgical margins were free of tumor.[15] Radiation therapy was recommended in the presence of residual disease or of a high-grade lesion. Others are more likely to employ radiation therapy, even after total excision.[3]

In one study, the overall 5-year survival of patients with olfactory neuroblastoma was 69%.[15] Despite resection and adjuvant therapy, progression or recurrence is common in the first 2 years; more than one third of tumors recur beyond 5 years of initial treatment.[15] Radiation therapy has been shown to be effective for recurrent or metastatic disease.[4] The same is true of chemotherapy, particularly platinum-based regimens.[10,18]

In the Mayo Clinic experience, histologic grade seems to be a particularly robust parameter.[15] In one series the 5-year survival was 80% with low-grade and 40% with high-grade tumors.[7, 15] Overexpression of wild-type p53 has been shown to be associated with recurrence and metastasis,[17] and abundance of S-100 protein–immunopositive sustentacular cells correlated with longer survival.[7]

## Papillary Endolymphatic Sac Tumor

This low-grade carcinoma is generally seen in adults as a destructive mass in the petrous portion of the temporal bone, often with extension into the cerebellopontine angle (Fig. 1–78).[2, 4–9] Some occur in the context of von Hippel–Lindau syndrome.[3, 10] Bilaterality has been observed.[6]

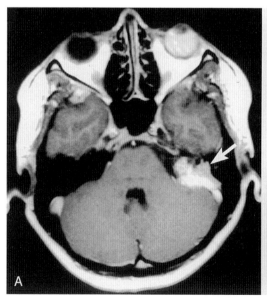 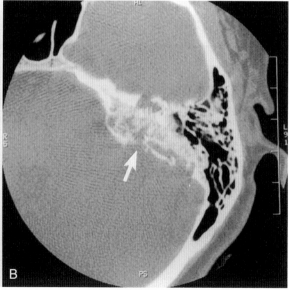

**FIGURE 1–78** PAPILLARY ENDOLYMPHATIC SAC TUMOR

As seen by MR (*A*) and CT (*B*), the lesion arises in, and erodes, the petrous bone. In *A*, note the ipsilateral ocular changes associated with a retinal hemangioblastoma in this patient with von Hippel–Lindau disease. (Courtesy of Dr. Marc K. Rosenblum, New York, NY.)

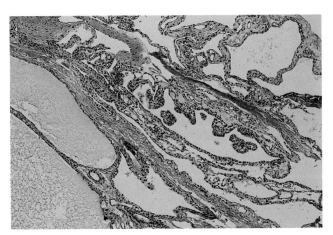

**FIGURE 1–79**    PAPILLARY ENDOLYMPHATIC SAC TUMOR

The papillary epithelium is extremely well differentiated.

Histologically, the lesion is a very well differentiated papillary carcinoma with only minimal cytologic atypia and mitotic activity (Fig. 1–79). Immunohistochemically, it reacts for cytokeratins, EMA, and carcinoembryonic antigen.[1, 3]

Given the papillary architecture of the lesion and the high degree of differentiation, the differential diagnosis logically includes *choroid plexus papilloma.* Plexus papillomas of the posterior fossa can extend into, or arise within, the lateral recess of the ventricle and then appear at the cerebellopontine angle. In contrast, papillary middle ear tumors arise in bone, as is well seen by radiologic studies. The carcinomas, in contrast to the papilloma, are strongly immunoreactive for cytokeratins and EMA but negative for S-100 and synaptophysin.

The treatment is surgical excision.[2, 9] Irradiation can be considered when resection is subtotal.[2, 8] Residual tumor may grow slowly for many years.

## Metastatic Neoplasms

Tumors metastatic to the skull seldom pass under the eye of the surgical pathologist, as most are the progeny of known primaries and have thus passed beyond the domain of remedial surgery. In adults, most originate in carcinoma of the lung and breast.[1, 2, 4] Thyroid[9] and renal cell carcinoma (Figs. 1–80 and 1–81) and malignant melanoma are also attracted to the skull, but as metastases they are numerically fewer given the lower incidence of their respective primaries. In children, neuroblastoma is the almost exclusive offender. Metastatic lesions to the base of the skull, as well as direct extensions from neoplasms of the nasopharynx and nasal sinuses, may symptomatically compress cranial nerves.[6,7] Among pituitary adenomas with extensive destruction of the skull base, prolactin cell adenomas are the most common. Adenoid cystic carcinoma is especially prone to traverse the skull along peripheral nerves (Figs. 1–82 and 1–83).[3, 5, 7, 10] Metastases in the vault may extend inward to elicit neurologic symptoms, but more often they remain clinically silent bone defects or elevations of the skull.

The malignant cells elicit different responses by bone, but focal osteolysis is the usual consequence (Figs. 1–84 to 1–86). The lytic reaction to metastases differs from that produced by benign lesions such as epidermoid cysts in that it is centrally incomplete and peripherally irregular. Their lack of a sclerotic rim is a further differential feature.

Osteoblastic metastases often originate from the prostate (Figs. 1–87 and 1–88) or, less commonly, the breast.

Neuroblastoma may be distinctive in its induction of radiating bone spicules (Figs. 1–89 to 1–92).[8, 12] Metastases involve any bone of the skull, but the affinity of breast carcinoma for the sella turcica is noteworthy.[11]

The histologic characteristics of most metastatic neoplasms are noncommittal with regard to the primary

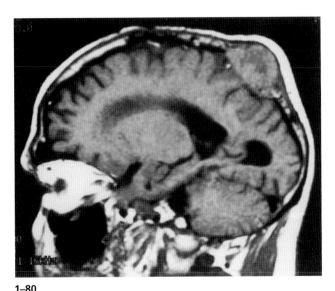

1–80

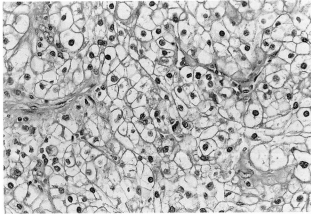

1–81

**FIGURES 1–80 AND 1–81**    METASTATIC CARCINOMA

A slowly enlarging scalp mass was noted by an 81-year-old man with a history of nephrectomy for renal cell carcinoma 6 years earlier (Fig. 1–80). Note postsurgical changes anterior to the lesion related to the previous resection of a skull metastasis 1 year earlier. Histologically, the lesion had the typical "clear cell" appearance of renal adenocarcinoma (Fig. 1–81).

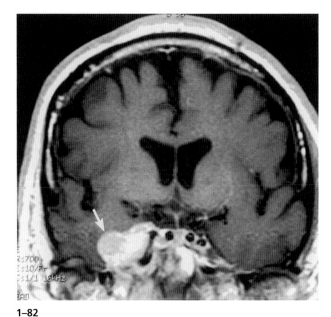

1–82

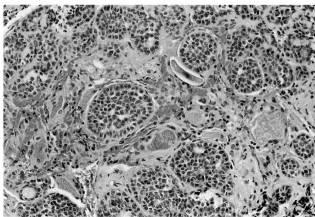

1–83

**FIGURES 1–82 AND 1–83**    ADENOID CYSTIC CARCINOMA

Adenoid cystic carcinomas have a distinctive tendency to spread along nerves and, by this route, can reach a cavernous sinus and/or a trigeminal ganglion. Such a result is seen here in a contrast-enhanced T1-weighted MR scan (Fig. 1–82). The primary lesion in this 61-year-old man arose in the hard palate. The tumor cells lie side by side with myelinated axons and neurons in the trigeminal ganglion (Fig. 1–83).

site of origin. Mammary, renal, and thyroid carcinomas,[9] as well as melanoma, are more informative in this regard.

Largely on the basis of their radiolucency, other lesions to be included in the differential diagnosis of metastasis include *epidermoid cyst, hemangioma, multiple myeloma*, osteoporosis circumscripta (focal Paget's disease), occasional lysis of bone in *meningioma*, and *congenital bone defects*.

## Multiple Myeloma

Multiple myeloma is a multicentric, neoplastic proliferation of plasma cells with a distinct tendency to focal destruction of bone, notably of vertebrae, ribs, and skull. The disorder is more common in men (2:1) and has a peak incidence during the fifth through seventh decades.

Metastases involving the cranial vault are no different from those affecting other bones. Most are multiple, discrete, and strikingly osteolytic. The neoplastic infiltrate first affects diploë and with time erodes outward through the bony cortex, sometimes appearing as a fleshy protuberance beneath the scalp. Less often, growth is directed inwardly in the form of an epidural mass that compresses the brain. Penetration of the dura is rare. Neoplastic growths at the base of the skull, particularly within the sphenoid bone or in the apices of its petrous portion, may produce cranial nerve deficits.[1]

Macroscopically, metastases are fleshy or jelly-like and vary from gray to red depending on their vascularity.

The distinction between an inflammatory and a neoplastic process is usually obvious at the histologic level.

Plasmacytoma, a localized form of plasma cell neoplasia, is discussed on pages 78 to 79.

## Other Malignant Neoplasms

Osteosarcoma occurs as a rare primary neoplasm of the skull[2, 13, 26] or in the setting of Paget's disease.[10, 17, 22–24, 30] It can also be a late sequela of therapeutic irradiation.[1, 4, 22, 24] Also observed as primary or metastatic lesions of the skull are angiosarcoma,[15] ceruminoma (middle ear adenoma),[21] chondrosarcoma (Figs. 1–93 to 1–95),[6, 11, 12, 14, 20, 27] malignant fibrous histiocytoma,[18] mesenchymal chondrosarcoma,[25] Ewing's sarcoma,[3, 8, 29] fibrosarcoma,[16] hemangiopericytoma,[5, 7] malignant lymphoma,[19, 28] and rhabdomyosarcoma.[9]

## DEVELOPMENTAL ANOMALIES

## Epidermoid and Dermoid Cysts

In the course of embryologic development, cells of cutaneous epithelium may be displaced into bone or the soft tissues of an osseous interspace such as a fontanelle. By a continuous process of cell proliferation, senescence, and desquamation, such nests may produce a cyst. Centrifugal enlargement then erodes bone to produce a lytic

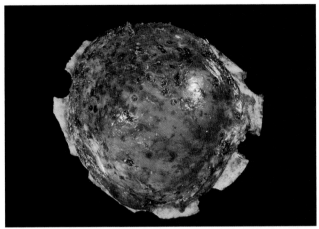

1–84

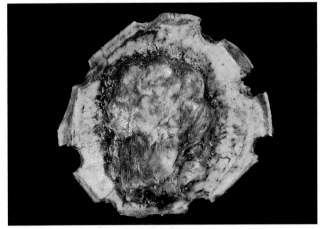

1–85

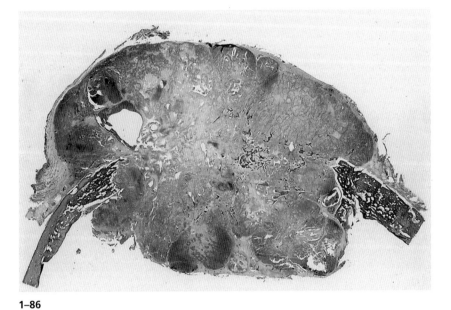

1–86

**FIGURES 1–84, 1–85, AND 1–86**   METASTATIC MALIGNANT MELANOMA

A cutaneous malignant melanoma was removed from the back of a 23-year-old man 5 years before the appearance of a lytic lesion in the right frontal bone. The excised tumor elevates the galea (Fig. 1–84) and extends inward to compress the brain (Fig. 1–85). In the whole-mount histologic section (Fig. 1–86), remnants of the calvarium appear as sequestered spicules of bone, the basis of the typical ragged, lytic radiographic appearance.

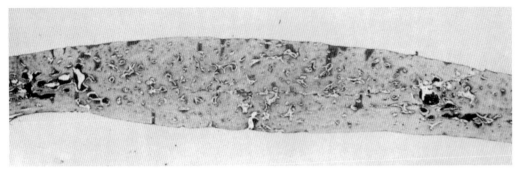

1–87

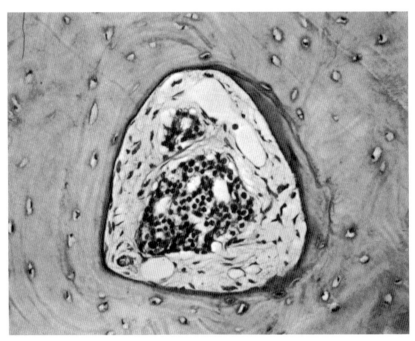

1–88

**FIGURES 1–87 AND 1–88    METASTATIC PROSTATE CARCINOMA**

In contrast to the osteolysis of most carcinomas metastatic to skull, an osteoblastic response is typically elicited by prostate carcinoma. This is evident in both a whole-mount histologic section (Fig. 1–87) and a photomicrograph (Fig. 1–88). In the latter, the small nest of neoplastic cells assumes the cribriform pattern commonly seen in prostatic cancer.

defect with a delicate, scalloped, and sclerotic rim (Figs. 1–96 to 1–98).[5] Epidermoid cysts may arise in any calvarial bone, variably involving the outer or inner table, or the diploë. In contrast to epidermoid cysts, so-called dermoids are more often midline and restricted to the scalp or to a fontanelle.[9, 11, 13–15]

Most dermoid and epidermoid cysts remain asymptomatic and are incidental radiographic findings. Less often, outward expansion produces a scalp mass or inward growth compresses the brain.[1–4, 6, 16, 17] Intracranial epidermoid and dermoid cysts are discussed in Chapter 2, pages 91 to 92, because they are usually located principally in the meninges.

Epidermoid cysts, also known as "pearly tumors," are distended with cheesy, keratinous debris (Figs. 1–99 and 1–100). Their lining is composed solely of kera-tinized squamous epithelial cells (Fig. 1–101), whereas the presence of adnexal structures characterizes the dermoid cyst (Fig. 1–102). Either lesion may be associated with a sinus tract.[12]

Incomplete removal of either an epidermoid or a dermoid cyst permits the development of a cystic recurrence.[16] The leisurely enlargement of either lesion is only rarely accelerated by malignant transformation.[7, 8, 10, 18]

## Meningocele and Encephalocele

Meningoceles and encephaloceles are, respectively, herniations of meninges alone or of meninges and nervous tissue through a defect in the skull. They are thus analo-

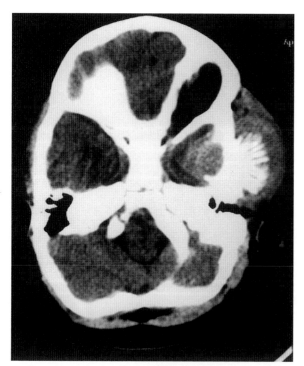

**FIGURE 1–89** METASTATIC NEUROBLASTOMA

This 1-year-old, previously asymptomatic girl presented with a 3-cm mass in the left temporal region. Computed tomography demonstrates the radiating spicules of bone occasionally seen in metastases of neuroblastoma. Isotope scanning of the skeleton disclosed abnormalities in both hips, one knee, and one ankle. A metaiodobenzylguanidine scan revealed a left adrenal mass.

gous to, but less frequent than, dysraphic malformations of the spine. A bony defect alone is known as "cranium bifidum," whereas herniation of meninges is a "meningocele" and herniation of meninges and brain is a "meningoencephalocele" or simply "encephalocele." Although failure of the neural tube to close or its subsequent rupture is a commonly cited explanation for the development, the concurrence of other malformations in some cases suggests a more complex pathogenesis.

Both meningocele and encephalocele occur as saccular outpouchings of variable size, most often in the occipital region (Figs. 1–103 and 1–104).[2, 4, 7, 8] Anterior,[1, 3, 9, 11, 14] lateral,[5, 12, 16] or basally situated[6, 12, 15] examples are less common. At their point of exit from the skull, the protuberances are encircled by a collar of hair-bearing skin that apically gives way to glabrous epidermis or translucent fibrous tissue, both being prone to ulceration. Thus, inflammatory cells are common in superficial layers and abound in the presence of ulceration. In meningoceles, loose fibrovascular tissue lies deep to the dermis (Fig. 1–105). Although in encephaloceles the nervous tissue may be fully formed cerebral cortex, more often it is structurally disorganized, with glioneuronal nests disposed in islands and masses demarcated by collagenous septa (Fig. 1–106). Ependyma and misshapen choroid plexus are occasionally included.

Heterotopic brain tissue may also be encountered as an incidental curiosity in the scalp.[10, 13]

Although even large meningoceles carry a good postoperative prognosis, those occurring in the occipital region are frequently accompanied by more profound abnormalities, including hydrocephalus, microcephaly, and mental as well as physical retardation. Anterior encephaloceles, more often a cosmetic than a neurologic problem, are less often linked to other cerebral abnormalities.

## Nasal Glial Heterotopia (Nasal "Glioma")

This non-neoplastic, congenital lesion results from anterior displacement of non-neoplastic neuroglial tissue. The commonly used designation "glioma" is therefore a misnomer. Similar, albeit smaller, heterotopias have been reported in occipital bone,[5] nasopharynx,[2] subcutaneous tissue of the temporoparietal area,[4] and as multiple scalp nodules.[8] In the nasal region, most glial heterotopias are encountered as a midline or parasagittal subcutaneous mass at the base of the nose (Fig. 1–107). Less commonly, some occur as an intranasal polyp.[3] Cosmetic complaints or nasal obstruction most often brings nasal lesions to medical attention. Cerebrospinal fluid rhinorrhea and meningitis are uncommon manifestations.

Neuroglial heterotopias are composed of disorganized neuroglial and fibrovascular tissue, the latter separating and encircling islands of the former (Fig. 1–108).[9] The glial element generally predominates and consists mainly of GFAP-positive astrocytes lying within an abundant fibrillar matrix.[6] Some astrocytes attain considerable size and often mimic neurons. Although less frequently present, neurons can be identified by their content of cytoplasmic Nissl substance as well as by the presence of axonal processes. The latter are demonstrated by silver stains (Bodian, Bielschowsky).[7] The organization of nasal glial heterotopia varies. Some do show vague cortical–white matter organization. Microcalcifications may be present.

Because the lesion is malformative rather than neoplastic, it is not surprising that simple excision is curative. "Recurrence" is rare.[1] Nasal gliomas, especially those occurring within the nose, may be attached either directly or via a fibrous stalk to the olfactory bulb or the inferior surface of the frontal lobe. The connection is typically via a defect in the cribriform plate. Nasal glial heterotopias are more than conceptually related to anterior encephalocele; as previously noted, their architecture at times approaches that of brain tissue. In either case, meningitis can be a serious complication if the connection of the extracranial element to an intracranial component is not appreciated. Although, to our knowledge, nasal lesions have not given rise to gliomas, tissue resembling oligodendroglioma has been reported in a nasopharyngeal heterotopia.[2]

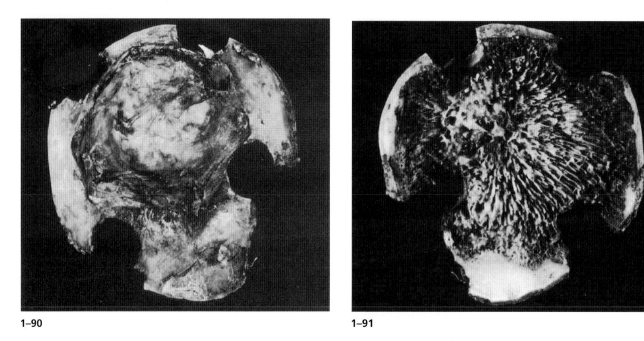

1–90

1–91

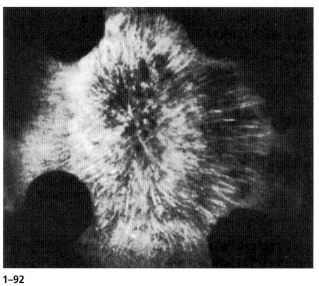

1–92

**FIGURES 1–90, 1–91, AND 1–92    METASTATIC NEUROBLASTOMA**

This section of calvarium was removed from a 10-year-old boy. It contains a metastatic deposit of neuroblastoma that elevates the galea (Fig. 1–90) and extends inward, where, as seen macroscopically (Fig. 1–91) and in a specimen radiograph (Fig. 1–92), radiating spicules are prominent.

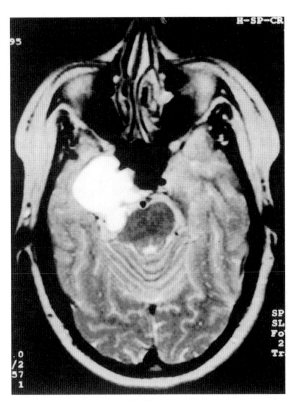

**FIGURE 1–93** CHONDROSARCOMA

This skull base chondrosarcoma displaces the brain stem and has entered the sphenoid sinus. In contrast to the chordoma, the tumor is unilateral. Unlike meningioma, it is bright, rather than dark, in a T2-weighted MR image.

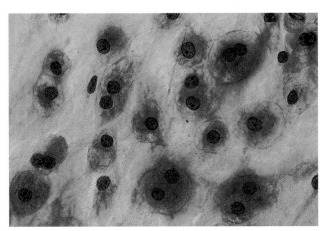

**FIGURE 1–95** CHONDROSARCOMA

As seen in a smear preparation from the lesion in Figure 1–94, the cells are not markedly atypical.

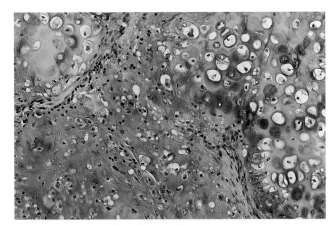

**FIGURE 1–94** CHONDROSARCOMA

The neoplasm in Figure 1–93 has the characteristic lobularity, cellular crowding, and subtle nuclear pleomorphism of well-differentiated chondrosarcoma.

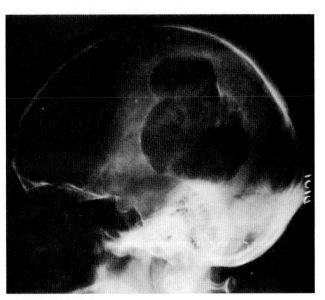

**FIGURE 1–96** EPIDERMOID CYST

This large asymptomatic lesion was an incidental radiographic finding in a 56-year-old man. The scalloped border and sclerotic rim are characteristic.

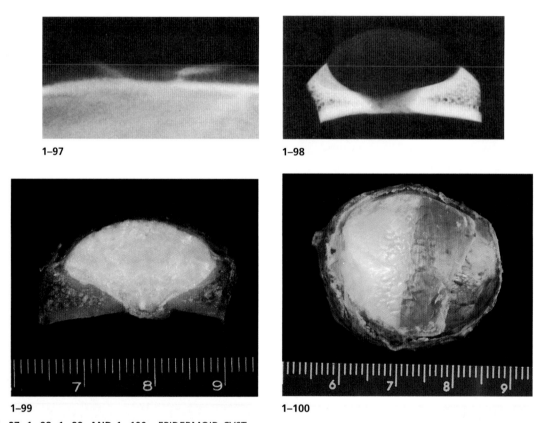

**1–97**

**1–98**

**1–99**

**1–100**

**FIGURES 1–97, 1–98, 1–99, AND 1–100**   EPIDERMOID CYST

A slowly enlarging scalp mass had been present for 5 years in a 7-year-old girl. Radiographs, both in situ (Fig. 1–97) and after excision (Fig. 1–98), show the remodeling effect of the mass on the frontal bone with the formation of a sclerotic rim. Seen in a cross section of the surgical specimen, the expanding sac-like lesion is filled with white keratin and lies against a surrounding lamina of dense, compact bone (Fig. 1–99). As viewed from above prior to bisection, the partly reflected, translucent dome on the lesion transmits the mother-of-pearl sheen typical of epidermoid cyst at any location (Fig. 1–100).

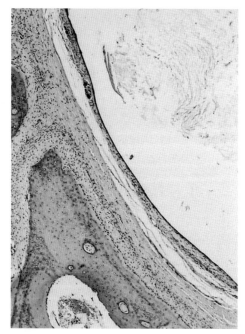

**1–101**

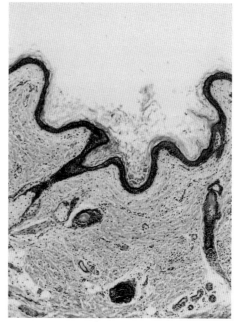

**1–102**

**FIGURES 1–101 AND 1–102**    EPIDERMOID AND DERMOID CYSTS

The epidermoid cyst is an expansile sac lined by a very thin layer of squamous epithelium and filled with keratinous debris (Fig. 1–101). In comparison, the wall of dermoid cysts contains cutaneous adnexae (Fig. 1–102).

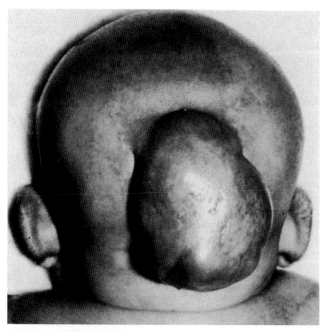

**FIGURE 1–103**    ENCEPHALOCELE

Most encephaloceles protrude from the occiput, as here in this 1-day-old girl.

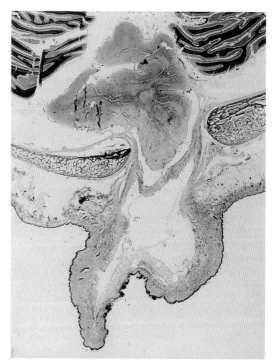

**FIGURE 1–104**    ENCEPHALOCELE

A whole-mount section of an encephalocele emphasizes the midline location of this occipital skull defect (cranium bifidum) and the outward herniation of both the meninges and dysplastic brain.

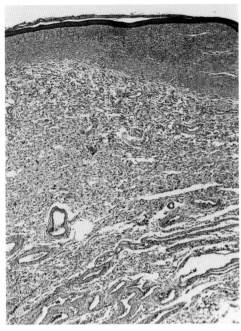

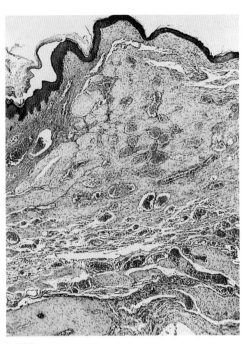

**1–105**                                                    **1–106**

**FIGURES 1–105 AND 1–106**   MENINGOCELE AND MENINGOENCEPHALOCELE

The subcutaneous portion of a meningocele consists of loose areolar connective tissue (Fig. 1–105). In contrast, the encephalocele contains malformed central nervous system tissue (Fig. 1–106), which is apparent as pale-staining subcutaneous bands and lobules. Multiple abnormal blood vessels are often present.

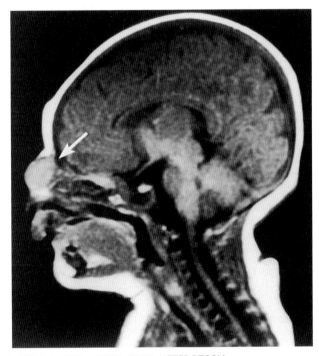

**FIGURE 1–107**   NASAL GLIAL HETEROTOPIA

As in this example in a 7-day-old girl, nasal glial heterotopias often present as a glabellar mass.

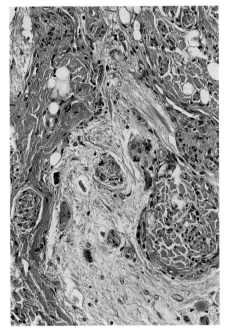

**FIGURE 1–108**   NASAL GLIAL HETEROTOPIA

The so-called "nasal glioma" consists of non-neoplastic glial or glioneuronal tissue separated into lobules by collagenous septa.

# REFERENCES

## Fibrous Dysplasia

1. Brown EW, Megerian CA, McKenna MJ, Weber A. Fibrous dysplasia of the temporal bone: imaging findings. AJR 1995;164:679–682.
2. Edgerton MT, Persing JA, Jane JA. The surgical treatment of fibrous dysplasia with emphasis on recent contributions from cranio-maxillo-facial surgery. Ann Surg 1985;202:459–479.
3. Fu Y-S, Perzin KH. Non-epithelial tumors of the nasal cavity, paranasal sinuses, and nasopharynx: a clinicopathologic study. II. Osseous and fibro-osseous lesions, including osteoma, fibrous dysplasia, ossifying fibro, osteoblastoma, giant cell tumor, and osteosarcoma. Cancer 1974;33:1289–1305.
4. Gurler T, Alper M, Gencosmanoglu R, Totan S, Guner U, Akin Y. McCune-Albright syndrome progressing with severe fibrous dysplasia. J Craniofac Surg 1998;9:79–82.
5. Jan M, Dweik A, Destrieux C, Djebbari Y. Fronto-orbital sphenoidal fibrous dysplasia. Neurosurgery 1994;34:544–547.
6. Katz BJ, Nerad JA. Ophthalmic manifestations of fibrous dysplasia: a disease of children and adults. Ophthalmology 1998;105:2207–2215.
7. Mark RJ, Poen J, Tran LM, Fu YS, Selch MT, Parker RG. Postirradiation sarcomas. A single-institution study and review of the literature. Cancer 1994;73:2653–2662.
8. Megerian CA, Sofferman RA, McKenna MJ, Eavey RD, Nadol JB Jr. Fibrous dysplasia of the temporal bone: ten new cases demonstrating the spectrum of otologic sequelae. Am J Otol 1995;16:408–419.
9. Morrissey DD, Talbot JM, Schleuning AJ. Fibrous dysplasia of the temporal bone: reversal of sensorineural hearing loss after decomposition of the internal auditory canal. Laryngoscope 1997;107:1336–1340.
10. Mortensen A, Bojsen-Moller M, Rasmussen P. Fibrous dysplasia of the skull with acromegaly and sarcomatous transformation. Two cases with a review of the literature. J Neurooncol 1989;71:25–29.
11. Nager GT, Kennedy DW, Kopstein E. Fibrous dysplasia: a review of the disease and its manifestations in the temporal bone. Ann Otol Rhinol Laryngol [Suppl] 1982;92:5–52.
12. Papay FA, Morales L Jr, Flaharty P, et al. Optic nerve decompression in cranial base fibrous dysplasia. J Craniofac Surg 1995;6:5–10.
13. Posnick JC, Wells MD, Drake JM, Buncic JR, Armstrong D. Childhood fibrous dysplasia presenting as blindness: a skull base approach for resection and immediate reconstruction. Pediatr Neurosurg 1993;19:260–266.
14. Sassin JF, Rosenberg RN. Neurologic complications of fibrous dysplasia of the skull. Arch Neurol 1968;18:363–369.
15. Schwartz DT, Alpert M. The malignant transformation of fibrous dysplasia. Am J Med Sci 1964;247:1–20.
16. Townsend GL, De Santo LW. Malignant change in sphenoid sinus fibrous dysplasia. Arch Otolaryngol 1970;92:267–271.
17. Unni KK. Dahlin's Bone Tumors. General Aspects and Data on 11,087 Cases. 5th ed. Philadelphia: Lippincott-Raven, 1996.

## Langerhans Cell Histiocytosis (Histiocytosis X, Eosinophilic Granuloma)

1. Brisman JL, Feldstein NA, Tarbell NJ, et al. Eosinophilic granuloma of the clivus: case report, follow-up of two previously reported cases, and review of the literature on cranial base eosinophilic granuloma. Neurosurgery 1997;41:273–278.
2. Ide F, Iwase BC, Saito I, Umemura S, Nakajima T. Immunohistochemical and ultrastructural analysis of the proliferating cells in histiocytosis X. Cancer 1984;53:917–921.
3. Lunardi P, Farah JO, Qhaso R, Puzzilli F, Siciliano P, Di Stefano D. Primary eosinophilic granuloma invading the skull base: case report and critical review of the literature. Tumori 1996;82:397–400.
4. Nezelof C. Histiocytosis X: a histological and histogenetic study. Perspect Pediatr Pathol 1980;5:153–178.
5. Williams JW, Dorfman RF. Lymphadenopathy as the initial manifestation of histiocytosis X. Am J Pathol 1979;3:405–421.
6. Willman CL, Busque L, Griffith BB, et al. Langerhans'-cell histiocytosis (histiocytosis X)—a clonal proliferative disease. N Engl J Med 1994;331:154–160.
7. Yu RC, Chu AC. Lack of T-cell receptor gene rearrangements in cells involved in Langerhans cell histiocytosis. Cancer 1995;75:1162–1166.

## Aneurysmal Bone Cyst

1. Alles JU, Schulz A. Immunocytochemical markers (endothelial and histiocytic) and ultrastructure of primary aneurysmal bone cysts. Hum Pathol 1986;17:40–45.
2. Bilge T, Coban O, Ozden B, Turantan I, Turker K, Bahar S. Aneurysmal bone cysts of the occipital bone. Surg Neurol 1983;20:227–230.
3. Cacdac MA, Malis LI, Anderson PJ. Aneurysmal parietal bone cyst: case report. J Neurosurg 1972;37:237–241.
4. Horvath D, Horvath Z, Horvath A, Illes T. Aneurysmal bone cyst of the occipital bone: case report. Surg Neurol 1993;40:332–335.
5. Hunter JV, Yokoyama C, Moseley IF, Wright JE. Aneurysmal bone cyst of the sphenoid with orbital involvement. Br J Ophthalmol 1990;74:505–508.
6. O'Brien DP, Rashad EM, Toland JA, Farrell MA, Phillips J. Aneurysmal cyst of the frontal bone: case report and review of the literature. Br J Neurosurg 1994;8:105–108.
7. Shah G, Doctor JR, Shah PS. Aneurysmal bone cyst of the temporal bone: MR findings. AJNR 1995;16:763–766.
8. Shimizu T, Ukai K, Hayashi T, Imanishi Y, Sakakura Y. Aneurysmal bone cyst of the temporal bone: magnetic resonance imaging as a valuable tool for preoperative diagnosis. Am J Otolaryngol 1998;19:379–382.

## Paget's Disease

1. Anderson JT, Dehner LP. Osteolytic form of Paget's disease. J Bone Joint Surg Am 1976;58:994–1000.
2. Chen J-R, Rhee SC, Wallach S, et al. Neurologic disturbances in Paget's disease of bone: response to calcitonin. Neurology 1979;29:448–457.
3. Clarke CRA, Harrison MJG. Neurological manifestations of Paget's disease. J Neurol Sci 1978;38:171–178.
4. Collins DH, Winn JM. Focal Paget's disease of the skull (osteoporosis circumscripta). J Pathol Bacteriol 1955;69:1–9.
5. Culebras A, Feldman RG, Fager CA. Hydrocephalus and dementia in Paget's disease of the skull. J Neurol Sci 1974;23:307–321.
6. Dohrmann PJ, Elrick WL. Dementia and hydrocephalus in Paget's disease: a case report. J Neurol Neurosurg Psychiatry 1982;45:835–837.
7. Fransen P, Mestdagh C, Dardenne G. Pagetic sarcoma of the calvarium: report of two cases. Acta Neurol Belg 1998;98:352–355.
8. Goldenberg RR. The skull in Paget's disease. J Bone Joint Surg Am 1951;33:911–922.
9. Goldenhammer Y, Braham J, Kosary IZ. Hydrocephalic dementia in Paget's disease of the skull: treatment by ventriculoatrial shunt. Neurology 1979;29:513–516.
10. Hens L, van den Bergh R. Hydrocephalus-dementia-complex in Paget's disease. Clin Neurol Neurosurg 1979;81:255–263.
11. Kasabach HH, Gutman AB. Osteoporosis circumscripta of the skull and Paget's disease: fifteen new cases and a review of the literature. Am J Roentgenol Radium Ther 1937;37:577–600.
12. McKenna RJ, Schwinn CP, Soong KY, Higinbotham NL. Osteogenic sarcoma arising in Paget's disease. Cancer 1964;17:42–66.
13. Merino S, Arrazola J, Saiz A, Blanco JA, Ortega L. Post-Paget telangiectatic osteosarcoma of the skull. Skeletal Radiol 1999;28:470–472.
14. Miller C, Rao VM. Sarcomatous degeneration of Paget's disease in the skull. Skeletal Radiol 1983;10:102–106.
15. Poretta CA, Dahlin DC, Janes JM. Sarcoma in Paget's disease of bone. J Bone Joint Surg Am 1957;39:1314–1329.
16. Salvati M, Cervoni L, Raguso M, Raco A. Post-Paget osteosarcomas of the skull. remarks on five cases. Tumori 1993;79: 363–366.
17. Salvati M, Ciappetta P, Capoccia G, Capone R, Raco A. Osteosarcoma of the skull. Report of a post-Paget and post-radiation case in an elderly woman. Neurosurg Rev 1994;17:73–76.

18. Young HA, Hardy DG, Ashleigh R. Osteogenic sarcoma of the skull complicating Paget's disease: case report. Neurosurgery 1983;12:454–457.

## Mucocele

1. Abla AA, Maroon JC, Wilberger JE Jr, Kennerdell JS, Deeb ZL. Intrasellar mucocele simulating pituitary adenoma: case report. Neurosurgery 1986;18: 197–199.
2. Arseni C, Chitescu M, Cioloca C. Intracerebral mucocele. Neurochirurgia 1973;16:50–54.
3. Chua R, Shapiro S. A mucopyocele of the clivus: case report. Neurosurgery 1996;39:589–591.
4. Diaz F, Latchow R, Duvall AJ III. Mucoceles with intracranial and extracranial extensions: report of two cases. J Neurosurg 1978;48:284–288.
5. Gore RM, Weinberg PE, Kim KS, Ramsey RG. Sphenoid sinus mucoceles presenting as intracranial masses on computed tomography. Surg Neurol 1980;13:375–379.
6. Hakuba H, Katsuyama J, Matsuoka Y, et al. Sphenoid sinus mucoceles: report of two cases. J Neurosurg 1975;43:368–373.
7. Lunardi P, Missori P, Di Lorenzo N, Fortuna A. Giant intracranial mucocele secondary to osteoma of the frontal sinuses: report of two cases and review of the literature. Surg Neurol 1993;39: 46–48.
8. Mamaka H, Tokoro K Sakata K, Ono A, Yamamoto I. Intradural extension of mucocele complicating frontoethmoid sinus osteoma: case report. Surg Neurol 1998;50:453–456.
9. Nugent GR, Sprinkle P, Bloor BM. Sphenoid sinus mucoceles. J Neurosurg 1970;32;443–451.
10. Perugini S, Pasquini U, Menichelli F, et al. Mucoceles in the paranasal sinuses involving the orbit: CT signs in 43 cases. Neuroradiology 1982;23:133–139.
11. Pool JL, Potanos JN, Krueger EG. Osteomas and mucoceles of the frontal paranasal sinuses. J Neurosurg 1962;19:130–135.
12. Smith GW, Chavez M. Giant mucocele of the frontal sinus. J Neurol Neurosurg Psychiatry 1960;23:179–181.
13. Tamas LB, Wyler AR. Intracranial mucocele mimicking arachnoid cyst: a case report. Neurosurgery 1985;16:85–86.

## Cholesterol Granuloma

1. Brodkey JA, Robertson JH, Shea JJ III, Gardner G. Cholesterol granulomas of the petrous apex: combined neurosurgical and otological management. J Neurosurg 1996;85:625–633.
2. Greenberg JJ, Oot RF, Wismer GL, et al. Cholesterol granuloma of the petrous apex: MR and CT evaluation. AJNR 1988;9: 1205–1214.
3. Griffin C, DeLaPaz R, Enzmann D. MR and CT correlation of cholesterol cysts of the petrous bone. AJNR 1987;8:825–829.

## Hemangioma

1. Bastug D, Ortiz O, Schochet SS. Hemangiomas in the calvaria: imaging findings. AJR 1995;164:683–687.
2. Bizzozero L, Solaining TC, Villa F, Brusamolino R, Collice M. Cavernous hemangioma of the skull. Case report and review of the literature. J Neurosurg Sci 1997;41:419–421.
3. Chow RW, Wilson CB, Olsen ER. Angiosarcoma of the skull: report of case and review of literature, cancer 1970;25:902–906.
4. Dorfman HD, Steiner GC, Jaffe HL. Vascular tumors of bone. Hum Pathol 1971;2:349–376.
5. Sargent EN, Reilly EB, Posnikoff J. Primary hemangioma of the skull: case report of an unusual tumor. Am J Roentgenol Radium Ther Nucl Med 1965;95:874–879.

## Glomus Tumor (Jugulotympanic Paraganglioma)

1. Beckerstaff ER, Howell JS. The neurological importance of tumours of the glomus jugulare. Brain 1953;76:576–593.
2. Capella C, Solcia E. Optical and electron microscopic study of cystoplasmic granules in human carotid body, carotid body tumours and glomus jugulare tumours. Virchows Arch [B] 1971;7:37–53.
3. DeLellis RA, Roth JA. Norepinephrine in a glomus jugulare tumor: histochemical demonstration. Arch Pathol 1971;92:73–75.
4. Gabriel EM, Sampson JH, Dodd LG, Turner DA. Glomus jugulare tumor metastatic to the sacrum after high-dose radiation therapy: case report. Neurosurgery 1995;37:1001–1005.

5. Karas DE, Kwartler JA. Glomus tumors: a fifty-year historical perspective. Am J Otol 1993;14:495–500.
6. Korat O, Trojanowski JQ, LiVolsi V, Merino MJ. Antigen expression in normal paraganglia and paragangliomas. Surg Pathol 1988;1:33–40.
7. Lack EE, Cubilla AL, Woodruff JM. Paragangliomas of the head and neck region. Apathologic study of tumors from 71 patients. Hum Pathol 1979;10:191–218.
8. Lack EE, Cubilla AL, Woodruff JM, Farr HW. Paragangliomas of the head and neck region: a clinical study of 69 patients. Cancer 1977;39:397–409.
9. Larner JM, Hahn SS, Spaulding CA, Constable WC. Glomus jugulare tumors. Long-term control by radiation therapy. Cancer 1992;69:1813–1817.
10. Matisak MZ, Symon L, Cheeseman A, Pamphlett R. Catecholamine-secreting paragangliomas of the base of the skull: report of two cases. J Neurosurg 1987;66:604–608.
11. Mukherji SK, Kasper ME, Tart RP, Mancuso AA. Irradiated paragangliomas of the head and neck: CT and MR appearance. AJNR 1994;15:357–363.
12. Olsen WL, Dillon WP, Kelly WM, Norman D, Brant-Zawadzki M, Newton TH. MR imaging of paragangliomas. AJNR 1986;7:1039–1042.
13. Patel SJ, Sekhar LN, Cass SP, Hirsch BE. Combined approaches for resection of extensive glomus jugulare tumors. J Neurosurg 1994;80:1026–1038.
14. Reddy EK, Mansfield CM, Hartman GV. Chemodectoma of glomus jugulare. Cancer 1983;52:337–340.
15. Robertson JH, Gardner G, Cocke EW. Glomus jugulare tumors. Clin Neurosurg 1994;41:39–61.
16. Spector GJ, Druck NS, Gado M. Neurologic manifestations of glomus tumors in the head and neck. Arch Neurol 1976;33:270–274.
17. Takahashi H, Nakashima S, Tumanishi T, Ikuta F. Paragangliomas of the craniocervical region. Acta Neuropathol 1987;73:227–232.
18. Whitfield PC, Grey P, Hardy DG, Moffat DA. The surgical management of patients with glomus tumours of the skull base. Br J Neurosurg 1996;10:343–350.

## Meningioma

1. Altinors N, Cetin A, Pak I. Scalp meningioma: case report. Neurosurgery 1985;16:379–380.
2. Crawford TS, Kleinschmidt-DeMasters BK, Lillehei KO. Primary intraosseous meningioma. J Neurosurg 1995;83:912–915.
3. Daugaard S. Ectopic meningioma of a finger: case report. J Neurosurg 1983;58:778–780.
4. Echlin F. Cranial osteomas and hyperostoses produced by meningeal fibroblastomas: a clinical pathologic study. Arch Surg 1934;28:357–405.
5. Farr HW, Gray GF Jr, Vrana M, Panio M. Extracranial meningioma. J Surg Oncol 1973;5:411–420.
6. Gaffey MJ, Mills SE, Askin FB. Minute meningothelial-like nodules: a clinicopathologic study of so-called pulmonary chemodectoma. Am J Surg Pathol 1988;12:167–175.
7. Geoffray A, Lee Y-Y, Jing B-S, Wallace S. Extracranial meningiomas of the head and neck. Am J Neuroradiol 1984;5:559–604.
8. Hallgrimsson J, Bjornsson A, Gudmundsson G. Meningioma of the neck: case report. J Neurosurg 1970;32:695–699.
9. Husaini TA. An unusual osteolytic meningioma. J Pathol 1970;101:57–58.
10. Ito H, Takagi H, Kawano N, Yada K. Primary intraosseous meningioma: case report. J Neurooncol 1992;13:57–61.
11. Kemnitz P, Spormann H, Heinrich P. Meningioma of lung: first report with light and electron microscope findings. Ultrastruct Pathol 1982;3:359–365.
12. Khanna SD, Singh G, Saigal RK. Ectopic meningioma in an infant. Arch Surg 1964;89:752–754.
13. Kjeldsberg CR, Minckler J. Meningiomas presenting as nasal polyps. Cancer 1972;29:153–156.
14. Kulali A, Ilcayto R, Rahmanli O. Primary calvarial ectopic meningiomas. Neurochirurgia (Stuttg) 1991;34:174–177.
15. Lopez DA, Silvers DN, Helwig EB. Cutaneous meningiomas—a clinicopathologic study. Cancer 1974;34:728–744.
16. McWhorter JM, Ghatak NR, Kelly DL Jr. Extracranial meningioma presenting as lytic skull lesion. Surg Neurol 1976;5:223–224.

17. Nochomovitz LE, Jannotta F, Orenstein JM. Meningioma of the scalp: light and electron microscopic observations. Arch Pathol Lab Med 1985;109:92–95.
18. Palma L, Mercuri S, Ferrante L. Epidural calvarial meningioma. Surg Neurol 1977;8:315–318.
19. Polpili A, Derome PJ, Visot A, Guiot G. Hyperostosing meningiomas of the sphenoid ridge—clinical features, surgical therapy, and long-term observations: review of 49 cases. Surg Neurol 1982;17:411–416.
20. Sadar ES, Conomy JP, Benjamin SP, Levine HL. Meningiomas of the paranasal sinuses, benign and malignant. Neurosurgery 1979;4:227–231.
21. Sibley DA, Cooper PH. Rudimentary meningocele: a variant of "primary cutaneous meningioma." J Cutan Pathol 1989;16:72–80.
22. So SC, Ngan H, Ong GB. Ectopic meningiomas: report of two cases and review of the literature. Surg Neurol 1978;9:231–237.
23. Taxy JB. Meningioma of the paranasal sinuses: a report of two cases. Am J Surg Pathol 1990;14:82–86.
24. Thompson LD, Gyure KA. Extracranial sinonasal tract meningiomas: A clinicopathologic study of 30 cases with a review of the literature. Am J Surg Pathol 2000;24:640–650.
25. Wagmann AD, Weiss EK, Riggs HE. Hyperplasia of the skull associated with intraosseous meningioma in the absence of gross tumor: report of three cases. J Neuropathol Exp Neurol 1960;19:111–115.
26. Wilson AJ, Ratliff JL, Lagios MD, Aguilar MJ. Mediastinal meningioma. Am J Surg Pathol 1979;3:557–562.
27. Wolff M, Rankow RM. Meningioma of the parotid gland: an insight into the pathogenesis of extracranial meningiomas. Hum Pathol 1971;2:453–459.

### Osteoma

1. Fu Y-S, Perzin KH. Non-epithelial tumors of the nasal cavity, paranasal sinuses, and nasopharynx: a clinicopathologic study. II. Osseous and fibro-osseous lesions, including osteoma, fibrous dysplasia, ossifying fibroma, osteoblastoma, giant cell tumor, and osteosarcoma. Cancer 1974;33:1289–1305.
2. Haddad FS, Haddad GS, Zaatari G. Cranial osteomas: their classification and management. A report on a giant osteoma and review of the literature. Surg Neurol 1997;48:143–147.
3. McNabb AA. Orbital osteoma in Gardner's syndrome. Aust N Z J Ophthalmol 1998;26:169–170.
4. Noterman J, Massager N, Vloeberghs M, Brotchi J. Monstrous skull osteomas in a probable Gardner's syndrome: case report. Surg Neurol 1998;49:302–304.
5. Pompili A, Caroli F, Iandolo B, Mazzitelli MR, Riccio A. Giant osteoma of the sphenoid sinus reached by an extradural transbasal approach: case report. Neurosurgery 1985;17:818–821.
6. Shady JA, Bland LI, Kazee AM, Pilcher WH. Osteoma of the frontoethmoidal sinus with secondary brain abscess and intracranial mucocele: case report. Neurosurgery 1994;34:920–923.
7. Terao H, Sato S, Kim S. Gardner's syndrome involving the skull, dura, and brain. J Neurosurg 1976;44:638–641.

### Giant Cell Tumor

1. Bertoni F, Unni KK, Beabout JW, Ebersold MJ. Giant cell tumor of the skull. Cancer 1992;70:1124–1132.
2. Coumbaras M, Pierot L, Felgeres AA, Boulin A, Gaillard S, Derome PJ. Giant-cell tumour involving the cranial vault: imaging and treatment. Neuroradiology 1999;41:826–828.
3. Lee HJ, Lum C. Giant-cell tumor of the skull base. Neuroradiology 1999;41:305–307.
4. Watkins LD, Uttley D, Archer DJ, Wilkins P, Path MRC, Plowman N. Giant cell tumors of the sphenoid bone. Neurosurgery 1992;30:576–581.
5. Wolfe JT, Scheithauer BW, Dahlin DC. Giant-cell tumor of the sphenoid bone: review of 10 cases. J Neurosurg 1983;59:322–327.
6. Yamamoto M, Fukushima T, Sakamoto S, Tomonaga M. Giant cell tumor of the sphenoid bone: long-term follow-up of two cases after chemotherapy. Surg Neurol 1998;49:547–552.

### Other Benign Neoplasms

1. Abdelhamid K, Camras LR, Nijensohn EM, Rosseau GL, Cerullo LJ. Intracranial chondroma arising from the cranial vault: CT and MR appearance. J Comput Assist Tomogr 1996;20:556–558.
2. Bakdash H, Alksne J, Rand RW. Osteochondroma of the base of the skull causing an isolated oculomotor nerve paralysis: case report emphasizing microsurgical techniques. J Neurosurg 1969;31:230–233.
3. Bertoni F, Unni KK, Beabout JW, Harner SG, Dahlin DC. Chondroblastoma of the skull and facial bones. Am J Clin Pathol 1987;88:1–9.
4. Bindal AK, Bindal RK, Van Loveren H, Sawaya R. Management of intracranial plasmacytoma. J Neurosurg 1995;83:218–221.
5. Caird J, McDermott M, Farrell M. March 2000: 5 month old boy with occipital bone mass. Brain Pathol 2000;10:317–318.
6. Dashti SR, Cohen ML, Cohen AR. Role of radical surgery for intracranial melanotic neuroectodermal tumor of infancy: case report. Neurosurgery 1999;45:175–178.
7. Du Preez JH, Branca EP. Plasmacytoma of the skull: case reports. Neurosurgery 1991;29:902–906.
8. Eisenberg MB, Al-Mefty O, DeMonte F, Burson TG. Benign nonmeningeal tumors of the cavernous sinus. Neurosurgery 1999;44:949–956.
9. Flowers CH, Rodriguez J, Naseem M, Reyes MM, Verano AS. MR of benign chondroblastoma of the temporal bone. AJNR 1995;16:414–416.
10. Frank E, Deruaz J-P, Tribolet N. Chondromyxoid fibroma of the petrous-sphenoid junction. Surg Neurol 1987;27:182–186.
11. Fu Y-S, Perzin KH. Non-epithelial tumors of the nasal cavity, paranasal sinuses, and nasopharynx: a clinicopathologic study. II. Osseous and fibroosseous lesions, including osteoma, fibrous dysplasia, ossifying fibroma, osteoblastoma, giant cell tumor, and osteosarcoma. Cancer 1974;33:1289–1305.
12. George JC, Edwards MK, Jakacki RI, Kho-Duffin J. Melanotic neuroectodermal tumor of infancy. AJNR 1995;16:1273–1275.
13. Ghogawala Z, Moore M, Strand R, Kupsky WJ, Scott RM. Clival chondroma in a child with Ollier's disease. Pediatr Neurosurg 1991–1992;17:53–56.
14. Han MH, Chang KH, Lee CH, Seo JW, Han MC, Kim C-W. Sinonasal psammomatoid ossifying fibromas: CT and MR manifestations. AJNR 1991;12:25–30.
15. Ito U, Hashimoto K, Inaba Y. Osteochondroma of the posterior clinoid process: report of a case with special reference to its histogenesis. Acta Neuropathol 1974;27:329–335.
16. Kapadia SB, Frisman DM, Hitchcock CL, Popek EJ. Clinicopathological, immunohistochemical, and flow cytometric study. Am J Surg Pathol 1993;17:566–573.
17. Karras SC, Wolford LM, Cottrell DA. Concurrent osteochondroma of the mandibular condyle and ipsilateral cranial base resulting in temporomandibular joint ankylosis: report of a case and review of the literature. J Oral Maxillofac Surg 1996;54:640–646.
18. LeMay DR, Sun JK, Mendel E, Hinton DR, Giannotta SR. Chondromyxoid fibroma of the temporal bone. Surg Neurol 1997;48:148–152.
19. Lorenzo ND, Palatinsky E, Bardella L, Maleci A. Benign osteoblastoma of the clivus removed by a transoral approach: case report. Neurosurgery 1987;20:52–55.
20. Maroon JC, Haines SJ, Phillips JG. Calvarial hemangioendothelioma with intracranial hemorrhage: case report. Neurosurgery 1979;4:178–180.
21. Mirich DR, Blaser SI, Harwood-Nash DC, Armstrong DC, Beckner LE, Posnick JC. Melanotic neuroectodermal tumor of infancy: clinical, radiologic, and pathologic findings in five cases. AJNR 1991;12:689–697.
22. Morimura T, Nakano A, Matsumoto T, Tani E. Chondromyxoid fibroma of the frontal bone. AJNR 1992;13:1262–1264.
23. Muntané A, Valls C, de Miguel MA, Pons LC. Chondroblastoma of the temporal bone: CT and MR appearance. AJNR 1993;14:70–71.
24. Nagashima C, Takahama M, Nakayama Y, Asano T. Giant occipital hemangioendothelioma with thrombocytopenia, anemia, and hypofibrinogenemia: case report. J Neurosurg 1975;43:74–79.
25. Nakagawa K, Takasato Y, Ito Y, Yamada K. Ossifying fibroma involving the paranasal sinuses, orbit, and anterior cranial fossa: case report. Neurosurgery 1995;36:1192–1195.
26. Nakase H, Nagata K, Yonezawa T, Morimoto T, Sakaki T. Extensive parasellar chondroma with Ollier's disease. Acta Neurochir 1998;140:100–101.
27. Ohkawa M, Fujiwara N, Tanabe M, et al. Benign osteoblastoma of the temporal bone. AJNR 1997;18:324–326.

28. Pierre-Kahn A, Cinalli G, Lellouch-Tubiana A, et al. Melanotic neuroectodermal tumor of the skull and meninges in infancy. Pediatr Neurosurg 1992;18:6–15.

29. Pikus HJ, Holmes B, Harbaugh RE. Teratoma of the cavernous sinus: case report. Neurosurgery 1995;36:1020–1023.

30. Provenzale JM, Schaefer P, Traweek ST, et al. Craniocerebral plasmacytoma: MR features. AJNR 1997;18:389–392.

31. Richardson RR, Deshpande VS, Thelmo WL, Rothballer A. Chondromyxoma of the middle cranial fossa: case report. Neurosurgery 1981;8:707–711.

32. Rossato RG, Timperly WR. Posterior fossa ceruminoma. Acta Neurochir 1973;28:315–322.

33. Salvati M, Cervoni L, Ciapetta P, Artico M, Raco A. Solitary plasmacytoma of the skull: report of two cases. Clin Neurol Neurosurg 1994;96:66–70.

34. Sato K, Kodera T, Kitai R, Kubota T. Osteochondroma of the skull base: MRI and histological correlation. Neuroradiology 1996;38:41–43.

35. Selfa-Moreno S, Arana-Fernández E, Fernández-Latorre F, Díaz-Ramón C, Ricart-Rodrigo M, Moreno-Flores A. Desmoplastic fibroma of the skull: case report. J Neurosurg 1995;82:119–120.

36. Sharma MC, Mahapatra AK, Gaikwad SB, Sarkar C. Solitary giant skull base schwannomas—report of four cases. Surg Neurol 1997;48:382–388.

37. Stowens D, Lin T-H. Melanotic progonoma of the brain. Hum Pathol 1974;5:105–113.

38. Terasaka S, Sawamura Y, Abe H. Surgical removal of a cavernous sinus chondroma. Surg Neurol 1997;48:153–159.

39. Tomabechi M, Sako K, Daita G, Yonemasu Y. Lipoma involving the skull. J Neurosurg 1992;76:312–314.

40. Tomita T, Huvos AG, Shah J, Sundaresan N. Giant ossifying fibroma of the nasal cavity with intracranial extension. Acta Neurochir 1981;56:65–71.

41. Villemure J-G, Meagher-Villemure K. Giant ossifying fibroma of the skull: case report. J Neurosurg 1983;58:602–606.

42. Wolf DA, Chaljub G, Maggio W, Gelman BB. Intracranial chondromyxoid fibroma. Arch Pathol Lab Med 1997;121:624–630.

## Chordoma

1. Borba LAB, Osma A, Mrak RE, Suen J. Cranial chordomas in children and adolescents. J Neurosurg 1996;84:584–591.

2. Chambers PW, Schwinn CP. Chordoma: a clinicopathologic study of metastasis. Am J Anat 1979;128:193–224.

3. Forsyth PA, Cascino T, Shaw EG, et al. Intracranial chordomas: a clinicopathological and prognostic study of 51 cases. J Neurosurg 1993;78:741–747.

4. Gay E, Sekhar LN, Rubinstein E, et al. Chordomas and chondrosarcomas of the cranial base: results and follow-up of 60 patients. Neurosurgery 1995;36:887–896.

5. Gessaga EC, Mair WGP, Grant DN. Ultrastructure of a sacrococcygeal chordoma. Acta Neuropathol 1973;25:27–35.

6. Heffelfinger MJ, Dahlin DC, MacCarty CS, Beabout JW. Chordomas and cartilaginous tumors at the skull base. Cancer 1973;32:410–420.

7. Horten BC, Montague SR. Human ecchordosis physaliphora and chick embryonic notochord: a comparative electron microscopic study. Virchows Arch [A] 1976;37:295–303.

8. Horten BC, Montague SR. In vitro characteristics of a sacrococcygeal chordoma maintained in tissue and organ culture. Acta Neuropathol 1976;35:13–25.

9. Hug EB, Loredo LN, Slater JD, et al. Proton radiation therapy for chordomas and chondrosarcomas of the skull base. J Neurosurg 1999;91:432–439.

10. Kaneko Y, Sato Y, Iwaki T, Shin R-W, Tateishi J, Fukui M. Chordoma in early childhood: a clinicopathological study. Neurosurgery 1991;29:442–446.

11. Kay S, Schatzki PF. Ultrastructural observations of a chordoma arising in the clivus. Hum Pathol 1972;3:403–413.

12. Meis JM, Giraldo AA. Chordoma: an immunohistochemical study of 20 cases. Arch Pathol Lab Med 1988;112:553–556.

13. Miettinen M. Chordoma: antibodies to epithelial membrane antigen and carcinoembryonic antigen in differential diagnosis. Arch Pathol Lab Med 1984;108:891–892.

14. Miettinen M, Karaharju E, Järvinen H. Chordoma with a massive spindle-cell sarcomatous transformation. Am J Surg Pathol 1987;11:563–570.

15. Miettinen M, Lehto V, Dahl D, Virtanen I. Differential diagnosis of chordoma, chrondroid and ependymal tumors as aided by anti–intermediate filament antibodies. Am J Pathol 1983;112:160–169.

16. Mitchell A, Scheithauer BW, Unni KK, Forsyth PJ, Wold LE, McGivney DJ. Chordoma and chondroid neoplasms of the spheno-occiput. An immunohistochemical study of 41 cases with prognostic and nosologic implications. Cancer 1993;72:2943–2949.

17. Nakamura Y, Becker LE, Marks A. S100 protein in human chordoma and human and rabbit notochord. Arch Pathol Lab Med 1983;107:118–120.

18. O'Connell JX, Renard LG, Liebsch NJ, Efird JT, Munzenrider JE, Rosenberg AE. Base of skull chordoma. A correlative study of histologic and clinical features of 62 cases. Cancer 1994;74:2261–2267.

19. Raffel C, Wright DC, Gutin PH, Wilson CB. Cranial chordomas: clinical presentation and results of operative and radiation therapy in twenty-six patients. Neurosurery 1985;17:703–710.

20. Rich TA, Schiller A, Suit HD, Mankin HJ. Clinical and pathologic review of 48 cases of chordoma. Cancer 1985;56:182–187.

21. Rosenberg AE, Brown GA, Bhan AK, Lee JM. Chondroid chordoma—a variant of chordoma. A morphologic and immunohistochemical study. Am J Clin Pathol 1994;101:36–41.

22. Rosenberg AE, Nielsen GP, Keele SB, et al. Chondrosarcoma of the base of the skull. A clinicopathologic study of 200 cases with emphasis on its distinction from chordoma. Am J Surg Pathol 1999;23:1370–1378.

23. Salisbury JR. Demonstration of cytokeratins and an epithelial membrane antigen in chondroid chordoma. J Pathol 1987;153:37–40.

24. Salisbury JR. The pathology of the human notochord. J Pathol 1993;171:253–255.

25. Salisbury JR, Isaacson PG. Demonstration of cytokeratins and an epithelial membrane antigen in chordomas and human fetal notochord. Am J Surg Pathol 1985;9:791–797.

26. Schoedel KE, Martinez AJ, Mahoney TM, Contis L, Becich MJ. Chordomas: pathological features; ploidy and silver nucleolar organizing region analysis. A study of 36 cases. Acta Neuropathol 1995;89:139–143.

27. Thodou E, Kontogeorgos G, Scheithauer BW, et al. Intrasellar chordoma mimicking pituitary adenoma. J Neurosurg 2000;92:976–982.

28. Toda H, Ankinori K, Iwasaki K. Neuroradiological characteristics of ecchordosis physaliphora: case report and review of the literature. J Neurosurg 1998;89:830–834.

29. Tomlinson FH, Scheithauer BW, Forsythe PA, Unni KK, Meyer FB. Sarcomatous transformation in cranial chordoma. Neurosurgery 1992;31:13–18.

30. Wolfe JT III, Scheithauer BW. "Intradural chordoma" or "giant ecchordosis physaliphora"?: report of two cases. Clin Neuropathol 1987;6:98–103.

31. Wyatt RB, Schochet SS Jr, McCormick WF. Ecchordosis physaliphora: an electron microscopic study. J Neurosurg 1971;34:672–677.

## Olfactory Neuroblastoma (Esthesioneuroblastoma, Esthesioneuroepithelioma)

1. Argani P, Perez-Ordoñez B, Xiao H, Caruana SM, Huvos AG, Ladanyi M. Olfactory neuroblastoma is not related to the Ewing family of tumors. Am J Surg Pathol 1998;22:391–398.

2. Choi H-SH, Anderson PJ. Olfactory neuroblastoma: an immunoelectron microscopic study of S-100 protein–positive cells. J Neuropathol Exp Neurol 1986;45:576–587.

3. Dulguerov P, Calcaterra T. Esthesioneuroblastoma: the UCLA experience 1970–1990. Laryngoscope 1992;102:843–849.

4. Foote RL, Morita A, Ebersold MJ, et al. Esthesioneuroblastoma: the role of adjuvant radiation therapy. Int J Radiat Oncol Biol Phys 1993;27:835–842.

5. Frierson HF, Mills SE, Fechner RE, Taxy JB, Levine PA. Sinonasal undifferentiated carcinoma. Am J Surg Pathol 1986;10: 771–779.

6. Frierson HF, Ross GW, Mills SE, Frankfurter A. Olfactory neuroblastoma. Additional immunohistochemical characterization. Am J Clin Pathol 1990;94:547–553.

7. Hirose T, Scheithauer BW, Lopes MBS, et al. Olfactory neuroblastoma. An immunohistochemical, ultrastructural, and flow cytometric study. Cancer 1995;76:4–19.

8. Hyams VJ. Special Tumors of the Head and Neck: Olfactory Neuroblastoma. Chicago: American Society of Clinical Pathologists, 1983, pp 24–29.

9. Li C, Yousem DM, Hayden RE, Doty RL. Olfactory neuroblastoma: MR evaluation. AJNR 1993;14:1167–1171.

10. McElroy EA Jr, Buckner JC, Lewis JE. Chemotherapy for advanced esthesioneuroblastoma: the Mayo Clinic experience. Neurosurgery 1998;42:1023–1027.

11. Meneses MS, Thurel C, Mikol J, et al. Esthesioneuroblastoma with intracranial extension. Neurosurgery 1990;27:813–820.

12. Mills SE, Fechner RE. "Undifferentiated" neoplasms of the sinonasal region: differential diagnosis based on clinical, light microscopic, immunohistochemical, and ultrastructural features. Semin Diagn Pathol 1989;6:316–328.

13. Mills SE, Frierson HF Jr. Olfactory neuroblastoma. A clinicopathologic study of 21 cases. Am J Surg Pathol 1985;9:317–327.

14. Mills SE, Gaffey MJ, Frierson FH Jr. Tumors of the Upper Aerodigestive Tract and Ear. Bethesda, MD: Armed Forces Institute of Pathology, 2000.

15. Morita A, Ebersold MJ, Olsen KD, Foote RL, Lewis JE, Quast LM. Esthesioneuroblastoma: prognosis and management. Neurosurgery 1993;32:706–714; discussion 14–15.

16. Ordonez NG, Mackay B. Neuroendocrine tumors of the nasal cavity. Pathol Annu 1993;28:77–111.

17. Papadaki H, Kounelis S, Kapadia SB, Bakker A, Swalsky PA, Finkelstein SD. Relationship of p53 gene alterations with tumor progression and recurrence in olfactory neuroblastoma. Am J Surg Pathol 1996;20:715–721.

18. Polin RS, Sheehan JP, Chenelle AG, et al. The role of preoperative adjuvant treatment in the management of esthesioneuroblastoma: the University of Virginia experience. Neurosurgery 1998;42:1029–1037.

19. Som PM, Lidov M, Brandwein M, Catalano P, Biller HF. Sinonasal esthesioneuroblastoma with intracranial extension: marginal tumor cysts as a diagnostic MR finding. AJNR 1994;15: 1259–1262.

20. Takahashi H, Ohara S, Yamada M, Ikuta F, Tanimura K, Hna Y. Esthesioneuroepithelioma: a tumor of true olfactory epithelium origin. An ultrastructural and immunohistochemical study. Acta Neuropathol 1987;75:147–155.

21. Tatagiba M, Samii M, Dankoweit-Timpe E, et al. Esthesioneuroblastomas with intracranial extension. Proliferative potential and management. Arq Neuropsiquiatr 1995;53:577–586.

22. Taxy JB, Hidvegi DF. Olfactory neuroblastoma: an ultrastructural study. Cancer 1977;39:131–138.

23. Vartanian RK. Olfactory neuroblastoma: an immunohistochemical, ultrastructural, and flow cytometric study [letter; comment]. Cancer 1996;77:1957–1959.

## Papillary Endolymphatic Sac Tumor

1. Gaffey MJ, Mills SE, Fechner RE, Intemann SR, Wick MR. Aggressive papillary middle-ear tumor. A clinicopathologic entity distinct from middle-ear adenoma. Am J Surg Pathol 1988;12: 790–797.

2. Heffner DK. Low-grade adenocarcinoma of probable endolymphatic sac origin. Cancer 1989;64:2292–2302.

3. Kerr D, Scheithauer BW, Weiland LH. Aggressive papillary middle ear tumor: a component of von Hippel–Lindau syndrome. J Neuropathol Exp Neurol 1992;51:367.

4. Meyer FB, Gebarski SS, Blaivas M. Cerebellopontine angle invasive papillary cystadenoma of endolymphatic sac origin with temporal bone involvement. AJNR 1993;14:1319–1323.

5. Mukherji SK, Albernaz VS, Lo WW, et al. Papillary endolymphatic sac tumors: CT, MR imaging, and angiographic findings in 20 patients. Radiology 1997;202:801–808.

6. Panchwagh J, Goel A, Shenoy A. Bilateral endolymphatic sac papillary carcinoma. Br J Neurosurg 1999;13:79–81.

7. Paulus W, Romstöck J, Weidenbecher M, Huk WJ, Fahlbusch R. Middle ear adenocarcinoma with intracranial extension. J Neurosurg 1999;90:555–558.

8. Polinsky MN, Brunberg JA, McKeever PE, Sandler HM, Telian S, Ross D. Aggressive papillary middle ear tumors: a report of two cases with review of the literature. Neurosurgery 1994;35: 493–497.

9. Roche P-H, Defour H, Figarella-Branger D, Pellett W. Endolymphatic sac tumors: report of three cases. Neurosurgery 1998;42:927–932.

10. Tibbs RE, Bowles AP, Raila FA, Fratkin JD, Hutchins JB. Should endolymphatic sac tumors be considered part of the von Hippel–Lindau complex? Pathology case report. Neurosurgery 1997;40:848–855.

## Metastatic Neoplasms

1. Arseni C, Constantinescu AI. Cerebral and cranial metastases from breast cancer. Neurochirurgia 1982;25:95–99.

2. Belal A Jr. Metastatic tumours of the temporal bone: a histopathological report. J Laryngol Otol 1985;99:839–846.

3. Dolan EJ, Schwartz ML, Lews AJ, Kassell EE, Cooper PW. Adenoid cystic carcinoma: an unusual neurosurgical entity. Can J Neurol Sci 1985;12:65–68.

4. Feinmesser R, Libson Y, Uziely B, Gay I. Metastatic carcinoma to the temporal bone. Am J Otol 1986;7:119–120.

5. Candour-Edwards R, Kapadia SB, Barnes L, Donald PJ, Janecka IP. Neural cell adhesion molecule in adenoid cystic carcinoma invading the skull base. Otolaryngol Head Neck Surg 1997;117: 453–458.

6. Ginsberg LE, DeMonte F. Imaging of perineural tumor spread from palatal carcinoma. AJNR 1998;19:1417–1422.

7. Gormley WB, Sekhar LN, Wright DC, et al. Management and long-term outcome of adenoid cystic carcinoma with intracranial extension: a neurosurgical perspective. Neurosurgery 1996;38: 1105–1113.

8. Kincaid OW, Hodgson JR, Dockerty MB. Neuroblastoma: a roentgenologic and pathologic study. Am J Roentgenol Radium Ther Nucl Med 1957;78:420–436.

9. Nagamine Y, Suzuki J, Katakura R, et al. Skull metastasis of thyroid carcinoma: study of 12 cases. J Neurosurg 1985;63:526–531.

10. Piepmeier JM, Virapongse C, Kier EZ, Kim J, Greenberg A. Intracranial adenocystic carcinoma presenting as a primary brain tumor. Neurosurgery 1983;12:348–352.

11. Roessmann U, Kaufman B, Friede RL. Metastatic lesions of the sella turcica and pituitary gland. Cancer 1970;25:478–480.

12. Sherman RS, Leaming R. The roentgen findings in neuroblastoma. Radiology 1953;60:837–849.

## Multiple Myeloma

1. Silverstein A, Doniger DE. Neurologic complications of myelomatosis. Arch Neurol 1963;9:534–544.

## Other Malignant Neoplasms

1. Amine ARC, Sugar O. Suprasellar osteogenic sarcoma following radiation for pituitary adenoma: case report. J Neurosurg 1976;44:88–92.

2. Ashkan K, Pollock J, D'Arrigo C, Kitchen ND. Intracranial osteosarcomas: report of four cases and review of the literature. J Neurooncol 1998;40:87–96.

3. Biousse V, Newman NJ, Lee AG, Eggenberger E, Patrinely JR, Kaufman D. Intracranial Ewing's sarcoma. J Neuroophthalmol 1998;18:187–191.

4. Carpentier AF, Chantelard J-V, Henin D, Poisson M. Osteosarcoma following radiation treatment for meningioma: report of a case and effective treatment with chemotherapy. J Neurooncol 1994;21:249–253.

5. Chin LS, Rabb CH, Hinton DR, Apuzzo MLJ. Hemangiopericytoma of the temporal bone presenting as a retroauricular mass. Neurosurgery 1993;33:728–731.

6. Coltrera MD, Googe PB, Harrist TJ, Hyams VJ, Schiller AL, Goodman ML. Chondrosarcoma of the temporal bone: diagnosis and treatment of 13 cases and review of the literature. Cancer 1986;58:2689–2696.

7. Cosentino CM, Poulton TB, Esguerra JV, Sands SF. Giant cranial hemangiopericytoma: MR and angiographic findings. AJNR 1993;14:253–256.

8. Fitzer PM, Steffey WR. Brain and bone scans in primary Ewing's sarcoma of the petrous bone: case report. J Neurosurg 1976;44: 608–612.

9. Fleischer AS, Koslow M, Rovit RL. Neurological manifestations of primary rhabdomyosarcomas of the head and neck in childhood. J Neurosurg 1975;43:207–214.

10. Fransen P, Mestdagh C, Dardenne G. Pagetic sarcoma of the calvarium: report of two cases. Acta Neurol Belg 1998;79:363–366.

11. Gay E, Sekhar LN, Rubinstein E, et al. Chordomas and chondrosarcomas of the cranial base: results and follow-up of 60 patients. Neurosurgery 1995;36:887–897.

12. Hug EB, Loredo LN, Slater JD, et al. Proton radiation therapy for chordomas and chondrosarcomas of the skull base. J Neurosurg 1999;91:432–439.
13. Huvos AG, Sundaresan N, Bretsky SS, Butler A. Osteogenic sarcoma of the skull: a clinicopathologic study of 19 patients. Cancer 1985;56:1214–1221.
14. Korten AG, ter Berg HJ, Spincemaille GH, van der Laan RT, Van de Wel AM. Intracranial chondrosarcoma: review of the literature. J Neurol Neurosurg Psychiatry 1998;65:88–92.
15. Lopes M, Duffau H, Fleuridas G. Primary spheno-orbital angiosarcoma: case report and review of the literature. Neurosurgery 1999;44:405–408.
16. Mansfield JB. Primary fibrosarcoma of the skull: case report. J Neurosurg 1977;47:785–787.
17. McKenna RJ, Schwinn CP, Soong KY, Higinbotham NL. Osteogenic sarcoma arising in Paget's disease. Cancer 1964;17:42–66.
18. Nakayama K, Nemoto Y, Inoue Y, et al. Malignant fibrous histiocytoma of the temporal bone with endocranial extension. AJNR 1997;18:331–334.
19. Parekh HC, Sharma RR, Keogh AJ, Prabhu SS. Primary malignant non-Hodgkin's lymphoma of cranial vault: a case report. Surg Neurol 1993;39:286–289.
20. Rosenberg AE, Nielson GP, Keel SB, et al. Chondrosarcoma of the base of the skull. A clinicopathologic study of 200 cases with emphasis on its distinction from chordoma. J Surg Pathol 1999;23:1370–1378.
21. Rossato RG, Timperly WR. Posterior fossa ceruminoma. Acta Neurochir 1973;28:315–322.
22. Salvati M, Cervoni L, Ciappetta P, Raco A. Radiation-induced osteosarcomas of the skull: report of two cases and review of the literature. Clin Neurol Neurosurg 1994;96:226–229.
23. Salvati M, Cervoni L, Raguso M, Raco A. Post-Pagetic osteosarcoma of the skull. Remarks on five cases. Tumori 1993;79:363–366.
24. Salvati M, Ciappetta P, Capuccia G, Capone R, Raco A. Osteosarcoma of the skull, report of a post-Paget and post-radiation case in an elderly woman. Neurosurg Rev 1994;17:73–76.
25. Seth HN, Singh M. Intracranial mesenchymal chondrosarcoma. Acta Neuropathol 1973;24:86–89.
26. Shinoda J, Kimura T, Funakosi T, et al. Primary osteosarcoma of the skull. J Neurooncol 1993;17:81–88.
27. Stapleton SR, Wilkins PR, Archer DJ, Uttley D. Chondrosarcoma of the skull base: a series of eight cases. Neurosurgery 1993;32:348–356.
28. Topolmicki W, White RJ. Primary reticulum cell sarcoma of the skull: response to irradiation. Cancer 1969;24:569–573.
29. Watanabe H, Tsubokawa T, Katayama Y, Koyama S, Nakamura S. Primary Ewing's sarcoma of the temporal bone. Surg Neurol 1992;37:54–58.
30. Young HA, Hardy DG, Ashleigh R. Osteogenic sarcoma of the skull complicating Paget's disease. Neurosurgery 1983;12:454–457.

## Epidermoid and Dermoid Cysts

1. Alpers BJ, Harrow R. Cholesteatoma originating in the skull bones causing symptoms of intracranial pressure. Am J Surg 1932;18:51–57.
2. Arana E, Latorre FF, Revert A, et al. Intradiploic epidermoid cysts. Neuroradiology 1996;38:306–311.
3. Canale DJ, Clarke HA, Pak YH, Burton WD. Giant primary intradiploic epidermoid tumor of the skull: case report. Surg Neurol 1974;2:51–54.
4. Constans JP, Meder JF, De Divitiis E, et al. Giant intradiploic epidermoid cysts of the skull: report of two cases. J Neurosurg 1985;62:445–448.
5. Garcia J, Lagier R, Hoessly M. Computed tomography–pathology correlation in skull epidermoid cyst. J Comput Assist Tomogr 1982;6:818–820.
6. Gormley WB, Tomecek FJ, Qureshi N, Malik GM. Craniocerebral epidermoid and dermoid tumours: a review of 32 cases. Acta Neurochir 1994;128:115–121.
7. Hig PV. Primary epidermoids of the skull: including a case with malignant changes. Am J Roentgenol Radium Ther Nucl Med 1956;76:1076–1080.
8. Hoeffel C, Heldt N, Chelle C, Claudon M, Hoeffel JC. Malignant change in an intradiploic epidermoid cyst. Acta Neurol Belg 1997;97:45–49.
9. Kanamaru K, Waga S. Congenital dermoid cyst of the anterior fontanel in a Japanese infant. Surg Neurol 1984;21:287–290.
10. Kveton JF, Glasscock ME III, Christiansen SG. Malignant degeneration of an epidermoid of the temporal bone. Otolaryngol Head Neck Surg 1986;94:633–636.
11. Martinez-Lage JF, Quinonez MA, Poza M, et al. Congenital epidermoid cysts over the anterior fontanelle. Childs Nerv Syst 1985;1:319–323.
12. Neblett CR, Caram PC, Morris R. Lateral congenital dermal sinus tract associated with an intradiploic dermoid tumor: case report. J Neurosurg 1970;33:103–105.
13. Ojikutu NA, Mordi VPN. Congenital inclusion dermoid cyst located over the region of the anterior fontanel in adult Nigerians: report of two cases. J Neurosurg 1980;52:724–727.
14. Pannell BW, Hendrick EB. Dermoid cysts of the anterior fontanelle. Neurosurgery 1982;10:317–323.
15. Reddick EJ, Ettinger D, Madauss WC. Dermoid cysts of the anterior fontanelle: case reports. Milit Med 1983;148:548–550.
16. Skandalakis JE, Godwin JT, Mabon RF. Epidermoid cyst of the skull: report of four cases and review of the literature. Surgery 1958;43:990–1001.
17 Swisher RC, Tesluk H. Epidermoid cyst of the skull causing displacement of brain. JAMA 1969;210:1280–1281.
18. Yanai Y, Tsuji R, Ohmori S, et al. Malignant change in an intradiploic epidermoid: report of a case and review of the literature. Neurosurgery 1985;16:252–256.

## Meningocele and Encephalocele

1. Bagger-Sjoback D, Bergstrand D, Edner G, Anggard A. Nasal meningoencephalocele: a clinical problem. Clin Otolaryngol 1983;8:329–335.
2. Caviness VS, Evrard P. Occipital encephalocele: a pathologic and anatomic analysis. Acta Neuropathol 1975;32:245–255.
3. David DJ, Sheffield L, Simpson D, White J. Fronto-ethmoidal meningoencephaloceles: morphology and treatment. Br J Plast Surg 1984;37:271–284.
4. Fisher RG, Uihlein A, Keith HM. Spina bifida and cranium bifidum: study of 530 cases. Proc Staff Meet Mayo Clin 1952;27:33–38.
5. Gray BG, Willinsky RA, Rutka JA, Tator CH. Spontaneous meningocele, a rare middle ear mass. AJNR 1995;16:20.
6. Hayashi T, Utsunomiya H, Hashimoto T. Transethmoidal encephalomeningocele. Surg Neurol 1985;24:651–655.
7. Ingraham FD, Swan H. Spina bifida and cranium bifidum. I. A survey of five hundred and forty-six cases. N Engl J Med 1943;228:559–563.
8. Karch SB, Urich H. Occipital encephalocele: a morphological study. J Neurol Sci 1972;15:89–112.
9. Larsen CE, Hudgins PA, Hunter SB. Skull-base meningoencephalocele presenting as a unilateral neck mass in a neonate. AJNR 1995;16:1161–1163.
10. Lee CM, McLaurin RL. Heterotopic brain tissue as an isolated embryonic rest. J Neurosurg 1955;12:190–195.
11. Mahapatra AK, Tandon PN, Dhawan IK, Khazanchi RK. Anterior encephaloceles: a report of 30 cases. Childs Nerv Syst 1994;10:501–504.
12. Nagulich I, Borne G, Georgevich Z. Temporal meningocele. J Neurosurg 1967;27:433–440.
13. Orkin M, Fisher I. Heterotopic brain tissue (heterotopic neural rest). Arch Dermatol 1966;94:699–708.
14. Raftopoulos C, David P, Allard S, Ickx B, Balériaux D. Endoscopic treatment of an oral cephalocele. J Neurosurg 1994;81:308–309.
15. Smith DE, Murphy MJ, Hitchon PW, et al. Transsphenoidal encephaloceles. Surg Neurol 1983;20:471–480.
16. Wilkins RH, Radtke RA, Burger PC. Spontaneous temporal encephalocele. J Neurosurg 1993;78:492–498.

## Nasal Glial Heterotopia ("Nasal Glioma")

1. Black BK, Smith DE. Nasal glioma: two cases with recurrence. Arch Neurol Psychiatry 1950;64:614–630.
2. Bossen EH, Hudson WR. Oligodendroglioma arising in heterotopic brain tissue of the soft palate and nasopharynx. Am J Surg Pathol 1987;11:571–574.

3. Choudhury AR, Bandey SQ, Haleem A, Sharif H. Glial heterotopias of the nose. A report of two cases. Childs Nerv Syst 1996;12:43–47.
4. Farhat SM, Hudson JS. Extracerebral brain heterotopia: case report. J Neurosurg 1969;30:190–194.
5. Goldring S, Hodges FH III, Luse SA. Ectopic neural tissue of occipital bone. J Neurosurg 1964;21:479–484.
6. Kindblom LG, Angervall L, Haglid K. An immunohistochemical analysis of S-100 protein and glial fibrillary acidic protein in nasal glioma. Acta Pathol Microbiol Immunol Scand 1984;92:378–389.
7. Mirra SS, Pearl GS, Hoffman JC, Campbell WG Jr. Nasal "glioma" with prominent neuronal component: report of a case. Arch Pathol Lab Med 1981;105:540–541.
8. Musser AW, Campbell R. Nasal glioma: report of an unusual case associated with multiple supragaleal nodules. Arch Otolaryngol 1961;73:732–736.
9. Patterson K, Kapur S, Chandra RS. "Nasal gliomas" and related brain heterotopias: a pathologist's perspective. Pediatr Pathol 1986;5:353–362.

# INTRACRANIAL MENINGES

2

As bland fibrous vestments of a magnificent organ, the meninges could be relegated easily to an insignificant status. However, as is emphasized in this chapter, they have an identity of their own and spawn a variety of distinctive and important pathologic lesions.

## BENIGN NEOPLASMS AND NON-NEOPLASTIC TUMORS

### Meningioma

**Definition.** A generally well-circumscribed, slowly growing neoplasm derived from meningothelial cells.

**General Comments.** The perception of meningioma has evolved in the space of several decades from that of a simple benign lesion with only a few histologic subtypes to that of a complicated and ever enlarging family. Grading has become standard practice. The following discussion is therefore more detailed than that of the previous edition. We apologize if we appear to make a simple lesion seem unnecessarily complex, but meningiomas are more heterogeneous than is often assumed.

There remains little reason to doubt that meningiomas take their origin from meningothelial cells that occur in greatest abundance in arachnoid villi but are also encountered as small clusters distributed diffusely in the arachnoid membrane of the craniospinal space. These cells become prominent during the later decades of life, when whorls emerge and psammoma bodies appear. Their cytologic and immunohistochemical features are replicated in the neoplasms they engender, thus giving insight into the origin of meningiomas and facilitating their recognition in histologic sections. The presence, normally, of meningothelial cells in the choroid plexus and tela choroidea explains the occurrence of meningiomas in these seemingly improbable locations. A related cell, the "arachnoid trabecular cell," has been suggested as a progenitor of meningiomas of the microcystic subtype.[59]

**Clinical Features.** Meningiomas are common intracranial neoplasms with biologic characteristics that distinguish them from most other intracranial tumors. They enlarge slowly, are reluctant to infiltrate brain, and, when favorably situated, are cured by simple excision. Most occur clinically after the third decade, but an occasional example is encountered during childhood,[28, 29, 41, 52, 56, 96, 129, 145, 146] and even neonates can be affected.[113]

Although it is not understood why the incidence of typical intracranial meningiomas in women exceeds that in men by a ratio of 3:2, this degree of biologic variation is not uncommon in the broad field of neoplasia. In contrast, atypical and malignant meningiomas are somewhat more frequent in males.[15, 54, 61, 63, 67, 95, 172] The growth of meningiomas may be accelerated during pregnancy.[10] An

explanation has been sought in the frequent presence of progesterone receptors.[15, 55, 76, 106]

Although the mystery concerning the etiology shadows most meningiomas, there are notable exceptions, such as those that occur after cranial radiation[35, 42, 49, 94, 132, 144, 151] or arise in the setting of neurofibromatosis 2 (NF2).[80] The rare occurrence of familial cases without NF2 gene mutations implicates other genes as well.[100,134] Trauma, an enduring suspect in rare cases, has avoided conviction in the presence of only circumstantial evidence.[4, 6, 131]

Although meningiomas occur throughout the craniospinal axis, certain sites are clearly favored (Fig. 2–1). These include the parasagittal area within several centimeters of the superior sagittal sinus (parasagittal meningioma), the cerebral convexities (free convexity meningioma), the wing of the sphenoid bone (sphenoid ridge meningioma), the tuberculum sella (suprasellar or sellar meningioma), the region of or adjacent to the cribriform plate (olfactory groove meningioma), the region surrounding the foramen magnum, the optic nerve,[117] and the tentorium.

For the embryologic reasons already described, the choroid plexus and tela choroidea of the ventricular system are the occasional sites of origin. Most intraventricular lesions arise in the lateral ventricles, where, for reasons unknown, the left is somewhat favored.[81, 97] Third ventricular examples occur primarily in children.[17, 56, 96, 136, 145] Fourth ventricular meningiomas are so unusual that a preoperative diagnosis is rarely made; choroid plexus tumors

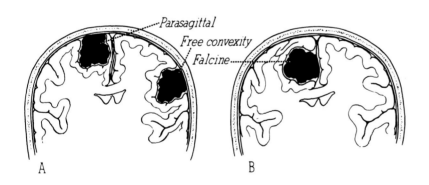

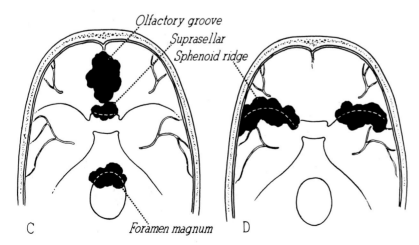

**FIGURE 2–1** MENINGIOMA

Common locations of meningiomas.

and ependymomas are statistically more likely in this locale.[128, 161]

Understandably, meningiomas arise within bone or pericranial soft tissues, but their occurrence in lung,[66, 87, 130] mediastinum,[169] brachial plexus,[21] skin,[90] parotid gland,[171] and sinonasal tract[156] is difficult to explain. The differentiating potential of germ cell neoplasia underlies a rare meningioma within a testicular tumor.[3]

Meningiomas are usually solitary but may be multiple in either the absence[36] or presence[80] of NF2. The NF2-associated lesions may be innumerable and diffusely stud the intracranial and intraspinal meninges. Almost by definition, they are accompanied by bilateral schwannomas of the vestibular, and often other intracranial and intraspinal sensory, nerves. In this setting, a meningioma and a schwannoma can arise concurrently in the cerebellopontine angle to form a single "mixed tumor." Molecular biologic studies suggest that some multiple meningiomas can be clonal and, therefore, represent subarachnoid dissemination of a single primary.[165] Similar studies suggest that recurrent meningiomas are also identical from a molecular perspective to the original tumor and are therefore a true recurrence and not a second primary.[166]

*Meningioangiomatosis*, a meningioma-like lesion occasionally associated with NF2, is discussed separately on pages 99 to 101.

In rare instances, meningiomas arise in association with an underlying glioma.[30, 99] Whether this is fortuitous or the result of a common oncogenic event is unknown. Some meningiomas are associated with systemic malignancies, particularly estrogen-dependent tumors such as carcinomas of the breast and ovaries.[11, 64] Carcinoma metastatic to meningiomas is also recognized; the primary site is usually the breast.[11]

**Radiologic Features.** Most meningiomas expand centrifugally and remain spherical or globular, even as they attain considerable size. An important exception is the flat, carpet-like *en plaque* meningioma that typically creeps over the sphenoid ridge (see Fig. 2–11). Most meningiomas are solid; cystic examples are relatively rare.[14, 31, 167, 174] Meningiomas can penetrate dura, occlude venous sinuses, and invade bone (see Figs. 1–45 to 1–47). They can also produce hyperostosis as a direct consequence of infiltration or by merely arising in the proximity.[50] Although infiltration of the skull may extend the lesion beyond the reach of surgery, this expansion is not necessarily indicative of malignancy. Occasional lesions arise primarily within diploë of bone.[83, 116] Meningiomas in, or of, the skull are discussed in Chapter 1 on page 21.

On magnetic resonance (MR) imaging scans, meningiomas are noted for the isointensity of their signal relative to cerebral cortex on T1- and T2-weighted images.[147] Most other central nervous system (CNS) lesions, whether neoplastic or not, are hyperintense, that is, white, in T2-weighted images. This darkness is carried to an extreme in some fibrous variants wherein collagen and calcification combine their effects to "shorten" the T2 signal and produce a black mass (Fig. 2–2).[37] Lipidized meningiomas are bright in precontrast

T1-weighted images to a degree proportional to the lesion's content of fat.[85, 139, 142]

Meningiomas are homogeneously and brightly contrast enhancing as viewed by both computed tomography (CT) and MR imaging. With MR, a distinctive feature is extension of enhancement from the periphery of the lesion onto the surrounding dural surface (Fig. 2–3). Such "dural tails," although nonspecific, are typical of meningiomas and, when combined with other signal characteristics, permit an accurate preoperative diagnosis in most instances.[13, 157] Histologically, the dural tail can be either a tongue of tumor or a wedge of reactive fibrovascular tissue.[44, 158]

Meningiomas of the optic nerve sheath surround the nerve to produce a characteristic "bull's-eye" profile by MR when seen "end on" (Figs. 2–4 to 2–7).

By the time they become symptomatic, intraventricular examples have become large contrast-enhancing masses (Fig. 2–8).

Some meningiomas incite a broad zone of vasogenic edema in the white matter of the adjacent brain. Although there are many exceptions, most edema-inducing tumors are large, have a high Ki-67 labeling index, are attached to or invade the brain, or derive their blood supply from the internal carotid artery system.[57, 58, 107, 143] Thus, the finding of edema suggests that the lesion may be atypical or malignant. An irregular interface with brain is additional, and more dependable, evidence that the lesion is more aggressive than the typical lesion (Fig. 2–9).

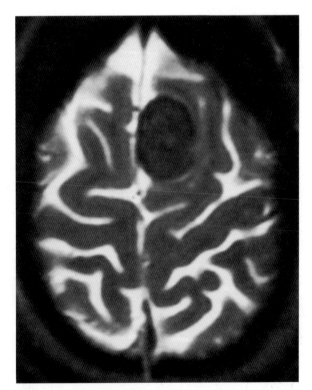

**FIGURE 2–2** MENINGIOMA

Unlike most intracranial tumors, which are hyperintense, or white, on T2-weighted MR images, meningiomas are isointense, if not hypointense, when compared with cortical gray matter. This fibrous meningioma was exceptionally dark because of its content of collagen and calcium.

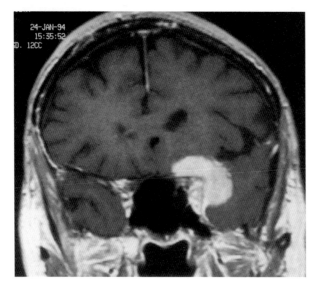

**FIGURE 2-3    MENINGIOMA**

Meningiomas are contrast enhancing, with a broad dural base and short extensions of enhancement along the dura ("dural tail" sign). A "tail" extends inferiorly from this sphenoid ridge tumor.

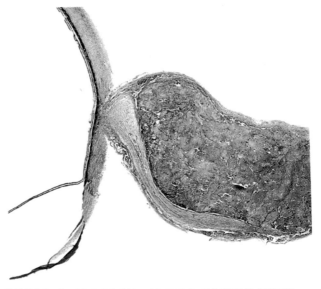

**FIGURE 2-5    MENINGIOMA OF THE OPTIC NERVE SHEATH**

Exophthalmos and visual loss were clinical expressions of this tumor situated immediately behind the globe of a 46-year-old woman. The discrete neoplasm expands within the optic sheath at the expense of the inferiorly displaced nerve.

**Macroscopic Features.** Intraoperatively, most meningiomas are globular discrete masses with a dural base (Fig. 2-10). The en plaque variant, which is usually found over the sphenoid wing, is a carpet-like mass (Fig. 2-11). The external contour of most meningiomas appears cobblestoned or bosselated, a feature reflected on cut section as characteristic lobularity (Fig. 2-12). Fibrous meningiomas, on the other hand, are often exceptionally smooth and well demarcated (Figs. 2-13 and 2-14).

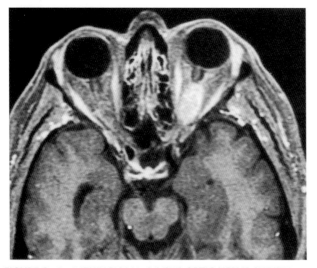

**FIGURE 2-4    MENINGIOMA OF THE OPTIC NERVE SHEATH**

Exophthalmos and visual loss drew attention to this contrast-enhancing mass that encased the optic nerve and displaced the globe anteriorly.

Tumor consistency varies from soft to tough or gritty, depending largely on the content of fibrous tissue and/or calcium. Color shades from tan to red reflect the tumor's vascularity. In some instances, a yellow-orange color is imparted by extensive xanthomatous change or frank lipidization. Although meningiomas of the optic nerve are usually intradural and surround the nerve in a tubular configuration, occasional examples are largely extradural.[98] Lastly, en plaque tumors often appear as a uniform or knobby sheet that, in following anatomic contours, defies gross total resection.

Although meningiomas are generally well-demarcated lesions that separate readily from the brain, some adhere to the pia and extend along cortical perivascular spaces. Removal of adherent or invasive tumors may avulse small fragments of cerebral cortex and leave behind a somewhat irregular "raw" cortical surface. Sampling of the tumor surface is then of importance to determine the presence or absence of brain invasion.

**Microscopic Features and Subtypes.** Meningiomas are histologically heterogeneous, with new subtypes added on what seems almost an annual basis. When individuality is given to minor variations, the family becomes large and complex. The classical monograph of Cushing and Eisenhardt listed 9 major types and 20 subtypes.[26] A simplified approach curtailed the family to five: syncytial, fibroblastic, transitional, angiomatous/angioblastic, and sarcomatous.[25] Never to be underestimated, however, the family recouped many of its losses and at the time of the World Health Organization (WHO) classification in 1993 had re-expanded to 11.[77] The present discussion considers 13, and it would be imprudent to predict that other variants will not be admitted. Most of the "new variants" are prognostically unfavorable. One of

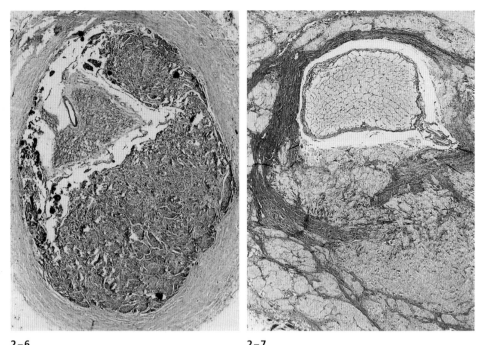

2–6                              2–7

**FIGURES 2–6 AND 2–7**    MENINGIOMA OF THE OPTIC NERVE SHEATH

Confined by the dura, the neoplasm in Figure 2–6 compressed the optic nerve into the triangular structure that is visible at the top of the illustration. Meningiomas in this location may also freely infiltrate the dura and extend outward into orbital soft tissues (Fig. 2–7).

the newer additions, the "rhabdoid" subtype, was one of the original 19 that was temporarily removed.[75, 124] Some meningioma variants occur most often in pure form,

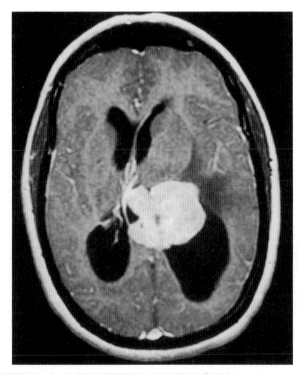

**FIGURE 2–8**    INTRAVENTRICULAR MENINGIOMA

Meningiomas uncommonly arise within a ventricle. The patient was a 61-year-old woman who presented with dementia.

whereas others, such as chordoid and rhabdoid, appear during tumor progression from well-differentiated to more anaplastic neoplasms. Meningothelial cells scattered throughout the arachnoid are a logical origin of meningiomas (Fig. 2–15).

There are many reasons to contest the meningothelial origin of the hemangiopericytoma (HPC) and hemangioblastoma, and these erstwhile "angioblastic meningiomas" are discussed separately on pages 76 and 78 to 83, respectively. The following discussion pertains to the principal meningioma variants. A number of minor variations are listed on pages 62 and 63.

1. *Meningotheliomatous (syncytial).* Meningothelial cells, with indistinct cellular borders aggregated into small sheets and large lobules, constitute this classical meningioma subtype (Fig. 2–16). The "syncytial" quality is explained ultrastructurally by interdigitating cell membranes that cannot be resolved by light microscopy into a distinct cell border (Fig. 2–17). The nuclei are pale and occasionally contain cytoplasmic invaginations (pseudoinclusions) that on occasion displace much of the intranuclear volume (see Fig. 2–16). Although these inclusions occur in other types of meningiomas, they are most typical of the meningotheliomatous type. The basophilic psammoma bodies are also diagnostically important and are often present in small numbers. Another colorful constituent, especially of the meningotheliomatous type, is xanthomatous change. As discussed in the following, the term *metaplastic* is sometimes applied to meningiomas with abundant adipose tissue, bone, or cartilage.

2. *Fibrous.* Macroscopically, such lesions appear as glistening, discrete masses without the surface lobularity

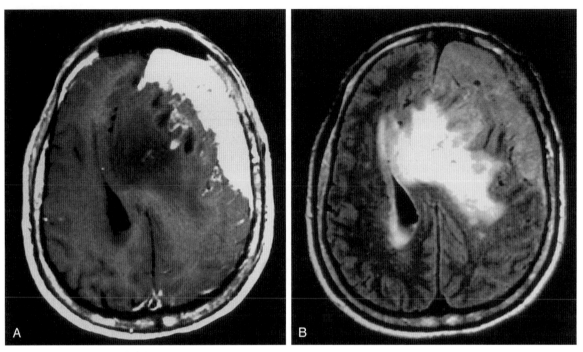

**FIGURE 2–9**   ATYPICAL MENINGIOMA

Atypical and malignant meningiomas often exhibit an irregular, or frankly ragged, interface with the brain, as is evident in this contrast-enhanced MR image (A). A T2-weighted image (B) records a broad zone of edema beneath the medial aspect of the lesion. Peritumoral edema is often elicited by atypical and malignant meningiomas but may be present with well-differentiated meningiomas as well.

so typical of meningiomas in general. The pattern can occur in transitions to other subtypes but often appears in "pure" form. It is characterized by sweeping, elongated cells accompanied by variably abundant intercellular collagen (Fig. 2–18). Architecturally, the lesion is vaguely fascicular and collagen rich, sometimes with a storiform pattern. The classical whorls are present only focally, if at all. Mineralization of collagen bands is a common feature; psammoma bodies are not. The elongated nuclei usually retain a meningothelial quality but

can have the spindle shape and density of chromatin that are more "fibroblastic" than meningothelial.

Ultrastructurally, fibroblastic meningiomas may not be obviously "meningothelial" because the cells, separated by collagenous stroma, show a paucity of desmosomes. Intermediate filaments may also be few. In some instances, there is abundant extracellular amorphous, basement membrane-like material (Fig. 2–19). The cells of fibrous meningioma differ from fibroblasts that typically exhibit far more rough endoplasmic reticulin and

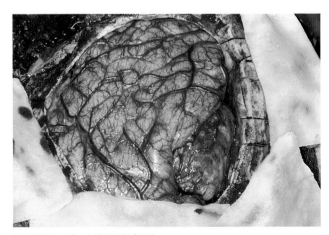

**FIGURE 2–10**   MENINGIOMA

The typical extra-axial position of most meningiomas is readily evident at surgery.

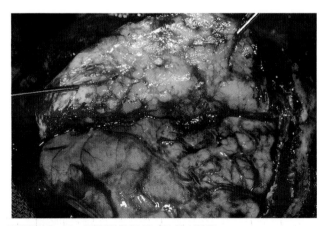

**FIGURE 2–11**   MENINGIOMA *EN PLAQUE*

Occurring most often in the temporal region and covering the sphenoid wing, *en plaque* meningiomas spread horizontally without the formation of a globular mass. (Courtesy of Dr. John C. D. Atkinson, Rochester, MN.)

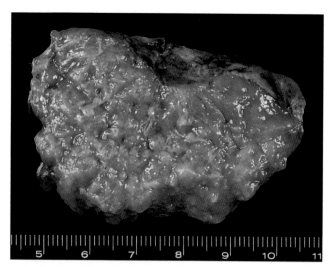

**FIGURE 2–12** MENINGIOMA

Meningiomas often appear lobular on cut section.

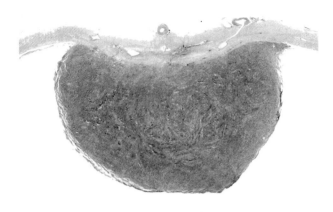

**FIGURE 2–14** MENINGIOMA

The smooth surface of fibrous meningiomas is well seen in this whole mount section. Note the "dural tail" (*right*), which in this lesion is a superficial extension of the neoplasm along the dura. In many cases, the tail consists simply of a wedge of loose fibrovascular tissue.

lack desmosomes. As is the case for other meningioma subtypes, epithelial membrane antigen (EMA) staining is the rule, but it may not be as conspicuous as in meningothelial tumors.

The differential diagnostic issue is usually to distinguish a fibrous meningioma from a schwannoma or solitary fibrous tumor. This is discussed on pages 71 to 73.

3. *Transitional.* Appropriately named, the transitional meningioma embodies features of both meningotheliomatous and fibroblastic tumors. Its cells often vary in arrangement and configuration, with nodules containing cores of syncytial cells surrounded by elongated fibroblas-

tic elements (Fig. 2–20). Psammoma bodies and whorls are thus frequent (Fig. 2–21).

4. *Psammomatous.* Most such tumors are simply whorl-rich transitional lesions with an abundance of psammoma bodies (Fig. 2–22). In some instances, the

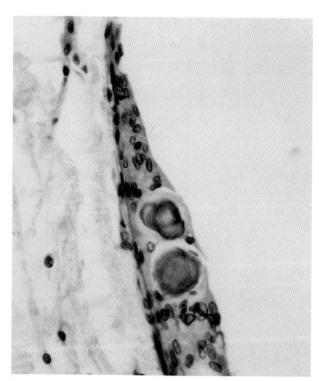

**FIGURE 2–15** NORMAL MENINGOTHELIAL CELLS

Scattered diffusely within the arachnoid membrane, normal meningothelial cells become prominent, and clustered, with age. Such aggregates show the classical features of meningioma, that is, oval nuclei that occasionally appear "empty" because of cytoplasmic invaginations, a whorled cellular pattern, and psammoma body formation.

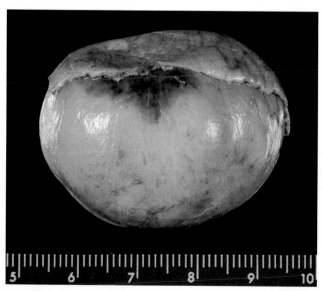

**FIGURE 2–13** MENINGIOMA

Fibrous meningiomas are often remarkably smooth surfaced.

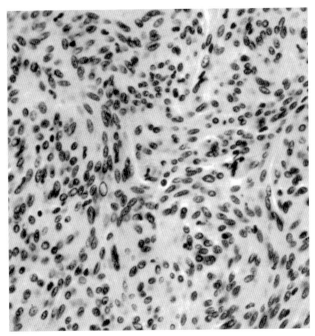

**FIGURE 2–16**   MENINGOTHELIOMATOUS MENINGIOMA

Whorls, lobules, indistinct cell borders, and intranuclear pseudoinclusions characterize meningotheliomatous meningiomas.

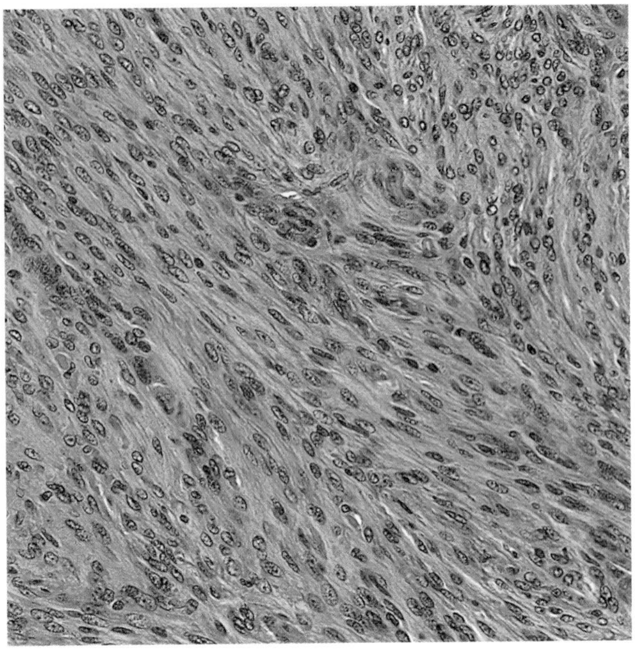

**FIGURE 2–18**   FIBROUS MENINGIOMA

This variant of meningioma is composed of markedly elongated cells. Whorls and psammoma bodies are infrequent.

lamellated, calcified structures are found in such profusion as to largely exclude intervening meningothelial cells. Some rock-hard examples are considered "burnt out" nonproliferative masses. Indeed, diffusely calcified meningiomas typically have a low MIB-1 index.[108] Intraspinal meningiomas are often densely psammomatous, as are some in the olfactory groove.

5. *Angiomatous.* This infrequently used designation refers not to a specific meningioma type but to any meningioma in which blood vessels are prominent (Fig. 2–23). The term is thus more a descriptor than a diagnosis and has no prognostic significance. Because of an unfortunate similarity in terms, it must be distinguished clearly from the old designation *angioblastic*

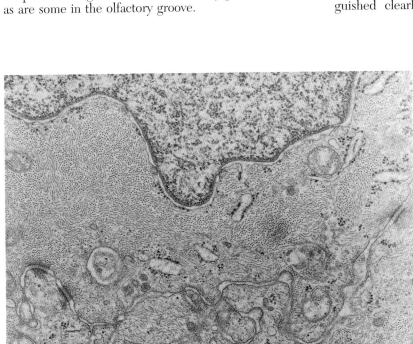

**FIGURE 2–17**   MENINGOTHELIOMATOUS (SYNCYTIAL) MENINGIOMA

Typical ultrastructural features of meningioma include (1) intermediate filaments, (2) interdigitation of cell membranes, and (3) desmosomes. A "syncytial" quality is often apparent at the magnification of light microscopy because interdigitated cell membranes cannot be resolved.

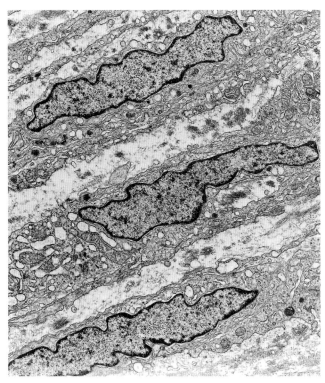

**FIGURE 2–19    FIBROUS MENINGIOMA**

This variant of meningioma is composed of elongated cells with abundant extracellular basement collagen deposition. In fibrous meningiomas, unlike syncytial and transitional lesions, desmosomes and intermediate filaments are sparse.

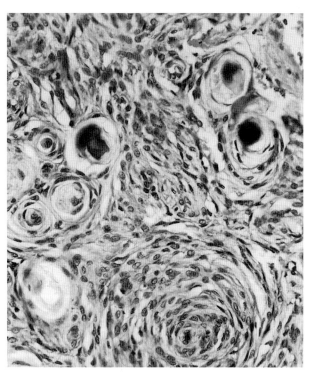

**FIGURE 2–20    TRANSITIONAL MENINGIOMA**

The transitional meningioma combines whorled meningothelial cells and elongated "fibroblastic" elements. The latter are most evident at the periphery of the whorls. Psammoma bodies are often prominent.

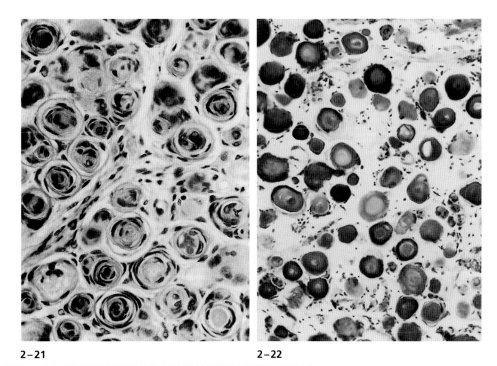

**2–21**                              **2–22**

**FIGURES 2–21 AND 2–22    TRANSITIONAL/PSAMMOMATOUS MENINGIOMAS**

Whereas some meningiomas are noted for the abundance of whorls (Fig. 2–21), little but psammoma bodies remains in others (Fig. 2–22).

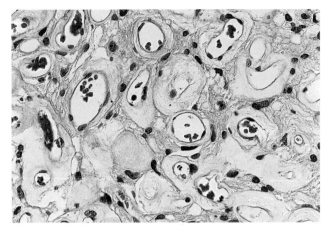

**FIGURE 2–23** ANGIOMATOUS MENINGIOMA

Blood vessels dominate some meningiomas. Elsewhere, this lesion had microcystic features.

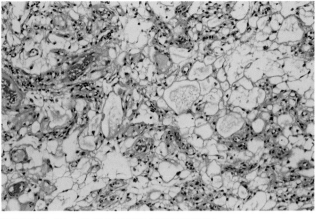

**FIGURE 2–25** MICROCYSTIC MENINGIOMA

Multiple intercellular spaces, scattered pleomorphic nuclei, and a paucity of whorls and psammoma bodies are typical features of this distinctive meningioma variant.

*meningioma,* which referred to what are now termed HPC and hemangioblastoma. The term *angioblastic* is best abandoned because it perpetuates the erroneous concept that the meningeal HPC is a variant of meningioma.

6. *Metaplastic.* Differentiation toward bone, cartilage, and adipose tissue (Fig. 2–24) are well known expressions of the meningioma repertoire. Such "metaplastic" elements are usually superimposed on otherwise conventional lesions in the meningotheliomatous-transitional-fibrous spectrum. On the basis of immunohistochemistry and electron microscopy, it is apparent that there is not a true metaplasia, that is, change of cell type, but only a progressive lipidization of meningothelial cells.[139] Meningiomas with lipomatous metaplasia should be distinguished from the microcystic meningioma variant with its pale mucin-containing, intercellular spaces delineated by encompassing cell processes. The rare

myxoid meningioma is less obviously meningothelial because its bipolar or vaguely stellate cells are dispersed in a mucoid stroma[8, 27, 48]; whorls and psammoma bodies are often absent. Myxoid meningiomas should be distinguished from *chordoid meningioma,* whose cells are more epithelial and cohesive.

7. *Microcystic.* The microcystic variant, among the most common of "nonclassical" meningiomas, occurs both in pure form and as an admixture with other meningioma patterns. More often it is pure. Its peculiar, rather nonmeningothelial, appearance creates diagnostic difficulty to those unfamiliar with its distinctive features.[78, 102, 109, 114] The latter include intercellular, pale, mucin-containing microcysts; vacuolated, and sometimes frankly xanthomatous, cells; scattered large dark nuclei; and hyalinized blood vessels (Figs. 2–25 and 2–26). As a rule, well-formed lobules, whorls, and psammoma bodies are lacking. Ultrastructural confirmation, by

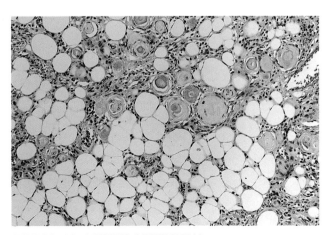

**FIGURE 2–24** LIPIDIZED MENINGIOMA

Lipid accumulation in meningiomas ranges from microvacuolar change to frank engorgement. The former produces cells with xanthomatous features; the latter creates cells that closely resemble adipocytes.

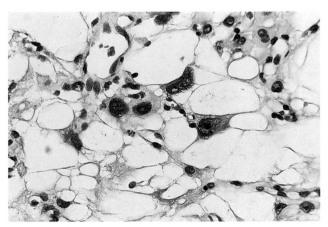

**FIGURE 2–26** MICROCYSTIC MENINGIOMA

The large nuclei and vacuolated cytoplasm create a close resemblance to hemangioblastoma.

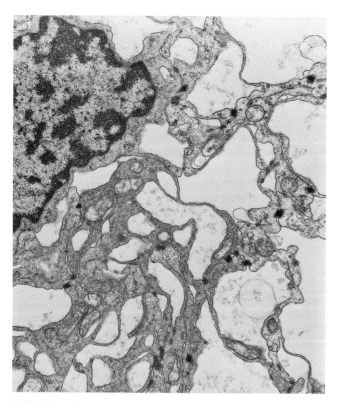

**FIGURE 2–27    MICROCYSTIC MENINGIOMA**

The cells of microcystic meningiomas are joined by desmosomes, a cardinal feature of all meningiomas. Microcysts consist of intercellular spaces between elongated cell processes.

demonstration of desmosomes, can be employed but is rarely necessary (Fig. 2–27).

There is no special prognostic significance to the microcystic pattern, although there may be a large cyst that adheres to and indents the brain.

8. *Secretory.* The secretory type is an esthetically appealing variant that is usually well differentiated and meningothelial-transitional in appearance.[2, 91, 133, 163] It is individualized by the presence of discrete, eosinophilic, strongly periodic acid–Schiff (PAS)–positive cytoplasmic inclusions, of which there may be more than one in a single cell (Fig. 2–28). The inclusions and their encircling cells are immunoreactive for carcinoembryonic antigen (CEA); the cells are also reactive for cytokeratins (Figs. 2–29 and 2–30).[110, 133, 155, 170] Serum and cerebrospinal fluid (CSF) elevations of CEA have been reported.[91,163]

Ultrastructurally, the inclusions consist of spaces lined by microvilli and filled with contents that are variably amorphous, particulate, lamellar, or vesicular (Fig. 2–31).[40, 70, 79] Secretory meningiomas are of no special prognostic significance. Although they are usually well differentiated, some are broadly attached to the brain. One study suggested that meningiomas of this histologic type are more often associated with peritumoral edema.[133]

9. *Clear cell.* This rare variant, long recognized as the "glycogen-rich" meningioma, is now known as the "clear cell" variant.[176] As a rule, such lesions appear pure

without admixtures of other patterns. Clear cell meningiomas arise at somewhat unorthodox locations such as the cerebellopontine angle and cauda equina region.

The lesions have three distinctive histologic features: a predominance of polygonal PAS-positive clear cells, a paucity of conventional meningioma features such as whorls and psammoma bodies (Fig. 2–32), and a patchwork of hyalinized vascular stroma that increases over time (Fig. 2–33). The clear cell appearance is due to intracellular PAS-positive, diastase-labile glycogen (Fig. 2–34). Bland in appearance, the nuclei differ from those of typical meningioma because of their roundness and absence of nuclear pseudoinclusions. One examines such tumors expectantly for whorls and psammoma bodies, but the former are elusive and poorly formed, at best, and a search for psammoma bodies is usually fruitless. Hyalinization, often striking, thickens vessel walls and fills the interstitium, leaving room for little if any neoplasm in areas where this substitution is most advanced.

Ultrastructurally, the clear cell variant is a typical meningioma, with massive cytoplasmic glycogen accumulation its only aberrant feature.[176] The immunohistochemical demonstration of EMA reactivity is confirmatory.

Despite the bland cytologic appearance and the paucity of mitoses, clear cell meningiomas are considerably more likely to recur than conventional counterparts; a smaller percentage even spread discontinuously in the subarachnoid space or give rise to a spinal "drop metastasis." The MIB-1 indices are generally higher than those of classical meningioma.[176]

10. *Chordoid.* Whereas the chordoid variant is rare in pure form, the pattern is not an uncommon focal feature in more aggressive atypical or malignant meningiomas (Fig. 2–35). Chordoid features can thus be acquired during progression from the typical to atypical or malignant phenotype, and the variant is thus more often a focal finding in an otherwise typical, if more

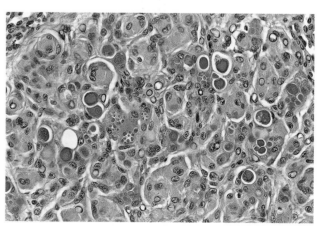

**FIGURE 2–28    SECRETORY MENINGIOMA**

Distinctively, this variant of meningioma is defined by its content of eosinophilic inclusions termed *pseudopsammoma bodies.* In contrast to true psammoma bodies, these inclusions have a clear halo about an eosinophilic noncalcified core. They are often multipartite and unencompassed by a whorl.

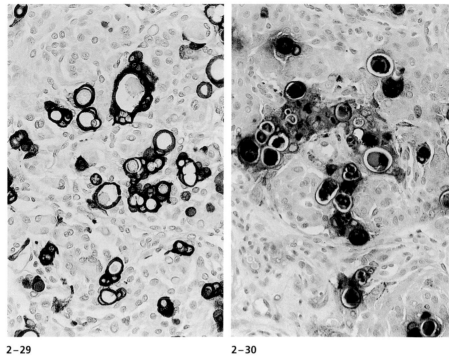

2-29                                    2-30

**FIGURES 2-29 AND 2-30    SECRETORY MENINGIOMA**

The cells that surround a pseudopsammoma body are immunoreactive for cytokeratin (Fig. 2-29) and carcinoembryonic antigen (Fig. 2-30), two antigens that are generally not detected in other forms of meningioma.

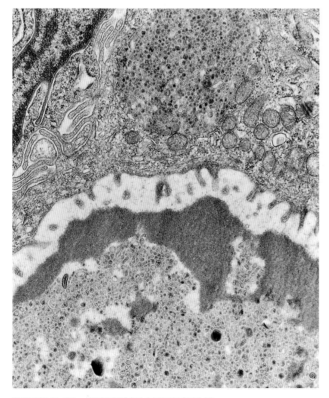

**FIGURE 2-31    SECRETORY MENINGIOMA**

The pseudopsammoma body (*left*) lies within a debris-filled space encompassed by cell surfaces that emit microvilli. A desmosome, characteristic of meningiomas, is present at the lower right.

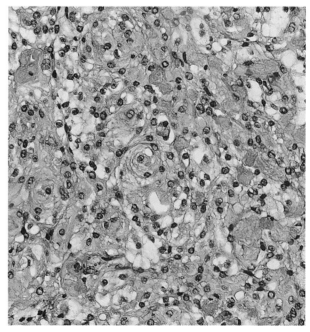

**FIGURE 2-32    CLEAR CELL MENINGIOMA**

Small, round to polygonal clear cells, without obvious meningothelial features, are typical of this uncommon meningioma variant. Whorls are poorly formed, and psammoma bodies are lacking. Nuclei are rounder and less "meningothelial" than those of other meningiomas. They are also devoid of intranuclear inclusions.

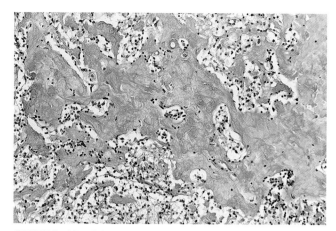

**FIGURE 2–33**   CLEAR CELL MENINGIOMA

Bands of collagen are a common feature. With time, they often crowd out tumor cells.

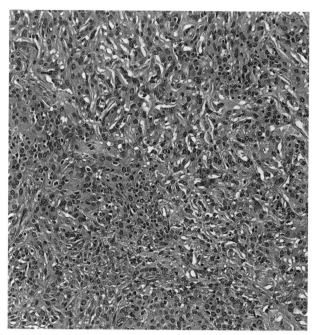

**FIGURE 2–35**   CHORDOID MENINGIOMA

Clusters and cords of polygonal cells in a mucinous matrix are more often only a focal feature.

aggressive, meningioma. As such, the lesions are generally prognostically unfavorable, with a recurrence rate that exceeds that of more traditional meningiomas. Although an early series reported its more frequent occurrence in young patients and an association with dense lymphoplasmacytic infiltrates and hypochromic anemia and/or dysgammaglobulinemia (Castleman's syndrome),[72] a subsequent report did not note this association.[23] The chordoid appearance results from the pattern created by epithelial-like cells strung out in short cords or disposed in aggregates within a basophilic mucoid matrix (Fig. 2–36).

11. *Rhabdoid.* The rhabdoid variant is an apparently recent addition to the meningioma family.[75, 124] The same lesion appears in Cushing and Eisenhart's text as "type I–variant 3."[26, 75] Usually encountered among higher grade meningiomas and seen to emerge in recurrences

during the process of malignant transition, this pattern is seen only infrequently in pure form.

Histologically, the descriptor *rhabdoid* refers to both the cytoplasm and nuclear configuration wherein gemistocytic-appearing eosinophilic cytoplasm often shows displacement of the nucleus by a spherical mass of intermediate filaments (Fig. 2–37). This change may be present diffusely throughout the lesion or focal in the background of a more classical meningioma pattern. The pattern often emerges during tumor progression and is therefore more obvious in recurrences than in the initial specimen. This

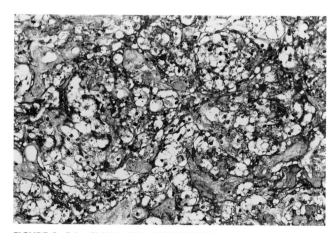

**FIGURE 2–34**   CLEAR CELL MENINGIOMA

The glycogen-rich cytoplasm is strongly periodic acid–Schiff (PAS) positive.

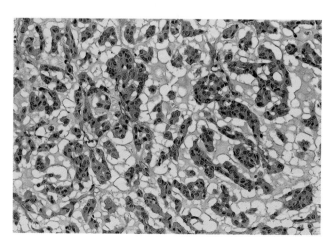

**FIGURE 2–36**   CHORDOID MENINGIOMA

A portion of the tumor illustrated in Figure 2–35 shows the "chordoid" architecture that is associated with an increased incidence of tumor recurrence.

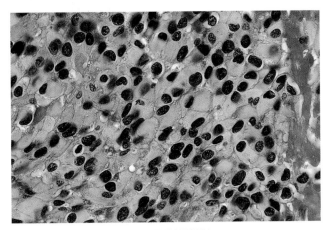

**FIGURE 2–37    RHABDOID MENINGIOMA**

Monomorphous sheets of cells that contain fibrillar to hyaline cytoplasmic inclusions characterize this rare, and aggressive, meningioma variant.

gradual transition is similar to that seen in the chordoid and papillary variants (see later). Although the cells themselves are not anaplastic, rhabdoid meningiomas as a whole are more likely to exhibit atypical or even malignant features. Thus, "sheeting," necrosis, atypia, elevated MIB-1 and mitotic rates, and brain invasion are likely to be seen in such tumors.[76, 127]

EMA staining is the rule but is variable in degree. Staining of cytoplasmic constituents, whether hyaline or finely fibrillar, generally shows reactivity for vimentin and to a lesser degree cytokeratins.[76, 127] Ultrastructurally, the spherical cytoplasmic accumulations consist of concentric whorls of intermediate filaments. The cytoplasmic interdigitations and desmosomes expected of a meningioma are also variably present.[76, 127]

*12. Lymphoplasmacyte-rich.* As a rule, meningiomas are remarkably free of inflammatory infiltrates,[7] but some cases attract chronic inflammatory cells in remarkable numbers, sometimes to the extent that the tumor is obscured by the inflammatory component (Fig. 2–38). Lymphoplasmacytic infiltrates with accompanying Russell bodies are seen most frequently.[38, 43, 53, 89] Obvious lobules of meningothelial cells may nestle in inflammatory infiltrates, or the neoplastic cells may be so intermingled that they are difficult to identify. A reticulin stain can be helpful by highlighting the nested neoplastic cells. Immunohistochemistry can be helpful, but both the tumor cells and the reactive plasma cells are EMA reactive.

*13. Papillary.* The papillary meningioma deserves special attention because of its reputation for locally aggressive behavior and the significant incidence of late distant metastases. It is of note that past descriptions of this subtype included cases of angioblastic meningioma, a nonmeningothelial tumor now classified as HPC.[93, 120] Thus, the literature contains few bona fide meningothelial tumors of papillary type on which to appraise their biologic behavior. In addition, the descriptions of even this restricted list do not clearly agree on criteria. Children appear to be affected preferentially.

Such neoplasms are composed of sheets of cytologically uniform cells with nuclei similar, yet not identical, to those of the typical meningioma. This distinctive tumor features a radial arrangement of neoplastic cells around blood vessels where cytoplasmic processes form a variant of perivascular pseudorosette (Fig. 2–39). Delicate but distinctive, radiating strands of reticulin may be abundant in these perithelial regions. Artifactual dehiscence of cell sheets during tissue processing contributes significantly to the appearance of pseudopapillae (Fig. 2–40). Despite the cytologic uniformity that typifies papillary meningioma, scattered mitotic figures are frequently observed. In most cases, whorls are not prominent and psammoma bodies are lacking. The meningothelial derivation of papillary meningioma could be challenged were it not for examples transitional to ordinary meningioma or instances in which electron microscopy shows filament-filled processes linked by well-formed desmosomes.[129]

In a child, the differential diagnosis of a papillary lesion includes the issue of *ependymoma* and *astroblastoma*. Both may be superficially situated and feature perivascular orientation of tumor cells. These lesions vary considerably in histologic appearances and, despite their usually obvious glial nature, can also have meningioma-like qualities. Ependymoma and astroblastoma are of course glial fibrillary acidic protein (GFAP) positive, but the extent of staining varies, particularly in the former. To confound the issue, GFAP positivity has been reported in an occasional papillary meningioma with HPC-like features.[16]

*14. Miscellaneous variants and tissue patterns.* Meningiomas are among the chameleons of CNS tumors with their various patterns, cell types, inclusions, and other individualizing features that seemingly appear and disappear at will. These include pseudogland formation,[74]

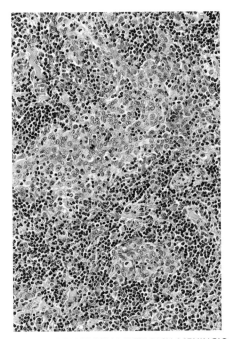

**FIGURE 2–38    LYMPHOPLASMACYTE-RICH MENINGIOMA**

Dense infiltrates of chronic inflammatory cells may obscure the underlying neoplasm.

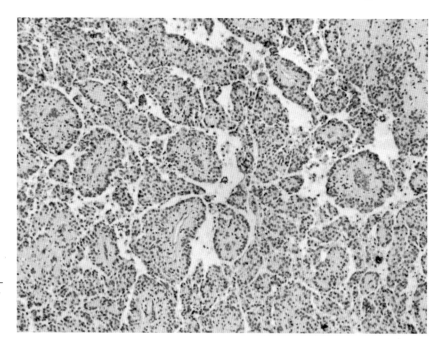

**FIGURE 2–39**   PAPILLARY MENINGIOMA

The pseudopapillary appearance is created by tissue dehiscence and an ependymoma-like radiation of cells around blood vessels. Meningiomas with this architecture are often aggressive.

palisading resembling that of schwannoma,[92, 150] oncocytic change,[138] actin-positive tumor cells,[162] intracytoplasmic inclusions,[69, 164] tyrosine-rich crystals,[24, 69, 164] and last, but not least, rheumatoid nodules.[73]

Carcinomas can metastasize to meningiomas, as discussed on page 51 (Fig. 2–41).[11]

Neuroradiologists can embolize the external carotid supply to a meningioma in an effort to devascularize the mass preoperatively. This can produce widespread necrosis that can prompt concern by the pathologist about "atypia" or "malignancy" because of perinecrotic reactive cellular atypia and elevated MIB-1 rate.[121]

**Grading.** Grading of meningiomas is now as much a part of specimen analysis as it is for gliomas. The procedure must consider both classical histologic features, such as mitotic index, and the tumor subtypes that have a higher rate of recurrence.

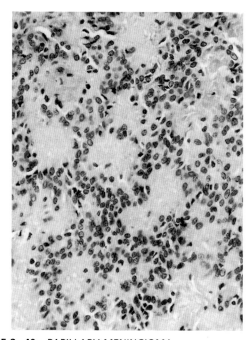

**FIGURE 2–40**   PAPILLARY MENINGIOMA

Perivascular, anucleate, fibrillar zones similar to those of an ependymoma characterize this rare meningioma variant. Reticulin stains often show a radiating perivascular pattern.

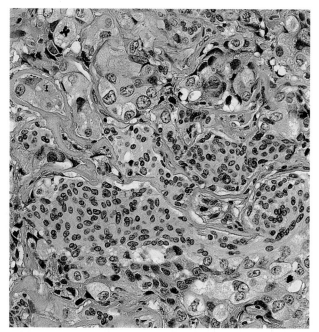

**FIGURE 2–41**   CARCINOMA METASTATIC TO MENINGIOMA

Lobules of adenocarcinoma were unexpected findings in a meningioma of a 52-year-old man with carcinoma of the lung.

Numerous studies have identified the negative prognostic factors that are illustrated in Table 2–1. These include tumor location, incomplete resection, loss of lobular pattern ("sheeting") (Fig. 2–42A), hypercellularity (Fig. 2–42A), cytologic atypia with macronucleoli (Fig. 2–42B), increased mitotic activity (its definition is discussed) (Fig. 2–42C), elevated MIB-1 labeling index (as defined subsequently) (Fig 2–42D), necrosis (in the absence of prior embolization) (Fig. 2–42E), small cell change (Fig. 2–42F), brain invasion (Fig. 2–42G–I), anaplasia (Fig. 2–42J), and absence of immunoreactivity for progesterone receptors.[32, 39, 55, 57, 61–63, 67, 68, 103, 105, 106, 115, 121, 122, 148, 154] Histologic types with negative prognostic significance include chordoid, rhabdoid, papillary, and clear cell variants.

**TABLE 2–1**
**Histologic and Immunohistochemical Features of Prognostic Significance in Meningiomas**

Loss of lobular pattern ("sheeting")
Hypercellularity
Cytologic atypia with macronucleoli
Increased mitotic rate ($\geq 4/10$ high-power field)
Necrosis (in the absence of prior embolization)
Elevated MIB-1 index
Small cell change
Invasion of the brain
Cellular anaplasia
Histologic subtype (rhabdoid, papillary, chordoid, clear cell)
Absence of immunoreactivity for progesterone receptors

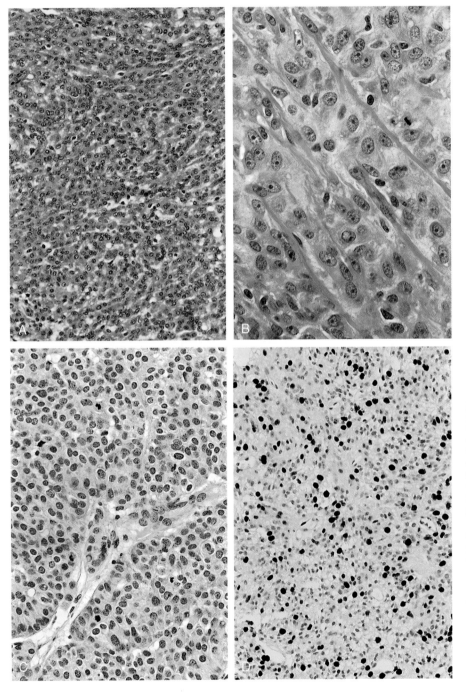

**FIGURE 2–42** HISTOLOGIC AND IMMUNOHISTOCHEMICAL FEATURES USED IN GRADING MENINGIOMAS

(A) *Hypercellularity and loss of lobular architecture (sheeting).* Hypercellular lesions such as this, with loss of lobularity and other features provided below, usually fall into the WHO grade II (atypical) category.
(B) *Cytologic atypia and prominent nucleoli.* Large nuclei with prominent nucleoli are common in atypical (grade II) and malignant (grade III) meningiomas.
(C) *Increased mitotic activity.* Mitoses are sparse in the classical grade I meningioma. The frequency here is excessive. The lesion also features lack of lobularity (sheeting).
(D) *Increased MIB-1 labeling index.* Levels greater than 4% have been associated with an increased rate of recurrence. The index here far exceeds that of the typical meningioma.

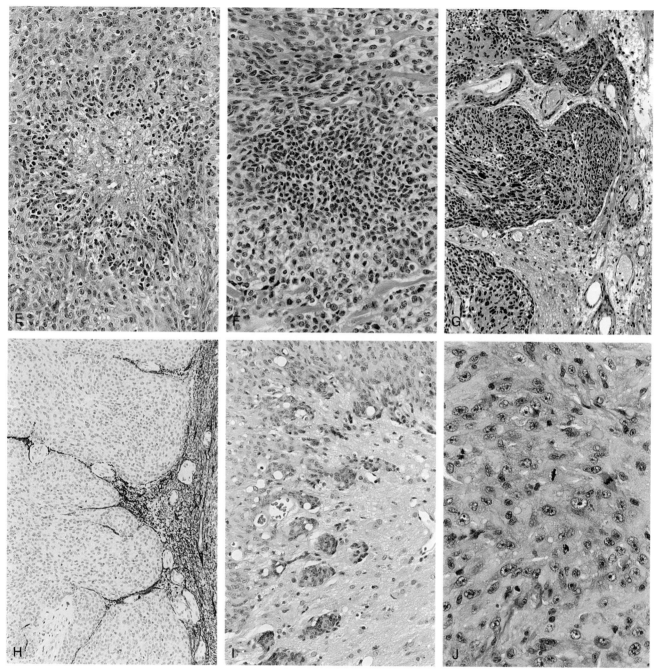

**FIGURE 2–42**   Continued.

*(E) Necrosis.* Necrosis is sometimes highlighted by peripheral "pseudopalisading." To be of prognostic significance, necrosis must be "spontaneous" and not be artifactually created by preoperative therapeutic embolization.

*(F) Small cell change.* Clusters or small aggregates of cells with small nuclei and scant cytoplasm are often seen in atypical and malignant meningiomas. The small cells are cytologically bland and not anaplastic.

*(G, H, I) Brain invasion.* Meningiomas often insinuate themselves into the subjacent cortex as small tongues or pegs of neoplastic tissue that follow the course of superficial blood vessels *(G)*. Note the small eosinophilic focus of necrosis in the larger tongue of tissue. Invasive meningiomas may be "atypical" or "malignant," but some are cytologically bland, whorl-rich lesions with few, if any, other prognostically adverse histologic features. As seen in *H*, immunohistochemistry for glial fibrillary acidic protein (GFAP) can be used to detect the extent to which a meningioma invades brain. Here, strands of GFAP-positive parenchyma are found well within the mass. Only uncommonly, as illustrated in *I*, do meningiomas infiltrate brain parenchyma as small nests or individual cells.

*(J) Anaplasia.* Overt cytologic malignancy is uncommon in meningiomas. Anaplasia in meningiomas is more often evident as a markedly elevated mitotic rate than as overt cytologic malignancy.

Among the histologic features, mitotic activity has been studied in greatest detail. Although there is overlap in the ranges of mitotic indices among different studies, there is a notable increase in the rate of recurrence of "totally resected" meningiomas when the mitotic index is four or more per 10 high-power fields.[126]

In regard to the cell cycle marker MIB-1, the results differ somewhat from study to study, but progressively higher indices are noted as one progresses from typical to atypical to malignant meningiomas.[57, 66, 75, 105, 122] More important, there is a relationship between the MIB-1 index and the likelihood of recurrence of well-differentiated lesions that were "totally resected." The mean index in the meningiomas that do not recur is reportedly about 1% or less, whereas that of lesions prone to recur has been in the 4% range.[127] No specific figure has been suggested as being a definite indicator of malignant meningioma. As in other neoplasms, one must consider MIB-1 indices in the context of histologic features. An artifactually increased rate occurs around zones of necrosis, as are produced by embolization.[121]

Immunoreactivity for progesterone receptors has also been correlated with outcome and histologic grade. In one study, the MIB-1 labeling index was significantly higher in the progesterone receptor–negative lesions.[106] In another study, "nonbenign" meningiomas, that is, atypical and malignant ones, were more frequently negative as well.[15] Yet another study reported an inverse relationship between the progesterone receptor staining score and the histologic grade as well as the mitotic index.[55] The postoperative progression-free intervals were shorter for patients with receptor-negative lesions. Immunostaining for estrogen receptors is generally negative.

Invasion of other tissues such as bone, or trapping of major vessels and cranial nerves, may render meningiomas unresectable. Nonetheless, in the absence of the requisite histologic features already noted, such lesions do not qualify as malignant on these criteria alone. Invasion of bone is a recognized property of meningiomas but in favorably situated lesions does not preclude total resection. However, it has been considered a factor that, overall, predicts a higher incidence of recurrence.[63] In contrast to brain invasion, nests of infiltrative cells may appear independent of the main mass. Although bone invasion is not a factor in histologic grading and does not relegate a meningioma to the atypical or malignant category, it may render a tumor unresectable and, in this context, be a prognostically unfavorable finding.

The interplay of clinical and prognostic variables in a population of patients with a meningioma is a paradise for the statistician but a bad dream for a pathologist studying an individual case. Attempting to synthesize multiple, sometimes only focal, and not always concordant pathologic features into an assured diagnosis, without overgrading or undergrading, can be difficult at best.

Recognizing that grading of meningiomas is an evolving subject, we recommend that meningiomas in the meningothelial-transitional-fibrous spectrum be assigned to one of three categories: well differentiated, atypical, or malignant, along the guidelines suggested by Perry and colleagues[125, 126] and adopted by the WHO.[77]

Grading issues that revolve around the four more aggressive meningioma subtypes are discussed on pages 59 to 63 and 67.

It is important to recognize that precise grading of meningiomas is not always possible and that the treatment planning will, in any case, consider clinical variables such as extent of resection, the patient's age, and the general medical condition. Given the uncertainties of grading in the inevitable borderline cases, one can forgo precise grading in certain instances, with the reasons for the uncertainty conveyed in a "See Comment" diagnosis.

The *well-differentiated meningioma* (WHO grade I) is a lobular, well-differentiated lesion, generally of the meningotheliomatous, psammomatous, fibrous, or microcystic type. Necrosis is absent in the absence of preoperative embolization. Mitoses may be present but are difficult to find. Nucleoli are small. Brain invasion is not seen. The MIB-1 index is usually less than 1%. Approximately 80% of meningiomas fulfill these criteria. The occasional, otherwise typical meningioma that does extend into the adjacent brain creates a diagnostic problem but, on the basis of invasion, is considered grade II by the WHO system.

The *atypical meningioma* (WHO grade II) demonstrates cytologic and histologic features expected of an intermediate grade lesion. The revised WHO classification recommends the designation when the lesion is mitotically active (four or more mitoses per high-power field) or demonstrates three or more of the following variables: loss of lobular architecture, prominent nucleoli, increased cellularity, small cells with high nuclear/cytoplasmic ratios, and foci of spontaneous necrosis. Because benign meningiomas with brain invasion behave biologically as do atypical meningiomas, the presence of invasion places the lesion in the atypical category.[77, 122] Although the finding of brain invasion by a histologically benign meningioma confers the same guarded prognoses as is implied by the term atypical meningioma, it does not worsen the prognosis to the level of malignant meningioma.[125] In the WHO system, brain invasion is, in itself, not sufficient evidence for a malignant meningioma (grade III).

In most situations, "invasion" is not infiltration by discontinuous single cells as in many systemic cancers but rather cohesive tongues of tumor that invade brain substance but remain contiguous with the parent tumor. Often, there is not even any broach of the pia and the invasion consists only of extension along perivascular spaces. Only infrequently do meningiomas truly invade brain. When the specimens are fragmented and the tumor-brain interface cannot be evaluated, GFAP stains may be useful in confirming the presence of overrun, trapped brain parenchyma (see Fig. 2–42I). Robust gliosis is conspicuous in such cases. In some specimens that have been avulsed from the brain, the invading pegs of tumor, still attached to the mass, are apparent, although largely devoid of attached brain parenchyma.

The features of atypia may be apparent throughout the mass or may be zonal in distribution. Nuclear pleomorphism and hyperchromasia alone are not indicative of atypia. As an isolated finding in the absence of mitoses, these features should be disregarded and considered a "degenerative" phenomenon. The MIB-1 labeling index in the atypical, that is, WHO grade II, meningioma is generally greater than 4%. Foci of necrosis, usually small and surrounded by palisades of cells, are frequent features.

Grading the clear cell meningioma is problematic because such tumors are cytologically bland and show little evidence, other than perhaps an elevated MIB-1 rate, of their greater tendency to recur. They are, in recognition of their biologic behavior, assigned grade II. The same is true for chordoid variants, which often have clear features of atypia in nonchordoid regions.

About 10% of all meningiomas are classified as atypical.

By definition, *malignant meningiomas* usually exhibit the atypical features already listed in addition to mitotic activity far exceeding that of most atypical lesions. The criterion of 20 or more mitoses per 10 high-power fields has been suggested as a threshold level.[125] The same study excluded brain invasion as an independent prognostic factor underlying recurrence and prognosis among meningiomas with atypical or malignant features. Meningiomas may appear malignant at the time of the first operation, or they may have been benign at their outset, acquiring anaplastic features over time.[20, 33, 60, 62, 84]

In the WHO system, both rhabdoid and papillary lesions are assigned grade III, although this may be done with reservation if the changes are only focal in a lesion that otherwise fits comfortably in the atypical category.

Only about 5% of meningiomas qualify for the designation malignant.

Cytogenics has begun to affect subtyping and grading of meningiomas. Although the precise molecular events underlying tumor progression are unknown, loss of heterozygosity of chromosomes 1, 6, 10, and 14 is associated with more aggressive lesions. The subject is discussed later in the section Cytogenetic and Molecular Biologic Findings.

**Features in Frozen Sections.** Given the broad and complex morphologic spectrum of meningioma, the surgeon's request for an intraoperative diagnosis provides the pathologist the stage on which to appear particularly inept by the misdiagnosis of what appears clinically as a straightforward meningioma. Frozen section artifacts and quirks of staining may distort and obscure histologic details and complicate the intraoperative diagnosis of meningioma (Figs. 2–43 and 2–44). An interpretative error by the pathologist may adversely affect the procedure. It is precisely for this reason that consultation with the neurosurgeon and an awareness of neuroimaging data are so important. Assessment of a representative tissue fragment free of cautery artifact and the concurrent use of cytologic preparations are important safeguards.

**Cytologic Features.** For all their histologic differences, meningiomas are remarkably similar in cytologic preparations. The cells have bland oval nuclei, occasional pseudoinclusions, and ample cytoplasm drawn out into wispy, terminally twisted extensions (Fig. 2–45). These features quickly obviate further consideration of malignant lesions, particularly carcinoma and high-grade gliomas. Nuclear atypia is often degenerative in nature. As an aside, the nuclei with their delicate chromatin provide ideal viewing conditions for the identification of Barr bodies in meningiomas in women (see Fig. 2–45). Pseudopsammoma bodies in secretory variants are also well seen (Fig. 2–46).[51]

**Immunohistochemical Findings.** The principal antibody used in the identification of meningiomas is EMA (Figs. 2–47 and 2–48). Although not a specific reagent, it often resolves differential diagnostic issues in the context of histologic findings.[5, 123] The typically diffuse and intense positivity for vimentin attests to the antigenicity of the meningioma tissue but offers little other diagnostic information. Meningiomas, as a whole, are only

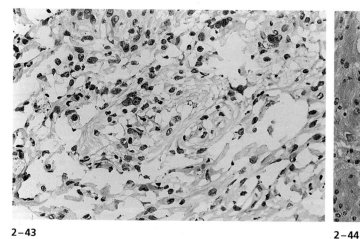

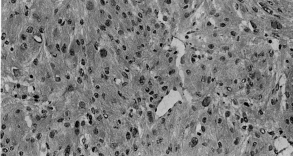

2–43

2–44

**FIGURES 2–43 AND 2–44**  MENINGIOMA—FROZEN SECTION

Artifacts of freezing obscure histologic and cytologic details. Although lobularity and whorl formation are often apparent, the lesion can easily be misinterpreted as a glioma (Fig. 2–43). Meningiomas with conspicuous cytoplasm are especially likely to be confused with a gemistocytic astrocytoma in frozen sections (Fig. 2–44).

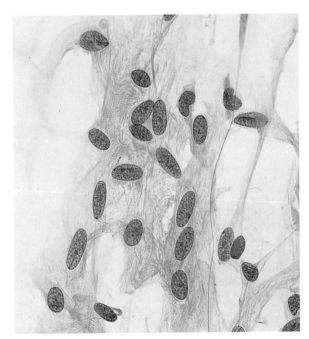

**FIGURE 2-45    MENINGIOMA—SMEAR PREPARATION**

Delicate chromatin, small precise nucleoli, and wispy cytoplasm are typical features of meningioma. Note the Barr bodies in this meningioma from a female patient.

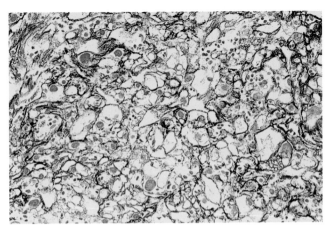

**FIGURE 2-47    MENINGIOMA**

As exemplified by this microcystic variant, cell surface staining for epithelial membrane antigen is characteristic of meningiomas.

weakly and focally S-100 positive. The uncommon fibrous variant is unique in that approximately 80% are immunoreactive for this marker. Although the incidence of staining for low- and high-molecular-weight keratins is reportedly as much as 50%,[5, 110] reactivity in our experience is a prominent feature only in tumors of the secretory type. Keratin staining in meningiomas does not approach the intensity and diffuseness seen in carcinoma, an important lesion in the differential diagnosis. In paraffin sections, somewhat over half of meningiomas are positive for progesterone receptors; staining for estrogen receptors is usually negative.[15, 39, 55, 76, 106] The prognostic significance of progesterone receptors was discussed earlier in the section on grading. The distinctive combination of cytokeratin and CEA staining in the secretory type was described earlier.

**Ultrastructural Features.** The two cardinal ultrastructural features are abundant cytoplasmic intermediate filaments and true desmosomes. Hemidesmosomes are also a common finding.[22] Interdigitation of cell membranes and processes, an ancillary feature, is prominent in meningotheliomatous (see Fig. 2–17), transitional, and microcystic tumors but less so in the fibrous variant (see Fig. 2–19), where stroma tends to separate cells.[46, 71]

**Cytogenetic and Molecular Biologic Findings.** A key in the molecular pathogenesis of many meningiomas is mutation of the *NF2* gene.[47, 101, 140, 168] This is usually associated with loss of the other allele because of loss of

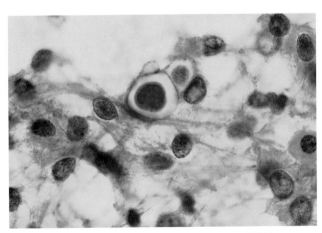

**FIGURE 2-46    MENINGIOMA—SMEAR PREPARATION**

Intensely eosinophilic, hyaline pseudopsammoma bodies are readily evident in this cytologic preparation from a secretory meningioma.

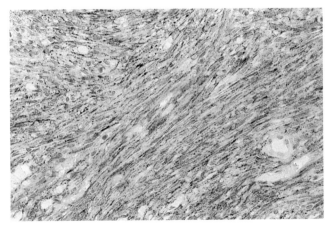

**FIGURE 2-48    MENINGIOMA**

Immunoreactivity of fibrous meningiomas for epithelial membrane antigen may be more restricted and less intense than in meningothelial and transitional tumors.

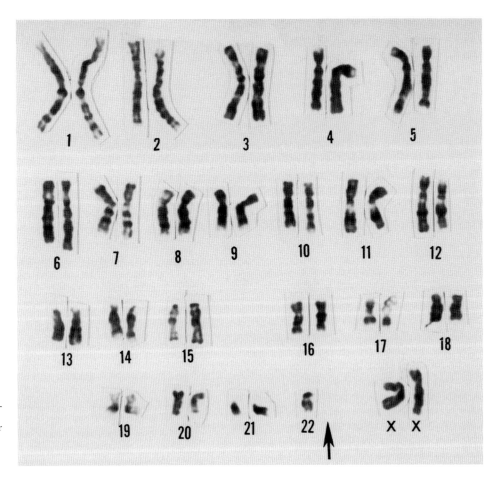

**FIGURE 2–49**   MENINGIOMA

Most meningiomas share a common chromosomal defect, a total or partial loss of one chromosome 22 (arrow). (Courtesy of Dr. Sandra H. Bigner, Durham, NC.)

the opposite chromosome, producing monosomy 22. The latter is the most common cytogenetic abnormality in meningiomas (Fig. 2–49).[34, 173] Monosomy 22 is most frequent in fibrous and transitional tumors and is less commonly present in the meningotheliomatous (syncytial) variant.[141, 168] In instances in which neither loss of chromosome 22 nor *NF2* mutations are observed, the molecular genetic basis of meningiomas remains unclear,[65] but it is likely to be resolved in the near future.

More complex karyotypes characterize atypical and malignant meningiomas. Among the nonrandom findings are loss of or losses on chromosomes 1p,[12, 34, 86] 6q,[34] 10q,[135] and 14q.[34, 160] A loss of the distal short arm of chromosome 1 is inferred when there is lack of immunohistochemical staining for alkaline phosphatase, whose gene lies in the deleted region.[112]

**Differential Diagnosis.** In permanent hematoxylin and eosin (H&E)–stained sections, most meningiomas, especially those of the meningotheliomatous-transitional spectrum, are recognized readily. Only a minority require immunohistochemistry or electron microscopy, both of which emphasize the lesion's epithelial features, that is, surface staining for EMA, interdigitating cell membranes, and well-formed desmosomes.

When "mesenchymal" in appearance, fibrous meningiomas prompt consideration of HPC, solitary fibrous tumor, and smooth muscle tumors as well as schwannoma and melanocytoma. On occasion, superficially situated gliomas undergo dural attachment to produce a discrete, meningioma-like mass of spindle cells.

Given its dense cellularity and distinctive histologic features, *hemangiopericytoma* is often summarily dismissed from the differential diagnosis. On occasion, however, visual similarities on H&E-stained sections alone create a diagnostic impasse (Fig. 2–50). Histochemistry for reticulin and particularly immunohistochemistry for EMA usually resolve the issue.[123] Electron microscopy can also be decisive by demonstrating cellular interdigitations and desmosomes in meningioma and extracellular basement membrane–like material in HPC.

Rare, but recognized increasingly, *solitary fibrous tumor* also enters into the differential because its cellularity and fascicular architecture resemble those of fibrous meningioma (see Fig. 2–53). One distinguishing feature is the meningioma's more uniform low-power histologic pattern; its thinner, more elongated nuclei; and the lesser degree of dense collagen deposition. Vague whorl formation and storiform cell arrangements are typical of fibrous meningioma, as is calcification of collagen deposits that are alien to solitary fibrous tumor. Although EMA staining may be only focal or weak in fibrous meningiomas, S-100 protein reactivity is present in the vast majority.[18] Lastly, solitary fibrous tumors show strong diffuse positivity for CD34; fibrous meningiomas react only to a limited extent.[18, 123] The distinction of solitary fibrous tumor from meningioma and other lesions is discussed in greater detail on page 72.

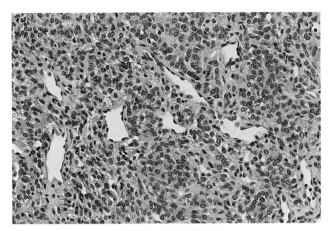

**FIGURE 2–50** MENINGIOMA RESEMBLING
HEMANGIOPERICYTOMA

Because of their high cellularity and slit-like vessels, some
meningiomas resemble hemangiopericytomas.

*Smooth muscle tumors*, benign and malignant, rarely
affect the meninges. As discussed on pages 79 and 83,
their association with immunosuppression and Epstein-
Barr virus infection is well recognized.

*Schwannoma* is a contender in the differential diagnosis of fascicular, collagen-rich lesions in the posterior
fossa, particularly those that reside in the cerebellopontine angle. Unlike fibrous meningioma, this nerve
sheath tumor generally features Antoni A and B patterns, Verocay bodies in some cases, pericellular
reticulin staining, and collagen IV or laminin immunoreactivity. Diffuse strong staining for S-100 protein
exceeds that seen in fibrous meningioma. Expansion of
the auditory canal and flaring of its meatus are gross expressions of the lesion's origin. Contrastingly, meningiomas often have a "dural tail" and are prone to induce
hyperostosis.

*Melanocytoma*, given its bland cytologic features, can
resemble either meningothelial or fibrous meningioma
(Fig. 2–51). The distinction is discussed on page 75.

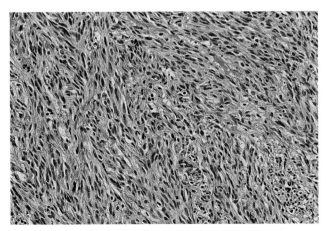

**FIGURE 2–51** MELANOCYTOMA RESEMBLING FIBROUS
MENINGIOMA

Melanocytomas can closely mimic meningiomas.

*Superficially positioned gliomas*, malignant astrocytomas, or oligodendrogliomas sometimes form firm discrete masses that, to both radiologist and surgeon,
mimic meningiomas. The spindle cell appearance of astrocytic examples and accompanying reactive fibroplasia
may deceive the pathologist as well. In this situation, the
issue is usually resolved by tissue sampling of the interface between the mass and the underlying brain. GFAP
staining quickly resolves the issue if doubts linger as to
the nature of the lesion.

The differential diagnosis of well-differentiated
meningiomas not in the meningothelial-transitional-
fibrous spectrum is generally straightforward and requires little more than familiarity with their distinctive
and often nonmeningothelial features.

*Microcystic meningiomas*, especially in pure form,
frequently cause diagnostic confusion. Because there
may be little in their appearance to suggest a meningothelial derivation, a pathologist may consider a diagnosis of *hemangioblastoma* or *angioblastic meningioma*.
The resemblance to hemangioblastoma is created by the
frequent presence of scattered pleomorphic nuclei as
well as cells resembling lipid-laden "stromal" cells. More
abundant than xanthoma cells, however, are innumerable, pale mucin-containing intercellular microcysts encircled by thin tumor cell processes. Particularly in
frozen sections or smear preparations, such processes
and microcysts may suggest an *astrocytoma* with microcyst formation. Again, awareness of radiologic and operative data is essential. Unlike hemangioblastoma and
glioma, microcystic meningiomas are immunoreactive for
EMA.

Especially in frozen sections or smears, microcystic
meningiomas may mimic *hemangioblastoma* as well as
microcyst-rich *pilocytic astrocytomas*. Uncertainty about
the nature of an individual lesion can be resolved simply
by immunohistochemistry; the meningothelial lineage of
a microcystic neoplasm is affirmed by EMA immunoreactivity and an absence of GFAP stainability.

*Clear cell meningiomas* are distinctive tumors readily recognized by their water-clear cells, bland cytologic
features, and predisposition to sclerosis. Whorl formation is vague. *Clear cell carcinomas*, such as those of renal origin, and *hemangioblastoma* both enter into the
differential diagnosis, but resolution is generally found in
the clinical history and, with the latter entity, in its
strong anatomic predilection for the cerebellum.

*Chordoid meningiomas*, in pure form, can resemble
chordoma, myxoid chondrosarcoma, and metastatic
carcinoma. Unlike *chordoma*, they lack the physaliphorous cells and are less keratin and EMA reactive. *Myxoid chondrosarcomas*, on the other hand, exhibit no reactivity for either antigen. Chordoid meningiomas lack
the anaplasia of *carcinoma*. Another chordoid lesion,
*chordoid glioma of the third ventricle*, is discussed on
pages 256 to 258.

*Papillary meningioma* presents both a practical and
a conceptual problem because its morphologic criteria
are not well defined. The differential diagnosis problem
arises particularly in children, an age group in which
*ependymoma* and *astroblastoma* are most common. Positive GFAP staining should resolve this problem except

for the claim that some papillary meningiomas are positive as well.[16]

In lymphoplasmacyte-rich examples, staining for κ and λ light chains may be needed to ensure the polyclonal nature of the infiltrate and to exclude *plasmacytoma*. The differential diagnosis also includes *inflammatory pseudotumors*. These are discussed on pages 93 to 98. Because reactive lymphoplasmacytic pseudotumors can trap nests of meningothelial cells, all efforts should be made to establish, by strict histologic, immunohistochemical, or ultrastructural criteria, that neoplastic meningothelial cells are present.

*Malignant meningiomas* vary in morphology and must be distinguished from metastatic carcinoma, meningeal sarcomas, melanocytic neoplasms, and superficial gliomas and gliosarcoma.

*Metastatic carcinoma*, if sufficiently patternless and formed of spindle cells ("sarcomatoid"), can closely mimic a malignant meningioma. Immunopositivity for cytokeratins and CEA is a marker for carcinoma. The issue must be decided with awareness that on rare occasions there is *metastasis to a meningioma*, often from a lung or breast primary.[9, 88, 119, 175]

A distinction between malignant meningioma and primary *meningeal sarcoma* may be difficult, particularly in the absence of a better differentiated meningioma component or a past history of meningioma. EMA staining would indicate meningioma. Most primary dural sarcomas have overtly mesenchymal features, such as a herringbone architecture, which is not generally seen in malignant meningiomas. In addition, meningiomas do not usually reach sarcomatoid states without historical evidence, that is, prior specimens with clearly defined meningothelial features, or immunohistochemical or ultrastructural evidence of a meningothelial cell of origin.

*Melanocytic neoplasms* must always be considered in the presence of a malignant or even benign-appearing mass. Immunohistochemistry for both S-100 protein and melanocytic markers, such as HMB-45, should be performed if a melanocytic neoplasm is suspected. Reactivity for S-100 protein alone does not reliably distinguish melanoma from meningioma.

### Diagnostic Checklist

- Have you excluded the possibility that this meningioma has some of the features associated with an increased incidence of recurrence?
- Is this "fibrous meningioma" not a solitary fibrous tumor or hemangiopericytoma?
- Is this meningioma not melanocytoma?

**Treatment and Prognosis.** Depending as it does on extent of resection, patient's age, histologic grade, molecular-cytogenic findings, and presence of other medical conditions, the ultimate prognosis for patients with meningioma can be considered only on a case-by-case basis. In one study, the recurrence-free rates at 5, 10, and 15 years were 93%, 80%, and 68%, respectively, after total resection.[105] Comparable figures after subtotal tumor removal were 63%, 45%, and 9%. In another study, atypical meningiomas were associated with 5- and

10-year survival rates of 95% and 79%[118]; the respective figures for malignant meningiomas were 64% and 34.5%. The role of radiation therapy in subtotally resected lesions has been difficult to determine, but an increased progression-free survival rate has been claimed.[45]

It seems a paradox that despite their frequent penetration of bone and intrusion into the dural venous sinuses, true meningiomas rarely metastasize. Such dissemination, most often to lungs, abdominal viscera, and bones, may be seen in meningiomas with either benign[1, 19, 104, 111, 148, 152, 159, 172] or malignant[1, 149, 172] histologic features and may occur before or after resection. Only rarely does a malignant meningioma spread within the subarachnoid space.[82]

## Solitary Fibrous Tumor

**Definition.** A discrete, collagen-rich, spindle cell neoplasm.

**General Comments.** This distinctive lesion is a new entry in the lexicon of meningeal tumors. The vast majority of solitary fibrous tumors (SFTs) occur at systemic sites.

**Clinical Features.** To date, intracranial examples have occurred only in adults, with the nonspecific effects of an intracranial mass. Spinal lesions are discussed briefly on page 534.

**Radiographic and Macroscopic Features.** Radiographically and macroscopically, the entity is a discrete, dural-based, meningioma-like mass (Fig. 2–52).[1–3, 8] Examples may appear in the orbit[5, 9, 11] and paranasal sinuses.[6]

**Microscopic Features.** Microscopically, the SFT is distinguished, oddly, by the absence of any single diagnostic feature. Pattern variation is the rule, wherein the most consistent feature is a composition of fascicles of moderately dense, elongated cells that alternate with paucicellular, collagen-rich tissue (Fig. 2–53). Dense bands of collagen appear in cross section as minute nodules that separate individual tumor cells. The cells that form straight and sometimes wavy fascicles are generally more plump than those of a fibrous meningioma. Whorls and storiform cell arrangements are absent, as are psammoma bodies. Mitotic figures are usually scant. Cellular, more mitotically active SFTs are less common, and histologically malignant examples are rare.

A diagnostically confusing aspect of some SFTs is a tissue pattern resembling that of HPC, that is, one with staghorn vessels and pericellular reticulin. Other cases replicate the vascular neoplasm less perfectly (Fig. 2–54).

**Immunohistochemical Features.** SFTs are diffusely positive for vimentin and CD34 (Fig. 2–55)[2, 6–9, 11] but are negative for EMA and S-100 protein. Like extracranial SFTs,[4, 10] the lesions are often positive for BCL-2.

**Ultrastructural Features.** Separated by collagen fibers, the cells of SFTs vary from fibroblastic to those that are

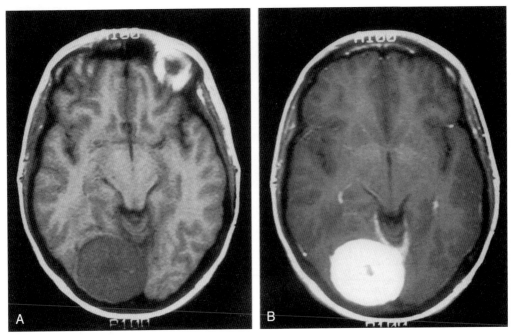

**FIGURE 2–52    SOLITARY FIBROUS TUMOR**

In every way counterfeiting meningiomas, solitary fibrous tumors are contrast enhancing and dura based. A solitary fibrous tumor is seen here in precontrast (*A*) and postcontrast (*B*) T1-weighted MR images.

rather nonspecific in their ultrastructural profile. Those resembling fibroblasts have well-developed rough endoplasmic reticulum. Cytoplasmic interdigitations and well-formed desmosomes, features seen in meningiomas, are lacking. The same is true of basement membrane–like material, which is such a prominent feature of HPCs.[2,8]

**Differential Diagnosis.** The "classical" SFT is readily recognized after one's exposure to several cases. The possibility of the entity then comes to mind in the presence of a meningeal mass with a fibrous tissue component. Thus fortified by experience, the diagnosis of

*fibrous meningioma* will be set aside because this common meningioma subtype lacks the plump cells and dense bands of collagen that characterize SFTs. As previously noted, EMA staining is absent in SFTs.[2,7] Although CD34 staining occurs in some meningiomas, it is not usually as diffuse and strongly positive as in SFTs, wherein its positivity is universal. A negative result would go far to exclude this uncommon entity. Ultrastructural differences between SFT and fibrous meningioma were discussed earlier.

The distinction from *hemangiopericytoma* can be problematic and is an important issue in light of the

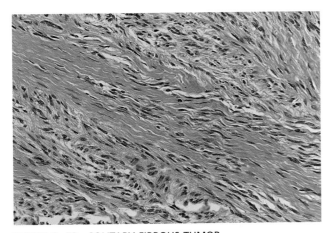

**FIGURE 2–53    SOLITARY FIBROUS TUMOR**

Fascicles of elongated undulating cells associated with collagenous bands are typical of solitary fibrous tumor.

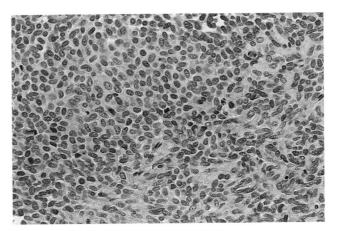

**FIGURE 2–54    SOLITARY FIBROUS TUMOR**

Cellular areas in solitary fibrous tumors may resemble hemangiopericytoma.

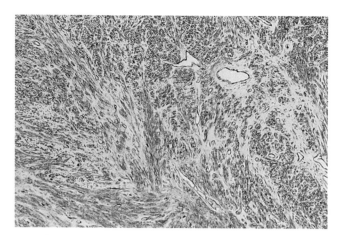

**FIGURE 2–55** SOLITARY FIBROUS TUMOR

The lesions are strongly and uniformly immunoreactive for CD34.

aggressive behavior of the latter neoplasm. As indicated before, the tissue patterns of these two lesions appear to coexist in occasional cases. It is the present consensus that small foci of HPC-like tissue can be accepted in SFT without prognostic consequences, but the histopathologic overlap, and prognostic ramifications thereof, between these two lesions is not yet clear. HPCs react less strongly and diffusely for CD34 than do SFTs.

**Treatment and Prognosis.** To date, meningeal SFTs have not recurred after complete resection despite occasional limited invasion of central or peripheral nervous system tissue. However, the ultimate biologic behavior of

SFTs has yet to be defined, as few reports define long-term follow-up.[2] The behavior of SFTs as a whole appears to be that of meningiomas; recurrence may follow subtotal resection.[2]

## Melanocytoma

**Definition.** A well-differentiated neoplasm arising from leptomeningeal melanocytes.

**General Comments.** Delicate, elongated melanocytes sparsely populate the normal leptomeninges. When sufficiently aggregated, as underneath the medulla and along the cervical cord, these neural crest derivatives are visible to the naked eye and even to the MR scanner.[3] Macroscopically, they appear as lacy patches with intensities of pigmentation that are roughly proportional to those of the patient's skin. Such melanocytes beget a family of pigmented lesions whose members exhibit variable cytoarchitectural and biologic characteristics.[1] Although the inevitable borderline cases confound precise definitions, both well-differentiated melanocytomas and malignant melanomas are represented. The latter are discussed on pages 85 to 87.

**Clinical Features.** Melanocytomas occur throughout the neuraxis but favor the posterior fossa, the region with the highest density of leptomeningeal melanocytes, and the spinal cord (Figs. 2–56 and 2–57).[1, 2, 4–12] Adults are most often affected. Intraspinal lesions are discussed on page 531.

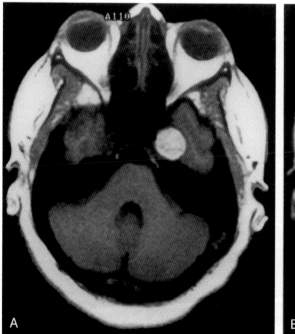
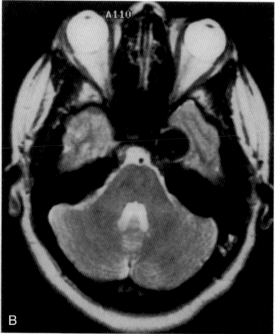

**FIGURE 2–56** MELANOCYTOMA

Heavily pigmented melanocytic neoplasms have a distinctive MR profile; they are bright on precontrast T1-weighted MR images (*A*) and dark on T2-weighted images (*B*). (From Brat DJ, Giannini C, Scheithauer BW, et al. Primary melanocytic neoplasms of the central nervous system. Am J Surg Pathol 1999;23:745–754.)

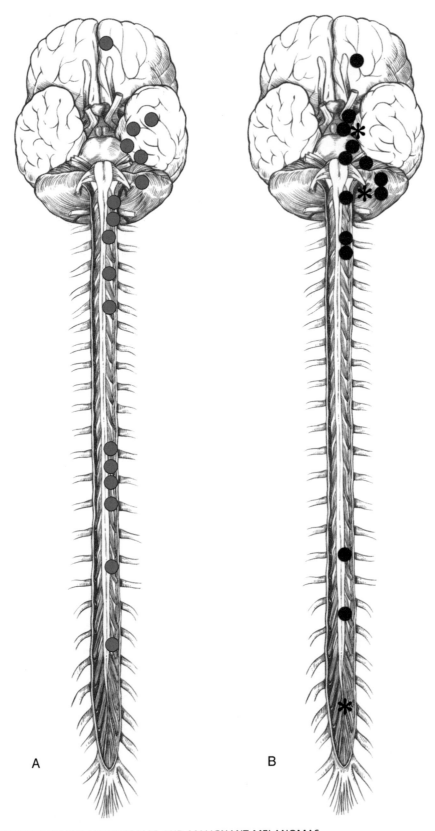

**FIGURE 2–57** DISTRIBUTION OF MELANOCYTOMAS AND MALIGNANT MELANOMAS

The distributions of individual melanocytomas (blue in *A*) and melanomas (red in *B*) are shown as a composite for the series of cases described in reference 1. Black asterisks in *B* mark the site of lesions of intermediate differentiation. Note the concentration of melanocytic neoplasms at the base of the brain and in the spinal canal. (Modified from Brat DJ, Giannini C, Scheithauer BW, et al. Primary melanocytic neoplasms of the central nervous system. Am J Surg Pathol 1999;23:745–754.)

**Radiologic Features.** When highly pigmented, melanocytomas appear on MR imaging as a mass with signaling characteristics of melanin, that is, bright, or hyperintense, on precontrast T1-weighted images and dark, or hypointense, on T2-weighted images (see Fig. 2–56).[9, 12] Many, however, are insufficiently melanotic to produce this distinctive signal combination.

**Macroscopic Features.** Melanocytomas are discrete, lobular masses that vary considerably in their degree of pigmentation.

**Microscopic Features.** The lesions vary considerably from those that are decidedly nested (Fig. 2–58) and those composed of patternless sheets. Some exhibit a fascicular growth pattern resembling that of "spindle A" melanomas of the eye (Fig. 2–59). Whereas some tumors are so pigmented that their cytoarchitecture is difficult to evaluate without resorting to melanin bleaching (Fig. 2–60), others are sparsely pigmented, if not amelanotic (see Fig. 2–59). Heavily pigmented cells at the periphery of such nests are found in some cases. Melanophages are often abundant and sometimes predominant in highly pigmented lesions. Necrosis is absent. Nucleoli are inconspicuous. Longitudinal nuclear grooves are common. Mitoses are rare, no more than one per 10 high-power fields if found at all.[1]

Invasion of the brain can be found in lesions that cytologically and histologically lack the obvious malignancy of melanoma. In one study, such lesions were assigned to an intermediate category between melanocytoma and melanoma.[1]

**Cytologic Features.** The nuclei of melanocytomas are bland, round to oval or bean shaped, and occasionally scored by a longitudinal groove. Nucleoli are usually present and, although they may be prominent, are seldom as conspicuous as in melanomas.

**Immunohistochemical Features.** The tumors are diffusely and unequivocally reactive for both S-100 protein and HMB-45. Without fail, the lesions are EMA negative despite the original designation "pigmented meningioma." In contrast to schwannomas, immunoreactivity for collagen type IV is confined to the vessels and does not diffusely surround individual tumor cells. The indolent behavior of these tumors is reflected in their low MIB-1 labeling index, usually less than 1%.[1]

**Differential Diagnosis.** The differential diagnosis of an amelanotic or only sparsely pigmented CNS lesion calls on the pathologist's past experience with amelanotic tumors at other anatomic sites and the observer's readiness to entertain the possibility of a melanocytic tumor when confronted by a rather uniform proliferation of spindle and/or epithelioid cells with somewhat prominent nucleoli. In the absence of this sensitivity, the lesions can be misinterpreted as *meningioma* or *schwannoma*. The meningioma is reactive for EMA and not for markers such as HMB-45. Schwannomas share the S-100 reactivity of melanocytic tumors but, unless they are melanocytic, are HMB-45 negative. Affirmation that the pigment is melanin and not iron narrows the differential to melanocytoma; malignant melanoma, with admission of a rare melanocytic neoplasm of intermediate grade; and melanotic schwannoma.

At this point, there are no histologic or cytologic criteria to divide what is a continuum into artificially discrete units, that is, melanocytoma and malignant melanoma. For practical purposes, melanomas are mitotically more active and more cytologically atypical. In one study, the MIB-1 index was 2% to 15% for melanomas but only 0% to 2% for melanocytomas.[1] Necrosis may be present in melanomas but not in melanocytomas. Melanomas are discussed on pages 85 to 87.

Distinguishing between melanocytoma and melanocytic schwannoma is discussed on page 543.

**Treatment and Prognosis.** The outlook for the patient with a melanocytoma is generally very favorable for melanocytomas defined rigidly as before, that is, lesions

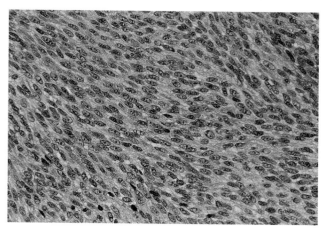

**FIGURE 2–59    MELANOCYTOMA**

When lightly pigmented, melanocytomas with a fascicular architecture can mimic fibrous meningiomas. This lesion resembles the "spindle A" variant of ocular melanoma, but mitoses are absent and the MIB-1 labeling index was only 1%.

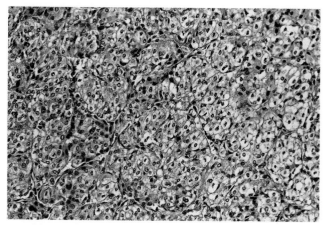

**FIGURE 2–58    MELANOCYTOMA**

Some melanocytomas have a prominent nested pattern.

with minimal if any mitotic activity, inconspicuous nucleoli, no evident CNS invasion, and a gross total resection. Subtotal resection leaves open the possibility of recurrence.[1] The value of radiotherapy remains uncertain, but the modality has been employed in some cases.

## Hemangioblastoma

Most intracranial neoplasms with the distinctive morphology of the hemangioblastoma occur in the cerebellum, brain stem (medulla), retina, or spinal cord. Only rarely do they arise in the cerebral meninges and then almost solely in the setting of von Hippel–Lindau disease.[2–4] A ventricle is yet another unusual site.[1]

    Supratentorial hemangioblastomas are globoid and highly vascular. Their microscopic appearance is indistinguishable from that of cerebellar hemangioblastoma as described on pages 329 to 335. Given the rarity of supratentorial examples, the burden of proof rests on the pathologist that a meningeal hemangioblastoma is not, in fact, a microcystic, xanthomatous, or clear cell meningioma.

## Lipoma

**Definition.** A mass of mature non-neoplastic adipose tissue.

**General Comments.** Although the meninges do not normally contain adipose tissue, yellow deposits of fat termed *lipomas* or *lipomatous hamartomas* are occasionally encountered in the intracranial and intraspinal spaces. Intracranially, most occur above the corpus callosum (Figs. 2–61 and 2–62),[2, 9, 12, 22] beneath the third ventricle,[2, 7, 8, 13, 14, 19, 22] in the third ventricle,[20] in the choroid plexus,[23] in the suprasellar region,[8, 19] over the quadrigeminal plate (Fig. 2–63),[1, 2] or in the cerebellopontine angle.[2–4, 11, 15, 16, 22] Other sites include the eighth

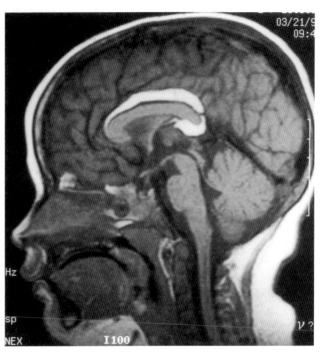

**FIGURE 2–61**   LIPOMA

Readily identified by its bright (hyperintense) MR signal in a precontrast T1-weighted image, this lipoma angles around the posterior end of the shortened corpus callosum. (Courtesy of Dr. Elias Melhem, Baltimore, MD.)

cranial nerve, sylvian-insular region,[5, 6, 10, 22] Meckel's cave,[16] thalamus,[18] and cerebellum.[17] The special variant on the eighth cranial nerve is discussed separately on page 342.

    The histologic appearance of lipomas, their often midline position, and the occasional association with developmental abnormalities such as agenesis of the corpus callosum (see Figs. 2–61 and 2–62) underscore the

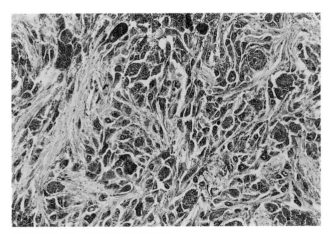

**FIGURE 2–60**   MELANOCYTOMA

Some melanocytomas are so heavily pigmented as to obscure cytologic detail.

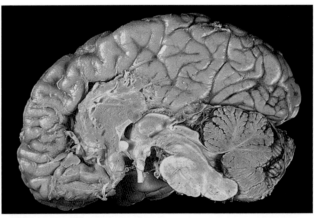

**FIGURE 2–62**   LIPOMA

This asymptomatic lipoma in the region of a congenitally absent corpus callosum occurred in a 56-year-old man who died of renal cell carcinoma. The lesion is canary yellow except for the small gray translucent nodule of cartilage just superior to the massa intermedia. Note the radiating sulci on the medial aspect of the frontal lobe that regularly accompany agenesis of the corpus callosum.

lesion's presumed embryonic basis.[2,22] Correlations of neuroradiologic findings with the events in normal embryogenesis have concluded that lipomas arise as a result of the persistence of the *meninx primativa* and reflect the latter's capacity for "mesenchymal" differentiation.[22] The meningeal "lipoma" is thus a non-neoplastic mass that is unlikely to appear as a surgical specimen.

**Clinical Features.** Although intracranial lipomas are usually incidental findings, some, such as those of the corpus callosum, are associated with seizures. Lesions of the tuber cinereum often produce hypothalamic disturbances, and those near the ventricular system may cause hydrocephalus. Cranial nerve dysfunction is one consequence of lipomas in the cerebellopontine angle.

**Radiologic Features.** Lipomas are characterized by a hyperintense signal on precontrast T1-weighted images similar to that of surrounding subcutaneous or intraorbital fat (see Fig. 2–61).[22] MR fat suppression sequences can be used for unambiguous identification.

**Macroscopic Features.** Color is the essence of the lesion that contrasts pleasurably with the functionally magnificent, but tinctorially drab, cerebrum.

**Microscopic Features.** Although much of this splendor is lost in tissue processing, it is supplanted by the curious presence in some lipomas of cranial nerve fascicles,[2,21,22] "hamartomatous" blood vessels,[2,18,24] bone,[2,8,19,20] and rarely cartilage (see Fig. 2–63).[2,17] These elements and the occasional presence of skeletal muscle or papillary epithelium lend a somewhat teratomatous appearance.[21] Peripherally situated calcifications often parenthesize lipomas that overlie the corpus callosum. Bone is a frequent component of suprasellar lesions (osteolipomas).[8,19]

**Treatment and Prognosis.** The central localization of most intracranial lipomas, their often irregular interface with brain, and their often considerable vascularity explain the difficulties in obtaining a complete, uncomplicated excision. Thus, although some lesions can be excised, the treatment is limited to shunting to relieve obstruction of cerebrospinal fluid flow.

## Fibroma and Fibromatosis

Only rarely do cellular fibrous masses reminiscent of fibroma appear in the meninges.[3,6] Myofibromatosis has been encountered in the CNS as well.[7] Lesions not readily classified, but loosely referred to as fibroma or fibromyxoma, have been reported to occur in the meninges of both children and adults.[4,6,8] Infiltrative, less cellular, fibrous lesions akin to fibromatosis or "desmoid tumors" are more frequent.[1,2,5] In some instances, prior surgery appears to have initiated this reactive but often aggressive process. Insofar as possible, wide local resection is indicated to control their potential for recurrence.[2]

## Chondroma, Osteochondroma, and Osteoma

The latent capacity of the meninges to form tissues such as cartilage and bone is occasionally expressed in exaggerated form as masses termed chondroma, osteochondroma, or as asymptomatic ossification (osteoma) of the falx and parasagittal meninges. Some lesions are betrayed by neurologic symptoms and thus pass from the hands of the surgeon into those of the pathologist.

Albeit rare, the most commonly excised of those lesions is the *chondroma* (Figs. 2–64 to 2–67). Most occur sporadically, but a minority arise in the setting of Ollier's disease[16] or Maffucci's syndrome.[2] Always discrete, and sometimes sizable, these bosselated, gray-white, semitranslucent masses usually arise over the cerebral convexities, where they are attached to the

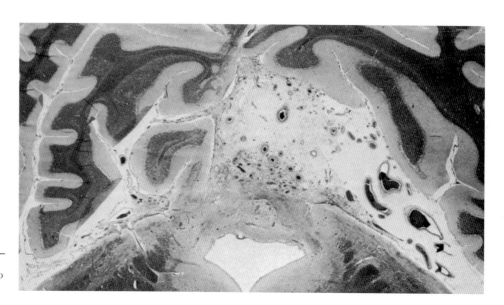

**FIGURE 2–63 LIPOMA**

Lipomas, as here over the tectal plate, can be intimately attached to the brain.

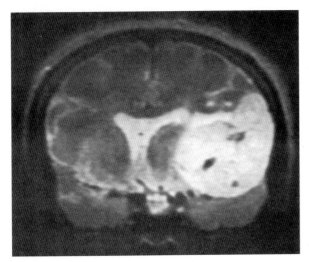

**FIGURE 2–64    CHONDROMA**

Intracranial chondromas can attain considerable size. As in this example occurring in a 69-year-old woman, they are discrete and dura based.

dura.[4, 6, 9, 11, 12, 14, 15, 17] Others are intraparenchymal, with no apparent relation to the pachymeninges.[1, 3] Excision is curative because hemispheric chondromas are both surgically accessible and noninfiltrative. The malignant counterpart, chondrosarcoma, is discussed on pages 84 to 85. Cartilaginous and osseous tumors of the skull are discussed on pages 21, 23, and 33.

Some meningeal lesions contain bone, either mixed with cartilage, as in *osteochondroma*,[8, 10, 13] or in pure form, as in asymptomatic ossification of the falx and parasagittal meninges.[7] The latter is usually an incidental autopsy finding in a patient with a history of chronic renal failure.[7] An occasional bony proliferation, possibly related to trauma, is loosely termed *osteoma*.[5]

## Plasmacytoma

**Definition.** A monoclonal proliferation of well-differentiated plasma cells.

**General Comments.** Masses composed of monoclonal, well-differentiated plasma cells not infrequently occur in the skull and paranasal sinuses[7, 10] or meninges.[2–5, 8, 9, 11] Examples arising in brain parenchyma are rare.[5, 12] Large examples occasionally involve both bone and meninges.[1] Skull lesions are discussed briefly on page 23.

**Clinical Features.** Plasmacytomas single out adults and often present as a meningioma-like mass. Almost none are associated with systemic manifestations of plasma cell neoplasia at the time of presentation.

**Macroscopic and Microscopic Features.** Soft and fleshy, the masses consist of a monomorphous proliferation of mature plasma cells that, by definition, are monoclonal. Amyloid deposits are occasionally noted. Intraparenchymal amyloidomas, only lately characterized

as a form of plasma cell neoplasia,[6] are discussed separately in Chapter 3 on pages 149 to 150.

**Differential Diagnosis.** At any anatomic site, the differential diagnosis of plasmacytoma quickly narrows to the exclusion of a plasma cell–rich inflammatory mass, that is, *plasma cell granuloma or inflammatory pseudotumor*, a lesion described later in this chapter on pages 95 to 96. Histologic features favoring the inflammatory lesions are the admixture of lymphocytes, germinal centers, a prominent connective tissue component, and, of course, polyclonality. Also in the differential diagnosis are *plasma cell–rich* or *lymphoplasmacytoid meningioma* and, at the skull base, *pituitary adenoma*. The latter is monomorphous and may closely resemble plasmacytoma, especially in frozen sections. It is synaptophysin, and usually chromogranin, positive. Attention to radiographic features such as sellar enlargement and the

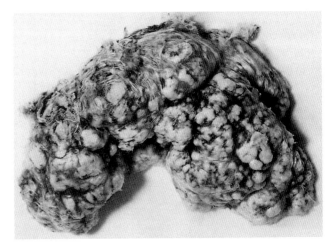

2–65

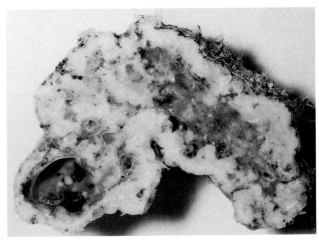

2–66

**FIGURES 2–65 AND 2–66    CHONDROMA**

Radiologic studies disclosed a large calcified mass in the right parieto-occipital region of a 16-year-old boy with a 2-year history of left-sided weakness. This knobby chondroma was firmly attached to the dura but separated readily from the brain (Fig. 2–65). The lesion has the typical translucent quality of hyaline cartilage (Fig. 2–66). There was no evidence of recurrence during 9 years of follow-up.

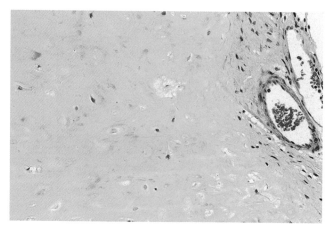

**FIGURE 2–67** CHONDROMA

The low cellularity, bland nuclei, and lack of mitoses distinguish this lesion from chondrosarcoma.

performance of smear preparations usually resolve the issue. Another basilar neoplasm, *olfactory neuroblastoma*, is a monomorphous, cytologically bland lesion that may resemble plasmacytoma. Once again, radiologic data (cribriform plate involvement) and cytologic findings aid in the distinction. Immunohistochemistry quickly resolves the issue.

**Treatment and Prognosis.** Radiation therapy has generally been employed in postoperative management of plasmacytomas.[1] Although plasmacytomas carry a risk of malignant transformation and dissemination,[10] this seems to be a most unusual occurrence in meningeal examples. Few develop into myeloma.

## Leiomyoma

Leiomyomas of the meninges or of brain are rare. Some arise in the setting of immunocompromise wherein the Epstein-Barr virus is the apparent oncologic agent.[1] The same is true of leiomyosarcomas, an entity discussed on pages 83 to 84.

## Vascular Malformations and Benign Vascular Neoplasms

As discussed in Chapter 7, the offending arteriovenous shunt of some intracranial arteriovenous malformations lies in the dura, not the brain. Occasional cavernous angiomas are leptomeningeal, but dura-based lesions are rare.[1, 3] The same is true of capillary hemangioma and hemangioendothelioma.[2, 4]

## PRIMARY MALIGNANT NEOPLASMS

In view of the unyielding volume of the intracranial space and the fundamental relationship of the brain to life, even the histologically benign meningeal lesions discussed up to this point are potentially lethal. The rare neoplasms described in the following section exhibit both histologic and biologic characteristics of malignancy.

## Hemangiopericytoma

**Definition.** A sarcoma attributed to neoplastic transformation of pericytes.

**General Comments.** Although intracranial HPC was at one time accepted as an "angioblastic" variant of meningioma, there is now little doubt that this distinctive mesenchymal neoplasm is unrelated to the meningioma's progenitor, the arachnoidal cell. This interpretation, long supported by histologic and immunohistologic differences, has now been confirmed by molecular studies that have failed to show either monosomy chromosome 22 or abnormalities in the *NF2* gene in HPCs.[8] These are present, however, in a significant percentage of meningiomas.

**Clinical Features.** Meningeal HPCs occur at all ages, but their peak incidence is the fourth through the sixth decades. In contrast to meningiomas, they occur somewhat more often in males.[6, 9] The sites of origin parallel those of meningiomas; most are dura based. Children are affected only occasionally by what may, in that setting, be a less aggressive lesion.[7]

**Radiologic Features.** On MR images, HPCs are similar to meningiomas in their dural attachment but are more likely to have a narrow pedicle rather than the broad base that anchors meningiomas to the dura (Fig. 2–68).[3] They are also more likely to erode the skull than to

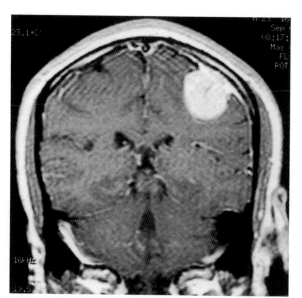

**FIGURE 2–68** HEMANGIOPERICYTOMA

As seen in a contrast-enhanced, T1-weighted MR image, this lesion of a 23-year-old man with headaches has a narrower dural attachment than is typical of meningiomas.

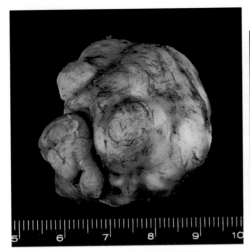
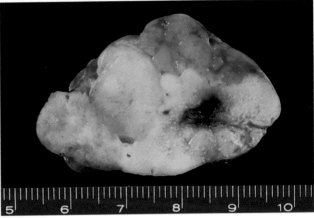

**FIGURES 2–69 and 2–70**    HEMANGIOPERICYTOMA

This bosselated, solid lesion was lifted from the parieto-occipital region of a 54-year-old man with headaches, seizures, and a visual field defect. Despite a gross total excision, local recurrence necessitated a second operation 3 years later. Complete resection was thereafter no longer possible.

produce hyperostosis, as is the case in meningioma. Unlike meningioma, HPCs are not calcified. The extensive arteriovenous shunting seen on arteriography should alert the surgeon and pathologist to the possible diagnosis.

**Macroscopic Features.** At surgery, the lobulated discrete mass usually adheres to the dura, but its vascular supply is provided directly by the carotid or vertebrobasilar system. Not surprisingly, copious bleeding follows incision of this soft, highly vascular tumor (Figs. 2–69 and 2–70).

**Microscopic Features.** The high cellularity and randomness of nuclear orientation impart a monotonous, yet chaotic, microscopic appearance that is sometimes relieved by rarified regions of reduced cellular density (Figs. 2–71 and 2–72), "staghorn" sinusoidal vessels (Fig. 2–73),[16] storiform architecture, tight clusters of neoplastic cells (Figs. 2–72 to 2–75), or foci of perivascular fibrosis. At higher magnification, the oval, plump,

and occasionally somewhat elongated nuclei are crowded and jumbled in sheets that are interrupted by vessels lined by flattened endothelial cells. Scant cytoplasm forms a background matrix without clearly defined cell boundaries. Mitotic figures are encountered in small to moderate numbers. Psammoma bodies, calcified collagen, and tight cell whorls are absent. Both low- and high-grade HPCs have been characterized,[9] their distinction being based upon mitotic index as well as other common cytologic and histologic features of malignancy (see the following).

Special stains are of diagnostic utility. A variably dense and pervasive network of reticulin is one of the lesion's most distinctive histochemical features. Its distribution ranges from pericellular to scant and sometimes highlights a nodular arrangement. Widespread deposition of reticulin around individual cells effectively excludes the common differential diagnosis—meningioma (Fig. 2–76). The utility of this still valuable technique is illustrated in Table 2–2.

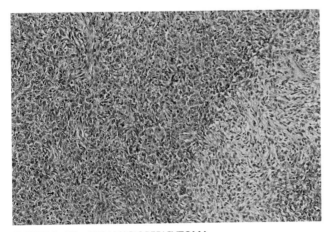

**FIGURE 2–71**    HEMANGIOPERICYTOMA

Hemangiopericytomas are, overall, highly cellular, but pale foci of reduced cellularity are common.

| TABLE 2–2 |
|---|
| **Utility of Reticulin Staining in Surgical Neuropathology** |
| Hemangiopericytoma and fibrosarcoma—extensive pericellular distribution not seen in meningioma |
| Schwannoma—extensive pericellular distribution not seen in meningioma |
| Pleomorphic xanthoastrocytoma—abundant, often at least focally pericellular in distribution, not found in most other gliomas |
| Primary central nervous system lymphoma—distinctive pericellular distribution in walls of blood vessels almost unique for this entity |
| Gliosarcoma—presence of pericellular reticulin identifies sarcomatous component |
| Hemangioblastoma—abundant deposition defining clusters and lobules not seen in most other central nervous system tumors |
| Pituitary adenoma—defines enlarged irregular lobules of the adenoma not found in the normal gland |

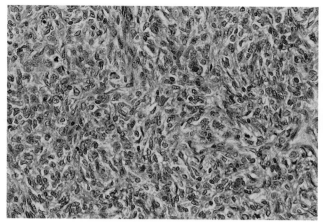

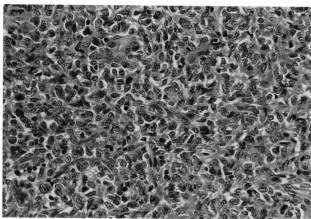

2–72                                    2–73

**FIGURES 2–72 AND 2–73**   HEMANGIOPERICYTOMA

Varying degrees of histologic turbulence are common.

**Features in Frozen Sections.** The identity of the lesion is not usually as clear as it is in permanent sections, but the histologic turbulence and staghorn vessels are often evident (Fig. 2–77).

**Cytologic Features.** The nuclei, with little visible attached cytoplasm, are ovoid, dark, and formed of evenly dispersed chromatin. Although in a sense nondescript, they are actually distinctive because of the uniformity in size and shape. They are larger and denser than those of meningioma (Fig. 2–78). Nucleoli are less conspicuous.

**Immunohistochemical Features.** The cells lining the vascular spaces are positive for CD31 and von Willebrand factor (factor VIII), but the neoplastic cells are not.[2] CD34 immunoreactivity of the neoplastic cells is present in less than half of cases and varies in extent (Fig. 2–79).[1, 2, 12] Scattered factor XIIIa–positive cells are also common.[10, 11] Despite the frequent assumption that pericytes are modified smooth muscle cells, the incidence of staining for muscle markers is low and does not help

identify the HPC.[13] Vimentin staining, aside from being a marker of immunoviability, is not diagnostically useful.

The MIB-1 index varies considerably from case to case, 1% to 39% in one series.[14] In that series there was little, if any, relationship to outcome.

**Ultrastructural Features.** The cells are separated by basement membrane–like material and lack the complex interdigitating processes and desmosomal attachments of meningioma (Fig. 2–80).[4, 15]

**Differential Diagnosis.** Some *meningiomas* with sinusoidal spaces simulate the HPC (see Fig. 2–50) except

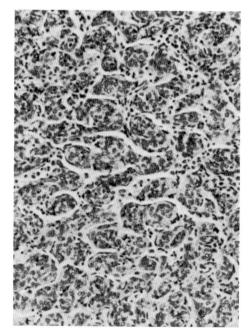

**FIGURE 2–75**   HEMANGIOPERICYTOMA

In some hemangiopericytomas, small lobules can resemble the whorls of a meningioma, although they are not as tightly wound nor do they contain psammoma bodies.

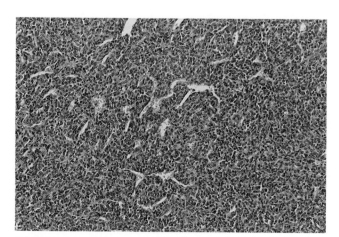

**FIGURE 2–74**   HEMANGIOPERICYTOMA

Lobules of neoplastic cells surrounding so-called staghorn vessels are a characteristic feature of hemangiopericytomas.

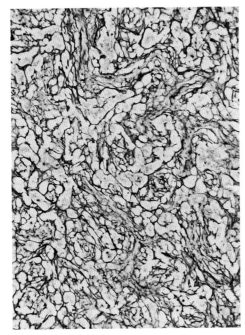

**FIGURE 2-76**  HEMANGIOPERICYTOMA

Investment of individual cells by reticulin is a hallmark of most, but not all, hemangiopericytomas.

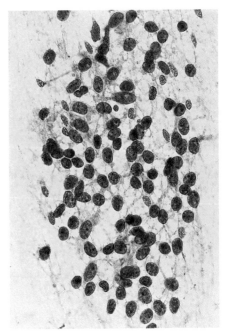

**FIGURE 2-78**  HEMANGIOPERICYTOMA—SMEAR PREPARATION

In smear preparations, the nuclei of hemangiopericytomas are somewhat darker and their chromatin is more uniformly distributed than in meningioma. The small discrete nucleoli of meningioma are also lacking.

for the latter's relative abundance of reticulin. This issue is discussed on pages 72 to 73.

The differential must also include a newcomer to meningeal neoplasms—*solitary fibrous tumor*. Uncertainty in this regard arises at the time of surgery because the globoid shape and the dural attachment are common to HPC, meningioma, and SFT. Resolution of the problem is achieved in most instances by routine light microscopy because the three are distinctive. The differential between HPC and SFT can be even more problematic in that densely cellular, HPC-like areas occur in

some SFTs and, conversely, occasional HPCs have focal spindle cells with associated collagen production and resemble SFT. Immunohistochemistry plays a role in differential diagnosis, but at this time there are no specific markers of HPC. Furthermore, the criteria are largely ones of exclusion, principally the lack of staining for EMA.[1, 12, 17] Staining of scattered cells in an HPC for factor XIIIa may be of some utility[10, 11] but has not been considered helpful in all studies.[12]

The differential diagnosis of the meningeal HPC, particularly anaplastic examples, must extend to *metastatic*

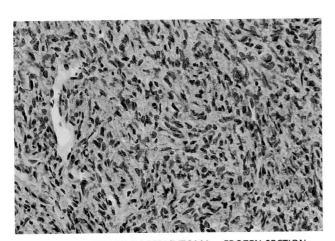

**FIGURE 2-77**  HEMANGIOPERICYTOMA—FROZEN SECTION

In frozen sections, cytologic agitation and staghorn vessels are clues to the diagnosis.

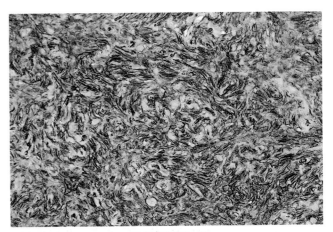

**FIGURE 2-79**  HEMANGIOPERICYTOMA

Approximately one half of meningeal hemangiopericytomas are immunopositive for CD34. The reaction is typically less than that seen in solitary fibrous tumor.

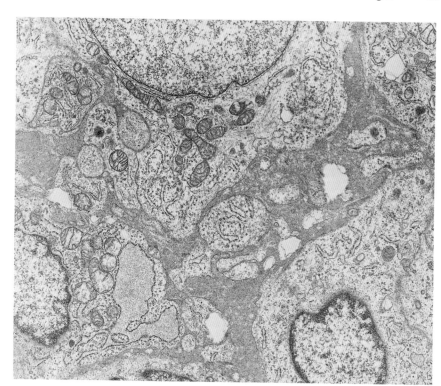

**FIGURE 2–80** HEMANGIOPERICYTOMA

Electron-dense extracellular material is the ultrastructural equivalent of the positive reticulin stain (see Fig. 2–76). The cells are devoid of desmosomes and lack the abundant intermediate filaments that characterize meningiomas (×9000).

*carcinoma.* This distinction is usually resolved by the absence of intercellular reticulin and the presence of epithelial markers, such as keratin and EMA, in carcinomas.

The small cell component of the rare *mesenchymal chondrosarcoma* of the meninges features a sinusoidal-staghorn vascular pattern similar to that of HPC, but the lesion is distinguished by its distinctive cartilaginous islands.

**Treatment and Prognosis.** The macroscopic similarity of HPC to meningioma, and the ease with which some are amenable to enucleation, belies the HPC's proclivity for multiple recurrence and metastasis, often after prolonged postoperative intervals. In one study, the 5-, 10-, and 15-year survival rates were 67%, 40%, and 23%, respectively.[6] Common metastatic sites include bone, liver, lymph nodes, lung, and the CNS.[6, 9] One study successfully stratified HPCs into differentiated and anaplastic lesions.[9] The latter were defined as tumors exhibiting brisk mitotic activity (greater than five mitoses per 10 high-power fields) and at least two of the following index features: moderate to high cellularity, moderate to marked nuclear atypia, and hemorrhage. Seventy-six percent of the differentiated lesions recurred in contrast to 85% in the anaplastic group. Histologic factors were not found to be predictive of outcome in other series, however.[6]

Gross total excision and postoperative radiotherapy are both favorable prognostic factors.[6, 9] Recurrent lesions are treated by surgery and, in some cases, radiation.[5]

## Fibrosarcoma and Leiomyosarcoma

*Fibrosarcoma* of the meninges may be incited by irradiation[5,12–14] or may occur de novo (Fig. 2–81).[2, 6, 7, 10, 11]

Those attributed to irradiation most often arise in the sellar region after treatment of a pituitary adenoma. These are discussed in Chapter 9 on page 483. Extensive involvement of the bone, dura, leptomeninges, and brain generally obscures a precise origin. Radiation-induced sarcomas must be distinguished from the

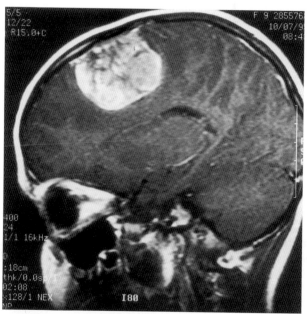

**FIGURE 2–81** FIBROSARCOMA

Fibrosarcomas are discrete, usually superficial to the brain, and contrast enhancing. This lesion produced signs and symptoms of increased intracranial pressure in a 9-year-old. It was resected but recurred locally 3 years thereafter despite craniospinal radiation and chemotherapy.

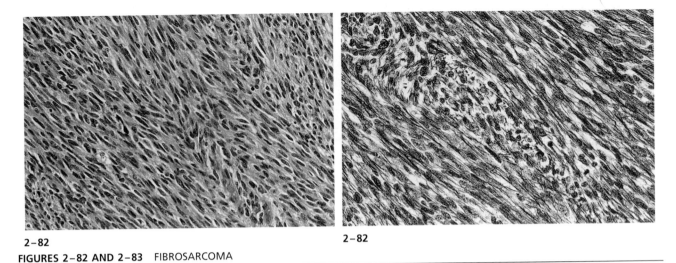

2-82                                        2-82

**FIGURES 2–82 AND 2–83    FIBROSARCOMA**

As with its extracranial counterparts, fibrosarcoma of the meninges is composed of densely packed fascicles of malignant cells in a "herringbone" pattern (Fig. 2–82). Note the abundant pericellular reticulin (Fig. 2–83).

malignant gliomas that can arise in this same post-therapy setting (see page 180).

Fibrosarcomas that appear de novo form a heterogeneous group in regard to patient's age, localization, and microscopic appearance. Some are discrete dural masses with a tendency to infiltrate adjacent bone, whereas others are diffuse leptomeningeal lesions. Some consist of interwoven herringbone-like arrangements of spindle cells accompanied by reticulin and collagen production and thus conform to the established prototype of fibrosarcoma (Figs. 2–82 and 2–83). Yet other lesions have less elongated, more pleomorphic cells associated with only a scant stroma. The latter appearance is more akin to that of the malignant fibrous histiocytoma.

The differential diagnosis of anaplastic lesions that are composed predominantly of spindle cells requires consideration of malignant meningioma and of the exuberant, sometimes neoplastic reaction that accompanies meningeal invasion by aggressive gliomas. Some malignant meningiomas acquire the histologic features of fibrosarcoma. In such instances, it is only the histologic presence of focal meningothelial features, or review of previous specimens with meningioma, that permits their distinction from ordinary sarcomas. The issue of *glial-meningeal interaction in the setting of gliomas* is discussed in Chapter 4 on page 189. Gliosarcomas are discussed in Chapter 4 on pages 196 to 198.

Only a rare primary meningeal sarcoma arises from smooth muscle.[1] Some of these *leiomyosarcomas* occur in the setting of immunosuppression and the presence of Epstein-Barr virus (Figs. 2–84 to 2–86).[3, 4, 8, 9]

Malignant fibrous histiocytoma in the CNS is discussed in Chapter 4 on page 317.

## Chondrosarcoma, Liposarcoma, and Osteosarcoma

Given the occurrence of well-differentiated meningeal neoplasms composed of hyaline cartilage, adipose tissue, or bone, it is not surprising that the literature records examples of meningeal chondrosarcoma, liposarcoma,[12] and osteosarcoma.[13] The spectrum of chondrosarcomas includes conventional (Fig. 2–87),[1–3, 5–8, 10, 11, 14, 15, 20] myxoid,[17, 19] and mesenchymal variants.

This intriguing mesenchymal chondrosarcoma makes its appearance during the first through the fifth decades of life.[4, 9, 16, 18] Although most arise in bone, the meninges

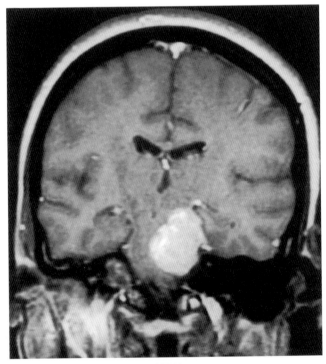

**FIGURE 2–84    LEIOMYOSARCOMA**

Most intracranial leiomyosarcomas arise in the meninges and occur in association with immunocompromise. This example appeared in the prepontine cistern of a 34-year-old woman with acquired immunodeficiency disease syndrome.

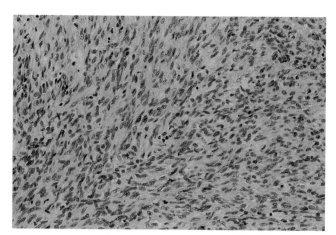

**FIGURE 2-85** LEIOMYOSARCOMA

Somewhat plump cells in fascicular arrangement are typical of leiomyosarcoma.

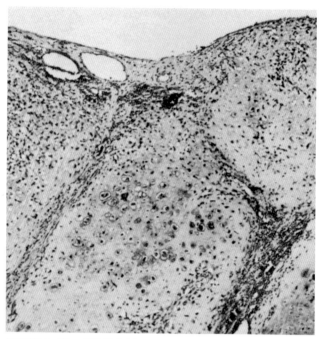

**FIGURE 2-87** CHONDROSARCOMA

The malignancy of this cartilaginous neoplasm is apparent because of its degree of cellularity, atypia, and, elsewhere in the specimen, invasion of dural veins. The lobular lesion was attached to the dura over the right parietal lobe of a 56-year-old man. (Courtesy of Dr. Dana D. Copeland, Raleigh, NC.)

are a preferred extraosseous site; where the lesions appear in discrete masses that compress or infiltrate brain, they often invade bone (Fig. 2–88).

Histologically, mesenchymal chondrosarcomas are formed of two discrete components whose extremes of nuclear density produce an appearance like that of clouds in the sky. The azure background is composed of crowded primitive cells with high nuclear/cytoplasmic ratios (Fig. 2–89) and variable degrees of mitotic activity. These cells are compacted into irregular or staghorn vascular channels, producing a resemblance to hemangiopericytoma (Fig. 2–90). The fleecy elements are pale-staining islands of hyaline cartilage that float within the small cell element. Delicate deposits of calcium in some chondroid nodules occasionally yield to prominent calcification that serves as the substrate of osseous metaplasia (see Fig. 2–90). The cartilaginous islands, although focal, are requisite for the diagnosis. As expected, they are immunoreactive for S-100 protein.[16]

Experience with the mesenchymal chondrosarcoma in the meninges is limited; elsewhere, the neoplasm is noted for local recurrence and late metastasis.[7] The same appears to be true for meningeal lesions.[16, 18] The tumor also affects the spinal meninges, where, presumably because of earlier detection, they appear to carry a more favorable prognosis.[18] These are discussed in Chapter 11 on pages 533 to 534.

## Malignant Melanoma

**Definition.** A malignant neoplasm derived from meningeal melanocytes.

**General Comments.** Malignant melanomas occur sporadically and, with greatly enhanced incidence, in the neurocutaneous melanosis syndrome or formes frustes thereof.[2, 5, 6, 9–11] This syndrome casts a shadow over the patient in the form of a large nevus preferentially affecting the head, neck, and trunk. A simultaneous diffuse proliferation of melanocytes in the meninges is at risk for malignant transformation.[11] In some instances, a more localized oculodermal melanosis, termed "nevus of Ota," is the superficial component.[3, 12] A meningeal cellular blue nevus has also been reported as a precursor of meningeal melanoma.[8] The meningeal element of neurocutaneous melanoses spans the spectrum from asymptomatic, cytologically benign sheets of melanocytes that are as intensely pigmented but substanceless as carbon

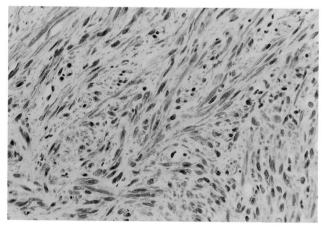

**FIGURE 2-86** LEIOMYOSARCOMA

Also illustrated in Figures 2–84 and 2–85, this tumor is immunoreactive for smooth muscle actin.

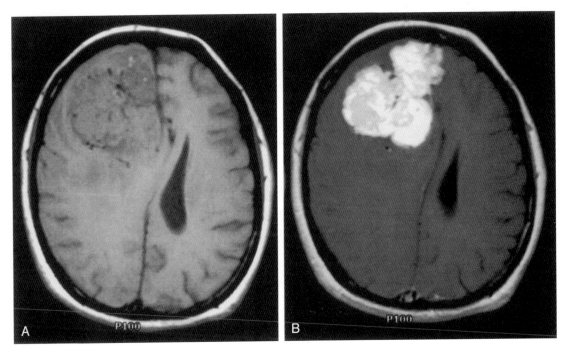

**FIGURE 2–88    MESENCHYMAL CHONDROSARCOMA**

As seen in precontrast (*A*) and postcontrast (*B*) T1-weighted MR images, the lesion is a superficial, dura-based mass.

paper to aggressively malignant neoplasms that overgrow the meninges, form tumorous masses, obstruct the flow of CSF, and invade the brain. Many lesions lie between these cytologic and architectural extremes.

**Clinical Features.** Despite well-recognized predisposing states, most melanomas arise de novo. Both adults and children are affected, the latter especially in the neurocutaneous syndrome. When malignant pigmented neoplasms are encountered in the absence of congenital cutaneous stigmata, it is difficult, if not impossible, to exclude the existence of a cryptic, extracranial primary lesion. This is particularly true of localized intracranial lesions. The case rests upon a careful postmortem

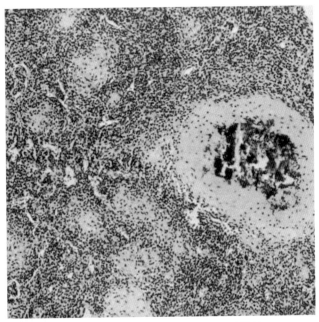

**FIGURE 2–89    MESENCHYMAL CHONDROSARCOMA**

Cartilaginous foci interrupt this otherwise densely cellular neoplasm. As is characteristic, calcium has been deposited in a cartilaginous island.

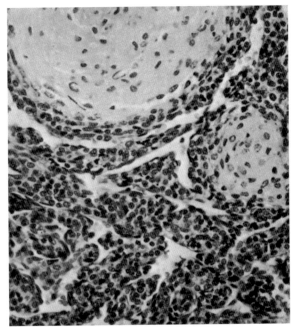

**FIGURE 2–90    MESENCHYMAL CHONDROSARCOMA**

Islands of cartilage drift in a sea of primitive cells. The intensely cellular areas can closely resemble hemangiopericytoma.

examination. By an incomplete study, many a pathologist has relinquished such information to the mortuary—and regretted it.

Isolated "sporadic" melanomas occur as discrete meningeal masses exhibiting the same general localization as their benign counterpart. The latter are discussed on pages 73 to 76.

**Macroscopic Features.** The lesions are variably pigmented, meningioma-like masses.

**Microscopic Features.** The histologic pattern is more likely to be sheet-like or fascicular than nested, as is often the case in melanocytomas. Considerable nuclear atypia is the rule (Fig. 2–91). Nucleoli are prominent and mitoses are generally found without difficulty—in one study with a mean frequency of 6 per 10 high-power fields.[4] Brain invasion is not uncommon. Focal necrosis is present in some lesions.

"Balloon cell" variants have been described.[1,7]

**Immunohistochemical Features.** The neoplasms show the expected immunoreactivity for S-100 protein and melanocyte markers such as HMB-45 and melan A (Fig. 2–92). The MIB-1 rate in one study ranged from 2% to 15%.[4]

**Differential Diagnosis.** The initial differential diagnosis of any cytologically bland mass, even in the apparent absence of pigmentation, should include the possibility of melanoma. Tumors with sheet-like architecture, uniform nuclei, and prominent nucleoli should be especially suspect. Once the melanocytic nature of a lesion is

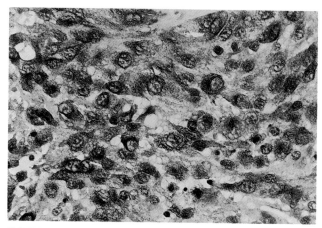

**FIGURE 2–92    MALIGNANT MELANOMA**

The cells illustrated in Figure 2–91 were HMB-45 immunoreactive.

established by immunohistochemistry or electron microscopy, the issue of its *primary versus metastatic nature* must be addressed, although most melanomas metastatic to the brain are intraparenchymal, not meningeal, masses. This distinction, of course, relies heavily upon a thorough clinical history together with exhaustive physical and radiologic examinations.

Distinguishing melanomas from their well-differentiated counterpart, the *melanocytoma*, can be straightforward at the extremes of these two lesions yet obviously can be problematic with lesions of intermediate grade. Although no sharp distinction can be drawn in all cases, melanomas are cytologically atypical and mitotically active and may be focally necrotic. Nesting, epithelioid cytologic features, a low MIB-1 labeling index, and perilobular collagen IV or laminin deposition that reflect the presence of basal lamina are features favoring a diagnosis of melanocytoma.

**Treatment and Prognosis.** Meningeal melanomas are generally aggressive lesions prone to local recurrence and dissemination through CSF pathways. As with many other relatively discrete malignant neoplasms in the intracranial and intraspinal compartments, a gross total resection with postoperative radiotherapy is curative in a subset of patients with primary meningeal melanoma.[4]

## Meningeal Glioma and Gliomatosis

It is not uncommon for gliomas to make contact with, and then seed, the leptomeninges.[3, 5, 8, 9, 11, 12] There are also occasional meningeal gliomas, either diffuse[4, 7] or localized,[6, 10] in which there is no recognized intraparenchymal element. Rare heterotopic nests of astroglia, sometimes with an ependymal component, are offered as potential precursors of these primary meningeal gliomas.[1, 2] However, even in cases studied after death, it may be difficult, if not impossible, to exclude an origin from a small undetected intraparenchymal focus.

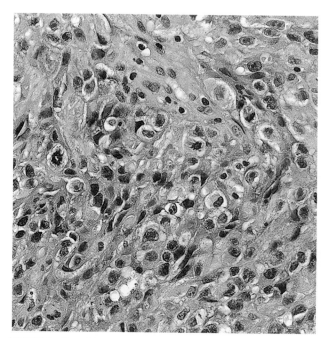

**FIGURE 2–91    MALIGNANT MELANOMA**

An extra-axial, mitotically active mass of cells with round nuclei and prominent nucleoli should prompt consideration of melanoma. This lesion was amelanotic.

# SECONDARY MALIGNANT NEOPLASMS

In the absence of lymphatic vessels within the CNS, leukemic, lymphomatous, and carcinomatous cells gain access to the meninges by one of two routes, that is, vascular embolization or direct extension from the skull or brain. Once they have penetrated these barriers, meningeal involvement may take the form of a discrete, often dura-based mass or of a diffuse proliferation typically involving the leptomeninges. Spread through the subarachnoid space is facilitated by the current of CSF.

## Metastatic Carcinoma

Because the intracranial dura is firmly adherent to the skull, symptomatic epidural carcinomas are rare. This stands in contrast to their frequent occurrence in the vertebral column, where the existence of an epidural space permits tumor growth and resultant spinal cord compression. Relatively few intracranial metastases are restricted to the dura (Figs. 2–93 and 2–94).[3] Most also involve bone, pia-arachnoid, or brain. The rare metastasis to a meningioma is discussed on page 51.

Parenchymal lesions that begin in the cerebral cortex may, by expansion, breach the pia and exfoliate into the subarachnoid compartment. Of particular interest are examples of widespread leptomeningeal dissemination, a process termed *meningeal carcinomatosis* (Fig. 2–95). The subarachnoid space is most receptive to adenocarcinoma, particularly those of the breast, lung, and stomach, as well as to malignant melanoma.[1, 4, 7, 9] Several studies have suggested that the neoplastic cells reach the meninges by way of extension along peripheral nerves.[5, 6, 8] Optimal sites for obtaining a positive biopsy include leptomeninges at the base of the brain and at the cerebellopontine angle.[2]

Meningeal carcinomatosis is evident in MR scans as diffuse meningeal contrast enhancement.[10]

The degree of meningeal clouding is proportional to the density of the malignant infiltrate. More often than not, it is so minimal as to be equivocal to the naked eye. When grossly visible, the aggregated cells "paint" the meninges tan or, in the case of melanoma, black.

Microscopically, the cancer cells follow the subarachnoid compartment to its limits as they follow the Virchow-Robin spaces along vessels into brain parenchyma. As in the case of leukemia and lymphoma, infiltration of cranial nerves is commonplace. The neoplastic cells are usually poorly differentiated.

The common symptoms of headache, change in mental status, and cranial nerve dysfunction are only shadows of the malignancy that is seen face to face in CSF cytologic preparations. Nurtured by this fluid, as if in tissue culture, the neoplastic cells proliferate rapidly. With aggressive treatment, reported median survivals vary but are generally in the range of 6 months.[1, 4, 9]

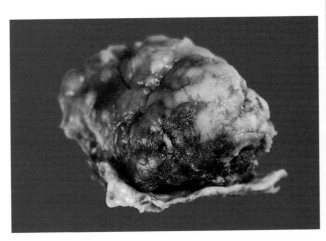

2–93

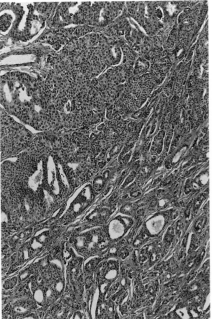

2–94

**FIGURES 2–93 AND 2–94   METASTATIC CARCINOMA MIMICKING MENINGIOMA**

A 71-year-old woman developed diplopia, right retro-orbital pain, and right facial numbness 7 years after a radical mastectomy for adenocarcinoma. Radiologic studies disclosed irregular destruction of the greater and lesser right sphenoid wings. This bosselated, discrete neoplasm was firmly attached to the dura (Fig. 2–93) and invaded the underlying sphenoid bone. On histologic examination, the glandular pattern of an adenocarcinoma was diagnostic (Fig. 2–94).

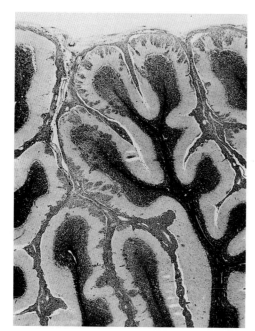

**FIGURE 2–95   MENINGEAL CARCINOMATOSIS**

Neoplastic cells fill the cerebellar subarachnoid space and extend along vessels into the superficial cortex.

## Myeloproliferative and Lymphoproliferative Diseases

Leukemia or lymphoma of dura does not usually produce a symptomatic mass. In the setting of acute myelogenous leukemia, however, a discrete tumefaction, so-called granulocytic sarcoma, may become clinically evident. A green hue may become apparent upon exposure to air, hence the descriptive term "chloroma."[3, 10, 15] Only rarely do such lesions occur in the absence of a recognized extracranial primary.[5]

Symptomatic involvement of the leptomeninges, however, is not uncommon in leukemia and lymphoma.[1, 13, 20–22] Plasma cell proliferations may also share this localization. Of the latter, well-differentiated types ("plasmacytomas") are discussed on pages 78 to 79. Multiple myelomas usually affect the skull but occasionally have a meningeal component[2, 11, 14, 18, 19] and are considered on page 33. Mycosis fungoides[4] and "lymphomatoid granulomatosis"[6, 12, 16, 17] may also involve the meninges. Lymphomatoid granulomatosis of the brain is discussed on page 324. Rare lymphomas appear to arise primarily at this site.[7–9]

Suspended in CSF, the malignant cells infiltrate the pia-arachnoid and opacify the membrane when the infiltration is dense. Neoplastic cells intimately relate to the walls of blood vessels. Like the cells of the primary cerebral lymphoma, those of leukemia and secondary lymphoma may be enmeshed in a perivascular network of reticulin. As in the case of meningeal carcinomatosis, involvement of Virchow-Robin spaces is often associated with an element of parenchymal invasion.

Neoplastic cells obstruct the flow of CSF and produce hydrocephalus. They may also symptomatically

infiltrate cranial nerves. Leptomeningeal leukemia or lymphoma is seldom diagnosed by open or stereotactic biopsy; rather, the diagnosis is based on cytologic examination of CSF (see Fig. 2–114).

## BENIGN CYSTIC LESIONS

### Arachnoid Cyst

**Definition.** A loculated collection of CSF.

**Clinical Features.** Arachnoidal or leptomeningeal cysts occur in both children and adults, with an incidence that is somewhat higher in males.[11, 16, 17] Some cysts are symptomatic, that is, as seizures or expressions of mass effects.[11, 16] Cerebellar or eighth nerve dysfunction often accompanies cerebellopontine examples.[2, 7, 13] Many cysts are only incidental radiologic findings in spite of their considerable size.[5, 11, 15]

The chronic expansion can produce craniomegaly in young children and erosion of the skull in older patients.[9, 11, 15] The observation that very large examples may be associated with little if any midline shift has suggested to some observers that the lesion may not be an expansile cyst at all but rather a compensatory expansion of the subarachnoid space over a hypoplastic or atrophic temporal lobe. In one instance, however, a postmortem study found that the two cerebral hemispheres were of equal weight,[14] and a CT study of another case found equivalent hemispheric volumes.[11]

Several supratentorial cases, examined in detail, have shown a cleaved arachnoid membrane totally surrounding the trapped fluid, thus supporting the developmental origin of these cysts.[5, 8, 12]

**Radiologic Features.** Whereas in the past arachnoid cysts were a welcome surprise to the surgeon who preoperatively anticipated a neoplasm, the satisfaction of discovery now falls to the radiologist. The contents of arachnoid cysts have the signal characteristics of CSF and are thus hyperintense on fluid attenuated inversion recovery (FLAIR) imaging. Other than the effects of displacement, the adjacent brain is unremarkable.[18] Remodeling of the skull is readily visualized.

In the sylvian fissure, the favored supratentorial site, large cysts splay the operculum to expose the insular cortex (island of Reil) (Figs. 2–96 and 2–97). Those in the middle fossa more often occur on the left.[11, 16, 17] In the posterior fossa, the cerebellopontine angle is most often affected.[2, 7, 13]

**Macroscopic Features.** At surgery, arachnoid cysts are filled with clear fluid and are delineated on their outer and inner aspects by a remarkably delicate, nearly transparent membrane (see Fig. 2–97). Despite their leptomeningeal derivation, the cysts show no macroscopic continuity with the subdural or subarachnoid spaces.

**Microscopic Features.** Arachnoid cysts readily collapse upon incision, and surgical specimens, if any, are usually limited to a portion of the outer wall. This diaphanous

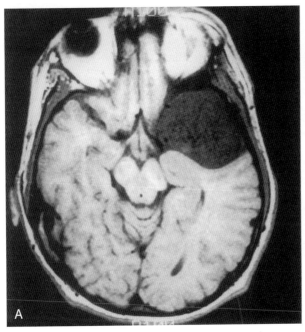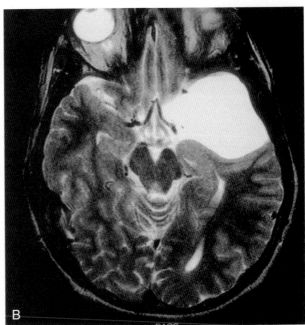

**FIGURE 2–96** ARACHNOID CYST

As seen in T1-weighted (A) and precontrast T2-weighted (B) MR studies, an arachnoid cyst expands the subarachnoid space and displaces the brain. Unlike those of most other meningeal cysts, its contents have the signal characteristics of cerebrospinal fluid. The sylvian fissure is a common site.

membrane of connective tissue is underwhelming when compared with the intact lesion in situ (Fig. 2–98). The delicate fibrovascular membrane often contains nests of meningothelial cells.

**Ultrastructural Features.** Ultrastructural studies support an arachnoidal origin.[3, 4, 8]

**Immunohistochemical Features.** In accord with ultrastructural findings, the lining is immunoreactive for EMA.[6]

**Treatment and Prognosis.** Arachnoid cysts are benign non-neoplastic lesions that can be drained, fenestrated, or partially resected. Without intervention, some

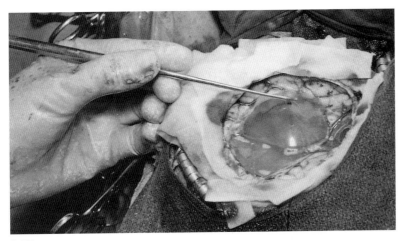

2–97

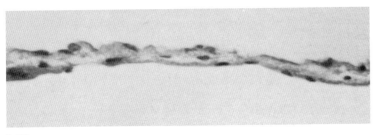

2–98

**FIGURES 2–97 AND 2–98** ARACHNOID CYST

The tip of the probe has been introduced into the dome of a transparent arachnoid cyst in the sylvian fissure (Fig. 2–97). The patient, a 45-year-old man, had experienced seizures and right facial weakness for 6 months. The outer wall consists of delicate arachnoid membrane sparsely populated by meningothelial cells (Fig. 2–98).

continue to enlarge. Others rupture spontaneously to produce a symptomatic subdural hygroma.[1, 10, 11] An occasional subdural hematoma appears to have been provoked in some way by an arachnoid cyst.[10]

## Epidermoid and Dermoid Cysts

**General Comments.** Epidermoid and dermoid cysts are developmental lesions that result from embryologic displacement of ectoderm into the meninges, ventricles, or rarely into the parenchyma of the brain. Rarely, the same lesions arise from implants of epithelium carried into the meninges during percutaneous aspiration of the subdural or subarachnoid space.[8]

Epidermoid cysts favor the cerebellopontine angle and parapontine region (Fig. 2–99)[17, 19, 21] but can occur at many other sites.[2] In contrast to that of epidermoids, the distribution of dermoid cysts is more restricted. Most of the latter occur in a fontanelle or the posterior fossa, where they occur either as midline lesions between the cerebellar hemispheres (Fig. 2–100) or within the fourth ventricle.[5, 9, 16]

**Clinical Features.** The symptoms of an epidermoid cyst, if any, are generally those of a slowly enlarging mass.[7] On occasion, leakage of cyst contents produces chemical irritation of the leptomeninges and/or ependyma.[15, 18] The fistulous tract that occasionally connects a dermoid cyst with the skin is a potential avenue for bacterial infection.[5, 9, 14, 16]

**Radiologic Features.** On precontrast T1-weighted MR images, the epidermoid cysts are isointense with CSF, whereas dermoid cysts can be either hyperintense (white) or hypointense (dark) depending on their content of lipid (see Fig. 2–99).[11, 20] Serpiginous borders are formed as the lesion insinuates itself among regional structures such as blood vessels and cranial nerves. In contrast to fluid-filled arachnoid cysts, epidermoid and dermoid cysts are usually hyperintense on FLAIR images.[12] Calcification may be noted around some dermoid cysts.

**Macroscopic Features.** To the surgeon or pathologist, the smooth, delicate, translucent capsule of the epidermoid cyst transmits the whiteness of its contents and glistens with the satisfying sheen of mother-of-pearl (Figs. 2–101 and 2–102). When opened, the cyst exudes its unpleasant flaky contents. The capsule of the dermoid cyst is thicker, and its cheesy pilosebaceous contents are even more disagreeable (Fig. 2–103; see Fig. 2–100).

**Microscopic Features.** The mundane histopathology of these lesions is familiar to the general pathologist (Figs. 2–104 and 2–105). It is only the ectopia of this epithelium that engenders special interest. In the dermoid cyst, the sweat and sebaceous glands seem especially inappropriate in juxtaposition to the scholarly brain. Both epidermoid and dermoid lesions produce anucleate squamae. Cell ghosts, or "shadow cells," reminiscent of the "wet keratin" of the adamantinomatous

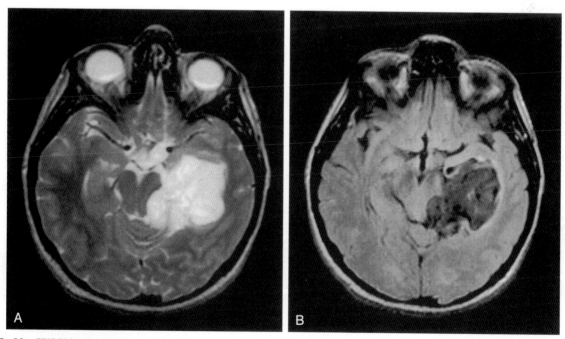

**FIGURE 2–99** EPIDERMOID CYST

Epidermoid cysts have an MR profile that in most cases is diagnostic. The lesions are bright in T2-weighted images (A) and dark in FLAIR images (B). Brightness on a diffusion image completed the triad of MR imaging features. As is typical, the lesion insinuates itself into the subarachnoid space. (Courtesy of Dr. Elias Melhem, Baltimore, MD.)

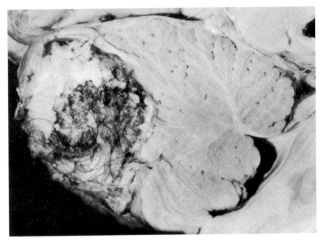

**FIGURE 2–100** DERMOID CYST

The fissure between the cerebellar hemispheres is a favored location of dermoid cysts, from which they often communicate with the cutaneous surface via a sinus in the occipital bone. The lesion shown here was an incidental finding in a 38-year-old woman. Its content of hair distinguishes this lesion from an epidermoid cyst.

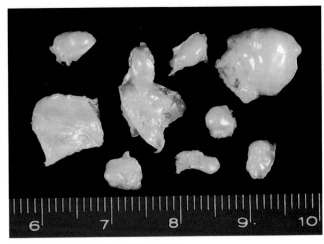

**FIGURE 2–102** EPIDERMOID CYST

This epidermoid cyst has a diagnostically pearly sheen. It lay in the left cerebellopontine angle of a 35-year-old woman with facial pain and numbness.

craniopharyngioma have been noted in the dermoid lesion and attributed to hair matrix differentiation.[10]

**Treatment and Prognosis.** The goal of surgery is total removal, but this may be precluded by the lesion's intimate relationship to vulnerable neurovascular structures trapped in the mass.[17, 19, 21] Overall, the postsurgical outlook is very favorable, especially after a gross total resection.[19,21] Subtotally resected lesions may recur, but many years may elapse before recurrence. Malignant degeneration of both epidermoid[1, 6, 13] and dermoid[4] cysts has been recorded (Figs. 2–106 to 2–108).

Reference is made to the rare and ostensibly primary squamous cell carcinoma without a recognized preexisting benign epidermoid or dermoid cyst.[3]

## Enterogenous Cyst

Leptomeningeal cysts composed of columnar epithelium occur most commonly in the spinal intradural space, as discussed on page 539. Only rarely do similar lesions appear in the intracranial meninges (Fig. 2–109).[1, 5] Variably referred to as enterogenous, neurenteric, bronchogenic, or respiratory cysts, they are lined by both mucin-producing and ciliated cells (Fig. 2–110). There

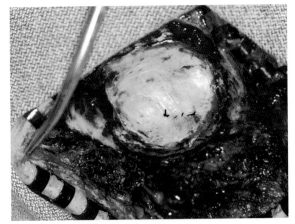

**FIGURE 2–101** EPIDERMOID CYST

As visualized in situ at surgery, the epidermoid cyst has a pearly quality. This was a recurrent lesion in the suprasellar region of a 47-year-old woman who initially presented with bitemporal hemianopsia and adrenal insufficiency. (Courtesy of Dr. Henry Brem, Baltimore, MD.)

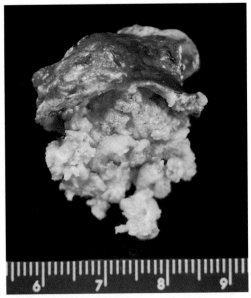

**FIGURE 2–103** DERMOID CYST

This dermoid cyst was situated superficially in the left temporal lobe of a 26-year-old woman with headaches. It has been opened to display its thin wall and cheesy content. The cyst's cavity communicated with the sphenoid sinus through a tract whose patency was evidenced by the cyst's content of air as seen on plain films of the skull.

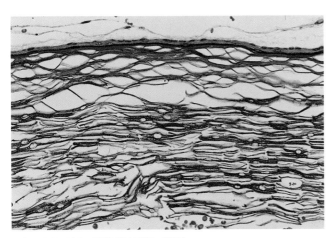

**FIGURE 2-104    EPIDERMOID CYST**

The attenuated epithelium sheds the anucleate "squames" that create the bulk of the mass.

are also basal cells, from which squamous metaplasia may evolve.[2, 3, 7, 8] Malignant degeneration is exceedingly rare,[4] as is seeding of epithelium throughout the neuraxis.[6]

# INFECTIOUS AND INFLAMMATORY DISORDERS

## Inflammatory Pseudoneoplasms

Inflammatory and infectious disorders of the meninges rarely come to the attention of the surgical pathologist. This is especially true of suppurative bacterial infections that are identified on the basis of their acute clinical

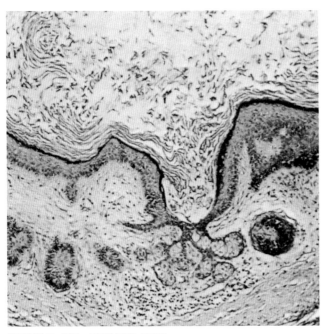

**FIGURE 2-105    DERMOID CYST**

The dermoid cyst is lined by well-differentiated keratinizing squamous epithelium with adnexal appendages.

course, the number and character of the inflammatory cells in CSF, and the visualization and culture characterization of the causative agent. Granulomatous inflammation, being more indolent in its clinical course and more tumefacient in its tissue reaction, may be approached surgically. In keeping with the anatomic orientation of this book, a number of lesions are discussed here, rather than in Chapter 3, because they are predominantly, although not always, meningeal processes.

## Sarcoidosis

**General Comments.** Intracranial sarcoidosis is a granulomatous inflammatory disease that shares with tuberculosis an affinity for the base of the brain (Fig. 2-111), particularly the region of the hypothalamus and optic chiasm (Fig. 2-112). Biopsy may be undertaken to establish the identity of a diffuse chronic leptomeningitis or the nature of a dura-based mass (Fig. 2-113). Whereas some cases occur in the setting of systemic sarcoidosis,[10] many are unassociated with recognized extracranial disease. The nosologic problems created by the latter lesions are self-evident.[3, 10]

**Clinical Features.** Consequences include obstruction of CSF flow, cranial nerve deficits, long tract signs, autonomic dysfunction, and hypothalamic-pituitary endocrine deficiency states.[8] Although the meninges are usually the predominant site of involvement, contiguous involvement of underlying parenchyma is common. The process may involve the subarachnoid space diffusely, including spinal levels.

**Macroscopic Features.** The lesions of intracranial sarcoidosis are usually either small nodular meningeal thickenings or large globular masses that simulate meningiomas.[2, 3, 5, 6, 7, 9, 10] Occasional lesions enlarge in the optic nerve sheath and may simulate a neoplasm such as a meningioma.[1, 2]

**Microscopic Features.** Sarcoidosis obviously shares many features with tuberculosis; both elicit epithelioid and giant cells, and both frequently target blood vessels (Fig. 2-114). Generally, the lesions in sarcoidosis are more nodular and richer in epithelioid cells that congregate in distinct tubercles. With time, the latter heal individually as the inflammatory component is gradually replaced by collagen (see Fig. 2-119). The finding of minute foci of necrosis within individual granulomas is entirely consistent with a diagnosis of sarcoidosis, but large, all-inclusive, geographic areas of necrosis are hallmarks of tuberculosis. Although necrosis prompts consideration of tuberculosis, cardinal features of the latter, namely tubercle bacilli and extensive geographic necrosis, are absent.

**Differential Diagnosis.** The differential diagnosis of CNS sarcoidosis is broad and covers virtually any of the granulomatous meningeal processes summarized in Table 2-3. Granulomatous inflammation in the suprasellar or pineal regions, especially in a youth, should bring

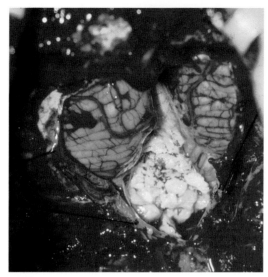

2–106

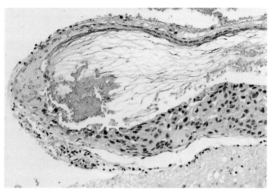

2–107

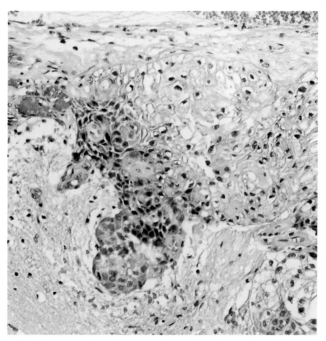

2–108

**FIGURES 2–106, 2–107, AND 2–108** MALIGNANT DEGENERATION OF AN EPIDERMOID CYST

A 53-year-old man complained of nausea and vomiting, postural unsteadiness, and diplopia. A solid and cystic lesion filled the fourth ventricle and extended into the cisterna magna (Fig. 2–106). Microscopically, it contained squamous epithelium of benign, malignant, and intermediate character. The delicate, well-differentiated epithelium of the typical epidermoid cyst is shown in the upper portion of Figure 2–107. This merges with a sector of carcinoma in situ at the lower left. Elsewhere, the malignant nature of the tumor is apparent by its invasive properties (Fig. 2–108).

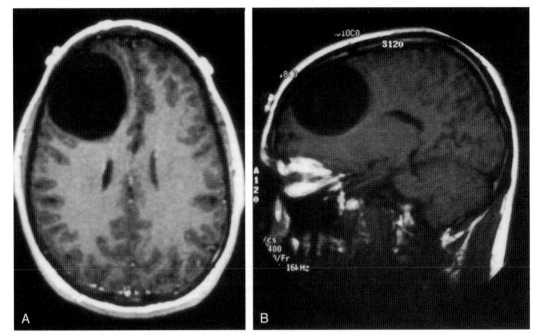

**FIGURE 2–109    ENTEROGENOUS CYST**

The expansile lesion creates a smoothly contoured, black void in a precontrast T1-weighted MR scan.

the possibility of *germinoma* to mind, even if the large round neoplastic cells are not present in the initial sections. The granulomatous and T-lymphocytic responses to germinomas can be the dominant, or even the exclusive, element in small specimens.[4]

**Treatment and Prognosis.** The tumoral lesions of sarcoidosis are generally treated with corticosteroids, which are effective in some instances.[3]

## Tuberculosis

The two forms of meningeal tuberculosis, tuberculoma and tuberculous meningitis, are discussed in Chapter 3 on pages 122 to 126.

## Other Inflammatory Pseudoneoplasms

A number of inflammatory masses arise in the CNS; most if not all have their systemic counterparts. Those

bound to the dura often form symptomatic, meningioma-like masses. The loose term *inflammatory pseudotumor* has been applied, although many are referred to by histologic or eponymous descriptors as follows.

*Plasma cell granuloma* is a term applied to masses, often dura based, that are composed of lymphocytes and plasma cells, the latter often with Russell bodies (Figs. 2–115 to 2–117).[1–3, 5, 6, 8, 11] Only rarely do equivalent lesions occur within the substance of the brain[7, 12] or in the choroid plexus.[10] The constituent cells are mature, polyclonal, and cytologically bland. Germinal centers may be present. The designation *inflammatory myofibroblastic pseudotumor* has been applied to variants rich in myofibroblasts. Nests of meningothelial cells

| TABLE 2–3 |
| :--- |
| **Meningeal Lesions with Granulomatous Inflammation** |

Sarcoidosis
Tuberculosis
Mycoses
Wegener's granulomatosis
Rheumatoid disease
Hypertrophic pachymeningitis
Germinoma with granulomatous inflammation

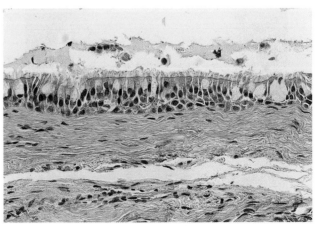

**FIGURE 2–110    ENTEROGENOUS CYST**

The benign epithelium is pseudostratified, ciliated, and mucus producing.

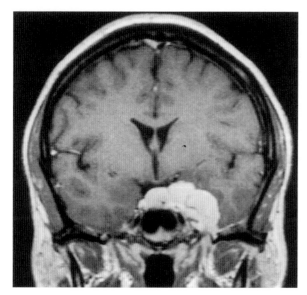

**FIGURE 2–111** SARCOIDOSIS

Meningeal sarcoidosis can present as solitary or multiple dura-based masses. This patient was a 44-year-old woman who experienced headaches, diplopia, and left facial pain and numbness as a consequence of cavernous sinus involvement. The preoperative diagnosis was meningioma.

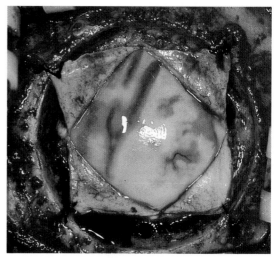

**FIGURE 2–113** SARCOIDOSIS

Leptomeningeal sarcoidosis may be approached surgically and is then visualized as thickened arachnoid.

are contained in some lesions,[8] but these primary inflammatory processes should not be confused with secondarily inflamed meningiomas (lymphoplasmacytoid meningioma). Extensive hyalinization of fibrous tissue characterizes some examples.[4, 9] Despite the designation *plasma cell granuloma*, these lesions are not granulomatous. They are benign and in most cases do not recur.[1]

*Rosai-Dorfman disease* is an idiopathic reactive lesion that in most instances arises in lymph nodes, especially those in the neck and mediastinum.[2, 8] Extranodal involvement, with or without concomitant lymph node disease, is not uncommon.[2, 3] In the meninges, meningioma is understandably the favored preoperative diagnosis (Fig. 2–118).[1–3, 5–7, 9, 10] As in systemic sites, CNS involvement affects patients of all ages; young adults are favored. Multiplicity has been observed.[10] A rare lesion is intraparenchymal.[4]

Macroscopically, the solitary or multiple, contrast-enhancing lesions are tan, rubbery masses with a broad dural base.

Microscopically, Rosai-Dorfman disease is a lymphoplasmacytic proliferation distinguished by its focal aggregates or larger sheets of pale, often multinucleated, histiocytes (Fig. 2–119). Fibrous connective tissue is present in variable amounts. A curious feature in most cases, although perhaps not as prominent as in classical nodal disease, is engulfment by histiocytes of viable lymphocytes and plasma cells (emperipolesis).

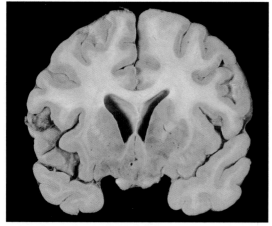

**FIGURE 2–112** SARCOIDOSIS

The base of the brain, notably the region of the optic chiasm and infundibulum, is a favored site of sarcoidosis. This lesion forms a large plaque-like mass beneath the frontal lobes.

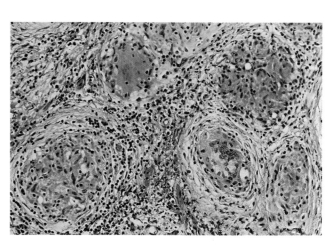

**FIGURE 2–114** SARCOIDOSIS

Small, discrete, noncaseating granulomas are typical.

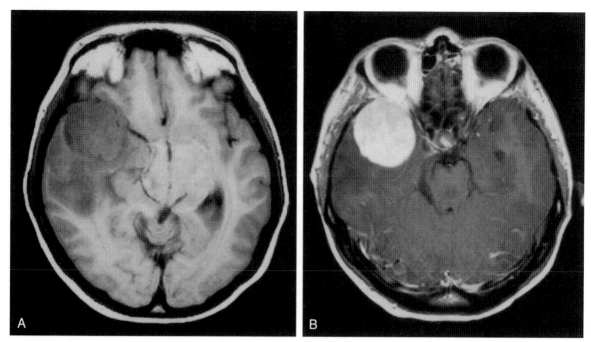

**FIGURE 2–115    PLASMA CELL GRANULOMA**

Meningeal inflammatory pseudotumors are often discrete, dura-based masses as seen here in precontrast (*A*) and postcontrast (*B*) T1-weighted MR scans.

Immunohistochemically, the striking positivity of the histiocytes for S-100 protein provides a diagnostic distinction of this lesion from most other inflammatory pseudotumors (Fig. 2–120).[2, 5, 7, 8] The lesion lacks the CD1a-positive Langerhans cells and the eosinophils of Langerhans cell histiocytosis.

Given the rarity of Rosai-Dorfman disease in the CNS, its biologic behavior has yet to be clarified. Nonetheless, gross total resection appears to be curative, and subtotally resected examples have grown little if at all.[2, 3, 6] Death caused by systemic CNS disease is unusual.[2, 3]

*Castleman's disease* is a rare lymphoproliferative disorder that, although classically confined to the mediastinum, occasionally appears as a meningeal mass, with or without associated lesions in more typical sites. Two histologic variants, both overtly follicular at low magnification, occur in mediastinal lesions. The so-called *hyaline vascular type* is characterized by hyalinized and usually proliferating vessels within lymphoid follicles. The

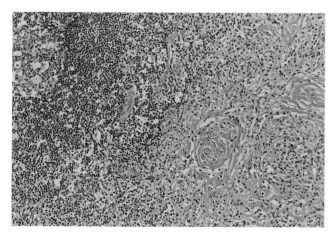

**FIGURE 2–116    PLASMA CELL GRANULOMA**

An intense lymphoplasmacytic infiltrate in a fibrous tissue background typifies the "plasma cell granulomatous" form of inflammatory pseudotumor.

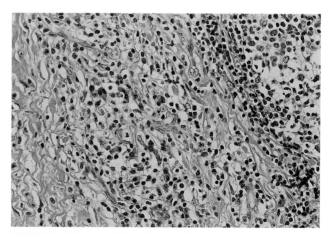

**FIGURE 2–117    PLASMA CELL GRANULOMA**

Mature plasma cells and lymphocytes are the typical components. Germinal centers are encountered in some cases.

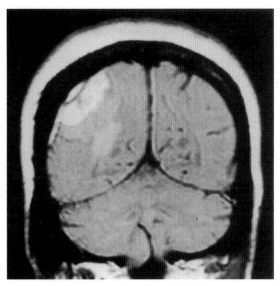

**FIGURE 2–118    ROSAI-DORFMAN DISEASE**

As in this 37-year-old woman, single or multiple discrete meningeal masses are the typical forms of intracranial involvement. There was no recurrence over a 6-year period of follow-up.

second form, the plasma cell variant, is noted for plasma cells that predominate in interfollicular zones.[2] Similar lesions have been reported rarely as dura-based masses.[1, 3, 4]

*Hypertrophic pachymeningitis* is an ill-defined entity that radiologically appears as extensive dural thickening and contrast enhancement.[1, 2] The spinal equivalent is discussed briefly in Chapter 11 on pages 539 to 540. Intracranial pachymeningitis is characterized by granulomatous inflammation in some reports,[2] but the diagnosis does not require a specific form of inflammation, rather the exclusion of a recognizable inflammatory process.

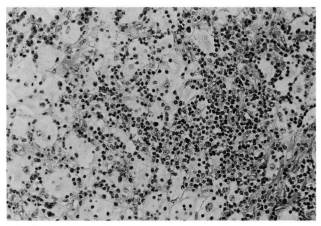

**FIGURE 2–119    ROSAI-DORFMAN DISEASE**

The lesion is a chronic inflammatory process containing large histiocytes, sometimes engaged in emperipolesis.

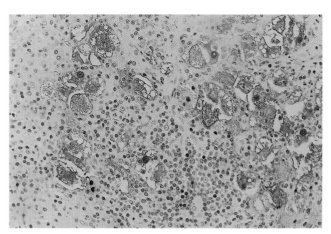

**FIGURE 2–120    ROSAI-DORFMAN DISEASE**

The large histiocytes are S-100 protein immunoreactive.

## Collagen-Vascular Diseases

*Wegener's granulomatosis* is often, but not invariably, associated with nearby sinus disease. The meninges are thickened either focally[5, 11, 17, 23] or more diffusely (Fig. 2–121).[12, 20, 24, 26, 28, 29] Cranial nerve deficits often accompany involvement of the basilar meninges.[7, 12, 18] Arteritis may result in parenchymal infarction.[7, 18, 21]

Microscopically, the lesion features necrobiosis of collagen and a smudgy, nonspecific chronic inflammation,

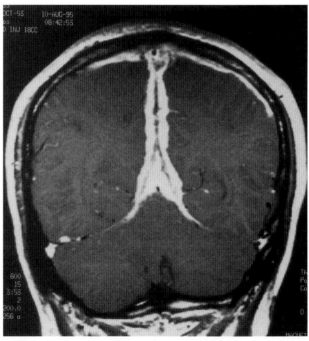

**FIGURE 2–121    WEGENER'S GRANULOMATOSIS**

A 41-year-old man had been treated for 4 years for Wegener's granulomatosis. He had initially presented with a saddle nose deformity, recurrent nasal discharge, and otitis. The recent complaint of double vision prompted MR studies that disclosed diffuse meningeal thickening and enhancement.

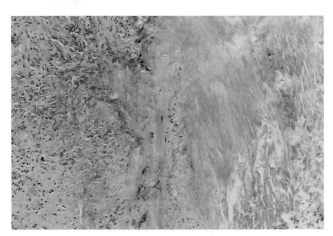

**FIGURE 2–122    WEGENER'S GRANULOMATOSIS**

Necrosis of collagen, often basophilic in character, and chronic inflammation are the principal histologic findings.

often with focal granulomatous inflammation, and vasculitis (Fig. 2–122).[12, 23, 24] The latter typically takes the form of capillaritis. Necrosis may extend across many microscopic fields, wherein inflamed as well as normal tissues, such as dura, are affected. Restricted to a few focal multinucleated giant cells, the granulomatous component is often inconspicuous (Fig. 2–123).

*Rheumatoid arthritis* occasionally affects the meninges of patients with long-standing systemic disease. Various localizing and diffuse symptoms are the consequence of inflammation that is usually limited to the meninges.[3] The meninges are affected in either a nodular and/or diffuse manner by nonspecific chronic inflammation. A diffuse dural thickening similar to that encountered in Wegener's granulomatosis has been reported.[3] Alternatively, classical rheumatoid nodules composed of focal or geographic zones of necrosis surrounded by slender palisaded epithelioid cells may be

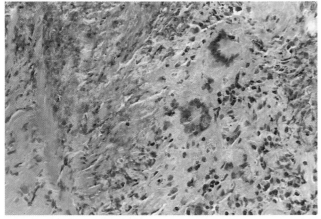

**FIGURE 2–123    WEGENER'S GRANULOMATOSIS**

Widely scattered giant cells may be the only expression of granulomatous inflammation.

present.[15, 19, 22, 27] There has been at least one report of a meningioma containing rheumatoid nodules.[14]

CNS symptoms are common in *systemic lupus erythematosus*.[8, 13] Multifocal lesions, as well as cerebral atrophy, may be seen on MR scans,[16, 25] but their etiology is unclear. Although a specific lupus vasculitis could be responsible, it is rare in our experience to find such changes around infarcts in postmortem specimens. More often, one finds infectious complications of corticosteroid therapy. The characteristic superficial spinal cord infarcts associated with systemic lupus erythematosus are described in Chapter 11 on page 545.

CNS involvement in *Sjögren's syndrome* includes focal intraparenchymal lesions similar to those seen in systemic lupus erythematosus.[1, 2] Chronic meningitis[1, 6] and vasculitis of large intracranial vessels[2, 9, 10] have also been reported. An inflammatory pseudotumor of the choroid plexus has prompted a report.[4]

# OTHER REACTIVE CONDITIONS AND NONINFLAMMATORY PSEUDONEOPLASMS

## Meningioangiomatosis

**Definition.** A plaque-like mass resulting from the downgrowth of meningothelial or fibroblast-like cells into the cerebral cortex.

**General Comments.** The name of this rare meningocortical entity is a tongue twister but descriptively captures its histopathologic features. The process is best conceptualized as a focal non-neoplastic proliferation of cells involving the subarachnoid space and underlying cerebral cortex. In the latter site, the lesion's perivascular distribution is its most distinctive feature. The origin of the lesion is not clear. A meningothelial source has been suggested because of (1) the meningothelial cytologic features in some cases, (2) the rare concurrence of a meningioma with underlying meningioangiomatosis,[1, 3] and (3) the occurrence of both meningiomas and meningioangiomatosis in the setting of NF2. Immunoreactivity of the cells for EMA is, however, sparse at best,[2, 15] and ultrastructural features are not compellingly meningothelial.[2, 15] Most cases do not arise in neurofibromatosis.[2, 10, 12, 15] Overall, meningioangiomatosis seems more reactive or hamartomatous than neoplastic, thus being more "-osis" than "-oma."

**Clinical Features.** Chronic seizures are understandable clinical expressions of this intracortical lesion that occurs in children and young adults.[6, 7, 15] Multifocality is likely in NF2, wherein the lesions are commonly asymptomatic and discovered only on postmortem examination.[13] The possibility that sporadic meningioangiomatosis is a forme fruste of NF2 has been entertained but has not been established convincingly. One study found no *NF2* mutations.[13] The concurrence of an oligodendroglioma in a single patient with meningioangiomatosis may be fortuitous.[8]

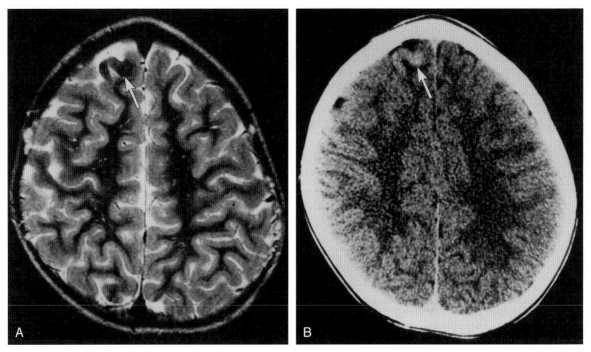

**FIGURE 2–124** MENINGIOANGIOMATOSIS

This plaque-like, intracortical frontal lobe lesion was an incidental finding in an 8-year-old child with amblyopia. A T2-weighted MR scan (*A*, arrow) discloses a dark, plaque-like mass associated with hyperintense edema in the subjacent white matter. The calcium content of the lesion is disclosed by the whiteness in the corresponding CT scan (*B*, arrow). (Courtesy of Dr. Marc K. Rosenblum, New York, NY.)

**Radiologic Features.** Meningioangiomatosis appears as a superficial mass that is distinctively hypointense on proton density and T2-weighted MR images because of its content of fibrous tissue and calcium (Fig. 2–124A).[14, 15] On CT, the calcified area is white (See Fig. 2–124B). There may be a small amount of vasogenic edema in the underlying white matter.

**Macroscopic Features.** At the time of surgery, the lesion consists of a firm, discrete, vascular, plaque-like intracortical mass that undulates with the contours of the cortical ribbon. In a minority of cases, a bosselated,

largely calcific mass (calcifying pseudoneoplasm, see pages 101 to 102) occupies an overlying sulcus.

**Microscopic Features.** Histologically, the affected cortex is variably replaced by fibrous tissue and perivascular sheaths of cells (Fig. 2–125). Islands of parenchyma may be all that is left of the cortex. Whereas the perivascular tissue element in some lesions appears meningothelial, it appears more fibroblastic in others. Scattered psammoma bodies are commonly encountered (Fig. 2–126). The subarachnoid space is typically filled with vessels that resemble a vascular malformation.

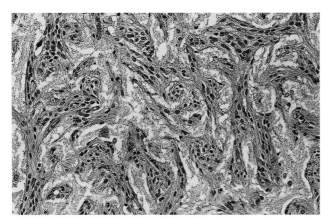

**FIGURE 2–125** MENINGIOANGIOMATOSIS

A population of spindle-shaped cells ensheathes vessels and encroaches upon the surrounding parenchyma.

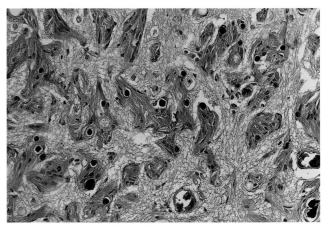

**FIGURE 2–126** MENINGIOANGIOMATOSIS

Psammoma bodies are often prominent in the perivascular tissue.

Spindle cells similar to those in underlying cortex may be abundant and, because of their occasional palisading, may mimic schwannoma.

The trapped cortical neurons are frequently marked by changes associated with Alzheimer's disease, that is, neurofibrillary change and, on occasion, granulovacuolar degeneration. The former are formed of bona fide paired helical filaments[5, 7, 9] immunoreactive for tau protein.[4,9] A4 amyloid appears to be absent.[4]

**Immunohistochemical Features.** Staining for EMA has been noted by some investigators,[4, 9, 11] but this may be slight or absent.[2, 15] As expected, the MIB-1 labeling index for cycling cells has been low, less than 1%.[11, 14]

**Differential Diagnosis.** Recognition of meningioangiomatosis requires awareness of the entity and a specimen sufficiently large to permit low-power recognition of its basic architectural features. Awareness of the lesion's localization to the cortex and its dark signal in T2-weighted images puts the lesion in context. In a limited specimen, the lesion may resemble *meningioma*, *schwannoma*, a *nonspecific mesenchymal proliferative reaction*, or even a *vascular malformation*. The entity can even be misconstrued as a *ganglion cell tumor* in light of its connective tissue component and the nests of seemingly abnormal neurons with neurofibrillary tangles.

**Treatment and Prognosis.** Meningioangiomatosis is cured by excision. Postoperatively, most patients have been reported to remain seizure free,[6,7] although in one series less than half became free of seizures postoperatively.[15]

## Calcifying Pseudoneoplasm ("Fibro-Osseous Lesion") of the Neuraxis

**Definition.** A reactive, polymorphous calcified mass.

**General Comments.** This rare and distinctive lesion appears along the neuraxis, potentially arising from not only the craniospinal meninges but also the bones of the spine. Both the terms *calcifying pseudoneoplasm*[1] and *fibro-osseous lesion*[2, 4, 5] have been applied, although it is not clear that the bony lesions are the same as those limited to the craniospinal meninges. Occasional examples arise in the setting of meningioangiomatosis,[3] but most are "sporadic" and arise without any clues to the pathogenesis.

**Clinical Features.** Osseous examples at the base of the skull can create cranial nerve deficits. Meningeal examples may be epileptogenic or remain asymptomatic.

**Radiologic Features.** The lesion is a discrete, densely calcified, bosselated "rock" in the leptomeninges when seen by CT (Fig. 2–127). Vasogenic edema may be present in the underlying white matter.

**Macroscopic Features.** The discrete, partially grumous, mass is knobby and gritty to rock hard (Fig. 2–128).

**Microscopic Features.** Histologically, calcifying pseudoneoplasms are a curious mélange of amorphous granular or fibrillar material with peripheral radial striation, calcification and even ossification, and an inconstant surface layer of what superficially resembles meningothelial cells (Figs. 2–129 and 2–130). A foreign body–type reaction may accompany osseous examples.

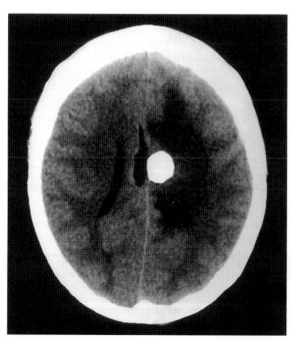

**FIGURE 2–127    CALCIFYING PSEUDONEOPLASM**

Adult-onset seizures called attention to this densely calcified meningeal mass that was situated between the two cerebral hemispheres. It was associated with agenesis of the posterior segment of the corpus callosum and a small regional "lipoma." In this CT scan, the latter is the dark area medial to the mass.

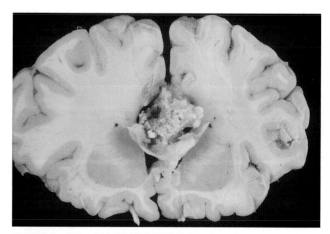

**FIGURE 2–128    CALCIFYING PSEUDONEOPLASM**

Positioned in the leptomeninges between the frontal lobes, the mass has a characteristic granular, grumous quality.

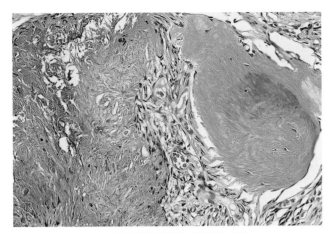

**FIGURE 2–129**    CALCIFYING PSEUDONEOPLASM

Microscopically, the lesion consists of fibrovascular tissue, amorphous stroma, calcification, fibrillar tissue, and mature bone.

Immunohistochemically, the peripheral cells have been noncommittal in regard to their origin.[5]

**Treatment and Prognosis.** This entirely benign lesion is cured by excision.

## Fibromatosis

Fibromatosis is discussed in the context of fibroma on page 77.

## Meningeal Response to Intracranial Hypotension

Reduction of intracranial pressure by CSF shunting, lumbar puncture, or surgery is followed in some cases by diffuse meningeal contrast enhancement that is located on

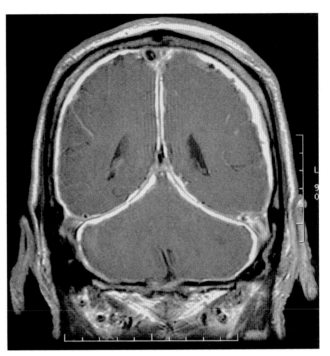

**FIGURE 2–131**    MENINGEAL RESPONSE TO INTRACRANIAL HYPOTENSION

Diffuse meningeal contrast enhancement followed by hydrocephalus in a 76-year-old man. Although there was no history of a malignancy, metastatic carcinoma was suspected.

the dura rather than the leptomeninges, as is the case with tumor dissemination in the subarachnoid space (Fig. 2–131).[1,3] Spontaneous intracranial hypotension can elicit the same response.[2] When hypotension occurs in the setting of a neoplasm, a biopsy may be performed to rule out disseminated tumor. Histologically, the surgical specimens are unimpressive, either being normal or demonstrating a thin layer of delicate new capillaries along the inner surface of the dura (Fig. 2–132).[1,3]

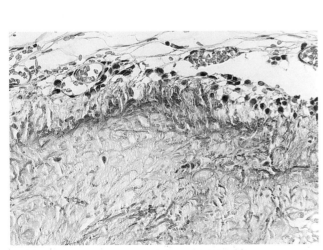

**FIGURE 2–130**    CALCIFYING PSEUDONEOPLASM

A narrow and inconstant row of plump cells surrounds a finely fibrillar, radiating peripheral zone.

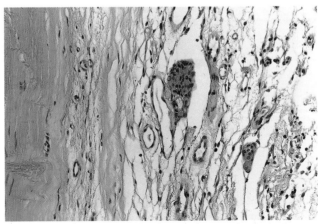

**FIGURE 2–132**    MENINGEAL RESPONSE TO INTRACRANIAL HYPOTENSION

The lesion is a layer of capillaries attached to the inner surface of the dura. Nests of meningothelial cells, sometimes prominent, should not be interpreted as meningioma.

# REFERENCES

## Meningioma

1. Adlakha A, Rao K, Adlakha H, et al. Meningioma metastatic to the lung. Mayo Clin Proc 1999;74:1129–1133.
2. Alguacil-Garcia A, Pettigrew NM, Sima AAF. Secretory meningioma: A distinct subtype of meningioma. Am J Surg Pathol 1986;10:102–111.
3. Allen EA, Burger PC, Epstein JI. Microcystic meningioma arising in a mixed germ cell tumor of the testis: a case report. Am J Surg Pathol 1999;23:1131–1135.
4. Annegers JF, Laws ER, Kurland LT, Grabow JD. Head trauma and subsequent brain tumors. Neurosurgery 1979;4:203–206.
5. Artlich A, Schmidt D. Immunohistochemical profile of meningioma and their histological subtypes. Hum Pathol 1990;21:843–849.
6. Barnett GH, Chou SM, Bay JW. Posttraumatic intracranial meningioma: a case report and review of the literature. Neurosurgery 1986;18:75–78.
7. Becker I, Roggendorf W. Immunohistological investigation of mononuclear cell infiltrates in meningiomas. Acta Neuropathol 1989;79:211–216.
8. Bégin LR. Myxoid meningioma. Ultrastruct Pathol 1990;14:367–374.
9. Bernstein RA, Grumet KA, Wetzel N. Metastasis of prostatic carcinoma to intracranial meningioma. Case report. J Neurosurg 1983;58:774–777.
10. Bickerstaff ER, Small JM, Guest IA. The relapsing course of certain meningiomas in relation to pregnancy and menstruation. J Neurol Neurosurg Psychiatry 1958;21:89–91.
11. Bonito D, Giarelli L, Galconieri G, et al. Association of breast cancer and meningioma. Report of 12 new cases and review of the literature. Pathol Res Pract 1993;189:399–404.
12. Boström J, Mühlbauer A, Reifenberger G. Deletion mapping of the short arm of chromosome 1 identifies a common region of deletion distal to D1S496 in human meningiomas. Acta Neuropathol 1997;94:479–485.
13. Bourekas EC, Wildenhain P, Lewin JS, et al. The dural tail sign revisited. AJNR 1995;16:1514–1516.
14. Bowen JH, Burger PC, Odom GL, et al. Meningiomas associated with large cysts with neoplastic cells in the cyst walls. J Neurosurg 1981;55:473–478.
15. Brandis A, Mirzai S, Tatgiba M, et al. Immunohistochemical detection of female sex hormone receptors in meningiomas: correlation with clinical and histological features. Neurosurgery 1993;33:212–218.
16. Budka H. Non-glial specificities of immunocytochemistry for the glial fibrillary acidic protein (GFAP). Acta Neuropathol 1986;72:43–54.
17. Cabezudo JM, Vaquero J, García-de-Sola R, et al. Meningioma of the anterior part of the third ventricle. Acta Neurochir 1981;56:219–231.
18. Carneiro SS, Scheithauer BW, Nascimento AG, et al. Solitary fibrous tumor of the meninges: a lesion distinct from fibrous meningioma. A clinicopathologic and immunohistochemical study. Am J Clin Pathol 1996;106:217–224.
19. Celli P, Palma L, Domenicucci M, et al. Histologically benign recurrent meningioma metastasizing to the parotid gland: case report and review of the literature. Neurosurgery 1992;31:1113–1116.
20. Cerdá-Nicolás M, López-Ginés C, Barcia-Salorio J, et al. Evolution to malignancy in a recurrent meningioma: morphological and cytogenetic findings. Clin Neuropathol 1998;17:210–215.
21. Coons SW, Johnson PC. Brachial plexus meningioma, report of a case with immunohistochemical and ultrastructural examination. Acta Neuropathol 1989;77:445–448.
22. Copeland DD, Bell SW, Shelburne JD. Hemidesmosome-like intercellular specializations in human meningiomas. Cancer 1978;41:2242–2249.
23. Couce ME, Aker FV, Scheithauer BW. Chordoid meningioma. A clinicopathologic study of 42 cases. Am J Surg Pathol 2000;24:899–905.
24. Couce ME, Perry A, Webb P, et al. Fibrous meningioma with tyrosine-rich crystals. Ultrastruct Pathol 1999;23:341–345.
25. Courville CB, Abbott KH. On the classification of meningiomas. A survey of ninety-nine cases in the light of existing schemes. Bull Los Angeles Neurol Soc 1941;6:21–31.
26. Cushing H, Eisenhardt L. Meningiomas: Their Classification, Regional Behavior, Life History and Surgical End Results. Springfield, IL: Charles C Thomas, 1938.
27. Dahmen HG. Studies on mucous substances in myxomatous meningiomas. Acta Neuropathol 1979;48:235–237.
28. Darling CF, Byrd SE, Reyes-Mugica M, et al. MR of pediatric intracranial meningiomas. AJNR 1994;15:435–444.
29. Davidson GS, Hope JK. Meningeal tumors of childhood. Cancer 1989;63:1205–1210.
30. Davis GA, Fabinyi GCA, Kalnins RM, et al. Concurrent adjacent meningioma and astrocytoma: a report of three cases and review of the literature. Neurosurgery 1995;36:599–605.
31. De Jesús O, Rifkinson N, Negrón B. Cystic meningiomas: a review. Neurosurgery 1995;36:489–492.
32. De La Monte SM, Flickinger J, Linggood RM. Histopathologic features predicting recurrence of meningiomas following subtotal resection. Am J Surg Pathol 1986;10:836–843.
33. De Vries J, Graf M, Scheremet R, et al. Case reports. Rapid dedifferentiating meningioma with repeated multifocal recurrences and pulmonary metastases. Clin Neurol Neurosurg 1994;96:58–65.
34. Deprez RHL, Riegman PH, van Drunen E, et al. Cytogenetic, molecular genetic and pathological analyses in 126 meningiomas. J Neuropathol Exp Neurol 1995;54:224–235.
35. Dweik A, Maheut-Lourmiere J, Lioret E, et al. Radiation-induced meningioma. Childs Nerv Syst 1995;11:661–663.
36. Eljamel MSM, Foy PM. Multiple meningiomas and their relation to neurofibromatosis. Review of the literature and report of seven cases. Surg Neurol 1989;32:131–136.
37. Elster AD, Challa VR, Gilbert TH, et al. Meningiomas: MR and histopathologic features. Radiology 1989;170:857–862.
38. Ferrara M, Bizzozero L, D'Aliberti G, et al. Inflammatory meningioma of the fourth ventricle. Case report. J Neurosurg Sci 1994;38:59–62.
39. Fewings PE, Battersby RD, Timperley WR. Long-term followup of progesterone receptor status in benign meningioma: a prognostic indicator of recurrence? J Neurosurg 2000;92:401–405.
40. Font RL, Croxatto JO. Intracellular inclusions in meningothelial meningioma: a histochemical and ultrastructural study. J Neuropathol Exp Neurol 1980;39:575–583.
41. Germano IM, Edwards MSB, Davis RL, et al. Intracranial meningiomas of the first two decades of life. J Neurosurg 1994;80:447–453.
42. Ghim TT, Seo J-J, O'Brien M, et al. Childhood intracranial meningiomas after high-dose irradiation. Cancer 1993;71:4091–4095.
43. Gi H, Nagao S, Yoshizumi H, et al. Meningioma with hypergammaglobulinemia. Case report. J Neurosurg 1990;73:628–629.
44. Goldsher D, Litt AW, Pinto RS, et al. Dural "tail" associated with meningiomas on Gd-DTPA-enhanced MR images: characteristics, differential diagnostic value, and possible implications for treatment. Radiology 1990;17:447–450.
45. Goldsmith BJ, Wara WM, Wilson CB, et al. Postoperative irradiation for subtotally resected meningiomas. A retrospective analysis of 140 patients treated from 1967 to 1990. J Neurosurg 1994;80:195–201.
46. Halliday WC, Yeger H, Duwe GF, et al. Intermediate filaments in meningiomas. J Neuropathol Exp Neurol 1985;44:617–623.
47. Harada T, Irving RM, Xuereb JH, et al. Molecular genetic investigation of the neurofibromatosis type 2 tumor suppressor gene in sporadic meningioma. J Neurosurg 1996;84:847–851.
48. Harrison JD, Rose PE. Myxoid meningioma: histochemistry and electron microscopy. Acta Neuropathol 1985;68:80–82.
49. Harrison MJ, Wolfe DE, Lau T-S, et al. Radiation-induced meningiomas: experience at the Mount Sinai Hospital and review of the literature. J Neurosurg 1991;75:564–574.
50. Heick A, Mosdal C, Jørgensen K, et al. Localized cranial hyperostosis of meningiomas: a result of neoplastic enzymatic activity? Acta Neurol Scand 1993;87:243–247.
51. Hinton DR, Kovacs K, Chandrasoma PT. Cytologic features of secretory meningioma. Acta Cytol 1999;43:121–125.
52. Hope JKA, Armstrong DA, Babyn PS, et al. Primary meningeal tumors in children: correlation of clinical and CT findings with histologic type and prognosis. AJNR 1992;13:1353–1364.

53. Horten BC, Urich H, Stefoski D. Meningiomas with conspicuous plasma cell–lymphocytic components. A report of five cases. Cancer 1979;43:258–264.

54. Hsu D, Pardo FS, Efird JT, et al. Prognostic significance of proliferative indices in meningiomas. J Neuropathol Exp Neurol 1994;53:247–255.

55. Hsu DW, Efird JT, Hedley-Whyte ET. Progesterone and estrogen receptors in meningiomas: prognostic considerations. J Neurosurg 1997;86:113–120.

56. Huang PP, Doyle WK, Abbott IR. Atypical meningioma of the third ventricle in a 6-year-old boy. Neurosurgery 1993;33: 312–316.

57. Ide M, Jimbo M, Yamamoto M, et al. MIB-1 staining index and peritumoral brain edema of meningiomas. Cancer 1996;78: 133–143.

58. Inamura T, Nishio S, Takeshita I, et al. Pertumoral brain edema in meningiomas–influence of vascular supply on its development. Neurosurgery 1992;31:179–185.

59. Ito H, Kawano N, Yada K, et al. Meningiomas differentiating to arachnoid trabecular cells: a proposal for histological subtype "arachnoid trabecular cell meningioma." Acta Neuropathol 1991;82:327–330.

60. Iwaki T, Takeshita I, Fukui M, et al. Cell kinetics of the malignant evolution of meningothelial meningioma. Acta Neuropathol 1987;74:243–247.

61. Jääskeläinen J. Seemingly complete removal of histologically benign intracranial meningioma: later recurrence rate and factors predicting recurrence in 657 patients. A multivariate analysis. Surg Neurol 1986;26:461–469.

62. Jääskeläinen J, Haltia M, Laasonen E, et al. The growth rate of intracranial meningiomas and its relation to histology. An analysis of 43 patients. Surg Neurol 1985;24:165–172.

63. Jääskeläinen J, Haltia M, Servo A. Atypical and anaplastic meningiomas: radiology, surgery, radiotherapy, and outcome. Surg Neurol 1986;25:233–242.

64. Jacobs DH, McFarlane MJ, Holmes FF. Female patients with meningioma of the sphenoid ridge and additional primary neoplasms of the breast and genital tract. Cancer 1987;60: 3080–3082.

65. Joseph JT, Lisle DK, Jacoby LB, et al. NF2 gene analysis distinguishes hemangiopericytoma from meningioma. Am J Pathol 1995;147:1450–1455.

66. Kaleem Z, Fitzpatrick MM, Ritter JH. Primary pulmonary meningioma. Report of a case and review of the literature. Arch Pathol Lab Med 1997;121:631–636.

67. Kallio M, Sankila R, Hakulinen T, et al. Factors affecting operative and excess long-term mortality in 935 patients with intracranial meningioma. Neurosurgery 1992;31:2-12.

68. Karamitopoulou E, Perentes E, Tolnay M, et al. Prognostic significance of MIB-1, p53, and bcl-2 immunoreactivity in meningiomas. Hum Pathol 1998;29:140–145.

69. Kawasaki K, Takahashi H, Kaneko H, et al. Novel eosinophilic intracytoplasmic inclusions in a meningioma. Cancer 1993;72: 2675–2679.

70. Kepes JJ. The fine structure of hyaline inclusions (pseudopsammoma bodies) in meningiomas. J Neuropathol Exp Neurol 1975; 34:282–289.

71. Kepes JJ. Meningiomas: Biology, Pathology, and Differential Diagnosis. New York: Masson, 1982.

72. Kepes JJ, Chen WY-K, Connors MH, et al. Chordoid meningeal tumors in young individuals with peritumoral lymphoplasmacellular infiltrates causing systemic manifestations of the Castleman syndrome. A report of seven cases. Cancer 1988;62:391–406.

73. Kepes JJ, Dunlap MD, O'Boynick P, et al. Meningioma with multiple rheumatoid nodules. A case report. Acta Neuropathol 1986;70:314–319.

74. Kepes JJ, Goldware S, Leoni R. Meningioma with pseudoglandular pattern. A case report. J Neuropathol Exp Neurol 1983;42: 61–68.

75. Kepes JJ, Moral LA, Wilkinson SB, et al. Rhabdoid transformation of tumor cells in meningiomas: a histologic indication of increased proliferative activity. Report of four cases. Am J Surg Pathol 1998;22:231–238.

76. Khalid H. Immunohistochemical study of estrogen receptor–related antigen, progesterone, and estrogen receptors in human intracranial meningiomas. Cancer 1994;74:679–685.

77. Kleihues P, Cavenee WK (eds). Pathology and Genetics of Tumours of the Nervous System. World Health Organization Classification of Tumours. Lyon: IARC Press, 2000.

78. Kleinman GM, Liszczak T, Tarlov E, et al. Microcystic variant of meningioma. A light-microscopic and ultrastructural study. Am J Surg Pathol 1980;4:383–389.

79. Kuratsu J, Matsukado Y, Sonoda H. Pseudopsammoma bodies in meningotheliomatous meningioma. A histochemical and ultrastructural study. Acta Neurochir 1983;68:55–62.

80. Lamszus K, Vahldiek F, Mautner VF, et al. Allelic losses in neurofibromatosis 2–associated meningiomas. J Neuropathol Exp Neurol 2000;59:504–512.

81. Lang I, Jackson A, Strang FA. Intraventricular hemorrhage caused by intraventricular meningioma: CT appearance. AJNR 1995;16:1378–1381.

82. Lee TT, Landy HJ. Spinal metastases of malignant intracranial meningioma. Surg Neurol 1998;50:437–441.

83. Lee W-H, Tu Y-C, Liu M-Y. Primary intraosseous malignant meningioma of the skull: case report. Neurosurgery 1988;23: 505–508.

84. LeMay DR, Bucci MN, Farhat SM. Malignant transformation of recurrent meningioma with pulmonary metastases. Surg Neurol 1989;31:365–368.

85. LeRoux P, Hope A, Lofton S, et al. Lipomatous meningioma—an uncommon tumor with distinct radiographic findings. Surg Neurol 1989;32:360–365.

86. Lindblom A, Ruttledge M, Collins VP, et al. Chromosomal deletions in anaplastic meningiomas suggest multiple regions outside chromosome 22 as important in tumor progression. Int J Cancer 1994;56:354–357.

87. Lockett L, Chiang V, Scully N. Primary pulmonary meningioma. Report of a case and review of the literature. Am J Surg Pathol 1997;21:453–460.

88. Lodrini S, Savoiardo M. Metastases of carcinoma to intracranial meningioma: report of two cases and review of the literature. Cancer 1981;48:2668–2673.

89. Loiseau H, Pedespan J-M, Vital A, et al. Lymphoplasmacyte-rich meningioma in a child. Case report. J Neurosurg 1995;83: 1075–1079.

90. Lopez DA, Silvers DN, Helwig EB. Cutaneous meningiomas—a clinicopathologic study. Cancer 1974;34:728–744.

91. Louis DN, Hamilton AJ, Sobel RA, et al. Pseudopsammomatous meningioma with elevated serum carcinoembryonic antigen: a true secretory meningioma. Case report. J Neurosurg 1991;74:129–132.

92. Louw D, Sutherland G, Halliday W, et al. Meningiomas mimicking cerebral schwannoma. J Neurosurg 1990;73:715–719.

93. Ludwin SK, Rubinstein LJ, Russell DS. Papillary meningioma: a malignant variant of meningioma. Cancer 1975;36:1363–1373.

94. Mack EE, Wilson CB. Meningiomas induced by high-dose cranial irradiation. J Neurosurg 1993;79:28–31.

95. Mahmood A, Caccamo DV, Tomecek FJ, et al. Atypical and malignant meningiomas: a clinicopathological review. Neurosurgery 1993;33:955–963.

96. Mallucci CL, Parkes SE, Barber P, et al. Paediatric meningeal tumours. Childs Nerv Syst 1996;12:582–589.

97. Mani RL, Hedgcock MW, Mass SI, et al. Radiographic diagnosis of meningioma of the lateral ventricle: review of 22 cases. J Neurosurg 1978;49:249–255.

98. Marquardt MD, Zimmerman LE. Histopathology of meningiomas and gliomas of the optic nerve. Hum Pathol 1982;13:226–235.

99. Matyja E, Kuchna I, Kroh H, et al. Meningiomas and gliomas in juxtaposition: casual or causal coexistence? Report of two cases. Am J Surg Pathol 1995;19:37–41.

100. Maxwell M, Shih SD, Galanopoulos T, et al. Familial meningioma: analysis of expression of neurofibromatosis 2 protein Merlin. Report of two cases. J Neurosurg 1998;88:562–569.

101. Mérel P, Hoang-Xuan K, Sanson M, et al. Predominant occurrence of somatic mutations of the NF2 gene in meningiomas and schwannomas. Genes Chromosomes Cancer 1995;13:211–216.

102. Michaud J, Gagné F. Microcystic meningioma. Clinicopathologic report of eight cases. Arch Pathol Lab Med 1983;107:75–80.

103. Miller D. Predicting recurrence of intracranial meningiomas. A multivariate clinicopathologic model–interim report of the New York University Medical Center Meningioma Project. Neurosurg Clin North Am 1994;5:193–200.

104. Miller DC, Ojemann RG, Proppe KH, et al. Benign metastasizing meningioma. Case report. J Neurosurg 1985;62:763–766.

105. Mirimanoff RO, Dosoretz DE, Linggood RM, et al. Meningioma: analysis of recurrence and progression following neurosurgical resection. J Neurosurg 1985;62:18–24.

106. Nagashima G, Aoyagi M, Wakimoto H, et al. Immunohistochemical detection of progesterone receptors and the correlation with Ki-67 labeling indices in paraffin-embedded sections of meningiomas. Neurosurgery 1995;37:478–483.

107. Nakasu S, Hirano A, Llena JF, et al. Interface between the meningioma and the brain. Surg Neurol 1989;32:206–212.

108. Nakasu S, Nakajima M, Matsumura K-I, et al. Meningioma: proliferating potential and clinicoradiological features. Neurosurgery 1995;37:1049–1055.

109. Ng H-K, Tse CCH, Lo STH. Microcystic meningiomas—an unusual morphological variant of meningiomas. Histopathology 1989;14:1–9.

110. Ng HK, Wong ATC. Expression of epithelial and extracellular matrix protein markers in meningiomas. Histopathology 1993; 22:113–125.

111. Ng THK, Wong MP, Chan KW. Benign metastasizing meningioma. Clin Neurol Neurosurg 1990;92:152–154.

112. Niedermayer I, Feiden W, Henn W, et al. Loss of alkaline phosphatase activity in meningiomas: a rapid histochemical technique indicating progression-associated deletion of a putative tumor suppressor gene on the distal part of the short arm of chromosome 1. J Neuropathol Exp Neurol 1997;56:879–886.

113. Niida H, Tanaka R, Takeda N, et al. Meningioma in a neonate: case report. Surg Neurol 1992;38:273–276.

114. Nishio S, Takeshita I, Fukui M. Microcystic meningioma: tumors of *arachnoid cap vs trabecular cells.* Clin Neuropathol 1994; 13:197–203.

115. Ohta M, Iwaki T, Kitamoto T, et al. MIB1 staining index and scoring of histologic features in meningioma. Indicators for the prediction of biologic potential and postoperative management. Cancer 1994;74:3176–3189.

116. Oka K, Hirakawa K, Yoshida S, et al. Primary calvarial meningiomas. Surg Neurol 1989;32:304–310.

117. Ortiz O, Schochet SS, Kotzan JM, et al. Radiologic-pathologic correlation. Meningioma of the optic nerve sheath. AJNR 1996; 17:901–906.

118. Palma L, Celli P, Franco C, et al. Long-term prognosis for atypical and malignant meningiomas: a study of 71 surgical cases. J Neurosurg 1997;86:793–800.

119. Pamphlett R. Carcinoma metastasis to meningioma. J Neurol Neurosurg Psychiatry 1984;47:561–563.

120. Pasquier B, Gasnier F, Pasquier D, et al. Papillary meningioma. Clinicopathologic study of seven cases and review of the literature. Cancer 1986;58:299–305.

121. Paulus W, Meixensberger J, Hofmann E, et al. Effect of embolisation of meningioma on Ki-67 proliferation index. J Clin Pathol 1993;46:876–877.

122. Perry A, Jenkins RB, Dahl RJ, et al. Cytogenetic analysis of aggressive meningiomas. Possible diagnostic and prognostic implications. Cancer 1996;77:2567–2573.

123. Perry A, Scheithauer BW, Nascimento AG. The immunophenotypic spectrum of meningeal hemangiopericytoma: a comparison with fibrous meningioma and solitary fibrous tumor of meninges. Am J Surg Pathol 1997;21:1354–1360.

124. Perry A, Scheithauer BW, Stafford SL, et al. "Rhabdoid" meningioma: an aggressive variant. Am J Surg Pathol 1998;22: 1482–1490.

125. Perry A, Stafford SL, Scheithauer BW, Lohse CM, Wollan PC. "Malignancy" in meningiomas: a clinicopathologic study of 116 patients with grading implications. Cancer 1999;85:2046–2056.

126. Perry A, Stafford SL, Scheithauer BW, Suman VJ, Lohse CM. Meningioma grading. An analysis of histologic parameters. Am J Surg Pathol 1997;21:1455–1465.

127. Perry A, Stafford SL, Scheithauer BW, Suman VJ, Lohse CM. The prognostic significance of MIB-1, p53, and DNA flow cytometry in completely resected primary meningiomas. Cancer 1998;82:2262–2269.

128. Perry DR, Parker GD, Hallinan JM. CT and MR imaging of fourth ventricular meningiomas. J Comput Assist Tomogr 1990; 14:276–280.

129. Piatt JH Jr, Campbell GA, Oakes J. Papillary meningioma involving the oculomotor nerve in an infant. Case report. J Neurosurg 1986;64:808–812.

130. Prayson RA, Farver CF. Primary pulmonary malignant meningioma. Am J Surg Pathol 1999;23:722–726.

131. Preston-Martin S, Paganini-Hill A, Henderson BE, et al. Case control study of intracranial meningiomas in women in Los Angeles County, California. J Natl Cancer Inst 1980;65:67–73.

132. Preston-Martin S, White SC. Brain and salivary gland tumors related to prior dental radiography: implications for current practice. J Am Dent Assoc 1990;120:151–158.

133. Probst-Cousin S, Villagran-Lillo R, Lahl R, et al. Secretory meningioma: clinical, histologic, and immunohistochemical findings in 31 cases. Cancer 1997;79:2003–2015.

134. Pulst S-M, Rouleau GA, Marineau C, et al. Familial meningioma is not allelic to neurofibromatosis 2. Neurology 1993;43: 2096–2098.

135. Rempel SA, Schwechheimer K, Davis RL, et al. Loss of heterozygosity for loci on chromosome 10 is associated with morphologically malignant meningioma progression. Cancer Res 1993;53:2386–2392.

136. Renfro M, Delashaw JB, Peters K, et al. Anterior third ventricle meningioma in an adolescent: a case report. Neurosurgery 1992;31:746–750.

137. Ron E, Modan B, Boice JD Jr, et al. Tumors of the brain and nervous system after radiotherapy in childhood. N Engl J Med 1988;319:1033–1039.

138. Roncaroli F, Riccioni L, Cerati M, et al. Oncocytic meningioma. Am J Surg Pathol 1997;21:375–382.

139. Roncaroli FSB, Scheithauer BW, Laeng RH, et al. "Lipomatous" meningioma: a clinicopathological study of 17 cases with special reference to the issue of metaplasia. Am J Surg Pathol, 2001;25: 769–775.

140. Ruttledge MH, Sarrazin J, Rangaratnam S, et al. Evidence for the complete inactivation of the NF2 gene in the majority of sporadic meningiomas. Nat Genet 1994;6:180–184.

141. Ruttledge MH, Xie Y-G, Han F-Y, et al. Deletions on chromosome 22 in sporadic meningiomas. Genes Chromosomes Cancer 1994;10:122–130.

142. Salibi SS, Nauta HJW, Brem H, et al. Lipomeningioma: report of three cases and review of the literature. Neurosurgery 1989;25: 122–126.

143. Salpietro FM, Alafaci C, Lucerna S, et al. Peritumoral edema in meningiomas: microsurgical observations of different brain tumor interfaces related to computed tomography. Neurosurgery 1994;35:638–642.

144. Salvati M, Cervoni L, Puzzilli F, et al. High-dose radiation–induced meningiomas. Surg Neurol 1997;47:435–442.

145. Sgouros S, Walsh AR, Barber P. Intraventricular malignant meningioma in a 6-year-old child. Surg Neurol 1994;42:41–45.

146. Sheikh BY, Siqueira E, Dayel F. Meningioma in children: a report of nine cases and review of the literature. Surg Neurol 1996;45:328–335.

147. Sheporaitis LA, Osborn AG, Smirniotopoulos JG, et al. Radiologic-pathologic correlation. Intracranial meningioma. AJNR 1992;13:29–37.

148. Simpson D. The recurrence of intracranial meningiomas after surgical treatment. J Neurol Neurosurg Psychiatry 1957;20: 22–39.

149. Slavin ML. Metastatic malignant meningioma. J Clin Neuroophthalmol 1989;9:55–59.

150. Sobel RA, Michaud J. Microcystic meningioma of the falx cerebri with numerous palisaded structures: an unusual histological pattern mimicking schwannoma. Acta Neuropathol 1985;68: 256–258.

151. Soffer D, Pittaluga S, Feiner M, et al. Intracranial meningiomas following low-dose irradiation to the head. J Neurosurg 1983; 59:1048–1053.

152. Som PM, Sacher M, Strenger SW, et al. "Benign" metastasizing meningiomas. AJNR 1987;8:127–130.

153. Stangl AP, Wellenreuther R, Lenartz D, et al. Clonality of multiple meningiomas. J Neurosurg 1997;86:853–858.

154. Takeuchi H, Kubota T, Kabuto M, et al. Prediction of recurrence in histologically benign meningiomas: proliferating cell nuclear antigen and Ki-67 immunohistochemical study. Surg Neurol 1997;48:501–506.

155. Theaker JM, Gatter KC, Esiri MM, et al. Epithelial membrane antigen and cytokeratin expression by meningiomas: an immunohistological study. J Clin Pathol 1986;39:435–439.

156. Thompson LD, Gyure KA. Extracranial sinonasal tract meningiomas: a clinicopathologic study of 30 cases with a review of the literature. Am J Surg Pathol 2000;24:640–650.

157. Tien RD, Yang PJ, Chu PK. "Dural tail sign": a specific MR sign for meningioma? J Comput Assist Tomogr 1991;15:64–66.
158. Tokumaru A, O'uchi T, Eguchi T, et al. Prominent meningeal enhancement adjacent to meningioma on Gd-DTPA–enhanced MR images: histopathologic correlation. Radiology 1990;175:431–433.
159. Tominaga T, Koshu K, Narita N, et al. Metastatic meningioma to the second cervical vertebral body: a case report. Neurosurgery 1994;34:538–540.
160. Tse JYM, Ng H-K, Lau K-M, et al. Loss of heterozygosity of chromosome 14q in low- and high-grade meningiomas. Hum Pathol 1997;28:779–785.
161. Tsuboi K, Nose T, Maki Y. Meningioma of the fourth ventricle: a case report. Neurosurgery 1983;13:163–166.
162. Tsuchida T, Matsumoto M, Shirayama Y, et al. Immunohistochemical observation of foci of muscle actin–positive tumor cells in meningiomas. Arch Pathol Lab Med 1996;120:267–269.
163. Tsunoda S, Takeshima T, Sakaki T, et al. Secretory meningioma with elevated serum carcinoembryonic antigen level. Surg Neurol 1992;37:415–418.
164. Utsuki S, Kawano N, Oka H, et al. Malignant meningioma with a new intracytoplasmic inclusion body. Clin Neuropathol 1998; 17: 216–220.
165. von Deimling A, Kraus JA, Stangl AP, et al. Evidence for subarachnoid spread in the development of multiple meningiomas. Brain Pathol 1995;5:11–14.
166. von Deimling A, Larson J, Wellenreuther R, et al. Clonal origin of recurrent meningiomas. Brain Pathol 1999;9:645–650.
167. Wasenko JJ, Hochhauser L, Stopa EG, et al. Cystic meningiomas: MR characteristics and surgical correlations. AJNR 1994;15: 1959–1965.
168. Wellenreuther R, Kraus JA, Lenartz D, et al. Analysis of the neurofibromatosis 2 gene reveals molecular variants of meningioma. Am J Pathol 1995;146:827–832.
169. Wilson AJ, Ratliff JL, Lagios MD, et al. Mediastinal meningioma. Am J Surg Pathol 1979;3:557–562.
170. Winek RR, Scheithauer BW, Wick MR. Meningioma, meningeal hemangiopericytoma (angioblastic meningioma), peripheral hemangiopericytoma, and acoustic schwannoma. A comparative immunohistochemical study. Am J Surg Pathol 1989;13:251–261.
171. Wolfe M, Rankow RM. Meningioma of the parotid gland: an insight into the pathogenesis of extracranial meningiomas. Hum Pathol 1971;2:453–459.
172. Younis GA, Sawaya R, De Monte F, et al. Aggressive meningeal tumors: review of a series. J Neurosurg 1995;82:17–27.
173. Zang KD. Cytological and cytogenetical studies on human meningioma. Cancer Genet Cytogenet 1982;6:249–274.
174. Zee CS, Chen T, Hinton DR, et al. Magnetic resonancy imaging of cystic meningiomas and its surgical implications. Neurosurgery 1995;36:482–488.
175. Zon LI, Johns WD, Stomper PC, et al. Breast carcinoma metastatic to a meningioma. Case report and review of the literature. Arch Intern Med 1989;149:959–962.
176. Zorludemir S, Scheithauer BW, Hirose T, et al. Clear cell meningioma. A clinicopathologic study of a potentially aggressive variant of meningioma. Am J Surg Pathol 1995;19:493–505.

**Solitary Fibrous Tumor**

1. Brunori A, Cerasoli S, Donati R, et al. Solitary fibrous tumor of the meninges: two new cases and review of the literature. Surg Neurol 1999;51:636–640.
2. Carneiro SS, Scheithauer BW, Nascimento AG, et al. Solitary fibrous tumor of the meninges: a lesion distinct from fibrous meningioma. Am J Clin Pathol 1996;106:217–224.
3. Challa VR, Kilpatrick SE, Ricci P, et al. Solitary fibrous tumor of the meninges. Clin Neuropathol 1998;17:73–78.
4. Chilosi M, Facchetti F, Dei Tos AP, et al. bcl-2 expression in pleural and extrapleural solitary fibrous tumours. J Pathol 1997;181:362–367.
5. Dorfman DM, To K, Dickersin GR, et al. Solitary fibrous tumor of the orbit. Am J Surg Pathol 1994;18:281–287.
6. Kim TA, Brunberg JA, Pearson JP, et al. Solitary fibrous tumor of the paranasal sinuses: CT and MR appearance. AJNR 1996; 17:1767–1772.
7. Perry A, Scheithauer BW, Nascimento AG. The immunophenotypic spectrum of meningeal hemangiopericytoma: a comparison with fibrous meningioma and solitary fibrous tumor of meninges. Am J Surg Pathol 1997;21:1354–1360.
8. Prayson RA, McMahon JT, Barnett GH. Solitary fibrous tumor of the meninges. Case report and review of the literature. J Neurosurg 1997;86:1049–1052.
9. Ramdial PK, Nadvi S. An unusual cause of proptosis: orbital solitary fibrous tumor: case report. Neurosurgery 1996;38: 1040–1043.
10. Suster S, Fisher C, Moran CA. Expression of bcl-2 oncoprotein in benign and malignant spindle cell tumors of soft tissue, skin, serosal surfaces, and gastrointestinal tract. Am J Surg Pathol 1998;22:863–872.
11. Westra WH, Gerald WL, Rosai J. Solitary fibrous tumor. Consistent CD34 immunoreactivity and occurrence in the orbit. Am J Surg Pathol 1994;18:992–998.

**Melanocytoma**

1. Brat DJ, Giannini C, Scheithauer BW, et al. Primary melanocytic neoplasms of the central nervous system. Am J Surg Pathol 1999;23:745–754.
2. Clarke DB, Leblanc R, Bertrand G, et al. Meningeal melanocytoma. Report of a case and a historical comparison. J Neurosurg 1998;88:116–121.
3. Gebarski SS, Blaivas MA. Imaging of normal leptomeningeal melanin. AJNR 1996;17:55–60.
4. Jellinger K, Böck F, Brenner H. Meningeal melanocytoma. Report of a case and review of the literature. Acta Neurochir 1988;94:78–87.
5. Kawaguchi T, Kawano T, Kazekawa K, et al. Meningeal melanocytoma in the left frontal region. Case report. Brain Tumor Pathol 1998;15:58–62.
6. Limas C, Tio FO. Meningeal melanocytoma ("melanotic meningioma"). Its melanocytic origin as revealed by electron microscopy. Cancer 1972;30:1286–1294.
7. Litofsky NS, Zee C-S, Breeze RE, et al. Meningeal melanocytoma: diagnostic criteria for a rare lesion. Neurosurgery 1992;31:945–948.
8. Maiuri F, Iaconetta G, Benvenuti D, et al. Intracranial meningeal melanocytoma: case report. Surg Neurol 1995;44:556–561.
9. Naul LG, Hise JH, Bauserman SC, et al. CT and MR of meningeal melanocytoma. AJNR 1991;12:315–316.
10. O'Brien TF, Moran M, Miller JH, et al. Meningeal melanocytoma. An uncommon diagnostic pitfall in surgical neuropathology. Arch Pathol Lab Med 1995;119:542–546.
11. Prabhu SS, Lynch PG, Keogh AJ, et al. Intracranial meningeal melanocytoma: a report of two cases and review of the literature. Surg Neurol 1993;40:516–521.
12. Uematsu Y, Yukawa S, Yokote H, et al. Meningeal melanocytoma: magnetic resonance imaging characteristics and pathological features. J Neurosurg 1992;76:705–709.

**Hemangioblastoma**

1. Diehl PR, Symon L. Supratentorial intraventricular hemangioblastoma: case report and review of literature. Surg Neurol 1981;15:435–443.
2. Hoff JT, Ray BS. Cerebral hemangioblastoma occurring in a patient with von Hippel–Lindau disease. Case report. J Neurosurg 1968;28:365–368.
3. Ishwar S, Taniguchi RM, Vogel FS. Multiple supratentorial hemangioblastomas. Case study and ultrastructural characteristics. J Neurosurg 1971;35:396–405.
4. Lee KR, Kishore PRS, Wulfsberg E, et al. Supratentorial leptomeningeal hemangioblastoma. Neurology 1978;28:727–730.

**Lipoma**

1. Baeesa SS, Higgins MJ, Ventureyra ECG. Dorsal brain stem lipomas: case report. Neurosurgery 1996;38:1031–1035.
2. Budka H. Intracranial lipomatous hamartomas (intracranial "lipomas"): a study of 113 cases including combinations with medulloblastoma, colloid and epidermoid cysts, angiomatosis and other malformations. Acta Neuropathol 1974;28:205–222.
3. Celik SE, Kocaeli H, Cordan T, et al. Trigeminal neuralgia due to cerebellopontine angle lipoma. Case illustration. J Neurosurg 2000;92:889.
4. Christensen WN, Long DM, Epstein JI. Cerebellopontine angle lipoma. Hum Pathol 1986;17:739–743.
5. Cserni G. Case report. Intracranial lipoma of the sylvian region. Neuropathol Appl Neurobiol 1993;19:282–285.
6. Dyck P. Sylvian lipoma causing auditory hallucinations: case report. Neurosurgery 1985;16:64–67.

7. Esposito S, Nardi P. Lipoma of the infundibulum: case report. J Neurosurg 1987;67:304–306.
8. Friede RL. Osteolipomas of the tuber cinereum. Arch Pathol Lab Med 1977;101:369–372.
9. Gastaut H, Regis H, Gastaut JL. Lipomas of the corpus callosum and epilepsy. Neurology 1980;30:132–138.
10. Hatashita S, Sakakibara T, Ishii S. Lipoma of the insula: case report. J Neurosurg 1983;58:300–302.
11. Jallo JI, Palumbo SJ, Buchheit WA. Cerebellopontine angle lipoma: case report. Neurosurgery 1994;34:912–914.
12. Kudoh H, Sakamoto K, Kobayashi N. Lipomas in the corpus callosum and the forehead, associated with a frontal bone defect. Surg Neurol 1984;22:503–508.
13. Lach B, Lesiuk H. Intracranial suprasellar angiolipoma: ultrastructural and immunohistochemical features. Neurosurgery 1994;34:163–167.
14. Mackenzie IRA, Girvin JP, Lee D. Symptomatic osteolipoma of the tuber cinereum. Clin Neuropathol 1996;15:60–62.
15. Rosenbloom SB, Carson BS, Wang H, et al. Cerebellopontine angle lipoma. Surg Neurol 1985;23:134–138.
16. Ruocco MJ, Robles HA, Rao KCVG, et al. Intratentorial lipomas with Meckel's cave and cerebellopontine angle extension. AJNR 1995;16:1504–1506.
17. Schmid AH. A lipoma of the cerebellum. Acta Neuropathol (Berl) 1973;26:75–80.
18. Shuangshoti S, Vajragupta L. Angiolipoma of thalamus presenting with abrupt onset suggestive of cerebrovascular disease. Clin Neuropathol 1995;14:82–85.
19. Sinson G, Gennarelli TA, Wells GB. Suprasellar osteolipoma: case report. Surg Neurol 1998;50:457–460.
20. Sperling SJ, Alpers BJ. Lipoma and osteolipoma of the brain. J Nerv Ment Dis 1936;83:13–21.
21. Tresser N, Parveen T, Roessmann U. Intracranial lipomas with teratomatous elements. Arch Pathol Lab Med 1993;117:918–920.
22. Truwit CL, Barkovich AJ. Pathogenesis of intracranial lipoma: an MR study in 42 patients. AJNR 1990;11:665–674.
23. Uchino A, Hasuo K, Matsumoto S, et al. Solitary choroid plexus lipomas: CT and MR appearance. AJNR 1993;14:116–118.
24. Wilkins PR, Hoddinott C, Hourihan MD, et al. Intracranial angiolipoma. Short report. J Neurol Neurosurg Psychiatry 1987;50:1057–1059.

### Fibroma and Fibromatosis

1. Friede RL, Pollak A. Neurosurgical desmoid tumors. Presentation of four cases with a review of the differential diagnoses. J Neurosurg 1979;50:725–732.
2. Mitchell A, Scheithauer BW, Ebersold MJ, et al. Intracranial fibromatosis. Neurosurgery 1991;29:123–126.
3. Mooney JE, Papasozomenos SC. Leptomeningeal fibroma. Clin Neuropathol 1996;15:92–95.
4. Palma L, Spagnoli LG, Yusuf MA. Intracerebral fibroma: light and electron microscopic study. Acta Neurochir 1985;77:152–156.
5. Quest DO, Salcman M. Fibromatosis presenting as a cranial mass lesion. J Neurosurg 1976;44:237–240.
6. Reyes-Mugica M, Chou P, Gonzalez-Crussi F, et al. Fibroma of the meninges in a child: immunohistogenesis and ultrastructural study. Case report. J Neurosurg 1976;44:237–240.
7. Rutigliano MJ, Pollack IF, Ahdab-Barmada M, et al. Intracranial infantile myofibromatosis. J Neurosurg 1994;81:539–543.
8. Yoshida D, Ikeda Y, Takahashi H, et al. Intracranial fibromyxoma in a four-year-old child. Surg Neurol 1993;39:191–195.

### Chondroma, Osteochondroma, and Osteoma

1. Ahyai A, Spoerri O. Intracerebral chondroma. Surg Neurol 1979;11:431–433.
2. Chakrabortty S, Tamaki N, Kondoh T, et al. Maffucci's syndrome associated with intracranial chondroma and aneurysm: case report. Surg Neurol 1991;36:216–220.
3. Chorobski J, Jarzymski J, Ferens E. Intracranial solitary chondroma. Surg Gynecol Obstet 1939;68:677–686.
4. De Coene B, Gilliard C, Grandin C, et al. Unusual location of an intracranial chondroma. AJNR 1997;18:573–575.
5. Dukes HT, Odom GL. Discrete intradural osteoma: report of a case. J Neurosurg 1962;19:251–253.
6. Dutton J. Intracranial solitary chondroma. Case report. J Neurosurg 1978;49:460–463.

7. Fallon MD, Ellerbrake D, Teitelbaum SL. Meningeal osteomas and chronic renal failure. Hum Pathol 1982;13:449–453.
8. Forsythe RW, Baker GS, Dockerty MB, et al. Intracranial osteochondroma. Proc Staff Meet Mayo Clin 1947;22:350–356.
9. Hadadian K, Abtahii H, Asil ZT, et al. Cystic falcine chondroma: case report and review of the literature. Neurosurgery 1991;29:909–912.
10. Haddad GF, Haddad FS, Zaatari G. Dural osteochondroma: case report, review of the literature and proposal of a new classification. Br J Neurosurg 1998;12:380–384.
11. Kretzschmar HA, Eggert HR, Beck U, et al. Intracranial chondroma. Case report. Surg Neurol 1989;32:121–125.
12. Luzardo-Small G, Mendez-Martinez O, Cardozo-Duran J. Cavitated (cystic) falcine chondroma: case report. Br J Neurosurg 1999;13:426–428.
13. Nagai S, Yamamoto N, Wakabayashi K, et al. Osteochondroma arising from the convexity dura mater. Case illustration. J Neurosurg 1998;88:610.
14. Nakazawa T, Inoue T, Suzuki F, et al. Solitary intracranial chondroma of the convexity dura: case report. Surg Neurol 1993;40:495–498.
15. Perriggo VHS-C, Oommen KJ, Sobonya RE. Silent solitary right parietal chondroma resulting in secondary mania. Clin Neuropathol 1993;12:325–329.
16. Traflet RF, Babaria AR, Barolat G, et al. Intracranial chondroma in a patient with Ollier's disease. Case report. J Neurosurg 1989;70:274–276.
17. Warnick RE, Raisanen J, Kaczmar T Jr, et al. Intradural chordoma of the tentorium cerebelli. Case report. J Neurosurg 1991;74:508–511.

### Plasmacytoma

1. Benli K, Inci S. Solitary dural plasmacytoma: case report. Neurosurgery 1995;36:1206–1209.
2. Gad A, Willén R, Willén H, et al. Solitary dural plasmacytoma. Acta Pathol Microbiol Scand Sect A 1978;86:21–24.
3. Kohli CM, Kawazu T. Solitary intracranial plasmacytoma. Surg Neurol 1982;17:307–312.
4. Krivoy S, González JE, CÇspedes G, et al. Solitary cerebral falx plasmacytoma. Surg Neurol 1977;8:222–224.
5. Krymholz A, Weiss HD, Jiji VH, et al. Solitary intracranial plasmacytoma: two patients with extended follow-up. Ann Neurol 1982;11:529–532.
6. Laeng RH, Altermatt HJ, Scheithauer BW, et al. Amyloidomas of the nervous system: a monoclonal B-cell disorder with monotypic amyloid light chain lambda amyloid production. Cancer 1998;82:362–374.
7. Losa M, Terreni MR, Tresoldi M, et al. Solitary plasmacytoma of the sphenoid sinus involving the pituitary fossa: a case report and review of the literature. Surg Neurol 1992;37:388–393.
8. Mancardi GL, Mandybur TI. Solitary intracranial plasmacytoma. Cancer 1983;51:2226–2233.
9. Mancilla-Jimenez R, Tavassoli FA. Solitary meningeal plasmacytoma. Report of a case with electron microscopic and immunohistologic observations. Cancer 1976;38:798–806.
10. Scully RE (ed). Case records of the Massachusetts General Hospital. Case 21-1992. N Engl J Med 1992;326:1417–1423.
11. Vaicys C, Schulder M, Wolansky LJ, et al. Falcotentorial plasmacytoma. Case report. J Neurosurg 1999;91:132–135.
12. Wisniewski T, Sisti M, Inhirami G, et al. Intracerebral solitary plasmacytoma. Neurosurgery 1990;27:826–829.

### Leiomyoma

1. Kleinschmidt-DeMasters BK, Mierau GW, Sze C-I, et al. Unusual dural and skull-based mesenchymal neoplasms: a report of four cases. Hum Pathol 1998;29:240–245.

### Vascular Malformations and Benign Vascular Neoplasms

1. McCormick WF, Boulter TR. Vascular malformations ("angiomas") of the dura mater: report of two cases. J Neurosurg 1966;15:309–311.
2. Phookan G, Davis AT, Holmes B. Hemangioendothelioma of the cavernous sinus: case report. Neurosurgery 1998;42:1153–1156.
3. Saldaña CJ, Zimman H, Alonso P, Mata PR. Neonatal cavernous hemangioma of the dura mater: case report. Neurosurgery 1991;29:602–605.

4. Willing SJ, Faye-Petersen O, Aronin P, et al. Capillary hemangioma of the meninges. AJNR 1993;14:529–536.

**Hemangiopericytoma**

1. Carneiro SS, Scheithauer BW, Nascimento AG, et al. Solitary fibrous tumor of the meninges: a lesion distinct from fibrous meningioma. A clinicopathologic and immunohistochemical study. Am J Clin Pathol 1996;106:217–224.
2. Chaubal A, Paetau A, Zoltick P, et al. CD34 immunoreactivity in nervous system tumors. Acta Neuropathol 1994;88:454–458.
3. Chiechi MV, Smirniotopoulos JG, Mena H. Intracranial hemangiopericytomas: MR and CT features. AJNR 1996;17:1365–1371.
4. D'Amore ESG, Manivel JC, Sung JH. Soft-tissue and meningeal hemangiopericytomas: an immunohistochemical and ultrastructural study. Hum Pathol 1990;21:414–423.
5. Galanis E, Buckner JC, Scheithauer BW, et al. Management of recurrent meningeal hemangiopericytoma. Cancer 1998;82:1915–1920.
6. Guthrie BL, Ebersold MJ, Scheithauer BW, et al. Meningeal hemangiopericytoma: histopathological features, treatment, and long-term follow-up of 44 cases. Neurosurgery 1989;25:514–522.
7. Herzog CE, Leeds NE, Bruner JM, et al. Intracranial hemangiopericytomas in children. Pediatr Neurosurg 1995;22:274–279.
8. Joseph JT, Lisle DK, Jacoby LB, et al. NF2 gene analysis distinguishes hemangiopericytoma from meningioma. Am J Pathol 1995;147:1450–1455.
9. Mena H, Ribas JL, Pezeshkpour GH, et al. Hemangiopericytoma of the central nervous system: a review of 94 cases. Hum Pathol 1991;22:84–91.
10. Molnar P, Nemes Z. Hemangiopericytoma of the cerebello-pontine angle. Diagnostic pitfalls and the diagnostic value of the subunit A of factor XIII as a tumor marker. Clin Neuropathol 1995;14:19–24.
11. Nemes Z. Differentiation markers in hemangiopericytoma. Cancer 1992;69:133–140.
12. Perry A, Scheithauer BW, Nascimento AG. The immunophenotypic spectrum of meningeal hemangiopericytoma: a comparison with fibrous meningioma and solitary fibrous tumor of meninges. Am J Surg Pathol 1997;21:1354–1360.
13. Porter PL, Bigler SA, McNutt M, et al. The immunophenotype of hemangiopericytomas and glomus tumors, with special reference to muscle protein expression: an immunohistochemical study and review of the literature. Mod Pathol 1991;4:46–52.
14. Probst-Cousin S, Bergmann M, Schroder R, et al. Ki-67 and biological behaviour in meningeal haemangiopericytomas. Histopathology 1996;29:57–61.
15. Scheithauer BW, Bruner JM. Central nervous system tumors. Clin Lab Med 1987;7:157–179.
16. von der Stein B, Schröder R. Three-dimensional reconstruction of some vessel types in meningeal hemangiopericytoma. Clin Neuropathol 1991;10:279–284.
17. Winek RR, Scheithauer BW, Wick MR. Meningioma, meningeal hemangiopericytoma (angioblastic meningioma), peripheral hemangiopericytoma, and acoustic schwannoma. A comparative immunohistochemical study. Am J Surg Pathol 1989;13:251–261.

**Fibrosarcoma and Leiomyosarcoma**

1. Asai A, Yamada H, Murata S. Primary leiomyosarcoma of the dura mater: case report. J Neurosurg 1988;68:308–311.
2. Bailey OT, Ingraham FD. Intracranial fibrosarcomas of the dura mater in childhood: pathological characteristics and surgical management. J Neurosurg 1945;2:1–15.
3. Bejjani GK, Stopak B, Schwartz A, et al. Primary dural leiomyosarcoma in a patient infected with human immunodeficiency virus: case report. Neurosurgery 1999;44:199–202.
4. Brown HG, Burger PC, Olivi A, et al. Intracranial leiomyosarcoma in a patient with AIDS. Neuroradiology 1999;41:35–39.
5. Chang SM, Barker FG II, Larson DA, et al. Sarcomas subsequent to cranial irradiation. Neurosurgery 1995;36:685–690.
6. Christensen E, Lara DE. Intracranial sarcomas. J Neuropathol Exp Neurol 1953;12:41–56.
7. Kernohan JW, Uihlein A. Sarcomas of the Brain. Springfield, IL: Charles C Thomas, 1962.
8. Kleinschmidt-DeMasters BK, Mierau GW, Sze C-I, et al. Unusual dural and skull-based mesenchymal neoplasms: a report of four cases. Hum Pathol 1998;29:240–245.

9. Litofsky NS, Pihan G, Corvi F, et al. Intracranial leiomyosarcoma: a neuro-oncological consequence of acquired immunodeficiency syndrome. J Neurooncol 1998;40:179–183.
10. Mena H, Garcia JH. Primary brain sarcomas: light and electron microscopic features. Cancer 1978;42:1298–1307.
11. Okeda R, Mochizuki T, Terad E, et al. The origin of intracranial fibrosarcoma. Acta Neuropathol 1980;52:223–230.
12. Scheithauer BW. Pathology of the pituitary and sellar regions: exclusive of pituitary adenoma. Pathol Annu 1985;20:67–155.
13. Schrantz JL, Araoz CA. Radiation induced meningeal fibrosarcoma. Arch Pathol 1972;93:26–31.
14. Waltz TA, Brownell B. Sarcoma: a possible late result of effective radiation therapy for pituitary adenoma; report of two cases. J Neurosurg 1966;24:901–907.

**Chondrosarcoma, Liposarcoma, and Osteosarcoma**

1. Adegbite ABO, McQueen JD, Paine KWE, Rozdilsky B. Primary intracranial chondrosarcoma: report of two cases. Neurosurgery 1985;17:490–494.
2. Alvira MM, McLaurin RL. Asymptomatic subdural chondrosarcoma: case report. J Neurosurg 1978;84:825–828.
3. Bernstein M, Perrin RG, Platts JE, et al. Radiation-induced cerebellar chondrosarcoma: case report. J Neurosurg 1984;61:174–177.
4. Bingaman KD, Alleyne CH Jr, Olson JJ. Intracranial extraskeletal mesenchymal chondrosarcoma: case report. Neurosurgery 2000;46:207–211; discussion 11–12.
5. Cybulski GR, Russell EJ, D'Angelo CM, et al. Falcine chondrosarcoma: case report and literature review. Neurosurgery 1985;16:412–415.
6. El-Gindi S, Abd-El-Hafeez M, Salanma M. Extracranial skeletal metastases from an extracranial meningeal chondrosarcoma: case report. J Neurosurg 1974;40:651–653.
7. Forbes RB, Eljamel MS. Meningeal chondrosarcomas, a review of 31 patients. Br J Neurosurg 1998;12:461–464.
8. Gerszten PC, Pollack IF, Hamilton RL. Primary parafalcine chondrosarcoma in a child. Acta Neuropathol 1998;95:111–114.
9. Harsh GR IV, Wilson CB. Central nervous system mesenchymal chondrosarcoma. Case report. J Neurosurg 1984;61:375–381.
10. Hassounah M, Al-Mefty O, Akhtar M. Primary cranial and intracranial chondrosarcoma: a survey. Acta Neurochir 1985;78:123–132.
11. Kernohan JW, Uihlein A. Sarcomas of the Brain. Springfield, IL: Charles C Thomas, 1962.
12. Kothandaram P. Dural liposarcoma associated with subdural hematoma: case report. J Neurosurg 1970;33:85–87.
13. Lam RMY, Malik CM, Chason JL. Osteosarcoma of meninges: clinical, light, and ultrastructural observations of a case. Am J Surg Pathol 1981;5:203–208.
14. Nagata S, Sawada K, Kitamura K. Chondrosarcoma arising from the falx cerebri. Surg Neurol 1986;25:505–509.
15. Roy S, Chopra P, Prakash BB, et al. Chondrosarcoma of the meninges. Acta Neuropathol 1972;22:272–274.
16. Rushing EJ, Armonda RA, Ansari Q, et al. Mesenchymal chondrosarcoma. A clinicopathologic and flow cytometric study of 13 cases presenting in the central nervous system. Cancer 1996;77:1884–1891.
17. Salcman M, Scholtz H, Kristt D, et al. Extraskeletal myxoid chondrosarcoma of the falx. Neurosurgery 1992;31:344–348.
18. Scheithauer BW, Rubinstein LJ. Meningeal mesenchymal chondrosarcoma. Report of 8 cases with review of the literature. Cancer 1978;42:2744–2752.
19. Smith TW, Davidson RI. Primary meningeal myxochondrosarcoma presenting as a cerebellar mass: case report. Neurosurgery 1981;8:577–581.
20. Waga S, Matsushima M, Ando K. Intracranial chondrosarcoma with extracranial metastases: case report. J Neurosurg 1972;36:790–794.

**Malignant Melanoma**

1. Adamek D, Kaluza J, Stachura K. Primary balloon cell malignant melanoma of the right temporo-parietal region arising from meningeal naevus. Clin Neuropathol 1995;14:29–32.
2. Allcutt D, Michowiz S, Weitzman S, et al. Primary leptomeningeal melanoma: an unusually aggressive tumor in childhood. Neurosurgery 1993;32:721–729.

3. Balmaceda CM, Fetell MR, Powers J, et al. Nevus of Ota and leptomeningeal melanocytic lesions. Neurology 1993;43:381–386.
4. Brat DJ, Giannini C, Scheithauer BW, et al. Primary melanocytic neoplasms of the central nervous system. Am J Surg Pathol 1999;23:745–754.
5. Kaplan AM, Itabashi HH, Hanelin LG, et al. Neurocutaneous melanosis with malignant leptomeningeal melanoma. Arch Neurol 1975;32:669–671.
6. Morris LL, Danta G. Malignant cerebral melanoma complicating giant pigmented naevus: a case report. J Neurol Neurosurg Psychiatry 1968;31:628–632.
7. Mowat R, Reid R, Mackie R. Balloon cell metastatic melanoma: an important differential in the diagnosis of clear cell tumours. Histopathology 1994;24:469–472.
8. Ochiai K, Nakano S, Miyahara S, et al. Magnetic resonance imaging of a malignant transformation of an intracranial cellular blue nevus. A case report. Surg Neurol 1992;37:371–373.
9. Reed WB, Becker SW Sr, Becker SW Jr, et al. Giant pigmented nevi, melanoma, and leptomeningeal melanocytosis. Arch Dermatol 1965;91:100–119.
10. Reyes-Mugica M, Chou P, Byrd S, et al. Nevomelanocytic proliferations in the central nervous system of children. Cancer 1993;72:2277–2285.
11. Slaughter JC, Hardman JM, Kempe LG, et al. Neurocutaneous melanosis and leptomeningeal melanomatosis in children. Arch Pathol 1969;88:298–304.
12. Theunissen P, Spincemaille G, Pannebakker M, et al. Meningeal melanoma associated with nevus of Ota: case report and review. Clin Neuropathol 1993;12:125–129.

### Meningeal Glioma and Gliomatosis
1. Bailey OT. Relation of glioma of the leptomeninges to neuroglia nests. Report of a case of astrocytoma of the leptomeninges. Arch Pathol 1936;21:584–600.
2. Cooper IS, Kernohan JW. Heterotopic glial nests in the subarachnoid space: histopathologic characteristics, mode of origin and relation to meningeal gliomas. Neuropathol Exp Neurol 1951;10:16–29.
3. Davila G, Dyckaerts C, Lazareth JP, et al. Clinical study. Diffuse primary leptomeningeal gliomatosis. J Neurooncol 1993;15:45–49.
4. Dietrich P-Y, Aapro MS, Rieder A, et al. Clinical study. Primary diffuse leptomeningeal gliomatosis (PDLG): a neoplastic cause of chronic meningitis. J Neurooncol 1993;15:275–283.
5. Grant R, Naylor B, Junck L, et al. Clinical outcome in aggressively treated meningeal gliomatosis. Neurology 1992;42:252–254.
6. Kakita A, Wakabayashi K, Takahashi H, et al. Case reports. Primary leptomeningeal glioma: ultrastructural and laminin immunohistochemical studies. Acta Neuropathol 1992;83:538–542.
7. Kitahara M, Katakura R, Wada T, et al. Diffuse form of primary leptomeningeal gliomatosis. Case report. J Neurosurg 1985;63:283–287.
8. Moonis M, Smith TW. Meningeal gliomatosis presenting as multiple cerebral infarcts: a case report. Neurology 1996;46:1760–1762.
9. Polmeteer FE, Kernohan JW. Meningeal gliomatosis. A study of forty-two cases. Arch Neurol Psychiatry 1947;57:593–616.
10. Sceats DJ Jr, Quisling R, Rhoton AL Jr, et al. Primary leptomeningeal glioma mimicking an acoustic neuroma: case report with review of the literature. Neurosurgery 1986;19:649–654.
11. Vertosik F Jr, Selker R. Brain stem and spinal metastases of supratentorial glioblastoma multiforme: a clinical series. Neurosurgery 1990;27:516–522.
12. Yung W-KA, Horten BC, Shapiro WR. Meningeal gliomatosis: a review of 12 cases. Ann Neurol 1980;8:605–608.

### Metastatic Carcinoma
1. Bokstein F, Lossos A, Siegal T. Leptomeningeal metastases from solid tumors. A comparison of two prospective series treated with and without intra-cerebrospinal fluid chemotherapy. Cancer 1998;82:1756–1763.
2. Cheng TM, O'Neill BP, Scheithauer BW, et al. Chronic meningitis: the role of meningeal or cortical biopsy. Neurosurgery 1994;34:590–595.
3. Fink LH. Metastasis of prostatic adenocarcinoma simulating a falx meningioma. Surg Neurol 1979;12:253–258.
4. Glantz MJ, Hall WA, Cole BF, et al. Diagnosis, management, and survival of patients with leptomeningeal cancer based on cerebrospinal fluid-flow status. Cancer 1995;75:2919–2931.
5. Gonzalez-Vitale JC, Garcia-Bunuel R. Meningeal carcinomatosis. Cancer 1976;37:2906–2911.
6. Herman DL, Courville CB. Pathogenesis of meningeal carcinomatosis: report of case secondary to carcinoma of cecum via perineural extension: with a review of 146 cases. Bull Los Angeles Neurol Soc 1965;30:107–117.
7. Jayson GC, Howell A, Harris M, et al. Carcinomatous meningitis in patients with breast cancer. Cancer 1994;74:3135–3141.
8. Kokkoris CP. Leptomeningeal carcinomatosis: how does cancer reach the pia-arachnoid? Cancer 1983;51:154–160.
9. Nakagawa H, Murasawa A, Kubo S, et al. Clinical study. Diagnosis and treatment of patients with meningeal carcinomatosis. J Neurooncol 1992;13:81–89.
10. Sze G, Soletsky S, Bronen R, et al. MR imaging of the cranial meninges with emphasis on contrast enhancement and meningeal carcinomatosis. AJNR 1989;10:965–975.

### Myeloproliferative and Lymphoproliferative Diseases
1. Azzarelli B, Roessmann U. Pathogenesis of central nervous system infiltration in acute leukemia. Arch Pathol Lab Med 1977;101:203–205.
2. Clarke E. Cranial and intracranial myelomas. Brain 1954;77:61–81.
3. Demaray MJ, Coladonato JP, Parker JC Jr, et al. Intracerebellar chloroma (granulocytic sarcoma): a neurosurgical complication of acute myelogenous leukemia. Surg Neurol 1976;6:353–359.
4. Gold JH, Shelburne JD, Bossen EH. Meningeal mycosis fungoides: cytologic and ultrastructural aspects. Acta Cytol 1976;20:349–355.
5. Ho DM-T, Wong T-T, Guo W-Y, et al. Primary cerebellar extramedullary myeloid cell tumor mimicking oligodendroglioma. Acta Neuropathol 1997;94:398–402.
6. Ironside JW, Martin JF, Richmond J, et al. Lymphomatoid granulomatosis with cerebral involvement. Neuropathol Appl Neurobiol 1984;10:397–406.
7. Jazy FK, Shehata WM, Tew JM. Primary intracranial lymphoma of the dura. Arch Neurol 1980;37:528–529.
8. Kumar S, Kumar D, Kaldjian EP, et al. Primary low-grade B-cell lymphoma of the dura. A mucosa associated lymphoid tissue-type lymphoma. Am J Surg Pathol 1997;21:81–87.
9. Lachance DH, O'Neill BP, Macdonald DR, et al. Primary leptomeningeal lymphoma: report of 9 cases, diagnosis with immunocytochemical analysis, and review of the literature. Neurology 1991;41:95–100.
10. Llena JF, Kawamoto K, Hirano A, et al. Granulocytic sarcoma of the central nervous system: initial presentation of leukemia. Acta Neuropathol 1978;42:145–147.
11. McCarthy J, Proctor SJ. Cerebral involvement in multiple myeloma: case report. J Clin Pathol 1978;31:259–264.
12. Michaud J, Banerjee D, Kaufmann JCE. Lymphomatoid granulomatosis involving the central nervous system: complication of a renal transplant with terminal monoclonal B-cell proliferation. Acta Neuropathol 1983;61:141–147.
13. Moore EW, Thomas LB, Shaw RK, et al. The central nervous system in acute leukemia: a postmortem study of 117 consecutive cases, with particular reference to hemorrhage, leukemic infiltrations, and the syndrome of meningeal leukemia. Arch Intern Med 1960;105:451–468.
14. Moran CC, Anderson CC, Caldemeyer KS, et al. Meningeal myelomatosis: CT and MR appearances. AJNR 1995;16:1501–1503.
15. Nickels J, Koivuniemi A, Heiskanen O. Granulocytic sarcoma (chloroma) of the cerebellum and meninges: a case report. Acta Neurochir 1979;46:279–301.
16. Pena CE. Lymphomatoid granulomatosis with cerebral involvement: light and electron microscopic study of a case. Acta Neuropathol 1977;37:193–197.
17. Schmidt BJ, Meagher-Villemure K, Del Carpio J. Lymphomatoid granulomatosis with isolated involvement of the brain. Ann Neurol 1984;15:478–481.
18. Schulman P, Sun T, Sharer L, et al. Meningeal involvement in IgD myeloma with cerebrospinal fluid paraprotein analysis. Cancer 1980;46:152–155.

19. Slager UT, Taylor WF, Opfell RW, et al. Leptomeningeal myeloma. Arch Pathol Lab Med 1979;103:680–682.
20. Stewart DJ, Smith TL, Keating MJ, et al. Remission from central nervous system involvement in adults with acute leukemia: effect of intensive therapy and prognostic factors. Cancer 1985;56: 632–641.
21. Viadana E, Bross ID, Pickren JW. An autopsy study of the metastatic patterns of human leukemias. Oncology 1978;35: 87–96.
22. Wolk RW, Masse SR, Conklin R, et al. The incidence of central nervous system leukemia in adults with acute leukemia. Cancer 1974;33:863–869.

## Arachnoid Cyst

1. Albuquerque FC, Giannotta SL. Arachnoid cyst rupture producing subdural hygroma and intracranial hypertension: case reports. Neurosurgery 1997;41:951–956.
2. Erdincler P, Kaynar MY, Bozkus H, et al. Posterior fossa arachnoid cysts. Br J Neurosurg 1999;13:10–17.
3. Go KG, Houthoff HF, Blaauw EH. Arachnoid cysts of the sylvian fissure: evidence of fluid secretion. J Neurosurg 1984;60: 803–813.
4. Go KG, Houthoff HJ, Blaauw EH, et al. Morphology and origin of arachnoid cysts: scanning and transmission electron microscopy of three cases. Acta Neuropathol 1978;44:57–62.
5. Golaz J, Bouras C. Frontal arachnoid cyst. A case of bilateral frontal arachnoid cyst without clinical signs. Clin Neuropathol 1993;12:73–78.
6. Inoue T, Matsushima T, Fukui M, et al. Immunohistochemical study of intracranial cysts. Neurosurgery 1988;23:576–581.
7. Jallo GI, Woo HH, Meshki C, et al. Arachnoid cysts of the cerebellopontine angle: diagnosis and surgery. Neurosurgery 1997;40: 31–38.
8. Krawchenko J, Collins GH. Pathology of an arachnoid cyst. Case report. J Neurosurg 1979;50:224–228.
9. Oberbauer RW, Haase J, Pucher R. Arachnoid cysts in children: a European co-operative study. Childs Nerv Syst 1992;8:281–286.
10. Parsch CS, Krauß J, Hofmann E, et al. Arachnoid cysts associated with subdural hematomas and hygromas: analysis of 16 cases, long-term follow-up, and review of the literature. Neurosurgery 1997;40:483–490.
11. Passero S, Filosomi G, Cioni R, et al. Arachnoid cysts of the middle cranial fossa: a clinical, radiological and follow-up study. Acta Neurol Scand 1990;82:94–100.
12. Rengachary SS, Watanabe I. Ultrastructure and pathogenesis of intracranial arachnoid cysts. J Neuropathol Exp Neurol 1981;40: 61–83.
13. Samii M, Carvalho GA, Schuhmann MU, et al. Arachnoid cysts of the posterior fossa. Surg Neurol 1999;51:376–382.
14. Shaw C-M. "Arachnoid cysts" of the sylvian fissure versus "temporal lobe agenesis" syndrome. Ann Neurol 1979;5:483–485.
15. Sommer IEC, Smit LME. Congenital supratentorial arachnoidal and giant cysts in children: a clinical study with arguments for a conservative approach. Childs Nerv Syst 1997;13:8–12.
16. Wester K. Peculiarities of intracranial arachnoid cysts: location, sidedness, and sex distribution in 126 consecutive patients. Neurosurgery 1999;45:775–779.
17. Wester K. Gender distribution and sidedness of middle fossa arachnoid cysts: a review of cases diagnosed with computed imaging. Neurosurgery 1992;31:940–944.
18. Wiener SN, Pearlstein AE, Eiber A. MR imaging of intracranial arachnoid cysts. J Comput Assist Tomogr 1987;11:236–241.

## Epidermoid and Dermoid Cysts

1. Cannon TC, Bane BL, Kistler D, et al. Primary intracerebellar osteosarcoma arising within an epidermoid cyst. Arch Pathol Lab Med 1998;122:737–739.
2. Catala M, Pradat P-F, Cornu P, et al. A case of epidermoid cyst arising from the rostral neuropore: case report. Neurosurgery 1998;43:374–376.
3. Garcia CA, McGarry PA, Rodriguez F. Primary intracranial squamous cell carcinoma of the right cerebellopontine angle: case report. J Neurosurg 1981;54:824–828.
4. Gluszcz A. A cancer arising in a dermoid of the brain: a case report. J Neuropathol Exp Neurol 1962;21:383–387.
5. Goffin J, Plets C, Van Calenbergh F, et al. Posterior fossa dermoid cyst associated with dermal fistula: report of 2 cases and review of the literature. Childs Nerv Syst 1993;9:179–181.
6. Goldman SA, Gandy SE. Squamous cell carcinoma as a late complication of intracerebroventricular epidermoid cyst. J Neurosurg 1987;66:618–620.
7. Gormley WB, Tomecek FJ, Qureshi N, et al. Craniocerebral epidermoid and dermoid tumours: a review of 32 cases. Acta Neurochir 1994;128:115–121.
8. Gutin PH, Boehm J, Bank WO, et al. Cerebral convexity epidermoid tumor subsequent to multiple percutaneous subdural aspirations. Case report. J Neurosurg 1980;52:574–577.
9. Higashi S, Takinami K, Yamashita J. Occipital dermal sinus associated with dermoid cyst in the fourth ventricle. AJNR 1995; 16:945–948.
10. Hitchcock MG, Ellington KS, Friedman AH, et al. Shadow cells in an intracranial dermoid cyst. Arch Pathol Lab Med 1995; 119:371–373.
11. Horowitz BL, Chari MV, James R, et al. MR of intracranial epidermoid tumors: correlation of in vivo imaging with in vitro $^{13}$C spectroscopy. AJNR 1990;11:299–302.
12. Ikushima I, Korogi Y, Hirai T, et al. MR of epidermoids with a variety of pulse sequences. AJNR 1997;18:1359–1363.
13. Knorr JR, Ragland RL, Smith TW, et al. Squamous carcinoma arising in a cerebellopontine angle epidermoid: CT and MR findings. AJNR 1991;12:1182–1184.
14. Logue V, Till K. Posterior fossa dermoid cysts with special reference to intracranial infection. J Neurol Neurosurg Psychiatry 1952;15:1–12.
15. Lunardi P, Missori P, Rizzo A, et al. Chemical meningitis in ruptured intracranial dermoid. Case report and review of the literature. Surg Neurol 1989;32:449–452.
16. Lunardi P, Missori P, Gagliardi FM, et al. Dermoid cysts of the posterior cranial fossa in children. Report of nine cases and review of the literature. Surg Neurol 1990;34:39–42.
17. Mohanty A, Venkatrama SK, Rao BR, et al. Experience with cerebellopontine angle epidermoids. Neurosurgery 1997;40: 24–30.
18. Smith AS, Benson JE, Blaser SI, et al. Diagnosis of ruptured intracranial dermoid cyst: value of MR over CT. AJNR 1991; 12:175–180.
19. Talacchi A, Sala F, Alessandrini F, et al. Assessment and surgical management of posterior fossa epidermoid tumors: report of 28 cases. Neurosurgery 1998;42:242–252.
20. Tampieri D, Melanson D, Ethier R. MR imaging of epidermoid cysts. AJNR 1989;10:351–356.
21. Vinchon M, Pertuzon B, Lejeune J-P, et al. Intradural epidermoid cysts of the cerebellopontine angle: diagnosis and surgery. Neurosurgery 1995;36:52–57.

## Enterogenous Cyst

1. Bejjani GK, Wright DC, Schessel D, et al. Endodermal cysts of the posterior fossa. Report of three cases and review of the literature. J Neurosurg 1998;89:326–335.
2. Del Bigio MR, Jay V, Drake JM. Prepontine cyst lined by respiratory epithelium with squamous metaplasia: immunohistochemical and ultrastructural study. Acta Neuropathol 1992;83:564–568.
3. Eynon-Lewis NJ, Kitchen N, Scaravilli F, et al. Neurenteric cyst of the cerebellopontine angle: case report. Neurosurgery 1998; 42:655–658.
4. Ho LC, Olivi A, Cho CH, et al. Well-differentiated papillary adenocarcinoma arising in a supratentorial enterogenous cyst: case report. Neurosurgery 1998;43:1474–1477.
5. Kim CY, Wang KC, Choe G, et al. Neurenteric cyst: its various presentations. Childs Nerv Syst 1999;15:333–341.
6. Perry A, Scheithauer BW, Zaias BW, et al. Aggressive enterogenous cyst with extensive craniospinal spread: case report. Neurosurgery 1999;44:401–404.
7. Schelper RL, Kagan-Hallet KS, Huntington HW. Brainstem subarachnoid respiratory epithelial cysts: report of two cases and review of the literature. Hum Pathol 1986;17:417–422.
8. Umezu H, Aiba T, Unakami M. Enterogenous cyst of the cerebellopontine angle cistern: case report. Neurosurgery 1991;23: 462–466.

## Sarcoidosis

1. Carmody RF, Mafee MF, Goodwin JA, et al. Orbital and optic pathway sarcoidosis: MR findings. AJNR 1994;15:775–783.
2. Clark WC, Acker JD, Dohan FC Jr, et al. Presentation of central nervous system sarcoidosis as intracranial tumors. J Neurosurg 1985;63:851–856.

3. Jackson RJ, Goodman JC, Huston DP, et al. Parafalcine and bilateral convexity neurosarcoidosis mimicking meningioma: case report and review of the literature. Neurosurgery 1998;42: 635–638.

4. Kraichoke S, Cosgrove M, Chandrasoma PT. Granulomatous inflammation in pineal germinoma. A cause of diagnostic failure at stereotaxic brain biopsy. Am J Surg Pathol 1988;12:655–660.

5. Ranoux D, Devaux B, Lamy C, et al. Meningeal sarcoidosis, pseudo-meningioma, and pachymeningitis of the convexity. J Neurol Neurosurg Psychiatry 1992;55:300–303.

6. Scully RE (ed). Case records of the Massachusetts General Hospital. Case 37-1996. N Engl J Med 1996;335:1668–1674.

7. Sherman JL, Stern BJ. Sarcoidosis of the CNS: comparison of unenhanced and enhanced MR images. AJNR 1990;11:915–923.

8. Stern BJ, Krumholz A, Johns C, et al. Sarcoidosis and its neurological manifestations. Arch Neurol 1985;42:909–917.

9. Stübgen J-P. Neurosarcoidosis presenting as a retroclival mass. Surg Neurol 1995;43:85–88.

10. Thomas G, Murphy S, Staunton H, et al. Pathogen-free granulomatous diseases of the central nervous system. Hum Pathol 1998;29:110–115.

## Plasma Cell Granuloma

1. Cannella DM, Prezyna AP, Kapp JP. Primary intracranial plasma-cell granuloma. Case report. J Neurosurg 1988;69:785–788.

2. Gangemi M, Maiuri F, Giamundo A, et al. Intracranial plasma cell granuloma. Neurosurgery 1989;24:591–595.

3. Gochman GA, Duffy K, Crandall PH, et al. Plasma cell granuloma of the brain. Surg Neurol 1990;33:347–352.

4. Han MH, Chi JG, Kim MS, et al. Fibrosing inflammatory pseudotumors involving the skull base: MR and CT manifestations with histopathologic comparison. AJNR 1996;17:515–521.

5. Le Marc'hadour F, Fransen P, Labat-Moleur F, et al. Intracranial plasma cell granuloma: a report of four cases. Surg Neurol 1994;42:481–488.

6. Maeda Y, Tani E, Nakano M, et al. Plasma-cell granuloma of the fourth ventricle. Case report. J Neurosurg 1984;60:1291–1296.

7. Makino K, Murakami M, Kitano I, et al. Primary intracranial plasma-cell granuloma: case report and review of the literature. Surg Neurol 1995;43:374–378.

8. Mirra SS, Tindall SC, Check IJ, et al. Inflammatory meningeal masses of unexplained origin. An ultrastructural and immunological study. J Neuropathol Exp Neurol 1983;42:453–468.

9. Nazek M, Mandybur TI, Sawaya R. Hyalinizing plasmacytic granulomatosis of the falx. Am J Surg Pathol 1988;12:308–313.

10. Pimentel J, Costa A, Tavora L. Inflammatory pseudotumor of the choroid plexus. Case report. J Neurosurg 1993;79:939–942.

11. Sitton JE, Harkin JC, Gerber MA. Intracranial inflammatory pseudotumor. Clin Neuropathol 1992;11:36–40.

12. Tresser N, Rolf C, Cohen M. Plasma cell granulomas of the brain: pediatric case presentation and review of the literature. Childs Nerv Syst 1996;12:52–57.

## Rosai-Dorfman Disease

1. Carey MP, Case CP. Case report. Sinus histiocytosis with massive lymphadenopathy presenting as a meningioma. Neuropathol Appl Neurobiol 1987;13:391–398.

2. Foucar E, Rosai J, Dorfman R. Sinus histiocytosis with massive lymphadenopathy (Rosai-Dorfman disease): review of the entity. Semin Diagn Pathol 1990;7:19–73.

3. Foucar E, Rosai J, Dorfman RF, et al. The neurologic manifestations of sinus histiocytosis with massive lymphadenopathy. Neurology 1982;32:365–371.

4. Gaetani P, Tancioni F, Di Rocco M, et al. Isolated cerebellar involvement in Rosai-Dorfman disease: case report. Neurosurgery 2000;46:479–481.

5. Kattner KA, Stroink AR, Roth TC, et al. Rosai-Dorfman disease mimicking parasagittal meningioma: case presentation and review of literature. Surg Neurol 2000;53:452–457.

6. Kim M, Provias J, Berstein M. Rosai-Dorfman disease mimicking multiple meningioma: case report. Neurosurgery 1995;36: 1185–1187.

7. Lopez P, Estes ML. Immunohistochemical characterization of the histiocytes in sinus histiocytosis with massive lymphadenopathy: analysis of an extranodal case. Hum Pathol 1989;20:711–715.

8. Rosai J, Dorfman RF. Sinus histiocytosis with massive lym-

phadenopathy: a pseudolymphomatous benign disorder. Cancer 1972;30:1174–1188.

9. Song SK, Schwartz IS, Strauchen JA, et al. Case report. Meningeal nodules with features of extranodal sinus histiocytosis with massive lymphadenopathy. Am J Surg Pathol 1989;13: 406–412.

10. Udono H, Fukuyama K, Okamoto H, et al. Rosai-Dorfman disease presenting multiple intracranial lesions with unique findings on magnetic resonance imaging. Case report. J Neurosurg 1999;91:335–339.

## Castleman's Disease

1. Gianaris PG, Leestma JE, Cerullo LJ, et al. Castleman's disease manifesting in the central nervous system: case report with immunological studies. Neurosurgery 1989;24:608–613.

2. Keller AR, Hochholzer L, Castleman B. Hyaline-vascular and plasma-cell types of giant lymph node hyperplasia of the mediastinum and other locations. Cancer 1972;29:670–683.

3. Lacombe M-J, Poirier J, Caron J-P. Intracranial lesion resembling giant lymph node hyperplasia. Am J Clin Pathol 1983;80: 721–723.

4. Severson GS, Harrington DS, Weisenburger DD, et al. Castleman's disease of the leptomeninges. Report of three cases. J Neurosurg 1988;69:283–286.

## Hypertrophic Pachymeningitis

1. Hatano N, Behari S, Nagatani T, et al. Idiopathic hypertrophic cranial pachymeningitis: clinicoradiological spectrum and therapeutic options. Neurosurgery 1999;45:1336–1342; discussion 42–44.

2. Mamelak AN, Kelly WM, Davis RL, et al. Idiopathic hypertrophic cranial pachymeningitis. J Neurosurg 1993;79:270–276.

## Collagen-Vascular Diseases

1. Alexander EL. Neurologic disease in Sjögren's syndrome: mononuclear inflammatory vasculopathy affecting central/peripheral nervous system and muscle. A clinical review and update of immunopathogenesis. Rheum Dis Clin North Am 1993;19: 869–908.

2. Alexander EL, Beall SS, Gordon B, et al. Magnetic resonance imaging of cerebral lesions in patients with the Sjögren syndrome. Ann Intern Med 1988;108:815–823.

3. Bathon JM, Moreland LW, DiBartolomeo AG. Inflammatory central nervous system involvement in rheumatoid arthritis. Semin Arthritis Rheum 1989;18:258–266.

4. Chang Y, Horoupian DS, Lane B, et al. Inflammatory pseudotumor of the choroid plexus in Sjögren's disease. Neurosurgery 1991;29:287–290.

5. Czarnecki EJ, Spickler EM. MR demonstration of Wegener granulomatosis of the infundibulum, a cause of diabetes insipidus. AJNR 1995;16:968–970.

6. de la Monte SM, Hutchins GM, Gupta PK. Polymorphous meningitis with atypical mononuclear cells in Sjögren's syndrome. Ann Neurol 1983;14:455–461.

7. Drachman DA. Neurological complications of Wegener's granulomatosis. Arch Neurol 1963;8:145–155.

8. Ellis SG, Verity MA. Central nervous system involvement in systemic lupus erythematosus: a review of neuropathologic findings in 57 cases, 1955–1977. Semin Arthritis Rheum 1979;8:212–221.

9. Ferreiro JE, Robalino BD, Saldana MJ. Primary Sjögren's syndrome with diffuse cerebral vasculitis and lymphocytic interstitial pneumonitis. Am J Med 1987;82:1227–1232.

10. Giordano MJ, Commins D, Silbergeld DL. Sjögren's cerebritis complicated by subarachnoid hemorrhage and bilateral superior cerebellar artery occlusion: case report. Surg Neurol 1995;43: 48–51.

11. Helmberger RC, Mancuso AA. Wegener granulomatosis of the eustachian tube and skull base mimicking a malignant tumor. AJNR 1996;17:1785–1790.

12. Jinnah HA, Dixon A, Brat DJ, et al. Chronic meningitis with cranial neuropathies in Wegener's granulomatosis. Arthritis Rheum 1997;40:573–577.

13. Johnson R, Richardson E. The neurological manifestations of systemic lupus erythematosus. Medicine (Baltimore) 1968;47: 337–369.

14. Kepes JJ, Dunlap MD, O'Boynick P, et al. Meningioma with multiple rheumatoid nodules. A case report. Acta Neuropathol 1986;70:314–319.

15. Maher JA. Dural nodules in rheumatoid arthritis. Report of a case. Arch Pathol 1954;58:354–359.

16. McCune WJ, MacGuire A, Aisen A, et al. Identification of brain lesions in neuropsychiatric systemic lupus erythematosus by magnetic resonance scanning. Arthritis Rheum 1988;31:159–166.

17. Miller KS, Miller JM. Wegener's granulomatosis presenting as a primary seizure disorder with brain lesions demonstrated by magnetic resonance imaging. Chest 1993;103:316–318.

18. Nishino N, Rubino FA, DeRemee RA, et al. Neurological involvement in Wegener's granulomatosis: an analysis of 324 consecutive patients at the Mayo Clinic. Ann Neurol 1993;33:4–9.

19. Ouyang R, Mitchell M, Rozdilsky B. Central nervous system involvement in rheumatoid disease. Report of a case. Neurology 1967;17:1099–1105.

20. Provenzale JM, Allen NB. Wegener granulomatosis: CT and MR findings. AJNR 1996;17:785–792.

21. Satoh J, Miyasaka N, Yamada T, et al. Case report. Extensive cerebral infarction due to involvement of both anterior cerebral arteries by Wegener's granulomatosis. Ann Rheum Dis 1988;47: 606–611.

22. Schachenmayr W, Friede RL. Dural involvement in rheumatoid arthritis. Acta Neuropathol 1978;42:65–66.

23. Scully RE (ed). Case records of the Massachusetts General Hospital. Case 12-1988. N Engl J Med 1988;318:760–768.

24. Scully RE (ed). Case records of the Massachusetts General Hospital. Weekly clinicopathological exercises. Case 9-1999. A 74-year-old woman with hydrocephalus and pleocytosis [clinical conference]. N Engl J Med 1999;340:945–953.

25. Sibbitt WL Jr, Haseler LJ, Griffey RH, et al. Analysis of cerebral structural changes in systemic lupus erythematosus by proton MR spectroscopy. AJNR 1994;15:923–928.

26. Spranger M, Schwab S, Meinck H-M, et al. Meningeal involvement in Wegener's granulomatosis confirmed and monitored by positive circulating antineutrophil cytoplasm in cerebrospinal fluid. Neurology 1997;48:263–265.

27. Spurlock RG, Richman AV. Rheumatoid meningitis. A case report and review of the literature. Arch Pathol Lab Med 1983;107: 129–131.

28. Tishler S, Williamson T, Mirra SS, et al. Wegener granulomatosis with meningeal involvement. AJNR 1993;14:1248–1252.

29. Weinberger LM, Cohen ML, Remler BF, et al. Intracranial Wegener's granulomatosis. Neurology 1993;43:1831–1834.

## Meningioangiomatosis

1. Blumenthal D, Berho M, Bloomfield S, et al. Childhood meningioma associated with meningioangiomatosis. Case report. J Neurosurg 1993;78:287–289.

2. Chakrabarty A, Franks AJ. Meningioangiomatosis: a case report and review of the literature. Br J Neurosurg 1999;13:167–173.

3. Giangaspero F, Guiducci A, Lentz FA, et al. Meningioma with meningioangiomatosis. A condition mimicking invasive meningiomas in children and young adults. Report of two cases and review of the literature. Am J Surg Pathol 1999;23:872–875.

4. Goates JJ, Dickson DW, Horoupian DS. Meningioangiomatosis: an immunocytochemical study. Acta Neuropathol 1991;82: 527–532.

5. Halper J, Scheithauer BW, Okazaki H, et al. Meningioangiomatosis: a report of six cases with special reference to the occurrence of neurofibrillary tangles. J Neuropathol Exp Neurol 1986;45:426–446.

6. Harada K, Inagawa T, Nagasako R. A case of meningioangiomatosis without von Recklinghausen's disease. Report of a case and review of 13 cases. Childs Nerv Syst 1994;10:126–130.

7. Liu SS, Johnson PC, Sonntag VKH. Meningioangiomatosis: a case report. Surg Neurol 1989;31:376–380.

8. López JI, Ereño C, Oleaga L, Areitio E. Meningioangiomatosis and oligodendroglioma in a 15-year-old boy. Arch Pathol Lab Med 1996;120:587–590.

9. Mokhtari K, Uchilhara T, Clémenceau S, et al. Atypical neuronal inclusion bodies in meningioangiomatosis. Acta Neuropathol 1998;96:91–96.

10. Ogilvy CS, Chapman PH, Gray M, et al. Meningioangiomatosis in a patient without von Recklinghausen's disease. J Neurosurg 1989;70:483–485.

11. Prayson RA. Meningioangiomatosis. A clinicopathologic study including MIB1 immunoreactivity. Arch Pathol Lab Med 1995;119:1061–1064.

12. Sakaki S, Nakagawa K, Nakamura K, et al. Meningioangiomatosis not associated with von Recklinghausen's disease. Neurosurgery 1987;20:797–801.

13. Stemmer-Rachamimov AO, Horgan MA, Taratuto AL, et al. Meningioangiomatosis is associated with neurofibromatosis 2 but not with somatic alterations of the NF2 gene. J Neuropathol Exp Neurol 1997;56:485–489.

14. Tien RD, Oakes JW, Madden JF, et al. Meningioangiomatosis: CT and MR findings. J Comput Assist Tomogr 1992;16:361–365.

15. Wiebe S, Munoz DG, Smith S, et al. Meningioangiomatosis. A comprehensive analysis of clinical and laboratory features. Brain 1999;122:709–726.

## Calcifying Pseudoneoplasm ("Fibro-Osseous Lesion") of the Neuraxis

1. Bertoni F, Unni K, Dahlin DC, et al. Calcifying pseudoneoplasms of the neural axis. J Neurosurg 1990;72:42–48.

2. Garen PD, Powers JM, King JS, et al. Intracranial fibro-osseous lesion. Case report. J Neurosurg 1989;70:475–477.

3. Halper J, Scheithauer BW, Okazaki H, et al. Meningioangiomatosis: a report of six cases with special reference to the occurrence of neurofibrillary tangles. J Neuropathol Exp Neurol 1986;45:426–446.

4. Jun C, Burdick B. An unusual fibro-osseous lesion of the brain. Case report. J Neurosurg 1984;60:1308–1311.

5. Qian J, Rubio A, Powers JM, et al. Fibro-osseous lesions of the central nervous system: report of four cases and literature review. Am J Surg Pathol 1999;23:1270–1275.

6. Rhodes RH, Davis RL. An unusual fibro-osseous component in intracranial lesions. Hum Pathol 1978;9:309–319.

## Meningeal Response to Intracranial Hypotension

1. Good DC, Ghobrial M. Pathologic changes associated with intracranial hypotension and meningeal enhancement on MRI. Neurology 1993;43:2698–2700.

2. Hochman MS, Naidich TP, Kobetz SA, et al. Spontaneous intracranial hypotension with pachymeningeal enhancement on MRI. Neurology 1992;42:1628–1630.

3. Mokri B, Parisi JE, Scheithauer BW, et al. Meningeal biopsy in intracranial hypotension: meningeal enhancement on MRI. Neurology 1995;45:1801–1817.

# THE BRAIN: INFLAMMATORY DISORDERS

3

In part because of the epidemic of acquired immunodeficiency syndrome (AIDS), but also as a consequence of the long, sure reach of stereotactically guided biopsy systems, inflammatory lesions are seen with increasing frequency among surgical specimens (Table 3–1). In some, the pathologist is rewarded with the gratifying identification of a treatable microorganism. In others, blatant and sometimes bizarre inflammatory reactions remain idiopathic. Still others, such as demyelinating disease, although not explainable, are at least sufficiently stereotypic as to be classifiable and useful in formulating a treatment plan.

## DEMYELINATING DISEASES

### Multiple Sclerosis and Unifocal Demyelinating Disease

Although demyelinating diseases share a selective loss of myelin, the disorders are diverse in localization, clinical expression, and presumed etiology. The pathologist's first duty is to recognize such a lesion for what it is and to avoid misinterpreting it as a neoplasm.[4, 31] Serious consequences may follow unintended radiation therapy for demyelinating diseases.[23] The second task is to distinguish such lesions from other macrophage-rich processes, such as cerebral infarcts. The third challenge is to subclassify the lesion among the sibling entities within the demyelinating disease family. Because demyelinating diseases are

**TABLE 3–1**
**Central Nervous System Inflammatory Diseases Classified by Predominant or Characteristic Cell Type and Tissue Response**

**Polymorphonuclear Leukocytes**

Abscess
Meningitis
   Bacterial
   Fungal
   Amebic (*Naegleria*)
Mycotic aneurysm
Mycoses, especially aspergillosis and phycomycosis
Toxoplasmosis
Acute hemorrhagic leukoencephalitis

**Lymphocytes and Plasma Cells**

Predominantly lymphocytes
   Meningitis
      Viral
      Bacterial
      Other
   Encephalitis
      Viral
      Rickettsial
      Bacterial–Lyme disease
      No organism identified
         Rasmussen's
         Postinfectious, perivenous
         Paraneoplastic
         Lymphocytic hypophysitis
         Behçet's disease
         Other
Predominantly plasma cells
   Syphilis
   Subacute sclerosing panencephalitis
   Plasma cell granuloma (inflammatory pseudotumor)
   Castleman's disease

**Epithelioid Cells, Giant Cells, Granulomas**

Tuberculosis
Sarcoidosis
Mycotic infections
Amebiasis (*Acanthamoeba*)
Human immunodeficiency virus (HIV)
Granulomatous angiitis
Temporal arteritis
Giant cell granuloma of adenohypophysis
Collagen-vascular disease
   Rheumatoid nodule
   Wegener's granulomatosis

Granulomatous inflammation accompanying germinoma
Textiloma
Other

**Macrophages**

Demyelinating diseases
Necrotizing myelopathy (including transverse myelitis and systemic lupus erythematosus myelitis)
Progressive multifocal leukoencephalopathy
Turberculosis (*Mycobacterium avium intracellulare*)
Whipple's disease
Malakoplakia
Histoplasmosis
Extramedullary sinus histiocytosis (Rosai-Dorfman disease)
Xanthomatous lesions
Primary central nervous system lymphomas treated with steroids

**Langerhans Cells**

Langerhans cell histiocytosis (histiocytosis X)

**Eosinophils**

Parasitic diseases
Eosinophilic granuloma (Langerhans cell histiocytosis)
Subdural hematoma

**Microglia**

Viral encephalitis (including HIV encephalitis)
Rickettsial infection
Rasmussen's encephalitis
Syphilis (general paresis)

**Coagulation Necrosis**

Tuberculosis
Toxoplasmosis
Wegener's granulomatosis
Radiation necrosis
Syphilis (gumma)
Sarcoidosis (focal, intragranuloma in some cases)
Mycoses

**Necrobiotic Collagen**

Rheumatoid nodule
Wegener's granulomatosis

---

classified largely on the basis of clinical and radiologic findings, this may not be possible on the basis of histologic findings alone. Unless otherwise specified, the following discussion refers to the pathologic features of the most common and prototypical demyelinating disease, multiple sclerosis. Solitary lesions with the same histologic appearances present a nosologic problem because the clinicopathologic term "multiple sclerosis" is not appropriate. The generic term "demyelinating disease" is a fitting designation.

The combination of spinal and visual pathway lesions, Devic's disease, is illustrated in Figure 11–52.

**Clinical Features.** Multiple sclerosis and unifocal (at least at onset) demyelinating diseases are generally disorders of youthful adults, with women affected more often. Children[7, 12, 26] or adolescents[21] are not totally exempt, nor are the elderly entirely free of risk. In nearly all instances in which multiple plaques are present, the diagnosis is established on clinicoradiologic evidence, supplemented by the electrophoretic finding of oligoclonal bands in cerebrospinal fluid. As a rule, brain biopsy is not necessary. On occasion, however, solitary, and sometimes even multiple, lesions are approached surgically, almost always with the presumptive diagnosis of neoplasia. Especially provocative are large lesions associated with considerable mass effect and edema.[11, 13, 25, 28]

Demyelinating lesions occur throughout the central nervous system (CNS), but many abut the ependyma at the angle of a lateral ventricle. Others lie immediately beneath the cortex.

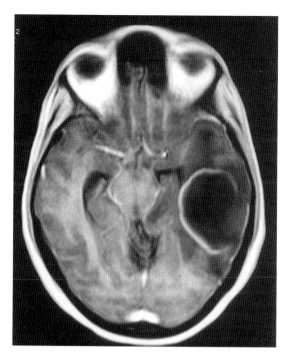

**FIGURE 3-1    DEMYELINATING DISEASE**

Demyelinating disease in its massive Marburg form is an expansile, contrast-enhancing lesion that simulates a glioma. The incomplete, horseshoe-shaped profile of enhancement is characteristic.

**Radiologic Features.** Acute and evolving demyelinating lesions are known for brightness in T2-weighted images and frequent contrast enhancement (Figs. 3–1 to 3–3).[20] The peripheral rim of enhancement is often incomplete, forming a horseshoe-shaped profile (see Fig. 3–1) that is usually seen best in the coronal plane.[16, 22] The incomplete segment faces inwardly toward the ventricle in ependyma-based lesions but opens outwardly, toward the surface, in superficial, subcortical plaques. Circumferential "rim" or "ring" enhancement is common to many CNS entities, but the horseshoe-shaped profile, open at one end, is strongly suggestive of a demyelinating disease.

Perilesional edema is variable around demyelinating disease plaques, but it may be pronounced in rapidly evolving lesions. The concentrically laminated pattern of the Baló variant is rarely seen.[6, 17, 19, 30]

**Microscopic Features.** The principal pathologic features of the demyelinating disease plaques are recorded in Figure 3–2. They are (1) discrete borders, (2) macrophage infiltrates, (3) loss of myelin, (4) perivascular lymphocytic infiltrates, and (5) reactive gliosis, often with so-called granular mitoses or Creutzfeldt cells.

The discreteness of a classical demyelinating lesion is seen best at low magnification in macroscopic specimens of the type not usually available to surgical pathologists. Understandably, this sharp border is present only in needle biopsy specimens taken from target points at the periphery of the lesion (Fig. 3–4).[5] In the more typical specimens, such as those retrieved stereotactically,

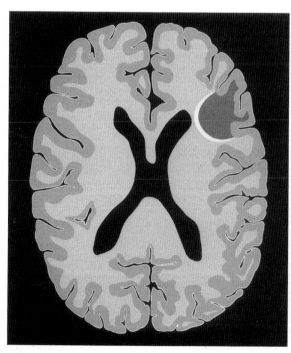

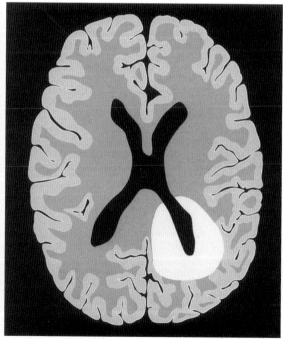

3-2                                3-3

**FIGURES 3-2 AND 3-3    DEMYELINATING DISEASE**

The two diagrams illustrate cardinal radiographic features of demyelinating disease. The horseshoe pattern of contrast enhancement is shown around a superficial demyelinating plaque in Figure 3–2. A paraventricular plaque is illustrated in Figure 3–3; note the lesion's brightness in this representation of a FLAIR image. (From Passe TJ, Beauchamp NJ, Burger PC. Neuroimaging in the identification of low-grade and non-neoplastic CNS lesions. The Neurologist 1999;5:293–299.)

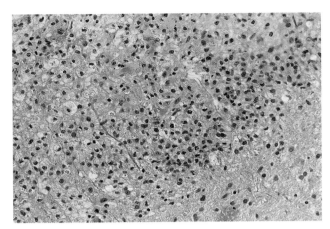

**FIGURE 3–4** DEMYELINATING DISEASE

Demyelinating lesions are cellular and are characterized by a relatively sharp interface with the surrounding brain.

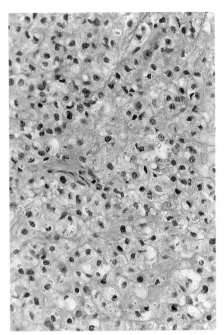

**FIGURE 3–6** DEMYELINATING DISEASE

Macrophages abound in the subacute plaque. Their foamy cytoplasm, discrete cell borders, and bland nuclei are distinctive cytologic features, although they may be subtle in suboptimal preparations.

this telltale feature may be inapparent. One can document the circumscription of demyelinating disease with the aid of myelin stain (Fig. 3–5), but the sharp borders of the lesions are often seen well after hematoxylin and eosin (H&E) staining alone (see Fig. 3–4). Such discreteness is unusual in the infiltrating gliomas, that is, oligodendrogliomas and astrocytomas, that are the principal differential diagnostic possibilities.

The second critical feature of an active demyelinating process, the predominance of macrophages, may be more obvious in cytologic preparations than it is in tissue sections (Fig. 3–6). In either setting, the cell has a bland nucleus, foamy or granular cytoplasm, and a discrete border. Once several macrophages have been identified, the rest usually become obvious and the nature of the process quickly becomes clear. Any lingering doubts can be dispelled by immunostains for macrophages, for example, HAM-56 or CD68 (see Fig. 3–13).[1, 10]

Although the descriptive term *demyelinating* is applied loosely to any lesion with myelin loss, it should be reserved for those wherein myelin is destroyed selectively and not where both myelin and axons are lost, as in a cerebral infarct. Selective demyelination is judged best in companion microsections, one stained for myelin (see Fig. 3–5) and the other for axons (Fig. 3–7). This is not to say that axon preservation is complete in a demyelinating focus, because some axons are acutely fragmented and ultimately lost.

To visualize myelin, we utilize the combined H&E–Luxol fast blue stain (see Fig. 3–5). For demonstrating axons, we recommend either the "silver-threads-

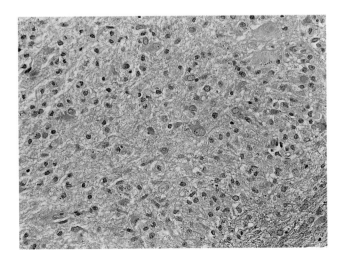

**FIGURE 3–5** DEMYELINATING DISEASE

Myelin stains, such as Luxol fast blue, here combined with hematoxylin and eosin, establish both the discreteness and the demyelinating character of the plaques. Blue, normally myelinated, white matter is seen at the lower right.

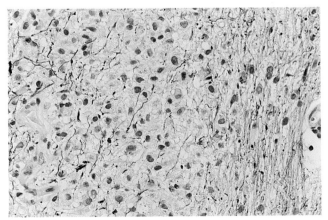

**FIGURE 3–7** DEMYELINATING DISEASE

As seen after immunohistochemical staining for neurofilament protein, axons are clearly preserved within demyelinating lesions (top left). Often, however, they are somewhat fragmented, show an occasional swelling, and are decreased in number. Normal white matter is present at the right.

among-the-gold" effect produced by a metallic method such as the Bielschowsky stain or immunostaining for neurofilament protein (see Fig. 3–7). Even without these techniques, although admittedly with less confidence, one can identify axons in H&E sections as they thread their way between the macrophages. Parenchymal cell loss in a demyelinating focus is generally limited to oligodendrocytes. There is no coagulative necrosis of parenchyma and vasculature. Histologic features of necrosis in CNS lesions are summarized in Table 4–6, page 188.

Perivascular lymphocytic infiltrates impart an inflammatory character to acute and subacute demyelinating lesions but vary in extent from specimen to specimen. The infiltrates are prominent in some lesions (Fig. 3–8) and absent in others. The lymphocytes, both perivascular and intraparenchymal, are largely T cells.[5]

The fifth essential component of the acute and subacute phase of a demyelinating lesion is gliosis, with enlargement of intralesional astrocytes. Only subtle changes are to be seen in astrocytes in the surrounding brain, even those a millimeter beyond the lesion's sharp border. With their expanded glassy cytoplasm, the reactive cells are easy to misinterpret as neoplastic. Glial fibrillary acidic protein (GFAP) staining highlights their size and, in so doing, may only increase the chance that they will be so misinterpreted as neoplastic (see Fig. 3–14). A discussion of gliosis and its distinction from glioma is provided on pages 174 to 175 and 553 to 554.

An interesting and easily overlooked finding of reactive gliosis in demyelinating disease is the curious astrocytic reaction known as granular mitosis or Creutzfeldt cell, a response that produces large, glassy, eosinophilic cells with nuclei fragmented into multiple, small, and seemingly viable micronuclei of varying size (Fig. 3–9).[28] The appearance mimics karyorrhexis and mitosis, but it is actually neither. The changes are to be distinguished from another alteration of reactive astrocytes in which chromosomes disperse or "explode" in a starburst pattern (see Fig. 3–12). Granular mitoses and Creutzfeldt cells are not unheard of in gliomas but are seen most often in reactive lesions, particularly demyelinating disease.

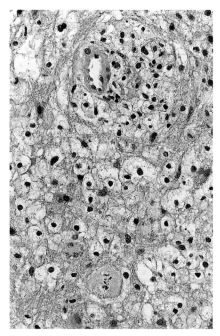

**FIGURE 3–9**    DEMYELINATING DISEASE

The presence of macrophages, particularly when concentrated in the perivascular region, is typical of demyelinating disease, as well as of cerebral infarcts. The presence of two Creutzfeldt cells at the bottom, with their multiple irregular nuclear fragments, supports the diagnosis of a reactive lesion such as demyelinating disease.

**Features in Frozen Sections.** The fine cytologic details by which macrophages can be identified may be effaced by the freezing process, and the lesions often appear as a glioma (Fig 3–10). Perivascular chronic inflammatory cells would be a clue that should bring the disorder into the differential diagnosis and prompt a search for macrophages that may otherwise be overlooked.

**Cytologic Features.** The classical features of macrophages are well seen (Fig. 3–11),[24] as are Creutzfeldt

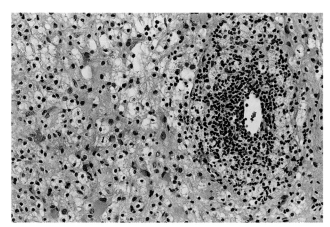

**FIGURE 3–8**    DEMYELINATING DISEASE

Perivascular lymphocytes are a frequent feature of demyelinating disease but are scant or lacking in some cases.

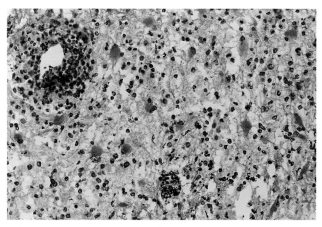

**FIGURE 3–10**    DEMYELINATING DISEASE

In either frozen sections (seen here) or permanent section, the highly cellular plaque can be misinterpreted as a neoplasm. The perivascular inflammation is a clue that the process is inflammatory and not neoplastic.

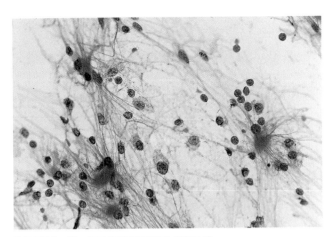

**FIGURE 3–11**    DEMYELINATING DISEASE

Macrophages are most easily identified in cytologic preparations, wherein their bland cytologic features and the full cell bodies with discrete borders are best seen. Reactive astrocytes with long processes are usually prominent.

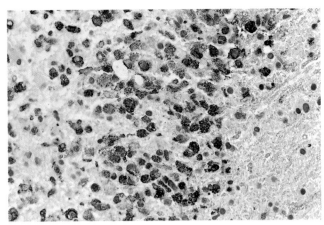

**FIGURE 3–13**    DEMYELINATING DISEASE

Immunostains such as HAM-56 resolve any doubt about the macrophage nature of the foamy cells. Note the border of the plaque at the lower right. The same area is seen in the H&E-stained section in Figure 3–4.

cells and "starburst" mitoses (Fig. 3–12). Large reactive astrocytes, often very conspicuous, with their radiating processes should not be interpreted as neoplastic.

**Immunohistochemical Features.** The overwhelming population of macrophages is readily disclosed by macrophage markers such as HAM-56 or CD68 (Fig. 3–13). GFAP-positive reactive astrocytes are usually prominent (Fig. 3–14).

**Differential Diagnosis.** Demyelinating disease must be distinguished from neoplasia, on the one hand, and from other reactive, macrophage-rich, lesions on the other. The former distinction is of critical importance; the latter is less essential and not always possible. In some instances, however, a simple diagnosis of "Demyelination, See Comment" must suffice.

The distinction from neoplasia begins with an awareness that demyelinating diseases are common and that biopsies are occasionally obtained. The neoplasms most readily mistaken for demyelinating disease are *oligodendroglioma, diffuse astrocytoma,* and *mixed oligoastrocytoma* (Table 4–9, page 213). Clues often reside in the radiographic findings. Infiltrative low-grade astrocytomas and oligodendrogliomas are not enhanced, especially in the horseshoe pattern typical of demyelinating disease.

In contrast to infiltrating gliomas, where there is normal brain in the background, demyelinating disease plaques consist of solid sheets of macrophages in abrupt transition to normal brain (Table 4–6, page 188). Microcysts, common in *oligodendrogliomas,* are not a part of demyelinating disease. On the other hand, clustering of macrophages about vessels is a distinctive feature of demyelinating disease but is alien to infiltrative gliomas. Cytologically, neoplastic oligodendrocytes and macrophages

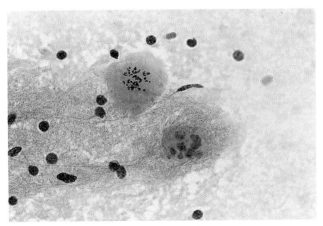

**FIGURE 3–12**    DEMYELINATING DISEASE

Two distinctive elements common in reactive lesions are so-called granular mitoses with a distinctive starburst-like appearance (top left) and Creutzfeldt cells with multiple micronuclei. Transitional forms suggest that the former may evolve into the latter.

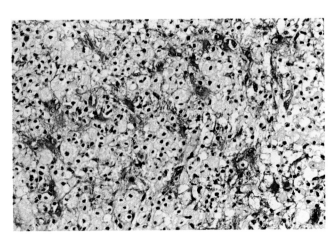

**FIGURE 3–14**    DEMYELINATING DISEASE

Immunohistochemistry for GFAP greatly increases the visibility of reactive astrocytes. Uniformly distributed and star shaped, they should not be misinterpreted as neoplastic.

differ, the latter having sharp cell borders and somewhat granular or foamy periodic acid–Schiff (PAS)–positive cytoplasm. In contrast, the cytoplasm of oligodendrocytes, as an artifact, often undergoes clear cell change. The cell borders of oligodendrocytes are generally indistinct if visible at all.

The *infiltrating fibrillary astrocytoma* enters into the differential diagnoses of demyelinating lesions. The conspicuous reactive cells in the latter are easily selected as a point of concern, while ignoring the predominant, and diagnostically telling, macrophages. In astrocytomas, neoplastic cells generally predominate and are not overshadowed by inflammatory cells, particularly macrophages. Only with great reservation should mitoses be interpreted as evidence of a grade III astrocytoma in the presence of a macrophage infiltrate.

*Granular cell astrocytoma*, a rare lesion, is discussed in Chapter 4 on pages 198 to 199.

A final, and seemingly improbable, entry in the differential diagnosis is a *primary CNS lymphoma* that has been treated previously with corticosteroids. The exquisite sensitivity of many lymphomas to steroids leaves many as little but seas of macrophages in post-treatment specimens. The often advanced age of the patient and the radiologic findings should raise high-level suspicion of lymphoma.

Once neoplasms have been excluded, the nature of non-neoplastic, macrophage-rich lesions must be explored.

Because *infarcts* have a destructive effect on neurons, the issue of infarct versus demyelinating disease is resolved quickly if gray matter is included in the specimen. Recently necrotic neurons are contracted, hypereosinophilic, and karyolytic (see Fig. 7–34). The classical "red neuron" of ischemia is discussed in Chapter 7 on pages 414 to 417. In infarcts, the cortex becomes somewhat granular and hypocellular. Small vessels become prominent and their pericytes and endothelial cells enlarged. Macrophages inundate the area by day 3 or 4. If only white matter is available, the distinction between demyelinating disease and infarction is not always clear-cut, although in many infarcts it is possible to document the loss and fragmentation of axons. Radiologically, infarcts almost always involve some gray matter, whereas demyelinating diseases are clearly based in the white matter.

Acute disseminated encephalomyelitis, progressive multifocal leukoencephalopathy, and herpes simplex encephalitis are discussed individually on pages 119, 129, and 127, respectively.

*Herpes simplex encephalitis* may exhibit some features of demyelinating disease, including macrophage infiltrates, but is an acute necrotizing process that involves gray matter, where both ischemic red neurons and inclusion bodies may be seen. Rather than selective demyelination, in the advanced lesion there is complete parenchymal necrosis that is more akin to infarction than demyelination. Necrosis in demyelinating disease is an event so fleeting and so exquisitely limited to oligodendrocytes as to escape detection in routine clinical material. Clinically and radiologically, the lesions of herpes simplex are often bilateral and frontotemporal in distribution. They feature cortical involvement with gyriform contrast enhancement. Given the heterogeneity of demyelinating diseases, the prognosis for individual patients varies considerably. Some individuals never develop another lesion, whereas other patients incrementally accrue additional neurologic deficits as additional lesions appear. In one study, the presence of concurrent, asymptomatic lesions at the time of initial presentation was strongly predictive of a progressive course, that is, multiple sclerosis.[18] Coincidence may explain the occurrence of infiltrating gliomas that arise in proximity to demyelinating foci.[3, 8, 25, 26, 29]

## Other Forms of Demyelinating Disease

*Demyelinating disease after 5-fluorouracil therapy* is a rare multicentric process that usually occurs in the setting of treatment of colon cancer.[9, 27] Although somewhat smaller and more numerous than those of multiple sclerosis, the lesions are histologically similar.

*Acute disseminated encephalomyelitis* is a poorly understood demyelinating process characterized by multiple lesions in the brain. Onset characteristically follows, by several days to several weeks, a viral syndrome.[2, 14] Numerous small, T2-bright foci are typically evident on magnetic resonance (MR) imaging.[3, 14, 15] Microscopically, the lesions have many of the features of classical demyelinating disease but are smaller, often less well defined, and generally associated with inflammatory infiltrates.

*Progressive multifocal leukoencephalopathy (PML)* is lytic for oligodendrocytes but not, at least initially, for axons. The latter are preserved in a macrophage-rich background. With few exceptions, the process affects immunosuppressed patients, commonly in the setting of AIDS. Astrocytes with bizarre, cytologically atypical if not overtly malignant nuclei may be present. Infected oligodendrocytes with their diagnostic "ground glass" nuclei help to distinguish PML from classic demyelinating diseases. PML is discussed in greater detail on pages 129 to 131.

Some macrophage-rich lesions defy precise classification, especially on the basis of histopathology alone. Indeed, one may have to settle for a descriptive diagnosis of a macrophage-rich lesion, with a discussion of the possibilities and probabilities. Final decisions concerning treatment must then be predicated on clinical and radiographic data. Some demyelinating lesions find no nosologic home, being clinically atypical for any entity. This is particularly true of a solitary lesion that may either represent a sentinel manifestation of what later proves to be multiple sclerosis or remain an isolated, unclassifiable lesion.

## BACTERIAL INFECTIONS

## Pyogenic Abscess

A pyogenic brain abscess is a localized focus of parenchymal suppuration that, with only rare exception, is bacterial in origin. Although the term *abscess* is sometimes loosely applied to a focus of toxoplasmosis, a tuberculoma, or syphilitic gumma, the latter lesions do not contain loculated, purulent liquid.

The organisms' portals of entry, although diverse, can often be inferred from the position and number of the lesions. An isolated focus in the anterior or inferior frontal lobe suggests extension from a paranasal sinus, whereas a lesion in the temporal lobe implicates the middle ear or mastoid sinus as the primary site of infection. Multiple and even single lesions in the superior aspect of the cerebrum strongly suggest hematogenous dissemination. Cerebellar lesions may arise from either otic or hematogenous sources.[18, 23] Lesions geographically related to the path of a penetrating wound or to a site of surgery are logically attributed to direct implantation.[1] Abscesses in the brain stem are variously related to direct extension or hematogenous spread.[11, 21, 22] Abscesses related to neighboring foci of suppuration often lie within the white matter and may be connected to the primary focus via a narrow, transcortical "neck." Curiously, such extensions into brain are usually unaccompanied by disseminated leptomeningitis, although meningitis or a subdural empyema may occur as an isolated finding.

Brain abscesses spare no age group. Although most occur in adults,[26] infants and children may be affected.[9, 15, 25] A primary extracranial site of infection, often the lung, may be apparent. Congenital heart disease with a septal defect enhances the incidence.[24] Although immunocompromised patients are affected occasionally,[12] brain abscesses are infrequent among the opportunistic infections that occur in AIDS. Only rarely do bacteria implant and flourish in infarcts and brain tumors.[19]

**Clinical Features.** The expansile quality of the abscess, as well as the accompanying edema, often results in early signs and symptoms of increased intracranial pressure.[16, 26] Although the clinical evolution of abscesses may be rapid, it can be so leisurely that a glioma, rather than an inflammatory process, is considered. Whereas open resection was often employed in the past, most lesions are now approached stereotactically for drainage and culture before antibiotic therapy.[2]

**Radiologic Features.** In contrast-enhanced images, the capsule is thinner and more uniform than the irregular shaggy rim or ring of enhancement in the glioblastoma (Fig. 3–15A). In addition, the capsule of an abscess is dark on T2-weighted images, in accord with its content of collagen. The cellular rim or ring of a malignant neoplasm such as glioblastoma is white (Fig. 3–15B).[13] A broad perilesional region of cerebral edema reflects the suppurative nature of the lesion. Proton MR spectroscopy may also be useful in diagnosis.[8]

**Macroscopic and Microscopic Features.** In the evolution of a brain abscess, interactions between the causative organism, inflammatory cells, and local fibroblasts are chronicled in a predictable sequence of gross and microscopic events that evolves into a mature encapsulated abscess (Figs. 3–16 and 3–17) Microscopically, cerebritis is seen as hyperemic, acutely inflamed tissue dotted by necrotic blood vessels and extravasated erythrocytes. Bacteria may be plentiful. This early stage of cerebritis is seen by computed tomography as an irregular area of low density with little or no contrast enhancement.[5, 6] Unlike the response to hemorrhage and

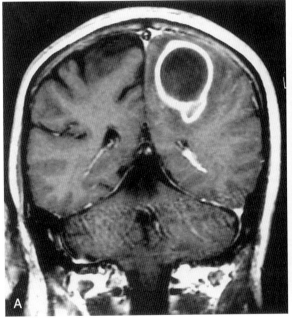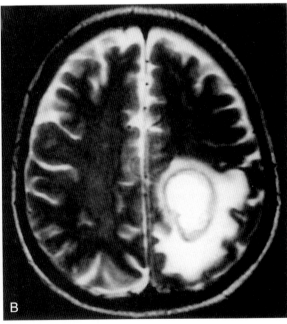

**FIGURE 3–15** PYOGENIC ABSCESS

A brain abscess has a circumferential isometric band of intense contrast enhancement (A) that differs from the coarse, "shaggy," enhancing rim of the glioblastoma. Because of its content of collagen, the capsule of an abscess is characteristically dark on T2-weighted MRI images (B). In contrast, the cellular rims of a glioblastoma and of most other neoplasms are bright. Note the extensive broad zone of perilesional edema in B that is typical of brain abscesses.

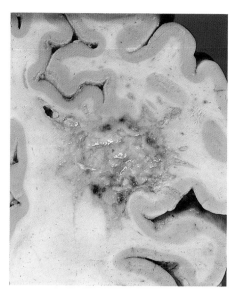

**FIGURE 3–16**   PYOGENIC ABSCESS

An 88-year-old man with mycosis fungoides developed *Listeria monocytogenes* sepsis. Subsequently, a mass became apparent in the right parietal region. Situated in white matter, the lesion is an early abscess characterized by an irregular area of suppuration and hemorrhage. At this early stage, there is no capsule.

infarction, cerebritis or cellulitis stimulates the proliferation and migration of fibroblasts from blood vessel walls. In a sometimes successful attempt to localize the process, these cells proceed to knit a widening, ever more substantial collagenous collar around the suppurative center.

At this stage, the region of the capsule becomes evident radiologically.[5, 6]

With advanced abscess formation, a firm fibrous capsule delineates the lesion and facilitates resection (Fig. 3–18; see Fig. 3–17). Intact excisions provide the pathologist with a saccular mass filled with purulent material. At this stage, lipid-laden macrophages and other inflammatory cells congregate around the purulent contents. The wall is replete with proliferating capillaries and fibroblasts, with accompanying collagen (Figs. 3–19 to 3–22). Although a small collagenous scar associated with scattered macrophages and lymphocytes constitutes the healed stage of an untreated abscess noted in experimental animals,[10] its counterpart in humans is not well documented. Although most abscesses are solitary, multiplicity can occur, especially in abscesses produced by *Nocardia* species (Figs. 3–23 and 3–24).

A potentially lethal consequence of a brain abscess is inherent in its propensity to extend inwardly as a new focus of cerebritis. With time, this new area of exudate evolves into a satellite lesion ("daughter" abscesses) that can rupture into a ventricle (Fig. 3–25).[27] Experimental work and clinical experience clearly demonstrate that encapsulation proceeds more slowly on the inner or white matter aspect of an abscess, a site less resistant to extension, than on the cortical face, where the rich vascularity provides the source for a dense fibrous stroma.[10] Systemic glucocorticoids have been experimentally shown to retard abscess encapsulation.[20]

**Bacterial Culture.** Traditionally, the offending agents have been *Staphylococcus aureus*, hemolytic streptococci, *Streptococcus viridans*, and various aerobic gram-negative rods.[3, 4, 7, 16] Anaerobic organisms often originate from paracranial sources.[14] In some instances, more than one organism is recovered. *Nocardia asteroides* is a gram-positive bacterium that may infect the CNS opportunistically or without compromising conditions.[12, 17]

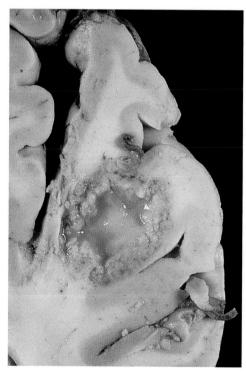

**FIGURE 3–17**   PYOGENIC ABSCESS

Encapsulation begins as a well-delineated rim of granulation tissue surrounding the lesion's purulent content.

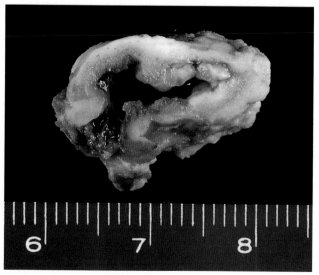

**FIGURE 3–18**   PYOGENIC ABSCESS

The capsule around this surgically excised abscess is well formed.

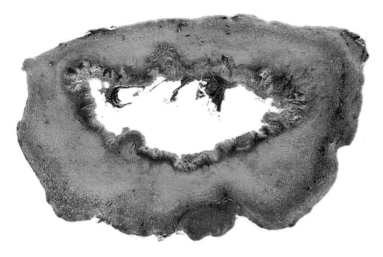

3–19

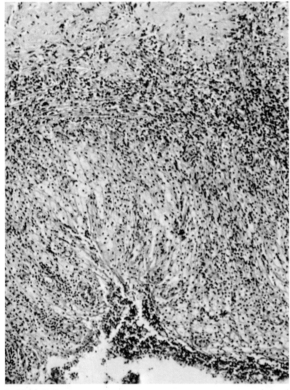

3–20

**FIGURES 3–19 AND 3–20    PYOGENIC ABSCESS**

This encapsulated abscess was excised with a margin of brain. The green-staining collagen in the evolving capsule is well seen in this Masson trichrome–stained section (Fig. 3–19). Higher magnification demonstrates lamination that progresses outward (from bottom to top in Fig. 3–20) from an inner layer of polymorphonuclear leukocytes, foamy macrophages, capillaries, and leukocytes to a peripheral layer of proliferating fibroblasts and collagen.

**Differential Diagnosis.** Given the findings of acute cellularity and prominence of reactive astrocytes, the differential diagnosis of an organizing abscess usually elicits concern about a *malignant glioma*. Histologically, the distinguishing features of an organizing abscess wall include abundant inflammation and collagen-producing fibroblasts.

## Tuberculosis

Tuberculosis occurs both as an intraparenchymal (tuberculoma) (Figs. 3–26 and 3–27) and a meningeal (tuberculous meningitis) form (Fig. 3–28). They are discussed together since the distinction is not always apparent in biopsy material.

**Tuberculoma.** The worldwide occurrence of tuberculosis introduces international intrigue into the bibliography of CNS *tuberculomas*, with its entries from such romantic quarters as Algiers,[6] Bombay,[5, 31] Madras,[29] Karachi,[28] Cairo,[19] Panama City,[12] Madrid,[11, 34] New Delhi,[30] Leeds,[10] Mexico City,[32] Santiago,[2] Seoul,[22] Bucharest,[1] and Columbus, Ohio.[8] Although in clinicopathologic terms, the tuberculoma is quite distinct from tuberculous leptomeningitis, these two expressions of the disease may coexist.

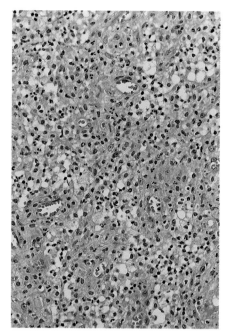

**FIGURE 3–21    PYOGENIC ABSCESS**

The wall of a subacute abscess consists of a mass of acute inflammatory cells, macrophages, and fibroblasts.

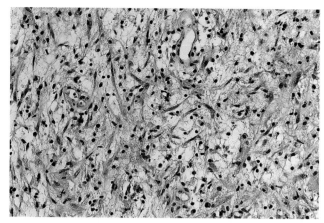

**FIGURE 3–22    PYOGENIC ABSCESS**

Proliferating fibroblasts contribute to the evolving capsule.

Tuberculomas are encountered in all age groups but occur most often in the first three decades of life. Recognized extracranial disease or a history of exposure to tubercle bacilli is a common, but not constant, feature. An association with human immunodeficiency virus (HIV) infection is noted in some cases.[9, 18, 35] Immunocompromise has also been associated with a histiocyte-rich mass related to *Mycobacterium avium* complex.[7, 27] Tuberculomas are diverse because the lesions can involve virtually any region, including the brain stem (see Fig. 3–26),[13, 15, 16, 32] hypothalamus,[20] meninges,[21, 23] and cavernous sinus.[14] The ratio of cerebellar to cerebral involvement is considerably higher than would be anticipated on the basis of the relative volumes of these two structures.

Signs and symptoms of tuberculomas include headache, seizures, papilledema, hemiplegia, and cerebellar dysfunction. Fever may intimate the inflammatory character of the lesion. On MR imaging, the most

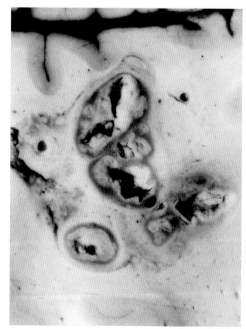

3–23

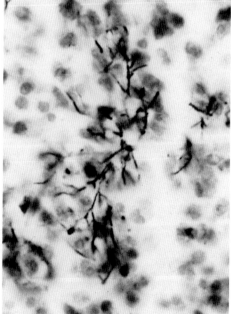

3–24

**FIGURES 3–23 AND 3–24    PYOGENIC ABSCESS (*NOCARDIA*)**

Cerebral abscesses related to *Nocardia* are noted for their white matter localization, multiplicity or multiloculation, variable encapsulation, and content of purulent exudate (Fig. 3–23). The organisms form delicate branching filaments that are readily evident on Grocott's methenamine-silver stain (Fig. 3–24, × 1000). The organism is also demonstrable with Gram stain.

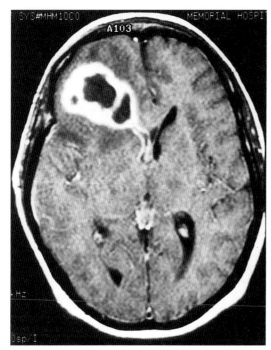

**FIGURE 3–25   PYOGENIC ABSCESS WITH VENTRICULAR EXTENSION**

Brain abscesses are prone to form smaller, more deeply situated satellite lesions. As seen here in the subjacent frontal horn, such secondary abscesses may rupture into a ventricle.

common profile is that of a single or multilocular lesion with a peripheral ring of contrast enhancement and a hypodense necrotic center.[22, 34] The lesions may be approached by stereotactically directed needle biopsy[24, 25] or open resection.

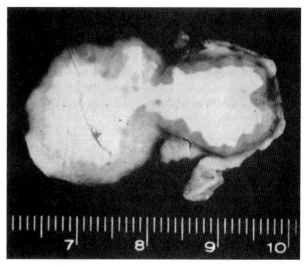

**FIGURE 3–27   TUBERCULOMA**

This expansile mass was resected from the cerebellum. The indurated rim of fibrous tissue contrasts sharply with the chalky interior of caseous necrosis.

Tuberculomas in situ are remarkable for their hard consistency relative to that of surrounding edematous brain. On section, these firm masses have a friable, caseous center that differs markedly from the purulent content of a pyogenic abscess, from the liquor of a cystic glioma, from the pultaceous material of a malignant glioma, and from the grumous center of some metastatic tumors. The indurated character of tuberculomas is imparted by a rim of woody, gray tissue from which nobs project into surrounding parenchyma.

Microscopically, the process of caseation culminates centrally as a core of amorphous, eosinophilic material

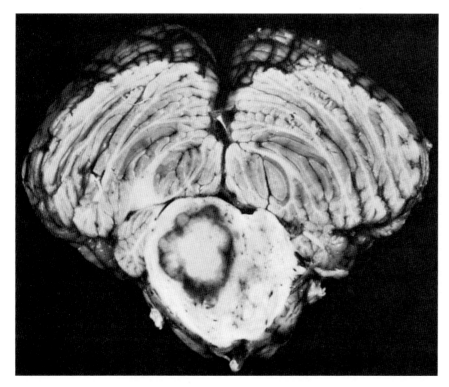

**FIGURE 3–26   TUBERCULOMA**

The typical tuberculoma is a discrete, expansile, bosselated lesion with central caseous necrosis and an outer margin of firm granulation tissue. This example in the pons of a 51-year-old man had produced slowly progressive cranial nerve palsies, as well as long tract signs, over a period of 14 months. There was an extracranial focus of active tuberculosis in a mesenteric lymph node.

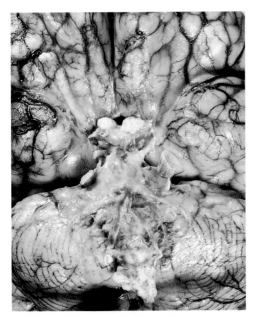

**FIGURE 3–28   TUBERCULOUS MENINGITIS**

The basal meninges are typically affected by the adhesive, tuberculous infiltrate.

surrounded by a basophilic band of karyorrhectic debris. It is in this outer zone that tubercle bacilli may be found in greatest number. The firm lamina that envelops this caseous core consists of chronically inflamed fibrous tissue containing scattered islands of lymphoid cells, granu-

lomas, and giant cells (Fig. 3–29). Polymorphonuclear leukocytes predominate in some lesions.

A tuberculoma variant seen in immunosuppression is composed of round or spindle-shaped histiocytes gorged with mycobacteria of the *M. avium* complex.[7, 27]

Fortunately, social and economic development and improved delivery of therapy have and will continue to lessen the incidence of tuberculomas. This might be "a matter of regret for the surgeon, who must view their passing somewhat wistfully, as he shifts his gaze to the barren prospect of ever-increasing gliomas."[5]

*Diffuse CNS tuberculosis*, a process characterized by macrophages filled with *Mycobacterium avium-intracellulare*, occurs in the setting of immunosuppression.[17]

**Tuberculous Meningitis.** Tuberculous meningitis may, because of its subacute course and the frequent difficulty of recovering the organism from spinal fluid, occasionally require a tissue diagnosis. This infection is usually leptomeningeal, but an occasional subdural tuberculous empyema has been reported.[33] Tuberculosis preferentially involves the base of the brain, where the leptomeninges are thickened and the subarachnoid space is filled with a thick exudate that clings to blood vessels, cranial nerves, and the pial surface (see Fig. 3–28).[4, 26] The tenacious reaction often extends laterally into the sylvian fissures, and in the posterior fossa it covers the cerebellar hemispheres. In areas removed from the main body of the exudate, isolated perivascular granulomas may appear as individual white granules. Vasculitis of the striate arteries is frequent and, on occasion, it initiates thrombosis with resultant infarction of the internal capsule.[36] Immunosuppression

**FIGURE 3–29   TUBERCULOMA**

Tubercles, multinucleated giant cells, lymphocytes, plasma cells, and caseous necrosis strongly suggest a tuberculous process. The definitive diagnosis awaits the demonstration of acid-fast organisms by stain or culture.

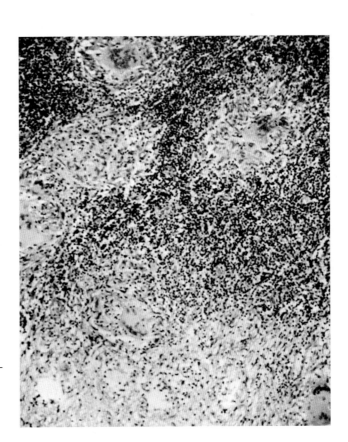

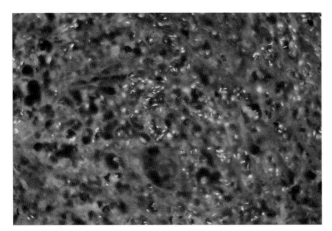

**FIGURE 3-30   TUBERCULOMA**

Fluorescence microscopy for tubercle bacilli using the auramine-rhodamine stain facilitates detection.

provides a setting that is favorable for CNS tuberculosis,[3, 34, 35] especially by *M. avium*.[17]

As in tuberculosis at extracranial sites, vascular involvement is often prominent in meningeal disease and, in association with meningitis, readily provides a presumptive diagnosis. The acid test, of course, is the demonstration of the organism. With Ziehl-Neelsen stain, or preferably the auramine-rhodamine fluorescent technique (Fig. 3-30), their visualization can be a time-consuming process. One becomes impressed that so violent and self-destructive a host response is elicited by so few organisms. The polymerase chain reaction method developed for detecting mycobacterial DNA sequences promises to be a useful diagnostic procedure,[21] especially when organisms cannot be found by conventional means.

## Other Bacterial Infections

**Syphilis.** The protean disease neurosyphilis occurs as acute syphilitic meningitis, meningovascular syphilis with stroke, myeloneuropathy (tabes dorsalis), general paresis, or as a mass lesion of tertiary syphilis—the gumma.[4, 10, 25] Meningovascular syphilis, with its associated vasculitis, is prone to produce parenchymal infarctions.[14] It is the gumma, a delayed hypersensitivity reaction to only scant treponemes, that is relevant to this discussion of parenchymal brain lesions. This now rare lesion may affect almost any organ or tissue and may arise in the setting of HIV infection.[3, 4, 13, 15] In most instances, large lesions are seen as a discrete, contrast-enhancing mass with a dark, necrotic center.[2-4, 15, 18, 26] Dense aggregates of lymphocytes, plasma cells, epithelioid histiocytes, and occasional giant cells occupy the zone that immediately surrounds the lesions' core of coagulative, "gummatous" necrosis. The process is further surrounded by a lymphoplasmacytic infiltrate and is totally encased in a dense layer of fibrous tissue.

**Whipple's Disease.** This rare multisystem disorder is caused by *Tropheryma whippelii*, which affects primarily the small intestine but occasionally occurs with coincident CNS involvement.[16, 23] Less often, it manifests itself as an

apparently isolated CNS process.[1, 5, 9, 11, 16, 19, 24] Some cases present with distinctive neurologic findings that are highly suggestive of the entity as it affects the CNS, that is, dementia, gaze palsy, and myoclonus.[16] Radiologically, focal enhancing and nonenhancing lesions have been seen.[15, 19, 23] At the histologic level, it is characterized by infiltrates of macrophages, mainly perivascular in distribution, filled with basophilic, intensely PAS-positive and diastase-resistant granular or sickle-shaped inclusions (Figs. 3-31 and 3-32). The bacillary content of the cells is evident at electron microscopic magnification (Fig. 3-33).[19]

**Actinomycosis.** Produced by a filamentous, fungus-like bacterium, the actinomycotic brain abscess is a rare cause of suppurative parenchymal lesions. The delicate organisms are gram positive and acid fast negative.[7] CNS infection is not increased in frequency in immunosuppressed hosts.

**Lyme Disease.** Caused by the tick-borne spirochete *Borrelia burgdorferi*, Lyme disease is a multisystem disorder in which manifestations of CNS involvement are highly varied, ranging from meningitis to radiculitis and encephalitis. Focal cerebral involvement is occasionally evident,[8, 12, 17, 20, 22] but biopsies are rarely performed. Histologic changes are reportedly nonspecific,[20, 22] but spirochetes compatible with *B. burgdorferi* have been found in some cases.[21]

**Cat-Scratch Disease.** A worldwide disease associated with proximity to cats, this zoonotic infection is caused by *Bartonella henselae*, an argyrophilic bacillus not

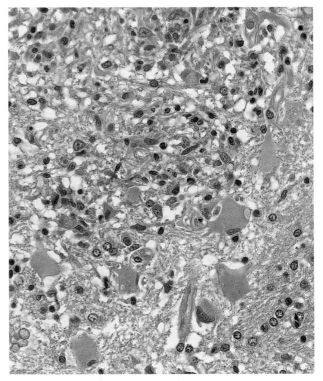

**FIGURE 3-31   WHIPPLE'S DISEASE**

The tissue response may appear rather nonspecific, as only gliosis and scattered macrophages.

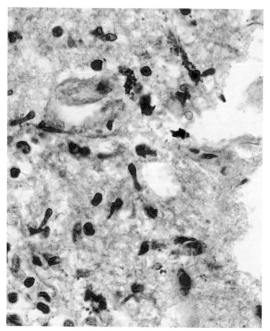

**FIGURE 3–32**  WHIPPLE'S DISEASE

Macrophages filled with PAS-positive, diastase-resistant bacilli are the hallmarks of Whipple's disease.

detectable with Gram stain. Occasional patients with this unusual disorder develop signs of peripheral or diffuse CNS involvement. Only rarely are focal lesions detected on neurologic examination or by imaging studies.[6] The histologic nature of such lesions is obscure because even in patients with systemic complications, most infections resolve without treatment. Infection can be confirmed by antibody titers. Culture methods have been developed for demonstrating the organism in affected tissue.

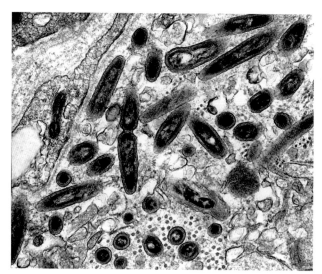

**FIGURE 3–33**  WHIPPLE'S DISEASE

The bacillary nature of the PAS-positive organisms is revealed by electron microscopy.

# VIRAL INFECTIONS

## Herpes Simplex Encephalitis

**General Comments.** The herpes simplex virus (HSV) is capable of producing lesions in all portions of the nervous system: peripheral nerves, spinal nerve roots and their ganglia, spinal cord, brain, and leptomeninges. It is possible that latent and subclinical infections of the brain obscure the true incidence of herpes simplex encephalitis. Nonetheless, herpes certainly underlies the most common and pernicious of CNS viral infections that frequently necessitate a diagnostic brain biopsy. Although occasional cases have been reported in the setting of AIDS,[22, 25] it is not usually associated with immunodeficiency states.

**Clinical Features.** Surgical pathologists are sometimes called upon to establish the diagnosis,[6, 11, 14] but herpes encephalitis is increasingly being treated on the basis of the clinical, laboratory, and radiologic findings alone. Indeed, polymerase chain reaction amplification of viral DNA in the cerebrospinal fluid offers a less invasive and more specific diagnostic method.[5, 12, 18, 24] In almost all cases, the responsible agent is the HSV-1 virus; only exceptional cases are due to HSV-2.[5] The disease occurs at any age but has its highest incidence in adolescence and young adulthood. More diffuse, "infarctive" forms of HSV infection have been reported in the setting of immunocompromise.[19] Early symptoms of fever, headache, seizures, and mental change may progress rapidly to coma and death.[26] The necrotic temporal lobe can exert a significant mass effect, with transtentorial herniation.[7]

The portal of viral entry and the role of latent CNS infection remain unsettled. That latency plays a role is suggested by the immunohistochemical detection of viral antigen[8,23] and the demonstration by polymerase chain reaction of HSV DNA sequences[13] in the olfactory bulbs and tract.[8] Occasional cases occur in reactivated form.[1]

**Radiologic Features.** Radiologically, herpes encephalitis is a unilateral or often bilateral temporal, insular, and inferior frontal lobe process with expansile zones of T2-bright signal (Fig. 3–34), sometimes with contrast enhancement in a cortical or gyriform pattern.[20]

**Macroscopic Features.** Macroscopically, the acute lesion consists of an expanding mass of necrotic, often hemorrhagic, parenchyma that is usually confined to one or both temporal lobes, the insular cortices, and the orbital surfaces of the frontal lobes.

**Microscopic Features.** Microscopically, the degree of necrosis often overshadows the inflammatory infiltrate. Indeed, in a limited biopsy, the process may easily be mistaken for an infarct (Fig. 3–35). Especially misleading are necrotic, "red dead" neurons of the sort generally seen in infarction, as discussed in Chapter 7 on pages 414 to 417. Further complicating the distinction from infarct is the frequent finding of macrophage infiltrates. Even in these areas, however, lymphocytic perivascular cuffing suggests an inflammatory process

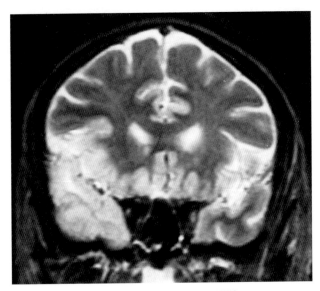

**FIGURE 3–34** HERPES SIMPLEX ENCEPHALITIS

As illustrated in this T2-weighted MRI image, herpes encephalitis preferentially involves the temporal and inferior frontal lobes, often bilaterally. In this case, a 1-week history of seizures and headache was followed by fever and progressive confusion. Both the localization of the disease and the clinical history are classic for herpes simplex encephalitis.

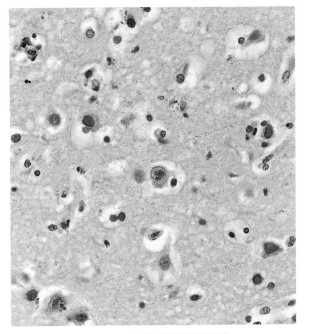

**FIGURE 3–36** HERPES SIMPLEX ENCEPHALITIS

Intranuclear viral inclusions appear either as discrete haloed eosinophilic masses (Cowdry A) or as homogeneous inclusion transformation of the entire nucleus. Both neurons and glia are affected.

(Fig. 3–35). As one examines less affected tissues, features clearly suggestive of viral infection usually become apparent. These include the finding of focal aggregates (microglial nodules) of elongated microglia (rod cells) or clusters of common leukocyte antigen–positive lymphocytes.

The most that one can hope for on light microscopy is to encounter intranuclear inclusion bodies—even one! Such bodies typically appear as round or irregular, eosinophilic, intranuclear masses surrounded by a zone that is free of chromatin, the latter being displaced toward the nuclear membrane (Cowdry A inclusions) (Fig. 3–36). More subtle, but no less esthetically pleasing, are homogeneous, wine-red nuclei with the translucent quality of stained glass. Although most conspicuous in neurons, inclusion bodies may also be abundant in glial cells.

In immunocompromised patients, herpes simplex encephalitis can be more diffuse and may affect multiple areas, including the brain stem. A form of the disease with little inflammation but many changes suggesting ischemia, such as red neurons, has been described.[19]

**Immunohistochemical Features.** As a diagnostic aid, immunostaining has generally supplanted electron microscopy and even viral culture (Fig. 3–37).[2, 3]

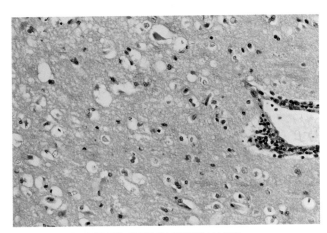

**FIGURE 3–35** HERPES SIMPLEX ENCEPHALITIS

Perivascular chronic inflammation and necrotic cortex containing red neurons are typical of the disease in its acute phase.

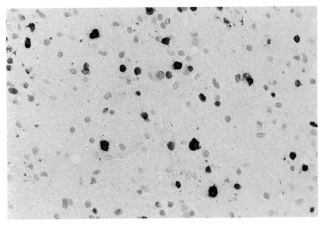

**FIGURE 3–37** HERPES SIMPLEX ENCEPHALITIS

Immunohistochemistry, here with antibodies to herpes simplex type 1, confirms the light microscopic impression.

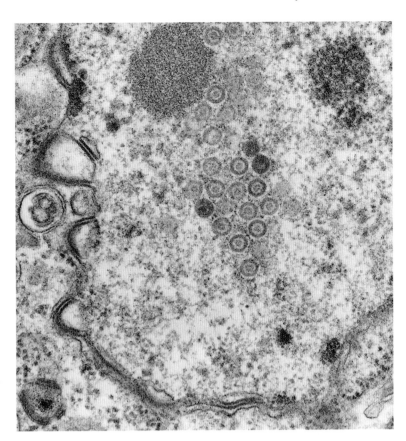

**FIGURE 3–38**   HERPES SIMPLEX ENCEPHALITIS

Electron microscopy of an inclusion-bearing astrocyte reveals an intranuclear core of viral particles
and clumps of nucleoprotein that create the
inclusion body.

**Ultrastructural Features.** The increment in resolution
provided by electron microscopy may be used to fortify
the diagnosis, because viral particles are remarkable in
number and distinctive in morphology. In the nucleus,
wherein they are assembled, they appear as subtly
hexagonal 90- to 100-nm capsids containing central nu-
cleoids (Figs. 3–38 and 3–39).[4, 21] Combined with a
dense matrix of nucleoprotein, they form the inclusion
body visible by light microscopy.[4] As viral particles penetrate the nuclear membrane, some acquire an envelope
that they retain when released from the cell (Fig. 3–40).

**Viral Culture.** The same virus (type 1) that produces
the oral herpetic lesion is usually identified in culture.
By contrast, HSV-2 affects newborns, their disseminated
disease being acquired at vaginal delivery.[15–17]

**Treatment and Prognosis.** Although it is gratifying to
the pathologist to establish a precise diagnosis, a high
mortality rate and the likelihood of serious sequelae remain. Nonetheless, a prompt diagnosis and the administration of new antiviral agents have considerably improved the outlook.[9, 26, 27] Smoldering postencephalitic
encephalitis has been reported in rare cases.[10]

## Progressive Multifocal Leukoencephalopathy

**General Comments.** The pathogenesis of PML, with
its possible clues to an association between a hypothetical

causative virus and CNS demyelination and neoplasia,
lends special interest to a lesion that already has intriguing morphologic features. Historically, PML was a rare
terminal complication of leukemia, lymphoma, or non-
neoplastic conditions treated with corticosteroids and/or
chemotherapeutic agents. In that setting, pathologists'
encounters with this entity occurred at postmortem examination. Biopsy was rarely considered.

The AIDS epidemic has introduced a new and large
population of immunologically compromised individuals
vulnerable to the pathologic consequences of this opportunistic agent.[14] In this present setting, intracranial
lesions may be approached surgically in order to distinguish them from other processes such as toxoplasmosis or
lymphoma. Application of the polymerase chain reaction
to the demonstration of JC virus DNA in cerebrospinal
fluid is now an alternative diagnostic procedure.[6, 8, 18, 19]
When the preexisting immunocompromise is not recognized, the diagnosis of grade II glioma is often entertained in the presence of a solitary lesion.

PML was first recognized as a clinicopathologic entity in 1958,[3] and its viral etiology was inferred shortly
thereafter from the presence of inclusion bodies.[7, 23] The
agent was demonstrated ultrastructurally in 1965 and
was likened to a virus of the papova group.[25, 32] Culture
studies subsequently confirmed this conclusion. The JC
variant of papovavirus is now the accepted etiologic
agent.[11, 12, 21, 24]

**Clinical Features.** The often multifocal nature of
JC virus infection may lead to a remarkable array of

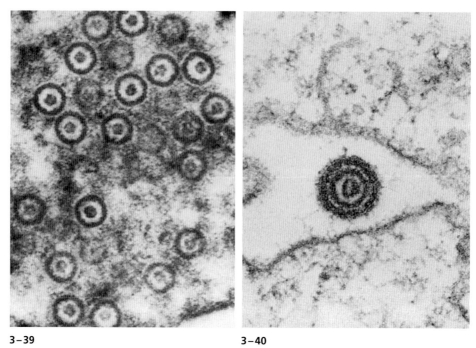

3–39                                     3–40

**FIGURES 3–39 AND 3–40**    HERPES SIMPLEX ENCEPHALITIS

Higher magnification of the cell in Figure 3–38 reveals viral particles (nucleocapsids) formed of a central nucleoid surrounded by a polygonal capsid (Fig. 3–39, ×86,000). Nucleocapsids released from the cell acquire an envelope derived from the membranes of the host cell. An enveloped virion lies in the extracellular space in Figure 3–40 (×108,000).

symptoms, including blindness, hemiparesis, intellectual decline, and signs of cerebellar and brain stem dysfunction. Only rare lesions present with mass effects.

**Radiologic Features.** A multifocal loss of myelin is produced by the virus' lytic action upon oligodendrocytes.

Replacement of the normally dark signal of myelin on T2-weighted MR images produces small foci and/or patches of brightness (Fig. 3–41).[13] Characteristically, there is little in the way of mass effect or contrast enhancement. Absence of the latter helps distinguish PML from toxoplasmosis and lymphoma because the latter

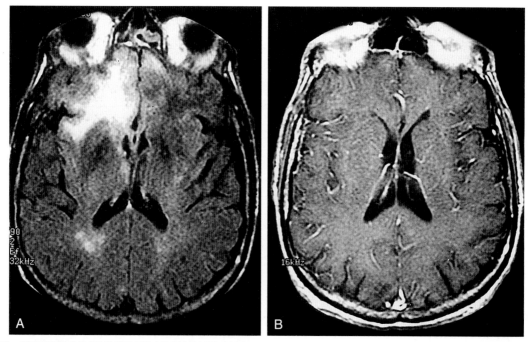

**FIGURE 3–41**    PROGRESSIVE MULTIFOCAL LEUKOENCEPHALOPATHY

As seen in a patient with AIDS, PML creates a white region with little mass effect in a FLAIR image (A). The usual absence of contrast enhancement (B) helps distinguish PML from toxoplasmosis and primary CNS lymphoma, the principal differentials in this clinical setting.

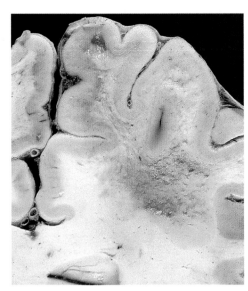

**FIGURE 3–42   PROGRESSIVE MULTIFOCAL
LEUKOENCEPHALOPATHY**

Confluent areas of necrosis in deep white matter and numerous small,
discrete, rather round lesions along the gray-white junction are typical
of PML. The patient, a 79-year-old woman, had none of the usual clinical syndromes predisposing to PML but did have a reduced CD4 lymphocyte count.

lesions are expanding, edema generating, and contrast
enhancing.[29] In the setting of immunocompromise, the
finding of one or more such nonenhancing lesions at an
unusual site, such as the cerebellum, is highly suggestive
of PML.

**Macroscopic Features.** PML is envisioned best as a
coalescence of many small, individual foci (Figs. 3–42 to
3–44).[4] By this mechanism, one or two principal lesions
assume sufficient size to produce focal neurologic
deficits. Whereas typical early lesions straddle the gray-
white junction, they may also appear disseminated in the
white matter throughout the brain. With time, large
necrotic lesions evolve deep within cerebral white
matter.

**Microscopic Features.** The lesions consist of rarefac-
tions in the myelin blanket, wherein axis cylinders and
neuronal cell bodies are spared (Fig. 3–45; see
Fig. 3–44). They are thus analogous to the plaques in
multiple sclerosis, although they are not as rich in
macrophages. They have, in addition, the distinctive
and diagnostic large, round hyperchromatic nuclei that
are found throughout the foci but are most numerous
around the circumference. Because of the presence of
transitional forms, these cells have been recognized as
altered oligodendroglia with megalic nuclei often so
dense as to obscure details of their internal structure
(Fig. 3–46; see Fig. 3–45). The nuclei of other cells
are transformed into purple homogeneous bodies with
a ground glass appearance classically associated with viral infection. More arresting, but uncommon, is the
owl's eye inclusion, wherein the pupil is more basophilic and less prominent than its counterpart in herpes encephalitis.

Particularly in the large lesions wherein necrosis
predominates, axons may degenerate, macrophages
emerge, and astroglia both become enlarged and acquire
atypical cytologic features (Fig. 3–47). Perivascular
leukocytic infiltration is typically scant.

Macrophages dot the background but can be a subtle finding, and there is usually not an outpouring of
these cells as there is in other demyelinating diseases
and cerebral infarction (see Fig. 3–47).

The diagnosis of PML is usually affirmed when a
myelin stain is applied to a specimen that includes the
edge of the lesion (see Fig. 3–45). Small biopsies that
capture only the core of the lesion may produce a specimen wherein macrophages and large astrocytes abound
and the oligodendroglia with viral cytopathic effects are
scant. Thus, PML must be considered in the differential
diagnosis of any macrophage-rich lesion, especially in
the setting of immunosuppression.

**Cytologic Features.** Both the macrophages and the
dark, infected oligodendroglia are well seen (Fig. 3–48).

**Immunohistochemical and In Situ Hybridization
Features.** Immunostaining for the JC virus reliably
identifies the infected dark cells (Fig. 3–49)[11]; both infected oligodendrocytes and large astrocytes are positive
on in situ DNA hybridization.[1, 2, 15, 24] Lastly, immunohistochemically demonstrable p53 protein accumulates in
cells of both types (Fig. 3–50).[2, 16]

**Ultrastructural Features.** Oligodendroglia are crowded with viral particles that appear as 30- to 40-nm
spheres often with associated 15- to 25-nm filamentous
forms (Fig. 3–51).[30–32] Virions are not ultrastructurally
apparent in the large bizarre astrocytes.

**Differential Diagnosis.** The diagnosis is elementary in
a large section if staining for myelin discloses multifocal
demyelinating foci with large dark cells. In the standard
H&E section of a small specimen, however, the lesion
often looks nonspecifically hypercellular or simulates a
glioma (see Figs. 3–46 and 3–47). *Astrocytoma* and, to
a lesser extent, *oligodendroglioma* are the principal considerations in light of the pleomorphism and hyperchromatism of the infected oligodendrocytes and the large,
bizarre astrocytes. Macrophages in the background
should caution, however, against the diagnosis of glioma.
Recognizing the infected oligodendrocytes, with their viral cytopathic effect, is critical.

**Treatment and Prognosis.** Our understanding of the
natural course of PML has been obscured by the concurrent presence of immunosuppression and the major
primary disease in the host. Although occasional long-
term survivals are recorded,[5, 10, 22, 27] most patients survive less than 6 months.[9, 14]

The narrow margin between the atypical astrogliosis
of PML and astrocytic neoplasia has been bridged only
rarely.[26] Such neoplastic transformation should not
be a surprise because viral isolates from PML have
been shown to induce brain tumors in experimental
animals.[17, 20, 28]

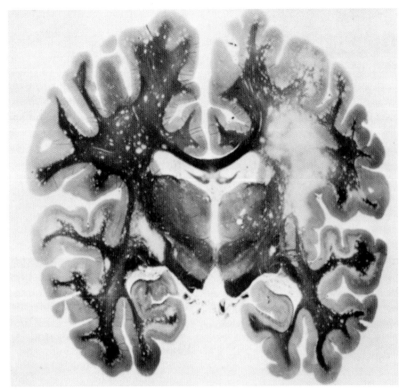

3–43

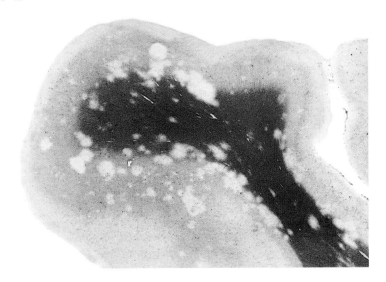

3–44

**FIGURES 3–43 AND 3–44**   PROGRESSIVE MULTIFOCAL LEUKOENCEPHALOPATHY

A 53-year-old man developed blindness and hemiparesis while receiving high-dose steroid therapy for systemic lupus erythematosus. An H&E–Luxol fast blue preparation emphasizes the multiplicity of lesions, which imparts a moth-eaten appearance, particularly along the gray-white junction (Fig. 3–43). The discrete character of the individual foci and their tendency to coalesce are apparent in Figure 3–44.

## Other Viral Infections

**Varicella-zoster encephalitis.** Varicella-zoster encephalitis is a clinically progressive, immunocompromise-associated, inflammatory-infarctive state that generally occurs with multiple lesions. Ventriculitis is common, as is vascular involvement with a stroke-like clinical picture.[2, 8, 9, 20] An episode of cutaneous zoster precedes CNS involvement in some cases.[8, 9, 11, 19]

Histologically, the lesions feature intranuclear viral inclusions of the Cowdry A type as well as variable amounts of inflammation and necrosis. The inclusions consist of discrete intranuclear eosinophilic bodies surrounded by a clear halo. Cells of all types, glial, neuronal, and vascular, can be visibly infected.

**Human Immunodeficiency Virus.** Most complications of this relatively common infection are due to the many

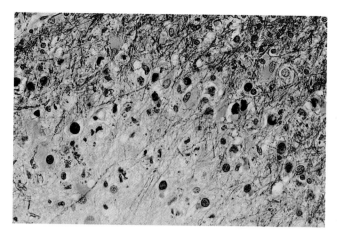

**FIGURE 3–45** PROGRESSIVE MULTIFOCAL LEUKOENCEPHALOPATHY

High magnification of an individual lesion discloses the large dark nuclei typical of PML. These are most abundant at the edge of the demyelinated focus (H&E–Luxol fast blue).

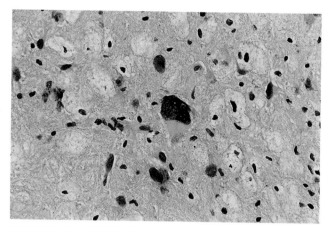

**FIGURE 3–47** PROGRESSIVE MULTIFOCAL LEUKOENCEPHALOPATHY

Large, markedly atypical astrocytes are common. Note the macrophages.

opportunistic infections individually discussed throughout this chapter. The direct effects of the virus on the brain are discussed under Acquired Immunodeficiency Syndrome on pages 145 to 146.

**Subacute Sclerosing Panencephalitis.** Subacute sclerosing panencephalitis (SSPE) represents a chronic infection by a defective measles virus. Clinically characterized by slowly progressive personality change, intellectual de-

terioration, and seizures,[5, 15, 22] it affects primarily children. Rare even when measles was endemic, SSPE is now a curiosity and unlikely to come to biopsy. On MR images, the process diffusely affects white matter and appears as a bright T2 signal.[3, 5] Cerebral atrophy is common in the advanced disease.

Histologically, the lesions exhibit all the features expected in viral encephalitis, including perivascular inflammatory cells, necrosis, and inclusion bodies.[6] Of the last, the most conspicuous is a large, discrete, brightly eosinophilic, haloed, intranuclear mass that occurs in consummate form within ganglion cells. Accompanying such cells are those with more subtle, intracytoplasmic inclusions. Especially numerous are translucent wine-colored, ground glass nuclear changes in oligodendroglia. Neurofibrillary change has also been noted.[12, 20] Measles virus antigen is readily demonstrated immunohistochemically.[1]

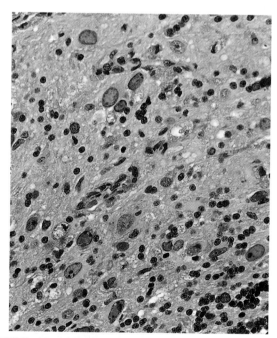

**FIGURE 3–46** PROGRESSIVE MULTIFOCAL LEUKOENCEPHALOPATHY

The process can easily be misinterpreted as a glioma because of its cellularity and nuclear pleomorphism. The viral cytopathic effect is seen at higher magnification as a ground glass alteration in the nuclei of the dark cells.

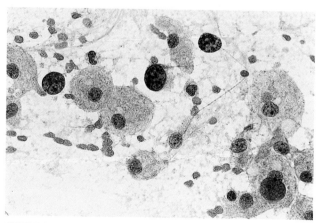

**FIGURE 3–48** PROGRESSIVE MULTIFOCAL LEUKOENCEPHALOPATHY—SMEAR PREPARATION

In a smear preparation, large, dark nuclei of infected oligodendroglia contrast with the small bland nuclei of macrophages.

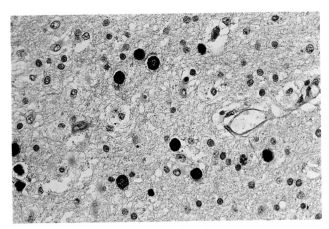

**FIGURE 3–49**    PROGRESSIVE MULTIFOCAL LEUKOENCEPHALOPATHY

Immunostaining for papovavirus aids in the identification of inclusion-bearing oligodendroglia.

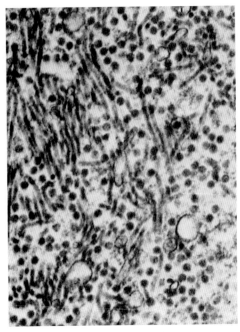

**FIGURE 3–51**    PROGRESSIVE MULTIFOCAL LEUKOENCEPHALOPATHY

Electron microscopy of the enlarged nucleus of an oligodendrocyte demonstrates its content of virions. Exhibiting features of the papova virus group, the virions appear as both 30- to 40-nm spheres and 15- to 25-nm filaments (×60,000).

Ultrastructurally, the nucleocapsids of SSPE are sinuous, 18- to 20-nm tubules that occupy the nucleus and perikaryon and are occasionally seen in neuronal processes.[16, 17, 21] Unlike the measles virus, which it otherwise resembles, the virus of SSPE does not bud from the cell surface. Mutations in the measles virus genome have been noted.[4]

SSPE is an indolent yet progressive disease that usually runs its lethal course in less than 2 years. Fortunately, effective vaccination for measles has reduced the incidence of both the natural disease and its rare late sequela, SSPE.[22]

**Miscellaneous Viral Encephalitides.** Although rarely the targets of a brain biopsy, cytomegalovirus infection,[10, 13, 18] eastern equine encephalitis,[7] and even rabies[14] must be considered when histologic changes suggest a viral etiology.

## FUNGAL INFECTIONS

### Aspergillosis

Encountered more often as domestic contaminants than as disease-producing organisms, fungi of the genus *Aspergillus* occur normally in soil and decaying organic material. Their spores, while able to germinate on a nutritious but biologically inert slice of bread, are generally unable to mature and proliferate in the immunocompetent human. Immunocompromised patients, on the other hand, provide a hospitable milieu readily exploited by this ubiquitous agent.[1–3, 7, 16, 17] Aspergillosis is not a frequent complication of AIDS, wherein the organisms that flourish are those normally held at bay by T cells, not polymorphonuclear leukocytes.[13] The respiratory tract (invasive pulmonary aspergillosis) is the most important portal of entry. Of the hundreds of species known, *Aspergillus fumigatus* is the most important pathogen. Cerebral aspergillosis rarely occurs in immunologically normal individuals, as a hematogenous infection in some cases related to mycotic endocarditis.[4] Infection may also extend directly to the brain from an adjacent paranasal sinus,[8, 11] through a skull fracture,[6] or from an infected surgical site.[8] In immunologically intact patients who are approached surgically, the intracranial lesion is usually a solitary expansile lesion.[9, 18, 19]

*Aspergillus* shares an affinity, together with the Zygomycetes, for blood vessels. In the immunologically deficient host, the organism proliferates without restraint

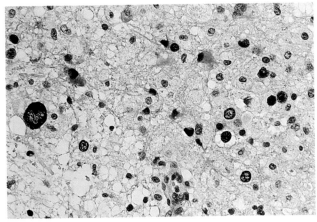

**FIGURE 3–50**    PROGRESSIVE MULTIFOCAL LEUKOENCEPHALOPATHY

Dark, infected oligodendrocytes and bizarre astrocytes are immunoreactive for p53 protein.

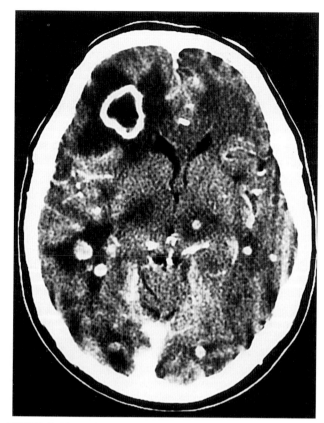

**FIGURE 3–52**     ASPERGILLOSIS

Multiple contrast-enhancing, centrally necrotic foci are typical of advanced disseminated cerebral aspergillosis, as seen in an immunocompromised patient.

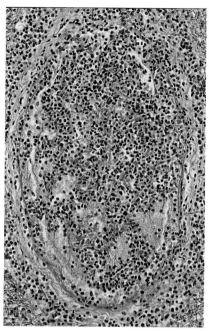

**FIGURE 3–53**     ASPERGILLOSIS

Hyphae are hidden in the wall of this inflamed, thrombosed vessel.

and produces multiple parenchymal infarcts. Even such major vessels as the carotid may be affected.[14, 19] Mycotic aneurysms are still another complication.[10] Radiologically, the lesions are widespread (Fig. 3–52) and are often seen in the basal ganglia and thalamus, often with imaging features suggesting hemorrhage.[5] Contrast enhancement is variable.

Parenchymal lesions appear not only as zones of necrosis in the distribution of a large vessel but also as spherical infarcts that include domains of more than one vessel. Some foci lack contrast enhancement, whereas others are peripherally delineated by an enhancing rim.[1, 12, 15]

The fungal organisms proliferate in the walls and lumens of vascular channels (Figs. 3–53 to 3–55) and can

**FIGURES 3–54 AND 3–55**
ASPERGILLOSIS

The organism can be elusive in surgical material. As seen in adjacent sections stained by H&E (Fig. 3–54) and the Grocott methenamine-silver method (Fig. 3–55), vascular involvement with parenchymal necrosis is typical of aspergillosis.

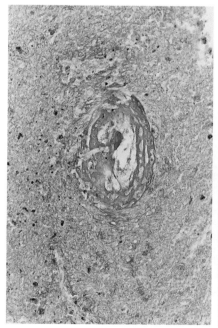

3–54

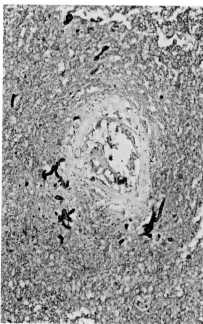

3–55

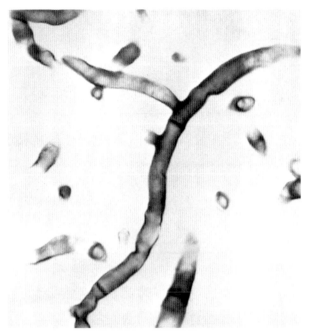

**FIGURE 3–56    ASPERGILLOSIS**

*Aspergillus* hyphae are acutely branching, septate, and uniform in caliber (Grocott methenamine-silver method).

fan out into the surrounding parenchyma. The intensity of the body's reaction to this intrusion is usually restrained and is often limited to polymorphonuclear leukocytes forming linear aggregates several cells deep along the hyphae. A granulomatous response with giant cells and fibrosis may be observed in noncompromised patients. The organisms form dichotomously branching septa 3 to 6 $\mu$m in diameter (Fig. 3–56). They are more slender and more uniform in contour than those of the nonsegmented Zygomycetes. Neither should be confused with normal large axons seen in some biopsy specimens (Fig. 3–57). Although not specific, methenamine

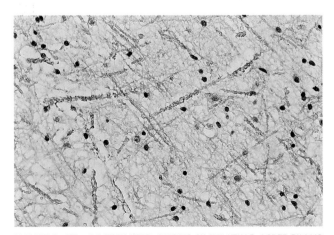

**FIGURE 3–57    MYELINATED AXONS SIMULATING ASPERGILLUS**

Large myelinated axons in edematous brain can be misinterpreted as hyphae. The uniformly slender myelin sheaths have a "bubbly" or beaded quality. Axons are not segmented and do not branch.

silver is an extremely sensitive method by which to visualize hyphae.

## Blastomycosis

*Blastomyces* encephalitis is usually a component of a systemic infection wherein pulmonary and/or cutaneous disease is primary.[1, 8] Nonetheless, solitary blastomycomas of the brain have been documented.[2, 4–9] The same is true of superinfection of a glioma.[3]

As the gross appearance of the lesions reflects their time course, they vary in consistency from soft to firm, the former being a manifestation of necrosis and suppuration (Fig. 3–58), the latter of fibrosis and gliosis. The inflammatory response features two dissimilar cell types: polymorphonuclear leukocytes and multinucleated giant cells. The former aggregate in microabscesses, sometimes encircled by epithelioid cells. Organisms are often contained within the cytoplasm of giant cells (Fig. 3–59).

The spherical to ovoid agent is variable in size. Organisms 8 to 12 $\mu$m in diameter predominate, but small, 2- to 4-$\mu$m "microforms" of *Blastomyces dermatitidis* are occasionally encountered. The larger types have a thick cell wall (Fig. 3–60). Budding from a broad base is characteristic (Figs. 3–61 and 3–62). The protoplasm of viable organisms appears as a lacy basophilic network but, with degeneration, condenses into a central or eccentric granule. Silver stains highlight the thick cell walls of this unencapsulated fungus.

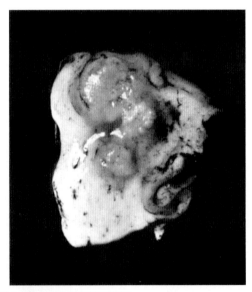

**FIGURE 3–58    BLASTOMYCOSIS**

This blastomycotic lesion was surgically removed from the left frontal lobe of a 13-year-old boy who, 3 years previously, had sustained a penetrating wound by a stick in the area. Although the incident was followed by transient fever and delirium, he remained asymptomatic for more than 2 years before developing right facial seizures. The lesion had destroyed gray and white matter over an area of approximately 2 × 3 cm. Despite postoperative recovery, the patient died of parenchymal and leptomeningeal blastomycosis 1 year thereafter. (From Fetter B, Klintworth GK, Hendry WS. Mycoses of the Central Nervous System. Baltimore: Williams & Wilkins, 1967.)

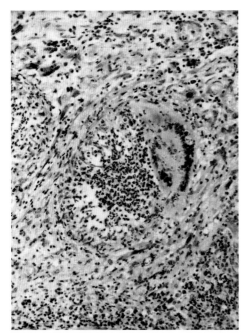

**FIGURE 3–59**  BLASTOMYCOSIS

Blastomyces organisms elicit both a suppurative and a granulomatous response, as illustrated here in the formation of both microabscesses and multinucleated giant cells, respectively.

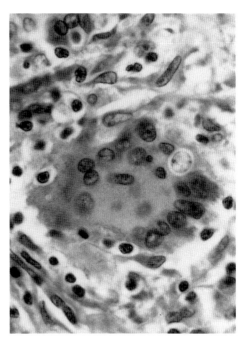

**FIGURE 3–60**  BLASTOMYCOSIS

This multinucleated giant cell contains a typical organism at 2 o'clock. Note its thick refractile wall and reticulated internal structure.

## Coccidioidomycosis

*Coccidioides immitis* exists in soil in certain arid climates of the Western Hemisphere. Acquired by inhalation of the spores, the disease is usually restricted to the lungs, and only in a minority of cases does dissemination to sites such as skin, brain, and meninges occur.[6] Systemic manifestations of the infection are as varied as those of

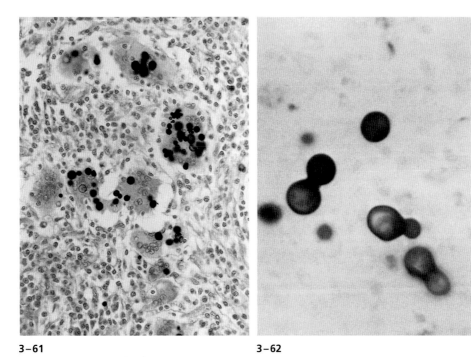

3–61                                                  3–62

**FIGURES 3–61 AND 3–62**  BLASTOMYCOSIS

The rounded organisms vary considerably in size. Here, some are sequestered within giant cells while others lie free in the inflammatory exudate (Fig. 3–61, Grocott methenamine-silver method). As is evident in Figure 3–62, *Blastomyces* buds from a broad base (Grocott methenamine-silver method).

syphilis. Intracerebral masses that require surgical intervention are rare.[1,4,7] The disorder usually affects immunocompetent individuals, but AIDS is a predisposing factor in some cases.[2,3,5]

Active lesions typically contain numerous organisms. As a rule, endosporulating spherules are readily identified, even in H&E-stained sections. Spherules range in size from 20 to 100 $\mu$m; endospores measure from 2 to 5 $\mu$m. Whereas the immature forms are conspicuous with Gomori's methenamine silver (GMS) and PAS stain, mature spherules may show little or no PAS reactivity. Typical lesions have a central suppurative response to released endospheres and a granulomatous reaction to mature spherules.

## Cryptococcosis

Cryptococci in the leptomeninges thrive in the setting of immunosuppression and produce symmetric, cyst-like expansions of perivascular spaces, particularly in the basal ganglia and thalamus.[1,2,4,6,8,9,11] The rare localized, solitary, parenchymal cryptococcoma germinates independent of immunosuppression.[3,5,7] It is such lesions that are likely to appear as surgical specimens. Intraventricular lesions have also been described.[10] Being encapsulated and often trabeculated by fibrous tissue, focal lesions are either firm or, less commonly, cystic. The organism's production of mucopolysaccharide imparts a gelatinous quality to the lesion's loculated or encysted contents (Fig. 3–63).

The inflammatory response is characteristically chronic and scant. In H&E-stained sections, the 2- to 15-$\mu$m, ovoid to spherical organisms are pale and translucent. As such, they are readily overlooked unless exposed in relief against surrounding structures by their invisible mucopolysaccharide capsules (Figs. 3–64 to 3–66). The full radiance of this corona is highlighted by

the alcian blue stain (Fig. 3–67). Most organisms are extracellular, but some lie sequestered within multinucleated giant cells. The India ink preparation can be applied to either cerebrospinal fluid or fluid expressed from a cryptococcoma (Fig. 3–68). In *Cryptococcus*, in contrast to *Blastomyces*, budding occurs with a narrow neck, the cell wall is thin, and a mucopolysaccharide capsule is thick (see Fig. 3–68).

## Candidiasis

In immunocompromised patients, CNS candidiasis indiscriminately affects the cerebral hemispheres, basal ganglia, and cerebellum with lesions that appear as microabscesses surrounded by areas with vasculitis. Symptomatic intraparenchymal masses may also occur in the setting of AIDS.[1,3] Only on rare occasions do mass lesions bring patients to surgery.[2]

The usual response to *Candida* infection is an acute inflammatory reaction. The H&E-stained sections reveal pale blue yeastlike bodies, often seriated in the form of pseudohyphae. The organisms are well seen on GMS and PAS preparations.

## Histoplasmosis

Acquired by inhalation of bird excreta as a contaminant in the soil, this global infection generally induces a systemic disease initiated by *Histoplasma capsulatum*.

Solitary, discrete parenchymal lesions are uncommon (Fig. 3–69).[2–7,9] Histoplasmosis occurs only occasionally in the setting of AIDS.[1,8] Mass lesions are often firm because of an abundance of fibrous tissue. Others are necrotic and soft.

Lymphocytes, plasma cells, and giant cells may be encountered (Fig. 3–70), but macrophages predominate

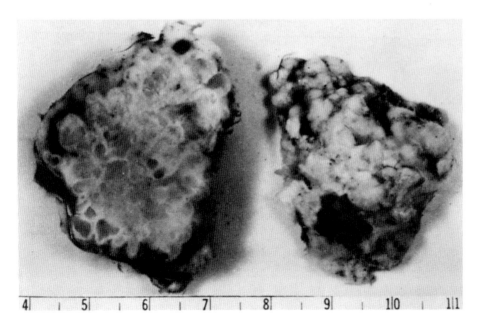

**FIGURE 3–63   CRYPTOCOCCOSIS**

This discrete, firm, knobby cryptococcoma was excised from the right frontal lobe of a 33-year-old man who presented with headaches and seizures. *Cryptococcus neoformans* was cultured. Radiographs disclosed an asymptomatic density in the apex of the left lung, which was viewed as a potential source of the cerebral infection. The patient's clinical course was uneventful over a 4-year period of follow-up. (From Dillon ML, Sealy WL. Surgical aspects of opportunistic fungal infections. Lab Invest 1962;11:1231–1236.)

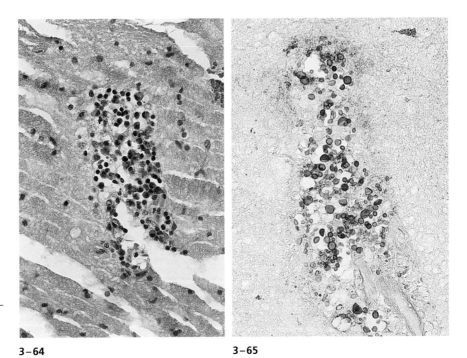

**FIGURES 3–64 AND 3–65**   CRYPTOCOCCOSIS

Cryptococci are aptly named. When sparse, they are difficult to recognize in H&E-stained sections (Fig. 3–64) but are readily identified after silver staining (Fig. 3–65, Grocott methenamine-silver method).

**3–64**          **3–65**

in the inflammatory response. Such cells gorge themselves on 1- to 5-μm round to oval organisms. These appear as small basophilic granules separated from surrounding cytoplasm by a narrow translucent halo. The latter is created by a capsule (Fig. 3–71) that stains strongly with methenamine silver (Fig. 3–72).

## Mucormycosis (Zygomycosis)

Mucormycosis is caused by fungi of the order Mucorales. The organism may be inhaled, ingested, or acquired directly as in burns. With reference to CNS involvement, the infection, which characteristically originates in the

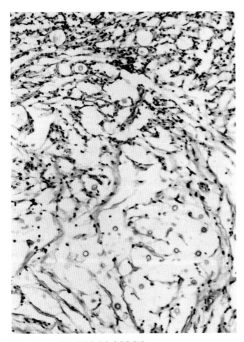

**FIGURE 3–66**   CRYPTOCOCCOSIS

The lesion of Figure 3–63 contained numerous spherical organisms, each highlighted by a clear capsule. The lymphocytic response is typically slight.

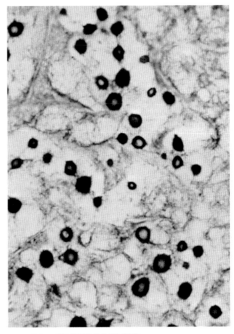

**FIGURE 3–67**   CRYPTOCOCCOSIS

The inner aspect of the capsule of the *Cryptococcus* organism stains positively for mucopolysaccharides (alcian blue).

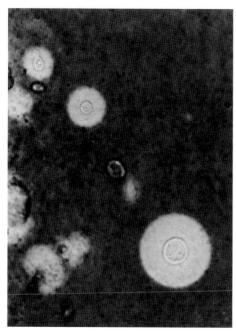

**FIGURE 3–68** CRYPTOCOCCOSIS

Whether derived from cerebrospinal fluid or the liquid expressed from a cryptococcal lesion, the organisms can be identified in India ink preparations that highlight their capsules. Here, multiple refractile yeast forms are surrounded by thick, clear capsules. At the upper left, an organism buds with the narrow base typical of *Cryptococcus* (×1000).

nose or sinuses, quickly finds its way to the orbit, meninges, and brain by vascular invasion.[1, 4, 8] Active infection at other sites is also known to undergo dissemination to brain by the hematogenous route.[5] Diabetic ketoacidosis provides the classical setting for this disease, but immunosuppression, hematologic malignancy, and other permissive states may also be responsible.[1, 8] An occasional case is associated with a skull fracture.[7]

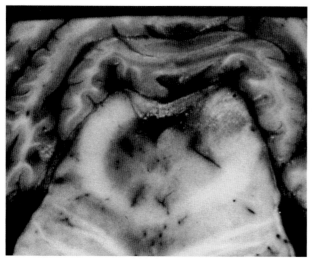

**FIGURE 3–69** HISTOPLASMOSIS

A 14-year-old boy with immune deficiency developed generalized histoplasmosis. Multiple ill-defined, granular lesions lie disseminated throughout the brain, as seen here in the tegmentum of the pons.

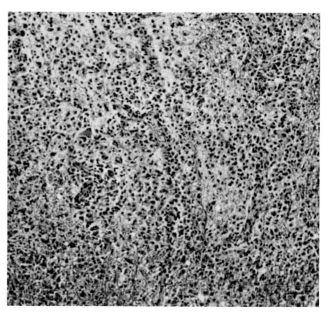

**FIGURE 3–70** HISTOPLASMOSIS

*Histoplasma* elicits a histiocytic response.

The affinity of this organism for blood vessels commonly produces thrombosis and darkened areas of infarction that may require débridement or exenteration. The infarctive cerebral lesions are usually widespread and lethal and are rarely approached surgically.[1, 3, 9]

The hyphae of *Mucor* are broad, ribbon-like, and somewhat irregular in caliber (5 to 20 $\mu$m in diameter) (Fig. 3–73). The organisms elicit only a mild inflammatory response. Although effective débridement and antifungal therapy have been reported,[1, 2, 6] mucormycosis is an aggressive and often lethal infection if it reaches the intracranial compartment.

## PROTOZOAL INFECTIONS

### Amebiasis

Although there are rare examples of cerebral involvement by the intestine-based *Entamoeba histolytica*, most cases of cerebral amebiasis result from infection by free-living amebae. Of these, *Naegleria* or *Acanthamoeba* species are most common.

Naeglerial infection is usually acquired in healthy individuals while swimming in warm water, an environment conducive to growth of the organisms. The protozoa come in contact with nasal mucosa, through which they gain access to the meninges and brain by way of the cribriform plate. Infected individuals present with a fulminating form of meningoencephalitis termed primary amebic meningoencephalitis.[1, 4] In fatal cases, the brain is soft and swollen with superficial areas of hemorrhage and necrosis. The purulent exudate typically contains the organisms.

Cerebral involvement with *Acanthamoeba*, on the other hand, usually occurs in patients immunologically

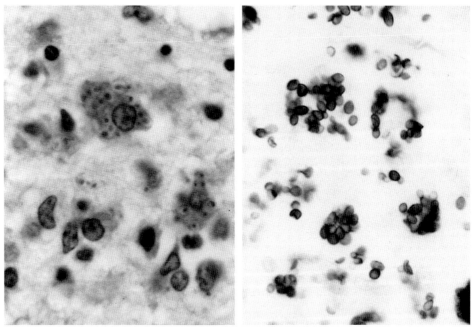

## FIGURES 3–71 AND 3–72
### HISTOPLASMOSIS

The cytoplasm of these histiocytes contains numerous encapsulated organisms 1 to 5 μm in diameter (Fig. 3–71, PAS, ×1000). On a Grocott methenamine-silver preparation, strong staining of the capsules greatly facilitates their detection (Fig. 3–72, ×1000).

**3–71**                                    **3–72**

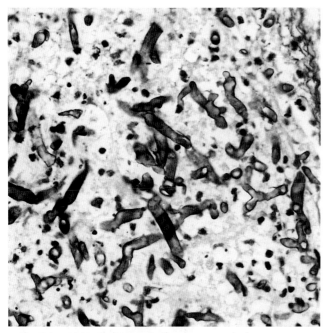

## FIGURE 3–73    ZYGOMYCOSIS (MUCORMYCOSIS)

A 65-year-old woman had undergone a 10-week course of high-dose glucocorticoid treatment for "interstitial plasma cell pneumonia." This was followed abruptly by left hemiparesis and a decreased level of consciousness. Computed tomography revealed a discrete area of low density in the right basal ganglia and internal capsule. Tissue obtained by needle biopsy reveals intravascular, broad, irregular, nonseptate hyphae typical of Zygomycetes (Grocott methenamine-silver method). Cultures were confirmatory.

predisposed to infection by chronic illness or debility. Single or multiple intraparenchymal lesions result (Fig. 3–74). Rare AIDS-associated cases have been reported.[2, 7] Acanthamoebic lesions take the form of a cerebritis wherein softened areas contain abundant organisms. Despite the designation "granulomatous amebic encephalitis," the inflammatory response is variable in degree and nature, occasionally being minimal and more often acute than granulomatous (Fig. 3–75).[3–6]

## Toxoplasmosis

Globally distributed, toxoplasmosis results from infection by *Toxoplasma gondii*, an intracellular protozoan with the capacity to infect humans and an almost universal realm of other mammals and birds. Biologically, the organism is a coccidian in cats within intestinal epithelium. The sexual stages develop through the formation of oocysts that are eliminated in cat feces. Infection is disseminated in nonfeline hosts.

When the fetal brain becomes infected by the transplacental route, *T. gondii* elicits a necrotizing and calcifying encephalitis, usually in a paraventricular distribution. In adults, the immunocompromised host, notably the patient with AIDS, is vulnerable to toxoplasmic encephalitis.[1, 2, 4–9, 11] In most instances, encephalitis results from recrudescence of chronic infection. In this setting, the infection creates masses that must be differentiated from other entities, particularly lymphoma. Both these processes are often multifocal.[3]

By MR or computed tomography, a central area of low density is encircled by a contrast-enhancing rim, which, in turn, is surrounded by a zone of edema whose magnitude reflects the activity of the process (Fig. 3–76).[2, 6, 7] Such lesions share a radiographic appearance

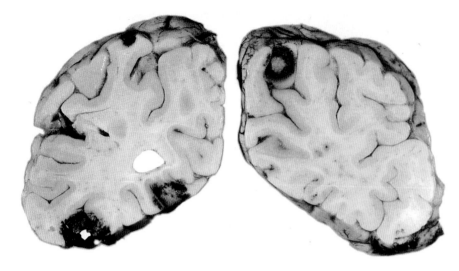

**FIGURE 3–74** AMEBIASIS— *ACANTHAMOEBA*

Multiple necrotic intraparenchymal masses characterize this *Acanthamoeba* infection, which occurred in the setting of immunocompromise. (Courtesy of Dr. A. Julio Martinez, Pittsburgh, PA.)

with primary CNS lymphomas and tuberculoma. A successful trial of antitoxoplasma therapy often establishes the diagnosis. Alternative diagnoses become more likely if this fails. *Toxoplasma* titers are not definitive in the setting of immunodeficiency because 15% of patients are seronegative.

Although the lesions are sometimes referred to as abscesses, their core is a dry granular coagulum that differs from necrotic material of most other cerebral lesions in which macrophages predominate.

Histologically, the lesion is a discrete area of granular coagulative necrosis with prominent necrotic blood vessels (Fig. 3–77). Inflammation may be rather scant, as determined in part by the immunocompromised state of the host. The organisms vary in concentration and are best seen at the margins of the lesion. Encysted organisms appear as spherical structures, 8 to 10 $\mu$m, filled with bradyzoites. Although Giemsa preparations are ordered frequently to assist in the visualization of the organisms, the contained bradyzoites are readily visible in the H&E-stained sections (Fig. 3–78). Identification of free-lying tachyzoites is more difficult because the individual organisms are minute and are difficult to distinguish from fragments of cell debris. In optimal preparations, they are visualized as slightly elongated,

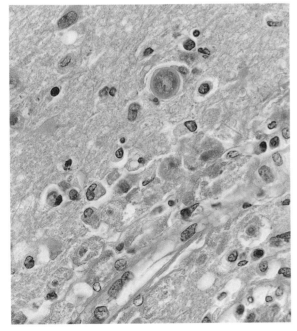

**FIGURE 3–75** AMEBIASIS—*ACANTHAMOEBA*

The organisms, both trophozoites and a cyst, are well seen in this H&E-stained section. The trophozoites may be mistaken for macrophages.

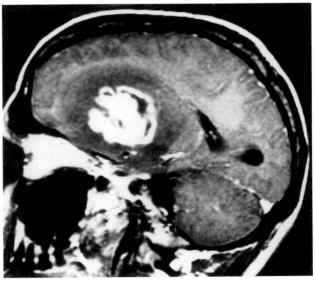

**FIGURE 3–76** TOXOPLASMOSIS

Toxoplasmosis produces a contrast-enhancing, edema-generating, centrally necrotic expansile mass. This example occurred in an HIV-positive patient.

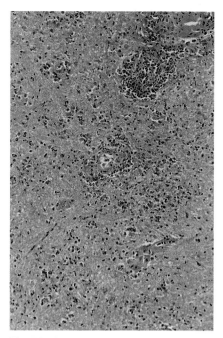

**FIGURE 3–77    TOXOPLASMOSIS**

The tissue response to toxoplasmosis is one of extensive necrosis with many necrotic blood vessels.

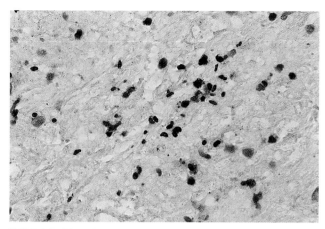

**FIGURE 3–79    TOXOPLASMOSIS**

Immunostains for toxoplasmosis assist in visualizing encysted organisms, but especially free-living tachyzoites.

nucleated structures. Immunohistochemistry is helpful in identifying these isolated tachyzoites (Fig. 3–79).[10]

The cyst and its brood of organisms can be dramatically visualized by electron microscopy (Fig. 3–80).

In its amorphous and seemingly nondescript state, the granular necrosis of toxoplasmosis is actually sugges-tive of the diagnosis. It is seen in few pathologic states other than radionecrosis and tumor necrosis. Necrosis in the brain usually elicits a macrophage response that is curiously absent in toxoplasmosis. Table 4–6, page 188, summarizes histologic features of necroses in CNS lesions. Cystic cavities have been described in the late stage of disease after treatment.[7]

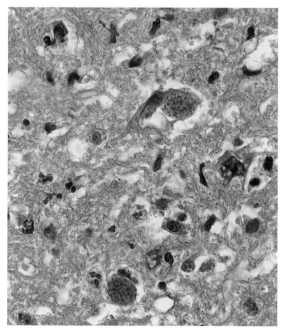

**FIGURE 3–78    TOXOPLASMOSIS**

As sacs filled with basophilic bradyzoites, the cysts of toxoplasmosis are readily visible with conventional stains.

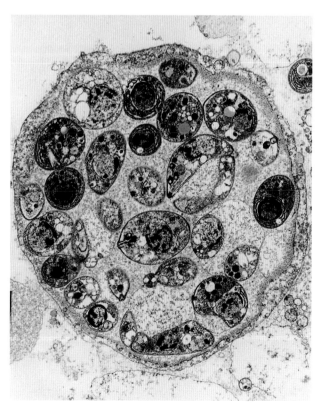

**FIGURE 3–80    TOXOPLASMOSIS**

The bradyzoites within a *Toxoplasma* cyst are dramatically illustrated by electron microscopy (×65,000). (Courtesy of Dr. Janet M. Bruner, Houston, TX.)

# PARASITIC INFECTIONS

## Cysticercosis

Immigration patterns have extended the geographic distribution of cysticercosis to include regions in which it was formerly regarded as a curiosity. The cerebral lesion is caused by larvae of the pork tapeworm *Taenia solium*. In the classics *Taenia*-human relationship, humans harboring the intestinal tapeworm are the definitive host and pigs infected by eggs from human stool are the intermediate hosts. For the pig, the result is disseminated larval taeniasis. As larvae in inadequately cooked pork infect the human gastrointestinal tract to form mature worms, the cycle continues. In cysticercosis, humans ingest the ova, not the larvae, to become intermediate hosts for a disseminated larval disease. Skeletal muscle and the brain are the sites primarily affected. The ova are ingested either in contaminated vegetables or by fecal-oral contamination.[10]

Within the intracranial compartment, the organisms grow within parenchyma or meninges. They may gain access to the ventricular system as free-floating cysts that "embolize" within the ventricular system to impede cerebrospinal fluid flow, particularly at the level of the aqueduct.[3, 9, 12, 16] Intraparenchymal lesions are generally confined to gray matter. Multiplicity is the rule, but solitary lesions are also encountered.[6, 11] The manifold consequences include neurologic deficits, seizures, and chronic meningitis.

MR imaging studies disclose the lesions with a variety of appearances. The spectrum extends from small, solid, calcified foci to large, cystic structures in the meninges or brain parenchyma.[4, 7, 8, 15] Small lesions with a delicate contrast-enhancing rim and an internal point of enhancement that represents the scolex are typical

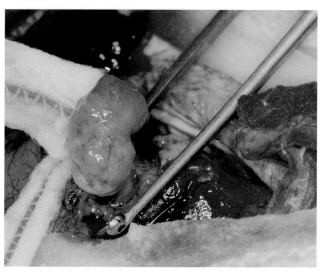

**FIGURE 3–82   CYSTICERCOSIS**

This cyst is being removed from the leptomeninges of a previously healthy 22-year-old woman who presented with a generalized seizure. She had lived in the Middle East for the 2 years prior to the onset of symptoms. (Courtesy of Dr. Henry Brem, Baltimore, MD.)

(Fig. 3–81). The so-called racemose form represents either a large cyst or grape-like masses of smaller, coalescent ones.[5] A solitary lesion that produces seizures or focal neurologic deficits frequently prompts a biopsy (Figs. 3–82 and 3–83).[1, 2, 11, 12]

In instances wherein affected brain is excised en bloc, the organism and a surrounding rim of gliotic, in-

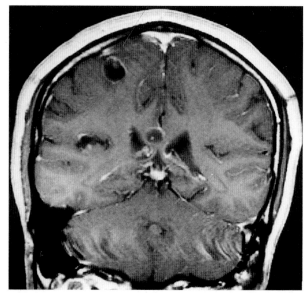

**FIGURE 3–81   CYSTICERCOSIS**

A delicately enhancing wall and a small central or eccentric focus of enhancement (the scolex) are typical features of cerebral cysticercosis.

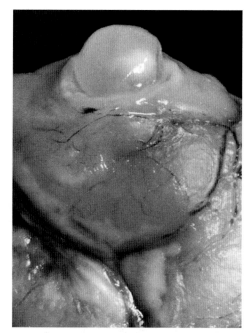

**FIGURE 3–83   CYSTICERCOSIS**

Characteristically discrete, the organism protrudes from the cut surface of the specimen. Distinctively, one pole of the cyst contains a white area, the scolex. An exudate fills the subarachnoid space in the lower portion of the illustration.

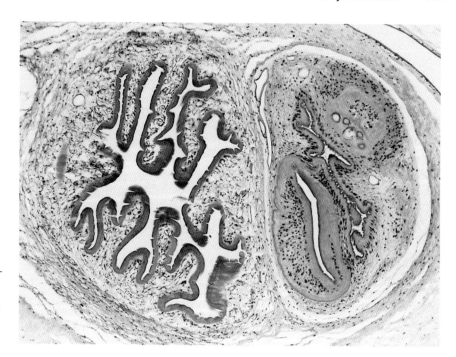

**FIGURE 3–84**   CYSTICERCOSIS

The organism consists of a branched tract on the left and a more rostral portion on the right. One of four muscular suckers protrudes from the latter. A line of four hooklets is evident in the upper right portion of the illustration.

durated parenchyma are readily palpable within the specimen. The cysts are remarkably resistant to the blade of the scalpel and may protrude intact when the specimen is bisected, like a chestnut from its husk (see Fig. 3–83). The glistening, translucent cyst with a white scolex at one pole is pathognomonic.

Microscopically, the exterior surface of the cyst is composed of a wavy, eosinophilic lamina whose inner aspect rests on a marginal cell layer containing scant nuclei. Internal to this cell layer, one encounters loose connective tissue.[10] Favorable sections disclose the organism armed with suckers and intimidating hooklets (Fig. 3–84). The larvae, particularly when degenerating, elicit marked acute and chronic inflammatory responses in the surrounding brain. Necrosis with peripheral palisading of monocytes may be seen, but giant cells are uncommon. In passing through progressive stages of degeneration, the lesion loses the complexity of the viable organism and terminates in a calcified fibrotic focus wherein the organism is no longer recognizable.[7, 14] A granulomatous response may still be apparent. Chronic seizures are a frequent consequence of such lesions.

There are effective anthelmintics to deal with viable organisms, but neurologic consequences, such as seizures, may persist.[4, 8, 13]

## Echinococcosis

Cerebral echinococcosis results from dissemination of the larvae of the tapeworm *Echinococcus granulosus.* The dog-sheep strain is more widely disseminated and virulent than those adapted to the dog-wolf and the dog-horse cycles. Adult worms reside in the intestines of dogs and, predictably, are passed through their feces to the ground. The worms, with their eggs, are ingested by grazing sheep, after which the eggs hatch in their hosts'

intestines. The resultant larvae penetrate capillaries in the bowel wall and are available for hematogenous dissemination, usually ending in the liver and lungs. In endemic regions, humans may unwillingly enter this cycle of infection and present with the mass lesions of intracerebral hydatids.[1–8] As a rule, hydatids are solitary and take the form of spherical cysts filled with clear fluid. Mass effects with increased intracranial pressure are the principal manifestations. Scolices may be grossly visible within the wall of the large cysts.

Microscopically, the cyst walls have an acellular band, the laminar layer, lined by a hypocellular, single-cell germinative layer. Some cysts are sterile and others fertile. Fertile cysts contain broad capsules to which the hooklets of scolices are often attached. Great care should be taken to avoid intraoperative rupture of such daughter cysts with resultant cerebrospinal dissemination of organisms.

## Other Parasitic Infections

Selected references provide accounts of cerebral infection in schistosomiasis,[1, 2, 6, 7, 10–14] sparganosis,[3, 4, 8, 16] paragonimiasis,[15] strongyloidiasis,[9] and trypanosomiasis.[5]

## ACQUIRED IMMUNODEFICIENCY SYNDROME

The epidemic of AIDS has produced a large population of immunosuppressed patients susceptible to a broad range of opportunistic agents. Notable among these are *T. gondii, Cryptococcus neoformans, M. avium-intracellulare,* papovavirus, cytomegalovirus, and varicella-zoster, to name but a few. Of these, *Toxoplasma* and JC virus, the papovavirus agent responsible for PML, are most

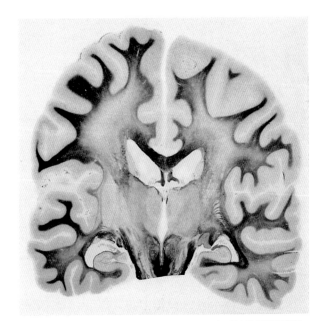

**FIGURE 3-85    ACQUIRED IMMUNODEFICIENCY SYNDROME**

Bilateral degeneration of cerebral white matter is sometimes a striking feature in the setting of AIDS. This patient was a 24-year-old woman with memory loss and other symptoms attributed to psychiatric disease. (From Kleihues P, Lang W, Burger PC, et al. Diffuse progressive leukoencephalopathy in patients with acquired immunodeficiency syndrome (AIDS). Acta Neuropathol 1986;68:333–339.)

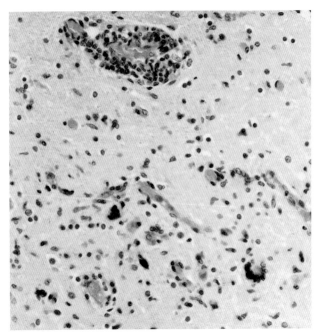

**FIGURE 3-86    ACQUIRED IMMUNODEFICIENCY SYNDROME**

Perivascular foci of inflammation, including prominent multinucleated giant cells, are the hallmarks of AIDS encephalopathy. Although numerous in the present case, such giant cells may be rare and unaccompanied by other evidence of inflammation.

frequently encountered in surgical material. These and other AIDS-related issues are summarized in several reviews.[5, 8, 13]

Although much attention has been given to these opportunistic infections, a diffuse encephalopathy caused by HIV is emerging as a clinical problem with a significance that is potentially greater than those of secondary infections. With a classical onset as mild cognitive changes, lethargy, and confusion in adults and as a delay or loss of developmental milestones in children, this subacute encephalopathy may progress to profound dementia, ataxia, and motor dysfunction.[5, 11] Cerebral atrophy and hydrocephalus ex vacuo have been noted in advanced cases.

The precise pathologic substrate for these clinical changes is unclear because there is not an absolute correlation between the types of radiographic changes, if any, and the presence of dementia.[4, 12] Nevertheless, diffuse degeneration of the cerebral white matter is a common finding (Fig. 3–85).[2, 3, 6, 14, 15] Typically, the centrum semiovale is histologically pale, vacuolated, edematous, and may be gliotic. Calcified blood vessels are present in the basal ganglia, especially in congenital AIDS. White and gray matter may contain perivascular chronic lymphocytic infiltrates and focal collections of macrophages. Less conspicuous, but considerably more diagnostic, is a population of perivascular multinucleated cells

(Fig. 3–86).[1, 10] These have been shown to contain the HIV-1 virus (Figs. 3–87 to 3–89).[7, 9, 10] These cells should receive paramount consideration during the examination of the brain of any AIDS patient.

## SARCOIDOSIS

Intracranial sarcoidosis is usually a superficial, meningioma-like mass, or masses, and only occasionally appears within the brain parenchyma[1-6, 8] or choroid plexus.[7] Sarcoidosis is discussed primarily in Chapter 2 on pages 93 to 95.

## OTHER INFLAMMATORY DISEASES

### Langerhans Cell Histiocytosis

The affinity of this disorder for the base of the brain and hypothalamic-pituitary axis is well known.[13, 30, 33, 45, 52] The pituitary stalk seems especially vulnerable. The disease can also occur in the parenchyma of the cerebral hemispheres (Figs. 3–90 and 3–91),[4, 7, 35] the choroid plexus,[27] and even the brain stem.[7] Langerhans cell histiocytosis and its apparent clonal nature are discussed primarily in Chapter 1 on pages 4 to 9.

**FIGURES 3-87, 3-88, AND 3-89    ACQUIRED IMMUNODEFICIENCY SYNDROME**

The multinucleated giant cells of AIDS encephalitis have the general features of macrophages (Fig. 3–87). Higher magnification discloses a budding organism at the upper portion of the illustration and a typical subplasmalemmal density on the left (Fig. 3–88, ×50,000). In Figure 3–89 (×25,000), the fully formed infectious particles of the HIV virus are free in the extracellular space. (From Mirra SS, del Rio C. The fine structure of acquired immunodeficiency syndrome encephalopathy. Arch Pathol Lab Med 1989;113:858–865).

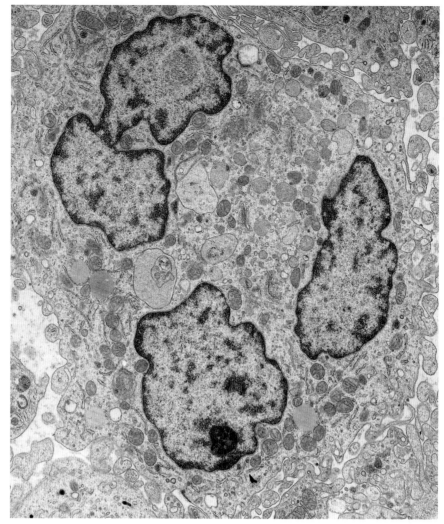

3–87

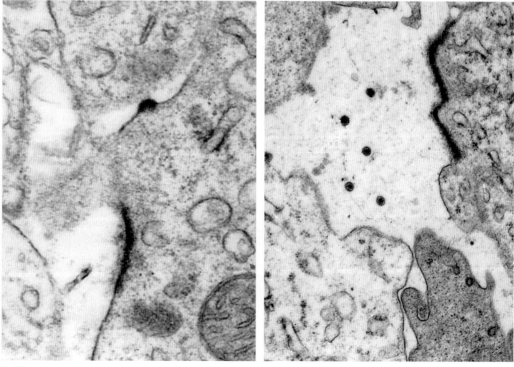

3–88

3–89

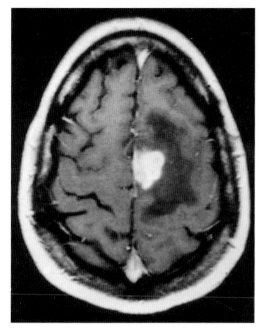

**FIGURE 3–90**    LANGERHANS CELL HISTIOCYTOSIS

This contrast-enhancing lesion was resected from the superficial brain and meninges of a 28-year-old man. There were no osseous lesions.

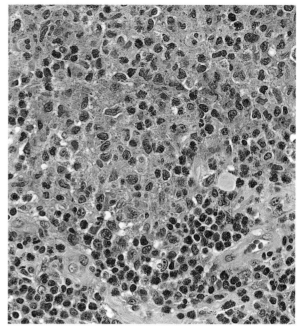

**FIGURE 3–91**    LANGERHANS CELL HISTIOCYTOSIS

The lesion seen in Figure 3–90 has the characteristic mixture of Langerhans cells and eosinophils.

## Rasmussen's Encephalitis

Rasmussen's encephalitis is a rare chronic inflammatory disorder of unknown etiology with a remarkable ten-dency toward unilateral involvement. Children afflicted with this progressive disorder lose motor function, language skills, and intellect.[25, 37, 39, 42, 56] A refractory form of seizures, epilepsy partialis continua, is the usual consequence. Substantial surgical resections are often

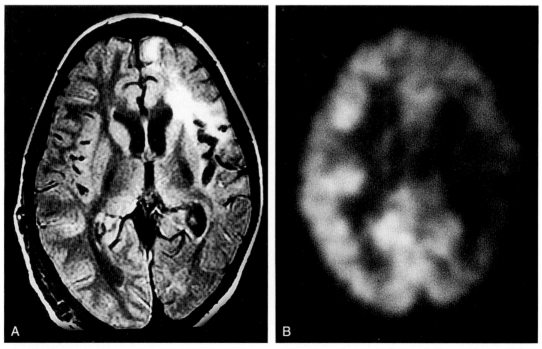

**FIGURE 3–92**    RASMUSSEN'S ENCEPHALITIS

The unilaterality of Rasmussen's encephalitis is apparent in a proton density MR scan (A) and an [18]F-deoxyglucose positron emission tomographic (PET) scan (B). MR imaging discloses a hyperintense signal in both white and gray matter of the atrophic left cerebral hemisphere. With PET, this region is dark, that is, metabolically "cold".

necessary, including hemispherectomy in some cases.[25, 37, 39, 56] Although such specimens are impressive, fully half of the brain is not removed because the deep gray matter structures, including the thalamus and basal ganglia, are preserved. Alternatively, the surgeon undercuts, and thereby electrically isolates, rather than excises the offending region.

Radiographically, advanced lesions are seen as a diffuse, unilateral hemispheric atrophy with attenuation of the cortex and compensatory ventricular dilation. In T2-weighted MR images, the normally dark white matter assumes a bright white signal in proportion to the degree of myelin loss (Fig. 3–92). Affected regions are metabolically "cold" on positron emission tomography (see Fig. 3–92).[51]

Although often unimpressive in a given section, the process, when taken in aggregate, is clearly capable of producing marked hemispheric atrophy. It features three basic tissue reactions: (1) chronic inflammation, (2) gliosis, and (3) neuronal loss.

The inflammatory infiltrate varies from case to case, and at times it is so minimal that the designation "encephalitis" is scarcely appropriate. In other instances, it is unmistakably apparent. Components of the infiltrate include lymphocytes, microglia, and macrophages (Fig. 3–93).[16, 25, 42] The lymphocytes, largely T cells, congregate in perivascular regions and infiltrate the parenchyma, where they may cluster about neurons. Leptomeningeal inflammation may also be present. Microglial cells, although inconspicuous and seemingly dormant in the normal brain, are awakened or activated, sometimes to a remarkable extent. Responding to the as yet unknown stimulus, they are evident with H&E stain as elongated nuclei (rod cells). These migrants can cluster in microaggregates confusingly referred to as both "microglial" and "glial" nodules that are sometimes centered around degenerating neurons, and they may simply loiter as individuals without obvious destination. During activation, microglia become HAM-56 and CD45 immunoreactive, their fuzzy bipolar processes with short ex-

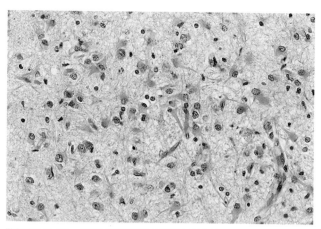

**FIGURE 3–94    RASMUSSEN'S ENCEPHALITIS**

Other areas of the brain, in the case of Figure 3–93, exhibit gliosis and depletion of neurons but little in the way of inflammation.

tensions becoming readily apparent. Although Rasmussen's encephalitis shares many histologic features with viral encephalitis, inclusion bodies are not present.

Gliosis can be either subtle and focal or marked and widespread, wherein it takes the form of the classical fibrillary gliosis, characterized by glassy cytoplasm and long, radiating cell processes (Fig. 3–94). In advanced cases, diffuse cortical microcystic change may be present.

In summary, the overall histologic appearance of Rasmussen's encephalitis is that of a chronic encephalitis with features suggestive of a viral origin. Nonetheless, attempts to find an etiologic agent have been unsuccessful.[57] An alternative hypothesis incriminates autoantibodies to the glutamate receptor GluR3.[43]

## Amyloidoma

Masses composed largely of amyloid appear occasionally within the brain substance,[11, 29, 48, 49, 53] at the base of the skull,[18, 31, 32, 54] and in cranial nerves. Among the last, the trigeminal is favored,[31, 32] sometimes bilaterally.[36] Neither systemic amyloidosis nor plasma cell dyscrasia is present.

The lesions are amorphous or concretion-filled masses with the flocculent or laminated appearance of amyloid (Fig. 3–95). Vascular involvement can be prominent, but the entity should be distinguished from the much more common cortex- or leptomeninges-oriented congophilic angiopathy discussed in Chapter 7. Birefringence with polarized light solidifies the diagnosis (Fig. 3–96). Immunohistochemical staining for $\lambda$ light chains suggested that the lesion is a well-differentiated clonal proliferation, that is, a neoplasm.[28, 55] The process is discussed here primarily in light of the inflammatory appearance in sections and the absence of evidence of systemic disease or local recurrence. Treatment has been by observation alone. Neither recurrence nor progression to a malignant plasma cell neoplasm has been observed.[48]

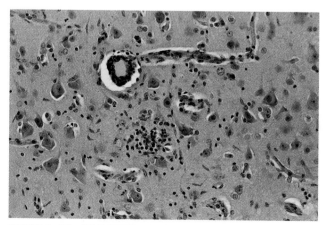

**FIGURE 3–93    RASMUSSEN'S ENCEPHALITIS**

Lymphocytes huddle around vessels, while microglial rod cells aggregate within the parenchyma. In this active area of inflammation, there is little gliosis or tissue loss.

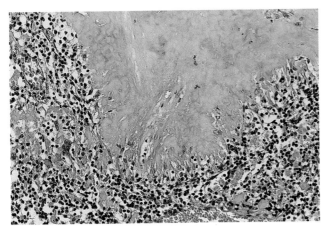

**FIGURE 3–95    AMYLOIDOMA**

A lymphocytic infiltrate surrounds a mass of eosinophilic material consistent with amyloid.

## Erdheim-Chester Disease

This rare intracranial inflammatory disorder is discussed in Chapter 9 on pages 488 to 489.

## Collagen-Vascular Diseases

The principal changes affect meninges and vessels in the subarachnoid space, and these lesions are described in Chapter 2 on pages 98 to 99. The myelopathy associated with systemic lupus erythematosus is discussed on page 545.

## Behçet's Disease

This is a rare systemic vasculitic process with recurrent ulcerations in the mouth and genital regions. Uveitis is common. CNS involvement is detected by MR in the form of T2-bright foci throughout the brain, including

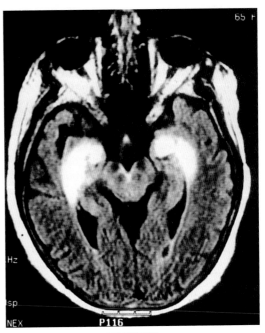

**FIGURE 3–97    LIMBIC ENCEPHALITIS**

As illustrated in this FLAIR MR image, the disease can be bilaterally symmetric. The abnormal white signal affects both medial temporal lobes. The patient, a 65-year-old woman, presented with severe recent memory loss and disorientation. No systemic neoplasm was detected. (Courtesy of Dr. Marc K. Rosenblum, New York, NY.)

the brain stem.[3, 15, 22, 26] Histologically, the nonspecific lesions contain lymphocytes, macrophages, and gliosis.[58] Large vessels may be affected.[2, 22]

## Paraneoplastic Disease (Limbic Encephalitis)

An occasional patient with systemic neoplasm, especially small cell carcinoma of the lung,[1, 8] develops cerebral lesions as a consequence of circulating anti-

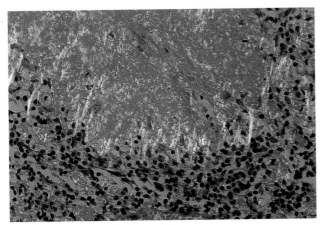

**FIGURE 3–96    AMYLOIDOMA**

The "apple green" birefringence of amyloid in a Congo red–stained section viewed with polarized light confirms the diagnosis.

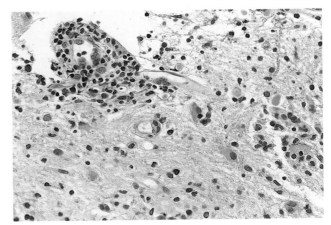

**FIGURE 3–98    LIMBIC ENCEPHALITIS**

The nonspecific histologic changes in the case illustrated in Figure 3–97 include perivascular lymphocyte infiltrates and gliosis.

neuronal antibodies, such as anti-Hu (Fig. 3–97).[12, 14, 44, 47] The neoplasm may not be apparent at the time the CNS expressions appear, and in some cases no tumor ever declares itself. The two most common conditions in the brain are cerebellar degeneration (especially Purkinje cell loss) and limbic encephalitis. Because the underlying neoplasm may not be recognized at the time of the initial cerebral symptoms, a rare case of the limbic encephalitis comes to biopsy.[9, 44] Personality change and memory disturbances are the common symptoms.[8, 9, 12, 20]

Limbic encephalitis classically appears on MR imaging as bilateral contrast-enhancing, T2-bright areas in the medial temporal lobes. Occasional cases are unilateral.[9] Histologically, foci of necrosis, perivascular lymphocytic infiltrates, and "glial," that is, microglial, nodules may be seen (Fig. 3–98).[12, 47, 50] Paraneoplastic disease of the spinal cord is described on pages 545 to 546.

## Malakoplakia

This rare chronic inflammatory lesion, with large phagolysosomes and laminated targetoid calcified concretions (Michaelis-Gutmann bodies), is only rarely seen in the brain.[5, 10, 21, 24]

## Textiloma (Muslinoma, Gauzoma)

An inflammatory reaction, often with foreign body giant cells, is induced by a fiber-containing substance that was used to wrap intracranial aneurysms.[6, 17, 19, 23, 34, 38, 40] A similar response to cotton balls left in the operative site can ensue.

## Graft-Versus-Host Disease

Focal lesions, either unilateral or bilateral, have been seen in the setting of bone marrow transplantation. It remains to be seen whether these are truly a graft response.[41, 46]

## Inflammatory Pseudoneoplasms

Because they are primarily meningeal lesions, often a meningioma-like mass, plasma cell granuloma, Rosai-Dorfman disease, Castleman's disease, hypertrophic pachymeningitis, and collagen-vascular diseases are discussed in Chapter 2 on pages 93 to 98.

## REFERENCES

**Demyelinating Diseases**

1. Adams CWM, Poston RN. Macrophage histology in paraffin-embedded multiple sclerosis plaques is demonstrated by the monoclonal pan-macrophage marker HAM-56: correlation with chronicity of the lesion. Acta Neuropathol 1990;80:208–211.
2. Adams RD, Kubik CS. The morbid anatomy of the demyelinative diseases. Am J Med 1952;12:510–546.
3. Atlas SW, Grossman RI, Goldberg HI, et al. MR diagnosis of acute disseminated encephalomyelitis. J Comput Assist Tomogr 1986;10:798–801.
4. Burger PC, Scheithauer BW, Lee RR, et al. An interdisciplinary approach to avoid the overtreatment of patients with central nervous system lesions. Cancer 1997;80:2040–2046.
5. Estes ML, Rudick RA, Barnett GH, et al. Stereotactic biopsy of an active multiple sclerosis lesion. Immunocytochemical analysis and neuropathologic correlation with magnetic resonance imaging. Arch Neurol 1990;47:1299–1303.
6. Gharagozloo AM, Poe LB, Collins GH. Antemortem diagnosis of Baló concentric sclerosis: correlative MR imaging and pathologic features. Radiology 1994;191:817–819.
7. Glasier CM, Robbins MB, Davis P, et al. Clinical, neurodiagnostic, and MR findings in children with spinal and brain stem multiple sclerosis. AJNR 1995;16:87–95.
8. Ho K-L, Wolfe DE. Concurrence of multiple sclerosis and primary intracranial neoplasms. Cancer 1981;47:2913–2919.
9. Hook CC, Kimmel DW, Kvols LK, et al. Multifocal inflammatory leukoencephalopathy with 5-fluorouracil and levamisole. Ann Neurol 1992;31:262–267.
10. Hulette CM, Downey BT, Burger PC. Macrophage markers in diagnostic neuropathology. Am J Surg Pathol 1992;16:493–499.
11. Hunter SB, Ballinger WE Jr, Rubin JJ. Multiple sclerosis mimicking primary brain tumor. Arch Pathol Lab Med 1987; 111:464–468.
12. Iannetti P, Marciani MG, Spalice A, et al. Primary CNS demyelinating diseases in childhood: multiple sclerosis. Childs Nerv Syst 1996;12:149–154.
13. Kepes JJ. Large focal tumor-like demyelinating lesions of the brain: intermediate entity between multiple sclerosis and acute disseminated encephalomyelitis? A study of 31 patients. Ann Neurol 1993;33:18–27.
14. Kesselring J, Miller DH, Robb SA, et al. Acute disseminated encephalomyelitis. MRI findings and the distinction from multiple sclerosis. Brain 1990;113:291–302.
15. Mader I, Stock KW, Ettlin T, et al. Acute disseminated encephalomyelitis: MR and CT features. AJNR 1996;17:104–109.
16. Masdeu JC, Moreira J, Trasi S, et al. The open ring. A new imaging sign in demyelinating disease. J Neuroimaging 1996;6:104–107.
17. Morre GRW, Neumann PE, Suzuki K, et al. Baló's concentric sclerosis: new observations on lesion development. Ann Neurol 1985;17:604–611.
18. Morrissey SP, Miller DH, Kendall BE, et al. The significance of brain magnetic resonance imaging abnormalities at presentation with clinically isolated syndromes suggestive of multiple sclerosis. A 5-year follow-up study. Brain 1993;116:135–146.
19. Nandini M, Gourie-Devi M, Shankar SK, et al. Case report. Baló's concentric sclerosis diagnosed intravitam on brain biopsy. Clin Neurol Neurosurg 1993;95:303–309.
20. Nesbit GM, Forbes GS, Scheithauer BW, et al. Multiple sclerosis: histopathologic and MR and/or CT correlation in 37 cases at biopsy and three cases at autopsy. Radiology 1991;180:467–474.
21. Osborn AG, Harnsberger HR, Smoker WRK, et al. Multiple sclerosis in adolescents: CT and MR findings. AJNR 1990; 11:489–494.
22. Passe TJ, Beauchamp NJ Jr, Burger PC. Neuroimaging in the identification of low-grade and nonneoplastic CNS lesions. Neurologist 1999;5:293–299.
23. Peterson K, Rosenblum MK, Power JM, et al. Effect of brain irradiation on demyelinating lesions. Neurology 1993;43:2105–2112.
24. Raisanen J, Goodman HS, Ghougassian DF, et al. Role of cytology in the intraoperative diagnosis of central demyelinating disease. Acta Cytol 1998;42:907–912.
25. Rieth KG, Chiro GD, Cromwell LD, et al. Primary demyelinating disease simulating glioma of the corpus callosum. J Neurosurg 1981;55:620–624.
26. Rusin JA, Vezina LG, Chadduck WM, et al. Tumoral multiple sclerosis of the cerebellum in a child. AJNR 1995;16:1164–1166.
27. Savarese DM, Gordon J, Smith TW, et al. Cerebral demyelination syndrome in a patient treated with 5-fluorouracil and levamisole. Cancer 1996;77:387–394.
28. Scully RE (ed). Weekly clinicopathological exercises: case 26-1998. N Engl J Med 1998;339:542–549.

29. Scully RE (ed). Weekly clinicopathological exercises; Case 12-1997. N Engl J Med 1997;336:1163–1171.
30. Shankar SK, Rao TV, Srivastav VK, et al. Baló's concentric sclerosis: a variant of multiple sclerosis associated with oligodendroglioma. Neurosurgery 1989;25:982–986.
31. Zagzag D, Miller DC, Kleinman GM, et al. Demyelinating disease versus tumor in surgical neuropathology. Am J Surg Pathol 1993;17:537–545.

## Pyogenic Abscess

1. Aarabi B, Taghipour M, Alibaii E, et al. Central nervous system infections after military missile head wounds. Neurosurgery 1998;42:500–509.
2. Barlas O, Sencer A, Erkan K, et al. Stereotactic surgery in the management of brain abscess. Surg Neurol 1999;52:404–410.
3. Beller AJ, Sahar A, Praiss I. Brain abscess. Review of 89 cases over a period of 30 years. J Neurol Neurosurg Psychiatry 1973;36:757–768.
4. Brewer NS, MacCarty CS, Wellman WE. Brain abscess: a review of recent experience. Ann Intern Med 1975;82:571–576.
5. Britt RH, Enzmann DR. Clinical stages of human brain abscesses on serial CT scans after contrast infusion. J Neurosurg 1983;59:972–989.
6. Britt RH, Enzmann DR, Yeager AS. Neuropathological and computerized tomographic findings in experimental brain abscess. J Neurosurg 1981;55:590–603.
7. Brook I. Bacteriology of intracranial abscess in children. J Neurosurg 1981;54:484–488.
8. Dev R, Gupta RK, Poptani H, et al. Role of in vivo proton magnetic resonance spectroscopy in the diagnosis and management of brain abscesses. Neurosurgery 1998;42:37–43.
9. Ersahin Y, Mutluer S, Güzelbag E. Brain abscess in infants and children. Childs Nerv Syst 1994;10:185–189.
10. Falconer MA, McFarlan AM, Russell DS. Experimental brain abscesses in the rabbit. Br J Surg 1943;30:245–260.
11. Fulgham JR, Wijdicks EFM, Wright AJ. Cure of a solitary brainstem abscess with antibiotic therapy: case report. Neurology 1996;46:1451–1454.
12. Gupta SK, Manjunath-Prasad KS, Sharma BS, et al. Brain abscess in renal transplant recipients: report of three cases. Surg Neurol 1997;48:284–287.
13. Haimes AB, Zimmerman RD, Morgello S, et al. MR imaging of brain abscesses. AJNR 1989;10:279–291.
14. Heineman HS, Braude AI. Anaerobic infection of the brain. Observations on eighteen consecutive cases of brain abscess. Am J Med 1963;35:682–697.
15. Krajewski R, Stelmasiak Z. Brain abscess in infants. Childs Nerv Syst 1992;8:279–280.
16. Mamelak AN, Mampalam TJ, Obana WG, et al. Improved management of multiple brain abscesses: a combined surgical and medical approach. Neurosurgery 1995;36:76–86.
17. Mamelak AN, Obana WG, Flaherty JF, et al. Nocardial brain abscess: treatment strategies and factors influencing outcome. Neurosurgery 1994;35:622–631.
18. Nadvi SS, Parboosing R, van Dellen JR. Cerebellar abscess: the significance of cerebrospinal fluid diversion. Neurosurgery 1997;41:61–67.
19. Nassar SI, Haddad FS, Hanbali FS, et al. Abscess superimposed on brain tumor: two case reports and review of the literature. Surg Neurol 1997;47:484–488.
20. Quartey GRC, Johnston JA, Rozdilsky B. Decadron in the treatment of cerebral abscess: an experimental study. J Neurosurg 1976;45:301–310.
21. Rajshekhar V, Chandy MJ. Successful stereotactic management of a large cardiogenic brain stem abscess. Neurosurgery 1994;34:368–371.
22. Ruelle A, Zerbi D, Zuccarello M, Andrioli G. Brain stem abscess treated successfully by medical therapy. Neurosurgery 1991;28:742–746.
23. Shaw MDM, Russell JA. Cerebellar abscess. A review of 47 cases. J Neurol Neurosurg Psychiatry 1975;38:429–435.
24. Takeshita M, Kagawa M, Yato S, et al. Current treatment of brain abscess in patients with congenital cyanotic heart disease. Neurosurgery 1997;41:1270–1279.
25. Tekkök IH, Erbengi A. Management of brain abscess in children: review of 130 cases over a period of 21 years. Childs Nerv Syst 1992;8:411–416.

26. Yang S, Zhao C. Review of 140 patients with brain abscess. Surg Neurol 1993;39:290–296.
27. Zeidman SM, Geisler FH, Olivi A. Intraventricular rupture of a purulent brain abscess: case report. Neurosurgery 1995;36:189–193.

## Tuberculosis

1. Arseni C. Two hundred and one cases of intracranial tuberculoma treated surgically. J Neurol Neurosurg Psychiatry 1958;21:308–311.
2. Asenjo A, Valladares H, Fierro J. Tuberculomas of the brain: report on one hundred and fifty-nine cases. Arch Neurol Psychiatry 1951;65:146–160.
3. Berenguer J, Moreno S, Laguna F, et al. Tuberculous meningitis in patients infected with the human immunodeficiency virus. N Engl J Med 1992;326:668–672.
4. Clark WC, Metcalf JC Jr, Muhlbauer MS, et al. *Mycobacterium tuberculosis* meningitis: a report of twelve cases and a literature review. Neurosurgery 1986;18:604–610.
5. Dastur HM, Desai AD. A comparative study of brain tuberculomas and gliomas based on 107 case records of each. Brain 1965;88:375–396.
6. Descuns P, Garré H, Phéline C. Tuberculomas of the brain and cerebellum. J Neurosurg 1954;11:243–250.
7. Di Patre PL, Radziszewski W, Martin NA, et al. A meningioma-mimicking tumor caused by *Mycobacterium avium* complex in an immunocompromised patient. Am J Surg Pathol 2000;24:136–139.
8. Evans HS, Courville CB. Calcification and ossification in tuberculoma of the brain: review of the literature and report of three cases. Arch Surg 1938;36:637–659.
9. Fischl MA, Pitchenik AE, Spira TJ. Tuberculous brain abscess and toxoplasma encephalitis in a patient with the acquired immunodeficiency syndrome. JAMA 1985;253:3428–3430.
10. Garland HG, Armitage G. Intracranial tuberculoma. J Pathol Bacteriol 1933;37:461–471.
11. González PRM, Herrero DV, Joachim GF. Tuberculous brain abscess. J Neurosurg 1980;52:419–422.
12. González-Revilla A. Intracranial tuberculomas: experience with ten consecutive cases. J Neurosurg 1952;9:555–563.
13. Gray F. Bacterial infections. Brain Pathol 1997;7:629–647.
14. Grayeli AB, Redondo A, Salama J, et al. Tuberculoma of the cavernous sinus: case report. Neurosurgery 1998;42:179–182.
15. Gropper MR, Schulder M, Duran HL, et al. Cerebral tuberculosis with expansion into brainstem tuberculoma. J Neurosurg 1994;81:927–931.
16. Gropper MR, Schulder M, Sharan AD, et al. Central nervous system tuberculosis: medical management and surgical indications. Surg Neurol 1995;44:378–385.
17. Gyure KA, Prayson RA, Estes ML. Symptomatic *Mycobacterium avium* complex infection of the central nervous system. A case report and review of the literature. Arch Pathol Lab Med 1995;119:836–839.
18. Harrison MJG, McArthur JC. Opportunistic infections—bacteria. In AIDS and Neurology. New York: Churchill-Livingstone, 1995, pp 151–170.
19. Higazi I. Tuberculoma of the brain: a clinical and angiographic study. J Neurosurg 1963;20:378–386.
20. Indira B, Panigrahi MK, Vajramani G, et al. Tuberculoma of the hypothalamic region as a rare case of hypopituitarism: a case report. Surg Neurol 1996;45:347–350.
21. Isenmann S, Zimmermann DR, Wichmann W, et al. Tuberculoma mimicking meningioma of the falx cerebri. PCR diagnosis of mycobacterial DNA from formalin-fixed tissue. Clin Neuropathol 1996;15:155–158.
22. Kim TK, Chang KH, Kim CJ, et al. Intracranial tuberculoma: comparison of MR with pathologic findings. AJNR 1995;16:1903–1908.
23. Lindner A, Schneider C, Hofmann E, et al. Isolated meningeal tuberculoma mimicking meningioma: case report. Surg Neurol 1995;43:81–84.
24. Mohanty A, Santosh V, Anandh B, et al. Diagnostic efficacy of stereotactic biopsies in intracranial tuberculomas. Surg Neurol 1999;52:252–257.
25. Mohanty A, Venkatarama SK, Vasudev MK, et al. Role of stereotactic aspiration in the management of tuberculous brain abscess. Surg Neurol 1999;51:443–446; discussion 6–7.

26. Molavi A, LeFrock JL. Tuberculous meningitis. Med Clin North Am 1985;69:315–330.
27. Morrison A, Gyure KA, Stone J, et al. Mycobacterial spindle cell pseudotumor of the brain: a case report and review of the literature. Am J Surg Pathol 1999;23:1294–1299.
28. Rab SM, Bhatti IH, Ghani A, et al. Tuberculous brain abscess: case report. J Neurosurg 1975;43:490–494.
29. Ramamurthi B, Varadarajan MG. Diagnosis of tuberculomas of the brain: clinical and radiologic correlation. J Neurosurg 1961;18:1–7.
30. Sandhyamani S, Roy S, Bhatia R. Tuberculous brain abscess. Acta Neurochir 1981;59:247–256.
31. Sinh G, Pandya SK, Dastur DK. Pathogenesis of unusual intracranial tuberculomas and tuberculous space-occupying lesions. J Neurosurg 1968;29:149–159.
32. Talamás O, Del Bruto OH, García-Ramos G. Brain-stem tuberculoma. An analysis of 11 patients. Arch Neurol 1989;46:529–535.
33. van Dellen A, Nadvi SS, Nathoo N, et al. Intracranial tuberculous subdural empyema: case report. Neurosurgery 1998;43:370–373.
34. Villoria MF, de la Torre J, Fortea F, et al. Intracranial tuberculosis in AIDS: CT and MRI findings. Neuroradiology 1992;34: 11–14.
35. Whiteman M, Espinoza L, Post MJD, et al. Central nervous system tuberculosis in HIV-infected patients: clinical and radiographic findings. AJNR 1995;16:1319–1327.
36. Winkelman NW, Moore MT. Meningeal blood vessels in tuberculous meningitis. Am Rev Tuberc 1940;42:315–333.

## Other Bacterial Infections

1. Adams M, Rhyner PA, Day J, DeArmond S, et al. Whipple's disease confined to the central nervous system. Ann Neurol 1987;21: 104–108.
2. Agrons GA, Han SS, Husson MA, et al. MR imaging of cerebral gumma. AJNR 1991;12:80–81.
3. Berger JR, Waskin H, Pall L, et al. Syphilitic cerebral gumma with HIV infection. Neurology 1992;42:1282–1287.
4. Brightbill TC, Ihmeidan IH, Donovan MJD, et al. Neurosyphilis in HIV-positive and HIV-negative patients: neuroimaging findings. AJNR 1995;16:703–711.
5. Brown AP, Lane JC, Murayama S, et al. Whipple's disease presenting with isolated neurological symptoms. Case report. J Neurosurg 1990;73:623–627.
6. Carithers HA, Margileth AM. Cat-scratch disease. Acute encephalopathy and other neurologic manifestations. Am J Dis Child 1991;145:98–101.
7. Dailey AT, LeRoux PD, Grady MS. Resolution of an actinomycotic abscess with nonsurgical treatment: case report. Neurosurgery 1993;32:134–136; discussion 6–7.
8. Fernandez RE, Rothberg M, Ferencz G, et al. Lyme disease of the CNS: MR imaging findings in 14 cases. AJNR 1990;11: 479–481.
9. Feurle GE, Volk B, Waldherr R. Cerebral Whipple's disease with negative jejunal histology. N Engl J Med 1979;300:907–908.
10. Gray F. Bacterial infections. Brain Pathol 1997;7:629–647.
11. Halperin JJ, Landis DMD, Kleinman GM. Whipple disease of the nervous system. Neurology 1982;32:612–617.
12. Halperin JJ, Luft BJ, Anand AK, et al. Lyme neuroborreliosis: central nervous system manifestations. Neurology 1989;39: 753–759.
13. Harrison MJG, McArthur JC. Opportunistic infections—bacteria. In AIDS and Neurology. New York: Churchill-Livingstone, 1995, pp 151–170.
14. Holmes MD, Brant-Zawadzki MM, Simon RP. Clinical features of meningovascular syphilis. Neurology 1984;34:553–556.
15. Horowitz HW, Valsamis MP, Wicher V, et al. Brief report: cerebral syphilitic gumma confirmed by the polymerase chain reaction in man with human immunodeficiency virus infection. N Engl J Med 1994;331:1488–1491.
16. Lewis DW, Tucker SH. Central nervous system involvement in cat scratch disease. Pediatrics 1986;77:714–721.
17. Logigian EL, Kaplan RF, Steere AC. Chronic neurologic manifestations of Lyme disease. N Engl J Med 1990;323:1438–1444.
18. Madsen FF, Pedersen KK, Stubbe-Teglbjaerg P. Short report. Cerebral gumma. Br J Neurosurg 1987;1:509–513.
19. Mendel E, Khoo LT, Go JL, et al. Intracerebral Whipple's disease diagnosed by stereotactic biopsy: a case report and review of the literature. Neurosurgery 1999;44:203–209.

20. Murray R, Morawetz R, Kepes J, et al. Lyme neuroborreliosis manifesting as an intracranial mass lesion. Neurosurgery 1992; 30:769–773.
21. Pachner AR, Duray P, Steere AC. Central nervous system manifestations of Lyme disease. Arch Neurol 1989;46:790–795.
22. Rafto SE, Milton WJ, Galetta SL, et al. Biopsy-confirmed CNS Lyme disease: MR appearance at 1.5 T. AJNR 1990;11:482–484.
23. Schnider P, Trattnig S, Kollegger H, et al. MR of cerebral Whipple disease. AJNR 1995;16:1328–1329.
24. Silbert SW, Parker E, Horenstein S. Whipple's disease of the central nervous system. Acta Neuropathol 1976;36:31–38.
25. Simon RP. Neurosyphilis. Arch Neurol 1985;42:606–613.
26. Vogl T, Dresel S, Lochmüller H, et al. Third cranial nerve palsy caused by gummatous neurosyphilis: MR findings. AJNR 1993;14:1329–1331.

## Herpes Simplex Encephalitis

1. Bourgeois M, Vinikoff L, Lellouch-Tubiana A, et al. Reactivation of herpes virus after surgery for epilepsy in a pediatric patient with mesial temporal sclerosis: case report. Neurosurgery 1999;44:633–635; discussion 5–6.
2. Budka J, Popow-Kraupp T. Rabies and herpes simplex virus encephalitis. An immunohistological study on site and distribution of viral antigens. Virchows Arch 1981;390:353–364.
3. Charpin C, Gambarelli D, Lavaut MN, et al. Herpes simplex virus antigen detection in human acute encephalitis: an immunohistochemical study using avidin-biotin-peroxidase complex method. Acta Neuropathol 1985;68:245–252.
4. Chou SM, Cherry JD. Ultrastructure of Cowdry type A inclusions. I. In human herpes simplex encephalitis. Neurology 1967; 17:575–586.
5. Dennett C, Cleator GM, Klapper PE. HSV-1 and HSV-2 in herpes simplex encephalitis: a study of sixty-four cases in the United Kingdom. J Med Virol 1997;53:1–3.
6. Di Sclafani A, Kohl S, Ostrow PT. The importance of brain biopsy in suspected herpes simplex encephalitis. Surg Neurol 1982;17:101–106.
7. Ebel H, Kuchta J, Balogh A, et al. Operative treatment of tentorial herniation in herpes encephalitis. Childs Nerv Syst 1999; 15:84–86.
8. Esiri MM. Herpes simplex encephalitis. An immunohistological study of the distribution of viral antigen within the brain. J Neurol Sci 1982;54:209–226.
9. Kaplan CP, Bain KP. Cognitive outcome after emergent treatment of acute herpes simplex encephalitis with acyclovir. Brain Inj 1999;13:935–941.
10. Koenig H, Rabinowitz SG, Day E, et al. Post-infectious encephalomyelitis after successful treatment of herpes simplex encephalitis with adenine arabinoside. N Engl J Med 1979;300: 1089–1093.
11. Kohl S, James AR. Herpes simplex virus encephalitis during childhood: importance of brain biopsy diagnosis. J Pediatr 1985; 107:212–215.
12. Lakeman FD, Whitley RJ. Diagnosis of herpes simplex encephalitis: application of polymerase chain reaction to cerebrospinal fluid from brain-biopsied patients and correlation with disease. J Infect Dis 1995;171:857–863.
13. Liedtke W, Opalka B, Zimmermann CW, Lignitz E. Age distribution of latent herpes simplex virus 1 and varicella-zoster virus genome in human nervous tissue. J Neurol Sci 1993;116:6–11.
14. Morawetz RB, Whitley RJ, Murphy DM. Experience with brain biopsy for suspected herpes encephalitis: a review of forty consecutive cases. Neurosurgery 1983;12:654–657.
15. Nahmias AJ, Roizman B. Infection with herpes-simplex viruses 1 and 2 (second of three parts). N Engl J Med 1973;289:719–725.
16. Nahmias AJ, Roizman B. Infection with herpes-simplex viruses 1 and 2 (third of three parts). N Engl J Med 1973;289:781–789.
17. Nahmias AJ, Roizman B. Infection with herpes-simplex viruses 1 and 2 (first of three parts). N Engl J Med 1973;289:667–674.
18. Rozenberg F, Lebon P. Amplification and characterization of herpesvirus DNA in cerebrospinal fluid from patients with acute encephalitis. J Clin Microbiol 1991;29:2412–2417.
19. Schiff D, Rosenblum MK. Herpes simplex encephalitis (HSE) and the immunocompromised: a clinical and autopsy study of HSE in the settings of cancer and human immunodeficiency virus-type 1 infection. Hum Pathol 1998;29:215–222.

20. Schroth G, Gawehn J, Thron A, Vallbracht A, Voigt K. Early diagnosis of herpes simplex encephalitis by MRI. Neurology 1987;37:179–183.
21. Swanson JL, Craighead JE, Reynolds ES. Electron microscopic observations on *Herpesvirus hominis* (herpes simplex virus) encephalitis in men. Lab Invest 1966;15:1966–1981.
22. Tan SV, Guiloff RJ, Scaravilli F, Klapper PE, Cleator GM, Gazzard BG. Herpes simplex type 1 encephalitis in acquired immunodeficiency syndrome. Ann Neurol 1993;34:619–622.
23. Tebas P, Nease RF, Storch GA. Use of the polymerase chain reaction in the diagnosis of herpes simplex encephalitis: a decision analysis model. Am J Med 1998;105:287–295.
24. Troendle-Atkins J, Demmler GJ, Buffone GJ. Rapid diagnosis of herpes simplex virus encephalitis by using the polymerase chain reaction. J Pediatr 1993;123:376–380.
25. Vital C, Monlun E, Vital A, et al. Concurrent herpes simplex type 1 necrotizing encephalitis, cytomegalovirus, ventriculoencephalitis and cerebral lymphoma in an AIDS patient. Acta Neuropathol 1995;89:105–108.
26. Whitley RJ. Herpes simplex virus infections of the central nervous system. A review. Am J Med 1988;85(Suppl 2A):61–66.
27. Whitley RJ, Alford CA, Hirsch MS, et al. Vidarabine versus acyclovir therapy in herpes simplex encephalitis. N Engl J Med 1986;314:144–149.

## Progressive Multifocal Leukoencephalopathy

1. Aksamit AJ, Mourrain P, Sever JL, Major EO. Progressive multifocal leukoencephalopathy: investigation of three cases using in situ hybridization with JC virus biotinylated DNA probe. Ann Neurol 1985;18:490–496.
2. Ariza A, Von Uexküll-Güldeband C, Mate JL, et al. Accumulation of wild-type p53 protein in progressive multifocal leukoencephalopathy: a flow cytometry and DNA sequencing study. J Neuropathol Exp Neurol 1996;55:144–149.
3. Åström K-E, Mancall EL, Richardson EP Jr. Progressive multifocal leuko-encephalopathy. A hitherto unrecognized complication of chronic lymphatic leukemia and Hodgkin's disease. Brain 1958;81:93–111.
4. Åström KE, Stoner GL. Early pathological changes in progressive multifocal leukoencephalopathy: a report of two asymptomatic cases occurring prior to the AIDS epidemic. Acta Neuropathol 1994;88:93–105.
5. Berger JR, Mucke L. Prolonged survival and partial recovery in AIDS-associated progressive multifocal leukoencephalopathy. Neurology 1988;38:1060–1065.
6. Bogdanovic G, Priftakis P, Hammarin AL, et al. Detection of JC virus in cerebrospinal fluid (CSF) samples from patients with progressive multifocal leukoencephalopathy but not in CSF samples from patients with herpes simplex encephalitis, enteroviral meningitis, or multiple sclerosis. J Clin Microbiol 1998;36: 1137–1138.
7. Cavanagh JG, Greenbaum D, Marshall AHE, Rubinstein LJ. Cerebral demyelination associated with disorders of the reticuloendothelial system. Lancet 1959;2:524–529.
8. Fong IW, Britton CB, Luinstra KE, Toma E, Mahony JB. Diagnostic value of detecting JC virus DNA in cerebrospinal fluid of patients with progressive multifocal leukoencephalopathy. J Clin Microbiol 1995;33:484–486.
9. Fong IW, Toma E. The natural history of progressive multifocal leukoencephalopathy in patients with AIDS. Clin Infect Dis 1995;20:1305–1310.
10. Garrels K, Kucharczyk W, Wortzman G, Shandling M. Progressive multifocal leukoencephalopathy: clinical and MR response to treatment. AJNR 1996;17:597–600.
11. Greenlee JE, Keeney PM. Immunoenzymatic labelling of JC papovavirus T antigen in brains of patients with progressive multifocal leukoencephalopathy. Acta Neuropathol 1986;71:150–153.
12. Hair LS, Nuovo G, Powers JM, et al. Progressive multifocal leukoencephalopathy in patients with human immunodeficiency virus. Hum Pathol 1992;23:663–667.
13. Hansman Whiteman ML, Donovan Post MJ, Berger JR, et al. Progressive multifocal leukoencephalopathy in 47 HIV-seropositive patients: neuroimaging with clinical and pathologic correlation. Radiology 1993;187:233–240.
14. Harrison MJG, McArthur JC. Opportunistic infections—viruses. In AIDS and Neurology. New York: Churchill-Livingstone, 1995, pp 133–150.
15. Hulette CM, Downey BT, Burger PC. Progressive multifocal leukoencephalopathy. Diagnosis by in situ hybridization with a biotinylated JC virus DNA probe using an automated histomatic code-on slide stainer. Am J Surg Pathol 1991;15:791–797.
16. Lammie GA, Beckett A, Courtney R, et al. An immunohistochemical study of p53 and proliferating cell nuclear antigen expression in progressive multifocal leukoencephalopathy. Acta Neuropathol (Berl) 1994;88:465–471.
17. London WT, Houff SA, Madden DL, et al. Brain tumors in owl monkeys inoculated with a human polyomavirus (JC virus). Science 1978;201:1246–1249.
18. McGuire D, Barhite S, Hollander H, et al. JC virus DNA in cerebrospinal fluid of human immunodeficiency virus–infected patients: predictive value for progressive multifocal leukoencephalopathy. Ann Neurol 1995;37:395–399.
19. Monforte Ad'A, Cinque P, Vago L, et al. A comparison of brain biopsy and CSF-PCR in the diagnosis of CNS lesions in AIDS patients. J Neurol 1997;244:35–39.
20. Nagashima K, Natsuda M, Ikeda K, et al. Induction of brain tumors experimentally by the JC virus. Prog Neuropathol 1986;6:145–163.
21. Padgett BL, Zu Rhein GM, Walker DL, et al. Cultivation of papova-like virus from human brain with progressive multifocal leucoencephalopathy. Lancet 1971;1:1257–1260.
22. Power C, Nath A, Aoki FY, et al. Remission of progressive multifocal leukoencephalopathy following splenectomy and antiretroviral therapy in a patient with HIB infection (Letter). N Engl J Med 1997;336:661–662.
23. Richardson EP Jr. Progressive multifocal leukoencephalopathy. N Engl J Med 1961;265:815–823.
24. Schmidbauer J, Budka H, Shah KV. Progressive multifocal leukoencephalopathy (PML) in AIDS and in the pre-AIDS era. Acta Neuropathol (Berl) 1990;80:375–380.
25. Silverman L, Rubinstein LJ. Electron microscopic observations on a case of progressive multifocal leukoencephalopathy. Acta Neuropathol (Berl) 1965;5:215–224.
26. Sima AAF, Finkelstein SD, McLachlan DR. Multiple malignant astrocytomas in a patient with spontaneous progressive multifocal leukoencephalopathy. Ann Neurol 1983;14:183–188.
27. Steiger MJ, Tarnesby G, Gabe S, et al. Successful outcome of progressive multifocal leukoencephalopathy with cytarabine and interferon. Ann Neurol 1993;33:407–411.
28. Walker DL, Padgett BL, Zu Rhein GM, et al. Human papovavirus (JC): induction of brain tumors in hamsters. Science 1973;181:674–676.
29. Whiteman MLH, Post MJD, Berger JR, et al. Progressive multifocal leukoencephalopathy in 47 HIV-seropositive patients: neuroimaging with clinical and pathologic correlation. Radiology 1993;187:233–240.
30. Woodhouse MA, Dayan AD, Burston J, et al. Progressive multifocal leukoencephalopathy: electron microscope study of four cases. Brain 1967;90:863–872.
31. Zu Rhein GM. Polyoma-like virions in a human demyelinating disease. Acta Neuropathol (Berl) 1967;8:57–68.
32. Zu Rhein GM, Chou S-M. Particles resembling papova viruses in human cerebral demyelinating disease. Science 1965;148: 1477–1479.

## Other Viral Infections

1. Allen IV, McQuaid S, McMahon J, et al. The significance of measles virus antigen and genome distribution in the CNS in SSPE for mechanisms of viral spread and demyelination. J Neuropathol Exp Neurol 1996;55:471–480.
2. Amlie-Lefond C, Kleinschmidt-DeMasters BK, Mahalingam R, et al. The vasculopathy of varicella-zoster virus encephalitis. Ann Neurol 1995;37:784–790.
3. Anlar B, Saatçi I, Köse G, et al. MRI findings in subacute sclerosing panencephalitis. Neurology 1996;47:1278–1283.
4. Baram TZ, Gonzalez-Gomez I, Xie Z-D, et al. Subacute sclerosing panencephalitis in an infant: diagnostic role of viral genome analysis. Ann Neurol 1994;36:103–108.
5. Brismar J, Gascon GG, Vult von Steyern K, et al. Subacute sclerosing panencephalitis: evaluation with CT and MR. AJNR 1996;17:761–772.
6. Dawson JR Jr. Cellular inclusions in cerebral lesions of lethargic encephalitis. Am J Pathol 1933;9:7–19.

7. Deresiewicz RL, Thaler SJ, Hsu L, et al. Clinical and neuroradiographic manifestations of eastern equine encephalitis. N Engl J Med 1997;336:1867–1874.

8. Gilden DH, Murray RS, Wellish M, et al. Chronic progressive varicella-zoster virus encephalitis in an AIDS patient. Neurology 1988;38:1150–1153.

9. Gray F, Bélec L, Lescs MC, et al. Varicella-zoster virus infection of the central nervous system in the acquired immune deficiency syndrome. Brain 1994;117:987–999.

10. Harrison MJG, McArthur JC. Opportunistic infections—viruses. In AIDS and Neurology. New York: Churchill-Livingstone, 1995, pp 133–150.

11. Jemsek J, Greenberg SB, Taber L, et al. Herpes zoster–associated encephalitis: clinicopathologic report of 12 cases and review of the literature. Medicine (Baltimore) 1983;62:81–97.

12. McQuaid S, Allen IV, McMahon J, et al. Association of measles virus with neurofibrillary tangles in subacute sclerosing panencephalitis: a combined in situ hybridization and immunocytochemical investigation. Neuropathol Appl Neurobiol 1994;20:103–110.

13. Morgello S, Cho E-S, Nielsen S, et al. Cytomegalovirus encephalitis in patients with acquired immunodeficiency syndrome: an autopsy study of 30 cases and a review of the literature. Hum Pathol 1987;18:289–297.

14. Mrak RE, Young L. Rabies encephalitis in humans: pathology, pathogenesis and pathophysiology. J Neuropathol Exp Neurol 1994;53:1–10.

15. Ohya T, Martinez J, Jabbour JT, et al. Subacute sclerosing panencephalitis. Correlation of clinical, neurophysiologic and neuropathologic findings. Neurology 1974;24:211–218.

16. Oyanagi S. Histopathology and electron microscopy of three cases of subacute sclerosing panencephalitis (SSPE). Acta Neuropathol (Berl) 1971;18:58–73.

17. Oyanagi S, Ter Meulen V, Katz M, et al. Comparison of subacute sclerosing panencephalitis and measles viruses: an electron microscope study. J Virol 1971;7:176–187.

18. Schmidbauer M, Budka H, Ulrich W, et al. Cytomegalovirus (CMV) disease of the brain in AIDS and connatal infection: a comparative study by histology, immunocytochemistry and in situ DNA hybridization. Acta Neuropathol (Berl) 1989;79:286–293.

19. Schmidbauer M, Budka H, Pilz P, et al. Presence, distribution and spread of productive varicella zoster virus infection in nervous tissues. Brain 1992;115:383–398.

20. Scully RE (ed). Case records of the Massachusetts General Hospital. Case 15-1998. N Engl J Med 1998;338:1448–1456.

21. Tellez-Nagel I, Harter DH. Subacute sclerosing leukoencephalitis: ultrastructure of intranuclear and intracytoplasmic inclusions. Science 1966;154:899–901.

22. Zilber N, Rannon L, Alter M, et al. Measles, measles vaccination, and risk of subacute sclerosing panencephalitis (SSPE). Neurology 1983;33:1558–1564.

## Aspergillosis

1. Boes B, Bashir R, Boes C, et al. Central nervous system aspergillosis. Analysis of 26 patients. J Neuroimaging 1994;4:123–129.

2. Carrazana EJ, Rossitch E Jr, Morris J. Isolated central nervous system aspergillosis in the acquired immunodeficiency syndrome. Clin Neurol Neurosurg 1991;93:227–230.

3. Chimelli L, Mahler-Araújo MB. Fungal infections. Brain Pathol 1997;7:613–627.

4. Dayal Y, Weindling HK, Price DL. Cerebral infarction due to fungal embolus. Neurology 1974;24:76–79.

5. DeLone DR, Goldstein RA, Petermann G, et al. Disseminated aspergillosis involving the brain: distribution and imaging characteristics. AJNR 1999;20:1597–1604.

6. Gupta R, Singh AK, Bishnu P, et al. Case report. Intracranial Aspergillus granuloma simulating meningioma on MR imaging. J Comput Assist Tomogr 1990;14:467–469.

7. Harrison MJG, McArthur JC. Opportunistic infections—fungi. In AIDS and Neurology. New York: Churchill-Livingstone, 1995, pp 119–132.

8. Kim DG, Hong SC, Kim HJ, et al. Cerebral aspergillosis in immunologically competent patients. Surg Neurol 1993;40:326–331.

9. Klein HJ, Richter H-P, Schachenmayr W. Intracerebral aspergillus abscess: case report. Neurosurgery 1983;13:306–309.

10. Kurino M, Kuratsu J, Yamaguchi T, et al. Mycotic aneurysm accompanied by aspergillotic granuloma: a case report. Surg Neurol 1994;42:160–164.

11. Kurita H, Shiokawa Y, Furuya K, et al. Parasellar Aspergillus granuloma extending from the sphenoid sinus: report of two cases. Surg Neurol 1995;44:489–494.

12. Miaux Y, Ribaud P, Williams M, et al. MR of cerebral aspergillosis in patients who have had bone marrow transplantation. AJNR 1995;16:555–562.

13. Minamoto GY, Barlam TF, Vander Els NJ. Invasive aspergillosis in patients with AIDS. Clin Infect Dis 1992;14:66–74.

14. Satoh H, Uozumi T, Kiya K, et al. Invasive aspergilloma of the frontal base causing internal carotid artery occlusion. Surg Neurol 1995;44:483–488.

15. Shuper A, Levitsky HI, Cornblath DR. Early invasive CNS aspergillosis. An easily missed diagnosis. Neuroradiology 1991;33:183–185.

16. Sparano JA, Gucalp R, Llena JF, et al. Clinical study. Cerebral infection complicating systemic aspergillosis in acute leukemia: clinical and radiographic presentation. J Neurooncol 1992;13:91–100.

17. Walsh TJ, Hier DB, Caplan LR. Aspergillosis of the central nervous system: clinicopathological analysis of 17 patients. Ann Neurol 1985;18:574–582.

18. Yanai Y, Wakao T, Fukamachi A, et al. Intracranial granuloma caused by Aspergillus fumigatus. Surg Neurol 1985;23:597–604.

19. Young RF, Gage G, Grinnell V. Surgical treatment of fungal infections in the central nervous system. J Neurosurg 1985;63:371–381.

## Blastomycosis

1. Chimelli L, Mahler-Araújo MB. Fungal infections. Brain Pathol 1997;7:613–627.

2. Craig W McK, Carmichael FA Jr. Blastomycoma of the cerebellum: report of a case. Proc Staff Meet Mayo Clin 1938;13:347–351.

3. Jay V, Laperriere N, Perrin R. Fulminant blastomycosis with blastomycotic infection of a cerebral glioma. Acta Neuropathol (Berl) 1991;82:420–424.

4. Mirra SS, Trombley IK, Miles ML. Blastomycoma of the cerebellum: an ultrastructural study. Acta Neuropathol 1980;50:109–113.

5. Morgan D, Young RF, Chow AW, et al. Recurrent intracerebral blastomycotic granuloma: diagnosis and treatment. Neurosurgery 1979;4:319–323.

6. Tang TT, Marsik FJ, Harb JM, et al. Cerebral blastomycosis: an immunodiagnostic study. Am J Clin Pathol 1984;82:243–246.

7. Waisbren BA, Ullrich D. An isolated blastomycetoma of the posterior cranial fossa treated successfully with surgery and amphotericin B. Am J Med 1962;32:621–624.

8. Ward BA, Parent AD, Raila F. Indications for the surgical management of central nervous system blastomycosis. Surg Neurol 1995;43:379–388.

9. Young RF, Gade G, Grinnell V. Surgical treatment for fungal infections in the central nervous system. J Neurosurg 1985;63:371–381.

## Coccidioidomycosis

1. Banuelos AF, Williams PL, Johnson RH, et al. Central nervous system abscesses due to Coccidioides species. Clin Infect Dis 1996;22:240–250.

2. Chimelli L, Mahler-Araújo MB. Fungal infections. Brain Pathol 1997;7:613–627.

3. Fish DG, Ampel NM, Galgiani JN, et al. Coccidioidomycosis during human immunodeficiency virus infection. A review of 77 patients. Medicine (Baltimore) 1990;69:384–391.

4. Mendel E, Milefchik EN, Ahmadi J, et al. Coccidioidomycotic brain abscess. Case report. J Neurosurg 1994;80:140–142.

5. Mischel PS, Vinters HV. Coccidioidomycosis of the central nervous system: neuropathological and vasculopathic manifestations and clinical correlates. Clin Infect Dis 1995;20:400–405.

6. Stevens DA. Coccidioidomycosis. N Engl J Med 1995;332:1077–1082.

7. Young RF, Gade G, Grinnell V. Surgical treatment for fungal infections in the central nervous system. J Neurosurg 1985;63:371–381.

## Cryptococcosis

1. Chimelli L, Mahler-Araújo MB. Fungal infections. Brain Pathol 1997;7:613–627.

2. Dillon ML, Sealy WC. Surgical aspects of opportunistic fungus infections. Lab Invest 1962;11:1231–1236.
3. Everett BA, Kusske JA, Rush JL, et al. Cryptococcal infection of the central nervous system. Surg Neurol 1978;9:157–163.
4. Garcia CA, Weisberg LA, Lacorte WSJ. Cryptococcal intracerebral mass lesions: CT-pathologic considerations. Neurology 1985;35:731–734.
5. Harper CG, Wright DM, Parry G, et al. Cryptococcal granuloma presenting as an intracranial mass. Surg Neurol 1979;11:425–429.
6. Harrison MJG, McArthur JC. Opportunistic infections—fungi. In AIDS and Neurology. New York: Churchill-Livingstone, 1995, pp 119–132.
7. Penar PL, Kim J, Chyatte D, et al. Intraventricular cryptococcal granuloma. Report of two cases. J Neurosurg 1988;68:145–148.
8. Popovich MJ, Arthur RH, Helmer E. CT of intracranial cryptococcosis. AJNR 1990;11:139–142.
9. Tien RD, Chu PK, Hesselink JR, et al. Intracranial cryptococcosis in immunocompromised patients: CT and MR findings in 29 cases. AJNR 1991;12:283–289.
10. Vender JR, Miller DM, Roth T, et al. Intraventricular cryptococcal cysts. AJNR 1996;17:110–113.
11. Wehn SM, Heinz ER, Burger PC, et al. Dilated Virchow-Robin spaces in cryptococcal meningitis associated with AIDS: CT and MR findings. J Comput Assist Tomogr 1989;13:756–762.

### Candidiasis

1. Chimelli L, Mahler-Araújo MB. Fungal infections. Brain Pathol 1997;7:613–627.
2. Ilgren EB, Westmoland D, Adams CBT, et al. Cerebellar mass caused by Candida species. Case report. J Neurosurg 1984;60:428–430.
3. Snider WD, Simpson DM, Nielsen S, et al. Neurological complications of acquired immune deficiency syndrome: analysis of 50 patients. Ann Neurol 1983;14:403–418.

### Histoplasmosis

1. Anaissie E, Fainstein V, Samo T, et al. Central nervous system histoplasmosis. An unappreciated complication of the acquired immunodeficiency syndrome. Am J Med 1988;84:215–217.
2. Bridges WR, Echols DH. Cerebellar histoplasmoma: case report. J Neurosurg 1967;26:261–263.
3. Greer HD, Geraci JE, Corbin KB, et al. Disseminated histoplasmosis presenting as a brain tumor and treated with amphotericin B: report of a case. Mayo Clin Proc 1964;39:490–494.
4. Klein CJ, Dinapoli RP, Temesgen Z, et al. Central nervous system histoplasmosis mimicking a brain tumor: difficulties in diagnosis and treatment. Mayo Clin Proc 1999;74:803–807.
5. Schochet SS, Sarwar M, Kelly PJ, et al. Symptomatic cerebral histoplasmoma: case report. J Neurosurg 1980;52:273–275.
6. Vakill ST, Eble JN, Richmond BD, et al. Cerebral histoplasmoma: case report. J Neurosurg 1983;59:332–336.
7. Venger BH, Landon G, Rose JE. Solitary histoplasmoma of the thalamus: case report and literature review. Neurosurgery 1987;20:784–787.
8. Wheat LJ, Batteiger BE, Sathapatayavongs B. Histoplasma capsulatum infections of the central nervous system. A clinical review. Medicine (Baltimore) 1990;69:244–260.
9. White HH, Fritzlen TJ. Cerebral granuloma caused by Histoplasma capsulatum. J Neurosurg 1962;19:260–263.

### Mucormycosis (Zygomycosis)

1. Adler DE, Milhorat TH, Miller JI. Treatment of rhinocerebral mucormycosis with intravenous, interstitial, and cerebrospinal fluid administration of amphotericin B: case report. Neurosurgery 1998;42:644–649.
2. Alleyne CH Jr, Vishteh AG, Spetzler RF, et al. Long-term survival of a patient with invasive cranial base rhinocerebral mucormycosis treated with combined endovascular, surgical, and medical therapies: case report. Neurosurgery 1999;45:1461–1463; discussion 3–4.
3. Bigner SH, Burger PC, Dubois PJ. Diagnosis of cerebral mucormycosis by needle aspiration biopsy: a case report. Acta Cytol 1982;26:699–704.
4. Chimelli L, Mahler-Araújo MB. Fungal infections. Brain Pathol 1997;7:613–627.

5. Gollard R, Rabb C, Larsen R, et al. Isolated cerebral mucormycosis: case report and therapeutic considerations. Neurosurgery 1994;34:174–177.
6. Hamill R, Oney LA, Crane LR. Successful therapy for rhinocerebral mucormycosis with associated bilateral brain abscesses. Arch Intern Med 1983;143:581–583.
7. Ignelzi RJ, Vanderark GD. Cerebral mucormycosis following open head trauma. Case report. J Neurosurg 1975;42:593–596.
8. Nussbaum ES, Hall WA. Rhinocerebral mucormycosis: changing patterns of disease. Surg Neurol 1994;41:152–156.
9. Watson DF, Stern BJ, Levin ML, et al. Isolated cerebral phycomycosis presenting as focal encephalitis. Arch Neurol 1985;42:922–923.

### Amebiasis

1. Carter RF. Primary amoebic meningo-encephalitis: clinical, pathological and epidemiological features of six fatal cases. J Pathol Bacteriol 1968;96:1–25.
2. Harrison MJG, McArthur JC. Opportunistic infections—parasites. In AIDS and Neurology. New York: Churchill-Livingstone, 1995, pp 171–181.
3. Martínez AJ, Guerra AE, García-Tamayo J, et al. Granulomatous amebic encephalitis: a review and report of a spontaneous case from Venezuela. Acta Neuropathol (Berl) 1994;87:430–434.
4. Martinez AJ, Visvesvara GS. Free-living, amphizoic and opportunistic amebas. Brain Pathol 1997;7:583–598.
5. Martinez JA. Acanthamoebiasis and immunosuppression. Case report. J Neuropathol Exp Neurol 1982;41:548–557.
6. Martínez JA, García CA, Halks-Miller M, et al. Granulomatous amebic encephalitis presenting as a cerebral mass lesion. Acta Neuropathol (Berl) 1980;51:85–91.
7. Wiley CA, Safrin RE, Davis CE, et al. Acanthamoeba meningoencephalitis in a patient with AIDS. J Infect Dis 1987;155:130–133.

### Toxoplasmosis

1. Bertoli F, Espino M, Arosemena VJR, et al. A spectrum in the pathology of toxoplasmosis in patients with acquired immunodeficiency syndrome. Arch Pathol Lab Med 1995;119:214–224.
2. Chang L, Cornford ME, Chiang FL, et al. Cerebral toxoplasmosis and lymphoma in AIDS. AJNR 1995;16:1653–1663.
3. Ciricillo SF, Rosenblum ML. Use of CT and MR imaging to distinguish intracranial lesions and to define the need for biopsy in AIDS patients. J Neurosurg 1990;73:720–724.
4. Gaston A, Gherardi R, Guyen JPN, et al. Cerebral toxoplasmosis in acquired immunodeficiency syndrome. A comparative assisted tomographic and neuropathological study of a case. Neuroradiology 1985;27:83–86.
5. Harrison MJG, McArthur JC. Opportunistic infections. In AIDS and Neurology. New York: Churchill-Livingstone, 1995, pp 171–181.
6. Laissy JP, Soyer P, Parlier C, et al. Persistent enhancement after treatment for cerebral toxoplasmosis in patients with AIDS: predictive value for subsequent recurrence. AJNR 1994;15:1773–1778.
7. Navia BA, Petito CK, Gold JWM, et al. Cerebral toxoplasmosis complicating the acquired immune deficiency syndrome: clinical and neuropathological findings in 27 patients. Ann Neurol 1986;19:224–238.
8. Porter SB, Sande MA. Toxoplasmosis of the central nervous system in the acquired immunodeficiency syndrome. N Engl J Med 1992;327:1643–1648.
9. Strittmatter C, Lang W, Wiestler OD, et al. The changing pattern of human immunodeficiency virus–associated cerebral toxoplasmosis: a study of 46 postmortem cases. Acta Neuropathol (Berl) 1992;83:475–481.
10. Sun T, Greenspan J, Tenenbaum M, et al. Diagnosis of cerebral toxoplasmosis using fluorescein-labeled antitoxoplasma monoclonal antibodies. Am J Surg Pathol 1986;10:312–316.
11. Tang TT, Harb JM, Dunne WM Jr, et al. Cerebral toxoplasmosis in an immunocompromised host. A precise and rapid diagnosis by electron microscopy. Am J Clin Pathol 1986;85:104–110.

### Cysticercosis

1. Colli BO, Martelli N, Assirati JA Jr, et al. Results of surgical treatment of neurocysticercosis in 69 cases. J Neurosurg 1986;65:309–315.

2. Couldwell WT, Zee C-S, Apuzzo MLJ. Definition of the role of contemporary surgical management in cisternal parenchymatous cysticercosis cerebri. Neurosurgery 1991;28:231–237.

3. Couldwell WT, Chandrasoma P, Apuzzo MLJ, et al. Third ventricular cysticercal cyst mimicking a colloid cyst: case report. Neurosurgery 1995;37:1200–1203.

4. Kim SK, Wang KC, Paek SH, et al. Outcomes of medical treatment of neurocysticercosis: a study of 65 cases in Cheju Island, Korea. Surg Neurol 1999;52:563–569.

5. La Mantia L, Costa A, Eoli M, et al. Case report. Racemose neurocysticercosis after chronic meningitis: effect of medical treatment. Clin Neurol Neurosurg 1995;97:50–54.

6. Lath R, Rajshekhar V. Solitary cysticercus granuloma of the brainstem. Report of four cases. J Neurosurg 1998;89:1047–1051.

7. Lotz J, Hewlett R, Alheit B, et al. Neurocysticercosis: correlative pathomorphology and MR imaging. Neuroradiology 1988;30:35–41.

8. Martinez HR, Rangel-Guerra R, Arredondo-Estrada JH, et al. Medical and surgical treatment in neurocysticercosis: a magnetic resonance study of 161 cases. J Neurol Sci 1995;130:25–34.

9. Neal JH. An endoscopic approach to cysticercosis cysts of the posterior third ventricle. Neurosurgery 1995;36:1040–1043.

10. Pittella JEH. Neurocysticercosis. Brain Pathol 1997;7:681–693.

11. Rajshekhar V, Chandy MJ. Enlarging solitary cysticercus granulomas. J Neurosurg 1994;80:840–843.

12. Saglado P, Rojas R, Sotelo J. Cysticercosis. Clinical classification based on imaging studies. Arch Intern Med 1997;157:1991–1997.

13. Sotelo J. Treatment of brain cysticercosis. Surg Neurol 1997;48:110–112.

14. Sotelo J, Guerrero V, Rubio F. Neurocysticercosis: a new classification based on active and inactive forms. Arch Intern Med 1985;145:442–445.

15. Teitelbaum GP, Otto RJ, Lin M, et al. MR imaging of neurocysticercosis. AJNR 1989;10:709–718.

16. Yang S, Wang M, Xue Q. Cerebral cysticercosis. Surg Neurol 1990;34:286–293.

## Echinococcosis

1. Coates R, von Sinner W, Rahm B. MR imaging of an intracerebral hydatid cyst. AJNR 1990;11:1249–1250.

2. Ersahin Y, Mutluer S, Güzelbag E. Intracranial hydatid cysts in children. Neurosurgery 1993;33:219–225.

3. Guo H-R, Lu Y-J, Bao Y-H, et al. Parasellar epidural hydatid cysts. Neurosurgery 1993;32:662–665.

4. Lunardi P, Missori P, Di Lorenzo N, et al. Cerebral hydatidosis in childhood: a retrospective survey with emphasis on long-term follow-up. Neurosurgery 1991;29:515–518.

5. Mascalchi M, Ragazzoni A, Dal Pozzo G. Pontine hydatid cyst in association with an acoustic neurinoma: MR appearance in an unusual case. AJNR 1991;12:78–79.

6. Nurchi G, Floris F, Montaldo C, et al. Multiple cerebral hydatid disease: case report with magnetic resonance imaging study. Neurosurgery 1992;30:436–438.

7. Taratuto AL, Venturiello SM. Echinococcosis. Brain Pathol 1997;7:673–679.

8. Topsakal C, Aydin Y, Aydin F, et al. Cerebral alveolar hydatidosis: case report. Surg Neurol 1996;45:575–581.

## Other Parasitic Infections

1. Bambirra EA, De Souza Andrade J, Cesarini I, et al. The tumoral form of schistosomiasis: report of a case with cerebellar involvement. Am J Trop Med Hyg 1984;33:76–79.

2. Cabral G, Pittella JEH. Tumoural form of cerebellar schistosomiasis mansoni. Report of a surgically treated case. Acta Neurochir 1989;99:148–151.

3. Chan S-T, Tse CH, Chan YS, et al. Sparganosis of the brain. Report of two cases. J Neurosurg 1987;67:931–934.

4. Chang KH, Cho SY, Chi JG, et al. Cerebral sparganosis: CT characteristics. Radiology 1987;165:505–510.

5. Chimelli L, Scaravilli F. Trypanosomiasis. Brain Pathol 1997;7:599–611.

6. Gjerde IO, Mörk S, Larsen JL, et al. Cerebral schistosomiasis presenting as a brain tumor. Eur Neurol 1984;23:229–236.

7. Mackenzie IR, Guha A. Manson's schistosomiasis presenting as a brain tumor. Case report. J Neurosurg 1998;89:1052–1054.

8. Mitchell A, Scheithauer BW, Kelly PJ, et al. Cerebral sparganosis. Case report. J Neurosurg 1990;73:147–150.

9. Morgello S, Soifer FM, Lin C-S, et al. Central nervous system *Strongyloides stercoralis* in acquired immunodeficiency syndrome: a report of two cases and review of the literature. Acta Neuropathol (Berl) 1993;86:285–288.

10. Pittella JEH. Neuroschistosomiasis. Brain Pathol 1997;7:649–662.

11. Pittella JEH, da Silva Gusmão SN, Carvalho GT, et al. Tumoral form of cerebral schistosomiasis mansoni. A report of four cases and a review of the literature. Clin Neurol Neurosurg 1996;98:15–20.

12. Preidler KW, Riepl T, Szolar D, et al. Cerebral schistosomiasis: MR and CT appearance. AJNR 1996;17:1598–1600.

13. Scrimgeour EM, Gajdusek DC. Involvement of the central nervous system in *Schistosoma mansoni* and *S. haematobium* infection. A review. Brain 1985;108:1023–1038.

14. Scully RE (ed). Case records of the Massachusetts General Hospital. Case 39-1996. N Engl J Med 1996;1906–1914.

15. Udaka F, Okuda B, Okada M, et al. CT findings of cerebral paragonimiasis in the chronic state. Neuroradiology 1988;30:31–34.

16. Yamashita K, Akimura T, Kawano K, et al. Cerebral sparganosis mansoni. Report of two cases. Surg Neurol 1990;33:28–34.

## Acquired Immunodeficiency Syndrome

1. Budka H. Multinucleated giant cells in brain: a hallmark of the acquired immune deficiency syndrome (AIDS). Acta Neuropathol (Berl) 1986;69:253–258.

2. Chrysikopoulos HS, Press GA, Grafe MR, et al. Encephalitis caused by human immunodeficiency virus: CT and MR imaging manifestations with clinical and pathological correlation. Radiology 1990;175:185–191.

3. Esiri MM. Viruses and rickettsiae. Brain Pathol 1997;7:695–709.

4. Glass JD, Wesselingh SL, Selnes OA, et al. Clinical-neuropathologic correlation in HIV-associated dementia. Neurology 1993;43:2230–2237.

5. Harrison MJG, McArthur JC. HIV-associated dementia complex. In AIDS and Neurology. New York: Churchill-Livingstone, 1995, pp 31–64.

6. Kleihues P, Lang W, Burger PC. Progressive diffuse leukoencephalopathy in patients with acquired immune deficiency syndrome (AIDS). Acta Neuropathol (Berl) 1985;68:333–339.

7. Koenig S, Gendelman HE, Orenstein JM, et al. Detection of AIDS virus in macrophages in brain tissue from AIDS patients with encephalopathy. Science 1986;233:1089–1093.

8. Lang W, Miklossy J, Deruaz JP, et al. Neuropathology of the acquired immune deficiency syndrome (AIDS): a report of 135 consecutive autopsy cases from Switzerland. Acta Neuropathol (Berl) 1989;77:379–390.

9. Meyenhofer MF, Epstein LG, Cho E-S, et al. Ultrastructural morphology and intracellular production of human immunodeficiency virus (HIV) in brain. J Neuropathol Exp Neurol 1987;46:474–484.

10. Mirra SS, del Rio C. The fine structure of acquired immunodeficiency syndrome encephalopathy. Arch Pathol Lab Med 1989;113:858–865.

11. Navia BA, Jordan BD, Price RW. The AIDS dementia complex: I. Clinical features. Ann Neurol 1986;19:517–524.

12. Navia BA, Cho E-S, Petito CK, Price RW. The AIDS dementia complex: II. Neuropathology. Ann Neurol 1986;19:525–535.

13. Petito CK, Cho E-S, Lemann W, et al. Neuropathology of acquired immunodeficiency syndrome (AIDS): an autopsy review. J Neuropathol Exp Neurol 1986;45:635–646.

14. Sharer LR. Pathology of HIV-1 infection of the central nervous system. A review. J Neuropathol Exp Neurol 1992;51:3–11.

15. Smith TW, DeGirolami U, Hénin D, et al. Human immunodeficiency virus (HIV) leukoencephalopathy and the microcirculation. J Neuropathol Exp Neurol 1990;49:357–370.

## Sarcoidosis

1. Branch EF, Burger PC, Brewer DL. Hypothermia in a case of hypothalamic infarction and sarcoidosis. Arch Neurol 1971;25:245–255.

2. Hayes WS, Sherman JL, Stern BJ, et al. MR and CT evaluation of intracranial sarcoidosis. AJR 1987;149:1043–1049.

3. Lasner TM, Sutton LN, Rorke LB. Multifocal infectious granulomatous encephalitis in a child. Case report. J Neurosurg 1997;86:1042–1045.

4. Lexa FJ, Grossman RI. MR of sarcoidosis in the head and spine: spectrum of manifestations and radiographic response to steroid therapy. AJNR 1994;15:973–982.

5. Powers WJ, Miller EM. Sarcoidosis mimicking glioma: case report and review of intracranial sarcoid mass lesions. Neurology 1981;31:907–910.

6. Stelzer KJ, Thomas CR Jr, Berger MS, et al. Radiation therapy for sarcoid of the thalamus/posterior third ventricle: case report. Neurosurgery 1995;36:1188–1191.

7. Strefling AM, Summerville JW, Urich H. Involvement of choroid plexuses in neurosarcoidosis. Acta Neuropathol (Berl) 1987;74:402–404.

8. Thomas G, Murphy S, Stannton H, et al. Pathogen-free granulomatous disease of the central nervous system. Hum Pathol 1998;29:110–115.

## Other Inflammatory Diseases

1. Alamowitch S, Graus F, Uchuya M, et al. Limbic encephalitis and small cell lung cancer. Clinical and immunological features. Brain 1997;120:923–928.

2. Bahar S, Çoban O, Gürvit IH, et al. Spontaneous dissection of the extracranial vertebral artery with spinal subarachnoid haemorrhage in a patient with Behçet's disease. Neuroradiology 1993;33:352–354.

3. Banna M, El-Ramahi K. Neurologic involvement in Behçet disease: imaging findings in 16 patients. AJNR 1991;17:791–796.

4. Bergmann M, Yuan Y, Bruck W, et al. Solitary Langerhans cell histiocytosis lesion of the parieto-occipital lobe: a case report and review of the literature. Clin Neurol Neurosurg 1997;99:50–55.

5. Blumbergs PC, Hallpike JF, McClure J. Cerebral malakoplakia. J Clin Pathol 1981;34:875–878.

6. Brady KM, Font RL, Lee AG. Muslin-induced intracranial sterile abscess: a cause of visual loss after aneurysm repair. Surg Neurol 1999;51:566–567.

7. Breidahl WH, Ives FJ, Khangure MS. Cerebral and brain stem Langerhans cell histiocytosis. Neuroradiology 1993;35:349–351.

8. Brennan LV, Craddock PR. Limbic encephalopathy as nonmetastatic complication of oat cell lung cancer. Am J Med 1983;75:518–520.

9. Burton GV, Bullard DE, Walther PJ, et al. Paraneoplastic limbic encephalopathy with testicular carcinoma. Cancer 1988; 62: 2248–2251.

10. Chandra R, Kapur S. Malakoplakia of the brain. A report of two cases occurring in childhood. Arch Pathol Lab Med 1979; 103:688–692.

11. Cohen M, Lanska D, Roessmann U, et al. Amyloidoma of the CNS. I. Clinical and pathologic study. Neurology 1992;42:2019–2023.

12. Corsellis JAN, Goldberg GJ, Norton AR. Limbic encephalitis and its association with carcinoma. Brain 1968;91:481–497.

13. Czech T, Mazal PR, Schima W. Resection of a Langerhans cell histiocytosis granuloma of the hypothalamus: case report. Br J Neurosurg 1999;13:196–200.

14. Dalmau J, Gultekin HS, Posner JB. Paraneoplastic neurologic syndromes: pathogenesis and physiopathology. Brain Pathol 1999; 9:275–284.

15. Devlin T, Gray L, Allen NB, et al. Neuro-Behçet's disease: factors hampering proper diagnosis. Neurology 1995;45:1754–1757.

16. Farrell MA, Droogan O, Secor DL, et al. Chronic encephalitis associated with epilepsy: immunohistochemical and ultrastructural studies. Acta Neuropathol (Berl) 1995;89:313–321.

17. Felsberg GJ, Tien RD, Haplea S, et al. Muslin-induced optic arachnoiditis ("gauzoma"): findings on CT and MR. J Comput Assist Tomogr 1993;17:485–487.

18. Ferreiro JA, Bhuta S, Nieberg RK, et al. Amyloidoma of the skull base. Arch Pathol Lab Med 1990;114:974–976.

19. Fuller GN, McCutcheon IE, Kumar AJ, et al. Textiloma (gossypiboma) mimicking recurrent brain tumor: evaluation of a series. Lab Invest 1997;76:150A.

20. Glantz MJ, Biran H, Myers ME, et al. The radiographic diagnosis and treatment of paraneoplastic central nervous system disease. Cancer 1994;73:168–175.

21. Grode ML, Borit A, Van De Velde RL, et al. Cerebral malakoplakia. Bull Los Angeles Neurol Soc 1978;43:6–11.

22. Hadfield MG, Aydin F, Lippman HR, et al. Neuro-Behçet's disease. Clin Neuropathol 1996;15:249–255.

23. Haisa T, Matsumiya K, Yoshimasu N, et al. Foreign-body granuloma as a complication of wrapping and coating an intracranial aneurysm. Case report. J Neurosurg 1990;72:292–294.

24. Ho K-L. Morphogenesis of Michaelis-Gutmann bodies in cerebral malacoplakia. Arch Pathol Lab Med 1989;113:874–879.

25. Honavar M, Janota I, Polkey CE. Rasmussen's encephalitis in surgery for epilepsy. Dev Med Child Neurol 1992;34:3–14.

26. Jager HR, Albrecht T, Curati-Alasonatti WL, et al. MRI in neuro-Behçet's syndrome: comparison of conventional spin-echo and FLAIR pulse sequences. Neuroradiology 1999;41:750–758.

27. Kim E-Y, Choi J-U, Kim T-S, et al. Huge Langerhans cell histiocytosis granuloma of choroid plexus in a child with Hand-Schüller-Christian disease. J Neurosurg 1995;83:1080–1084.

28. Laeng RH, Altermatt HJ, Scheithauer BW, et al. Amyloidomas of the nervous system: a monoclonal B-cell disorder with monotypic amyloid light chain lambda amyloid production. Cancer 1998; 82:362–374.

29. Lee J, Krol G, Rosenblum M. Primary amyloidoma of the brain: CT and MR presentation. AJNR 1995;16:712–714.

30. Maghnie M, Aricò M, Villa A, et al. MR of the hypothalamic-pituitary axis in Langerhans cell histiocytosis. AJNR 1992;13:1365–1371.

31. Matsumoto T, Tani E, Maeda Y, et al. Amyloidomas in the cerebellopontine angle and jugular foramen. Case report. J Neurosurg 1985;62:592–596.

32. Matsumoto T, Tani E, Fukami M, et al. Amyloidoma in the gasserian ganglion: case report. Surg Neurol 1999;52:600–603.

33. Mazal PR, Hainfellner JA, Preiser J, et al. Langerhans cell histiocytosis of the hypothalamus: diagnostic value of immunohistochemistry. Clin Neuropathol 1996;15:87–91.

34. McFadzean RM, Hadley DM, McIlwaine GG. Optochiasmal arachnoiditis following muslin wrapping of ruptured anterior communicating artery aneurysms. J Neurosurg 1991;75:393–396.

35. Montine TJ, Hollensead SC, Ellis WG, et al. Solitary eosinophilic granuloma of the temporal lobe: a case report and long-term follow-up of previously reported cases. Clin Neuropathol 1994; 13:225–228.

36. O'Brien TJ, McKelvie PA, Vrodos N. Bilateral trigeminal amyloidoma: an unusual case of trigeminal neuropathy with a review of the literature. Case report. J Neurosurg 1994;81:780–783.

37. Oguni H, Andermann F, Rasmussen TB. The syndrome of chronic encephalitis and epilepsy. A study based on the MNI series of 48 cases. Adv Neurol 1992;57:419–433.

38. Parmar DN, Sharr MM. Cotton gauze foreign body granuloma following microvascular decompression. Br J Neurosurg 1999; 13:87–89.

39. Piatt JH Jr, Hwang PA, Armstrong DC, et al. Chronic focal encephalitis (Rasmussen syndrome): six cases. Epilepsia 1988; 29:268–279.

40. Prabhu SS, Keogh AJ, Parekh HC, et al. Optochiasmal arachnoiditis induced by muslin wrapping of intracranial aneurysms. A report of two cases and a review of the literature. Br J Neurosurg 1994;8:471–476.

41. Provenzale JM, Graham ML. Reversible leukoencephalopathy associated with graft-versus-host disease: MR findings. AJNR 1996; 17:1290–1294.

42. Rasmussen T, Olszewski J, Lloyd-Smith D. Focal seizures due to chronic localized encephalitis. Neurology 1958;8:435–445.

43. Rogers SW, Andrews I, Gahring LC, et al. Autoantibodies to glutamate receptor GluR3 in Rasmussen's encephalitis. Science 1994;265:648–651.

44. Rosenblum MK. Paraneoplasia and autoimmunologic injury of the nervous system: the anti-Hu syndrome. Brain Pathol 1993;3:199–212.

45. Rosenfield NS, Abrahams J, Komp D. Brain MR in patients with Langerhans cell histiocytosis: findings and enhancement with Gd-DTPA. Pediatr Radiol 1990;20:433–436.

46. Rouah E, Gruber R, Shearer W, et al. Single case reports. Graft-versus-host disease in the central nervous system: a real entity? Am J Clin Pathol 1988;89:543–546.

47. Scaravilli F, An SF, Groves M, et al. The neuropathology of paraneoplastic syndromes. Brain Pathol 1999;9:251–260.

48. Schröder R, Linke RP, Voges J, et al. Intracerebral A λ amyloidoma diagnosed by stereotactic biopsy. Clin Neuropathol 1995;14:347–350.

49. Spaar FW, Goebel HH, Volles E, et al. Tumor-like amyloid formation (amyloidoma) in the brain. J Neurol 1981;224:171–182.

50. Stern RC, Hulette CM. Paraneoplastic limbic encephalitis associated with small cell carcinoma of the prostate. Mod Pathol 1999;12:814–818.
51. Tien RD, Ashdown BC, Lewis DV Jr, et al. Rasmussen's encephalitis: neuroimaging findings in four patients. AJR 1992;158:1329–1332.
52. Tien RD, Newton TH, McDermott MW, et al. Thickened pituitary stalk on MR images in patients with diabetes insipidus and Langerhans cell histiocytosis. AJNR 1990;11:703–708.
53. Townsend JJ, Tomiyasu U, MacKay A, et al. Central nervous system amyloid presenting as a mass lesion. J Neurosurg 1982;56:439–442.
54. Ünai F, Hepgül K, Bayindir Ç, et al. Skull base amyloidoma. Case report. J Neurosurg 1992;76:303–306.
55. Vidal RG, Ghiso J, Gallo G, et al. Amyloidoma of the CNS. II. Immunohistochemical and biochemical study. Neurology 1992;42:2024–2028.
56. Vining EPG, Freeman JM, Brandto J, et al. Progressive unilateral encephalopathy of childhood (Rasmussen's syndrome): a reappraisal. Epilepsia 1993;34:639–650.
57. Vinters HV, Wang R, Wiley CA. Herpesviruses in chronic encephalitis associated with intractable childhood epilepsy. Hum Pathol 1993;24:871–879.
58. Yamamori C, Ishino H, Inagaki T, et al. Neuro-Behçet disease with demyelination and gliosis of the frontal white matter. Clin Neuropathol 1994;13:208–215.

# THE BRAIN—TUMORS

4

Other Germ Cell Neoplasms

### Hemangioblastoma

### Atypical Teratoid/Rhabdoid Tumor

### Tumors of Intracranial Peripheral Nerves

Schwannoma and Malignant Peripheral Nerve Sheath Tumors

Other Tumors of Intracranial Peripheral Nerves

### Benign Cystic Lesions

Colloid Cyst

Ependymal Cyst

Choroid Plexus Cyst

Other Cysts

## METASTATIC NEOPLASMS

## REFERENCES

Tumors of the brain constitute a remarkably diverse group of both neoplastic and non-neoplastic conditions that can occur at virtually any site and in patients of any age. They can be (1) primary neoplasms in all degrees of differentiation, derived from any of the many normal cellular constituents; (2) non-neoplastic tumorous masses arising from normal constituents (hamartomas); (3) neoplasms derived from embryologically misplaced tissues; or (4) secondary neoplasms metastatic from a variety of primary sites (Fig. 4–1). Any classification that grapples with this multitude of entities is prone to complexity, redundancy, and controversy. Fortunately, molecular and cytogenetic features are being uncovered that may well be the basis of more objective means of tumor classification. Distinctive molecular features, on the verge of being classifying features in their own right, are increasingly used to identify or subclassify oligodendroglioma, glioblastoma, atypical teratoid/rhabdoid tumor, and medulloblastoma. Despite rapid progress with these contemporary methods, brain tumors are still characterized largely by their histologic features, often with a presumption about the "cell of origin." This is done here as well, but with the disclaimer that, aside from lesions such as ependymomas and choroid plexus tumors, cytogenesis is more a theoretical concept than a definitive basis for tumor classification.

The classification used here is similar to that of the 2000 World Health Organization (WHO) system summarized in Table 4–1, p. 163.[61] Table 4–2, p. 164 lists central nervous system (CNS) tumors by anatomic region. Figure 4–2 emphasizes the important distinction between CNS tumors that are infiltrative and those that are relatively discrete.

## PRIMARY NEOPLASMS

### Astrocytic Neoplasms

Normal astrocytes are stellate cells with thread-like processes that attach to blood vessels, approximate neurons, and permeate the interstices of the neuropil. Like fibrocytes, they play a stromal role, seemingly dormant until stimulated by injury to undergo hypertrophy or

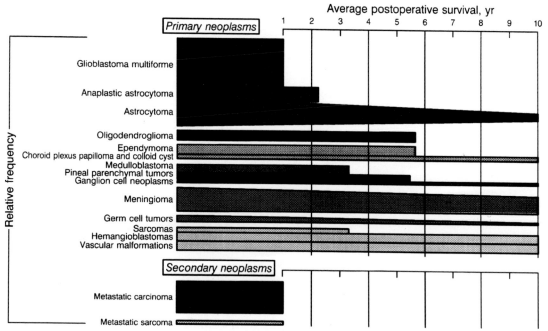

**FIGURE 4–1**    PRIMARY AND METASTATIC TUMORS OF THE BRAIN: INCIDENCE AND SURVIVAL RATES

Relative incidence and mean postoperative survival rates are indicated by the width and length of the individual arms, respectively.

## TABLE 4–1
## WHO Classification of Tumors of the Nervous System

### Tumors of Neuroepithelial Tissue

#### Astrocytic Tumors

| | |
|---|---|
| Diffuse astrocytoma | 9400/3° |
| Fibrillary astrocytoma | 9420/3 |
| Protoplasmic astrocytoma | 9410/3 |
| Gemistocytic astrocytoma | 9411/3 |
| Anaplastic astrocytoma | 9401/3 |
| Glioblastoma | 9440/3 |
| Giant cell glioblastoma | 9441/3 |
| Gliosarcoma | 9442/3 |
| Pilocytic astrocytoma | 9421/1 |
| Pleomorphic xanthoastrocytoma | 9424/3 |
| Subependymal giant cell astrocytoma | 9384/1 |

#### Oligodendroglial Tumors

| | |
|---|---|
| Oligodendroglioma | 9450/3 |
| Anaplastic oligodendroglioma | 9451/3 |

#### Mixed Gliomas

| | |
|---|---|
| Oligoastrocytoma | 9382/3 |
| Anaplastic oligoastrocytoma | 9382/3† |

#### Ependymal Tumors

| | |
|---|---|
| Ependymoma | 9391/3 |
| Cellular | 9391/3 |
| Papillary | 9393/3 |
| Clear cell | 9391/3 |
| Tanycytic | 9391/3 |
| Anaplastic ependymoma | 9392/3 |
| Myxopapillary ependymoma | 9394/1 |
| Subependymoma | 9383/1 |

#### Choroid Plexus Tumors

| | |
|---|---|
| Choroid plexus papilloma | 9390/0 |
| Choroid plexus carcinoma | 9390/3 |

#### Glial Tumors of Uncertain Origin

| | |
|---|---|
| Astroblastoma | 9430/3 |
| Gliomatosis cerebri | 9381/3 |
| Chordoid glioma of the third ventricle | 9444/1 |

#### Neuronal and Mixed Neuronal-Glial Tumors

| | |
|---|---|
| Gangliocytoma | 9492/0 |
| Dysplastic gangliocytoma of cerebellum (Lhermitte-Duclos) | 9493/0 |
| Desmoplastic infantile astrocytoma/ ganglioglioma | 9412/1 |
| Dysembryoplastic neuroepithelial tumor | 9413/0 |
| Ganglioglioma | 9505/1 |
| Anaplastic ganglioglioma | 9505/3 |
| Central neurocytoma | 9506/1 |
| Cerebellar liponeurocytoma | 9506/1 |
| Paraganglioma of the filum terminale | 8680/1 |

#### Neuroblastic Tumors

| | |
|---|---|
| Olfactory neuroblastoma (aesthesioneuroblastoma) | 9522/3 |
| Olfactory neuroepithelioma | 9523/3 |
| Neuroblastomas of the adrenal gland and sympathetic nervous system | 9500/3 |

#### Pineal Parenchymal Tumors

| | |
|---|---|
| Pineocytoma | 9361/1 |
| Pineoblastoma | 9362/3 |
| Pineal parenchymal tumor of intermediate differentiation | 9362/3 |

#### Embryonal Tumors

| | |
|---|---|
| Medulloepithelioma | 9501/3 |
| Ependymoblastoma | 9392/3 |
| Medulloblastoma | 9470/3 |
| Desmoplastic medulloblastoma | 9471/3 |
| Large cell medulloblastoma | 9474/3 |
| Medullomyoblastoma | 9472/3 |
| Melanotic medulloblastoma | 9470/3 |
| Supratentorial primitive neuroectodermal tumor (PNET) | 9473/3 |
| Neuroblastoma | 9500/3 |
| Ganglioneuroblastoma | 9490/3 |
| Atypical teratoid/rhabdoid tumor | 9508/3 |

### Tumors of Peripheral Nerves

#### Schwannoma

| | |
|---|---|
| Neurilemmoma, neurinoma | 9560/0 |
| Cellular | 9560/0 |
| Plexiform | 9560/0 |
| Melanotic | 9560/0 |

#### Neurofibroma

| | |
|---|---|
| | 9540/0 |
| Plexiform | 9550/0 |

#### Perineurioma

| | |
|---|---|
| | 9571/0 |
| Intraneural perineurioma | 9571/0 |
| Soft tissue perineurioma | 9571/0 |

#### Malignant Peripheral Nerve Sheath Tumor (MPNST)

| | |
|---|---|
| | 9540/3 |
| Epithelioid | 9540/3 |
| MPNST with divergent mesenchymal and/or epithelial differentiation | 9540/3 |
| Melanotic | 9540/3 |
| Melanotic psammomatous | 9540/3 |

### Tumors of the Meninges

#### Tumors of Meningothelial Cells

| | |
|---|---|
| Meningioma | 9530/0 |
| Meningothelial | 9531/0 |
| Fibrous (fibroblastic) | 9532/0 |
| Transitional (mixed) | 9537/0 |
| Psammomatous | 9533/0 |
| Angiomatous | 9534/0 |
| Microcystic | 9530/0 |
| Secretory | 9530/0 |
| Lymphoplasmacyte-rich | 9530/0 |
| Metaplastic | 9530/0 |
| Clear cell | 9538/1 |
| Chordoid | 9538/1 |
| Atypical | 9539/1 |
| Papillary | 9538/3 |
| Rhabdoid | 9538/3 |
| Anaplastic meningioma | 9530/3 |

**TABLE 4–1**
**WHO Classification of Tumors of the Nervous System** *Continued*

### Tumors of the Meninges *Continued*

#### Mesenchymal, Nonmeningothelial Tumors

| | | | |
|---|---|---|---|
| Lipoma | 8850/0 | Osteochondroma | 9210/0 |
| Angiolipoma | 8861/0 | Hemangioma | 9120/0 |
| Hibernoma | 8880/0 | Epithelioid hemangioendothelioma | 9133/1 |
| Liposarcoma (intracranial) | 8850/3 | Hemangiopericytoma | 9150/1 |
| Solitary fibrous tumor | *8815/0* | Angiosarcoma | 9120/3 |
| Fibrosarcoma | 8810/3 | Kaposi's sarcoma | 9140/3 |
| Malignant fibrous histiocytoma | 8830/3 | **Primary Melanocytic Lesions** | |
| Leiomyoma | 8890/0 | | |
| Leiomyosarcoma | 8890/3 | Diffuse melanocytosis | 8728/0 |
| Rhabdomyoma | 8900/0 | Melanocytoma | 8728/1 |
| Rhabdomyosarcoma | 8900/3 | Malignant melanoma | 8720/3 |
| Chondroma | 9220/0 | Meningeal melanomatosis | 8728/3 |
| Chondrosarcoma | 9220/3 | **Tumors of Uncertain Histogenesis** | |
| Osteoma | 9180/0 | | |
| Osteosarcoma | 9180/3 | Hemangioblastoma | 9161/1 |

### Lymphomas and Hematopoietic Neoplasms

| | |
|---|---|
| Malignant lymphoma | 9590/3 |
| Plasmacytoma | 9731/3 |
| Granulocytic sarcoma | 9930/3 |

### Germ Cell Tumors

| | | | |
|---|---|---|---|
| Germinoma | 9064/3 | Mature | 9080/0 |
| Embryonal carcinoma | 9070/3 | Immature | 9080/3 |
| Yolk sac tumor | 9071/3 | Teratoma with malignant transformation | 9084/3 |
| Choriocarcinoma | 9100/3 | Mixed germ cell tumors | 9085/3 |
| Teratoma | 9080/1 | | |

### Tumors of the Sellar Region

| | | | |
|---|---|---|---|
| Craniopharyngioma | 9350/1 | Papillary | *9352/1* |
| Adamantinomatous | *9351/1* | Granular cell tumor | *9582/0* |

### Metastatic Tumors

*Morphology code of the International Classification of Diseases for Oncology (ICD-O) and the Systematized Nomenclature of Medicine (SNOMED). Behavior is coded /0 for benign tumors, /1 for low or uncertain malignant potential or borderline malignancy, (/2 for in situ lesions), and /3 for malignant tumors.

†The italicized numbers are provisional codes proposed for the third edition of ICD-O. They should, for the most part, be incorporated into the next edition of ICD-O, but they are subject to change.

From Kleihues P, Cavenee WK (eds). World Health Organization Classification of Tumours: Pathology and Genetics of Tumours of the Nervous System. Lyon, France: IARC Press, 2000, pp 6–7.

hyperplasia. However, in view of their abundance, their intimate relationship to blood vessels, and their specialized cell contacts, it is clear that astroglia play a vital and dynamic role in the traffic of the normal brain.

Neoplastic transformation of astrocytes begets a heterogeneous family of new growths that, by virtue of clinical and biologic diversity, overshadows all other primary intracranial neoplasms. Evaluation of such a formidable array is facilitated by certain predictable relations among the anatomic location, the histopathology of the lesion, the age of the patient, and the anticipated clinical course.

### Infiltrative Astrocytic Neoplasms

Although it is sport to criticize the grading of astrocytomas, the process is, like other arbitrary creations such as geographic time zones, a system born of need. The schema used here differs somewhat from that of the WHO,[61] which is itself a modification of the Ste. Anne–Mayo grading scheme proposed by Daumas-Duport and colleagues.[32] The latter computes grades based on the presence or absence of four histologic parameters: nuclear atypia, mitoses, microvascular proliferation, and necrosis. Lesions with three or four variables are grade IV (glioblastoma multiforme), whereas those with two features are grade III ("anaplastic" or "malignant" astrocytoma), and tumors with one parameter are assigned grade II. There is, in concept, an astrocytoma grade I, but such an entity would require a lack of even cytologic atypia, a rare lesion that most observers would be hesitant to identify as neoplastic. As is discussed on page 170, we do not always apply this system strictly, because we are

**TABLE 4–2**
**Brain Tumors by Location**

| | |
|---|---|
| **Cerebral Hemispheres** | **Craniopharyngioma** |
| Diffuse astrocytoma grades II, III, IV | Adamantinomatous |
| Pilocytic astrocytoma | Papillary |
| Pleomorphic xanthoastrocytoma | Chordoid glioma |
| Oligodendroglioma | Germ cell tumor |
| Ependymoma | Dysembryoplastic neuroepithelial tumor |
| Astroblastoma | **Fourth Ventricle** |
| Primary CNS lymphoma | Ependymoma |
| Metastatic carcinoma | Subependymoma |
| Ganglion cell tumor | Exophytic brain stem pilocytic astrocytoma |
| "Parenchymal" neurocytic neoplasm | Choroid plexus tumor |
| Hemangioblastoma | Medulloblastoma |
| Dysembryoplastic neuroepithelial tumor | Hemangioblastoma |
| Small cell embryonal tumor (PNET) | **Suprasellar Region** |
| Atypical teratoid/rhabdoid tumor | Pituitary adenoma |
| **Corpus Callosum** | Pilocytic astrocytoma |
| Diffuse astrocytoma grades II, III, IV | Craniopharyngioma |
| Oligodendroglioma | Germ cell tumor |
| Primary CNS lymphoma | Rathke's cleft cyst |
| **Cerebellum** | Epidermoid cyst |
| Medulloblastoma | Meningioma |
| Pilocytic astrocytoma | Chordoma |
| Hemangioblastoma | Olfactory neuroblastoma |
| Ependymoma | Pituicytoma/granular cell tumor |
| Metastatic carcinoma | **Cranial Nerves** |
| Atypical teratoid/rhabdoid tumor | Schwannoma |
| **Brain Stem** | Lipoma (cranial nerve VIII) |
| Diffuse astrocytoma grades II, III, IV | **Thalamus** |
| Pilocytic astrocytoma | Diffuse astrocytoma grades II, III, IV |
| Ependymoma | Pilocytic astrocytoma |
| Ganglion cell tumor | Primary CNS lymphoma |
| **Pineal Region** | **Cerebellopontine Angle** |
| Germ cell tumor | Schwannoma |
| Pineal parenchymal tumor | Meningioma |
| Pineal cyst | Epidermoid cyst |
| **Lateral Ventricle** | Cholesterol granuloma |
| Choroid plexus neoplasm | Glomus jugulare tumor |
| Subependymoma | Ependymoma |
| Ependymoma | Choroid plexus papilloma |
| Central neurocytoma | Papillary endolymphatic sac tumor |
| Subependymal giant cell astrocytoma | **Meninges** |
| **Third Ventricle** | Meningioma |
| Pilocytic astrocytoma | Hemangiopericytoma |
| Colloid cyst | Solitary fibrous tumor |

CNS, central nervous system; PNET, primitive neuroectodermal tumor.

reluctant to assign lesions to the grade III category solely on the basis of an isolated mitosis.

When this, or almost any other, system is applied, a close relation is immediately seen between the tumor grade and the patient's age. As a general rule, patients with grade II astrocytomas are in the third or fourth decade of life, those with grade III lesions are in the fifth decade, and those with glioblastomas are in the sixth decade and beyond. There are, of course, many exceptions. However, among astrocytomas of the cerebral hemispheres in adults, the relationship between tumor grade and patient age is close and of great practical significance. One does not, for example, anticipate a well-differentiated astrocytoma in an elderly individual. The apparent finding of such a lesion in this setting should raise concern about the adequacy of tissue sampling and should prompt review of the neuroimaging findings. Dif-

fuse astrocytomas of any grade of the pons are typically tumors of childhood.

The cause is unknown, except for rare high-grade examples that arise after radiotherapy for an unrelated neoplasm or in the setting of an inherited cancer syndrome, discussed on page 180.

### Diffuse Astrocytoma (Grade II)

**Definition.** A well-differentiated, infiltrating neoplasm with astrocytic cytologic features.

**Clinical Features.** Young adults are affected primarily, generally in the third and fourth decades of life; most lesions are in the cerebral hemispheres. In children, some diffuse astrocytomas occur in this location, but more often they arise in the brain stem[14, 34] or thalamus.[15, 113]

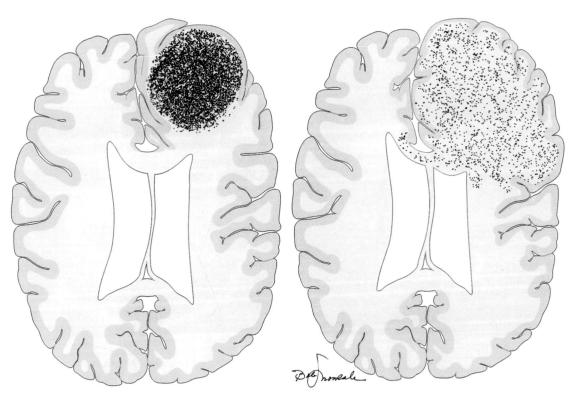

**FIGURE 4-2**    GROWTH PATTERNS OF CENTRAL NERVOUS SYSTEM TUMORS

Most central nervous system tumors express one of two growth patterns: diffuse infiltration (*right*) or relative discreteness (*left*). Diffuse neoplasms are contrast enhancing only in the higher grades, whereas enhancement is typically robust in discrete lesions, with the few nonenhancing exceptions noted with an asterisk in the following list.

| **Infiltrative** | **Discrete** |
|---|---|
| Diffuse astrocytoma, grades II,° III, and IV | Pilocytic astrocytoma |
| Oligodendroglioma, grades II,° III, and IV | Ganglion cell tumor |
| Gliomatosis cerebri° | Pleomorphic xanthoastrocytoma |
| Primary central nervous system lymphoma | Astroblastoma |
| | Ependymoma |
| | Dysembryoplastic neuroepithelial tumor° |
| | Subependymoma° |
| | Choroid plexus papilloma and carcinoma |
| | Central neurocytoma† |
| | Hemangioblastoma |
| | Pituicytoma and granular cell tumor |
| | Hypothalamic neuronal hamartoma° |

°Usually little if any contrast enhancement is present.
†Enhancement is present, but the extent is variable.

A specific form of brain stem glioma is a slowly growing, periaqueductal, nonpilocytic form of "tectal glioma" whose relationship to diffuse astrocytomas is not clear.[9, 14] Those in the thalamus often occur in children.[15, 113, 142] Brain stem examples are uncommon in adults.[71] The cerebellum is affected infrequently in all age groups.[47, 66] Seizures and expressions of mass effect are common initial manifestations of cerebral lesions, whereas patients with brain stem tumors present with a distinctive combination of long tract and brain stem signs.[34] Sixth nerve dysfunction is common among the latter.

**Radiologic Features.** On magnetic resonance imaging (MRI) scans, cerebral hemispheric lesions appear as T2- and fluid-attenuated inversion recovery (FLAIR)-bright regions, largely confined to the white matter (Fig. 4–3). Mass effect varies from case to case, being trivial in some and pronounced in others. Astrocytomas may appear diffuse, with ill-defined margins, but some look surprisingly well circumscribed, given their reputation for infiltration.

Thalamic lesions can be so strikingly symmetric as to suggest a bilateral origin.[15, 65, 113]

Diffuse astrocytomas of the brain stem permeate the long tracts and overrun nuclei to produce distinctive, diffuse enlargement ("hypertrophy") and a radiographic whiteout in T2-weighted and FLAIR images.[14, 34] The epicenter of the lesion is usually the pons. By ventral expansion, the lesion often partially engulfs the basilar artery and creates an almost pathognomonic radiologic image (Fig. 4–4). Radiologically "diffuse" but biologically

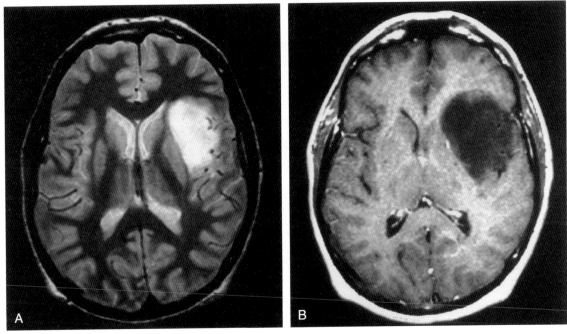

**FIGURE 4–3** ASTROCYTOMA

As visualized in a T2-weighted magnetic resonance imaging scan, the grade II astrocytoma is a rather discrete area of increased signal intensity (A) and does not demonstrate contrast enhancement (B). The patient was a 36-year-old man. As illustrated in Figure 4–31, the lesion progressed to glioblastoma over the next 4 years.

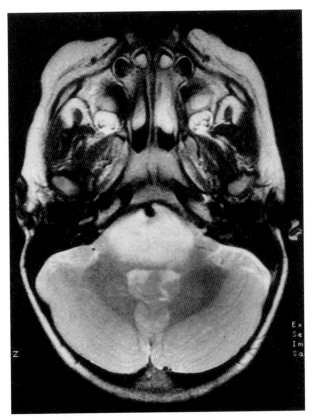

**FIGURE 4–4** ASTROCYTOMA

In this T2-weighted image, a symmetrically enlarged pons engulfs the basilar artery. This radiologic profile is almost pathognomonic of a pontine astrocytoma of the diffuse type.

indolent astrocytomas occur in the setting of neurofibromatosis 1 (NF1). Tectal gliomas include both well-circumscribed, contrast-enhancing pilocytic astrocytomas and nonenhancing, often periaqueductal, lesions that grow slowly if at all.[9, 14]

Characteristically, grade II astrocytomas do not enhance in the absence of secondary changes (see Fig. 4–3), such as those produced by anaplastic transformation (see Fig. 4–31) or prior radiotherapy. In the absence of prior treatment, foci of contrast enhancement are thus prima facie evidence of malignant transformation and should alert the pathologist to the possibility of inadequate tissue sampling if only a grade II tumor is evident histologically. The presence of contrast enhancement in a "low-grade" astrocytoma should also alert one to the possibility of a pilocytic astrocytoma (see Tables 4–6, p. 188 and 4–8, p. 211).

Gliomatosis cerebri, a diffuse form of glioma that spans multiple lobes, is discussed later in a separate section.

**Macroscopic Features.** At surgery, there may be little or no external abnormality in the case of a small, deep-seated cerebral hemispheric lesion; larger, more superficial tumors may expand gyri. The infiltrative nature of a diffuse astrocytoma is apparent to the surgeon, as its boundaries are usually difficult or impossible to define (Fig. 4–5). Indeed, the tumor often appears more ill defined and diffuse to the surgeon than MRI scans suggest. Which of these two perceptions more accurately reflects the true boundaries of the lesion is unclear. Typically, astrocytomas are gray, sometimes with a hint

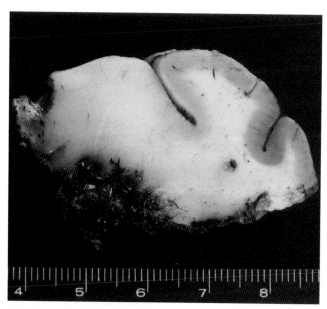

**FIGURE 4–5**    ASTROCYTOMA

Macroscopically, grade II diffuse or infiltrating astrocytomas are poorly defined. This seizure-associated example, in the temporal lobe of a 38-year-old man, expands a gyrus and obscures the gray-white junction.

cles the basilar artery. Anaplastic transformation of an astrocytoma to a glioblastoma typically produces a more discrete mass that is often gelatinous, hemorrhagic, and necrotic.

**Microscopic Features.** Astrocytomas at low magnification appear as palely staining, rather well-circumscribed regions (Fig. 4–6). In some well-differentiated astrocytomas, the cell density only minimally exceeds that of normal white matter, and the diagnosis, if possible at all, is based on cytologic features alone. Fortunately, most astrocytomas are hypercellular by a factor of two or more (Figs. 4–7 to 4–9).

The infiltrative nature of diffuse astrocytomas is apparent in the permeation of the neoplastic cells into the brain parenchyma, where they intermingle with normal CNS elements. When edema is present, the neoplastic cells are well seen interposed between myelinated axons; the latter should not be misinterpreted as fungal hyphae (see Figs. 4–9 and 3–57). Immunostains for neurofilament protein assist in recognizing axons and substantiating the degree of tissue infiltration (Fig. 4–10).

The cells of diffuse astrocytomas are usually marked by nuclear hyperchromasia and pleomorphism, often with variations in polarity (see Figs. 4–6 to 4–9). Their nuclei are thus larger, more irregular, and more coarsely textured than those of normal astrocytes. As a rule, the degree of nuclear atypia in astrocytomas exceeds that in oligodendrogliomas—the principal differential diagnostic consideration.

The extent to which the neoplastic cells conform to one's expectations of astrocytic differentiation varies considerably, both from case to case and from area to area within an individual lesion. In most instances—particularly in zones of infiltration, where isolated cells lie in intact parenchyma—the cytoplasm is inconspicuous, and nuclei appear "naked" (see Figs. 4–6 to 4–9). With increased cellularity, greater numbers of cells acquire the astrocytic phenotype, with eosinophilic cytoplasm and

of yellow, and they vary in consistency from soft to almost gelatinous; some are described as stringy or tough. Cysts, usually small, may be encountered.

As previously noted, grade II diffuse astrocytomas in the brain stem produce enlargement, or hypertrophy, without creating a discrete mass. Subtle architectural details are typically effaced, whereas major landmarks are often preserved. Continued growth fills the cerebello-pontine angle or interpeduncular fossa and elevates the floor of the fourth ventricle. Like a growing tree meeting the obstruction of a barbed wire fence, the tumor encases as well as displaces, so ventral extension encir-

**FIGURE 4–6**    ASTROCYTOMA

Diffuse astrocytomas usually arise in cerebral white matter, as does this large lesion that expands the temporal lobe. The malignant degeneration that occurred at a more rostral plane of section is illustrated in Figure 4–32. The 35-year-old patient had a 3-year history of seizures.

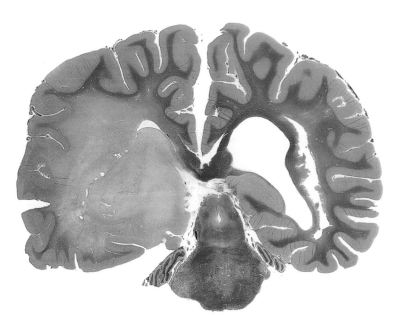

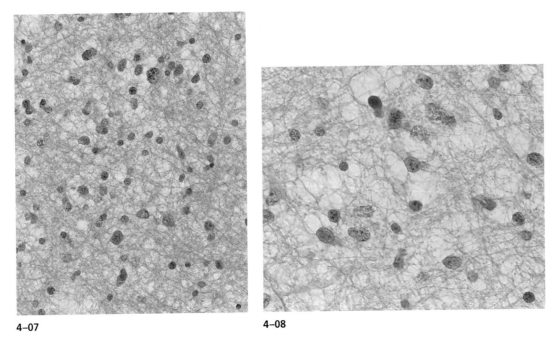

4–07                                          4–08

**FIGURES 4–7 AND 4–8**    ASTROCYTOMA

Grade II astrocytomas diffusely infiltrate brain tissue and generally create a two- to threefold increase in cellularity (Fig. 4–7). Nuclei are moderately pleomorphic and, in nongemistocytic lesions, often appear "naked" or devoid of cytoplasm (Fig. 4–8).

processes that create a fibrillar background. Perinuclear halos are not uncommon in astrocytomas and always raise the possibility of oligodendroglioma (Fig. 4–11).

Most diffuse astrocytomas consist of cells with small perikarya and variously disposed processes, but others are constructed primarily of plump cells with abundant eosinophilic, hyaline cytoplasm and an asymmetric corona of short processes (Figs. 4–12 and 4–13). Referred to as "gemistocytic astrocytomas," these variants rarely occur in pure form. Perivascular infiltrates of lymphocytes, occasionally associated with germinal centers, are common.[131]

On occasion, gemistocytic astrocytomas show condensation of their fibril-rich cytoplasm into brightly eosinophilic bodies resembling the Rosenthal fibers that, ordinarily, characterize pilocytic astrocytomas. CNS tumors and nonneoplastic lesions with gemistocytes or gemistocyte-like cells are listed in Table 4–3, p. 169.

Because gemistocytic astrocytomas often contain small cells with dense nuclei, scattered mitoses, and a high MIB-1 labeling index, they usually fall into the grade III malignant or anaplastic astrocytoma category, as described later. Scattered, often widely, throughout

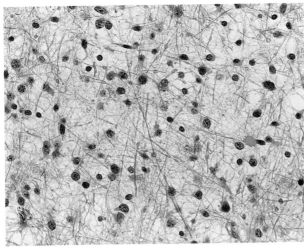

**FIGURE 4–9**    ASTROCYTOMA

Cells of the astrocytoma are clearly more numerous, more hyperchromatic, and larger than normal astrocytes. Note the myelinated axons between the infiltrating tumor cells.

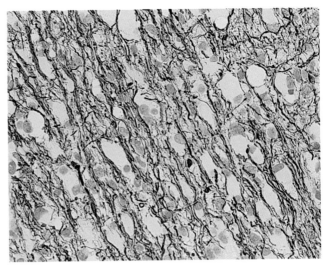

**FIGURE 4–10**    ASTROCYTOMA

The infiltrating quality of diffuse astrocytoma is best demonstrated with immunohistochemistry for neurofilament protein. Tumor cells crowd the interstices between the thread-like neuronal processes.

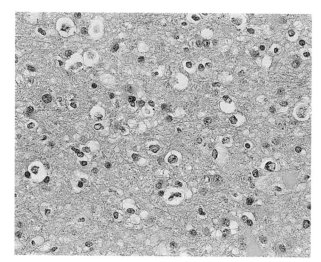

**FIGURE 4–11 ASTROCYTOMA**

There may be a degree of nuclear roundness and perinuclear halo formation in grade II astrocytomas, but the degree of nuclear pleomorphism and the absence of distinct nucleoli distinguish this lesion from oligodendroglioma.

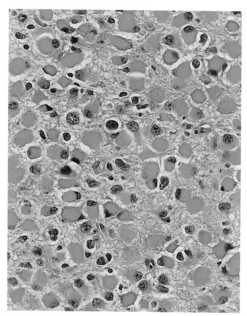

**FIGURE 4–13 GEMISTOCYTIC ASTROCYTOMA**

Although scattered gemistocytes are common in astrocytomas, only a minority of lesions consist predominantly or exclusively of such cells.

the neoplasm are large, dark nuclei with little if any apparent cytoplasm (Fig. 4–14). They represent the main proliferating element of this variant of astrocytoma and have, accordingly, a high MIB-1 index, whereas that of the gemistocytes themselves is low (Fig. 4–15).

A vexing issue with regard to gemistocytes is their distinction from the "minigemistocytes" commonly encountered in oligodendrogliomas but occasionally present in astrocytomas as well. In concept, the minigemistocyte has an eccentric, spherical, glial fibrillary acidic protein (GFAP)–positive intracytoplasmic mass. Similar to an inclusion body, it has a hyaline or faintly fibrillar appearance. In contrast, gemistocytes are larger, more diffusely eosinophilic, and less sharply circumscribed, often with a partial fringe of short processes. In contrast to the minigemistocyte, GFAP positivity is confined to the periphery of the cell, with the central portion remaining negative or only weakly reactive. There is considerable

overlap in the appearances of these two cells, and neither is absolutely diagnostic of either tumor entity.

Microcystic change, even when inconspicuous, is a generally reliable indicator of glioma (Figs. 4–16 and 4–17); it rarely occurs in gliosis (Table 4–4, p. 171), except in a chronic setting wherein the process is contractile and the likelihood of a neoplasm is not an issue.

To some extent, neoplastic astrocytes in cortical gray matter cluster about neurons in a configuration known as "satellitosis." It should be recalled, however, that two or three oligodendroglia normally orbit neurons, especially in deeper cortical layers. Neoplastic cells of astrocytomas may also accumulate beneath the pia, but these "secondary structures" are more typical of oligodendrogliomas.

Amorphous or lamellar grains of calcium are encountered in somewhat less than 10% of diffuse astrocytomas. As in oligodendrogliomas, they are functionally passive but play an active role in diagnosis, because their presence strongly supports a diagnosis of glioma rather than gliosis. Dense aggregates in the cortex, particularly when aligned to capillaries, are more common in oligodendrogliomas than in astrocytomas.

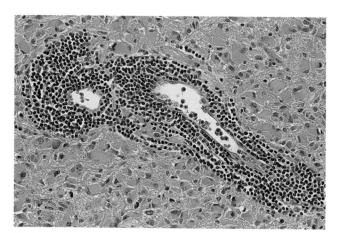

**FIGURE 4–12 GEMISTOCYTIC ASTROCYTOMA**

Gemistocytic astrocytomas are composed largely of cells with abundant eosinophilic cytoplasm and eccentric nuclei. Perivascular lymphocytic infiltrates are frequently present.

**TABLE 4–3**
**Central Nervous System Lesions with Gemistocytes or Gemistocyte-Like Cells**

Gemistocytic astrocytoma
Minigemistocyte-rich oligodendroglioma
Subependymal giant cell astrocytoma
Astroblastoma
Ependymoma
Demyelinating disease with astrogliosis

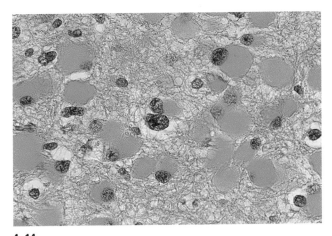

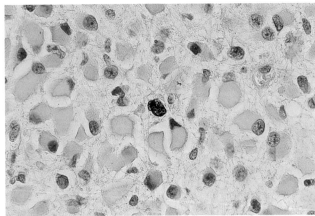

4–14

4–15

**FIGURES 4–14 AND 4–15**    GEMISTOCYTIC ASTROCYTOMA

Cells with hyperchromatic nuclei and scant cytoplasm are the principal proliferative component of this astrocytoma subtype (Fig. 4–14). MIB-1 immunoreactivity is confined largely to these elements (Fig. 4–15).

Cartilaginous metaplasia is a striking finding in a rare astrocytoma. Even more striking is the discovery that the "chondrocytes" within their lacunae are GFAP positive.[58]

As originally proposed, the Ste. Anne–Mayo grading scheme stipulated that the finding of any mitoses must be factored into the grading formula.[32] Based on this premise, an astrocytoma with a solitary mitosis was designated grade III. Almost from the onset, there was reluctance to accept this imperative, and it has been clearly demonstrated that grade III astrocytoma with a solitary mitosis in a generous tissue sample does not behave less favorably than a tumor lacking evident mitotic activity.[42] As assessed by another perspective, patients with grade III astrocytomas in which more than 10 mi-

croscopic fields must be examined before a mitosis is identified do only slightly less well than those in which no dividing cells are encountered.[29] We thus accept a solitary mitosis in a well-sampled grade II astrocytoma.

Neither necrosis nor microvascular proliferation is expected in grade II astrocytomas. Both are features of grade IV lesions, glioblastomas. It must be emphasized, however, that although necrosis is usually indicative of malignancy in a diffuse astrocytic neoplasm, neither it nor vascular proliferation should, as an individual finding, be the sole determinant of malignancy when unaccompanied by other diagnostic features such as increased cellularity, cytologic atypia, and mitoses. It is possible, but unusual, that a rare well-differentiated as-

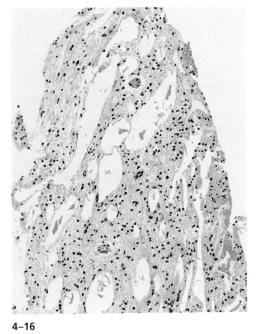

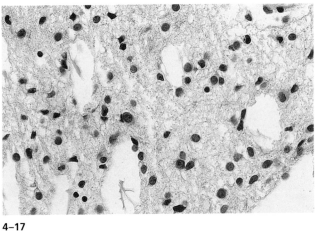

4–16

4–17

**FIGURES 4–16 AND 4–17**    ASTROCYTOMA

The presence of microcystic change points strongly to a neoplastic process (Fig. 4–16). In this case, the hypercellularity and nuclear pleomorphism secure the diagnosis of astrocytoma (Fig. 4–17).

**TABLE 4–4**
**Gliosis versus Glioma**

|  | Gliosis | Glioma |
|---|---|---|
| Cytology | Stellate cells | Variable |
| Cellularity | Mild | Increased |
| Distribution | Uniform | Irregular |
| Gray-white junction | Preserved | Lost |
| Mitoses | Rare | Uncommon |
| Microcysts | Rare | Common |
| Calcifications | No | Occasional |

trocytoma might show focal necrosis due to vascular compression and ischemia.

**Features in Needle Biopsy Specimens.** Establishing a diagnosis of a well-differentiated astrocytoma based on a needle biopsy specimen can pose a challenge, particularly in frozen sections (see Figs. 5–29 to 5–31). In these often minute specimens, it is difficult to assess a lesion's infiltrative quality and to exclude reactive gliosis. Microcysts, a feature more evident in the larger specimens obtained by open biopsy, are helpful diagnostic features of glioma (see Figs. 4–16 and 4–17).

**Features in Frozen Sections.** Edematous white matter, such as that overrun by an infiltrating glioma, is prone to develop a mosaic of ice crystals that is difficult to prevent (Fig. 4–18). The cortex fares better, because it is only minimally affected by vasogenic edema (Fig. 4–19). Seen as clear spaces that compress parenchyma, the crystals, when numerous, make it difficult to estimate the degree of cellularity and cytologic atypia. Such vacuities must be distinguished from true microcysts, which are round rather then polygonal and, in many cases, filled with a faintly basophilic or eosinophilic material. In frozen sections, nuclei in astrocytomas are often contorted and contracted and often appear almost karyolytic. The instantaneous freezing necessary to capture the cells in their native configuration is achieved only in the most superficial portion of the specimen, where nuclei retain their natural shape.

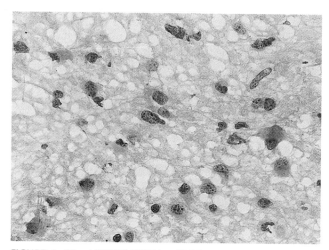

**FIGURE 4–19   ASTROCYTOMA—FROZEN SECTION**

The nuclear hyperchromasia and angulation that typify astrocytomas are best evaluated in the cortex, where ice crystal artifact is usually minimal.

Perineuronal satellitosis is a valuable finding, because it is not a feature of cortical gliosis. As a rule, it is distinguished readily from the attentive clustering of normal oligodendrocytes about cortical neurons by the hypercellularity and cytologic atypia that are the hallmarks of neoplasia. Prominent satellitosis, especially when accompanied by another form of so-called secondary structure (e.g., subpial aggregation of tumor cells), should raise the suspicion of oligodendroglioma.

A note of caution is in order. The assessment of tissue previously used for a frozen section should be done with the realization that artifactual nuclear angulation and hyperchromatism can cause (1) normal or gliotic brain to appear neoplastic, (2) an oligodendroglioma to resemble an astrocytoma (see Figs. 5–26 and 5–27), and (3) a grade II lesion to appear as if it were grade III.

**Cytologic Features.** Neoplastic diffuse astrocytes show considerable morphologic variation, both in quantity and quality of cytoplasm and in degree of nuclear pleomorphism (Fig. 4–20; see also Fig. 5–22). As noted previously, some cells are nearly devoid of cytoplasm ("naked nuclei"). When cytoplasmic processes are evident, they may extend asymmetrically or radiate away from a centrally placed nucleus. In other instances, they simply contribute to a common fibrillar background. In any case, the findings suggest a glioma, specifically an astrocytoma. Attention to cytoplasmic configuration, to processes, and to nuclear features aids in the distinction between astrocytoma and oligodendroglioma, because the cells of an oligodendroglioma typically have scant, process-poor cytoplasm and uniformly round nuclei. Reactive astrocytes exuberantly project their processes radially so as to fill a circular domain larger and more complete than that of their neoplastic counterparts (see Figs. 3–11 and 5–21). As a rule, the processes of neoplastic astrocytes are fewer, shorter, and asymmetrically disposed (see Fig. 4–20). Smear preparations of normal gray and white matter are illustrated in Figures 5–23 and 5–24.

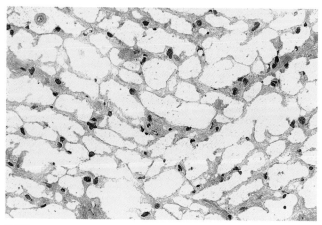

**FIGURE 4–18   ASTROCYTOMA—FROZEN SECTION**

Ice crystals confound the interpretation of frozen sections of astrocytomas residing in edematous white matter.

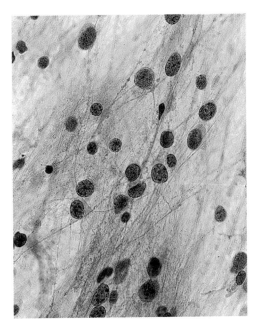

**FIGURE 4–20    ASTROCYTOMA**

Nuclear pleomorphism is well seen in smear preparations. Note also the finely fibrillar background created by tumor cell processes.

**Immunohistochemical Features.** Although the processes of the astrocytes may be evident by hematoxylin and eosin (H&E) staining, especially in the presence of edema, they are seen most easily after immunohistochemistry for GFAP.

The central portion of the ample cell body of gemistocytes is relatively poor in intermediate filaments. As a consequence, it is often weakly reactive or even negative for GFAP (Fig. 4–21). Only subplasmalemmal filament aggregates at the cell periphery are well stained. Because the cells of many astrocytomas have little cytoplasm ("naked nuclei"), GFAP staining is not as useful in tumor classification as it might appear. Often the procedure does little but accentuate coexisting reactive astrocytes.

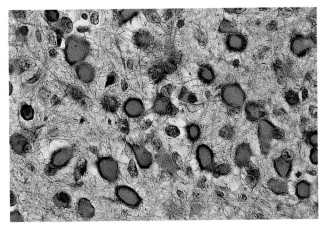

**FIGURE 4–21    GEMISTOCYTIC ASTROCYTOMA**

In keeping with their ultrastructural features (illustrated in Fig. 4–24), immunoreactivity for glial fibrillary acidic protein is more intense in the subplasmalemmal region.

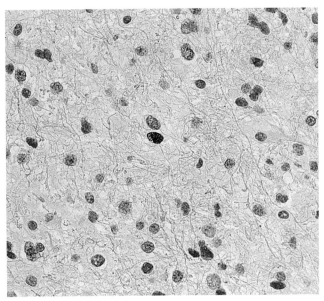

**FIGURE 4–22    ASTROCYTOMA**

The MIB-1 index in grade II astrocytomas is usually in the 1% to 2% range.

Immunostaining for phosphorylated neurofilament protein is useful in defining the infiltrating property that is so central to this form of astrocytoma (see Fig. 4–10). MIB-1 staining, usually 2% or less (Fig. 4–22), is discussed later in the section on differential diagnosis.

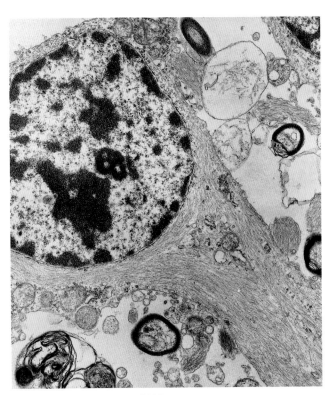

**FIGURE 4–23    ASTROCYTOMA**

Broad processes filled with intermediate ("glial") filaments radiate from the perikarya of neoplastic astrocytes ($\times$ 11,000).

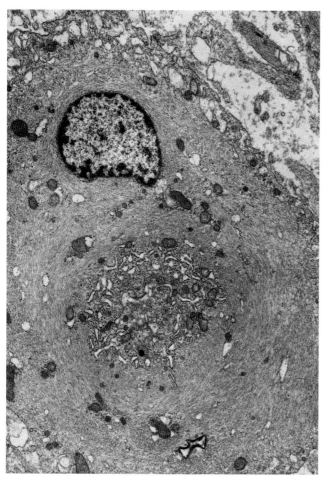

**FIGURE 4–24**   GEMISTOCYTIC ASTROCYTOMA

In gemistocytic astrocytomas, cytoplasmic intermediate filaments are excluded from the core of the cell, which is filled instead with organelles such as mitochondria and rough endoplasmic reticulum (× 5000).

Some grade II astrocytomas are immunoreactive for p53, especially the gemistocytic lesions.[63]

**Ultrastructural Features.** Electron microscopy plays little or no role in the diagnosis of diffuse astrocytoma. When isolated neoplastic astrocytes are observed ultrastructurally in intact parenchyma, they often contain no intermediate filaments (Fig. 4–23). With increased cellularity, intermediate filaments become variably abundant. The central core of gemistocytes is generally occupied by organelles and is relatively devoid of filaments, compared with the peripheral regions (Fig. 4–24).[64, 121] On rare occasion, miniature Rosenthal fibers may be encountered in such cells. Interestingly, a layer of basement membrane covers astrocytes that have an extended stromal contact.

**Molecular and Cytogenetic Features.** Some grade II astrocytomas, especially the gemistocytic variant, exhibit mutations in the p53 tumor suppressor gene.[60, 63, 114] This may represent a prodromal event in the "secondary" or "progression" pathway to glioblastoma (see pages 191 to

**TABLE 4–5**
**Algorithm for Analysis of Central Nervous System Tumors**

1. Is the tissue abnormal?
2. Is the tissue neoplastic?
3. If the tissue is neoplastic, is it an infiltrating or relatively discrete mass?
4. Is it primary or metastatic?
5. What is the grade of the lesion?
6. Does the histologic diagnosis fit with the clinical and radiologic data?

192). Gain of chromosome 7q is seen in some grade II astrocytomas.[96]

**Differential Diagnosis.** The differential diagnosis of astrocytoma should adhere rigidly, and without exception, to an algorithm that, sequentially, (1) establishes the presence of an abnormality, (2) confirms its neoplastic nature, (3) classifies the lesion, and (4) assigns a grade (Table 4–5).

The recognition of astrocytoma and its distinction from *normal brain* (Figs. 4–25 and 4–26) hinges largely on two factors: cellularity and nuclear atypia. Hypercellularity is definitively ascertained only after a twofold or greater increase. Anything less should prompt caution regarding the diagnosis. Exceptions include both hypocellular well-differentiated astrocytomas and the periphery of anaplastic lesions, where widely separated cells do not produce an increase in cellularity but are clearly atypical. A diagnosis may not be possible in this situation. Positivity of these scattered, atypical nuclei for

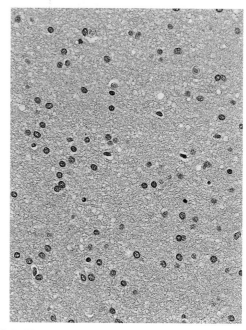

**FIGURE 4–25**   NORMAL WHITE MATTER

Small, round, dark nuclei of oligodendroglia predominate numerically over the larger, paler nuclei of astrocytes.

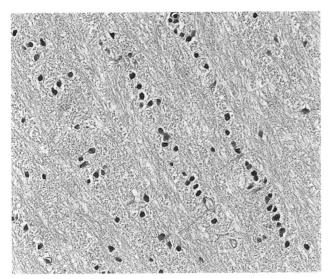

**FIGURE 4–26    NORMAL WHITE MATTER**

Fortuitous sections capture rows of oligodendrocytes aligned between fascicles of axons. These normal formations should not be misinterpreted as columns of infiltrating tumor cells.

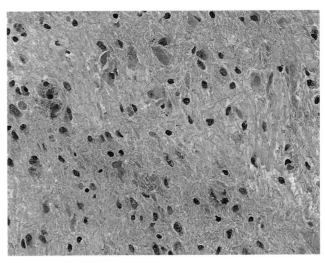

**FIGURE 4–27    PILOID GLIOSIS**

Composed of densely fibrillar tissue with Rosenthal fibers, this form of gliosis is a common response to long-standing tumors in the hypothalamus (especially craniopharyngioma), in the cerebellum (typically hemangioblastoma and pilocytic astrocytoma), and in the spinal cord (any chronic expansile process lesion, including syrinx).

MIB-1 antigen suggests that a neoplasm may be present but is not definitive evidence, because reactive elements can be immunopositive as well. At present, a firm diagnosis of neoplasia still rests on histologic criteria—specifically, cellularity and cytologic features—not on immunohistochemistry. Tumor-specific markers are eagerly awaited.

Additional features that establish the presence of an abnormality include uneven cell distribution, nuclear pleomorphism, and, in some instances, mitoses. The nuclei of normal astrocytes are round to slightly oval and uniformly distributed (see Fig. 4–25). Their chromatin pattern is delicate. In comparison, normal oligodendroglia are somewhat less regular in distribution and, in favorable sections, are aligned in rows along fiber pathways (see Fig. 4–26). Their nuclei are smaller and more hyperchromatic than those of normal astrocytes.

If abnormality is ascertained, the algorithm should proceed to a consideration of *reactive gliosis*. This requires an understanding of the two types of gliosis and the histologic features they share with astrocytoma (see Table 4–4, p. 171).

*Piloid gliosis* is a chronic process that occurs intracranially, principally in the hypothalamus around a craniopharyngioma or in the cyst wall of a cerebellar hemangioblastoma (Fig. 4–27). Piloid gliosis is therefore not a common issue in the differential diagnosis of cerebral hemispheric diffuse astrocytoma, but it is seen occasionally around or within the superficial cortex adjacent to chronic lesions. Although the changes of this variant of gliosis overlap with those of infiltrating astrocytoma, it is a distinctive process—paucicellular, highly fibrillar, and often rich in Rosenthal fibers.

The more common and more difficult task is to distinguish diffuse astrocytoma from *subacute gliosis* of the "fibrillary" type (i.e., hypertrophy) and, to a lesser extent, hyperplasia of resident astrocytes (Figs. 4–28 to 4–30). This differential must address cellularity, archi-

tectural features, and cytologic qualities, as well as the presence of microcysts, calcification, and mitoses. Subacute gliosis features nuclear and cytoplasmic enlargement in responding cells but does not appreciably increase their number. Such reactive astrocytes are hypertrophic and conspicuous, even after H&E staining. Being no more numerous than in their "resting" state, they remain evenly distributed.

The gliosis that occurs in association with demyelinating disease can closely mimic an astrocytoma or mixed "oligoastrocytoma," as is discussed in detail on pages 116 to 119. It is essential that the specimen be analyzed in

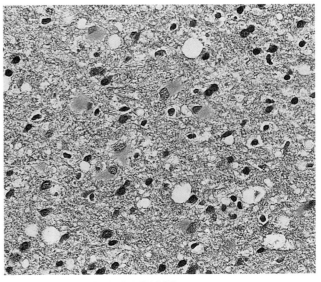

**FIGURE 4–28    FIBRILLARY GLIOSIS**

In contrast to astrocytoma, the gemistocytes appearing in subacute gliosis are uniformly spaced and only minimally increased in number.

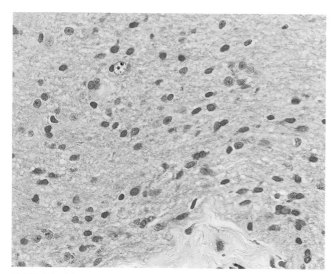

**FIGURE 4–29    FIBRILLARY GLIOSIS**

Although the tissue is somewhat hypercellular, there is no cytologic atypia in this gliotic response to a cavernous angioma.

such a way that reactive, non-neoplastic conditions are excluded before the diagnosis of a neoplasm is entertained (see Tables 4–5, p. 173 and 4–9, p. 213). In the "active" phase of demyelination, reactive astrocytes within a plaque are difficult to ignore because of their sometimes alarming cytologic atypia and hypertrophy. GFAP staining only reinforces the misperception that these cells are neoplastic (see Fig. 3–14). However, in spite of the cytologic features, the cells are widely separated, with neither proliferative activity nor abnormal clustering. The abundant crop of long, radiating cytoplasmic processes typical of reac-tive astrocytes is seen as well. As the situation defervesces and gliosis becomes chronic, cytoplasm shrinks, processes withdraw, and a fine background fibrillarity emerges. Unlike astrocytoma, this end-stage gliosis is not expansile, and it is typically contractile. Table 4–3, p. 169 summarizes CNS lesions with gemistocytes and gemistocyte-like cells.

Reactivity of astrocytes for p53 outside the setting of progressive multifocal leukoencephalopathy, where infected cells are known to be immunoreactive, has been suggested as indicative of neoplasia.[150] Caution is indicated, however, because the legitimacy of this approach has not yet been established. Negative staining certainly does not exclude astrocytoma.

Microcyst formation and calcification can be helpful features in the distinction of gliosis from astrocytoma, because both are foreign to gliosis. But neither per se establishes a diagnosis of glioma. Care must be taken not to interpret edema and mechanical tissue disruption as microcystic change, particularly in frozen tissues. "Bone dust" in a needle biopsy specimen may mimic tumoral calcification (see Fig. 5–28).

If reactive conditions can be excluded, the process of differential diagnosis moves to step two: what category of neoplasm is it? This question is generally best answered by determining whether the lesion is an "infiltrative glioma"—namely, astrocytoma, gliomatosis, or

oligodendroglioma—or a more localized lesion such as *pilocytic astrocytoma* or *pleomorphic xanthoastrocytoma*. See Figure 4–2 for the members of these two groups.

Although there is little prognostic significance in the distinction between *gliomatosis cerebri* and diffuse astrocytoma grade II, the opposite is true concerning *pilocytic astrocytoma*. Mistaking a pilocytic astrocytoma for a diffuse, even anaplastic astrocytoma can have serious therapeutic and prognostic ramifications, and every effort should be made to draw a distinction. At least initially, pilocytic lesions are often treated as surgical entities, whereas diffuse astrocytomas are viewed as nonresectable lesions with a tendency to recur, often with increased anaplasia. Diagnoses such as "astrocytoma" and "low-grade astrocytoma" do not adequately distinguish the two lesions and should be avoided unless qualified by a comment that clarifies the ambiguity.[11]

The distinction between pilocytic and diffuse astrocytoma begins by reviewing clinical and radiologic features. Pilocytic tumors are typically discrete and contrast enhancing, whereas grade II diffuse astrocytomas are often ill defined and, almost by definition, nonenhancing. The histologic finding of a well-differentiated astrocytoma in the face of contrast enhancement is prima facie evidence of either a pilocytic astrocytoma or some other well-circumscribed grade I lesion such as ganglioglioma or subependymal giant cell astrocytoma. In other words, in the absence of prior radiotherapy, a diagnosis of grade II diffuse astrocytoma is inconsistent with the finding of a contrast-enhancing mass.

As a rule, histologic distinction between a diffuse and a pilocytic astrocytoma is not difficult. Classic pilocytic astrocytomas have a biphasic pattern, Rosenthal fibers, eosinophilic granular bodies, and hyalinized vessels. A reassuring realization is that the tissue is entirely neoplastic, as befits a neoplasm more prone to push the brain aside than to invade it. Nonetheless, in small specimens, such as those obtained from the brain stem, even a classic

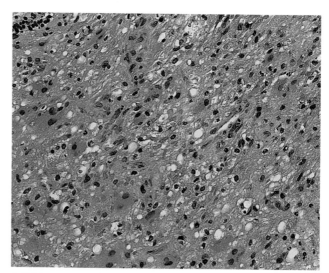

**FIGURE 4–30    FIBRILLARY GLIOSIS**

Vessels and evenly spaced hypertrophic astrocytes create the hypercellularity of this subacute response to a hematoma. In contrast to an astrocytoma, cytologic atypia is minimal.

pilocytic neoplasm may resemble a diffuse astrocytoma. Staining for neurofilament protein can provide evidence of the infiltrative capacity of a given tumor by documenting the extent to which overrun axons are present in the lesion. In diffuse astrocytomas, tumor cells are often found interposed among axons to an extent not seen in conventional pilocytic neoplasms. The fact that some pilocytic astrocytomas are somewhat infiltrative further complicates their distinction from diffuse astrocytomas, even when a sizable specimen is available.

Thus, if a lesion appears obviously infiltrative on the basis of the finding of trapped brain parenchyma, both diffuse astrocytoma and oligodendroglioma become prime diagnostic candidates. Gliomatosis cerebri, a remarkably widespread infiltrative glioma, is discussed in a separate section later.

The distinction between diffuse astrocytoma grade II and *oligodendroglioma grade II* is important and may be difficult, particularly with suboptimal histologic preparations. A molecular-cytogenetic distinction appears to be at hand, as is discussed on pages 237 to 238. This common diagnostic dilemma typically arises in young adults with nonenhancing tumors. The correct diagnosis becomes especially critical if mitoses are found, because their presence, particularly in small specimens, indicates that the astrocytoma is a grade III malignancy. In contrast, low-level mitotic activity can be tolerated in grade II oligodendroglioma. Thus, when mitoses are seen in an infiltrative glioma, one must determine whether the tumor is a grade III (or anaplastic) astrocytoma, which is a tumor with a grim prognosis that necessitates radiotherapy, or an oligodendroglioma, which in most instances is a slowly growing mass that can be followed with periodic MRI scans.

It is difficult to know where to begin a discussion of the differential diagnosis of astrocytoma and oligodendroglioma, but it is probably best to turn to the section on oligodendrogliomas and to be aware that astrocytomas can, because of perinuclear halos and a degree of nuclear roundness, resemble oligodendrogliomas (see Fig. 4–30). It is thus clear that the currently used criteria are rather subjective. Indeed, the decision often depends on one's willingness to diagnose oligodendroglioma in the absence of such classic findings as closely packed monotonous cells with round nuclei and cleared cytoplasm, calcification, and chicken wire vasculature. Extensive cortical infiltration with obvious secondary structures, such as subpial accumulation of neoplastic cells and perineuronal satellitosis, completes the archetype. Many grade II gliomas fall short of this prototype but at the same time are formed of cells cytologically rounder and more uniform than those of the textbook astrocytoma. Although smear preparations are valuable in making the distinction, that may not be possible in frozen sections alone, and they are not infallible; some lesions exhibit cytologic features between those of astrocytoma and oligodendroglioma.

When the features of a lesion are so frustratingly ambiguous that one cannot assign it to either category, it is perfectly acceptable to admit defeat and find refuge in the diagnosis of "well-differentiated infiltrating glioma (see comment)." This problem usually occurs in specimens obtained from patients in the third and fourth decades of life. In this setting, simple observation may be the treatment of choice, and the distinction may have to await the results of a future biopsy at the time of recurrence.

In almost all instances, the radiographic and histologic features of astrocytoma provide a clear distinction from *ependymoma*. Nonetheless, foci resembling astrocytic differentiation are not uncommon in ependymomas of the cellular and tanycytic varieties.

### Diagnostic Checklist

- Is this an astrocytoma or simply chronic gliosis?
- Have active or subacute reactive lesions such as demyelinating disease been excluded?
- Is what appears to be a diffuse astrocytoma really a pilocytic astrocytoma?
- Is the diagnosis of astrocytoma grade II consistent with the neuroimaging findings?

**Treatment and Prognosis.** Given the observation that, like with many other CNS tumors, the extent of the resection is prognostic in both children and adults,[6, 39, 95, 109] the treatment of diffuse astrocytomas has increasingly focused on surgery initially. Other prognostic factors include patient age[95] and neurologic status at presentation (Karnofsky score).[95, 142]

The prognostic value of the MIB-1 labeling index, a measure of cell cycling, has been validated in many studies of diffuse astrocytomas.[42, 52, 80, 84, 110, 142] Nonetheless, values vary considerably and often overlap with those of tumors of higher grade, so it is difficult to apply standards to individual laboratories and specific cases. Reported values (in mean percent) have been 0.05,[110] 0.88,[52] 2.3,[42] 3.1,[84] and 3.8.[142] One study that included astrocytomas at multiple anatomic sites and from patients of all ages suggested a less favorable prognosis when the levels were above 2%.[80] An index of 1.5% is another proposed division separating astrocytoma grades II and III.[52]

The value of radiation therapy has been a subject of debate. In individual cases, the decision depends on the experience of the physician, the presence of symptoms, the wishes of the patient, and the volume of radiologically apparent residual tumor. Strong biases in favor of, or opposed to, radiation therapy at the time of the original diagnosis have made it difficult to study the issue objectively.

The life history of a well-differentiated or grade II diffuse astrocytoma of a cerebral hemisphere takes one of two courses. The lesion may remain well differentiated, permitting survival for many years, or it may undergo anaplastic transformation, augmenting the neurologic deficit and hastening death (Figs. 4–31 and 4–32). In one study of adult patients, grade II lesions were lethal only after anaplastic transformation.[138] The interval to transformation varies. The mean time to progression to grade IV (glioblastoma) has been estimated at between 3 and 5 years.[97] As previously noted, progression is especially likely in gemistocytic astrocytomas.[145]

In adults, overall median survival time was 12 years in one series,[108] 7 years[79] and 7.5 years[73] in two others, and 4 years in a series from the Mayo Clinic.[32]

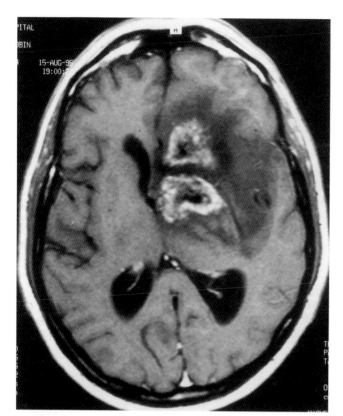

**FIGURE 4–31**   MALIGNANT TRANSFORMATION OF ASTROCYTOMA

Two areas of contrast enhancement corresponding to glioblastoma appeared 4 years after the magnetic resonance imaging scan in Figure 4–3 was taken.

The prognosis of children with grade II diffuse astrocytomas of the cerebral hemispheres may not be as unfavorable as assumed. It is not yet clear whether pediatric lesions are biologically different or more amenable to excision, but one study of nonpilocytic low-grade astrocy-

tomas in the cerebral hemispheres recorded a 10-year survival rate of 82%.[109] Optimism has been expressed about control of these lesions by surgery alone.[39, 109] Removal of the T2-bright area has been associated with excellent tumor control, at least over the time course studied to date.[39, 109]

The outlook for children with grade II astrocytoma of the pons is especially poor, because the lesion is neither surgically resectable nor responsive to therapy, even high doses of irradiation. Most patients succumb within 12 months.[34] Thalamic astrocytomas also carry a poor prognosis.[65, 113]

### Anaplastic Astrocytoma (Grade III)

**Definition.** A biologically aggressive astrocytoma characterized by cytologic atypia and mitotic activity.

**Clinical Features.** It is not surprising that grade III astrocytomas of adults, like well-differentiated or grade II astrocytomas, show a proclivity for the cerebral hemispheres. However, they generally occur a decade later in life and a full decade earlier than glioblastoma. In children, the pons and sometimes the thalamus are additional sites of predilection. Only rarely is the visual system (optic nerves and chiasm), cerebellum, or spinal cord affected.

**Radiologic Features.** Owing to problems in tissue sampling and the conflicting criteria with which the diagnosis is often made, precise histologic-radiologic correlations have been difficult to determine. Although grade III lesions often enhance in a focal or patchy pattern, this is not always the case, and mitotically active lesions may be nonenhancing. The latter is particularly true for lesions at the lower end of the grade III spectrum, where cellularity and mitotic activity are less pronounced. Lesions termed grade III astrocytomas but

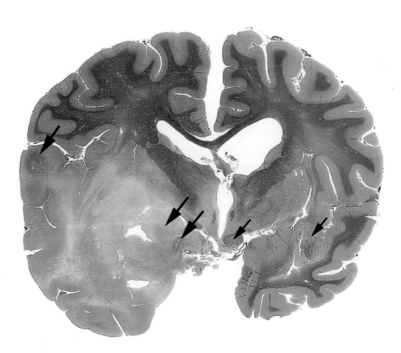

**FIGURE 4–32**   MALIGNANT TRANSFORMATION OF ASTROCYTOMA

Progression to glioblastoma can be multifocal, as in this temporal lobe astrocytoma previously illustrated in Figure 4–6. Separate areas of glioblastoma (*large arrows*) arose within the grade II precursor and seeded the subarachnoid space (*small arrows*).

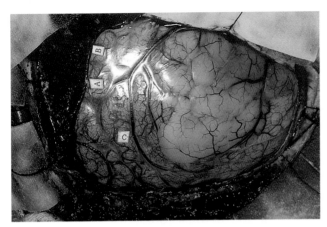

**FIGURE 4–33**   GRADE III ASTROCYTOMA

Astrocytic neoplasms with this degree of mass effect and cortical extension are usually grade III. This lesion, which was focally contrast enhancing, produced seizures at age 35. It contained grade II and III astrocytoma, as well as tumor tissue with advanced cellularity and pleomorphism, but with neither microvascular proliferation nor necrosis. (Courtesy of Dr. Allan H. Friedman, Durham, NC.)

that feature a rim or ring configuration of enhancement about a central area of necrosis are almost certainly inadequately sampled and undergraded glioblastomas.

**Macroscopic Features.** The neoplasm is generally overtly expansile (Fig. 4–33).

**Microscopic Features.** Depending on the individual pathologist's definition, the diligence with which mitoses are sought, and the adequacy of tissue sampling, the designation of grade III astrocytoma covers a broad histologic spectrum. This includes both high-grade gliomas with the anaplasia and cellularity of glioblastomas but

without the requisite necrosis or vascular proliferation, and well-differentiated astrocytomas designated grade III on the basis of a single mitosis found only after a determined search. The real grade III astrocytoma is difficult to define, but it obviously lies between these two extremes.

At the lower end of the spectrum are grade III astrocytomas that at first glance differ little from grade II lesions, except for the mitoses and nuclei that are darker, more angulated, and more atypical, often with so little cytoplasm as to appear "naked." Although cellularity is usually higher and nuclei are often more hyperchromatic and irregular (Figs. 4–34 and 4–35), lesions of low cellularity with scant mitotic activity and a high MIB-1 labeling index (usually greater than 3% to 4%) also qualify. From here, the spectrum advances to include lesions that are more cellular, more cytologically atypical, and more mitotically active (Figs. 4–36 and 4–37).

Whereas purely gemistocytic astrocytomas often exhibit few or no mitoses, others readily fall into the grade III category, with a component of small hyperchromatic cells featuring mitoses and a high MIB-1 labeling index.

As in grade II tumors, the extent to which cytoplasm is expressed in grade III astrocytomas varies considerably. It is often so scant as to be inconspicuous in isolated, widely infiltrative tumor cells. Such cells with their atypical, naked-appearing nuclei lie isolated in a fibrillar background of intact parenchyma. In contrast, cells in more intimate contact possess varying quantities of cytoplasm, with gemistocytic or even giant cells representing the extremes.

By definition, the essential features of glioblastoma (i.e., microvascular proliferation and necrosis) are absent in grade III astrocytomas.

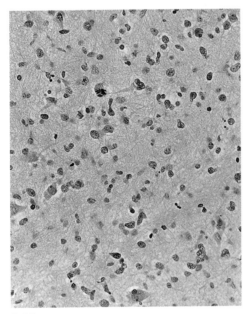

4–34

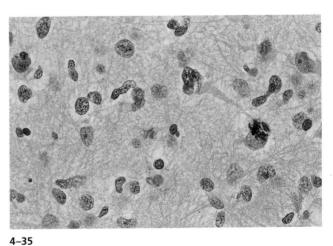

4–35

**FIGURES 4–34 AND 4–35**   GRADE III ASTROCYTOMA

In contrast to its grade II counterpart, this tumor shows greater nuclear pleomorphism. Scattered mitoses are present.

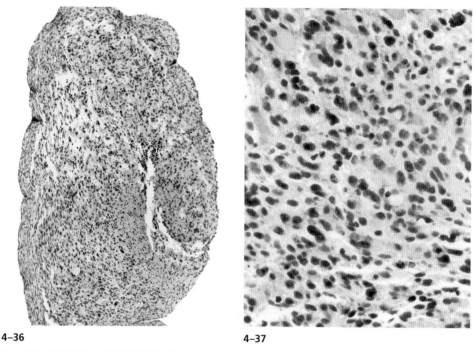

4-36                                    4-37

**FIGURES 4–36 AND 4–37   GRADE III ASTROCYTOMA**

The possibility of glioblastoma should be entertained when a specimen obtained by needle biopsy demonstrates this degree of anaplasia.

Last, one must be cautious in evaluating tissue previously subject to frozen section, because this process produces nuclear hyperchromatism and angulation. As a result, the once round nuclei that characterize well-differentiated oligodendrogliomas come to resemble those of astrocytomas (see Figs. 4–188, 5–26, and 5–27).

**Immunohistochemical Features.** Reported labeling indices for the cell cycling marker MIB-1 vary considerably. Mean values of 4.1,[110] 60,[42] 8.75,[52] and 18.4[142] have been reported, making it difficult to generalize regarding

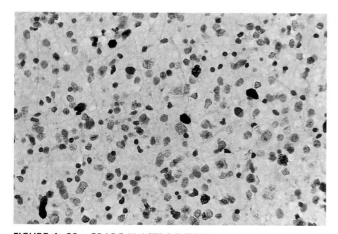

**FIGURE 4–38   GRADE III ASTROCYTOMA**

The MIB-1 labeling index of grade III astrocytomas almost always exceeds 3%. The index here, of approximately 6%, is well within the range of the intermediate-grade lesion.

indices of specific tumor grades. Almost by definition, however, the rate is above 3% (Fig. 4–38).

**Molecular Features.** Although precise molecular correlations have been difficult to determine, given definitional and sampling problems, it appears that the loss of chromosome 10 and amplification of the epidermal growth factor receptor (EGFR) are pivotal events as the lesion passes from grade III to IV. These common cytogenetic-molecular findings should be absent in grade III lesions, although they could be observed focally (e.g., by fluorescence in situ hybridization) as a molecular step to glioblastoma in a lesion that is still, histologically, grade III astrocytoma.

**Differential Diagnosis.** The resolution of a differential diagnosis of grade III astrocytoma begins by establishing that it is indeed a neoplasm and not a reactive condition such as a *demyelinating disease* (Table 4–9, p. 213). This critical distinction is discussed on pages 116 to 119 and 174 to 175. Having confirmed neoplasia, it is helpful to consider two broad classes of gliomas: (1) infiltrating entities that include diffuse astrocytoma, oligodendroglioma, and oligoastrocytoma; and (2) more discrete neoplasms such as pilocytic astrocytoma, pleomorphic xanthoastrocytoma, subependymal giant cell astrocytoma, and ganglion cell tumors. Attention to neuroimaging helps focus this differential (see Table 4–7, p. 205).

If a diagnosis of infiltrating glioma is established, one must determine whether it is astrocytic or oligodendroglial. If astrocytic, the principal differential lies among *astrocytoma grades II, III, and IV*. A discussion of astrocytoma grade II versus grade III appears on page 176. The differential between astrocytomas grade III and IV is simplified in the WHO system, which assigns a malignant astrocytoma to grade IV (i.e., glioblastoma) when either microvascular proliferation or necrosis is present. When a tumor's cellularity, mitotic index, and degree of differentiation are commensurate with those of glioblastoma but these features are unaccompanied by microvascular proliferation or necrosis, the diagnosis of astrocytoma grade III can be made with a qualifying comment regarding the likelihood that the lesion is, in reality, a glioblastoma. Except when a precise diagnosis of glioblastoma is required for eligibility in a treatment protocol, this distinction is often not of great therapeutic significance. In practice, the treating physician can refer to the neuroimaging appearances when faced with such discordance. A ring-enhancing neoplasm of the diffuse or infiltrative type that is histologically grade III is without question a glioblastoma.

One must exclude nondiffuse astrocytic neoplasms, generally low-grade entities such as *pilocytic astrocytoma*, *pleomorphic xanthoastrocytoma*, and *astroblastoma*. The common distinguishing feature of these lesions is their compact, largely noninfiltrating nature, as well as a number of cytologic and histologic features that characterize each entity.

### Diagnostic Checklist

- Have you excluded a non-neoplastic condition, such as demyelinating disease?
- Are you certain that the grade III astrocytoma is not a well-differentiated glioma such as pilocytic astrocytoma or pleomorphic xanthoastrocytoma?

**Treatment and Prognosis.** The prognosis of patients with grade III astrocytoma is poor, because such tumors are prone to anaplastic or glioblastomatous transformation. Death occurs within 2 to 4 years in most patients,[29, 32, 42, 59, 107] but longer survival is not uncommon in younger patients, especially if the grade III status is determined by the presence of a solitary mitosis.[42, 107] Those few patients whose grade III astrocytomas feature ring enhancement on computed tomography (CT) or MRI scan can be expected to succumb within the temporal limits imposed by glioblastoma.

### Glioblastoma Multiforme (Grade IV)

**Definition.** The fully malignant, WHO grade IV, infiltrating or "diffuse" astrocytoma.

**General Comments.** Glioblastoma multiforme, the most common primary brain neoplasm, represents the most malignant end of the diffuse astrocytoma spectrum, being preceded immediately by astrocytoma grade III and foreshadowed more distantly by astrocytoma grade II. Some astrocytic neoplasms, by passing sequentially through this spectrum, evolve over time into glioblastomas (see Figs. 4–3 and 4–31). The process is evident when well-differentiated astrocytoma is found to coexist with glioblastoma in the same specimen (see Fig. 4–32). Such lesions were referred to by Scherer as "secondary" glioblastomas.[60, 122] Other glioblastomas appear clinically

to arise sui generis, often in later life, with no compelling histologic evidence of a well-differentiated precursor lesion. These lesions were designated "primary" glioblastomas.[60, 122] Subsequent histologic studies supported the concept that some glioblastomas evolve from lower-grade astrocytomas, whereas others are poorly differentiated from the onset.[18]

Recently, the concept of two glioblastoma pathways has been approached from the perspective of molecular genetics, using the terms "type II," or "de novo," and "type I," or "progressive," to refer to primary and secondary types, respectively, as discussed later in the section on molecular and cytogenetic features. Although the overall incidence of glioblastoma is slightly higher in men, secondary tumors show a somewhat higher incidence in women. It remains to be seen how closely the histologic, clinical, and molecular concepts correspond.

**Clinical Features.** Glioblastomas occur throughout the brain, including the cerebrum, brain stem, and cerebellum. In the cerebral hemispheres, it shows a peak incidence in the fifth and sixth decades. Although not striking, an overall male predominance of 3:2 persists throughout large series. Most examples in the brain stem occur in children. The cerebellum is an unusual site at any age.[23, 47, 67, 74] Very rarely do glioblastomas affect the optic nerve, a preferential location for pilocytic astrocytomas.[2, 51, 78, 83]

Although in the vast majority of cases the cause of glioblastoma is unknown, irradiation appears to be responsible for rare examples.[10, 111, 120, 128] Genetic predisposition is a factor in Turcot's syndrome,[45] Ollier's disease, and Maffucci's syndrome.[26, 36, 49, 81, 112, 136] High-grade astrocytomas consistent with glioblastomas occasionally arise in the setting of NF1.[135] Germline mutations in p53, in some cases in the setting of Li-Fraumeni syndrome,[76] are thought to be underlying predisposing factors in some cases in which tumor multifocality seems to be more common.[68, 69] Distinct p53 mutations in the initial tumor and in a second geographically distinct tumor suggest true multicentricity without a predisposing germline p53 mutation.[115] It remains to be seen whether the rare glioblastoma occurring in patients with acquired immunodeficiency syndrome (AIDS) is due to anything other than chance.[88] The occasional association of glioblastoma with meningioma is discussed on page 51. Astrocytomas arising in association with demyelinating disease are described on page 119.

The symptoms one associates with cerebral hemispheric lesions include mental change, expressions of increased intracranial pressure, focal neurologic deficits, and seizures. An occasional glioblastoma presents with intracranial hemorrhage. The typically short duration of the preoperative symptoms is in keeping with the well-recognized relationship between the degree of histologic malignancy and the rate of symptom progression in patients with diffuse astrocytomas.

Glioblastomas of the pons present with a combination of long tract and cranial nerve signs. With the support of neuroimaging, the scenario is sufficiently characteristic that radiotherapy is usually prescribed without a tissue diagnosis.

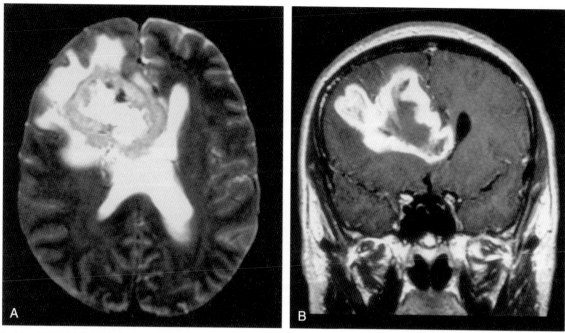

**FIGURE 4–39**   GLIOBLASTOMA MULTIFORME

As evident in the axial plane of a T2-weighted image, this typical glioblastoma forms a ring-shaped mass surrounded by a broad zone of T2-bright cerebral edema (*A*). As seen in the frontal plane, the tumor has a necrotic center that is delineated by an irregular, shaggy rim of contrast enhancement (*B*). The 44-year-old patient had a 3-month history of altered mood, a 3-day history of headache, and a 1-day history of nausea and vomiting.

**Radiologic Features.** As seen on CT or MRI, the typical glioblastoma is an expansile, contrast-enhancing mass configured as a bright, doughnut-shaped ring around a central hypodense area of necrosis (Fig. 4–39).[17] As a reflection of its aggressive expansion and rapid growth, a peripheral zone of tumor infiltration and edema extends well beyond the contrast-enhancing rim. Although these findings are by no means specific for glioblastoma, they are highly characteristic. A diagnosis of grade II or even grade III astrocytoma is inconsistent with such an image. The radiologic differences between this profile and that of abscess is discussed on page 120.

Chapter 5 discusses the issues with regard to stereotactic needle biopsy—in particular, that in some cases, few if any neoplastic cells are found outside of the contrast-enhancing rim.

Although the facility with which glioblastomas permeate brain parenchyma and form satellite lesions makes it difficult to calculate the frequency of multicentric tumors, convincing evidence supports multicentricity in some instances.[5, 68, 69, 102]

**Macroscopic Features.** When large and superficial in location, glioblastomas often expand gyri and recruit a supply of blood through dilated vessels visible on the surface of the brain (Fig. 4–40). Small, thrombosed, "black" veins are a common and ominous finding.

Despite the false impression of circumscription gained from viewing MRI scans, individual glioblastoma cells often extend far afield by following fiber tracts that act as circuits of superconductivity. Such dispersed cells lie within and often extend beyond the zone of peritumoral edema that floods peritumoral white matter. Infiltration

along white matter tracts is best illustrated in association with glioblastomas nearby the corpus callosum, a structure used frequently as a conduit to the contralateral hemisphere. In advanced lesions, the wings of neoplasm that unfold into the two hemispheres from the body of the corpus callosum have been likened to those of a butterfly. It is ironic that this delicate creature serves as an analogy for such a malignant lesion. This likeness of glioblastoma to the Lepidoptera extends also to coloration, especially in fresh specimens, where areas of necrosis and hemorrhage variegate the neoplasm with yellows, reds, and browns

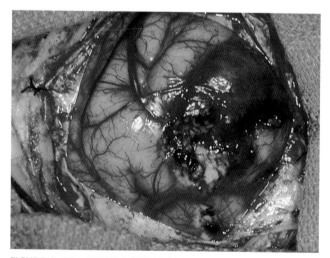

**FIGURE 4–40**   GLIOBLASTOMA MULTIFORME

Exposed at surgery, this superficial lesion expands a gyrus and reaches the surface as a hypervascular mass.

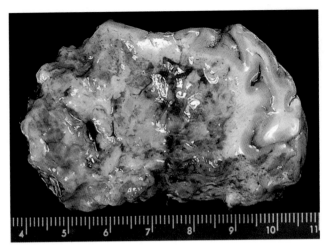

**FIGURE 4–41    GLIOBLASTOMA MULTIFORME**

The white matter localization, infiltrative properties, necrosis, and hemorrhage strongly suggest glioblastoma. This tissue was excised from the left parieto-occipital region of a 65-year-old woman with right facial numbness.

(Fig. 4–41). In the occasional glioblastomas that are almost entirely necrotic, it may be only in the cortex where viable proliferating cells form a ribbon of neoplastic tissue delineating the outer surface of the lesion.

Although in surgical specimens most glioblastomas are not well circumscribed, demarcation is a feature of some giant cell glioblastomas, and the surgeon often suspects metastatic carcinoma (Fig. 4–42).[77] More conventional glioblastomas that reach the subarachnoid space may become so desmoplastic and discrete that the surgeon has difficulty accepting any diagnosis other than meningioma.

**Microscopic Features.** At low magnification, the glioblastoma is a rim of densely cellular tissue—the contrast-enhancing component—about a necrotic core (Figs. 4–43 and 4–44). As is illustrated in Figure 5–5, the margins may be so focally discrete that there are problems in tissue sampling in the case of stereotactic biopsy that does not sample the cellular, contrast-enhancing component.

The cytologic composition of glioblastomas is remarkably diverse, and there is virtually no limit to the scope of their histologic and cytologic appearance within the viable regions (Figs. 4–45 to 4–47). The tumors range from monotonous, small cell neoplasms to "monstrocellular" tumors with a variety of grotesque forms. It is not surprising, given the tendency of lower-grade astrocytic neoplasms to transform, that tissue patterns of well-differentiated and anaplastic astrocytoma, as well as glioblastoma, may coexist in the same specimen. This variation is the hallmark of secondary glioblastoma, which often arises multifocally in a background of well-differentiated astrocytoma. Mitoses vary from frequent to sparse. Although the profile of the contrast-enhancing rim suggests circumscription, glioblastomas are, with the exception of some giant cell variants, highly infiltrating. In the cortex, secondary structures such as satellitosis (Fig. 4–48), perivascular accumulation, and subpial aggregation of tumor cells may be prominent.

Although the histologic and cytologic variations of glioblastoma are endless, several patterns are sufficiently frequent or distinctive to deserve mention.

A common pattern consists of a somewhat jumbled mixture of cells with pleomorphic, hyperchromatic nuclei and a variable amount of glassy cytoplasm (Fig. 4–49). Scattered large pleomorphic cells with glassy, "astrocytic" cytoplasm are a frequent finding.

Another distinctive variant is the small cell glioblastoma, a tumor that carries monomorphism to the extreme (Figs. 4–50 and 4–51). Their rather bland nuclei can appear either elongated, as the cells journey through compact fiber tracts, or round, when viewed in cross section. GFAP immunoreactivity is often scant, being proportional to the meager amount of cytoplasm. Nonetheless, some small cell glioblastomas have enough processes to create a fibrillary background, usually with a somewhat fascicular architecture. Although the small, uniform cells may create a low-power likeness to oligodendroglioma, enhanced in some cases by calcification, high magnification discloses the variation in nuclear shape, albeit limited in degree, that characterizes this glioblastoma variant. The nuclei of a small cell glioblastoma lack the uniform nuclear roundness of oligodendroglioma, even those of higher grade. Perivascular pseudorosettes, generally subtle, in some small cell glioblastomas resemble those in ependymoma (see Fig. 4–69). As small cell glioblastomas diffuse into surrounding tissues, individual isolated cells stand alone, and it can be very difficult to distinguish them from normal glia and to determine a surgical margin by histologic or cytologic criteria (Fig. 4–52).

At the opposite cytologic extreme from the small cell lesion is an entity termed giant cell glioblastoma, a tumor composed primarily of extremely large cells with multilobed, or even multiple, nuclei. A lesser number of small

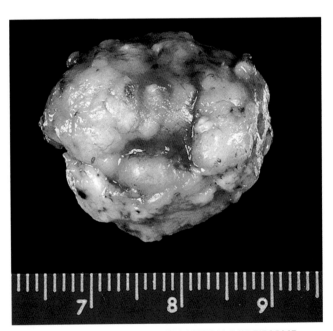

**FIGURE 4–42    GIANT CELL GLIOBLASTOMA MULTIFORME**

This unusual variant of glioblastoma is characteristically discrete and firm because of its collagen content. Radiologically and macroscopically, this lesion often mimics a metastasis.

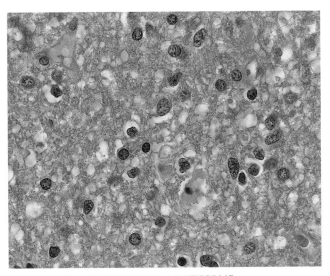

**FIGURE 4-52**    GLIOBLASTOMA MULTIFORME

Small, cytologically bland tumor cells can be difficult to identify as neoplastic when they are individually dispersed in the sparsely cellular, infiltrative edge of the tumor. Nonetheless, the MIB-1 labeling index will be high.

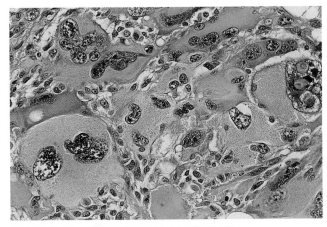

**FIGURE 4-53**    GLIOBLASTOMA MULTIFORME

Grotesque forms, with interposed small neoplastic cells and lymphocytes, typify the giant cell glioblastoma variant.

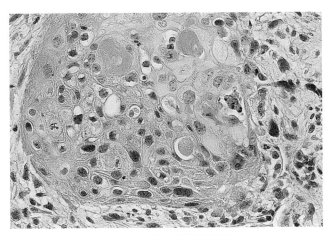

**FIGURE 4-54**    GLIOBLASTOMA MULTIFORME

Squamous differentiation is a rare, eye-catching feature in glioblastoma and gliosarcoma.

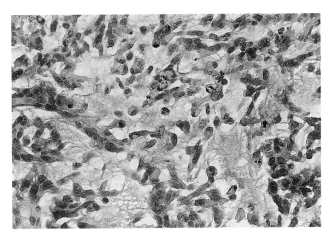

**FIGURE 4-55**    GLIOBLASTOMA MULTIFORME

Cellular elongation in a myxoid background lends a mesenchymal appearance to some glioblastomas.

subdued, nonglomeruloid form in which the response is more hypertrophy than hyperplasia (see Fig. 7-35).

Necrosis is a hallmark of glioblastoma. Its presence in an untreated diffuse astrocytoma, or the finding of microvascular proliferation, distinguishes glioblastoma from grade III or anaplastic astrocytoma. Foci, or zones, of necrosis are typically of the coagulative type, without prominent macrophages or other tissue responses such as granulation tissue. The necrosis may involve not only the neoplastic tissue but its vasculature as well. Table 4-6, p. 188 summarizes the histologic characteristics of necrosis in CNS lesions.

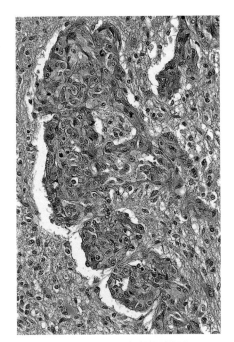

**FIGURE 4-56**    GLIOBLASTOMA MULTIFORME

Vascular proliferation, a cardinal diagnostic feature of glioblastoma multiforme, is usually prominent in the viable tissue adjacent to the neoplasm's necrotic core. Note the orientation of the vascular response, which was directed toward an area of necrosis off the left of the illustration.

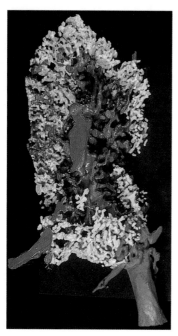

**FIGURE 4–57**   GLIOBLASTOMA MULTIFORME

This wax model of a large conglomerate of glomeruloid vessels in a glioblastoma demonstrates a feeder vessel (*red*) entering at the bottom right. This afferent channel then branches into collagen-containing intermediate vessels (*green*). In turn, these give rise to capillaries (*yellow*). The model was constructed from wax templates of serial histologic sections.

**TABLE 4–6**
**Characteristics of Necrosis in Central Nervous System Lesions**

Glioblastoma multiforme. Affects both parenchyma and vasculature; granular, coagulative, few macrophages

Metastatic carcinoma. Spares isometric perivascular zone of viable tumor; coagulative, necrotic cell "ghosts" prominent, few macrophages

Malignant lymphoma. Affects both parenchyma and vasculature; coagulative, usually extensive in the setting of immunosuppression

Radionecrosis. Usually limited to white matter and sometimes deeper cortical laminae; affects both parenchyma and vasculature; discrete areas, coagulative, "fibrinoid" necrosis of vessels, few macrophages

Toxoplasmosis. Similar to radionecrosis but not localized to white matter; inflammation sparse, necrotic vessels common

Abscess. Purulent, liquefactive, granulation tissue in capsule

Herpes simplex encephalitis. Affects both white and gray matter; coagulative, vessels necrotic, "red neurons" present

Demyelinating disease. Involves white matter with relative sparing of axons; necrosis limited to oligodendrocytes (but fleeting and rarely captured in histologic sections); macrophages, not coagulative, no cavitation

Infarct. Affects both gray and white matter, but gray matter involvement is predominant; vasculature often spared; "red neurons" prominent in acute lesions, hypertrophy of cells in microvasculature, macrophage response as lesion evolves, axons lost, cavitation in chronic lesions

In many glioblastomas, a distinct and classic peripheral concentration of neoplastic cells outlines the zones of necrosis (Fig. 4–59). The descriptive terms "palisading" and "pseudopalisading" are well-known descriptors of this helpful diagnostic feature. It is not always present, however, and necrosis may emerge abruptly or even imperceptibly without any peripheral cellular corona. Among the palisading cells, one often finds apoptotic bodies in variable numbers.[130] When they are abundant, the impression is often that the necrosis is really a zone of confluent apoptosis rather than zonal necrosis. For diagnostic purposes, bona fide coagulation necrosis must be seen, not simply single-cell necrosis or apoptosis.

Perivascular lymphocytes and rarely plasma cells are present in some glioblastomas, particularly those rich in gemistocytic astrocytes or the giant cell variant.[119, 131] It has been suggested that such lesions are associated with a more favorable prognosis,[101] but this was not confirmed by a subsequent study.[12] If it truly portends a better prognosis, it may reflect the fact that lymphocytes are usually present in gemistocyte-rich "secondary" glioblastomas that occur more often in younger patients.

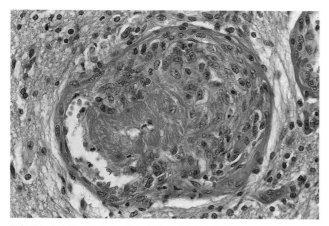

**FIGURE 4–58**   GLIOBLASTOMA MULTIFORME

The second variant of vascular proliferation—the intraluminal proliferation of endothelial cells—is more restricted to high-grade gliomas than is the glomeruloid type.

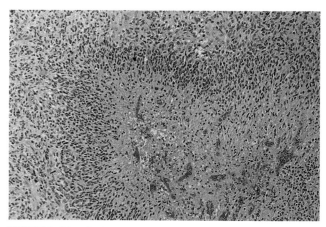

**FIGURE 4–59**   GLIOBLASTOMA MULTIFORME

Palisading around zones of necrosis is a classic feature of glioblastoma multiforme.

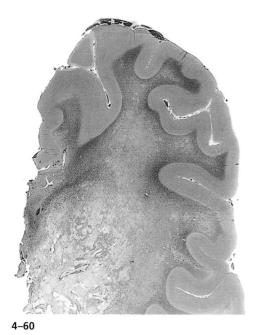

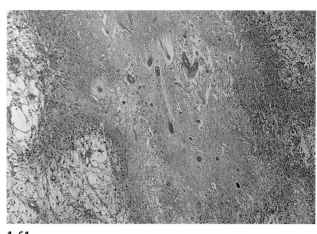

4-60                                    4-61

**FIGURES 4-60 AND 4-61     REOPERATION SPECIMEN OF PREVIOUSLY IRRADIATED GLIOBLASTOMA**

An extensive mosaic pattern of radionecrosis is present in this "recurrent" occipital glioblastoma (Fig. 4-60). Microscopically, the viable tissue in such postradiation tumors often lacks the anaplastic component of the original pretreatment tissue, consisting instead of better differentiated tissue that may be difficult to characterize definitively as either neoplastic or reactive (Fig. 4-61).

When glioblastomas infiltrate meninges, particularly the dura, or even the adventitia of blood vessels, the resultant fibroplasia may be so exuberant that a discrete mass is produced. In such cases, the neoplastic cells often retain their astrocytic features and form aggregates amidst the proliferating connective tissue. Alternatively, they may commingle with the collagen- and reticulin-forming cells to such an extent as to be almost undetectable. Nonetheless, although the two phenotypes may appear indistinguishable in H&E-stained sections, the glial component can be identified by immunostaining for GFAP. Gliosarcomas are discussed in a later section.

**Effects of Prior Radiotherapy.** Reoperation to debulk a mass of expansile contrast-enhancing tissue is not uncommon in glioblastoma patients, particularly those who are younger and therefore more likely to benefit by decompression. Both recurrent neoplasm and radionecrosis produce a similar clinical and radiologic picture of an expanding, edema-producing, and contrast-enhancing mass. Although positron emission tomography and magnetic resonance (MR) spectroscopy may aid in the distinction of these two very different processes, the decision to proceed with further adjuvant treatment, usually chemotherapy, often awaits histopathologic confirmation that the lesion is recurrent neoplasm and not radionecrosis. The pathologist is then left with the challenge of sorting out what is often a confusing melange of cellular and proliferating "active" tumor, residual paucicellular "quiescent" neoplasm with radiation effects, and spontaneous tumor necrosis. In this endeavor, there is often no dichotomy between clearly defined recurrent, "active" neoplasm, responsible in itself for the clinical

and radiologic recurrence, and pure radionecrosis (Figs. 4-60 and 4-61).

Radiotherapy is often effective in eradicating undifferentiated cells, thus leaving behind only the better-differentiated or paucicellular tissue that contains large, bizarre cells with abundant pink cytoplasm (Fig. 4-62).[16, 19, 41] In such cases, the original cellular, mitotically active neoplasm may no longer be evident. Although the pleomorphic cells are neoplastic, their proliferative capacity seems to be minimal, and the cells should be interpreted as "persistent" or "quiescent,"

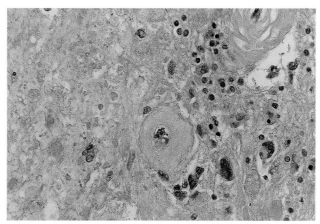

**FIGURE 4-62     PREVIOUSLY IRRADIATED GLIOBLASTOMA MULTIFORME**

Following radiotherapy, glioblastomas are often extensively necrotic, but without the pseudopalisading seen in the untreated tumor. Low cellularity and widely dispersed, large pleomorphic cells are typical findings. Highly cellular, actively proliferating neoplasm, as seen in the pretreatment lesion, is either absent or present only focally.

rather than "recurrent." Because glioblastomas are rarely cured, active proliferating cells must lurk in the tissue, presumably as small, isolated forms that are not readily identifiable in histologic sections and that contribute only minimally to the mass. Discrete foci of parenchymal necrosis are typical of radiation effect, as seen within the bed of an irradiated neoplasm. Similar necrosis is seen in some cases as an unwanted treatment effect. In true recurrence of the tumor, the neoplasm reappears in or around the original tumor bed as a largely undifferentiated, mitotically active, small cell neoplasm. Whereas spontaneous tumor necrosis often features pseudopalisading, radionecrosis does not (see Table 4–6, p. 188).

Although necrosis typifies irradiated neoplasms and represents a desired treatment effect, a large volume of radionecrosis in and around the neoplasm may require surgical debulking. As discussed earlier, a sharp distinction often cannot be made among the disease, the desired effects of treatment, and a complication (e.g., parenchymal radionecrosis). The issue of "pure" radionecrosis (i.e., that following radiation for an extracranial primary neoplasm) is discussed later in the section on differential diagnosis.

**Features in Needle Biopsy Specimens.** Although stereotactic needle biopsy is common, the diagnosis of glioblastoma by this method is sometimes a trying task (see Chapter 5). Under optimal conditions, it is an expeditious and definitive technique, but in other instances, it is neither. One can be left with a largely necrotic specimen that suggests that a neoplasm may be present but provides little objective evidence that this is so. The small size and fragmentation of some specimens, as well as inadequate tissue sampling, often prolong the procedure and increase the likelihood that a nondiagnostic sample has been obtained. As discussed in Chapter 5, it is important that the pathologist be familiar with the radiologic features of the lesion. With glioblastoma, it is usually the contrast-enhancing rim of the lesion that is targeted for biopsy (see Figs. 5–4 to 5–8). As illustrated in Figure 4–43, this zone varies not only from case to case but also within a given neoplasm. In some instances, it is so narrow that a needle that skirts its target by a millimeter or two yields tissue that is normal or contains only rare, isolated tumor cells.[17, 18, 31] A biopsy from the center of the lesion may obtain only necrotic tissue. Although the coagulative nature may help exclude an infarct, which is usually rich in macrophages, there may be so few tumor cells that a secure diagnosis is not possible. Deeper sectioning is usually in order in an attempt to find viable tumor that, if present, is most likely to be found in perithelial domains.

In addition to their occasional failure to obtain diagnostic tissue, needle biopsies may result in tumor undergrading. This is especially true in glioblastomas of the secondary type, wherein anaplastic foci arise in the background of a preexisting, better-differentiated astrocytoma. For example, a small specimen that samples only a non–contrast-enhancing area may yield tissue with the characteristics of a grade II or III astrocytoma. Chapter 5 presents guidelines for smear preparation and speci-

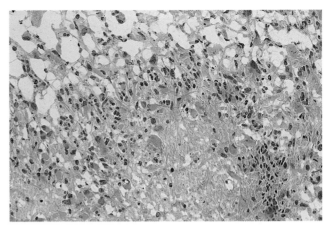

**FIGURE 4–63**    GLIOBLASTOMA MULTIFORME—FROZEN SECTION

The fibrillar processes of tumor cells are often more evident in frozen tissues than they are in permanent sections.

men handling, as well as the evaluation of specimens obtained by stereotactically directed needle biopsy.

**Features in Frozen Sections.** Although the cytologic findings of cell processes and a fibrillar background help in the diagnosis, tissue sections better demonstrate a lesion's hypercellularity and invasiveness. The fibrillar background created by the neoplastic cells is often more evident in frozen than in permanent sections (Fig. 4–63). Invasiveness is evidenced by incorporation of neurons and reactive astrocytes. The finding of microvascular proliferation or necrosis with pseudopalisading solidifies the diagnosis. One must be cautious in interpreting what appear to be foci of necrosis when there is no pseudopalisading, because normal gray matter, in comparison with tumor, appears oligocellular and hence necrotic. Microvascular proliferation is detected best under low magnification (Fig. 4–64).

**Cytologic Features.** Smear preparations of glioblastomas faithfully mirror the variability in nuclear size and

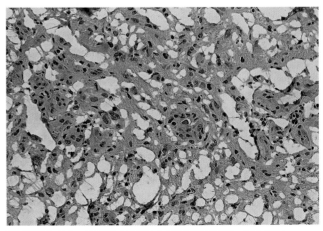

**FIGURE 4–64**    GLIOBLASTOMA MULTIFORME—FROZEN SECTION

Vascular proliferation may be a subtle finding in frozen sections.

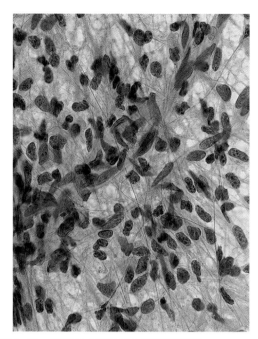

**FIGURE 4-65    GLIOBLASTOMA MULTIFORME**

In smear preparations, small, cytologically bland cells immersed in a delicate fibrillar background distinguish glioblastoma from primary central nervous system lymphoma and metastatic carcinoma. Other glioblastomas exhibit larger, more pleomorphic, and patently "astrocytic" cells.

shape, as well as in cytoplasmic volume and conformation. In many instances, however, most of the cells are small and bipolar (Fig. 4–65; see also Fig. 5–6). Nucleolar prominence is uncommon. Mitoses are found in most instances, albeit often with difficulty. Scanty cytoplasm extends away from opposite poles of the cell, and the processes, in aggregate, create a fibrillar background. As a rule, nuclear features readily establish the neoplastic nature of the lesion. The presence of fine cytoplasmic processes exculpates both lymphoma and carcinoma.

**Immunohistochemical Features.** The presence of glial filaments within neoplastic cells can be established readily by immunohistochemical stains for GFAP (Fig. 4–66). Reactivity for this filamentous protein highlights much of the cytoplasm of spindle cells and the periphery of gemistocytes. In small cell components, staining is often scant within processes or perikarya. Immunoreactive cells may be limited to, or most abundant in, perivascular regions, but caution is advised, because reactive astrocytes and their processes frequent these zones. Finally, a negative GFAP stain does not exclude a diagnosis of glioma, because glioblastomas may be devoid of reactivity. The possibility that vagaries of tissue processing underlie the loss of immunoreactivity must be considered if the specimen is negative for antibodies to vimentin. The latter are good as "controls" for the staining technique and the antigenicity of the tissue but have little other diagnostic utility. When used to distinguish anaplastic glioma from metastatic carcinoma, antibodies to cytokeratin can be misleading. AE1-AE3 antisera, particularly, may stain astrocytomas and ependymomas.[30, 94]

Reactive astrocytes are intensely labeled, sometimes better than by antibodies to GFAP. This cross-reactivity is less likely with the antibody CAM 5.2. Immunoreactivity of the epithelioid glioblastoma subtype is discussed later in the section on differential diagnosis.

Although the finding of numerous macrophages should always prompt consideration of demyelinating diseases or infarction, these cells are occasionally numerous in glioblastomas. The same is true of large, activated microglia. In their normal state, the latter are nonreactive with such macrophage immunomarkers as HAM-56 or KP-1, but when activated by any number of local stimuli, their long, bipolar, typically fuzzy processes stain prominently.[117]

The glioblastoma MIB-1 staining index varies considerably from report to report, with mean percentages of 9.1,[42] 9.12,[52] 18.9,[84] and 31.6.[142] Higher levels have been noted in glioblastomas with CDKN2 (p16) deletions than in those without[100] and in those amplified for EGFR.[134] Given their considerable regional variation and the occasional lack of staining altogether, MIB-1 indices are of little use in prognostication.[28, 42, 116]

**Ultrastructural Features.** Electron microscopy is an infrequently used adjunct in the diagnosis of glioblastoma. Only in selected instances is it useful in demonstrating the nonepithelial nature of the lesion. Although poorly formed junctions are commonly encountered, glioblastoma cells lack well-formed desmosomes with inserting tonofilaments. Although suggestive of a glioma, the finding of cytoplasmic intermediate filaments is not diagnostic of glioma, because the various intermediate filament subtypes are ultrastructurally indistinguishable. Basement membrane may be seen at the interface of glioma cells and stroma.

**Molecular and Cytogenetic Features.** Not surprisingly, the designation multiforme is as applicable to the cytogenetic and molecular profile of glioblastomas as it is to their histologic features. Attempts are ongoing to establish order among this complexity and to identify

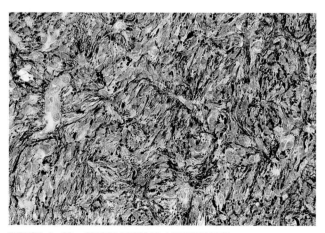

**FIGURE 4-66    GLIOBLASTOMA MULTIFORME**

With rare exceptions, glioblastomas are immunoreactive, at least in part, for glial fibrillary acidic protein.

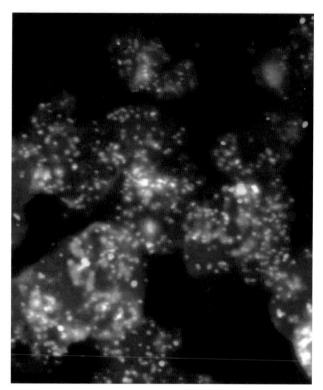

**FIGURE 4–67    GLIOBLASTOMA MULTIFORME**

In this fluorescence in situ hybridization (FISH) preparation, the large number of red signals for epidermal growth factor receptor indicates gene amplification, as occurs in glioblastomas of the primary type. (Courtesy of Dr. Robert B. Jenkins, Rochester, MN.)

features of prognostic or therapeutic value. Although a coherent picture has yet to emerge, recent molecular parameters have been used to subclassify glioblastomas into "primary" and "secondary" types. Giant cell glioblastoma has intermediate features. Other subtypes or prognostically useful combinations of genetic abnormalities undoubtedly await description.

The most common molecular subtype of glioblastoma has been referred to as the primary, de novo, or type II lesion, in which several abnormalities are commonly seen.[7, 60, 61] These include EGFR amplification or overexpression (Fig. 4–67), mutations in the tumor suppressor gene *PTEN*, and homozygous deletions of *CDKN2A* (p16).[7, 46, 60, 61, 114, 132, 140] Mutations in p53 are uncommon, but the common amplification of *MDM2* is another means for the cells to avoid p53-regulated growth control.[8] Primary glioblastomas generally occur later in life than the secondary or progressive lesions, in which mutations of the p53 gene are an early event. EGFR amplification or overexpression and p53 mutations appear to be almost mutually exclusive.[60, 114, 141, 144] Loss of heterozygosity on chromosome 10 is in many cases linked with EGFR amplification,[72, 139, 140] but it can occur in the secondary pathway as well, where it is more likely to be restricted to the long arm.[38] Loss of heterozygosity on chromosome 19q is common in secondary but not primary glioblastomas.[91]

One series disclosed that the demographics of these two groups are different, with women more often affected by secondary lesions and men by primary lesions.[60, 144] Given the predominance of primary lesions, men are more affected by glioblastomas as a whole.

The genetics of pediatric high-grade astrocytomas appear to be somewhat different, with a considerably lower incidence of *EGFR* amplification in one study.[27] An additional investigation also found a high incidence of p53 mutations but found a lack of *EGFR* amplification.[129] There may also be evidence of DNA mismatch repair, in the form of microsatellite instability, in a minority of pediatric cases.[27, 129] Astrocytomas of the brain stem have a high incidence of p53 mutations.[27, 75]

The demonstration of these various abnormalities may be useful, especially in needle biopsy specimens, for distinguishing astrocytoma grade III from grade IV (glioblastomas). Loss of chromosome 10 and *EGFR* amplification are common in glioblastoma multiforme, and the former may be the cytogenetic lesion underlying the transition from grade III to grade IV.[1, 89, 98] Abnormalities in the *p16/RB/CDK4* pathway might be markers of neoplasms in the astrocyte series and may be useful, along with study of chromosomes 1p and 19q, in distinguishing glioblastomas from high-grade oligodendrogliomas.[106]

Correlations between molecularly and clinically defined primary and secondary glioblastoma multiforme are incomplete, although glioblastomas arising in the histologic background of a better-differentiated precursor astrocytoma are well described.[18, 122] The composition of the primary glioblastoma is less clear, although both large "geographic" areas of necrosis[133] and a small cell architecture have been described.[13] It remains to be seen whether identification of chromosome 1p loss, as occurs in oligodendrogliomas, portends a better prognosis in high-grade gliomas without oligodendroglioma features.[54]

It is a matter of debate whether these molecular features are significant to treatment, interval to recurrence, or the extent to which primary and secondary lesions are clearly defined entities. Indeed, one study found no correlation between survival and the altered expression of p53, EGFR, CDKN2 (p16), MDM2, or Bcl-2 genes.[92] It also questioned the distinction of glioblastomas into primary and secondary types on the basis of molecular features alone. Nonetheless, several studies have reported poorer survival rates among patients whose tumors featured EGFR amplification or overexpression.[123, 134] One study noted shorter survival times in younger patients without p53 mutations.[4] Amplification of *EGFR* is usually accompanied by a mutation.[37]

The giant cell glioblastoma partially overlaps with both the secondary type, because of a high incidence of p53 mutation, and the primary type, because of the significant incidence of *PTEN* mutation.[60, 82] In common with the primary lesion, there is a short clinical history, absence of a precursor lesion, and a 30% incidence of *PTEN* mutation. Giant cell glioblastoma shares with the secondary type a younger patient age and a substantial (greater than 70%) incidence of p53 mutation.[104] *EGFR* amplification is less common than in supratentorial "primary" glioblastomas.[104, 105]

**Differential Diagnosis.** Although most specimens of glioblastomas clearly reveal a neoplastic process, it is still appropriate to pause and ask whether the lesion in question could be reactive rather than neoplastic. For example, an *evolving infarct* may mimic a malignant glioma both clinically and radiologically, thus prompting surgical intervention (see Figs. 5–14 and 7–30). Owing to the influx of macrophages, these vascular lesions can be highly cellular, and the microvasculature may be hypertrophic and even somewhat hyperplastic (see Fig. 7–35). It is of note, however, that infarction generally spares large vessels, whereas those in the glioma are often necrotic. The necrosis is also macrophage rich and "liquefactive," not coagulative (see Figs. 5–16 and 5–17). The histopathologic features of infarcts are discussed in Chapter 7.

Although *demyelinating disease* is not known for geographic areas of necrosis, its cellularity and reactive astrocytosis, in the context of a contrast-enhancing lesion, can be deceptive and create the appearance of a high-grade glioma (see Figs. 3–1 to 3–4 and Table 4–9, p. 213). Its constituent macrophages diffusely infiltrate the lesion and crowd about vessels in company with lymphocytes. Distinctively, astrocytes are uniformly distributed and feature long stellate processes. Demyelinating lesions are discussed in detail in Chapter 3.

Some glioblastomas are so overrun with polymorphonuclear leukocytes as to appear part of an abscess (Fig. 4–68). Multiple sections may be necessary to identify the neoplastic tissue.

Once non-neoplastic lesions have been excluded, one can focus on neoplasms that simulate glioblastoma. The distinction of glioblastoma from astrocytoma grade III is discussed on pages 179 to 180.

Given the polymorphism of glioblastoma, its cytologic and histologic profile encroaches on that of many other tumors. Although distinguishing it from other malignant gliomas is certainly important, it is less important than the distinction of glioblastoma from low-grade lesions, particularly pleomorphic xanthoastrocytoma and pilocytic astrocytoma.

The distinction from *pleomorphic xanthoastrocytoma* is accomplished largely by awareness of the latter

entity and its radiologic features. It is generally an enhancing, solid, superficially situated mass, sometimes occurring as a mural nodule in a cyst. The features that contribute to a misdiagnosis of high-grade astrocytoma include cellular pleomorphism, nuclear atypia, occasional mitotic activity, and the infrequent occurrence of necrosis. The difficult issue of distinguishing glioblastoma from malignant pleomorphic xanthoastrocytoma is considered on page 220.

Although it seems counterintuitive, one confronts the occasional necessity of distinguishing glioblastoma from *pilocytic astrocytoma*. The therapeutic and prognostic ramifications of this issue need no elaboration. As discussed on pages 209 to 210, some pilocytic astrocytomas are sufficiently cellular and pleomorphic that they resemble grade III or IV astrocytomas. Although glomeruloid vasculature is a well-known feature of pilocytic tumors, proliferation of endothelial cells within large vessels is seen only occasionally. This latter form of vascular proliferation is closely associated with glioblastoma. Last, faced with occasional necrosis, even without pseudopalisading, the temptation to make a diagnosis of glioblastoma is ever present. These features and those of a rare, truly malignant pilocytic astrocytoma are discussed on page 211.

The differential diagnosis of glioblastoma multiforme and *malignant oligodendroglioma* and *malignant ependymoma* is of practical importance and, to some extent, a philosophical issue. As previously noted, and in keeping with the WHO definition, the term "glioblastoma" refers only to the highest grade (IV) of diffuse astrocytic tumor. Given the molecular biologic and therapeutic differences between glioblastoma and the other anaplastic glial neoplasms, limited use of the term is appropriate. The differentials of glioblastoma versus malignant oligodendroglioma and malignant ependymoma are discussed on pages 240 and 246, respectively.

Although most glioblastomas are astrocytic, an occasional tumor, usually a small cell variant, has features reminiscent of *malignant ependymoma* (Fig. 4–69). Unless there is unequivocal and widespread evidence of

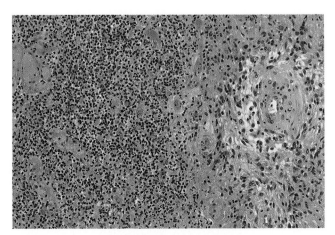

**FIGURE 4–68   GLIOBLASTOMA MULTIFORME**

A dense infiltrate of polymorphonuclear leukocytes can be misinterpreted as an abscess. Neoplastic tissue is evident on the right.

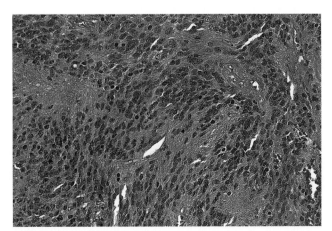

**FIGURE 4–69   GLIOBLASTOMA MULTIFORME**

Focal perivascular pseudorosettes of small cell glioblastomas may create a resemblance to ependymoma.

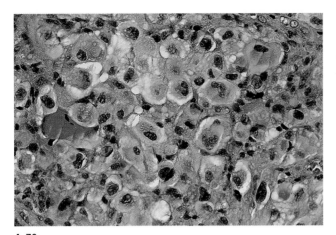

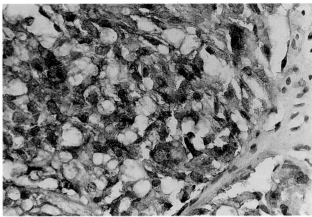

4-70                                                                  4-71

**FIGURES 4-70 AND 4-71**    GLIOBLASTOMA MULTIFORME

Occasionally, epithelioid cells in a glioblastoma may imitate those of metastatic carcinoma (Fig. 4-70). The mimicry is enhanced when the lesion is immunoreactive for epithelial membrane antigen (Fig. 4-71), although the staining is diffusely cytoplasmic rather than linearly membranous, as occurs in truly epithelial neoplasms.

ependymal differentiation, it is our practice to designate these infiltrating neoplasms as glioblastoma. Attention to tumor architecture and neuroimaging is helpful in drawing the distinction. Most high-grade ependymomas are solid, well circumscribed, and devoid of overrun parenchyma.

Of greater practical importance than the exclusion of other malignant gliomas is the distinction of glioblastoma from metastatic carcinoma and primary CNS lymphoma. Aids in the differential diagnosis of *metastatic carcinoma* are the following: (1) the infiltrative properties of most glioblastomas contrast with the discreteness of metastatic deposits; (2) the background of fibrillated glial processes that characterizes glioblastomas differs from the collagenous stroma, cohesive cellularity, and discrete cell borders that characterize most metastatic carcinomas; (3) the pattern of necrosis of gliomas is often random and encircled by pseudopalisading, whereas that of metastatic carcinomas generally spares viable cuffs of tumor tissue in perivascular zones; (4) the microvascular proliferation is exuberant within and about glioblastomas but is usually restrained in metastases and confined to tissue surrounding the alien lesions; and (5) unlike glioblastomas, the cells of metastatic carcinomas are usually larger and more clearly epithelial, with prominent nucleoli as well as frequent mitoses. One glioblastoma variant, the epithelioid lipid-rich subtype, may have focal immunoreactivity for epithelial membrane antigen (EMA), although not in the membranous pattern typical of truly epithelial neoplasms (Figs. 4-70 and 4-71). The adenoid variant also simulates a carcinoma (Fig. 4-72).

Immunohistochemistry for EMA and cytokeratins can be helpful, although some antisera, particularly AE1-AE3, show significant staining of astrocytes. On occasion, the reaction is even more impressive than that for GFAP. Thus, interpretation of stains for cytokeratins should be done in conjunction with the results of antibodies to EMA and GFAP.

*Primary* or *secondary malignant lymphomas* may appear to the neurosurgeon as infiltrative masses resembling glioblastomas. Radiographically, however, primary CNS lymphoma, because it occurs sporadically, should be a strong suspect, given its homogeneous pattern of enhancement (i.e., one without dark, nonenhancing areas). The most helpful diagnostic characteristic of lymphoma in H&E-stained sections is the perivascular and intramural accumulation of neoplastic cells, a pattern highlighted by a reticulin stain (see Table 2-2, p. 80 for other uses of this enduring diagnostic method). The percolation of isolated lymphoma cells within brain parenchyma may pose a problem, but the distinction from glial cells is readily made by (1) attention to cytologic features such as large vesicular nuclei, indented membranes, and prominent nucleoli; and (2) immunostaining for leukocyte common antigen (CD45) and with markers for specific lymphoid subsets.

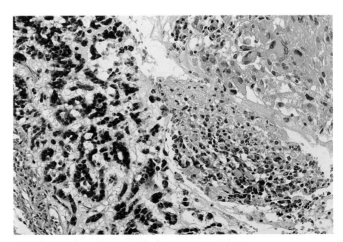

**FIGURE 4-72**    GLIOBLASTOMA MULTIFORME

An adenoid pattern in some glioblastomas, particularly in gliosarcomas, can be confused with metastatic carcinoma. In this tumor, neoplastic tissue that is obviously glial is present on the right.

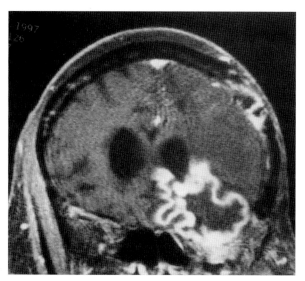

**FIGURE 4–73    RADIATION NECROSIS SIMULATING GLIOBLASTOMA**

Glioblastoma multiforme was suspected in this expansile, contrast-enhancing lesion that arose in the left temporal lobe of a 56-year-old man. An ipsilateral mandibular ameloblastoma had been irradiated 15 months earlier.

A final differential diagnostic consideration is *radionecrosis,* which occasionally follows radiotherapy for a neoplasm of the head or neck (Fig. 4–73). This usually occurs when total doses exceed 50 Gy, after an interval of 1 year or more. The edema-producing, contrast-enhancing mass closely simulates glioblastoma, although the rim of enhancement is often thinner, more isometric, and more aligned to the gray-white junction than it is in malignant glioma. Histologically, radionecrosis is a curious form of coagulation necrosis that favors the white matter, although it may focally creep into the deeper cortical laminae. The cellularity around the edge

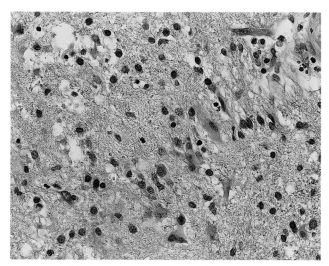

**FIGURE 4–74    GLIOSIS ASSOCIATED WITH RADIONECROSIS**

Reactive gliosis, sometimes with radiation-induced atypia, should not be misinterpreted as an astrocytic neoplasm.

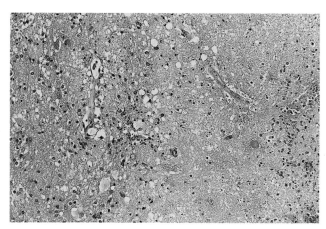

**FIGURE 4–75    RADIONECROSIS**

Radionecrosis is a granular coagulative lesion with few, if any, macrophages. Both parenchyma and vasculature are affected.

is not that of glioblastoma, but when combined with a degree of cytologic atypia, it can simulate that of glioma (Fig. 4–74). Distinguishing features of radionecrosis include its distinctive mosaic of confluent coagulative necrosis unaccompanied by peripheral pseudopalisading (Fig. 4–75), as well as microcalcifications, particularly in subcortical white matter. Unlike the proliferative vascular changes that typify glioblastoma, those associated with radionecrosis are largely degenerative or dystrophic in nature. They feature fibrinoid necrosis (Fig. 4–76), telangiectases, and hyaline thickening of vessels. True vasoproliferative changes are uncommon. Table 4–6, p. 188 compares the histologic features of necrosis in CNS lesions.

## Diagnostic Checklist

- Have you ruled out a reactive condition such as cerebral infarct and demyelinating disease?
- Have you excluded the possibility that the tumor is well differentiated, for example, pleomorphic xanthoastrocytoma or pilocytic astrocytoma?

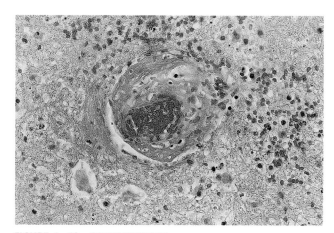

**FIGURE 4–76    RADIONECROSIS**

Fibrinoid necrosis of blood vessels is a common feature of radionecrosis.

- Have you excluded the possibility that the "glioblastoma" is not a malignant astrocytic neoplasm, such as pleomorphic xanthoastrocytoma?
- Have carcinoma and lymphoma been considered?

**Treatment and Prognosis.** The intrinsic malignancy of glioblastoma is appreciated best by considering the median postoperative survival—a brief 14 weeks in cases in which therapeutic efforts are limited to surgery and supportive care.[21, 143] Although radiation therapy may extend survival to 2 years in some cases, there has been little progress in prolonging survival beyond this point in all but a very small number of patients. In one series, only 22 (5%) of 449 patients had survived 5 years after diagnosis.[25] Chemotherapy, either alone or in combination with radiotherapy, has not greatly improved the outlook. Thus, despite many clinical trials of new and old agents, the general outlook is essentially what it was more than 2 decades ago. Cure, although accomplished from time to time, is at this point an unrealistic expectation.

As with any rule, there are always exceptions in the form of individuals who become long-term survivors.[125] Thus far, molecular studies have failed to identify anything unique about the tumors in these fortunate few.[85] Factors associated with prolongation of life include young patient age,[20, 147] long duration of preoperative symptoms, favorable neurologic status at diagnosis, and presence of a better-differentiated component.[125] Among these prognostically favorable features, the age of the patient is by far the most significant.

Although it is difficult to establish a cause-and-effect relationship, the extent of resection also appears to influence survival.[3, 22, 35, 56, 147, 148] The giant cell variant has been viewed as conferring a somewhat better prognosis,[21, 62] although recent studies have cast doubts about even this small glimmer of favoritism.[53]

Whether there is any prognostic significance to the primary versus secondary designation is unclear. The history of a prior low-grade astrocytoma both has[147] and has not[33] been associated with a somewhat better outlook.

Seeding of glioblastoma within the cerebrospinal pathways, although an unusual event, is well documented.[43, 48, 99, 124, 137] Direct extension into pericranial structures is also uncommon.[50, 126] The lesion sometimes spreads extensively in the subependymal regions. Particularly unusual is tumor emigration to systemic sites such as lung, pleura, lymph nodes, liver, or bone.[103] Such spread usually follows surgical intervention[48, 70, 90, 149] or shunting[93] and may thus be mechanically aided. Only rarely is systemic spread a presenting manifestation.[40] It remains to be seen whether the incidence of systemic metastases will increase when the primary disease is better controlled.

The cause of death in some cases is explained by the local effects of the tumor, but in many instances, it cannot be explained readily, even when the brain is studied post mortem.[19, 55] Progressive neurologic deterioration, unassociated with significant mass effects, is seen in some patients. Expansile masses of tumoral and parenchymal radiation necrosis and edema explain other cases. In many instances, the cause of death is multifactorial.[127]

## Gliosarcoma

**Definition.** A malignant (grade IV) neoplasm with both glial and phenotypically mesenchymal components.

**General Comments.** Despite initial acceptance of the mixed tumor concept as applied to gliosarcoma, recent studies have shown that both glial and mesenchymal components share cytogenetic abnormalities[3] or an identical p53 mutation.[2] This evidence of clonality suggests that the "sarcoma" is only an expression of metaplasia within the glioma, not an independent neoplasm. This observation, and the fact that the prognosis of gliosarcoma is the same as that of glioblastoma, makes the identification of gliosarcoma less of an issue than it was in the past. Nevertheless, gliosarcomas' distinctive and often confusing histologic features justify a separate discussion.

In most glioblastomas, the mesenchymal tissue represents a conventional desmoplastic reaction, usually in the presence of meningeal invasion. However, an occasional glioma exhibits a mesenchymal component that has all the histologic attributes of a distinct neoplasm. Admittedly, there are many tumors in which mesenchymal tissue is difficult to assign to either the reactive or the neoplastic category. The "mesenchymal" component of gliosarcomas varies in nature from case to case, as discussed later, and may not be limited to fibrous tissue. Nonetheless, it has been suggested that, even by histologic criteria, there is no such entity as gliosarcoma distinct from glioblastoma—only glioblastomas with varying degrees of desmoplasia.[6]

**Macroscopic Features.** At least in part, gliosarcomas are firm and discrete and thus often appear to the surgeon as a metastatic tumor or, when superficial, a meningioma (Fig. 4–77).

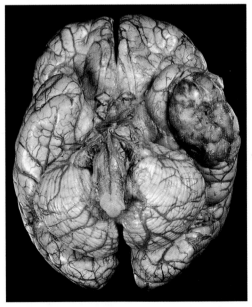

**FIGURE 4–77    GLIOSARCOMA**

This uncommon variant of glioblastoma usually forms a well-circumscribed mass. The temporal lobe is most often affected.

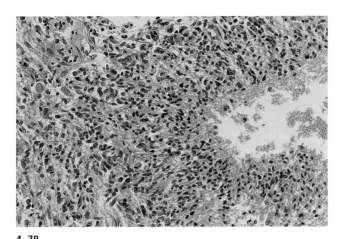

4–78

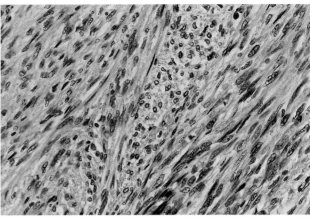

4–79

**FIGURES 4–78 AND 4–79    GLIOSARCOMA**

The infiltrating component of gliosarcomas is almost always a conventional glioblastoma, seen here as pleomorphic cells with glial processes in association with necrosis with peripheral palisading (Fig. 4–78). The sarcomatous component resembles fibrosarcoma, with woven fascicles of spindle-shaped cells (Fig. 4–79).

**Microscopic Features.** The morphologic spectrum of gliosarcomas varies widely in accord with the ratio of gliomatous (Fig. 4–78) and "sarcomatous" (Fig. 4–79) components. In some instances, the latter streams through the glioma like chocolate in a marble cake (Fig. 4–80); in others, it is focal and more segregated from the glial element. In most cases, the mesenchymal component resembles typical fibrosarcoma, with a prominent network of intercellular reticulin (Fig. 4–81). Alternatively, it may be less organized and exhibit the degree of pleomorphism seen in malignant fibrous histiocytoma. In some instances, the distinction between glial and mesenchymal components requires immunohistochemistry. In any variant, there usually is a florid microvascular proliferation, with vessels generating laminae of spindle-shaped cells. Where reactivity ends and neoplasia begins is often difficult to determine.

Cartilaginous,[5, 11] angiosarcomatous,[13] and rhabdomyosarcomatous[1] components have been described. Foci of adenoid and squamous differentiation raise the issue of metastatic carcinoma.[7, 10]

**Immunohistochemical Features.** GFAP is present in the gliomatous component (Fig. 4–82). Although it is generally absent in the sarcomatous element,[8, 12] isolated GFAP-positive spindle cells may be seen in some tumors (Fig. 4–83). The mesenchymal cells generally do not stain for CD34,[14] although some react with antibodies to actin.[4, 6, 12]

**Differential Diagnosis.** If one accepts the interpretation of the molecular evidence concerning clonality described earlier, the distinction between gliosarcoma and glioblastoma no longer exists. There remains, however, the obligation to identify the presence of a glial component to distinguish the lesion from other spindle cell

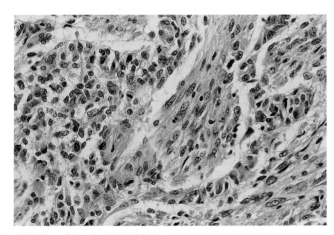

**FIGURE 4–80    GLIOSARCOMA**

The glial and "sarcomatous" elements of gliosarcomas are often intimately intermixed. At low magnification, ribbons of disordered glial cells crowd the interstices of the fibrosarcoma-like component.

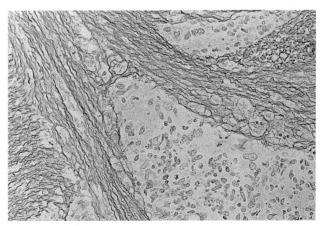

**FIGURE 4–81    GLIOSARCOMA**

Reticulin is abundant in sarcomas and scant in gliomas.

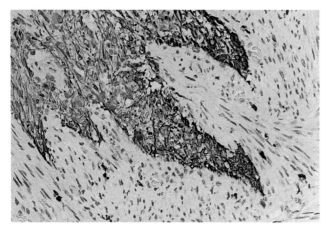

**FIGURE 4–82   GLIOSARCOMA**

Islands of glial tissue are marked by immunohistochemistry for glial fibrillary acidic protein.

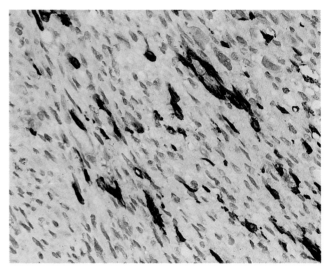

**FIGURE 4–83   GLIOSARCOMA**

Scattered spindle-shaped, sarcoma-appearing cells are often immunoreactive for glial fibrillary acidic protein.

entities such as *malignant meningioma* and pure *fibrosarcoma*. Immunohistochemistry for GFAP is ideally suited for this task. In a very young patient, *desmoplastic infantile ganglioglioma* must be excluded, using the guidelines discussed on page 270.

**Treatment and Prognosis.** Gliosarcomas are neither more nor less aggressive than glioblastoma.[9, 12]

### Granular Cell Astrocytoma of the Cerebrum

**Definition.** An infiltrating astrocytoma with prominent granular cytoplasm due to lysosome accumulation.

**General Comments.** Rare infiltrating neoplasms formed of coarsely discrete, granulated cells have been termed "granular cell tumors." These lesions must be distinguished from the discrete infundibular lesions discussed in Chapter 9. Although the nature of the granular cells in infiltrating granular cell neoplasms was once debated, there is now little question that they are composed of astrocytes with abundant autophagocytic vacuoles. Their identity is inferred from the transition zones in some cases between granulated areas and conventional astrocytoma, immunohistochemical reactions for GFAP, and the ultrastructural demonstration of intermediate filaments. Usually of high grade, such tumors are best considered as granular cell variants of diffuse astrocytomas. In light of their distinctive appearance, these tumors are separately discussed here.

**Clinical Features.** Because these tumors occur during the fifth through eighth decades of life, the patients generally fall into the same age group as those with infiltrating astrocytomas of grades III and IV. Symptoms of mass effect generally predominate.[1–3, 6]

**Radiologic Features.** As in the case of high-grade fibrillary astrocytomas, contrast enhancement and edema are the rule (Fig. 4–84).[1, 3, 6]

**Microscopic Features.** Infiltrative, often mitotically active, and sometimes necrotic, these lesions consist to a variable extent of cells with coarse granules (Figs. 4–85 and 4–86). Lipidized cells may be present as well. In some instances, only sheets of granular cells are present; in others, such cells blend and merge with those of classic fibrillary astrocytoma, usually of high grade. Granules often distend the cytoplasm and displace the nucleus peripherally. Although the discrete borders of the cells and their granular cytoplasm create a macrophage-like appearance, the cells of granular cell tumors are somewhat larger, and their nuclei are often atypical. A nested architecture may be present. As expected of lysosomes, the granules are variably periodic acid–Schiff (PAS) positive (Fig. 4–87). Reticulin deposition may be a prominent feature.[3]

**Cytologic Features.** The granules are well seen, as are cell processes, in accord with the lesion's astrocytic derivation (Fig. 4–88).

**Immunohistochemical Features.** Whereas the central portion of the granule-filled cytoplasm is weakly GFAP positive at best, the periphery may be strongly stained (Fig. 4–89).[1–4] Macrophage markers such as HAM-56, MAC-386, and CD68 are variably positive, but this does not indicate a derivation from macrophages.[3, 6]

**Ultrastructural Features.** Membrane bound, the granules are filled with the heterogeneous, amorphous to lamellar, electron-dense material expected of lysosomes and autophagosomes.[1, 2, 4, 5] In some instances, bundles of intermediate (glial) filaments course among the granules.

**Differential Diagnosis.** Because granulated astrocytes look very much like macrophages, and because macrophages may be present in some high-grade astrocytomas, reactive lesions enter into the differential diagnosis. These include *demyelinating disease* and *infarct*. Transitions to conventional fibrillary astrocytoma must

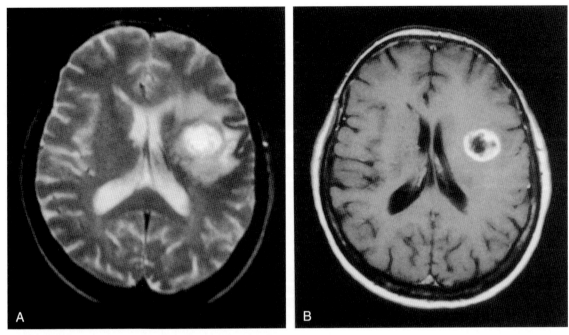

**FIGURE 4–84**   GRANULAR CELL ASTROCYTOMA OF THE CEREBRUM

This malignant lesion is commonly edema generating (A) and contrast enhancing (B).

be sought, and the nature of the cells should be confirmed by immunohistochemistry. Granular neoplastic astrocytes are GFAP positive, but this may be only focal and often occurs in only a subplasmalemmal band of reactivity.

### Diagnostic Checklist

- Have you excluded a macrophage-rich non-neoplastic lesion such as infarct or demyelinating disease?

**Treatment and Prognosis.**  Despite radiotherapy, granular cell astrocytomas recur or progress in the time frame expected of a lesion that is, in essence, a high-

grade astrocytoma.[1, 3] Most of the few reported patients were dead within 2 years.

### Gliomatosis Cerebri

**Definition.**  A diffusely infiltrating glioma, involving two or more contiguous cerebral lobes or anatomic compartments.

**General Comments.**  Gliomatosis cerebri is an entity that is difficult to define, because its recognition depends heavily on both histologic and radiologic features, neither of which is specific. Involvement of at least two contiguous lobes is a reasonable requirement. Many

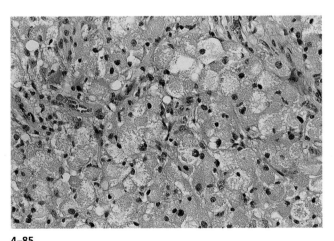

4–85                              4–86

**FIGURES 4–85 AND 4–86**   GRANULAR CELL ASTROCYTOMA OF THE CEREBRUM

Cells with faint granules and distinct cytoplasmic borders constitute this aggressive lesion.

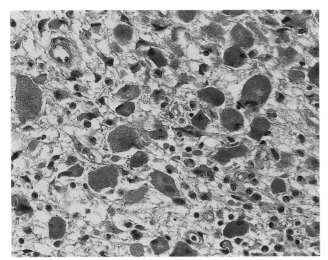

**FIGURE 4–87    GRANULAR CELL ASTROCYTOMA OF THE CEREBRUM**

The cells are periodic acid–Schiff positive.

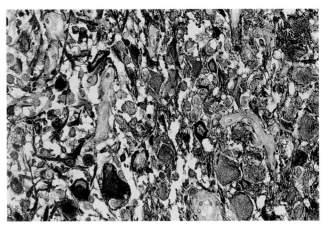

**FIGURE 4–89    GRANULAR CELL ASTROCYTOMA OF THE CEREBRUM**

The cells are immunopositive for glial fibrillary acidic protein, particularly in areas of transition between granular cell tumor and conventional diffuse astrocytoma.

examples of gliomatosis are bilateral or multicompartmental. Spanning of the corpus callosum is common but does not, in itself, warrant the designation "gliomatosis." Necrosis may supervene during the process of tumor progression, but it is not a component of the initial lesion. Although the typically astrocytic neoplasm is often grade III in the WHO system, some are cytologically bland and behave like grade II lesions. Some are extremely indolent.

**Clinical Features.** Given the diffuse nature of the lesion, it is not surprising that nonlocalizing deficits such

as alterations in behavior and mentation are frequent clinical expressions. Seizures, headaches, and multifocal neurologic deficits are also apparent in some cases.[9]

**Radiologic Features.** Although extensive T2- or FLAIR-bright regions are the essential neuroimaging findings, there is considerable variation in the localization of these changes. Some lesions pervade the white matter of one entire cerebral hemisphere, others infiltrate bilaterally (Fig. 4–90), and still others center on the basal ganglia and thalamus.[5, 6] Cortical gray matter may be expanded in others. Mass effects may be subtle.[11] At presentation, contrast enhancement is not a property of classic gliomatosis, but it can appear later as a correlate of malignant progression.[11]

**Macroscopic Features.** Although gliomatosis may result in diffuse enlargement of the affected structures, macroscopic findings may be little more than a subtle suggestion of white matter edema, with blurring of the gray-white junction.

**Microscopic Features.** The "typical" lesion is an infiltrating glioma characterized by monomorphic, often elongated, tumor cells that diffuse freely through the brain parenchyma (Figs. 4–91 and 4–92).[1, 6, 7, 10, 12, 13] In some cases, the presence of a neoplastic infiltrate is obvious. When cellularity is low, however, a diagnosis may not be possible, in spite of an impressive area of T2 abnormality and insistence by the surgeon that a glioma must be present. In many cases, the neoplastic cells appear undifferentiated, because a relative lack of cytoplasm renders the nuclei "naked." In other instances, there may be just the slightest cytoplasmic differentiation. Most examples of gliomatosis are considered astrocytic, but occasional lesions exhibit oligodendrogliomatous features.[2]

As the neoplastic cells in gliomatosis permeate the cerebral cortex, they are arrested in their movement by natural barriers such as the subpial zones, perineuronal

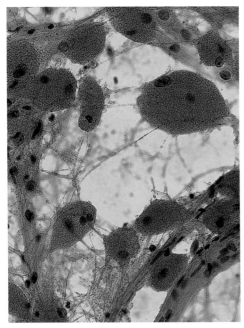

**FIGURE 4–88    GRANULAR CELL ASTROCYTOMA OF THE CEREBRUM—SMEAR PREPARATION**

Cytoplasmic processes help confirm the glial nature of the granular cells, which in tissue sections resemble macrophages.

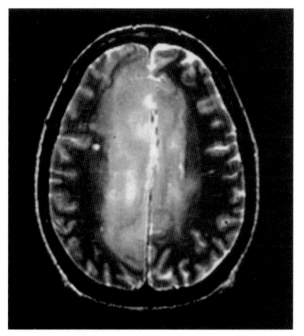
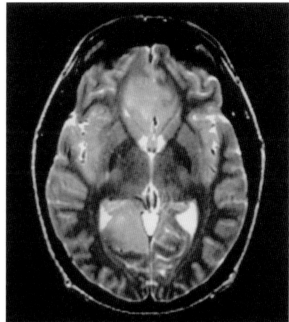

**FIGURE 4–90    GLIOMATOSIS CEREBRI**

Bilateralism is not uncommon in gliomatosis. All lobes were involved in this 25-year-old man with a recent history of seizures.

regions, and perivascular domains. Because similar "secondary structures," or concentrations of cells, can be seen in other infiltrating gliomas, such as fibrillary astrocytomas and oligodendrogliomas, they aid in the diagnosis of tumor but are not specific for gliomatosis.

A frequent but not universal feature of gliomatosis, particularly at the margins of infiltration, is the elongation of neoplastic nuclei, sometimes to the same degree as in microglial "rod" cells. This accounts for the original misnomer "microgliomatosis" for some lesions that today would be considered gliomatosis. This nuclear feature is characteristic of gliomatosis and may serve as a point of distinction from glioblastoma; the cells of the latter are

generally incapable of assuming this degree of polarized slenderness, even when squeezed between the most compact fiber tracts.

**Grading.** Gliomatosis is difficult to grade. Given the often low cellularity of these tumors, mitoses are understandably sparse. Because microvascular proliferation and necrosis are late to develop and are seen only in some cases, one generally assigns the designation of grade II or III. Even this issue may be difficult to resolve, unless one accepts a solitary, hard-won mitosis as evidence of a grade III lesion. Calculating a meaningful MIB-1 (Ki-67) labeling index also poses a problem. In

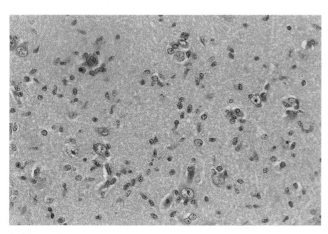
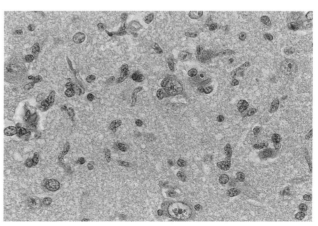

4–91                                                            4–92

**FIGURES 4–91 AND 4–92    GLIOMATOSIS CEREBRI**

Low and high magnifications illustrate the minimal degree of cellularity and cytologic atypia that characterizes many cases of gliomatosis. Other examples exhibit more cytologic atypia.

one study of 16 patients, it ranged from zero to 7.5%.[9] Obviously, it would be higher in the presence of anaplastic transformation. However, very high levels should generate concern that the tissue was taken from the edge of a glioblastoma. Correlation with radiologic features may help distinguish this tumor from the far less common and generally more widespread gliomatosis.

**Features in Needle Biopsy Specimens.** The difficult combination of a small specimen and a low cell density means that only a few neoplastic cells will be seen. One must look carefully for subtle cytologic clues or the finding of vague secondary structure formation. Paucity of cells also frustrates the assessment of smear preparations.

**Cytologic Features.** In well-differentiated examples, small cells with bland nuclei sit in a finely fibrillar background (Fig. 4–93).

**Immunohistochemical Features.** Immunoreactivity of the neoplastic cells for GFAP is occasionally noted, but the small infiltrating cells are usually negative for all antibodies except S-100 protein.

**Ultrastructural Features.** The largely undifferentiated nature of the cells is readily apparent at the ultrastructural level.[3]

**Differential Diagnosis.** The initial issue is to distinguish gliomatosis from *normal brain* and *reactive gliosis* and then to exclude other infiltrative gliomas. The H&E features of gliomatosis may be so minimal as to preclude a diagnosis (Fig. 4–94). Scattered MIB-1–positive cells

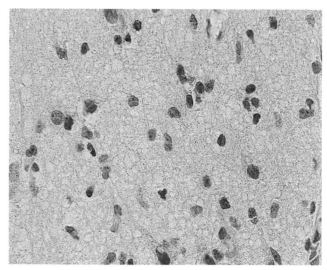

**FIGURE 4–94    GLIOMATOSIS CEREBRI**

Tissue from the lesion in Figure 4–90 illustrates the marginal increase in cellularity seen in many cases of gliomatosis.

may be seen, raising the index of suspicion, but these alone are not necessarily diagnostic of a neoplasm. Pressure will no doubt be exerted by the surgeon if the neurologic and imaging findings are substantial but the pathology report is negative or noncommittal. Although such a clinicoradiologic scenario leaves few diagnostic options other than infiltrating glioma, the pathologist should confirm the diagnosis on the basis of histology alone. The reader is referred to pages 174 to 175 for a discussion of the differential between astrocytoma and gliosis.

The exclusion of gliomatosis from *fibrillary astrocytomas of grade II, III, or IV* hinges in large part on restricted definitions in which radiologic parameters play an important role. Although gliomatosis may be suspected when seemingly unrestrained percolation of cells produces a very diffuse lesion, there are no specific histologic criteria for the diagnosis. In other words, the diagnosis is made only in conjunction with supportive radiographic findings. Thus, if at presentation a "gliomatosis" histologic pattern occurs in conjunction with ring enhancement, the tumor is almost certainly a glioblastoma.

True *microgliomatosis*, a very rare entity, is a diffusely infiltrative process comprising markedly elongated rod cells that are immunohistochemically reactive for macrophage markers.[8] This lesion is discussed on page 324.

### Diagnostic Checklist

- Is this "gliomatosis" really nothing more than gliosis?
- Is only a slight increase in cellularity insufficient for a specific diagnosis?
- Is this highly infiltrative lesion actually gliomatosis or just the infiltrative edge of a glioblastoma?

**Treatment and Prognosis.** The duration of life from first symptom to death has been variable, ranging from

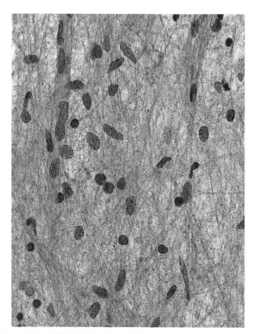

**FIGURE 4–93    GLIOMATOSIS CEREBRI—SMEAR PREPARATION**

Smear preparations illustrate both the cytologic blandness and the fine cytoplasmic processes of gliomatosis in its common form.

weeks to decades.[4, 9] Because almost all cases have been diagnosed post mortem, there is little evidence regarding the benefits of adjuvant therapy. Nonetheless, small series suggest efficacy.[4] In one small study, the MIB-1 index was prognostically significant on univariate analysis.[9] In a small series limited to six cases, median survival was 9 months, and 1-year survival was 37.5%, when the MIB-1 labeling indices were greater than 1%. No deaths occurred in five cases in which indices were below 1%.[9]

## Protoplasmic Astrocytoma

**Description.** A superficial, extensively microcystic, well-differentiated astrocytoma composed of loosely textured, poorly fibrillated astrocytes.

**General Comments.** Conceptually, the protoplasmic astrocytoma takes its origin from "protoplasmic astrocytes" resident within gray matter. These normal cells are distinguished from the "fibrillary astrocytes" of the white matter by their more lush domain of velvety processes. There is, however, no established identity for the protoplasmic astrocyte, nor is there agreement about the criteria for the derivative neoplasm. There is, however, a subset of superficially situated, monomorphous, extensively microcystic lesions that is sufficiently distinctive to justify a separate description, although not with the assurance that it is a clearly defined clinicopathologic entity.[1]

**Macroscopic Features.** Protoplasmic astrocytomas generally present as superficial, variably cystic masses.

**Microscopic Features.** The lesion is characterized by cysts, both small and large (Fig. 4–95), that macro- and microscopically appear to represent a continuum. With

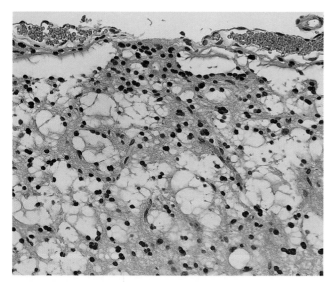

**FIGURE 4–95** PROTOPLASMIC ASTROCYTOMA

Monotonous cells with cobweb-like, poorly fibrillated processes, as well as microcysts, are key features of protoplasmic astrocytomas. This lesion's resemblance to oligodendrogliomas, the spongy component of pilocytic astrocytomas, and occasional tumors with transitional features makes the diagnosis of protoplasmic astrocytoma a tenuous one.

confluence, they form macroscopic fluid-filled spaces and, on occasion, a large solitary cavity. The neoplastic cells have round to oval nuclei, not notably distinctive from other members of the astrocytic family, but the appearance of their cytoplasm is distinctive. Its extension into short, faltering processes is responsible for the tumor's loose texture.

**Treatment and Prognosis.** Because of the difficulties in defining the lesion, it is problematic to describe its clinical course, but total excision appears to be beneficial for patients with this relatively well-circumscribed and slowly growing lesion.[1]

## Localized Astrocytic Neoplasms

### Pilocytic Astrocytoma

**Definition.** A generally well-circumscribed, often cystic astrocytoma composed of variable proportions of loose and compact tissue. It is WHO grade I.

**General Comments.** The descriptor "pilocytic" refers to the frequent presence within these tumors of hair-like cells with long, bipolar processes best seen in cytologic preparations. The origin of these lesions is unclear, but a reasonable candidate is a bipolar astrocyte prone to produce Rosenthal fibers. Although inconspicuous in the normal CNS, such a cell becomes evident in long-standing gliosis induced by lesions such as craniopharyngioma, pineal cyst, hemangioblastoma, and intramedullary (spinal) lesions (see Figs. 4–27 and 11–78, page 557).

Depending on their anatomic site and macroscopic appearance, pilocytic astrocytomas have a number of pseudonyms, including "optic nerve glioma," "hypothalamic glioma," "cerebellar astrocytoma," "exophytic" or "discrete brain stem glioma," and "cystic astrocytoma." All refer to the same entity, but the terms invite confusion with diffuse astrocytoma grade II and certain other low-grade gliomas. Thus, use of these designations is discouraged.[4]

**Clinical Features.** Pilocytic astrocytomas typically present in the first 2 decades of life; only the inevitable exception occurs later, usually in the cerebral hemispheres or cerebellum. NF1 predisposes to the development of pilocytic astrocytomas at any site, especially in the optic nerve. What follows are brief descriptions of the clinical features of this tumor at various locations.

*Intraorbital optic nerve* (Fig. 4–96): Although visual loss is common in pilocytic astrocytomas of the optic nerve, the deficit often goes unreported by very young patients, who accept the insidious decrement without notice or complaint. Large examples produce proptosis. "Optic nerve gliomas" arising in the setting of NF1 are often bilateral.[29]

*Hypothalamus and adjacent visual pathways (intracranial optic nerves, optic chiasm, and optic tracts)* (Fig. 4–97): These lesions usually impair vision, but their proximity to the hypothalamus and pituitary gland add signs and symptoms of hypothalamic and pituitary dysfunction in some cases.[38] Obstruction of cerebrospinal fluid (CSF) flow, with resultant hydrocephalus, complicates large lesions.

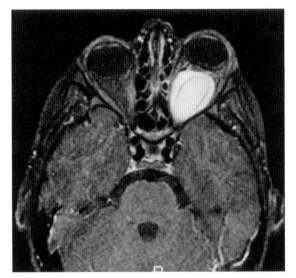

**FIGURE 4–96**    PILOCYTIC ASTROCYTOMA OF THE OPTIC NERVE

Pilocytic astrocytomas of the optic nerve (optic nerve gliomas) have a distinctive profile on magnetic resonance imaging scans. As visualized in a contrast-enhanced image, a central enlarged nerve is delineated by a thin nonenhancing lamina and a peripheral outer region that corresponds to the tumor's extension into the leptomeninges. Visual loss was discovered incidentally in this 4-year-old boy when acuity was tested after a bee sting near the left eye. Proptosis was present. There was no evidence of neurofibromatosis 1.

*Thalamus and basal ganglia:* These lesions encroach on the nearby internal capsule to produce weakness. Large tumors can produce increased intracranial pressure.[31]

*Cerebral hemispheres:* Mass effects, and sometimes seizures, are the presenting features of cerebral lesions.[8, 15, 36]

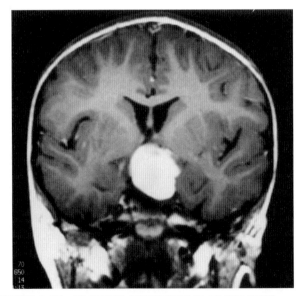

**FIGURE 4–97**    PILOCYTIC ASTROCYTOMA OF THE OPTIC CHIASM AND HYPOTHALAMUS

The suprasellar, hypothalamic region is a common location for pilocytic astrocytomas. This patient was a 23-month-old girl who presented with proptosis as a consequence of a large mass that involved the optic nerve, optic chiasm, and hypothalamus. The tumor, with the histologic features of "pilomyxoid" astrocytoma, enlarged rapidly, severely compromised vision, and required subsequent surgical debulkings.

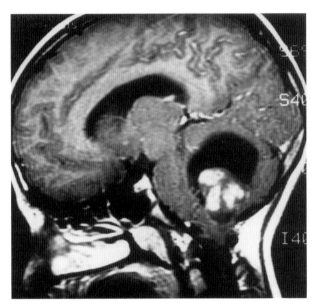

**FIGURE 4–98**    PILOCYTIC ASTROCYTOMA OF THE CEREBELLUM

Pilocytic astrocytomas of the cerebellum are often contrast-enhancing mural nodules in the wall of a cyst. This 8-year-old boy had a 1-month history of headache and a 1-week period of nausea and vomiting.

*Cerebellum* (Fig. 4–98): The classic cerebellar lesion expands into the fourth ventricle and blocks CSF flow. In many cases, such obstruction is accompanied by signs and symptoms of cerebellar dysfunction.[1, 12]

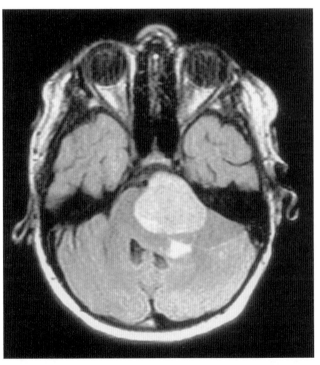

**FIGURE 4–99**    PILOCYTIC ASTROCYTOMA OF THE BRAIN STEM

As in most other sites, pilocytic astrocytomas of the brain stem are discrete, contrast-enhancing masses that displace rather than infiltrate. This lesion produced left-sided arm and leg weakness in a 7-year-old boy. Contrast this largely extrinsic mass with the intrinsic diffuse astrocytoma of the pons illustrated in Figure 4–4.

## TABLE 4–7
## Radiologic Features of "Low-Grade" Brain Tumors

Cystic architecture, especially with mural nodule—pleomorphic
xanthoastrocytoma, pilocytic astrocytoma, ganglion cell tumors, hemangioblastoma, ependymoma (supratentorial)
Superficial location—pleomorphic xanthoastrocytoma, dysembryoplastic neuroepithelial tumor, ganglion cell tumor, oligodendroglioma (small)
Paucity of mass effect—dysembryoplastic neuroepithelial tumor, ganglion cell tumor, pilocytic astrocytoma, subependymal giant cell astrocytoma
Paucity of cerebral edema—dysembryoplastic neuroepithelial
tumor, ganglion cell tumor, pilocytic astrocytoma, pleomorphic xanthoastrocytoma, subependymal giant cell astrocytoma
Skull erosion—dysembryoplastic neuroepithelial tumor, pleomorphic xanthoastrocytoma, oligodendroglioma
Calcification—oligodendroglioma, astrocytoma (diffuse, pilocytic, subependymal giant cell), ganglion cell tumor, neurocytoma, ependymoma

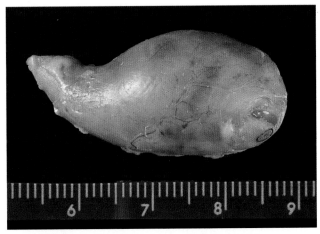

**FIGURE 4–100**    PILOCYTIC ASTROCYTOMA OF THE
OPTIC NERVE

As seen in a surgical specimen resected just posterior to the globe, a
pilocytic astrocytoma produces fusiform enlargement.

*Brain stem* (Fig. 4–99): Pilocytic astrocytomas of
the brain stem are discrete, often exophytic masses that,
in many instances, block CSF flow. The dorsal midbrain
and cerebellopontine angle are common sites. Because
most lesions are superficial in location, signs of brain
stem dysfunction are less common than with intrinsic
diffuse astrocytomas of the pons.[14, 24]

**Radiologic Features.** Discreteness, contrast enhancement, and lack of surrounding cerebral edema are the
cardinal radiologic features of intracranial pilocytic astrocytomas[27] (see Figs. 4–96 to 4–99). A cyst of varying
size is a fourth feature in some cases. This appearance
differs markedly from that of an infiltrating grade II diffuse astrocytoma, which is neither discrete nor contrast
enhancing. Pilocytic astrocytomas do, however, share
many radiologic features with other circumscribed
gliomas such as pleomorphic xanthoastrocytoma, ganglioglioma, ependymoma, and astroblastoma (Table 4–7).

Pilocytic astrocytomas of the optic nerve are also
contrast enhancing, but they are more likely to diffuse
along contiguous neural pathways (e.g., optic nerves,
tracts, and radiations) than are pilocytic lesions in other
sites. Optic nerve tumors are particularly prone to escape the confines of the nerve and grow expansively
within the subarachnoid space. The resultant two
components—enlarged nerve and circumferential leptomeningeal sleeve—are seen well on MRI scans. Although it has been suggested that leptomeningeal extension is a feature limited to tumors associated with
NF1,[45] there are many exceptions (see Fig. 4–96). Leptomeningeal extension characterizes many pilocytic astrocytomas of the cerebellum as well.

Pilocytic astrocytomas of the brain stem are discrete,
enhancing masses that are usually more extrinsic than
intrinsic.[5, 14, 24] Most arise from the medulla or midbrain,
in contrast with most diffuse astrocytomas, which originate in the base of the pons. The few pilocytic tumors
that are intraparenchymal are often cystic. Pilocytic
astrocytomas of the superior or dorsal midbrain are a

distinct subset of the so-called tectal gliomas.[3, 5] Other
tectal astrocytomas are non–contrast enhancing, notably
the circumaqueductal tumors that are more closely related to diffuse astrocytomas.[2, 5, 41]

**Macroscopic Features.** As previously noted, pilocytic
astrocytomas of the optic nerve grow within the cylindric
confines of the optic sheath to produce a fusiform enlargement reminiscent of an egg in a black snake (Figs.
4–100 and 4–101). The cross-sectional anatomy of these
anterior visual pathway tumors recounts a tale so vivid
and distinctive as to be almost pathognomonic—a neoplasm infiltrating and greatly expanding the optic nerve
while transgressing the pia and proliferating beneath the
optic sheath. The result is a megalic optic nerve surrounded by a white corona of neoplastic astrocytes and
reactive mesodermal elements, all wrapped by a dural
envelope (Figs. 4–101 and 4–102).

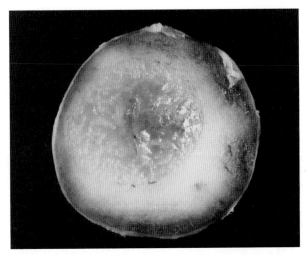

**FIGURE 4–101**    PILOCYTIC ASTROCYTOMA OF THE OPTIC
NERVE

Viewed in cross section, the soft, gelatinous, enlarged nerve is surrounded by the pale extension of the neoplasm in the leptomeninges.

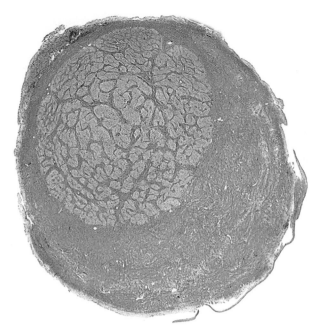

**FIGURE 4–102** PILOCYTIC ASTROCYTOMA OF THE OPTIC NERVE

A whole mount histologic section illustrates a neoplasm that infiltrates and enlarges the septated nerve and expands within the leptomeninges.

Hypothalamic and chiasmal tumors are large, often cystic, soft, and gray. Those in the cerebral hemispheres and cerebellum are discrete masses (Fig. 4–103), associated in many cases with a cyst. Pilocytic astrocytomas of the brain stem are fastened firmly to the surface but are only minimally invasive.

**Microscopic Features.** As one scans classic pilocytic astrocytomas at low magnification, two organizational patterns usually become apparent: loose glial tissue reticulated by extensive cystic change, and dense piloid tissue. Combined in the classic "biphasic pattern," the result is a distinctive and readily recognized neoplasm (Figs. 4–104 and 4–105). The loose tissue features minute vacuoles, microcysts, and even larger spaces filled with eosinophilic fluid (Fig. 4–106). It is easy to believe that these microscopic lacunae coalesce into macroscopic cavities visible to the naked eye. Cytologically, the cells constituting this loose tissue possess round to oval nuclei contained within cytoplasm that radiates into short, webby, afibrillar processes.

The second tissue pattern consists of islands or sheets of compact, elongated cells that are markedly fibrillated and often contain Rosenthal fibers. The latter are discussed later. This compact tissue may be interposed between the microcystic spongy tissue or, less often, is the exclusive element (Figs. 4–107 and 4–108). The nuclei of the bipolar cells usually share the benign appearance of those within stellate cells, but they are often somewhat elongated. Hyperchromasia and "degenerative atypia" are common in long-standing tumors (see the later section on atypia in pilocytic astrocytomas).

Although dramatic and instantly recognizable, the combination of these two patterns in so-called biphasic lesions characterizes only a minority of cases. Thus, it is not essential to the diagnosis. Indeed, if this pattern were required, many pilocytic lesions would be forced artificially into other tumor categories such as diffuse astrocytoma, protoplasmic astrocytoma, or simply the generic low-grade astrocytoma. Though technically correct, the last designation may be misinterpreted by clinicians as a diffuse grade II astrocytoma. The result is a simultaneous misclassification and overgrading.

Eye-catching clusters or ribbons of cells (Fig. 4–109) are occasionally encountered in tumors that are otherwise typical pilocytic astrocytomas. The same is true of organoid and diffusely spongy patterns.

Only a minority of pilocytic astrocytomas are calcified, but those that are can be impressively mineralized.

Ganglion cells are present within some pilocytic astrocytomas, especially those of the cerebellum. In most cases, they are clearly trapped normal neurons—notably, Purkinje's cells or neurons of the dentate nucleus or roof nuclei. In other instances, they are dysmorphic and give every

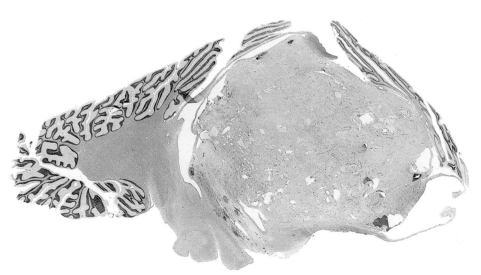

**FIGURE 4–103** PILOCYTIC ASTROCYTOMA OF THE CEREBELLUM

Cerebellar pilocytic astrocytoma is a discrete mass that is often amenable to total excision.

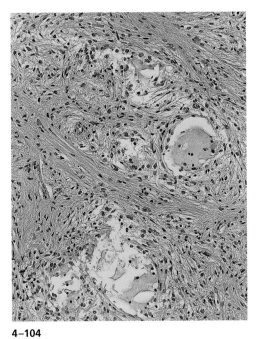

4–104

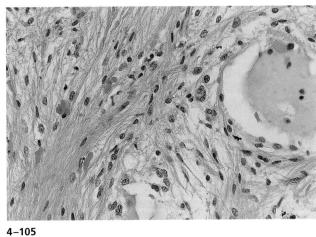

4–105

**FIGURES 4–104 AND 4–105**   PILOCYTIC ASTROCYTOMA

Microcysts intermingled with compact piloid tissue create the classic "biphasic" pattern. Rosenthal fibers are prominent in the compact areas.

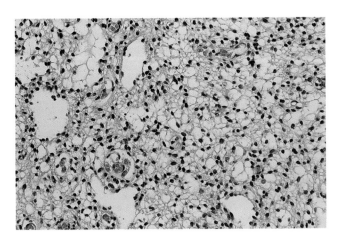

**FIGURE 4–106**   PILOCYTIC ASTROCYTOMA

Some pilocytic astrocytomas are largely or exclusively spongy.

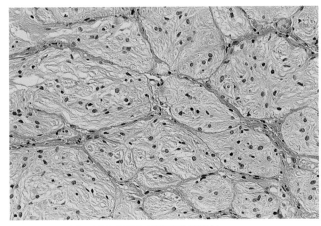

**FIGURE 4–108**   PILOCYTIC ASTROCYTOMA

Dense, nonspongy tissue in pilocytic astrocytomas is sometimes septated.

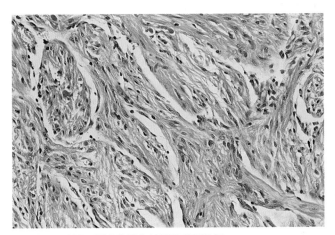

**FIGURE 4–107**   PILOCYTIC ASTROCYTOMA

Piloid tissue assumes many forms, including dense fascicular tissue. Rosenthal fibers are often numerous.

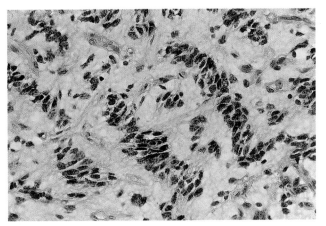

**FIGURE 4–109**   PILOCYTIC ASTROCYTOMA

Distinctive ribbons of cells enliven some pilocytic astrocytomas.

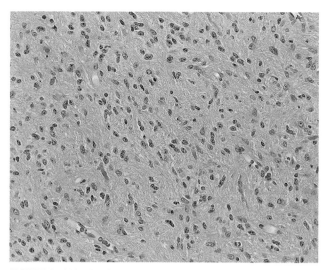

**FIGURE 4–110   PILOCYTIC ASTROCYTOMA**

Although some pilocytic astrocytomas superficially resemble diffuse astrocytomas, they are compact, noninfiltrating, and rich in Rosenthal fibers.

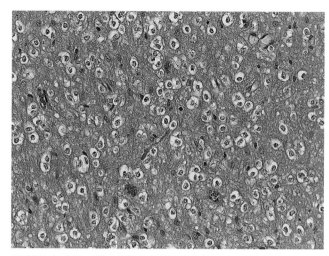

**FIGURE 4–113   PILOCYTIC ASTROCYTOMA**

Pilocytic astrocytomas, especially those of the cerebellum, may closely resemble oligodendrogliomas.

evidence of being part of the neoplasm.[51] Strictly speaking, such tumors warrant a diagnosis of ganglioglioma.

Occasional pilocytic astrocytomas of the cerebellum are somewhat "diffuse" in appearance. Their nuclei are very uniform and extremely bland. Despite a resemblance to infiltrating diffuse astrocytomas, many are relatively solid masses containing little or no trapped brain tissue (Fig. 4–110). Classic features of pilocytic astrocytoma (e.g., microcysts and eosinophilic granular bodies and/or compact spindle cells with Rosenthal fibers) may be found focally,[20] and neither axons nor reactive astrocytes are found in appreciable numbers. Conversely, some cerebellar astrocytomas do appear diffuse and may incorporate axons, as seen with immunostaining for neurofilament protein (Figs. 4–111 and 4–112). Some of

these are cystic lesions that can reasonably be assumed to be pilocytic variants. Other "diffuse" cerebellar gliomas deceptively resemble oligodendrogliomas, sometimes remarkably so. One can usually find typical pilocytic areas, but there are cases that closely resemble oligodendrogliomas (Fig. 4–113). Radiologically, these diffuse neoplasms are usually solid, contrast enhancing, and cyst associated, as would be expected of a pilocytic astrocytoma. Others are nonenhancing but rather well circumscribed. Diffuse astrocytomas affecting the cerebellum are uncommon and are usually high grade.

A histologic pattern often assigned to the pilocytic category conforms to what has been called "pilomyxoid astrocytoma,"[47] or the "infantile" form of pilocytic astrocytoma.[10]

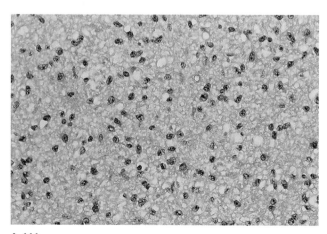

4–111

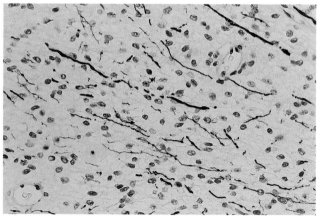

4–112

**FIGURES 4–111 AND 4–112   PILOCYTIC ASTROCYTOMA**

The infiltrating quality of some cerebellar pilocytic astrocytomas is apparent in H&E sections (Fig. 4–111) but is even more obvious with staining with antibodies to neurofilament protein. Tumor cells lie between passing axons (Fig. 4–112). Such lesions simulate "diffuse" astrocytomas but often have features of pilocytic astrocytomas elsewhere in the specimen. In this case, there was extensive extension into the subarachnoid space.

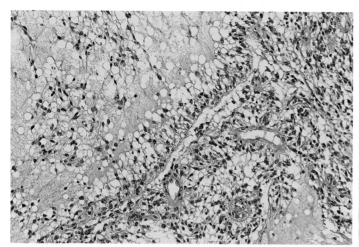

**FIGURE 4–114**   PILOMYXOID/PILOCYTIC ASTROCYTOMA

The pilomyxoid lesion exhibits uniformly small, bipolar cells in a mucinous background. Note the absence of Rosenthal fibers and eosinophilic granular bodies.

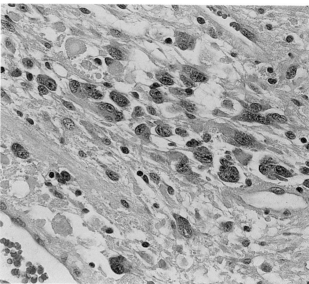

**FIGURE 4–116**   PILOCYTIC ASTROCYTOMA

The presence of nuclear pleomorphism and hyperchromatism alone should not be accepted as evidence of anaplasia. The same is true of an occasional mitotic figure. Note the eosinophilic granular bodies.

Although it is unclear whether this truly represents a pilocytic subtype or a distinct morphologic entity, it is discussed here because of its often piloid features. Most patients with this lesion, or variant, present in the first 2 decades of life with a mass in the frequent sites of conventional pilocytic astrocytomas, particularly the hypothalamus. Occasional examples occur in the cerebellum. The neoplasm is distinctive for its monotonous composition of small, elongated GFAP-positive cells that sit in a mucoid background (Fig. 4–114). The neoplastic cells may orient about vessels to produce an ependymoma-like appearance (Fig. 4–115), but the texture is more mucoid and piloid than ependymal. Mitoses, and even necrosis, may be present. These tumors are more likely to recur locally or seed the CSF spaces than are classic pilocytic astrocytomas.[47]

Although large, hyperchromatic nuclei (Fig. 4–116) or multinucleated cells with nuclei arranged in a "pennies on a plate" fashion sometimes raise concerns about anaplasia, this change is degenerative and of no prognostic significance (Fig. 4–117). If need be, one can find reassurance in their typical clinical evolution, radiographic appearance, hyalinized vessels, and lack of proliferative activity. Lesions with degenerative nuclear atypia most often occur in "older" individuals—those having reached the advanced age of 25 or greater. Other senescent features include vascular hyalinization, hemosiderin deposits, and chronic inflammation. Closely packed sclerotic vessels resembling a cavernous angioma are not uncommon (Fig. 4–118).

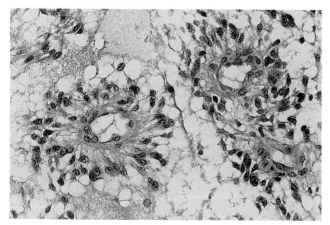

**FIGURE 4–115**   PILOMYXOID/PILOCYTIC ASTROCYTOMA

The radial orientation of tumor cells about vessels produces a resemblance to ependymoma.

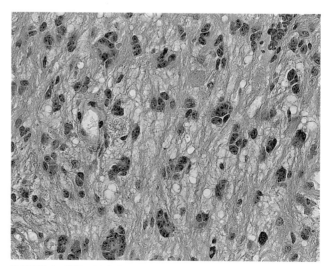

**FIGURE 4–117**   PILOCYTIC ASTROCYTOMA

The presence of multinucleated cells with a "pennies on a plate" configuration is a common "degenerative" change that is usually seen in long-standing pilocytic astrocytomas.

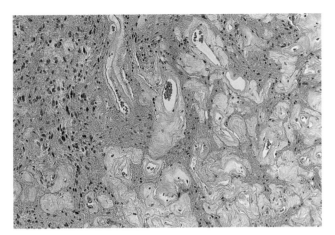

**FIGURE 4–118    PILOCYTIC ASTROCYTOMA**

Aggregates of hyalinized vessels may simulate cavernous angioma.

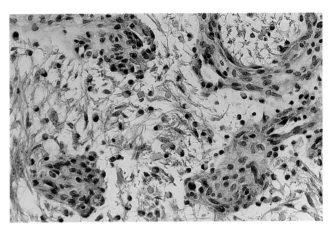

**FIGURE 4–120    PILOCYTIC ASTROCYTOMA**

Glomeruloid microvascular proliferation is common in pilocytic tumors and, as a solitary feature, should not prompt an erroneous diagnosis of high-grade astrocytoma. The second form of microvascular proliferation—hyperplasia of endothelial cells within larger vessels—is rarely seen in pilocytic tumors.

Extension of tumor into the subarachnoid space is a common and diagnostically helpful feature that is particularly prominent in lesions of the optic nerve (see Fig. 4–102) and cerebellum (Fig. 4–119). Counterintuitively, it is not a harbinger of aggressive behavior or leptomeningeal seeding and is, in fact, a common finding in grade I and II gliomas such as ganglion cell tumors and pleomorphic xanthoastrocytomas.

Microvascular proliferation is seen occasionally (Fig. 4–120), but this is more often a feature of the cyst wall, where it forms a subluminal layer of hyperplastic capillaries. Typically glomeruloid in pattern, such a uniform lamina of vascular proliferation is presumptive evidence of a low-grade rather than a high-grade neoplasm. Less common but more troubling is microvascular proliferation of endothelial cells within larger vessels, as is frequent in glioblastomas. Its prognostic significance in pilocytic astrocytomas is discussed later in the section on grading.

Necrosis is seen in up to 8% of pilocytic astrocytomas[17] and is usually infarct-like in a typically paucicellular neoplasm with scant mitotic activity (Fig. 4–121). Clearly defined perinecrotic palisading is rare (see the discussion of grading).

Eosinophilic granular bodies (EGBs) or "protein droplets" are a common feature of pilocytic astrocytomas, as they are in gangliogliomas and pleomorphic xanthoastrocytomas (see Figs. 4–116 and 4–117). These structures are nonspecific but in most instances mark slow-growing, low-grade, prognostically favorable lesions (Table 4–8, p. 211).[22, 23] The structures vary in appearance from aggregates of minute, spherical, eosinophilic droplets to single sizable spheres. Their PAS positivity can be exploited for detection in cases in which EGBs are inconspicuous in H&E-stained sections.

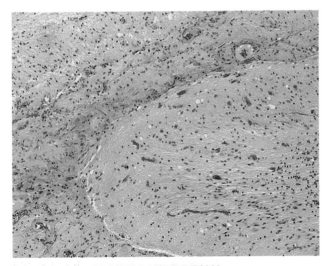

**FIGURE 4–119    PILOCYTIC ASTROCYTOMA**

The common extension of cerebellar pilocytic astrocytomas into the subarachnoid space is not an expression of malignancy.

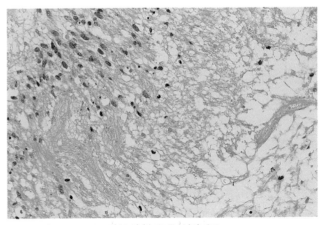

**FIGURE 4–121    PILOCYTIC ASTROCYTOMA**

Zones of necrosis, in some cases with an inflammatory response, may be present in some large pilocytic lesions. These infarct-like areas usually do not elicit pseudopalisading.

**TABLE 4-8**
**Central Nervous System Neoplasms with Eosinophilic Granular Bodies**

Ganglion cell tumor
Pilocytic astrocytoma
Pleomorphic xanthoastrocytoma

Rosenthal fibers are beaded, sausage- to corkscrew-shaped hyaline bodies of varying size (see Figs. 4–105, 4–107, and 4–110). They occur principally in compact areas of pilocytic tumors, where they may be scant to abundant. Though a "signature" feature, they are neither specific nor requisite. Indeed, Rosenthal fibers are a common feature of long-standing "piloid" gliosis, as is discussed on pages 174 and 554. Although Rosenthal fibers are easily seen after H&E staining, they are bright red on Masson trichrome preparations and blue with the Luxol fast blue method.

**Grading.** Fortunately for both patient and pathologist, grading is generally not an issue in pilocytic astrocytomas. With only rare exceptions, these lesions begin and remain grade I. Although the descriptors "atypical" and "malignant" may be applied when worrisome histologic features are encountered, no consensus has been reached regarding the utility of grading or the criteria on which it could be based.

In one small study of cerebellar lesions, "atypical" and "malignant" subtypes were identified, but the designations bore little relation to survival.[48] "Atypical" lesions were defined as those with a low mitotic index but with increased cellularity and/or vascular proliferation. All six patients with such lesions were alive 13 to 24 years after resection. The term "malignant" was applied to four lesions with brisk mitotic activity—that is, one or more mitosis per high power ($\times$ 250) microscopic field; vascular proliferation was common, and necrosis was uniformly present. Of these patients, two succumbed, one was alive without detectable disease at 5 years, and one was lost to follow-up.

A larger study of pilocytic astrocytomas occurring in various anatomic locations found vascular proliferation in 18% and necrosis without pseudopalisading in 8%.[17] There was no relationship between these or other histologic variables and eventual outcome. The mean, median, and range of MIB-1 labeling indices were 1.1, 0.9, and up to 3.9, respectively.[17] Again, no relationship with survival was noted for this variable. Although rare mitoses are seen in up to 30% of pilocytic astrocytomas, MIB-1 labeling indices rarely exceed 10%.[17, 19]

The validity of grading pilocytic astrocytomas by a system in which "high grade" is defined largely in terms of mitotic activity, rather than overt anaplasia, is doubtful. There are, nevertheless, rare lesions that feature high cellularity, brisk mitotic activity, microvascular proliferation, and/or necrosis with pseudopalisading for which the term "malignant" is inescapable (Figs. 4–122 and 4–123). Although such lesions can occur either de novo or in previously irradiated patients, most arise in the latter setting.[34, 44, 48] Such histologically malignant lesions behave in a malignant fashion.

**Features in Frozen Sections.** Unfortunately, this frequently used method may obscure telltale histologic features of pilocytic astrocytomas. Many lesions look less obviously pilocytic and more closely resemble generic

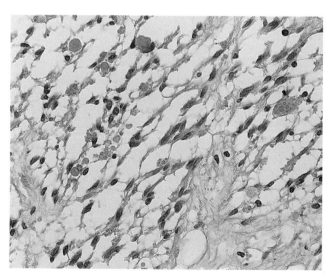
4-122

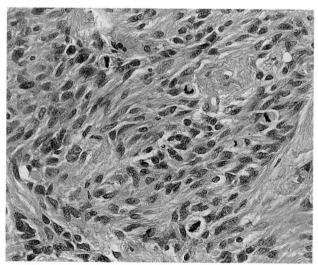
4-123

**FIGURES 4-122 AND 4-123**   PILOCYTIC ASTROCYTOMA WITH MALIGNANT DEGENERATION

It is rare for a pilocytic astrocytoma (Fig. 4–122) to show concomitant anaplastic features. In such exceptions, anaplasia is often expressed as "spindle cells" in a fascicular arrangement (Fig. 4–123). Mitoses are frequent; microvascular proliferation and necrosis with pseudopalisading may be present.

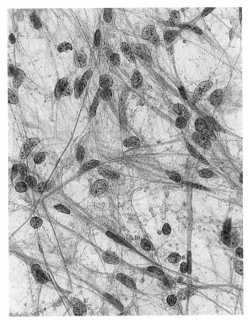

**FIGURE 4–124**   PILOCYTIC ASTROCYTOMA—SMEAR PREPARATION

*The hair-like processes and cytologically bland nuclei of pilocytes are well seen in smear preparations.*

"astrocytomas" in frozen than in permanent sections. Clues to the pilocytic nature of a tumor may be found in the presence of microcysts, although this feature is found in occasional infiltrating astrocytomas and is infrequently present in oligodendrogliomas. Hyalinized vessels are a helpful clue. Rosenthal fibers and EGBs withstand freezing and are additional features. The radiologic images of a rather discrete, contrast-enhancing mass in the face of a "low-grade" astrocytoma should prompt consideration of the diagnosis. Grade II diffuse astrocytomas do not enhance.

**Cytologic Features.**   The cells of pilocytic astrocytomas typically appear elongated and hair-like. This is true not only of compact lesions composed of obviously bipolar cells but also, to some extent, of spongy microcystic lesions in which histologic sections show little cellular elongation. The long, fine processes extend far away from the nuclei, with little change in caliber except around Rosenthal fibers or EGBs (Fig. 4–124). The nuclei are typically oval to elongated, uniform, and notably bland. They may, however, be hyperchromatic and irregular in the face of degenerative atypia, which often includes cytoplasmic pseudoinclusion formation.

**Immunohistochemical Features.**   Pilocytic astrocytomas are strongly GFAP positive in compact fibrillar areas and less so in loose-textured, spongy regions. Rosenthal fibers are negative for GFAP[25] but positive for the lens protein $\beta$-crystallin.[18] EGBs are positive for $\beta$-crystallin, ubiquitin, serine protease inhibitors, $\alpha_1$-antichymotrypsin, and $\alpha_1$-antitrypsin.[23, 33]

The results of immunostaining for the cell cycle marker MIB-1 are described earlier in the section on grading. Investigations using the DNA S-phase marker bromodeoxyuridine and the cell cycling marker MIB-1 suggest that pilocytic astrocytomas are most proliferative in the young.[19, 21] Labeling indices decline thereafter to about the age of 20.[21] As with MIB-1, labeling does not correlate with outcome.

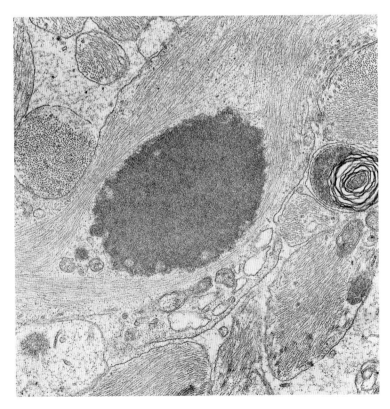

**FIGURE 4–125**   PILOCYTIC ASTROCYTOMA

*Rosenthal fibers are electron-dense, intracellular masses intimately associated with glial filaments.*

Immunohistochemistry for neurofilament protein can be used to assess the degree to which an infiltrative growth pattern is present.

**Ultrastructural Features.** Whether contained in neoplastic or reactive astrocytes, Rosenthal fibers are masses of amorphous, electron-dense material embedded in glial filaments within fibril-rich cell processes (Fig. 4–125).[42] Although similarly situated, EGBs consist of membrane-bound dense bodies.[23, 33] The spongy component carries its microcystic change to the electron microscopic level. Intermediate, "glial" filaments are uncommon.

**Molecular and Cytogenetic Features.** As anticipated from the occurrence of pilocytic astrocytomas in NF1, loss of genetic material has been found in the region 17q11.2.[52] There is little other evidence, however, that the NF1 gene is involved in their pathogenesis.[39] Few consistent cytogenetic abnormalities have been documented, and no molecular "marker" of this lesion is known, as yet. Despite immunoreactivity for p53 protein in some cases,[48] mutations in the p53 gene are very uncommon.[26]

**Differential Diagnosis.** As for almost all brain tumors, the differential diagnosis begins with the exclusion of non-neoplastic conditions (see Table 4–5, p. 173). *Piloid gliosis* is therefore of primary concern, because its densely fibrillar tissue and accompanying Rosenthal fibers closely resemble the compact tissue composition of a pilocytic astrocytoma of the dense variant. Supratentorially, piloid gliosis typically occurs in the hypothalamic region around such lesions as craniopharyngiomas (see Fig. 9–101). The distinction between piloid gliosis and the traditional fibrillary or gemistocytic gliosis is discussed on page 174. In the cerebellum, it can surround any long-standing process, including hemangioblastoma and even pilocytic astrocytoma itself. Piloid gliosis is uncommon in the cerebral cortex, but it appears occasionally in the subpial zone around any number of chronic lesions. No absolute criteria distinguish piloid gliosis from pilocytic astrocytoma, but the reactive process generally lacks a microcystic component, shows little vascular hyalinization and cytologic atypia, and is more likely to contain large numbers of Rosenthal fibers. Piloid gliosis is further discussed on pages 174 and 554.

If gliosis is excluded, the differential diagnosis turns to compact, generally discrete, contrast-enhancing neoplasms that histologically mimic pilocytic astrocytoma. These include ganglioglioma and pleomorphic xanthoastrocytoma. The discreteness and other radiologic features of this important class of CNS tumors are summarized in Table 4–7, p. 205. These are the same neoplasms in which EGBs are common (see Table 4–8, p. 211). The diagnosis of an infiltrating or "diffuse" form of glioma in the setting of certain radiologic features should be a cautionary alert that the diagnosis may be incorrect (Table 4–9).

*Ganglioglioma* is a principal differential entity because, like pilocytic astrocytoma, it is relatively solid and noninfiltrative, is associated with cysts, and often has either compact or microcystic patterns or both. As a result,

---

**TABLE 4–9**
**Scenarios Suggesting that the Proposed Histologic Diagnosis May Be Incorrect**

Grade II diffuse astrocytoma or oligodendroglioma in the face of a contrast-enhancing lesion. Such lesions do not enhance.

Grade II or III diffuse astrocytoma or oligodendroglioma in the face of a solidly ("homogeneously") enhancing mass. Solidly enhancing lesions are usually prognostically favorable tumors, such as the nodular portion of pilocytic astrocytomas, ganglion cell tumors, and pleomorphic xanthoastrocytomas, or malignant cellular tumors, such as primary central nervous system lymphomas or metastatic carcinomas.

Grade III or IV diffuse astrocytoma in the face of a superficial, homogeneously enhancing nodule in the wall of a cyst. This is the image of such well-differentiated lesions as pilocytic astrocytoma, pleomorphic xanthoastrocytoma, and ganglion cell tumor.

Oligodendroglioma for an intraventricular mass at the foramen of Monro. This is the radiologic profile of central neurocytoma.

Oligodendroglioma for an intracortical nodular lesion with skull erosion, particularly in a young adult with a long-standing history of partial complex seizures. These are features of dysembryoplastic neuroepithelial tumor.

Grade II or III diffuse astrocytoma, oligodendroglioma, or mixed glioma for a periventricular or superficial lesion with a "horseshoe" pattern of contrast enhancement. This is the radiologic profile of demyelinating disease.

---

Rosenthal fibers and EGBs are commonly seen. Gangliogliomas with prominent microcystic change can closely simulate pilocytic lesions, and one must search carefully for dysmorphic neurons while remembering that normal overrun ganglion cells may be trapped in the substance of a pilocytic astrocytoma. Although the immunophenotype of ganglion cells facilitates their recognition, dysmorphism continues to be the most reliable diagnostic feature of neoplastic neurons.

Excluding *pleomorphic xanthoastrocytoma* is usually not difficult. Its greater cellularity, exaggerated pleomorphism, partially fascicular architecture, perivascular lymphocytic infiltrates, reticulin deposition, and lack of Rosenthal fibers are distinguishing features. Spongy, microcystic tissue is rare in pleomorphic xanthoastrocytoma.

*Diffuse astrocytomas* of grade II or III are the principal and clinically most important differential diagnosis (Figs. 4–126 and 4–127). As discussed later, grade IV lesions also need to be considered. This conundrum arises when a pilocytic astrocytoma lacks classic features such as compact and microcystic architecture, Rosenthal fibers, and EGBs. Attention to radiologic findings is obviously helpful, especially when faced with a small specimen. Contrast enhancement unassociated with perilesional edema, as well as the presence of a cystic component, strongly suggests a pilocytic rather than a diffusely infiltrating astrocytoma.[7]

Although grade II diffuse astrocytomas are radiologically distinct from pilocytic astrocytomas, histologic similarities create diagnostic dilemmas in some cases. These issues arise most frequently in small specimens of cerebellar lesions, particularly of the "diffuse" form of

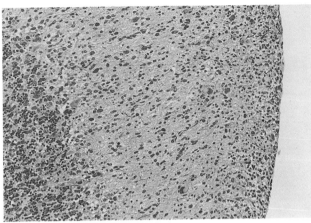

4–126

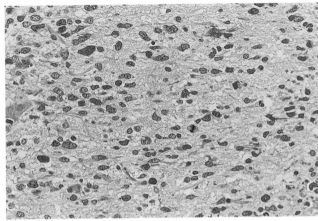

4–127

**FIGURES 4–126 AND 4–127**    FIBRILLARY OR "DIFFUSE" ASTROCYTOMA OF THE CEREBELLUM

Diffuse infiltration and anaplasia distinguish this rare form of cerebellar astrocytoma from the common pilocytic type.

pilocytic astrocytoma. It cannot be overstressed that the diagnosis of pilocytic astrocytoma is largely architectural and that nonrepresentative biopsies invite misdiagnosis. Attention to the radiologic features is useful in identifying a circumscribed, discrete lesion that is unlikely to be a malignant glioma.

Although the solid, relatively noninfiltrative nature of pilocytic astrocytomas is a helpful diagnostic feature, there is still a zone of infiltration. One correlative radiologic-morphologic study found a degree of parenchymal invasion in the majority.[9] Thus, the finding of overrun normal brain elements such as axons, reactive astrocytes, and neurons in peripheral portions of the tumor does not exclude a diagnosis of pilocytic astrocytoma. This is particularly true in the "diffuse" variant that frequents the cerebellum (see Figs. 4–126 and 4–127). In this lesion, the nuclei are evenly distributed, uniform, and cytologically bland, whereas those of diffuse astrocytomas are more pleomorphic and less evenly distributed. EGBs and Rosenthal fibers are typically a focal finding in these unusual pilocytic tumors. As a result, thorough sampling is required. As previously noted, pilocytic astrocytomas occasionally exhibit an oligodendroglial-like component that can be impressive. Again, sampling usually demonstrates a more typical pilocytic component, and a reassuring cyst or mural nodule architecture is present in some cases.

The differential diagnosis between pilocytic astrocytoma with vascular proliferation, and sometimes necrosis, and *glioblastoma* is discussed on page 193.

Last, regimentation of cells in palisades is occasionally seen in pilocytic astrocytomas. This uncommon finding introduces into the differential diagnosis *primitive polar spongioblastoma*, an entity that may or may not exist.[43] Such palisading in pilocytic tumors is generally focal and histologically benign.

### Diagnostic Checklist

- Is this "pilocytic astrocytoma" nothing more than piloid gliosis?
- Is this "pilocytic astrocytoma" a ganglion cell tumor?

**Treatment and Prognosis.** Owing to considerable variation in tumor location, it is difficult to generalize about the optimal treatment of pilocytic astrocytomas. The principal therapy, however, is surgery. The reason for its success in tumor control lies in the discreteness of these lesions, their slow rate of growth, and the stability of residual disease in cases of subtotal resection. In many cases, apparent recurrence is due to expansion of a tumoral cyst rather than proliferation of the residual solid component. Occasional tumors even regress.[28, 46]

Postoperative treatment of residual tumor varies considerably from one institution to another and from case to case. Although symptomatic residual neoplasm occasionally prompts postoperative adjuvant therapy, in our institutions, one or even two recurrences are generally required before radiation, and sometimes chemotherapy, is administered. Other institutions are quicker to use those modalities.

The prognosis of *optic nerve* or *chiasmal pilocytic astrocytoma* depends on a number of variables, including tumor location, extent of resection, patient age, and presence or absence of NF1. Lesions of the optic nerve often go untreated unless the lesion enlarges and threatens to involve the optic chiasm. Many lesions do not enlarge over long periods of observation, especially in the setting of NF1.[29] Some even regress.[37] As expected, patients with high-grade "diffuse" astrocytomas do poorly.[11]

Tumors of the *optic chiasm* and *hypothalamus* often grow slowly but inexorably and can become massive. In some cases, recurrent cysts contribute more to the mass than does regrowth of the solid component.

The prognosis of patients with *cerebellar pilocytic astrocytoma* is excellent, as total excision is possible in most cases.[1, 13] In one series, the 5-, 10-, and 20-year survival rates were 85%, 81%, and 79%, respectively.[20] Complete resection was associated with a 100% 5-year survival rate in another study.[19] Although the numbers were limited, there was a suggestion in the same investigation that patients with "mixed" lesions (i.e., those with classic pilocytic and more diffuse-appearing astrocytomas) did less

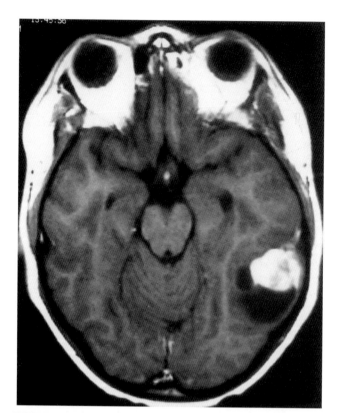

**FIGURE 4–128**  PLEOMORPHIC XANTHOASTROCYTOMA

As in this temporal lobe tumor in a 12-year-old boy with a 3-month history of seizures, pleomorphic xanthoastrocytomas are usually superficial in location and often cystic.

## Pleomorphic Xanthoastrocytoma

**Definition.** A generally superficial, rather circumscribed astrocytic tumor noted for cellular pleomorphism and, in some cases, xanthomatous change. The lesion is usually grade II. The issue of higher-grade examples is discussed below in the section in grading.

**Clinical Features.** Although most pleomorphic xanthoastrocytomas (PXAs) present with seizures during the second decade of life, some remain subclinical until well into adulthood.[5] Precipitous hemorrhage heralds an exceptional case.[12] Multicentricity has manifested rarely after an initial surgery.[6]

**Radiologic Features.** On CT and MRI scans, a PXA classically appears as a discrete, contrast-enhancing mass that, in about half of cases, is a nodule in the wall of a cyst (Fig. 4–128). The temporal lobe is the classic site, but examples have been reported throughout the brain, including the cerebellum[20] and even the retina.[23] Whether a mural nodule or not, the mass is generally superficial and in contact with the leptomeninges; the dura is usually unaffected.[5, 13, 22] As a result of chronic pressure, some superficial PXAs "remodel" or "scallop" the inner table of the skull. Radiologic features of low-grade CNS tumors, many exemplified by PXA, are summarized in Table 4–7, p. 205.

**Macroscopic Features.** The superficial position of many PXAs (Fig. 4–129), with contiguous involvement of the leptomeninges, creates a sharp interface with the underlying brain over at least part of its circumference (Fig. 4–130). Although lipidized cells are generally few, their abundance in some lesions imparts a yellow hue.

**Microscopic Features.** The histologic features of PXA vary, depending on the portion of the tumor submitted

well. Although most tumors are radiologically stable over a long interval, recurrence may be seen after partial resection, sometimes necessitating multiple excisions and occasionally radiotherapy as well.[1, 13, 35] Malignant change is rare.[49]

In both adults and children, *pilocytic astrocytomas of the cerebral hemispheres* are associated with an excellent outlook.[15, 36] In one series, 10-year survival was 100% after gross total or radical subtotal resection; it was 74% for cases in which resection or biopsy was performed.[1] The overall 10-year survival was 95% in one series of pediatric patients.[40]

Although there are few data regarding outcome in cases of *pilocytic astrocytoma of the brain stem*, 5-year survival rates of 80% or more have been reported.[6, 14] At the authors' institutions, multiple reoperations for debulking are generally undertaken before chemotherapy or radiotherapy is used. The outlook is vastly improved over that of the more "diffuse" astrocytoma of the brain stem.[14]

Exceptional tumors that were considered pilocytic astrocytomas have recurred rapidly and seeded the neuraxis.[16, 30, 32, 50] The so-called pilomyxoid astrocytoma, usually situated in the hypothalamus, is overrepresented among such aggressive lesions.[10, 47] On occasion, classic pilocytic astrocytomas also recur quickly or disseminate in cerebrospinal pathways. Surprisingly, despite neuroimaging findings of multiple drop metastases, some patients do well for years with this increased and disseminated tumor burden.[30]

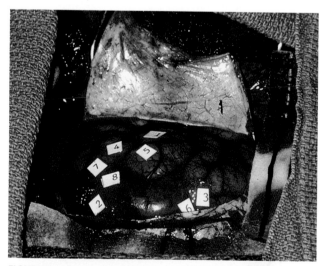

**FIGURE 4–129**  PLEOMORPHIC XANTHOASTROCYTOMA

As is typically the case, the tumor is a superficial, well-defined mass. The patient, a high school football player, was having difficulty kicking as a consequence of the lesion's proximity to the motor cortex. (Courtesy of Dr. Allan H. Friedman, Durham, NC.)

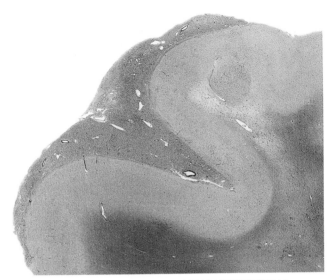

**FIGURE 4–130**    PLEOMORPHIC XANTHOASTROCYTOMA

Although pleomorphic xanthoastrocytomas have an element of parenchymal involvement, much of the mass often expands within the subarachnoid space, creating a sharp border between the leptomeningeal component of the neoplasm and the underlying brain.

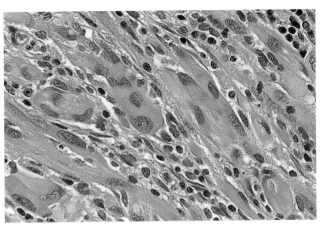

**FIGURE 4–132**    PLEOMORPHIC XANTHOASTROCYTOMA

Although pleomorphism is the hallmark, it is not always extreme.

for study. Superficial components lying on the surface of the brain expand within the subarachnoid space (Figs. 4–131 and 4–132) and extend secondarily into the cerebral cortex along perivascular (Virchow-Robin) spaces. The diagnostically important superficial position may not be obvious initially in small or fragmented specimens but can often be inferred from the presence of large, muscularized arteries within the substance of the lesion. Such vessels occur normally within the subarachnoid space but not the parenchyma of the brain.

The most consistent feature is its compact and largely noninfiltrating architecture, which it shares with other well-differentiated neoplasms that grow slowly and, to a large extent, noninvasively—namely, pilocytic astrocytoma, astroblastoma, and ganglion cell tumors (see Fig. 4–2). The result is a solid tumor mass containing only a minor amount of incorporated brain parenchyma.

In addition to discreteness, several features are of diagnostic utility, although they may be variably present in individual cases. These include (1) a fascicular arrangement of neoplastic cells, often at the periphery of the tumor; (2) pleomorphic astrocytic cells with bizarre cytologic features; (3) lipidization of astrocytes; (4) perivascular lymphocytes; (5) reticulin staining about single or grouped tumor cells; and (6) EGBs.

To some extent, most PXAs create a fascicular pattern that often appears as a rather subtle interweaving of cell bundles (Fig. 4–133) but, on occasion, is so conspicuous and storiform as to mimic the pattern of a fibrohistiocytic neoplasm.

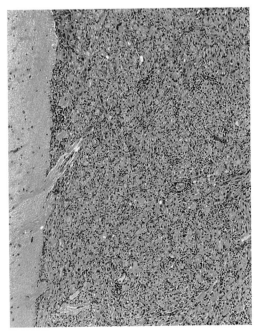

**FIGURE 4–131**    PLEOMORPHIC XANTHOASTROCYTOMA

Characteristically, the tumor is compact, largely leptomeningeal in location, and marked by a mild lymphocytic infiltrate.

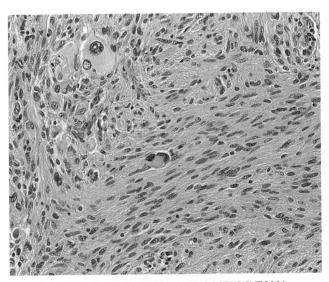

**FIGURE 4–133**    PLEOMORPHIC XANTHOASTROCYTOMA

A fascicular architecture is common in pleomorphic xanthoastrocytomas, particularly at the periphery of the leptomeningeal component.

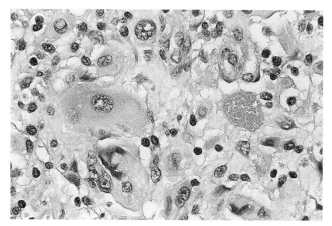

**FIGURE 4–134**    PLEOMORPHIC XANTHOASTROCYTOMA

Most pleomorphic xanthoastrocytomas contain not only large pleomorphic cells but also eosinophilic granular bodies, such as those usually encountered in well-differentiated, macroscopically discrete glial or glioneuronal neoplasms.

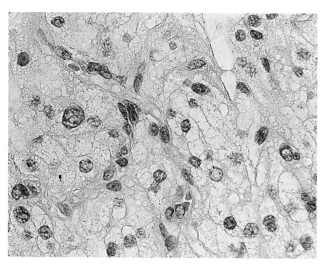

**FIGURE 4–136**    PLEOMORPHIC XANTHOASTROCYTOMA

In spite of the tumor's name, xanthomatous change may be only focal.

Pleomorphic cells are present almost by definition (Fig. 4–134), but they vary in number. Although pleomorphic cells dominate the landscape in some cases, they are inconspicuous in others. They also vary considerably in size and configuration. Large cells with moderate pleomorphism are the rule, and truly monstrous forms are less common. In some cases they simulate the somewhat more polar large cells of malignant fibrous histiocytoma. In the appropriate milieu (i.e., in the absence of mitoses and the presence of abundant reticulin), such cells are actually a comforting diagnostic feature with regard to the biologic behavior of the lesion.

The astrocytic quality of PXA is lent by the glassy and variably fibrillar cytoplasm, GFAP positivity, and the presence in some cases of an infiltrating component resembling that of a diffuse astrocytoma (Fig. 4–135).

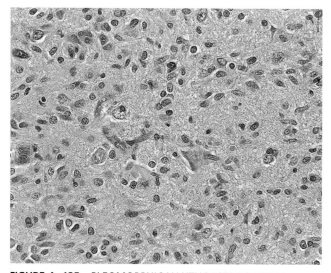

**FIGURE 4–135**    PLEOMORPHIC XANTHOASTROCYTOMA

Taken out of context, cortical infiltration by pleomorphic xanthoastrocytomas may be misinterpreted as evidence of a diffuse, infiltrative form of astrocytoma.

In PXAs, the "X" is generally the least prominent component, the most difficult to confirm, and the least important diagnostically. Whereas lipid may vacuolate the cytoplasm of the larger cells (Fig. 4–136), it is so scant in some instances as to require confirmation by special stains such as oil red O applied to frozen sections.

Lymphocytes are typically present perivascularly, but only loosely so, and they show little hesitation to diffuse into surrounding tumor parenchyma. These T lymphocytes are sometimes accompanied by plasma cells.

Reticulin is usually most abundant around vessels but is generally present in the solid regions of maximal pleomorphism, where it invests individual cells or clusters of cells, at least focally (Fig. 4–137). Reticulin is not always abundant, but the diagnosis should be considered carefully in its absence.

The presence of EGBs is an important diagnostic feature. As is evident in Table 4–8, p. 211, EGBs characteristically frequent discrete, low-grade lesions for which surgical resection is the principal treatment. EGBs are found in most PXAs, and we are hesitant to make the diagnosis in their absence. These are small aggregates of eosinophilic, hyaline material (see Fig. 4–134). Localization of these droplets to the processes of astrocytes is well visualized in smear preparations. The PAS stain facilitates the detection of these sometimes elusive structures (Fig. 4–138). Interestingly, Rosenthal fibers are not a component of PXA, and when present, they are usually situated in the surrounding parenchyma of the brain.

In addition to the pleomorphic, compact, subarachnoid component, PXAs usually have an infiltrative element that may closely resemble diffuse astrocytoma. Taken out of context, it may be interpreted erroneously as a negative prognostic factor. Although the number of PXAs studied to date is limited, such infiltrative growth has not emerged as a predictor of later recurrence.[5] Even in instances of malignant transformation, infiltration is generally less widespread than in diffuse astrocytomas.

PXAs themselves are uncommonly calcified, but calcospherites are not unusual in the adjacent cortex.

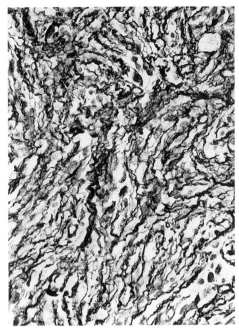

**FIGURE 4–137**    PLEOMORPHIC XANTHOASTROCYTOMA

Reticulin is prominent, at least focally, in most pleomorphic xanthoastrocytomas. In this instance, it is more abundant and more pericellular
in distribution than usual.

Large ganglion cells are present in some PXAs (Fig.
4–139). Distinguishing trapped non-neoplastic ganglion
cells from those that are a true component of the lesion
is not always elementary and may require the presence
of telltale cytologic features such as binucleation. Immunohistochemistry may be necessary when neurons occur as isolated cells or in very small clusters, but it may
not be necessary in the less common situation in which
such cells are abundant or occupy large regions of the
tumor.[4, 16, 17] In some instances, neurons are seen in the
recurrence but not in the original specimen.[16] Although

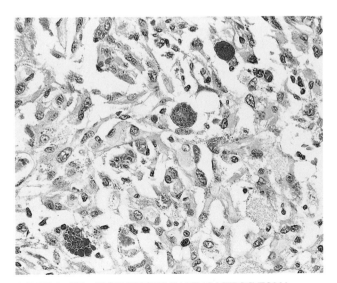

**FIGURE 4–138**    PLEOMORPHIC XANTHOASTROCYTOMA

Eosinophilic granular bodies are periodic acid–Schiff positive.

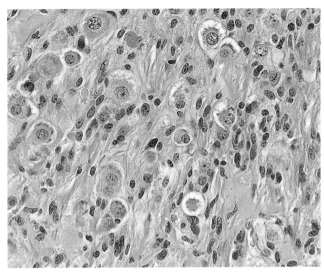

**FIGURE 4–139**    PLEOMORPHIC XANTHOASTROCYTOMA

Well-formed ganglion cells are an infrequent component of pleomorphic xanthoastrocytomas. Note the binucleated form.

PXAs with a neuronal component are, in effect, a form
of ganglioglioma, we consider them grade II PXAs with
ganglionic differentiation, rather than simply grade I
gangliogliomas. This approach is justified by their biologic behavior. One ganglioglioma recurred as a PXA.[17]

Rare PXAs produce melanosomal melanin.[7]

**Grading.**  Discounting the "smoke but no fire" cellularity and pleomorphism, classic PXAs are clearly low-grade
processes—mitoses are hard to find, necrosis is absent,
and EGBs are present. Even the minority of PXAs with
conspicuous mitotic activity or the presence of necrosis
are not as overtly malignant as anaplastic astrocytomas
or glioblastomas. The diagnostic difficulty presented by
PXAs with anaplastic features is discussed later in the
section on differential diagnosis.

Although a favorable outlook is the rule, it is clear
that PXAs recur in a minority of patients and that some
become histologically malignant with the passage of
time. Even primary tumors occasionally show anaplastic
features (Fig. 4–140). The relationship between histologic attributes and outcome is of great importance, but
there have been few comprehensive studies that addressed the issue of grading critically. Not surprisingly,
one retrospective study found that "anaplastic" PXAs
(i.e., tumors with high mitotic activity, vascular proliferation, and necrosis) are prognostically less favorable.[14] A
much larger study, with enough patients to permit multivariate analysis, suggested that the extent of resection
and the degree of mitotic activity were the principal predictive variables.[5] Specifically, it found that 5 or more
mitoses per ten high-power fields was associated with a
significantly higher incidence of recurrence. The presence of necrosis, deemed prognostically insignificant in
one investigation,[15] was not independently predictive.
Nonetheless, necrosis is not a feature in the typical PXA,
and its presence should be viewed with concern and
should prompt a search for mitoses.

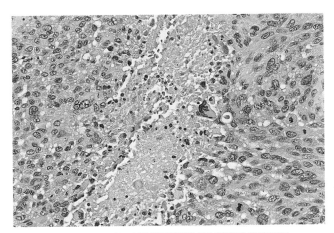

**FIGURE 4–140   PLEOMORPHIC XANTHOASTROCYTOMA**

High mitotic activity, often with associated necrosis, defines pleomorphic xanthoastrocytomas with a greater likelihood of recurrence.

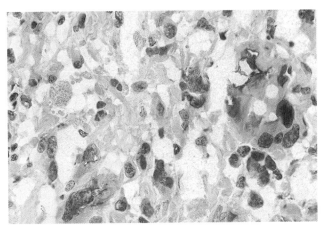

**FIGURE 4–141   PLEOMORPHIC XANTHOASTROCYTOMA— FROZEN SECTION**

The presence of an eosinophilic granular body (*left*) in a pleomorphic astrocytic tumor is an alert that one is dealing with a well-differentiated rather than a high-grade neoplasm.

Although PXAs with mitotic activity above the arbitrary value of 5 or more per 10 fields can be considered of "higher grade" than the classic grade II lesion, one must be cautious in assigning the unqualified designation of "anaplastic" or "malignant" to such tumors. These terms are often used to justify aggressive adjuvant therapy that may not be necessary for a completely excised lesion.

Whether grade IV PXAs exist is somewhat of a philosophic issue. Admittedly, it is hard to resist the designation when faced with a pleomorphic, discrete, and superficially situated astrocytic tumor with EGBs but also with ample mitoses and necrosis. As a rule, high-grade PXAs lack the microvascular proliferation common to glioblastomas. Attention to cytologic details is helpful, because PXAs undergoing malignant change generally become more monomorphous than pleomorphic. The predominance of epithelioid cells differs from the composition of giant cell glioblastomas, in which the large cells with bizarre mitoses are obviously anaplastic and are regularly accompanied by small, undifferentiated cells. Thus, in compliance with the prognostic considerations discussed later, we avoid the term "glioblastoma" for a grade IV PXA.

**Features in Frozen Sections.** When the possibility of a well-differentiated ("low-grade") lesion is indicated by the clinical or radiologic features, cellular pleomorphism is not taken at face value as evidence of a high-grade lesion. EGBs are reassuring evidence of the possibility of PXA (Fig. 4–141).

**Cytologic Features.** The cells are glial, as evidenced by their cytoplasmic processes, with a degree of nuclear pleomorphism that varies from case to case.

**Immunohistochemical Features.** Although the staining for GFAP may be weak and focal, PXAs are positive for GFAP.[9] S-100 protein immunoreactivity is regularly widespread. Participating ganglion cells are immunoreactive for synaptophysin and/or neurofilament protein.[16, 17]

Double labeling of individual cells for both neurofilament protein and GFAP has been reported.[17] Large cells with astrocytic features of indeterminate nature, as well as ganglion cells, may also show immunoreactivity for class III β-tubulin and for various neuropeptides.[5]

**Ultrastructural Features.** Astrocytes, with variable contents of intermediate filaments, are the principal component. In favorable sections, the cell bodies and processes of the astrocytic cells may be invested by basement membrane material (Fig. 4–142).[8, 10]

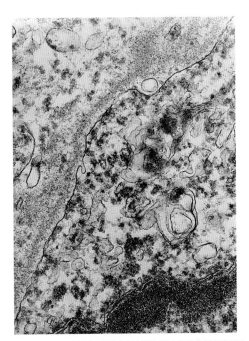

**FIGURE 4–142   PLEOMORPHIC XANTHOASTROCYTOMA**

Well-defined basement laminae are common ultrastructural features, particularly in superficial portions of the tumor. As in a number of gliomas, they are most readily seen covering the interface between neoplastic cells and tumor stroma.

Well-developed rough endoplasmic reticulum, microtubules, and dense core granules are features of ganglion cells.[4]

**Differential Diagnosis.** The histologic features create an Alice-in-Wonderland scene in which cellularity, pleomorphism, and even the mitotic figure or two are not what they seem. Just the opposite, they suggest a "benign" rather than a "malignant" lesion. The differential diagnosis therefore hinges conceptually and practically on the distinction of this neoplasm from other pleomorphic and often more aggressive astrocytic neoplasms.[11] The algorithm presented in Table 4–5, p. 173 is especially useful. The importance of the radiographic features and the age of the patient cannot be overemphasized.[1–3] With these in mind, one cannot take cellularity and pleomorphism at face value in a superficially situated, solidly enhancing lesion, especially one that is accompanied by a cyst. Such a neoplasm is very unlikely to be a glioblastoma or any other malignant neoplasm. Lesions such as ganglioglioma and pilocytic astrocytoma should be excluded, but these distinctions pale in comparison to the importance of ruling out a diffuse astrocytoma of any grade.

Distinguishing PXA from *glioblastoma multiforme* is usually elementary if the possibility of PXA is entertained and the pathologist takes a "prove it to me" attitude when faced with clinical and radiographic data that appear to contradict the initial histologic impression. Discrete, superficial growth of a compact tumor featuring little infiltration, pleomorphism, EGBs, abundant reticulin, and a paucity of mitoses should fortify the position in favor of PXA (see Table 4–9, p. 213).

In high-grade PXAs, however, one is dealt a more challenging hand—namely, the distinction from *giant cell glioblastoma*. The diagnosis of glioblastoma is strengthened by the presence of widespread pleomorphism among giant cells, bizarre mitoses, a paucity of reticulin, and an absence of EGBs. More consistent with PXA are (1) involvement of the subarachnoid space by giant cells lacking mitoses, (2) the emergence of prominent small cells, (3) an epithelioid component, (4) a relatively noninvasive growth pattern, (5) a fascicular architecture, and (6) the presence of EGBs.

*Pilocytic astrocytomas* have the compact, largely noninfiltrating architecture of PXAs but are much more likely to be microcystic, at least in part. They are generally less cellular and pleomorphic than PXAs, and lipidization is usually lacking. Rosenthal fibers are common in pilocytic astrocytomas, whereas they are infrequent in PXAs and, if found, occur primarily in peritumoral tissue.

*Ganglioglioma* also enters into the differential diagnosis, given the often young age of the patient, the presence of cellular pleomorphism, a propensity for cyst formation, and a common location in the temporal lobe. Compact regions of both lesions are often characterized by pleomorphism, a vague fascicular architecture, a content of reticulin, and the presence of lymphocytic infiltrates. Gangliogliomas are, however, only rarely as pleomorphic as PXAs. The distinction between PXA and ganglioglioma is blurred by the occurrence of PXAs with ganglion cells, as discussed earlier.

*Malignant fibrous histiocytoma* shares the compactness, cellular pleomorphism, and lymphocytic infiltrates with PXA. The PXA's immunoreactivity for GFAP readily settles the issue.

**Diagnostic Checklist**

- Is this "PXA" really a ganglioglioma or a pilocytic astrocytoma?
- Is this mitotically active "PXA" really a giant cell glioblastoma?

**Treatment and Prognosis.** Surgery is the principal treatment, and long survivals and cures are expected in most instances. In one study of 71 patients, the overall 5- and 10-year survival rates were 81% and 70%, respectively.[5] The extent of resection and the mitotic index were the two most significant predictors of outcome. PXAs are not universally benign, however, and in approximately 15% to 20% of cases, anaplastic features are present in the initial specimen or evolve during the follow-up period. The result can be a monomorphous, small cell, often epithelioid neoplasm with many of the features of glioblastoma.[5, 9, 18, 19, 21]

The differences in biologic behavior between PXAs with overt anaplastic features and glioblastomas are not clear, but in our experience, the former can be considerably less aggressive. It sometimes lends itself to local control, at least in the short term, by repeated surgical debulking, usually after an initial course of radiotherapy.

## Subependymal Giant Cell Astrocytoma

**Definition.** A discrete, large cell astrocytoma arising near the foramen of Monro, almost always in the setting of tuberous sclerosis. It is WHO grade I.

**General Comments.** In the CNS, morphologic expressions of tuberous sclerosis include cerebral cortical tubers, white matter heterotopias, and subependymal hamartomatous nodules. Peripheral manifestations include lesions of the kidneys and lymph nodes (angiomyolipoma), heart (rhabdomyoma), lung (lymphangioleiomyomatosis), and skin (sebaceous adenoma, hypomelanotic macules, shagreen patches, and subungual fibromas).[9]

Subependymal hamartomas are elevated, often calcified nodules that, owing to their shape, are referred to as "candle drippings." Formed of large cells with abundant eosinophilic cytoplasm, the nodules are indistinguishable from subependymal giant cell astrocytomas (SEGAs) except for their small size. On occasion, one or more such nodules near the foramen of Monro enlarge into a mass sufficient to obstruct the flow of CSF. More posteriorly placed hamartomas rarely enlarge into symptomatic masses and remain as calcified lesions that are typical of tuberous sclerosis.

**Clinical Features.** Clinical or radiographic features of tuberous sclerosis are present in nearly all cases, but histologically typical SEGAs occasionally occur in the absence of tuberous sclerosis or radiologic evidence of the syndrome. Clinical manifestations of SEGA usually

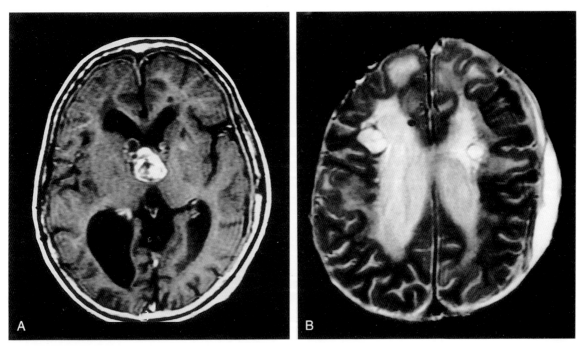

**FIGURE 4–143**    SUBEPENDYMAL GIANT CELL ASTROCYTOMA

Subependymal giant cell astrocytomas are discrete, contrast-enhancing, obstructing masses adjacent to the foramen of Monro (A). As part of the complex of tuberous sclerosis, they are typically accompanied by asymptomatic subependymal hamartomas elsewhere in the lateral ventricles (B). In the T2-weighted image (B), the small hamartoma in the right frontal lobe is darkened by calcification.

appear during the second decade of life,[7, 10, 12] but congenital examples have been encountered in premature infants.[3] It is not uncommon to document the slow evolution of an asymptomatic lesion during routine radiologic screening of patients with the tuberous sclerosis complex.[12]

**Radiologic Features.** Whether solitary or bilateral, these contrast-enhancing masses are solid and sharply demarcated from the underlying caudate head. Their obstructive effects at the foramen of Monro are evident on CT and MRI scans (Fig. 4–143).[11] The other cerebral components of cerebral tuberous sclerosis are usually evident as well. These include (1) calcified subependymal nodules in the lateral ventricles (see Fig. 4–143); (2) cortical tubers with either subjacent rarefaction or cyst formation,[8] evident as hyperintensity in T2-weighted images; and (3) linear abnormalities that reflect hypomyelination of the underlying white matter.

**Macroscopic Features.** SEGAs are discrete masses (Fig. 4–144) that are well vascularized and thus pink; they are sometimes calcified and gritty.

**Microscopic Features.** The low-power histologic appearance of SEGAs is characterized by solid growth demarcation from brain parenchyma and considerable pattern variation. Although certainly large, the cells of SEGAs are rarely "giant." In combination, their glassy cytoplasm, round vesicular nuclei, and distinct nucleoli often give the cells the appearance of both gemistocytic

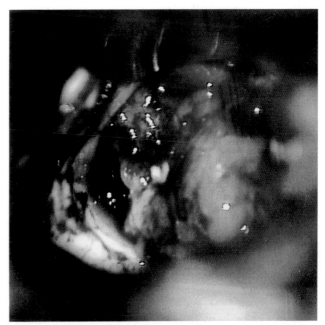

**FIGURE 4–144**    SUBEPENDYMAL GIANT CELL ASTROCYTOMA

At surgery, the tumor appears as a discrete, gray, intraventricular mass near the foramen of Monro. The 14-year-old patient with tuberous sclerosis experienced headaches and had papilledema. (Courtesy of Dr. Jon D. Weingart, Baltimore, MD.)

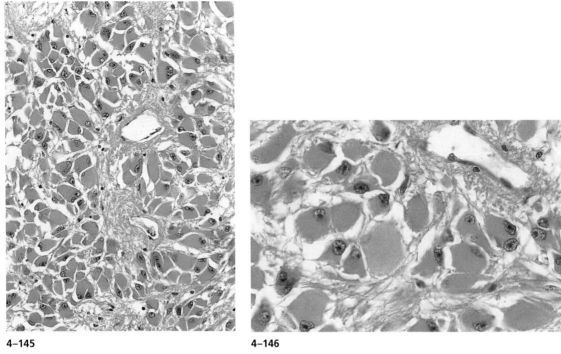

**4–145**                                    **4–146**

**FIGURES 4–145 AND 4–146**    SUBEPENDYMAL GIANT CELL ASTROCYTOMA

The cells of the prototypical lesion resemble large neurons because of the abundant glassy cytoplasm and prominent nucleoli. Perivascular fibrillar zones are larger and more irregular than the perivascular pseudorosettes of ependymomas.

astrocytes and ganglion cells (Figs. 4–145 and 4–146). In addition to these sizable, plump cells, smaller spindle cells may be present in large numbers (Fig. 4–147). Unlike the large cells, which often lie clustered, the spindle cells, with their long processes, tend to be loosely gathered into fascicles that either contribute to a coarse fibrillar background or sweep from vessels to form pseudorosettes that are larger than those of most ependymomas. On occasion, more epithelioid cells also form pseudorosettes that can be similar to those of ependymoma.

Histologic benignity, though belied by considerable nuclear pleomorphism in some cases, is evidenced by the paucity of mitotic figures, although mitotically active examples replete with necrosis have been reported.[7] Calcification is only occasionally prominent. Mast cells may be present in some numbers. Table 4–10 summarizes the short list of mast cell–containing CNS tumors.

**Cytologic Features.** The glassy, somewhat elongated cells of SEGAs project processes from either pole of the cell, whereas those of gemistocytes often originate around the entire circumference (Fig. 4–148).[1] The eccentric position of the nucleus is well visualized, as are cytoplasmic nuclear inclusions and occasional mast cells.

**Immunohistochemical Features.** The plump, as well as spindle, cells of SEGAs show reactivity for GFAP (Fig. 4–149) and for neuronal markers such as synaptophysin, neurofilament protein (Fig. 4–150), class III β-tubulin, and neuropeptides.[5, 13] Most often, clusters of

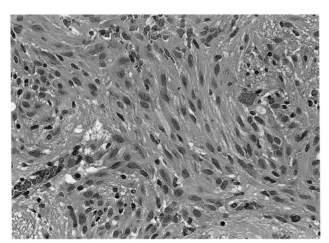

**FIGURE 4–147**    SUBEPENDYMAL GIANT CELL ASTROCYTOMA

Some subependymal giant cell tumors have fascicles of fusiform cells.

**TABLE 4–10
Central Nervous System Neoplasms with Mast Cells**

Meningioma
Hemangioblastoma
Subependymal giant cell astrocytoma (tuberous sclerosis)

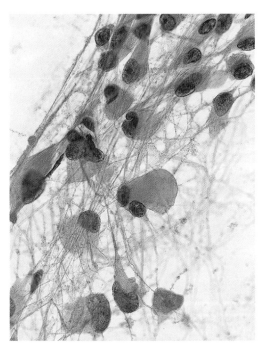

**FIGURE 4–148**   SUBEPENDYMAL GIANT CELL ASTROCYTOMA

Cell processes are readily apparent in smear preparations.

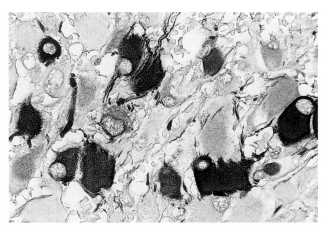

**FIGURE 4–150**   SUBEPENDYMAL GIANT CELL ASTROCYTOMA

A minor cell population is often immunoreactive for neuronal markers such as neurofilament protein (illustrated here), as well as synaptophysin, chromogranin, and a variety of other neurotransmitter substances.

cells stain for either glial or neuronal markers, although rare cells are positive for both.[13] The MIB-1 labeling index is usually low, about 1% in one series.[4]

**Ultrastructural Features.** The cells are characterized by accumulated intermediate filaments, both among organelles and within cell processes. Cytoplasmic lysosomes are common and occasionally encompass distinctive membrane-bound crystalloids. Common features suggesting neuronal differentiation include microtubules and stacks of rough endoplasmic reticulum, but "hard evidence" in the form of neurosecretory granules and synapses is less often apparent.[5]

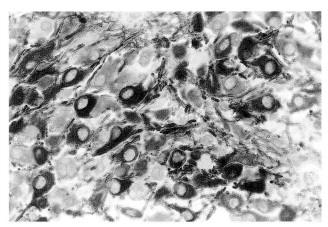

**FIGURE 4–149**   SUBEPENDYMAL GIANT CELL ASTROCYTOMA

Many, but not all, cells are immunoreactive for glial fibrillary acidic protein.

**Differential Diagnosis.** Given their association with tuberous sclerosis and their distinctive localization, the differential diagnosis of SEGAs is limited. It includes *gemistocytic astrocytoma,* an infiltrative glioma occurring in older individuals and differing in cytologic appearance, as well as *giant cell glioblastoma,* also an intraparenchymal tumor. The latter is composed of truly giant cells with anaplastic features. Glioblastoma would be a most unusual lesion in this anatomic location and age group. CNS lesions with gemistocytes and gemistocyte-like cells are summarized in Table 4–3, p. 169.

**Treatment and Prognosis.** SEGAs are treated principally by surgery, repeated if necessary. The prognosis is good following total or even subtotal resection.[10] Patients typically survive for years without evidence of recurrence,[10] albeit often with other manifestations of tuberous sclerosis. The finding of anaplastic features in SEGAs does not appear to affect patient survival.[7] On rare occasion, conventional malignant gliomas have also been reported to occur in the setting of tuberous sclerosis.[2, 6]

### *Pituicytoma and Infundibuloma*

These infundibular and neurohypophysial lesions are discussed in Chapter 9 on pages 473 to 475.

## Oligodendroglioma and Mixed Glioma (Oligoastrocytoma)

**Definition.** Infiltrating gliomas thought to originate by neoplastic transformation of oligodendrocytes. "Mixed" lesions have phenotypic features of both oligodendroglioma and astrocytoma. The neoplasms range from WHO grade II to IV.

**General Comments.** The emergence of oligodendroglioma as a frequent representative among gliomas is

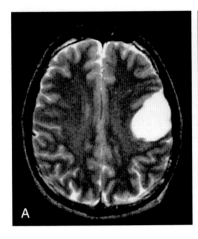
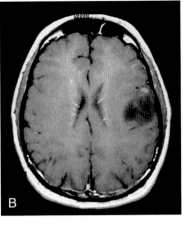

**FIGURE 4–151    OLIGODENDROGLIOMA**

Well-differentiated (grade II) oligodendrogliomas often are superficially situated, involve the cortex, and have a well-delineated deep interface with the brain. These features are well illustrated in the T2-weighted magnetic resonance image (A). Contrast enhancement is absent or minimal (B).

a recent development in neuro-oncology. This entity, somewhat of a curiosity in the past, has become commonplace. Barnyard similes involving "fried eggs" and "chicken wire" have even found their way into the vocabulary. Aware that oligodendrogliomas are less aggressive than diffuse astrocytomas of comparable grade, both patients and treating physicians encourage pathologists to identify this glioma, either in pure form or as a component, however small, of a "mixed glioma." Patients are even beginning to ask for molecular genetic characterization of their tumors. The availability of relatively specific chemotherapy for high-grade tumors and the spectrum of oligodendroglioma look-alikes, many with very favorable prognoses, make an understanding of these lesions even more important.

The present section includes descriptions of both "pure" oligodendrogliomas and the problematic "oligoastrocytomas." The two are not only linked conceptually but are usually treated similarly.

**Clinical Features.** Oligodendrogliomas account for about 10% to 15% of all gliomas, thus approximating the frequency of well-differentiated diffuse astrocytomas. By one set of criteria (which we consider extreme), many if not most grade II diffuse astrocytomas are considered oligodendrogliomas.[9, 10] Oligodendrogliomas occur primarily in adults, although a rare lesion presents in childhood.[43, 54] Seizures often punctuate a relatively long but otherwise asymptomatic latent period. It is not surprising that oligodendrogliomas predominate in the cerebral hemispheres. Cerebellar[40] or brain stem examples[23] are rare. Radiotherapy has been incriminated causally in at least one case.[19]

**Radiologic Features.** On MRI scans, the tumors present as T2- or FLAIR-bright regions with variable degrees of mass effect (Fig. 4–151). Others are rather superficial in the cerebral hemispheres, have relatively circumscribed borders, and exhibit minimal edema.[31] Still others are corticocentric and expand the cortical ribbon over lengthy segments. Others are deep-seated and occasionally cross the corpus callosum in a usually nonenhancing variant of "butterfly glioma." Grade III oligodendrogliomas often contrast enhance but usually do not have the "rim" or "ring" pattern so characteristic of glioblastomas.

Calcification, a common feature seen best on CT scan, is usually restricted to the cortex and thereby assumes a curvilinear, "gyriform" distribution that is nearly diagnostic of this form of glioma (Fig. 4–152). "Scalloping," "erosion," or "remodeling" of the inner table of the skull may occur in long-standing, superficial examples,[31] but caution must be exercised to rule out dysembryoplastic neuroepithelial tumor (DNT) in any "oligodendroglioma" that erodes the skull.

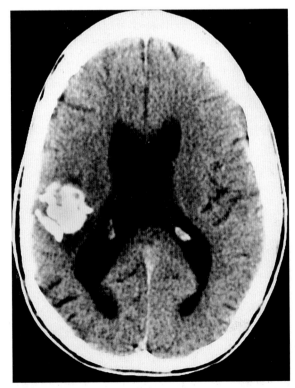

**FIGURE 4–152    OLIGODENDROGLIOMA**

Computed tomography discloses most clearly the curvilinear profiles of intracortical calcification. This lesion occurred in a 23-year-old graduate student with seizures.

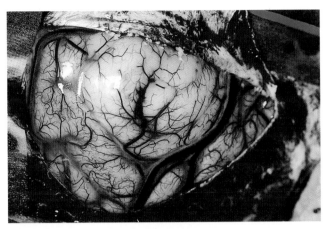

**FIGURE 4–153    OLIGODENDROGLIOMA**

As visualized during surgery, superficial oligodendrogliomas expand the cerebral cortex. The patient was a 32-year-old woman with a 9-month history of left focal motor seizures. (Courtesy of Dr. Henry Brem, Baltimore, MD.)

**Macroscopic Features.** Oligodendrogliomas are gelatinous to soft, gray to pink masses that thicken the cerebral cortex and obscure architectural details, particularly the gray-white junction (Figs. 4–153 and 4–154). Occasional tumors are gritty, but few are densely calcified. Some high-grade examples are well circumscribed (Fig. 4–155).

**Microscopic Features.** Like pornography, in the observation by Supreme Court Justice Stewart, the oligodendroglioma is easy to recognize but may be difficult to define. Although there are objective histologic features that aid in recognition, only one or two may be found in a given microsection.

One of the oligodendroglioma's most prominent features is its affinity for cerebral cortex, where perineuronal

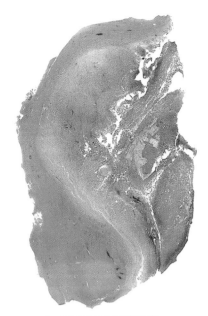

**FIGURE 4–155    OLIGODENDROGLIOMA**

Although they are infiltrating neoplasms, oligodendrogliomas may in part be well circumscribed. This is especially true of grade III lesions.

satellitosis, perivascular aggregation of tumor cells, and subpial accumulation are distinctive (Figs. 4–156 and 4–157). Perineuronal satellitosis must be distinguished from the normal oligodendrocyte-neuron relationship, in

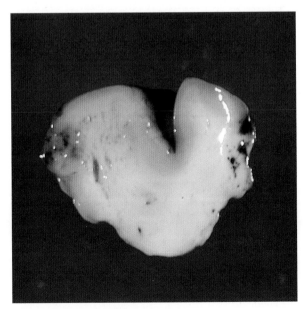

**FIGURE 4–154    OLIGODENDROGLIOMA**

Infiltrating gliomas, both oligodendroglial and astrocytic, macroscopically obscure the gray-white junction. Small cysts are prominent in this case.

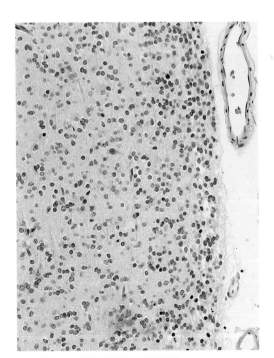

**FIGURE 4–156    OLIGODENDROGLIOMA**

Oligodendrogliomas that infiltrate the overlying cerebral cortex can exhibit perineuronal satellitosis, perivascular aggregation, and subpial accumulation. These "secondary structures" are helpful diagnostic features of both oligodendrogliomas and astrocytomas but are more prominent in the former.

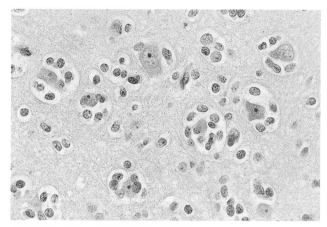

**FIGURE 4–157    OLIGODENDROGLIOMA**

Clustering of tumor cells around neurons (satellitosis) is a common feature of oligodendrogliomas.

which satellite oligodendrocytes orbit large cortical neurons. The distinction is accomplished on the basis of cell number and the presence of cytologic atypia of the perineuronal cells. Both are greater in tumors than in the normal state. The corticocentrism and the highly infiltrative nature of oligodendroglioma ensure that preexisting normal ganglion cells are usually included in the neoplasm. The ganglion cells should not, because of their seeming increase in number, size, and uniformity, be interpreted as part of the neoplasm (i.e., "ganglioglioma"; see Fig. 4–197). This important issue is discussed in the context of gangliogliomas on pages 269 to 270.

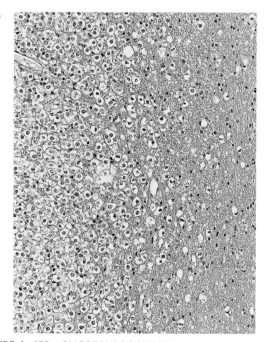

**FIGURE 4–158    OLIGODENDROGLIOMA**

The infiltrating borders of some oligodendrogliomas are rather discrete as they interface with normal parenchyma, particularly in the white matter.

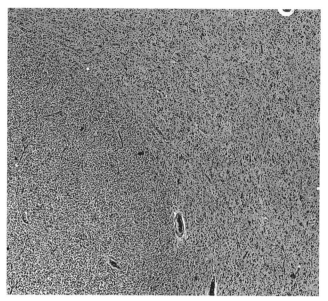

**FIGURE 4–159    OLIGODENDROGLIOMA**

Discrete "clonal" nodules with increased cellularity and mitotic activity appear in some oligodendrogliomas.

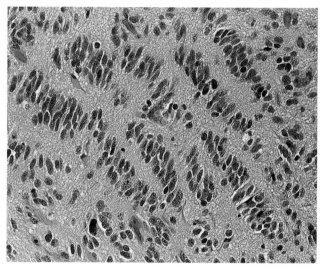

**FIGURE 4–160    OLIGODENDROGLIOMA**

Particularly in high-grade oligodendrogliomas, the cells may advance in enfilades.

**TABLE 4–11**
**Central Nervous System Tumors with Cellular Ribboning or Palisading**

Glioblastoma multiforme (around foci of necrosis)
Oligodendroglioma
Medulloblastoma
Neuroblastoma
Pilocytic astrocytoma
Medulloepithelioma
Primitive polar spongioblastoma°

°This lesion may be only a tissue pattern and not a distinct entity.

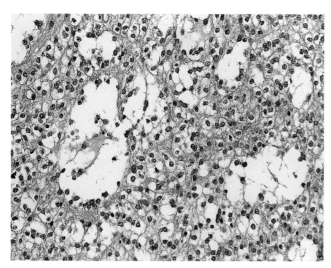

**FIGURE 4–161  OLIGODENDROGLIOMA**

Microcysts are more common in oligodendrogliomas than in diffuse astrocytomas.

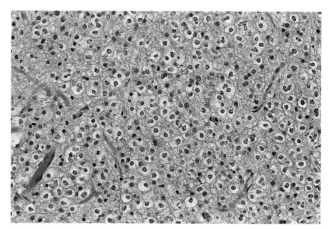

**FIGURE 4–163  OLIGODENDROGLIOMA**

The patternless sheets of oligodendrocytes are relieved visually by delicate arcuate capillaries.

Gangliogliomas are characteristically masses with a considerable glial stroma, often with a mesenchymal element and chronic inflammatory cells.

Although the neoplasm is a decidedly infiltrating process, the border with the uninvolved brain may be rather abrupt (Fig. 4–158).

Unlike in astrocytomas, where anaplastic cells originating in a better-differentiated precursor lesion diffuse into the surrounding tissues, cells of an oligodendroglioma that have been upgraded in terms of the degree of anaplasia often stay close to home in homogeneous "clonal" nodules where cellularity, mitotic activity, and cytologic atypia are all increased (Fig. 4–159). A similar phenomenon occurs in ependymoma. The results in either setting are circular basophilic foci that are visible, sometimes to the naked eye, in microsections.

A startling feature in some oligodendrogliomas, particularly those of higher grade, is the presence of palisaded neoplastic cells marching through the cortex in regimented enfilades (Fig. 4–160). Rosette-like structures are imaged when these cell arrangements are viewed in cross section. CNS tumors with ribboning or palisading are listed in Table 4–11, p. 226.

Microcysts, usually intracortical, are prominent in some oligodendrogliomas (Fig. 4–161). The eosinophilia or slight basophilia of their contents, their PAS positivity, and peripheral vacuolization all clearly indicate that these structures are not merely frozen section artifacts. In some tumors, a faintly basophilic, mucinous matrix also permeates the cortex. Such lesions must be distinguished from DNT.

Calcification is more frequent in oligodendrogliomas than in ependymomas or astrocytomas, attaining an incidence of approximately 90% (Fig. 4–162). Both tumor-bearing and unaffected brain, usually cerebral cortex, may be mineralized. The laminated calcific grains may also be accompanied by structureless mineralization of blood vessels. Bone is a purposeless constituent of some highly calcified lesions.

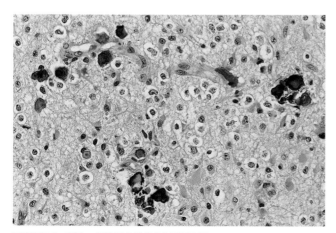

**FIGURE 4–162  OLIGODENDROGLIOMA**

Perivascular or intraparenchymal calcospherites are common in oligodendrogliomas. The cortex is principally affected.

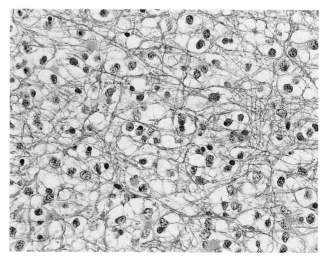

**FIGURE 4–164  OLIGODENDROGLIOMA**

Artifactual halos highlight the uniform round nuclei. Note the thread-like axons that have been overrun by infiltrating tumor cells.

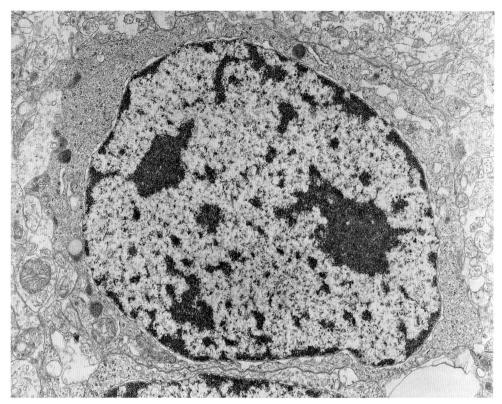

**4–165**

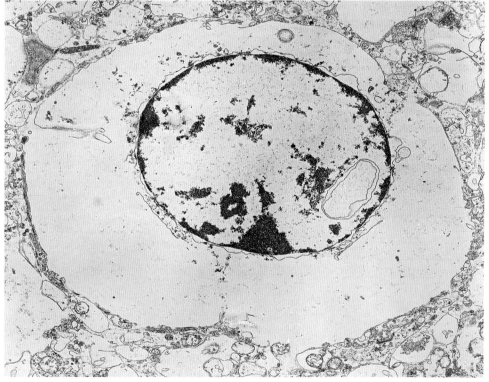

**4–166**

**FIGURES 4–165 AND 4–166    OLIGODENDROGLIOMA**

Autolysis creates the perinuclear halos of oligodendrogliomas. This artifact is absent in specimens that are promptly fixed (Fig. 4–165) but is present when the specimen is incubated in warm saline before fixation and processing (Fig. 4–166).

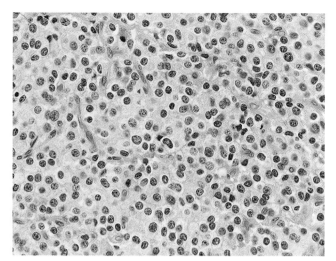

**FIGURE 4–167    OLIGODENDROGLIOMA**

In the absence of perinuclear halos, cytologic monotony is a helpful diagnostic feature.

Likened to "chicken wire," the delicate blood vessels of both low- and high-grade oligodendrogliomas intertwine to marginate lobules of tumor tissue (Fig. 4–163). Typically, the delicate capillaries form short arcs and angulated segments. In exaggerated form, arborizing and occasionally hyalinized vessels link to circumscribe large, lobular islands of neoplastic cells.

Paired features that unify oligodendrogliomas are round nuclei and uniform cell density. Together, they create the monomorphism for which the lesion is well known. Nuclei in better-differentiated lesions have delicate chromatin and small nucleoli, whereas those in higher-grade lesions often show cytologic atypia, particularly in the form of coarse chromatin and increased variation in nuclear size. Nevertheless, they still project an overall uniformity in nuclear size and shape. Relative cellular uniformity, roundness, and nucleoli remain, however, and karyomegaly is usually restricted to scattered large, round, hyperchromatic cells.

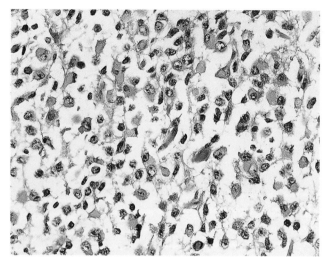

**FIGURE 4–169    OLIGODENDROGLIOMA**

Regionally, the tumor cells of some otherwise typical oligodendrogliomas contain enough eosinophilic cytoplasm to resemble astrocytes. The classic features of oligodendroglioma were present elsewhere in this lesion, as illustrated in Figure 4–158.

Perinuclear halos are a distinctive (Fig. 4–164) but potentially misleading feature, because they are neither uniformly present nor limited to this glioma. As artifacts of delayed fixation, halos are absent in tissues that are fixed promptly (Fig. 4–165) and are prominent in those that are not (Fig. 4–166). Nevertheless, this alteration is eye-catching and is so consistent as to be of great diagnostic significance. It is often the first feature to suggest oligodendroglioma. Oligodendrogliomas without halos can be difficult to diagnose (Fig. 4–167), especially in zones of infiltration (Fig. 4–168).

A number of other neoplasms contain cells with an "astrocyte" appearance created by prominent pink cytoplasm and, sometimes, cell processes (Figs. 4–169 to 4–174). Many descriptive terms have been applied to

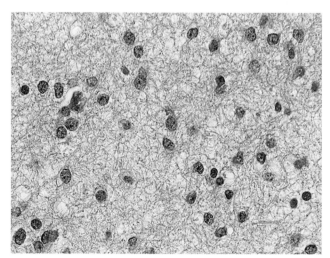

**FIGURE 4–168    OLIGODENDROGLIOMA**

Diffusely infiltrating oligodendrogliomas without perinuclear halos can be difficult to distinguish from astrocytomas. Elsewhere, this lesion had the classic features of oligodendroglioma.

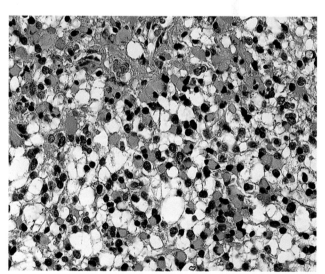

**FIGURE 4–170    OLIGODENDROGLIOMA**

"Minigemistocytes" have the round nuclei of oligodendrocytes and the intracytoplasmic mass of eosinophilic hyaline material. A few fine processes may be present.

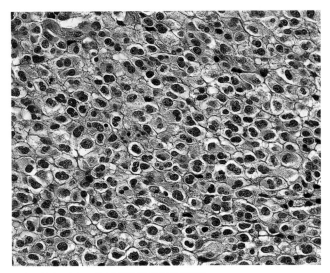

**FIGURE 4–171**   OLIGODENDROGLIOMA

"Gliofibrillary oligodendrocytes," a second form of astrocyte-like cell in oligodendrogliomas, form sheets. The cells have well-defined cell borders and few, if any, processes.

such cells. "Minigemistocyte" refers to small gemistocytes with oligodendrocytic nuclei and plump, hyaline cell bodies (see Fig. 4–170). Such cells are smaller than conventional gemistocytes and lack process formation. Disposed in a pavement fashion, so-called gliofibrillary oligodendrocytes also possess a moderate quantity of cytoplasm, but their fibrillarity is less obvious. Again, processes are sparse, if present at all (see Fig. 4–171). The term "transitional cell" has also been used to refer to all these cell types, because they form a cytologic bridge between typical astrocytes and oligodendrocytes. Transitional cells may be admixed with classic neoplastic oligodendrocytes or may form homogeneous sheets or lobules. Such large aggregates are more common in higher-grade lesions (see Figs. 4–172 to 4–174).[30] Transitional cells tend to be more prominent about vessels. On occasion, the cells contain minute, intracytoplasmic bodies that resemble Rosenthal fibers (see Fig. 4–174).[42] Neoplasms and reactive conditions with gemistocytes and gemistocyte-like cells are summarized in Table 4–3, p. 169.

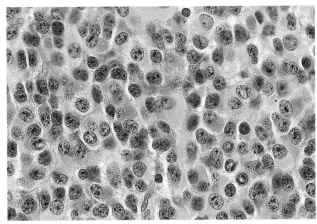

4–172

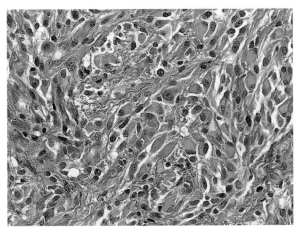

4–173

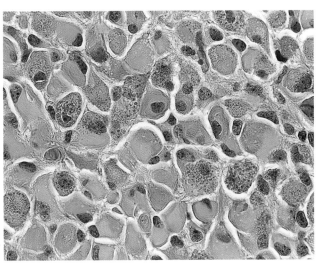

4–174

**FIGURES 4–172, 4–173, AND 4–174**   MALIGNANT OLIGODENDROGLIOMA

Malignant oligodendrogliomas may show considerable intratumoral variation with respect to "astrocytic" features (pink cytoplasm, cytoplasmic fibrillarity, process formation). The illustrated lesion has the nuclear roundness and cytologic monotony of oligodendroglioma, but there are scattered cells with a distinctive rim of eosinophilic cytoplasm (Fig. 4–172). Elsewhere, the cytoplasm is even more prominent and extends into processes (Fig. 4–173). In still other areas, tumor cells with glassy or fibrillar cytoplasm contain minute, brightly eosinophilic bodies (Fig. 4–174).

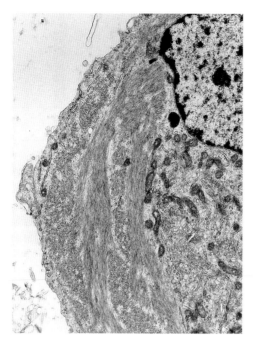

**FIGURE 4–175**    OLIGODENDROGLIOMA

Masses of intermediate filaments are the ultrastructural correlate of the glassy or fibrillar cytoplasm of cells seen in some oligodendrogliomas.

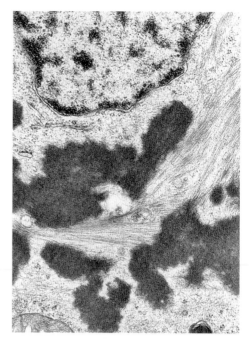

**FIGURE 4–176**    MALIGNANT OLIGODENDROGLIOMA

Ultrastructurally, the eosinophilic cytoplasmic bodies illustrated in Figure 4–174 are electron dense and are closely associated with glial filaments. Both features are characteristic of Rosenthal fibers.

Ultrastructurally, the astrocyte-like cells are rich in intermediate filaments (Fig. 4–175).

The small cytoplasmic bodies are electron-dense deposits similar to Rosenthal fibers (Fig. 4–176).

Unfortunately, astrocyte-like cell types are not distinct cytologic entities but merge with one another along a spectrum that bridges astrocytes and oligodendrocytes. A gamut of oligodendrocytes, transitional cells, and "astrocytes" may be seen in some oligodendrogliomas, especially higher-grade lesions that are prone to shift toward "astrocytic" differentiation. In principle, gemistocytes have processes and a hyaline cytoplasm without any cytoplasmic hyaline mass. In contrast to a typical transitional cell, the central portion of a gemistocyte is GFAP negative. There are, however, many exceptions.

The issue of "mixed glioma," or "oligoastrocytoma," is likely to arise when astrocytes or cells with comparable features make their appearance. Unfortunately, aside from those tumors in which distinct fields of classic oligodendroglioma and diffuse astrocytoma coexist (Figs. 4–177 and 4–178),[16] there are no firm histologic criteria for the diagnosis of mixed glioma. Most tumors designated mixed gliomas are grade II or III neoplasms that contain cells with the rounded nuclei of an oligodendrocyte but the cytoplasm of an "astrocyte," that is, transitional cells. Although this may be inappropriate termi-

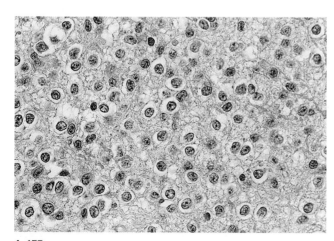

4–177

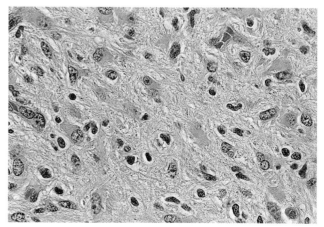

4–178

**FIGURES 4–177 AND 4–178**    MIXED GLIOMA

Geographically distinct populations of oligodendrocytes and astrocytes justify the diagnosis of mixed glioma, or oligoastrocytoma. The present lesion contained both oligodendroglioma (Fig. 4–177) and astrocytoma (Fig. 4–178). In routine practice, however, most oligoastrocytomas are more hybrid than biphasic in their cellular makeup.

nology, it is difficult to be critical, because some lesions with oligodendrocytes and many transitional cells have areas that are, by nuclear or cytoplasmic criteria, "astrocytic." We reserve the "mixed" designation for truly biphasic tumors with fibrillary or frankly gemistocytic elements. Some tumors contain cells with neither the nuclear nor the cytoplasmic features of either oligodendroglia or astrocytes. Although these are sometimes labeled "mixed glioma," they are not really "mixed" in composition but rather "intermediate" or "hybrid" in nature. The nosologic and therapeutic problems created by these neoplasms are obvious.

Some observers require a certain threshold percentage of "astrocytes" before a diagnosis of mixed glioma is rendered. A commonly quoted figure is 20%. Beyond this arbitrary approach, there are no consensus criteria for a diagnosis of mixed glioma. As a result, the lesion is endemic in some institutions but is almost a reportable disease in others. The cytogenetics of mixed gliomas is discussed later.

Fortunately, at present, the distinction between oligodendroglioma and mixed glioma makes little initial therapeutic difference, because oligoastrocytomas and pure oligodendrogliomas are treated similarly. For the patient, however, the difference can be highly significant, given the more aggressive nature of diffuse astrocytic neoplasms. The designation of an astrocytic neoplasm as a mixed glioma may generate undeserved prognostic optimism. One might expect mixed gliomas with a 1p/19q loss to behave in the "benign" fashion of an oligodendroglioma, whereas those without this profile would be expected to act biologically like astrocytic tumors, that is, more aggressive and more prone to high-grade transformation.

In addition to the key features presented here, several less specific qualities complete the histologic repertoire of oligodendrogliomas. These include (1) the presence of a mucinous background, (2) vascular proliferation and necrosis in high-grade lesions, and (3) apoptosis.

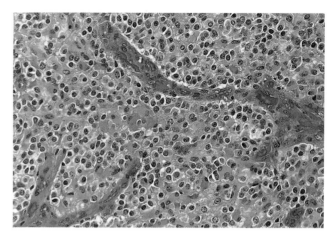

**FIGURE 4–180**   MALIGNANT OLIGODENDROGLIOMA

Vascular elements in high-grade oligodendrogliomas are more often hypertrophic than hyperplastic.

Microvascular proliferation can assume the "glomeruloid" pattern seen in other gliomas, but it is usually somewhat more restrained (Figs. 4–179 and 4–180).

Necrosis is often present in anaplastic oligodendrogliomas but is usually unassociated with conspicuous "pseudopalisading" (Fig. 4–181).

Apoptosis may be quite evident in oligodendrogliomas, particularly those of higher grade. It has not been shown to be an independent prognostic indicator.[57]

**Grading.**   Most oligodendrogliomas are well-differentiated, grade II lesions, but these merge gradually and imperceptibly with examples that demonstrate unequivocal anaplasia. As the spectrum descends into histologic malignancy, the cells become more closely packed, nuclear-cytoplasmic ratios increase, and mitotic figures become readily evident if not abundant (Figs. 4–182 to 4–184). More transitional cells often appear. Although nuclei have coarser chromatin and more prominent nucleoli, they typically retain a nuclear roundness and uniformity not generally seen in other malignant gliomas. The

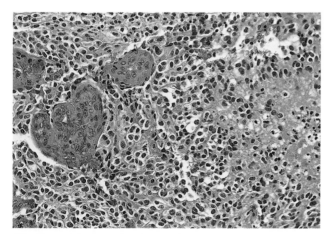

**FIGURE 4–179**   MALIGNANT OLIGODENDROGLIOMA

Microvascular proliferation is an unfavorable prognostic feature in oligodendrogliomas and is one diagnostic criterion for grade III or IV lesions. As illustrated here, the response is usually most prominent in perinecrotic regions.

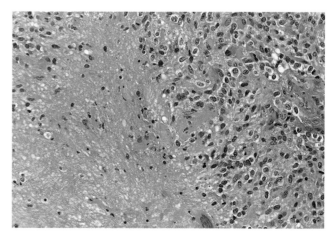

**FIGURE 4–181**   MALIGNANT OLIGODENDROGLIOMA

Necrosis, often without pseudopalisading, is common in malignant oligodendrogliomas.

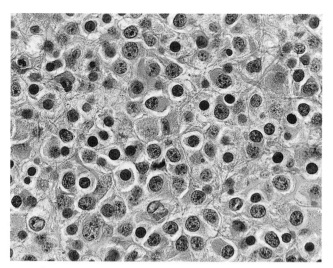

**FIGURE 4–182    MALIGNANT OLIGODENDROGLIOMA**

This "typical" malignant oligodendroglioma retains features of oligodendroglioma—namely, uniform cell distribution, rounded nuclei, and perinuclear halos. Sharply defined cell borders and a rim or crescent of pink cytoplasm are commonly present.

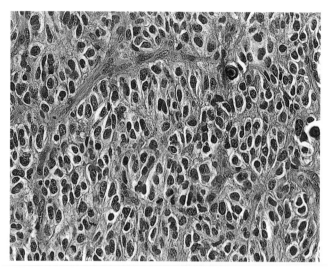

**FIGURE 4–184    MALIGNANT OLIGODENDROGLIOMA**

Although these cells have the polarity and the nuclear pleomorphism that suggest glioblastoma, there is also the monotony, the even cell distribution, and the calcification of oligodendroglioma. Elsewhere, this neoplasm had prototypical features of a malignant oligodendroglioma.

incremental nature of the process is well seen in the cellular nodules discussed earlier, where tumor grade is often half a step higher than that of the surrounding tumor.

At the extreme of anaplasia, oligodendrogliomas, like other gliomas, lose all evidence of their cellular origins. Indeed, their heritage may be surmised only on finding better-differentiated foci. Even in anaplastic oligodendrogliomas, the typical geometric vascularity is usually retained. In some tumors, the vascular pattern is exaggerated so as to impart an organoid appearance. In the process of malignant transformation, vascular hypertrophy and proliferation, and sometimes necrosis, are often acquired. Transitional cells may become prominent. In rare instances, mesenchymal metaplasia evolves into gliosarcoma.[12]

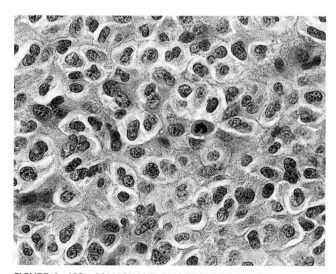

**FIGURE 4–183    MALIGNANT OLIGODENDROGLIOMA**

In more cellular areas, the nuclei's angulation and polarity may overlap with those of glioblastoma. Elsewhere, this lesion had clearly defined features of oligodendroglioma.

Attempts to systematize grading have successfully identified morphologic parameters of prognostic significance. Microcysts are a "favorable" feature, whereas cytologic atypia, high cellularity, pleomorphism, vascular proliferation, and necrosis are the converse.[5, 36] A large study involving seven neuropathologists identified six unfavorable prognostic factors by univariate analysis: older age, high cellularity, presence of mitoses, endothelial hypertrophy, microvascular proliferation, and necrosis.[13, 14] Multivariate analysis reduced the significant variables to two: age and and microvascular proliferation. For technical reasons, mitoses were not significant for the group of pathologists as a whole, but they were significant when most of the pathologists' analyses were considered individually. Although these parameters are similar to those of prognostic importance in diffuse astrocytomas, it remains unclear how to use these features in a dependable grading scheme. Unfortunately, factors found to be of prognostic significance in one study are often not validated in another.[5, 36, 52] Furthermore, no published study of grading has yet considered molecular and cytogenetic features, such as 1p and 19q loss, as entry criteria or in a multivariate analysis. The prognostic significance of MIB-1 labeling indices is discussed on pages 234 to 235.

A widely quoted study from the Armed Forces Institute of Pathology assigned tumors to one of four grades on the basis of a binary (yes-no) assessment of the presence of five variables.[52] These variables were proliferation, necrosis, nuclear-cytoplasmic ratio, cell density, and pleomorphism.[52] Not surprisingly, significant differences in survival were noted between patients with neoplasms of low and high grades ("A" and "D"), but the survival curves overlapped for patients with the two intermediate grades ("B" and "C"). The effect was a three-tiered system with a skewed distribution of grades (A—23%, B plus C—71%, and D—6%). Pleomorphism was the only histologic variable closely correlated with patient survival.

This system yielded similar results when applied at another institution.[27]

The WHO system identifies two grades—oligodendroglioma grades II and III—using the general criteria discussed later.[22]

In the practical world of tumor grading, there are frequent discrepancies in individual cases that complicate histologic analyses. Examples of these include (1) a grade II lesion with a high MIB-1 index, (2) a well-differentiated tumor with necrosis, (3) a cellular and/or somewhat pleomorphic tumor with only sparse mitotic activity, and (4) an anaplastic tumor with a high mitotic index but without vascular proliferation.

We suggest the following approach to oligodendroglioma grading.

*Grade II oligodendrogliomas* form a large group that extends from very well differentiated tumors to ones that are almost grade III. Most show low to moderate cellularity, mild nuclear atypia, and infrequent mitoses. Although early vascular hypertrophy may be present, frank microvascular proliferation and necrosis are not. Multifocal nodules with increased cellularity, nuclear atypia, and mitotic activity are permitted. Microcystic change may be prominent. Within this group are those infrequent oligodendrogliomas with only minimal atypia, no or only rare mitoses, and no vessel alterations or necrosis. Most of these very well differentiated tumors occur in children and young adults, where the main differential diagnosis is DNT. Although it is tempting to assign these cases to a separate category—namely, grade I oligodendroglioma—this is not accepted for an infiltrating oligodendroglioma or diffuse astrocytoma. One study of grade II oligodendrogliomas found that a subdivision was possible. Patients whose tumors had no mitoses or had MIB-1 indices less than 5% did better than patients whose tumors exceeded those values.[45]

*Grade III oligodendrogliomas* are decidedly "bluer" after H&E staining owing to their greater cellularity and show greater cytologic atypia and mitotic activity. Vascular hypertrophy and proliferation are present, as is necrosis in some cases.[9] The grade III designation is appropriate in the absence of vascular proliferation if cellularity, atypia, and mitotic activity are pronounced.

*Grade IV oligodendrogliomas* are relatively rare and controversial. These tumors have grade III features with obvious microvascular proliferation, frequently combined with necrosis with palisading, but they are more anaplastic (Figs. 4–185 and 4–186). Clearly defined oligodendrogliomatous features must be present, usually in the form of uniform, round nuclei and other features of grade II or III oligodendrogliomas described earlier. The mere presence of perinuclear halos or a vague sense that the tumor might be oligodendroglial is not a sufficient criterion. In many cases, nuclear features become decisive. Those of diffuse astrocytomas show granular irregularity and feature more coarse chromatin. In doubtful cases, a comment regarding some "oligodendroglioma qualities" is appropriate. These qualities may be taken into consideration by clinicians in formulating a treatment plan.

**Proliferation Indices in Grading.** MIB-1 indices vary considerably from study to study but are related to grade. Not surprisingly, a wide range of values has been reported for grade II oligodendrogliomas.[11, 26, 45, 57] In one study, the median value for grade II lesions was 1.7%, with a range from 0 to 21.3%.[8] In another study, the mean for WHO grade II tumors was 1.91%, and for grade III lesions it was 7.87%.[57]

There have been several detailed studies of the prognostic utility of MIB-1 labeling indices as forms of "objective grading" independent of histopathologic features. Most reports describe significantly shorter survival times in patients whose tumors showed a higher percentage of immunopositive nuclei. Technical differences in tissue processing and immunostaining methods, quantification of reactions, and format of expressing results make it difficult to summarize reports without commenting on the specifics of individual studies.

One study found that patients with oligodendrogliomas having MIB-1 labeling indices of 5% or less

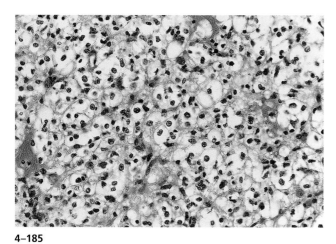

4–185

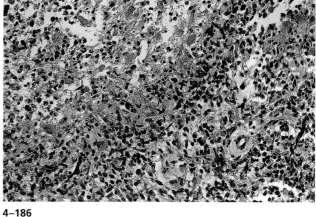

4–186

**FIGURES 4–185 AND 4–186    GRADE IV OLIGODENDROGLIOMA**

Tumors with clearly defined features of oligodendroglioma (Fig. 4–185) but with advanced anaplasia, as noted here by necrosis with pseudopalisading (Fig. 4–186), qualify as grade IV oligodendroglioma.

had a median survival of 1718 days, whereas those in which the index was above 5% had a median survival of 452 days.[8] Another investigation found that the 5-year survival rate was 35% for patients with tumors having labeling indices less than 10%, 30% with tumors staining at a 10% to 20% level, and 14% at values greater than 20%.[26] A cutoff point of 3% was determined by a third study, in which the mean survival time for patients with tumors whose indices were less than 3% was 72.5 months; for those with indices above 3%, mean survival was 23.5 months.[17] In yet another study, the 5-year survival rate was 83% for patients whose tumors had MIB-1 values less than 5%, but only 24% for those whose indices were greater than 5%.[11] Within the grade II category, one report described a significantly better outlook for patients whose tumors had MIB-1 indices less than 5%.[45]

**Features in Stereotactic Biopsy Specimens.** The diagnosis of oligodendroglioma can be difficult in small specimens, because they are often fixed rapidly. As a result, perinuclear halos are usually absent or only slightly formed. Although prominent cortical involvement may be seen, this alone is not a definitive feature. The uniform roundness of oligodendroglial nuclei, seen to greatest advantage in cytologic preparations, is often the distinguishing feature.

**Features in Frozen Sections.** By denying the tumor cells their "fried egg" appearance, but adding artifactual nuclear angulation and hyperchromasia, the freezing process blurs the distinction of oligodendroglioma from diffuse astrocytoma. The inevitable ice crystals that arise in edematous white matter further cloud the issue. The latter may so dominate the scene that the biopsy is almost uninterpretable with respect to the degree of cytologic atypia and even cellularity. Identifying gray matter then becomes helpful, because with little edema and therefore few crystals, both cellularity and cytologic atypia can be evaluated more accurately. Prominent perinuclear satellitosis is a clue to the nature of the lesion (Fig. 4–187).

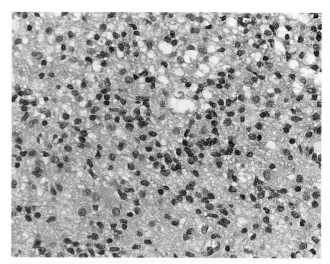

**FIGURE 4–188    OLIGODENDROGLIOMA**

Oligodendrogliomas that were used previously for frozen sections have the artifactual nuclear hyperchromatism and angulation that simulate cytologic features of astrocytomas.

Because the distinction between oligodendroglioma and diffuse astrocytoma is of little significance at surgery, it is prudent to render a tentative diagnosis of "well-differentiated infiltrating glioma" and to reserve precise classification until review of permanent sections. Bolder pathologists may wish to seek perineuronal satellitosis, mucin-filled microcysts, calcifications, and characteristic cytologic features in smear preparations. For most of us, however, reaching the diagnosis of a grade II infiltrating glioma is challenging enough.

As noted earlier, permanent sections of a previously frozen oligodendroglioma acquire artifactual nuclear hyperchromatism and angulation, the combined effects of which simulate grade II or III diffuse astrocytoma (Fig. 4–188; see also Figs. 5–26 and 5–27). Thus, it is important that one reserve some unfrozen tissue for permanent sections.

**Cytologic Features.** Although oligodendrogliomas and astrocytomas should, and in most instances do, have distinguishing features, there is considerable cytologic overlap. Thus, one should not be surprised to find that a lesion that appeared "astrocytic" in a smear preparation looks more "oligodendroglial" in permanent sections. Smear preparations emphasize nuclear roundness, a rather open chromatin distribution, a small but distinct nucleolus, and a paucity of cell processes (Fig. 4–189). Round, "naked" nuclei with small nucleoli sit in a background that is less fibrillar than that of astrocytomas. This is particularly true in more cellular tumors, where there is less background parenchyma to contribute to the appearance of fibrillarity. The glassy or fibrillar cytoplasm of the GFAP-positive transitional cells is also well seen in smears (Fig. 4–190). Nuclei of higher-grade tumors, although still generally uniform in size and shape, have coarser chromatin and greater mitotic activity. In some instances, these nuclei resemble those of metastatic carcinoma.

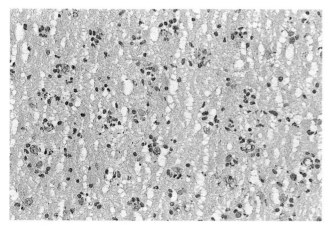

**FIGURE 4–187    OLIGODENDROGLIOMA—FROZEN SECTION**

On frozen section examination, extensive cortical involvement with perineuronal satellitosis should suggest the likelihood of oligodendroglioma.

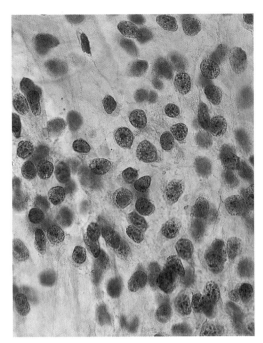

**FIGURE 4–189    OLIGODENDROGLIOMA**

As seen in a smear preparation, cells of an oligodendroglioma have nuclei that are rounder than those of an astrocytoma, and the background is less fibrillar. Generally, nucleoli are more prominent in oligodendrogliomas.

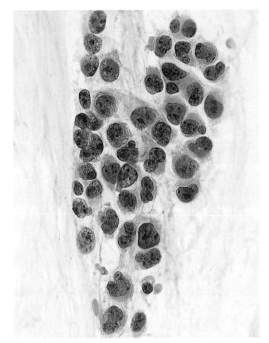

**FIGURE 4–190    OLIGODENDROGLIOMA—SMEAR PREPARATION**

The brightly eosinophilic, fibrillar cytoplasm of "minigemistocytes" is well seen in smear preparations.

**Immunohistochemical Features.** Although oligodendrogliomas might be expected to express diagnostically useful antigens that reflect their cell lineage (e.g., myelin basic protein or myelin-associated glycoprotein), investigations to date have been singularly unsuccessful in confirming the utility of such markers.[48] This lack of a specific marker is regrettable, and the diagnosis of oligodendroglioma continues to rest on cytologic and histologic criteria. There is light on the horizon, however, in the form of a molecular and cytogenetic profile, discussed later.

Although the cells of a well-differentiated oligodendroglioma are inherently immunonegative for GFAP, the transitional cells, as discussed earlier, have astrocytic characteristics and are GFAP positive (Fig. 4–191). Because oligodendrogliomas also incite reactivity in normal astrocytes, the latter are prominent after GFAP staining.

Neuronal markers are frequently applied to oligodendrogliomas in an effort to distinguish them from neurocytic or neuroblastic neoplasms, as well as gangliogliomas. Although synaptophysin stains the cortex overrun by an oligodendroglioma, it does not stain the neoplastic cells themselves in most cases. There are rare cases, however, that do stain focally. Antibodies to "neuronal proteins" such as N-methyl-D-aspartate receptor do stain oligodendrogliomas.[58] Markers such as NeuN have not been demonstrated,[58] and only a single tumor has been immunopositive for human antineuronal antibodies (anti-Hu).[15] These observations, and the finding of neurosecretory granule-like structures in some oligodendrogliomas,[39] sustain a debate centered on how closely oligodendrocytes might be related to neurons. A heretical notion, expressed from time to time, is that neoplasms of oligodendrocytes may not exist at all, given the lack of any accepted immunohistochemical marker. The occasional expression of ultrastructural features distinctive of oligodendrocytes, as well as the unique cytogenetic features (see later), appear to relieve the uncertainty and establish oligodendrogliomas as neoplasms distinct from neuronal tumors and other gliomas. The concepts of cytogenesis, as applied to many CNS tumors, are vague, however, and the last word on the interrela-

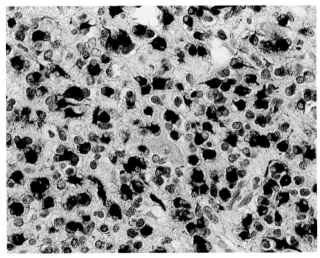

**FIGURE 4–191    OLIGODENDROGLIOMA**

The small cells with eosinophilic cytoplasm are immunoreactive for glial fibrillary acidic protein.

tionships between gliomas and neuronal tumors has not been heard.

**Ultrastructural Features.** A number of studies of the fine structure of oligodendrogliomas have been reported.[25, 35, 47] Although an exceptional finding, electron microscopic studies have demonstrated lamellated cytoplasmic processes that seemingly recapitulate the role of the oligodendrocyte in the formation and maintenance of myelin sheaths.[47] A feature of the well-differentiated oligodendroglioma that helps distinguish it from the astrocytoma is the presence of microtubules, rather than glial filaments, within cell processes (see Fig. 4–165).

Ultrastructurally and philosophically, the difference between the astrocytoma and the oligodendroglioma is less clearly defined among oligodendrogliomas with GFAP-positive transitional cells and in mixed gliomas. Not surprisingly, transitional cells contain an abundance of intermediate filaments (see Figs. 4–175 and 4–176).[18, 25, 28] In concept, and in contrast to the large gemistocytes of gemistocytic astrocytomas, filaments in gliofibrillary oligodendrocytes and minigemistocytes are disposed in compact, tight fascicles rather than dispersed in small numbers throughout the cytoplasm or concentrated at the cell periphery.[28] In an occasional lesion, cells may contain small, brightly eosinophilic cytoplasmic particles that ultrastructurally consist of amorphous electron-dense material surrounded by intermediate filaments. In essence, these are mini Rosenthal fibers. As previously noted, neurosecretory granule-like structures are sometimes seen in oligodendrogliomas; their distinction from small lysosomes is not always possible.

**Molecular and Cytogenetic Features.** Although precise correlations remain to be established, loss of both the entire short arm of one chromosome 1 and the entire long arm of one chromosome 19 is closely correlated with the oligodendroglioma phenotype (Fig. 4–192).[3, 7, 24, 44, 46, 50, 55] Not all "oligodendrogliomas" have this chromosomal deficiency, and the occasional "astrocytoma" does. Nonetheless, the association is strong, and the finding appears to be prognostically significant for both low- and high-grade lesions, as discussed later. Because the sought-after tumor suppressor genes on these chromosomes have not been identified, it is possible that some oligodendrogliomas could have undetected small deletions or point mutations rather than extensive chromosomal loss, or perhaps important abnormalities on other chromosomes. In the meantime, one might be skeptical about those "oligodendrogliomas" without the expected cytogenetic profile. In one study of grade II oligodendrogliomas and oligoastrocytomas, the survival experience for patients with the 1p/19q loss was considerably more favorable than for those with tumors without these two genetic losses.[51] On retrospective review, such tumors appear less "oligodendrogliomatous" in terms of histopathologic features than do oligodendrogliomas with the 1p/19q loss.[4]

Not surprisingly, the genetics of the mixed glioma (oligoastrocytoma) are less clear. Some have the aforementioned double loss, whereas others have a more "astrocytic" genotype.[33] It thus remains to be seen whether so-called mixed gliomas are mixed in the cytogenetic or molecular sense. One very small study found that they were not, as determined by study of tissues obtained by

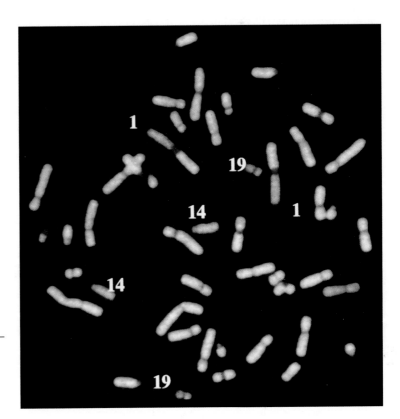

**FIGURE 4–192**   OLIGODENDROGLIOMA

As detected by comparative genomic hybridization, oligodendrogliomas characteristically lose chromosomal arms 1p and 19q. In this preparation loss of chromosomal material is seen as a red signal. In this neoplasm, chromosomal arm 14q is also lost. (Courtesy of Dr. Burt G. Feuerstein, San Francisco, CA.)

microdissection of the oligodendrogliomatous areas and the "astrocytic" areas. In each of three cases, both tissue patterns had the 1p and 19q loss.[24]

Staining for p53 is present in some oligodendrogliomas, but it is usually not the diffuse, dark staining one often sees when mutations are present. Mutations of the p53 gene appear to be uncommon in oligodendrogliomas.[56] Whether the presence of mutations or widespread strong p53 immunoreactivity has any value in classification (astrocytoma versus oligodendroglioma) or grading (grade II versus grade III oligodendroglioma) is unclear.[4]

**Differential Diagnosis.** The differential diagnosis of oligodendrogliomas can be challenging. If you are thinking of the diagnosis of oligodendroglioma, you should probably be thinking of something else, and if you are not thinking of oligodendroglioma, you probably should be (see Table 4–9, p. 213). There are, in other words, many oligodendroglioma-like lesions, and not all oligodendrogliomas exhibit classic morphologic features. This heterogeneous group is summarized in Table 4–12. Neoplasms with enfilades similar to those in some oligodendrogliomas are listed in Table 4–11, p. 226.

Exclusion of *macrophage-rich lesions* such as demyelinating disease, infarct, and progressive multifocal leukoencephalopathy is an essential first step in the evaluation of lesions with oligodendrogliomatous features. To the unwary, lipid-filled macrophages can be mistaken for neoplastic glial cells, although the cytoplasm of neoplastic oligodendrocytes is water-clear, whereas that of macrophages is granular and somewhat refractile (Fig 4–193). Although "traditional" stains, such as PAS or Luxol fast blue, can be used to highlight cytoplasmic contents of macrophages, most pathologists now bypass these methods and move directly to immunohistochemical markers such as HAM-56 or KP-1 (CD68).

Of the three macrophage-rich lesions, *demyelinating diseases* are the most problematic, and consequential, in the face of diagnostic error. This disorder must always be considered before rendering the diagnosis of oligodendroglioma, mixed glioma, or even diffuse astrocy-

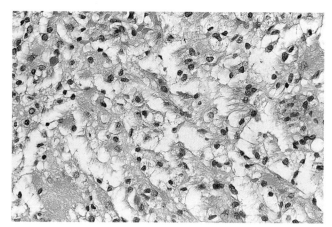

**FIGURE 4–193**   DEMYELINATING DISEASE RESEMBLING OLIGODENDROGLIOMA

The active phase of demyelinating disease can closely resemble oligodendroglioma, although the debris-filled cytoplasm of the macrophage is granular rather than water-clear.

toma grade II or III. Attention to radiologic findings is a helpful adjunct. Many demyelinating plaques biopsied in the active phase are contrast enhancing, often with a distinctive U- or horseshoe-shaped profile. In the setting of this or any other contrast-enhancing mass, the diagnosis of a grade II oligodendroglioma, astrocytoma, or mixed glioma represents a discrepancy that must be resolved before a pathology report is signed. Grade II oligodendrogliomas or diffuse astrocytomas are not contrast enhancing. Diffuse gliomas enhance only in high-grade form. Even then, they rarely do so in the distinctive manner of the class of demyelinating diseases discussed on pages 113 to 119.

*Cerebral infarct* must also be excluded, although this entity is usually recognized by its clinical presentation, phased evolution on neuroimaging scans, cortical involvement, distinctive capillary reaction in the early stages, content of macrophages, and presence of ischemic "red" or "red-dead" neurons (see pages 414 to 417). The macrophage infiltrate in *progressive multifocal leukoencephalopathy* can be misinterpreted as oligodendroglioma or mixed glioma if the distinctive inclusion-bearing oligodendrocytes, atypical large astrocytes, and numerous macrophages are not recognized. Again, the clinical setting of immunosuppression and the usually distinctive imaging abnormality, which does not include cortical involvement, provide valuable clues to the diagnosis.

Although *gliosis* is an astrocytic process, and technically it does not fall into the differential diagnosis of oligodendroglioma, the low cellularity of many grade II oligodendrogliomas overlaps with that of gliosis and requires exclusion of the latter, using the guidelines discussed earlier for diffuse astrocytomas. An interesting phenomenon with overtones of gliosis is the *apparent increase in the number of oligodendroglia around arteriovenous malformations*.[38] Another is the *apparent hypercellularity of oligodendrocytes in white matter and the deeper cortical laminae*. This is created when several layers of cells align along the vessels and about cor-

**TABLE 4–12**
**Oligodendroglioma and Oligodendroglioma-Like Lesions**

Oligodendroglioma
Diffuse astrocytoma
Clear cell ependymoma
Neurocytic neoplasms
    Central neurocytoma
    Extraventricular neurocytic tumor
Nodular medulloblastoma
Dysembryoplastic neuroepithelial tumor
Pilocytic astrocytoma
Clear cell meningioma
Non-neoplastic macrophage-rich lesions
    Demyelinating disease
    Infarct
    Progressive multifocal leukoencephalopathy

tical neurons. This pattern is seen most often in lobectomy specimens removed to control seizures, but it is occasionally evident in fortuitous cuts of apparently normal brain (see Fig. 6–19). It is also encountered from time to time in other specimens as an apparent variation of normal. These changes are not a neoplastic or preneoplastic state.

Among gliomas, grade II oligodendrogliomas must be distinguished principally from *diffuse astrocytomas*. Although always subjective and often challenging, this distinction has significant implications for grading, treatment, and prognosis. To underscore the problem, occasional mitoses are tolerated in grade II oligodendroglioma, but their presence is often used as the basis for a grade III designation if encountered in a diffuse astrocytoma. It is our opinion that pathologists have become overly sensitive to nuclear roundness and perinuclear halos, so that many astrocytomas are being unjustifiably catalogued as oligodendrogliomas. In the absence of perinuclear clearing and the presence of equivocal fibrillarity, the distinction rests largely on nuclear characteristics. The nuclei of diffuse astrocytoma tend toward elongation, angulation, and hyperchromasia, whereas those of oligodendroglioma are more prone to roundness and uniformity, open chromatin being the exception (Fig. 4–194). Nucleoli are more prominent in oligodendrogliomas. In individual cases, however, such generalizations fail to distinguish these two closely related gliomas, even when specimens are optimally fixed, processed, and stained.

An additional issue is *clear cell ependymoma*. Both lesions consist of monotonous populations of cells prone to the formation of artifactual perinuclear halos. There are several points of distinction. As a rule, the cells of ependymomas are more compact, and their nuclei, unlike those of oligodendrogliomas, are more hyperchromatic. The solid, displacing nature of the ependymoma contrasts sharply with the infiltrating quality of the oligo-

dendroglioma, wherein there is trapping of normal elements. Neurofilament protein–positive axons pervade oligodendrogliomas but are sparse in ependymomas. Lastly, oligodendrogliomas lack the GFAP-positive perivascular fibrillar zones (pseudorosettes). Ependymomas have occasional dot-like paranuclear or intercellular EMA staining (diminutive true rosettes). Electron microscopy may be required to demonstrate the latter, which contain microvilli and cilia and are bounded by complex intercellular junctions. Radiologically, clear cell ependymoma and oligodendroglioma are clearly different. The ependymoma is a discrete, sometimes cyst-associated, contrast-enhancing mass.

The distinction between oligodendroglioma and *neurocytic neoplasms* also poses a problem (Fig. 4–195; see also Table 4–9, p. 213). Reports of oligodendrogliomas staining for "neuronal" markers[58] such as paranuclear synaptophysin, and the ultrastructural observation of scattered neurosecretory granule-like structures in classic oligodendrogliomas, compound the confusion.[39] Neurocytic neoplasms and oligodendrogliomas differ in their growth patterns and imaging profiles. Whereas grade II oligodendrogliomas are infiltrative and nonenhancing, neurocytic neoplasms are discrete, enhancing masses. This is particularly true of intraventricular, "central" neurocytomas. The distinction between oligodendrogliomas and extraventricular neurocytomas can be more problematic, because the latter are often looser and more fibrillar and therefore resemble gliomas.

A particularly complex, and not always resolvable, differential diagnosis involves the *dysembryoplastic neuroepithelial tumor* (Fig. 4–196). This benign, multinodular, intracortical entity typically presents in childhood or adolescence with partial complex seizures. When the classic features of DNT are lacking, one may be left with a well-differentiated oligodendroglioma-like lesion that cannot be assigned to either the oligodendroglioma or the DNT category. An ambivalent, noncommittal report to the clinician is not as unhelpful as it may appear. The clinical presentation, when coupled with the radiologic profile, can be used to arrive at a working diagnosis. An

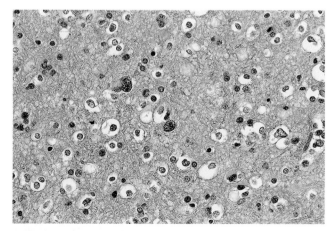

**FIGURE 4–194    ASTROCYTOMA RESEMBLING OLIGODENDROGLIOMA**

Perinuclear halos and a degree of nuclear roundness are insufficient criteria for the diagnosis of oligodendroglioma. The illustrated degree of nuclear pleomorphism is more consistent with astrocytoma than with oligodendroglioma.

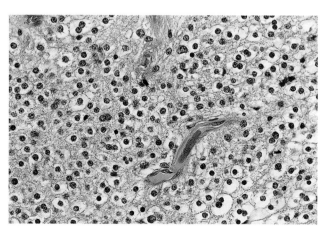

**FIGURE 4–195    EXTRAVENTRICULAR NEUROCYTOMA RESEMBLING OLIGODENDROGLIOMA**

Neurocytes can deceptively resemble oligodendrocytes.

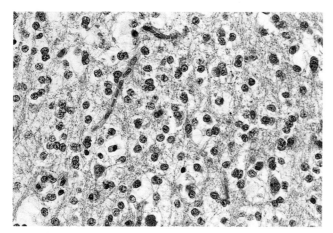

**FIGURE 4–196**   DYSEMBRYOPLASTIC NEUROEPITHELIAL TUMOR RESEMBLING OLIGODENDROGLIOMA

Viewed at high magnification, dysembryoplastic neuroepithelial tumors closely resemble oligodendrogliomas.

oligodendrogliomatous lesion with intracortical nodules on MRI scans is almost certainly a DNT. Even in the absence of this classic feature, a superficial, discrete, oligodendroglioma-like mass, at least at the authors' institutions, is usually followed after surgery without adjuvant therapy. Reoperation with histologic reassessment may be undertaken at the time of progression or recurrence.

Although oligodendrogliomas and *pilocytic astrocytomas* vary in their biologic properties, their histologic appearances can be quite similar (see Fig. 4–113). Thus, the burden of proof lies squarely on the pathologist who entertains a diagnosis of oligodendroglioma for a cerebellar mass in a child. Generally, such oligodendroglioma-like tumors have, at least focally, classic features of pilocytic astrocytoma. Typical radiographic features, such as cyst and nodule formation, are usually apparent as well.

An occasional oligodendroglioma traverses the leptomeninges and adheres to dura. Often somewhat desmoplastic, such tumors may mimic *meningioma*, particularly the clear cell variety. The differential between a potentially resectable meningioma and an infiltrative glioma is critical at surgery, when confusion is most likely to arise. In frozen section, the calcospherites of oligodendroglioma may be misinterpreted as psammoma bodies. The absence of whorls, thick-walled vessels, or collagenous stroma favors a diagnosis of glioma. Cytologic features distinguish the two lesions.

Given the lesion's affinity for the cerebral cortex, normal ganglion cells are trapped in many cases (Fig. 4–197). These cells should not be interpreted as part of the neoplasm. The diagnosis of ganglioglioma would be at odds with the usual understanding of that entity as a discrete, contrast-enhancing mass.

The presence of high cellularity, hyperchromasia, microvascular proliferation, and necrosis may prompt consideration of *small cell glioblastoma multiforme*. The latter appears monomorphous at low magnification but not at high magnification, where the nuclei of this glioblastoma variant are somewhat elongated, mildly pleomor-

phic, and jumbled in orientation (see Fig. 4–51). In oligodendroglioma, the pattern of microvascular proliferation rarely includes glomeruloid vessel proliferation.

High-grade oligodendrogliomas pose a somewhat different diagnostic challenge. This primary lesion must be distinguished not only from a metastatic neoplasm but also from other anaplastic gliomas, particularly glioblastoma. The similarity to *metastatic carcinoma* is greatest among poorly differentiated oligodendrogliomas, particularly those with prominent transitional cells. The resemblance is enhanced when the highly cellular glioma is macro- or microscopically discrete. Resolution should be sought in the more highly differentiated areas that are often present in high-grade oligodendrogliomas. Such features as infiltrative properties, calcification, "chicken wire" vasculature, vascular hypertrophy or microvascular proliferation, and some degree of GFAP immunoreactivity generally resolve the issue. It is important to recall that reactivity with wide-spectrum keratin antibodies, particularly AE1-AE3, parallels that with GFAP.

### Diagnostic Checklist

- Have you ruled out reactive processes such as demyelinating disease and infarct?
- Are you sure you have ruled out a reactive lesion?
- Is your "oligodendroglioma" possibly one of the low-grade neoplasms listed in Table 4–7, such as neurocytic neoplasm or DNT?
- Is this "oligodendroglioma" really an astrocytoma or glioblastoma with perinuclear halos?
- Could this grade III oligodendroglioma really be a clear cell ependymoma?
- Is this "mixed glioma" really just an astrocytoma?

**Treatment and Prognosis.** Although grade II oligodendrogliomas are infiltrative neoplasms once thought to be not fully resectable, this issue has never been resolved, and total resection of the radiologic abnormality

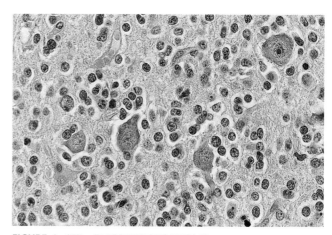

**FIGURE 4–197**   OLIGODENDROGLIOMA

The cortical ganglion cells frequently trapped in an oligodendroglioma should not be misinterpreted as neoplastic and evidence of a ganglioglioma.

(i.e., the T2-bright area) is attained in some cases. Postoperative treatment varies from case to case, depending on (1) the extent of resection, (2) the treatment philosophy of the physician, and (3) the wishes of the patient. In many centers, patients with totally or largely excised, well-differentiated oligodendrogliomas are only observed, and additional therapies are withheld until the time of recurrence, which may take a decade or more. Patients with grade III and IV lesions are generally treated postoperatively by radiation and chemotherapy. The utility and appropriate timing of radiation therapy have been the subject of ongoing debate. The perception is evolving that such treatment may not be necessary at initial diagnosis, especially for completely resected or asymptomatic low-grade lesions.[41]

There has been recent recognition that high-grade oligodendrogliomas often respond to chemotherapy.[6, 7, 41] The success of the PCV (procarbazine, CCNU, vincristine) combination is now well established for oligodendrogliomas,[6, 7] but other regimens are beneficial as well. Although this multiagent combination is efficacious for high-grade oligodendrogliomas,[6, 7] it may be applicable to grade II lesions as well.[34, 53] Of particular interest in high-grade oligodendrogliomas is the observation that favorable responses appear to be restricted to those with a chromosomal 1p loss, a regular feature of the 1p/19q combination.[7] Malignant oligodendrogliomas without this loss apparently do not respond. A similar prognostic advantage for tumors with this molecular criterion seems to hold for grade II oligodendrogliomas as well.[51] The nature of these "oligodendrogliomas" without the 1p/19q loss is, however, not clear.

Although well-differentiated oligodendrogliomas carry a better prognosis than do diffuse astrocytomas of comparable grade, past studies indicate that the outlook for patients with low-grade oligodendrogliomas is still guarded. Their prognosis is difficult to evaluate at present, because only a few preliminary studies have followed patients with respect to the molecular and cytogenetic profiles of their tumors.

For tumors of grades I and II as defined by the Kernohan and the St. Anne–Mayo systems, the median survival was approximately 10 years; 5- and 10-year survival rates were 75% and 46%, respectively.[49] For grade III and IV lesions combined, the median survival was 3.9 years; the respective 5- and 10-year survival rates were 41% and 20%. Although other retrospective series have revealed similar results, the different grading systems applied and various methods of presenting data make comparisons difficult.[27, 29, 32, 52] The issue of prognosis in mixed gliomas is difficult to evaluate, given the imprecise diagnostic criteria. In one study, the median survival for combined grade I and II lesions was 6.3 years, and the 5- and 10-year survival rates were 58% and 32%, respectively.[49] For combined tumors of grades III and IV, the median survival was 2.8 years, and the respective 5- and 10-year survival rates were 36% and 9%.

Recent studies done in the context of molecular and cytogenetic findings offer a more encouraging view of the biologic behavior of low-grade oligodendrogliomas and of the response to therapy of their high-grade counterparts. For example, in the study of Smith and colleagues, no relapses were noted in cytogenetically positive (1p/19q deletion) oligodendrogliomas in a group of patients followed as long as 10 years.[51] Patients with high-grade lesions with the same cytogenetic profile also did better than historical experience would have suggested. Earlier studies may well have contained "oligodendrogliomas" without the molecular and cytogenetic marker.

Although oligodendroglial tumors, like diffuse astrocytomas, may become increasingly malignant with the passage of time[2], their propensity for "dedifferentiation" is less pronounced. Oligodendrogliomas sometimes spread via CSF pathways[1, 37] and, on rare occasion, even undergo extracranial metastasis.[20, 21]

## Tumors of Ependyma and Related Cells

### Ependymoma

**Definition.** A variably fibrillar and/or epithelial-appearing neoplasm attributed to neoplastic transformation of ependymal cells.

**Clinical Features.** Ependymomas of the brain can present at any age but do so mainly during the first 2 decades of life.[2, 9, 20, 24] The fourth ventricle is the most common site of origin. Ependymomas in adults are more often spinal, but intracranial examples occur as well.[31] Rare extraneural sites are the mediastinum,[6, 23] lung,[16] and ovary.[10]

Ependymomas of the fourth ventricle usually produce symptoms referable to obstruction of CSF flow and cranial nerve dysfunction.[5, 20] Cerebral hemispheric lesions present with any of the generic expressions of an expanding intraparenchymal mass.

**Radiologic Features.** Ependymomas of the fourth ventricle often protrude from the floor as discrete, exophytic, contrast-enhancing masses that relate to the brain much as a villous adenoma does to the wall of the colon (Fig. 4–198). A minority of tumors in this region arise more laterally in the foramen of Luschka or superiorly in the ventricular roof. A peculiar feature of some ependymomas of the posterior fossa is the "plasticity" they express as they ooze out of the foramina and encircle the brain stem.[34] Supratentorial ependymomas are frequently cystic and often para- rather than intraventricular (Fig. 4–199).[18, 34] Some even arise near the surface of the brain.

**Macroscopic Features.** Ependymomas at any site are sharply demarcated, soft, and fleshy (Fig. 4–200). Only occasional examples are gritty due to calcification. Lateral extension of some fourth ventricular ependymomas brings them to the subarachnoid space, where they may encase cranial nerves and blood vessels.

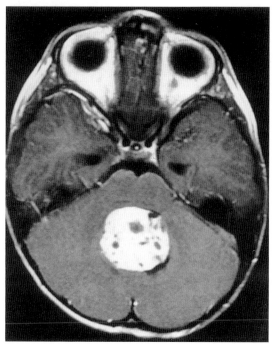

**FIGURE 4–198   EPENDYMOMA**

Intracranial ependymomas arise most often in the posterior fossa as discrete contrast-enhancing masses attached to the floor of the fourth ventricle. This lesion obstructed the flow of cerebrospinal fluid in a 3-year-old boy with a 4-month history of morning vomiting.

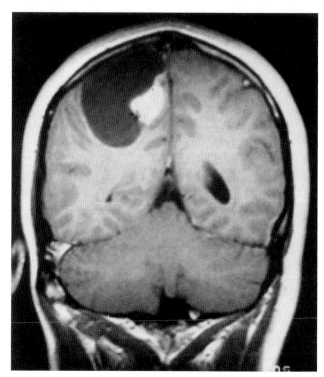

**FIGURE 4–199   EPENDYMOMA**

Supratentorial ependymomas are often cystic and frequently arise in a para- rather than intraventricular locus.

**Microscopic Features.** In its normal state, ependyma consists of a delicate veneer of focally ciliated cells on the ventricular surface. Although this epithelial quality is retained in some tumors, more often, glial features prevail, in the form of cellular processes and a GFAP-positive background fibrillarity. Some tumors have both glial and epithelial features.

Ependymomas are known for their lobulation and discrete interface with surrounding brain (Figs. 4–201 and 4–202). Particularly in fourth ventricular examples,

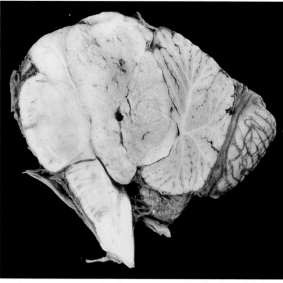

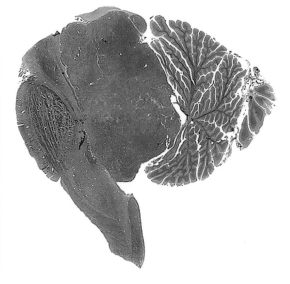

**FIGURE 4–200   EPENDYMOMA**

This ependymoma was an incidental finding in a 9-year-old drowning victim. The lesion filled the fourth ventricle and retained a broad attachment to the ventricular floor. As is characteristic of ependymomas, the lesion is well circumscribed.

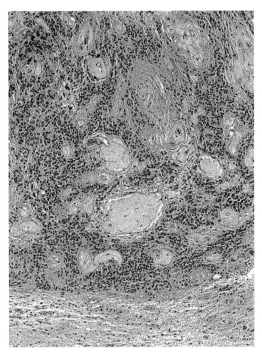

**FIGURE 4–201   EPENDYMOMA**

Ependymomas are well demarcated, with only a limited capacity for brain invasion. This lesion arose from the floor of the fourth ventricle.

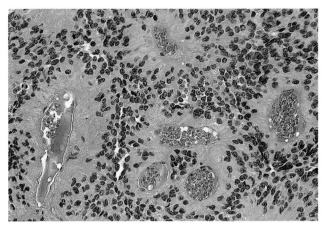

**FIGURE 4–203   EPENDYMOMA**

The dense cellularity of this classic "cellular" ependymoma is interrupted by perivascular "nuclear-free zones" composed of radiating processes (perivascular pseudorosettes).

a delicate covering layer of ependyma is still apparent. Occasional high-grade lesions are in part infiltrative, but this is exceptional.

"Glial" features predominate in the most common, "cellular" variant of ependymoma, which consists of a

monomorphous proliferation of neoplastic cells unpatterned except for the presence of nuclei-free process-rich zones around blood vessels (Figs. 4–203 and 4–204). Termed "perivascular pseudorosettes," these diagnostically critical structures are best appreciated at low magnification. It is imperative in the case of a high-grade lesion to distinguish these structures from rudimentary orientation of cells about vessels and from nonspecific perivascular deposition of collagen. The distinction is made expeditiously using immunohistochemistry for GFAP. Histochemical stains can be helpful. In Masson trichrome preparations, the gray-green of glial fibers is easily differentiated from the bright green of collagen.

Some ependymomas are predominantly glial in appearance, and perivascular pseudorosettes are faint or absent (Fig. 4–205). They consist of paucicellular, highly fibrillar tissue that often contains scattered, small, more full-bodied GFAP-positive cells (Fig. 4–206). Perivascular pseudorosettes can still be found but may be inconspicuous. Such highly fibrillar neoplasms may suggest

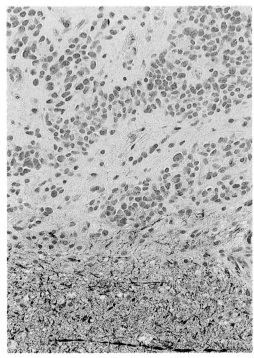

**FIGURE 4–202   EPENDYMOMA**

Staining of axons for neurofilament protein emphasizes the pushing rather than infiltrating nature of ependymomas.

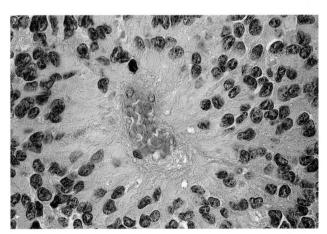

**FIGURE 4–204   EPENDYMOMA**

Perivascular pseudorosettes are formed of tumor cell processes.

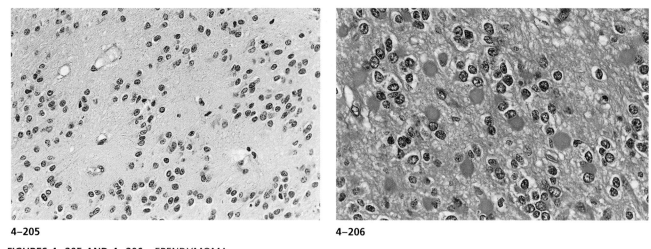

4–205                                          4–206

**FIGURES 4–205 AND 4–206   EPENDYMOMA**

Ependymomas of the fourth ventricle often contain paucicellular regions where perivascular pseudorosettes are ill defined (Fig. 4–205) or highly fibrillar areas with gemistocyte-like cells (Fig. 4–206).

the diagnosis of "mixed glioma," or "ependymoastrocytoma." Although this diagnosis may be defensible on purely histologic grounds, it is misleading, because such tumors are—clinically, radiologically, and biologically—ependymomas.

Epithelial properties are clearly evident in only a minority of ependymomas but, when present, do much to distinguish this neoplasm from other gliomas. The cells are disposed in arrangements of variable sizes and configurations, from papillae with smooth-contoured surfaces to closed glands or canals (Fig. 4–207). The latter, termed "true ependymal rosettes," are frequently intermingled with more glial-appearing ependymal cells. True rosettes are distinguished from perivascular pseudorosettes by their well-defined lumens marked by the apical surfaces of the constituent cells. Such rosettes may be large and immediately apparent, or they may be so

tiny as to require critical focusing through different planes in small and ostensibly solid clusters of cells. Various combinations of patterns are often encountered in the same lesion and may include the pattern of subependymoma, discussed in the next section.

An uncommon but prognostically important variant is the clear cell ependymoma, in which prominent perinuclear halos impart an oligodendroglial appearance[17, 19] (Figs. 4–208 and 4–209). Calcospherites may round off the similitude. Perivascular pseudorosettes, however, are present and help establish the diagnosis. Electron microscopy supports the ependymal nature of these clear cells, as is discussed later. Clear cell ependymomas are usually supratentorial and generally grade III, as judged by cytologic atypia, mitotic activity, and microvascular proliferation.

A rare variant with both epithelial and fibrillar features is the papillary ependymoma. In this lesion, redundant epithelial surfaces cover cores of fibrillar GFAP-positive cells.

Also rare is the so-called tanycytic ependymoma. This entity deserves special attention, because its composition of elongated cells creates a microscopic picture remarkably similar to that of an astrocytoma (Fig. 4–210).[8] Being a highly fibrillated tumor of low to moderate cellularity, it has a vaguely fascicular architecture. Nuclear pleomorphism is mild to moderate, and mitoses are often absent. As compared with the classic ependymoma, perivascular pseudorosettes are rudimentary and easily overlooked. True ependymal rosettes are typically absent.

The myxopapillary ependymoma and the pleomorphic "giant cell" ependymoma are indigenous to the lumbar spinal cord and filum terminale but may occasionally present as a primary intracranial lesion.[3]

Whereas calcification is not unusual in ependymoma, cartilaginous and osseous metaplasia are exceptional (Fig. 4–211). Trivial but eye-catching features in an occasional ependymoma are cells that contain small eosinophilic granules,[14] clear vacuoles,[11] or melanin.[27] Rare lesions are lipidized.[28]

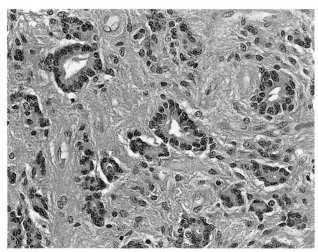

**FIGURE 4–207   EPENDYMOMA**

"True" ependymal rosettes, or even larger versions termed "canals," appear in only a minority of ependymomas.

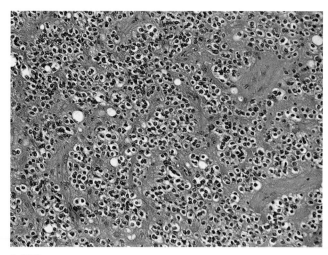

4–208

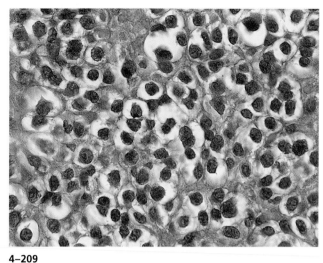

4–209

**FIGURES 4–208 AND 4–209**  CLEAR CELL EPENDYMOMA

Because of their perinuclear halos, "clear cell" ependymomas resemble oligodendrogliomas. This uncommon ependymoma variant is usually supratentorial and grade III.

**Grading.** Although ependymomas can be graded, it has been difficult to document a clear relationship between histologic factors and outcome. The issue is discussed later in the section on treatment and prognosis. We use the following grading schema.

*Grade II ependymomas* vary considerably in cellularity, possess no or infrequent mitoses, and show only slight or mild cellular pleomorphism. Perivascular pseudorosettes are often prominent, as are large, confluent fibrillar zones. Cellular pleomorphism or necrosis, without pseudopalisading, may be present. Nodules with greater cellularity and mitotic activity are permitted, as long as they are not the dominant component.

*Grade III ependymomas* are usually supratentorial in location, exhibit moderate to high cellularity, have brisk mitotic activity, and almost always show microvascular proliferation (Fig. 4–212). Most contain extensive necrosis, but this feature is of little significance, because it is common even in low-grade ependymomas of the posterior fossa. One study found necrosis to be a negative prognostic factor among supratentorial ependymomas.[30] Grade III ependymomas retain traces of their ependymal heritage, usually in the form of perivascular pseudorosettes. Lacking these, the diagnosis of ependymoma is suspect and requires immunohistochemical or ultrastructural support.

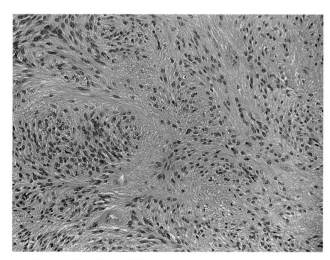

**FIGURE 4–210**  TANYCYTIC EPENDYMOMA

The highly fibrillar "tanycytic" ependymoma is easily mistaken for a pilocytic astrocytoma. Distinguishing features are the ependymoma's fascicular architecture and vague perivascular pseudorosettes.

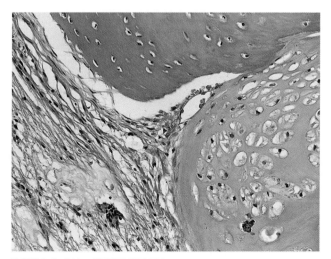

**FIGURE 4–211**  EPENDYMOMA

Osseous and cartilaginous metaplasia can occur in ependymomas.

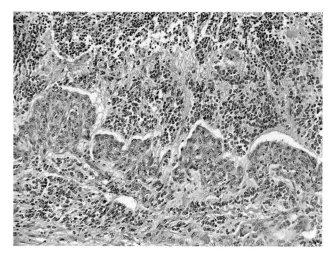

**FIGURE 4–212   ANAPLASTIC EPENDYMOMA**

Although the grading of ependymomas remains controversial, most ependymal tumors with microvascular proliferation and increased mitotic activity are classified as grade III lesions.

*Intratumoral variations in tumor grade* may be present. Ependymomas show case-to-case variation in differentiation, as well as intralesional gradations. This usually takes the form of one or more hypercellular nodules with increased cytologic atypia and mitotic activity (Figs. 4–213 and 4–214). These are analogous to the nodules occasionally seen in oligodendrogliomas (see Fig. 4–159). Such cellular foci often fall short of grade III, but their cytologic features and proliferative activity are too atypical for the lesion to be placed comfortably in the grade II category. Violating the general rule of grading based on the most anaplastic area, we designate ependymomas as anaplastic only when this feature is dominant or exclusive.

Although we believe that focal areas of atypia or anaplasia do not elevate a lesion to grade III, or anaplastic, status, they have been reported to convey a somewhat less favorable prognosis.[20]

The *relationship between ependymoma and glioblastoma* is problematic and largely semantic. Unlike glioblastoma, very high grade ependymomas usually exhibit a solid, noninfiltrating growth pattern. In contrast, glioblastomas rarely show unequivocal ependymomatous features, and then only in the form of focal and vague perivascular pseudorosettes. Nevertheless, some high-grade ependymomas are infiltrative, and occasional well-circumscribed glioblastomas satisfy the minimal criteria for ependymoma. How these lesions should be categorized is problematic but should be based on the predominant tissue pattern. As a rule of thumb, malignant infiltrating gliomas with focal perivascular pseudorosettes in adults are best considered glioblastomas rather than malignant ependymomas.

**Features in Frozen Sections.** Recognizing ependymomas in frozen sections can be challenging, especially if the epithelial features are absent, as they usually are, and perivascular pseudorosettes are inconspicuous, as is often the case. The freezing process exacerbates the problem by overemphasizing fibrillarity and the gemistocyte-like quality of the cells. As a result, ependymomas often appear distinctly astrocytic. Perivascular pseudorosettes, appreciated best at low magnification, are usually decisive findings (Fig. 4–215).

**Cytologic Features.** The cells of ependymomas resist disaggregation because of their hold on blood vessels, as is apparent in the form of perivascular pseudorosettes. Tissue fragments, rather than abundant individual cells, are therefore characteristic (Fig. 4–216). Aggregation

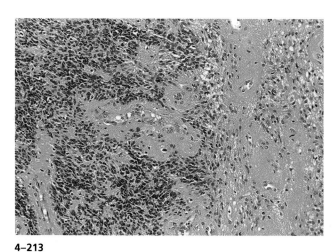

4–213

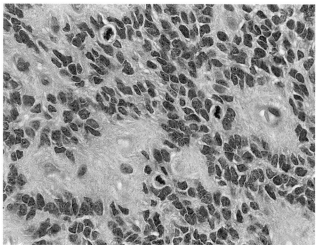

4–214

**FIGURES 4–213 AND 4–214   EPENDYMOMA**

Confounding the grading of ependymomas is the fact that many tumors contain islands of increased cellularity where nuclear-cytoplasmic ratios, cytologic atypia, and mitotic activity are all increased over those of the background lesion.

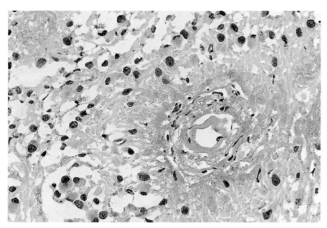

**FIGURE 4–215    EPENDYMOMA—FROZEN SECTION**

The cellular processes that constitute the perivascular pseudorosettes are often more apparent in frozen tissues than in permanent sections.

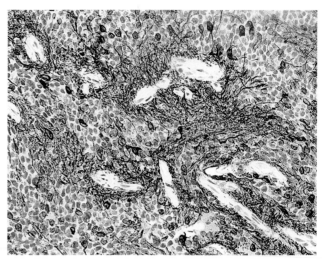

**FIGURE 4–217    EPENDYMOMA**

Tumor cell processes in perivascular pseudorosettes are immunopositive for glial fibrillary acidic protein.

around vessels may be conspicuous. The nuclei are uniform, are round to oval, and often feature a distinct nucleolus. In contrast to other gliomas, cuboidal, epithelial-like cells may be a common finding.[22]

**Immunohistochemical Features.** To varying degrees, the processes that constitute the perivascular rosettes are

GFAP positive (Fig. 4–217). In addition, luminal surfaces, such as those of true rosettes, canals, and even papillae, can be EMA positive (Fig. 4–218).[7, 13, 35] Ependymomas show widespread vimentin and S-100 protein reactivity.

With respect to cell proliferation, the MIB-1 labeling index has been found to correspond to regional mitotic activity, nuclear atypia, necrosis, and cell density; it varies considerably in different areas within the tumor.[29] Overall indices are higher in grade III tumors (mean, 34%), compared with grade II lesions (mean, less than 2%).[29] Grade III lesions are also more likely to be immunoreactive for p53.[29]

**Ultrastructural Features.** Electron microscopy emphasizes the similarity between normal and neoplastic

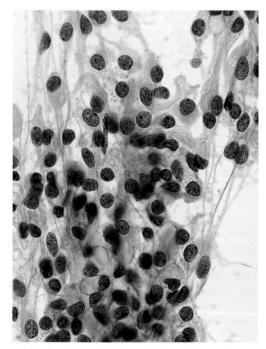

**FIGURE 4–216    EPENDYMOMA—SMEAR PREPARATION**

Smear preparations of ependymomas often contain tissue fragments in which cytoplasmic "glial" processes—some of which radiate relative to vessels—are a conspicuous feature. Typically, the nuclei are small, uniform, and ovoid and contain distinct micronucleoli.

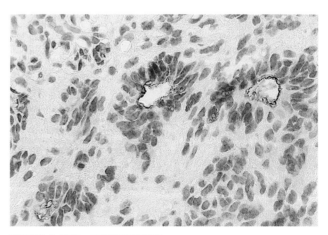

**FIGURE 4–218    EPENDYMOMA**

Antibodies to epithelial membrane antigen stain the cell surfaces of "true" rosettes. Some rosettes are so small that they are nearly invisible in routine H&E stained sections.

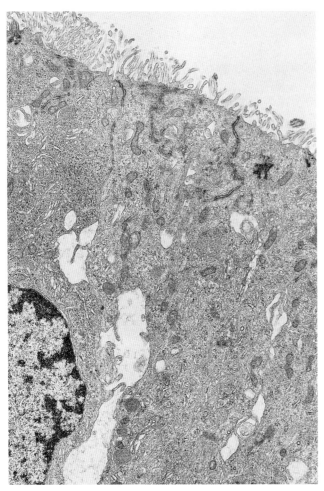

**FIGURE 4-219    EPENDYMOMA**

Ependymal "true" rosettes are formed of neoplastic cells joined apically by complex, "zipper-like," intermediate junctions. The small central lumen is filled with microvilli, scattered cilia, and cellular debris (× 8000).

ependyma. Decisive features include (1) gland-like lumens containing microvilli and cilia with basal bodies, (2) intracytoplasmic intermediate filaments, and (3) long, multipart "zipper-like" cell junctions (Figs. 4–219 and 4–220). The junctions are often extensive and, as robust structures, are well seen even in deparaffinized material. Single cells can also express their epithelial phenotype in the form of intracellular "lumens" with cilia and microvilli (Fig. 4–221).[12] Clear cell ependymomas exhibit all the ultrastructural features of more conventional ependymomas.[14] When the tumors show a conspicuous glial pattern of growth, the abundance of filament-containing processes may overshadow subtle, more diagnostic features.

**Differential Diagnosis.** The differential diagnosis of ependymoma must be formulated with knowledge of the location of the lesion. In the posterior fossa, *medulloblastoma* is the main pretender, although its cellularity and mitotic activity generally exceed that of

ependymoma. *Pilocytic astrocytoma* of the cerebellum or brain stem usually poses few diagnostic problems because it is less cellular, more piloid, and frequently micro- as well as macrocystic. Rosenthal fibers, which are classic features of pilocytic astrocytomas, can be seen in ependymomas and subependymomas, particularly those with a decidedly glial pattern of growth. *Diffuse astrocytomas* of the brain stem may project into the fourth ventricle, but their infiltrative nature, more so than their fibrillar quality and degree of nuclear atypia, usually facilitates a diagnosis. The prominent fibrillarity of some ependymomas was discussed earlier.

In the cerebral hemispheres, the alternative diagnosis of *oligodendroglioma* may arise when one is confronted with a clear cell ependymoma. Distinguishing the two lesions is the solid, noninfiltrating nature of the ependymoma, which is expressed as a shoving front relative to surrounding brain. Thus, sections stained for neurofilament protein record the absence or paucity of axons within the boundaries of the neoplasm (see Fig. 4–202). Also typical of clear cell ependymomas are GFAP-positive perivascular pseudorosettes, in at least some areas. Electron microscopy readily settles the issue (see earlier).

The rare papillary ependymoma may resemble the more common *choroid plexus papilloma*, but the distinction is usually not difficult. The fibrous stroma of choroid plexus papilloma mimics that of normal choroid plexus, whereas glia form the "stroma" beneath epithelial surfaces of the ependymoma. It is of note that focal ependymal differentiation is seen in some papillomas.

The differential diagnosis of an ependymoma in the suprasellar region and third ventricle, an uncommon site for this lesion, includes pituitary adenoma and "pilomyxoid glioma," discussed on pages 208 to 209, and central neurocytoma. The clinical and radiologic localization of a primary lesion in the sella turcica virtually excludes consideration of ependymoma—or any glial neoplasm, for that matter. Furthermore, *pituitary adenomas* lack GFAP positivity and are uniformly synaptophysin immunoreactive. *Pilomyxoid gliomas* may show perivascular pseudorosette formation resembling that seen in ependymoma (see Fig. 4–115), but these lesions are less cellular, looser in texture, and more myxoid than ependymomas. A *central neurocytoma* arising in the region of the foramen of Monro, or rarely in the third ventricle proper, is highly cellular and features a form of perivascular pseudorosette. Its cells, best seen in smear preparations, are more monomorphous than those of ependymoma. This focal expression of processes does not center on vessels. Both the crowded cells and the fibrillar areas react with antibodies to synaptophysin. GFAP staining may be localized to scattered cells, but overall, it is either negative or weak.

## Diagnostic Checklist

- Is an "ependymoma" near the foramen of Monro really a central neurocytoma?

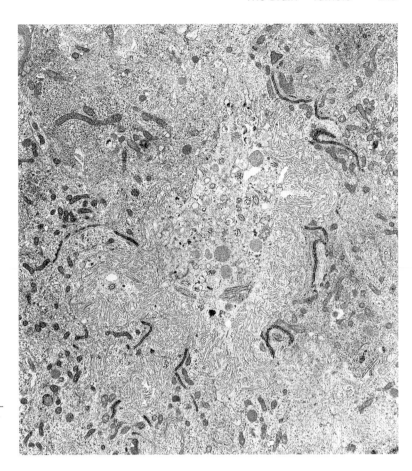

**FIGURE 4-220    EPENDYMOMA**

The luminal surface of a "true" ependymal rosette is defined by cells with prominent microvilli and scattered cilia. Note the complex intercellular junctions that join the apex of one cell to another.

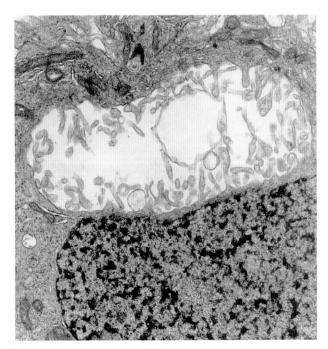

**FIGURE 4-221    EPENDYMOMA**

Minute, apparently intracellular "lumens" attest to the epithelial character of some ependymomas.

- Is the posterior fossa mass arising from the floor of the fourth ventricle of a child really an "ependymoastrocytoma" (a diagnosis that may confuse clinicians), or is it just an ependymoma with fibrillar zones?
- Is the high-grade glioma with focal perivascular pseudorosettes really malignant ependymoma, or are the overall neuroimaging and histologic features more consistent with glioblastoma?

**Treatment and Prognosis.** Many studies have affirmed the extent of surgical excision as the key prognostic factor.[2, 20, 24, 26, 31] Complete resection is possible in approximately 50% of cases, and the 5-year survival rate of approximately 50% may well be rising.[2, 20, 24, 26, 31]

There have been numerous studies of histologic grading as it relates to prognosis for patients with ependymomas. Some failed to find a relationship between grade and outcome[9], whereas others noted less favorable outcomes for patients with "anaplastic" tumors.[2, 15, 25, 30–32] Approaching the problem somewhat differently, one study found a higher incidence of craniospinal dissemination when the primary tumor was high grade (i.e., high mitotic activity, microvascular proliferation, and necrosis).[25]

The inconsistency between grading and outcome is not surprising, given the various definitions of "anaplasia" and "malignancy." There may also be site-dependent differences that relate to prognosis. In one study, for example, a high mitotic index was a predictive factor for supratentorial tumors but not for those in the posterior fossa.[30] Not to be underemphasized is the fact that many ependymomas are completely excised, histologically high grade or not. Resectability clearly reduces the predictive power of histologic features, as it does for other discrete and potentially excisable lesions such as meningioma, choroid plexus tumor, and PXA.

Although radiotherapy is generally administered for both low- and high-grade ependymomas, it has been suggested that it might not be needed when complete resection is well documented.[2]

When ependymomas recur, they usually do so locally and within several years after surgery. Only occasionally do they seed the subarachnoid space. The reported incidence of the latter ranges from 10% to 20%, but the median is approximately 10%.[2, 24, 25] Metastasis outside of the CNS is most unusual.[21] Recurrent lesions pose a therapeutic problem, as they are often more difficult to excise than the original tumors and no more sensitive to radiation and chemotherapy.

An interesting concept, Collin's law, suggests that the interval between surgery and symptomatic recurrence should not exceed the interval between conception and initial clinical presentation.[4, 33] This is relevant mainly for pediatric patients. Thus, a 6-year-old patient with a resected ependymoma might be viewed as being past the period of risk of recurrence after a postoperative tumor-free survival of 81 months. This hypothesis, of course, assumes that the postoperative growth rate of the neoplasm is no greater than that during the preoperative period, a supposition that ignores the capacity of ependymomas to become increasingly anaplastic over time. Anaplastic progression in ependymomas has not been as well documented as that in astrocytomas. Nonetheless, there is evidence of such a tendency.[1]

## Subependymoma

**Definition.** A well-differentiated, nodular, and highly fibrillar ependymal tumor generally situated within a ventricle. It is WHO grade I.

**General Comments.** The subependymoma has been viewed variously as a neoplasm of subependymal glia, astrocytes, ependymal cells, or an admixture thereof. In favor of an astrocytic derivation is its abundance of long processes rich in glial filaments. Supporting an ependymal origin are its circumscription, nuclear characteristics, ultrastructural features, and, particularly in fourth ventricular lesions, the coexistence of a conventional ependymoma component in some cases. Both suggestions may therefore be true.

**Clinical Features.** Subependymomas are most often encountered as incidental findings (see Fig. 4–225). Only rarely are they sufficiently bulky to obstruct the flow of CSF or to produce focal neurologic deficits.[6, 9] Presentation with intratumoral hemorrhage has been recorded (see Fig. 4–226).[2] Whether incidental or

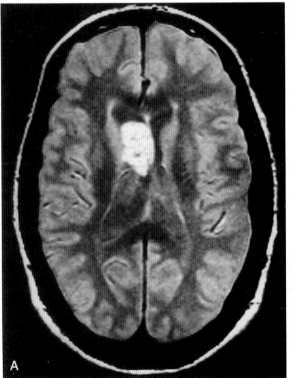
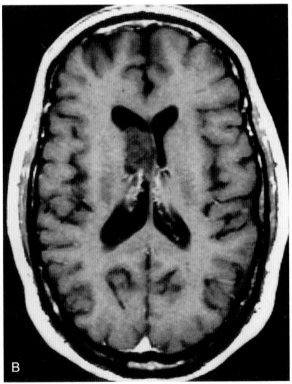

**FIGURE 4–222** SUBEPENDYMOMA

Subependymomas in the lateral ventricles usually arise near the foramen of Monro. Unlike most neoplasms that appear in this region, subependymomas distinctively show little or no contrast enhancement. This example, which appears bright in a proton-density image (*A*), showed no enhancement after administration of gadolinium (*B*).

symptomatic, they occur far more often in adults than in adolescents or children. Familial cases have been observed.[3, 14]

The lateral ventricle near the caudate nucleus[2, 9, 11, 12, 16, 18] and the floor of the fourth ventricle[1, 3, 5, 6, 9, 16] are the two most common locations. Like ependymomas, occasional examples occur near the surface of the brain.[8]

**Radiologic Features.** Most supratentorial subependymomas lie near the foramen of Monro as discrete masses fixed to the ventricle wall (Fig. 4–222). Among other regional neoplasms (central neurocytomas, choroid plexus tumors, and subependymal giant cell astrocytomas), they have the distinction of showing little if any contrast enhancement.[4, 7] Fourth ventricular examples grow from the floor (Fig. 4–223) and may, like ependymomas, extend laterally via the foramen of Luschka to reach the subarachnoid space. Dense calcification is common in subependymomas of the posterior fossa (Fig. 4–224). Contrast enhancement is minimal, if not absent, but it may be more prominent in fourth ventricle than in lateral ventricle lesions.[4, 7]

**Macroscopic Features.** As bosselated, flat-based tumors, subependymomas are firmly attached to their site of origin (Figs. 4–224 to 4–226). Secondarily, adherence may be established to adjacent ventricular surfaces. Although basically soft, tan, and solid, the texture of long-standing lesions may be modified by calcification, hemorrhage (see Fig. 4–226), or cyst formation.

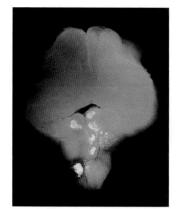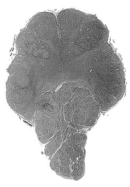

**FIGURE 4–224    SUBEPENDYMOMA**

A specimen radiograph and a whole mount histologic section illustrate the typical origin of these lobular, frequently calcified subependymomas from the floor of the fourth ventricle. Compare with Figure 4–223.

**Microscopic Features.** Although all subependymomas are paucicellular, highly fibrillar, and noted for clustering of nuclei, there are histologic peculiarities that are somewhat site specific.

Subependymomas near the foramen of Monro are individualized by the presence of microcysts that are often filled with a faintly basophilic material (Figs. 4–227 and 4–228). Some clustering of nuclei is present, but microcysts are often the dominant histologic feature. Cytoplasm is glassy, albeit scant, and the cells therefore appear more "astrocytic" than ependymal. In most instances, cells are cytologically bland, but scattered pleomorphic nuclei are

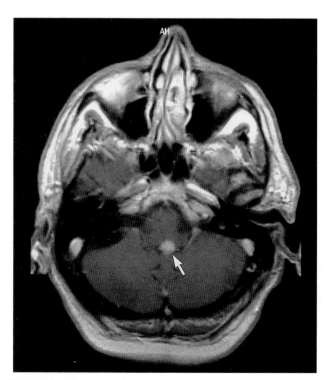

**FIGURE 4–223    SUBEPENDYMOMA**

Subependymomas in the fourth ventricle (*arrow*) usually arise from the medulla.

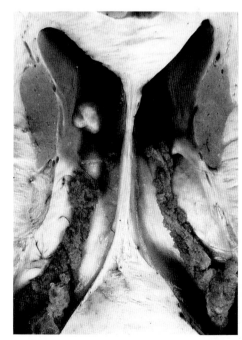

**FIGURE 4–225    SUBEPENDYMOMA**

Subependymomas of the lateral ventricle are usually incidental postmortem findings.

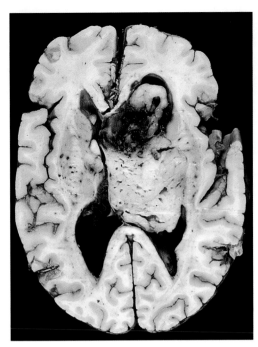

**FIGURE 4–226**    SUBEPENDYMOMA

Subependymomas arising near the foramen of Monro can be sizable and symptomatic. In this case, acute hemorrhage was responsible for an abrupt increase in intracranial pressure in a 46-year-old woman.

common in large, long-standing lesions. Occasional mitoses may be seen. Hyalinized vessels, with or without hemosiderin deposits, are also frequently seen. Lateral ventricular lesions are usually not calcified.

Subependymomas of the fourth ventricle are more closely related to ependymomas. They largely lack microcystic change and are more notable for a clustering of nuclei in a highly fibrillar background (Figs. 4–229 and 4–230). Calcification is common. Monotonous nuclei with elliptic outlines and uniform chromatin density are reminiscent of those of normal ependymal cells. Mitoses are rare. Rosenthal fibers are present in some cases.

Unusual features include a "sarcomatous" proliferation of the vasculature,[10] a rhabdomyosarcomatous component,[17] and melanosis.[15]

**Immunohistochemical Features.** Subependymomas are intensely GFAP positive, in accord with their high content of glial filaments. Vimentin and S-100 protein staining is widespread. Although in one study the MIB-1 staining index was virtually 0, occasional tumors show definite, albeit low, levels of reactivity. A low MIB-1 index, with a mean of 0.3%, was recorded in one study.[13]

**Ultrastructural Features.** In view of the highly fibrillar background of subependymomas, it is not surprising that electron microscopy demonstrates an abundance of closely packed cell processes filled with intermediate (glial) filaments (Fig. 4–231). Ependymal features, such as inter- or intracellular clusters of microvilli, cilia, and multipart "zipper-like" junctions, are most frequent in fourth ventricular tumors.[1, 5]

**Differential Diagnosis.** The differential diagnosis of a fourth ventricular subependymoma focuses naturally on *ependymoma*, from which a sharp distinction cannot always be drawn. Focally and at high magnification, the

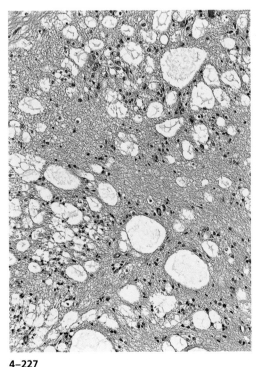

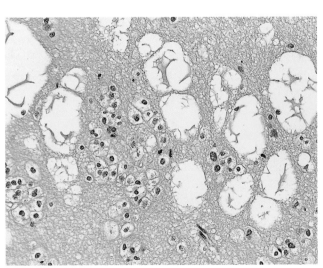

4–227                                 4–228

**FIGURES 4–227 AND 4–228**    SUBEPENDYMOMA

Subependymomas that arise near the foramen of Monro are lobular, sparsely cellular, and prone to microcystic change.

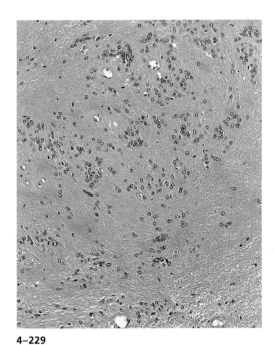

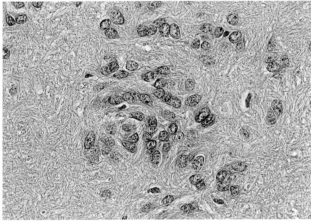

4–229                    4–230

**FIGURES 4–229 AND 4–230**  SUBEPENDYMOMA

As exemplified by this fourth ventricular lesion, subependymomas are lobular masses with a distinctive clustering of nuclei (Fig. 4–229). High magnification resolves the intervening fine fibrillar background and the typically bland nuclei (Fig. 4–230).

two neoplasms may be remarkably similar. Indeed, foci closely resembling subependymoma are commonly seen in fourth ventricular ependymomas. Ependymomas, however, occur primarily in children, are usually more cellular, and contain prominent perivascular pseudo-rosettes and, in some cases, true ependymal rosettes. Fourth ventricular subependymomas occur later in life and are usually more homogeneously subependymomal in appearance.

With their gross appearance, nodularity, clustering of nuclei, background fibrillarity, and microcysts, subependymomas of the lateral ventricle are distinctive and are unlikely to be confused with other lesions.

**Treatment and Prognosis.** Whereas subependymomas of the lateral ventricle may be resected with relative ease, total excision may not be as feasible when the tumor arises from the floor of the fourth ventricle.

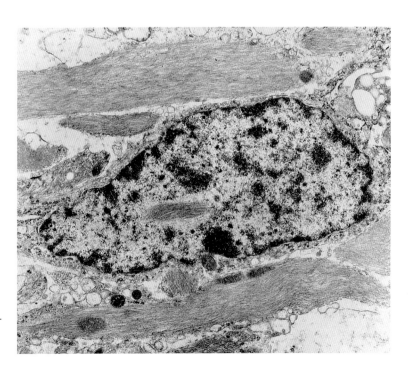

**FIGURE 4–231**  SUBEPENDYMOMA

The predominance of cellular processes is recorded at the ultrastructural level, where one nucleus is nestled among processes that are filled with glial filaments.

Nevertheless, the outlook is excellent.[13] Here, debulking and re-establishment of CSF flow suffice, in that these lesions grow slowly, and residual tumor may take years or decades to re-form a symptomatic mass. In contrast to ependymomas, radiotherapy is not recommended, even for incompletely resected, asymptomatic lesions.[9, 11]

## Other Gliomas

### Astroblastoma

**Definition.** A well-circumscribed, solid or cystic, often superficially situated tumor with a distinctive perivascular orientation of epithelioid neoplastic cells.

**General Comments.** As originally defined, the "astroblastoma" was a grade of diffuse astrocytoma intermediate between the well-differentiated astrocytoma and the spongioblastoma (later glioblastoma) multiforme.[3] The term was applied subsequently in a nonspecific manner to a disparate group of tumors linked only by the presence of glial cells that radiate about blood vessels ("astroblast formation"). We endorse the preceding restricted definition of "astroblastoma," because it is the one that the literature defines as a clinicopathologic entity.[2, 3] Ironically, it possesses a number of ependymomal features, at both light and electron

microscopic levels. Whatever its cellular derivation, astroblastoma poses a diagnostic problem to anyone unfamiliar with its distinctive architectural and histologic features.

**Clinical Features.** Astroblastomas can be found throughout the brain, and most occur during the first 3 decades of life and present with any element of the triad of mass effect, seizures, and focal neurologic deficit.[2, 3, 10] The cerebral hemispheres are far more often affected than is the posterior fossa.[2, 3] Congenital examples have been reported.[8]

**Radiologic Features.** Discreteness, superficial location, and contrast enhancement are common findings that, though nonspecific, clearly distinguish astroblastomas from diffuse astrocytomas with astroblast formation (Fig. 4–232).[1] As previously noted, some astroblastomas are cystic.

**Microscopic Features.** Although high-grade astroblastomas may show focal infiltration of brain parenchyma, most are solid, smoothly contoured, and noninfiltrating (Fig. 4–233). Little if any overrun brain tissue is found within the tumor substance. Astroblastomas therefore share fundamental architectural features with ependymomas, ganglion cell tumors, well-demarcated pilocytic astrocytomas, and PXAs (see Fig. 4–2).

One distinctive histologic attribute is a variant of perivascular pseudorosette, formed as tumor cell processes converge on vessels. The cellular processes are shorter and broader than those of ependymomas and are sometimes so short and stout that the cells have a decidedly epithelial appearance (Figs. 4–234 and 4–235).

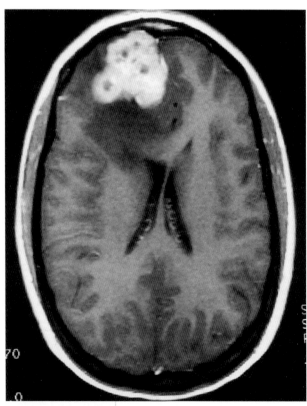

**FIGURE 4–232  ASTROBLASTOMA**

Astroblastomas generally appear in the cerebral hemispheres as discrete masses. This lesion in a 24-year-old woman was well differentiated, although it was associated with considerable peritumoral edema, as seen in a contrast-enhanced magnetic resonance imaging scan.

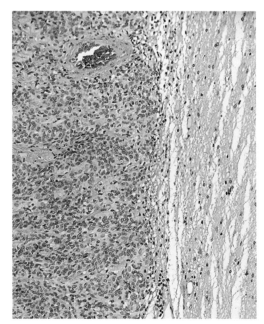

**FIGURE 4–233  ASTROBLASTOMA**

Astroblastomas typically have sharp borders, making them resectable in many cases.

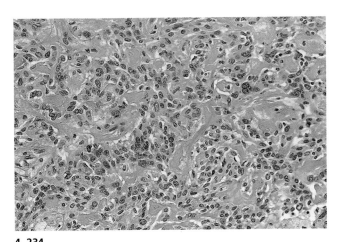

4-234

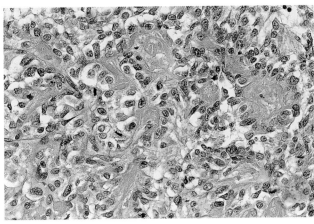

4-235

**FIGURES 4–234 AND 4–235    ASTROBLASTOMA**

Astroblastomas are compact, largely noninfiltrating masses with a form of perivascular pseudorosette reminiscent of that in ependymomas. Distinguishingly, the perithelial processes are thicker, shorter, and more epithelioid than fibrillar in appearance.

Given the generally single cell layer constituting the pseudorosettes and its short corona of processes, astroblastic pseudorosettes are commensurably smaller than those of ependymoma. They are also more uniform and more precisely defined. Large areas of the tumor may be devoid of pseudorosettes, however, and offer only solid, unrelieved sheets of tumor cells or the hyalinized tissue discussed later. Tissue dehiscence in rosette-rich areas produces pseudopapillae.

Another distinctive feature of astroblastoma is vascular thickening and progressive hyalinization that, when advanced, can crowd out the intervening tumor cells (Fig. 4–236). Little if any viable neoplastic tissue remains where this process has evolved to completion. Dystrophic calcification may be superimposed on this hyalinized tissue.

**Grading.** In terms of their histologic malignancy, astroblastomas reside along a continuum that has yet to be clearly linked to prognosis. Nuclear pleomorphism and mitotic activity are restrained in lower-grade lesions, whereas the latter feature is particularly conspicuous in higher-grade versions (Fig. 4–237). Necrosis and microvascular proliferation may also be present.[2, 3, 10]

**Immunohistochemical Features.** Intense GFAP positivity is expected in some, but not all, of the vessel-based cells (Fig. 4–238).[3, 5, 7] Staining for S-100 protein and vimentin is widespread. As in ependymoma, focal EMA reactivity is not uncommon but does not approach the degree or extent seen in carcinomas. MIB-1 labeling varies greatly.

**Ultrastructural Features.** The ependymomatous appearance of the lesion has its counterpart at the fine structural level, where cell surfaces may have microvilli and occasional cilia, and juxtaposed cell surfaces may be joined by zipper-like junctions.[2, 9] Whereas these

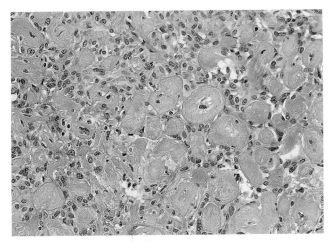

**FIGURE 4–236    ASTROBLASTOMA**

Vascular hyalinization is often prominent.

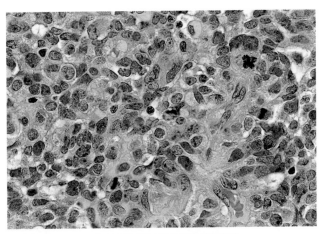

**FIGURE 4–237    MALIGNANT ASTROBLASTOMA**

Increased cellularity, mitotic activity, and cytologic atypia are indices of malignancy that may be focal in a lesion that is well differentiated elsewhere.

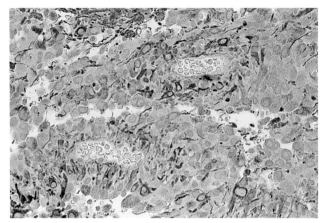

**FIGURE 4–238    ASTROBLASTOMA**

Typically, some of the perivascular glial processes are strongly immunopositive for glial fibrillary acidic protein, whereas others lack reactivity.

findings suggest an origin from subependymal glia,[2, 9] other studies reported less specific findings.[5–8]

**Molecular and Cytogenetic Features.** The cytogenetic changes are incompletely characterized. The most common findings in an initial small study were gains of chromosomes 19 and 20q—changes that are not common in ependymomas.[3]

**Differential Diagnosis.** Practically and conceptually, astroblastoma should be distinguished from *ependymoma*, a lesion that, in the cerebrum, can also occur near the brain surface. Distinguishing features are (1) the short, robust nature of the processes that construct perivascular pseudorosettes in astroblastoma (Fig. 4–239); (2) the often sizable portions of tumor that are devoid of these structures; and (3) the distinctive hyalinization of vessels. Whereas the pseudorosettes of ependymoma are diffusely GFAP positive, those of

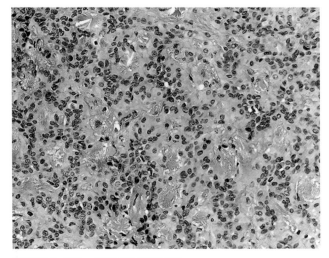

**FIGURE 4–239    ASTROBLASTOMA**

Although astroblastomas resemble ependymomas, the cytoplasm of the tumor cells that orient to vessels is more epithelioid than fibrillar.

astroblastoma often contain cells that are either very positive or immunonegative.

*Papillary meningioma* is another diagnostic consideration, because it too can mimic ependymoma based on uniformity in nuclear size and shape, as well as the formation of perivascular pseudorosettes. Such meningiomas often have an element of conventional meningioma and are far more immunoreactive for EMA than the occasional ependymoma and its true rosettes and epithelial surfaces. Inexplicably, immunopositivity for GFAP has been reported to occur in an occasional papillary meningioma.[4]

The discreteness and contrast enhancement of astroblastoma make an erroneous diagnosis of *diffuse astrocytoma* unlikely, although an astroblastic pattern is seen in some astrocytic tumors.

**Diagnostic Checklist**

- Is this "astroblastoma" really an ependymoma?
- Is this "astroblastoma" just a diffuse astrocytic neoplasm with astroblast formation?
- Is this "astroblastoma" really a papillary meningioma?

**Treatment and Prognosis.** Given the infrequent occurrence of astroblastoma, there is no consensus regarding its optimal treatment. A logical goal is gross total removal, in view of the lesion's solid, demarcated nature. Resection is possible in many instances, especially with low-grade tumors. Many fortunate patients may be cured.[2, 3, 10] Less frequently, resectable high-grade lesions may be fatal; nonetheless, even some of these patients survive after gross total resection and radiotherapy.[2, 3, 10]

### Chordoid Glioma of the Third Ventricle

**Definition.** A discrete, chordoma-like glioma typically occurring in the third ventricle.

**General Comments.** Chordoid glioma is a recently described entity that, to date, has been reported only in the third ventricle.[1, 2, 4, 5] Its cellular derivation has been debated. The possibility that the lesion is derived from a specialized form of ependyma in the subcommissural organ is discussed later in the section on ultrastructural features. We placed the tumor in the glioma group because of its immunoreactivity for GFAP and its content of intermediate (glial) filaments. Thus far, there is no convincing immunohistochemical, ultrastructural, or molecular evidence that chordoid glioma is linked to chordoid meningioma or chordoma.[1, 2, 4, 5]

**Clinical Features.** The lesion presents in adults with the generic symptoms attributable to any obstructing third ventricular mass. Females are more frequently affected.[1, 2, 4, 5]

**Radiologic Features.** The lesions are remarkably similar from case to case; all are discrete, smooth-contoured, contrast-enhancing, third ventricular masses that obstruct CSF flow and produce hydrocephalus (Fig. 4–240).[3]

**Macroscopic Features.** The solid, lobulated lesion often distends the third ventricle and adheres to its wall (Fig. 4–241).

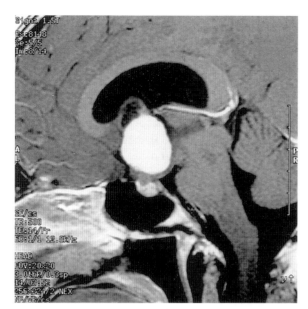

**FIGURE 4–240    CHORDOID GLIOMA OF THE THIRD VENTRICLE**

This typical lesion forms a well-circumscribed mass within the third ventricle.

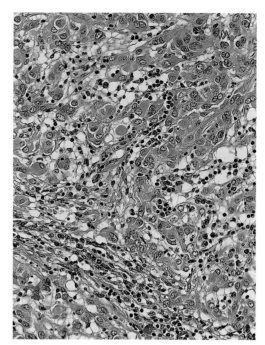

**FIGURE 4–242    CHORDOID GLIOMA OF THE THIRD VENTRICLE**

Cords of neoplastic epithelioid cells and a chronic inflammatory infiltrate are the essential features of this distinctive lesion.

**Microscopic Features.** In accord with the radiologic and macroscopic findings, the lesion has a sharp interface with surrounding brain parenchyma. Its substance consists of ribbons, cords, and lobules of uniform, epithelial-like cells in a faintly basophilic, mucinous matrix (Fig. 4–242). Nuclei are uniform, nucleoli are small, and mitoses are absent to rare. A prominent lymphoplasmacytic infiltrate is often interposed between the neoplastic cells. Perhaps unique to primary glial neoplasms, Russell bodies may be prominent (Fig. 4–243).

**Immunohistochemical Features.** The epithelioid tumor cells are positive for GFAP (Fig. 4–244) and focally may exhibit surface staining for EMA.

**Ultrastructural Features.** Two studies failed to find specific features,[1, 5] but one found similarities to modified ependymal cells of the subcommissural organ.[2]

**Differential Diagnosis.** The lesion must be distinguished from two other chordoid lesions—chordoid meningioma and chordoma—neither of which is GFAP positive. The lesion can be separated from *chordoid meningioma* by the absence of any meningioma-associated features, such as whorls and psammoma bodies, as well as interdigitating cell membranes and desmosomes at the ultrastructural level. Chordoid glioma lacks physaliphorous cells, as well as the cartilaginous quality of some *chordomas*.

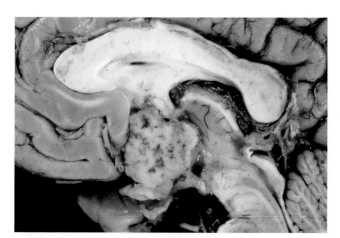

**FIGURE 4–241    CHORDOID GLIOMA OF THE THIRD VENTRICLE**

Although macroscopically discrete, the lesion is unfavorably situated and difficult to resect.

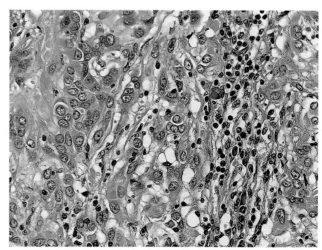

**FIGURE 4–243    CHORDOID GLIOMA OF THE THIRD VENTRICLE**

This tumor is almost unique among central nervous system neoplasms; the lymphoplasmacytic infiltrate contains Russell bodies.

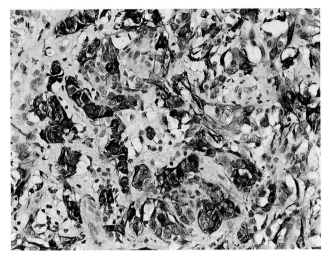

**FIGURE 4-244**   CHORDOID GLIOMA OF THE THIRD VENTRICLE

The tumor cells are immunoreactive for glial fibrillary acidic protein.

**Treatment and Prognosis.** Total resection has not been possible without serious residual neurologic deficits in most cases reported to date. Residual tumor has remained stable or grown only slowly.[1]

## Choroid Plexus Papilloma and Carcinoma

**Definition.** Papillary epithelial neoplasms derived from choroid plexus.

**General Comments.** Choroid plexus papilloma is an uncommon neoplasm, with satisfying macroscopic qualities that are complemented by the microscopic precision with which it reproduces its parent tissue. It is remarkable how much literature has been generated by this uncommon tumor, for which simple excision is almost always curative.

**Clinical Features.** Choroid plexus papillomas occur most frequently in the first decade of life. Rare cases are

diagnosed prenatally[3, 40] or at birth.[7, 8] Choroid plexus carcinomas usually present by age 3 years.[6, 15, 33, 35, 36] Any segment of the plexus is a potential site of origin, but there are certain general relationships between age and site. Thus, the lateral and, to a lesser extent, third ventricles[10] are favored during childhood for both papilloma and carcinoma, whereas the fourth ventricle most often plays host to papillomas in adults.[24] The lateral recess and cerebellopontine angle may be sites for papillomas.[39] Bilaterality has been observed.[19] Rare cases occur in Aicardi's syndrome, which includes psychomotor retardation, infantile spasms, corpus callosum agenesis, and chorioretinal abnormalities.[42] Germline mutations in p53 may also be a predisposing factor.[17, 43, 45]

Symptoms referable to choroid plexus papilloma include increased intracranial pressure due to obstruction to flow or overproduction of CSF.[6] Cerebrospinal seeding by carcinomas, and rarely by papillomas, may produce symptoms at various levels of the neuraxis.

**Radiologic Features.** Choroid plexus tumors, both benign and malignant, are intraventricular, intensely enhancing, discrete, and often obviously papillary (Fig. 4-245). Large and occasionally multiloculate cysts are commonly associated with large lesions of the lateral ventricle. Some tumors, mainly papillomas of the fourth ventricle, are densely calcified.

**Macroscopic Features.** Grossly, the fluid environment and the papillary architecture of these lesions call to mind coral (Figs. 4-246 and 4-247). Papillomas are often cinnamon colored. Some choroid plexus tumors bleed profusely.

**Microscopic Features.** In terms of differentiation, choroid plexus tumors span a broad spectrum that ranges from entirely benign grade I papillomas to anaplastic tumors with only focal epithelial features.

A striking microscopic feature of many papillomas is their virtual lack of architectural or cytologic abnormalities. Indeed, their uniform epithelial cells and stroma faithfully counterfeit the fronds of normal choroid plexus, sometimes replete with concretions and xanthomatous change. In such tumors, the neoplastic

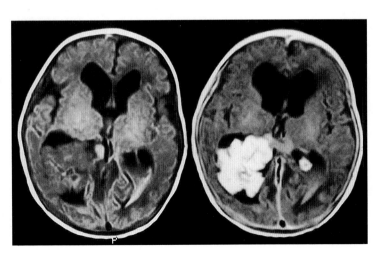

**FIGURE 4-245**   CHOROID PLEXUS PAPILLOMA

As seen here before and after the administration of gadolinium, papillomas of the choroid plexus are discrete, lobulated, papillary, intraventricular, and intensely contrast enhancing.

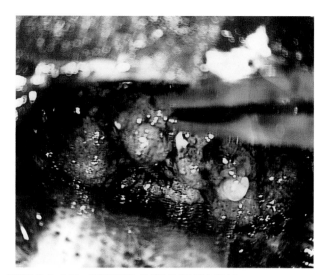

**FIGURE 4–246**   CHOROID PLEXUS PAPILLOMA

Papillomas of the choroid plexus are discrete, gray, and papillary. This lesion, in a lateral ventricle of a 6-month-old, was detected during a workup for increased head circumference. Limitation of upward gaze was a consequence of the hydrocephalus. (Courtesy of Dr. Jon D. Weingart, Baltimore, MD.)

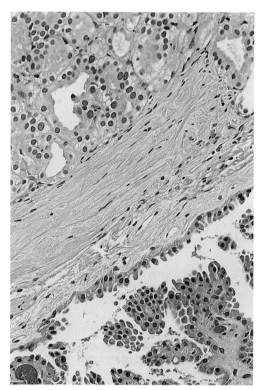

**FIGURE 4–248**   CHOROID PLEXUS PAPILLOMA AND NORMAL CHOROID PLEXUS

The distinction between papilloma (*top*) and normal choroid plexus (*bottom*) is apparent even at low magnification.

columnar cells are strikingly regular, squarely seated on underlying fibrovascular stroma, and lack mitotic activity. In most papillomas, however, the counterfeit is less than perfect, their cells being more crowded, more columnar, and more pleomorphic than the "cobblestoned" cells of the normal choroid plexus (Figs. 4–248 to 4–252).

Osseous[13, 14] or cartilaginous metaplasia, oncocytic change,[38] and acinar or tubular architecture (Fig. 4–253)[1, 4] are points of "scenic interest" in rare cases. Unusual cases have distinctive foci of "chondroid" differentiation. Only a rare lesion is pigmented with a brown, Fontana-positive substance that is neuromelanin in some instances (Fig. 4–254)[37, 44] and neural crest melanin (melanosome associated) in others.[26] The neoplasm

occasionally expresses glial properties in the form of "ependymal differentiation" expressed as the production of long, fibrillar, GFAP-positive processes (Figs. 4–255 and 4–256).

The point of distinction between papilloma and low-grade carcinoma is arbitrary, but the diagnosis of carcinoma is unambiguous in the face of marked architectural complexity; partially solid, nonpapillary growth; marked cytologic atypia; brisk mitotic activity; atypical mitoses; and obvious necrosis (Figs. 4–257 and 4–258). Although differing in degree, invasion of surrounding parenchyma may be seen in both papillomas and carcinomas but is more common in the latter.[41] Most carcinomas express their epithelial phenotype, at least focally, as poorly formed papillations or nests of epithelial cells with defined borders (Fig. 4–259). At the extremes of anaplasia, the neoplasms are largely small cell neoplasms (Fig. 4–260), although almost all contain better-differentiated areas with at least a suggestion of epithelial differentiation.

High-grade carcinomas have few if any papillary qualities and are recognized as epithelial only by the zonal uniformity of plump cells with defined borders. Areas rich in undifferentiated, pleomorphic, or giant cells are seen in some cases. In occasional high-grade lesions, sheets of small cells with perinuclear halos create the appearance of an oligodendroglioma (see Fig. 4–260). Hyaline droplet formation may be a prominent feature of pleomorphic carcinomas of infancy (Fig. 4–261).

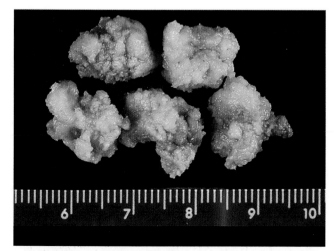

**FIGURE 4–247**   CHOROID PLEXUS PAPILLOMA

The papillary nature of the excised lesion often permits a presumptive gross diagnosis.

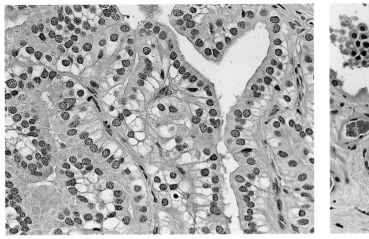

4–249

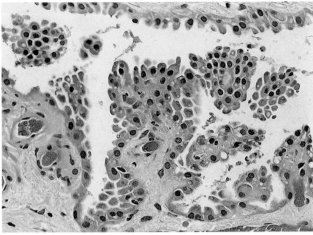

4–250

**FIGURES 4–249 AND 4–250**    CHOROID PLEXUS PAPILLOMA

The epithelium of the choroid plexus papilloma is columnar (Fig. 4–249), whereas the normal choroid plexus has a low cuboidal, "cobblestone" profile (Fig. 4–250).

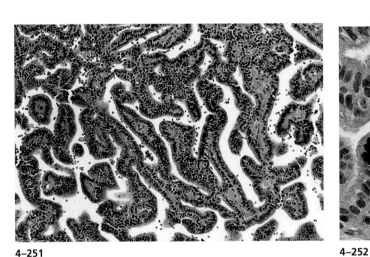

4–251

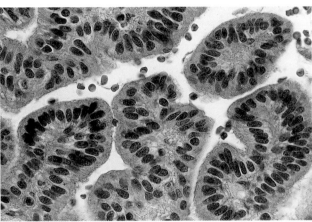

4–252

**FIGURES 4–251 AND 4–252**    CHOROID PLEXUS PAPILLOMA

Most choroid plexus tumors are papillomas with very well differentiated columnar epithelia.

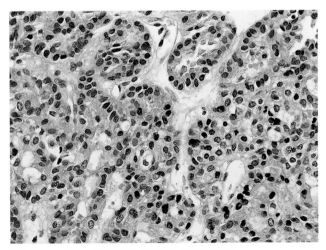

**FIGURE 4–253**    CHOROID PLEXUS PAPILLOMA

Some choroid plexus tumors are more adenomatous than papillary.

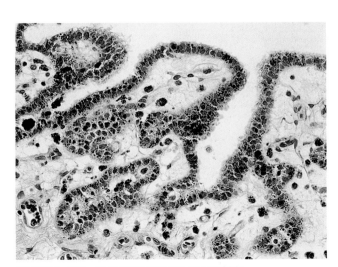

**FIGURE 4–254**    CHOROID PLEXUS PAPILLOMA

A rare papilloma is melanotic.

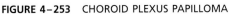

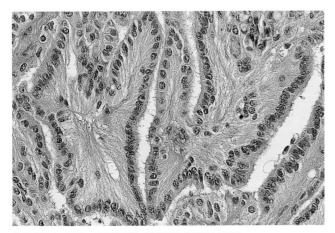

**FIGURE 4–255**   CHOROID PLEXUS PAPILLOMA

Expansion of tumor cell cytoplasm with formation of linear processes is termed "ependymal differentiation."

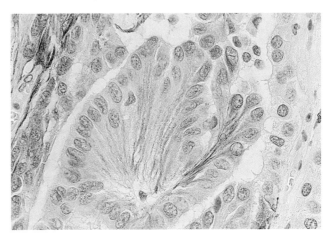

**FIGURE 4–256**   CHOROID PLEXUS PAPILLOMA

The linear cell processes in ependymal differentiation are well seen after staining for glial fibrillary acidic protein.

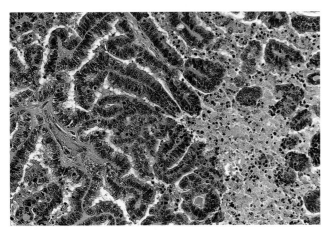

**FIGURE 4–257**   CHOROID PLEXUS CARCINOMA

The illustrated degree of mitotic activity and cytologic atypia exceeds that of papilloma or "atypical papilloma." The presence of necrosis, though occasionally seen in papilloma, lends support to the diagnosis of carcinoma.

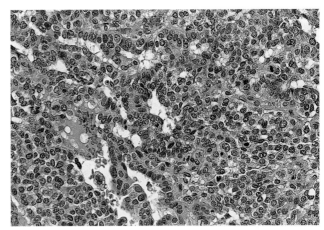

**FIGURE 4–258**   CHOROID PLEXUS CARCINOMA

Solid, nonpapillary areas are common in carcinomas.

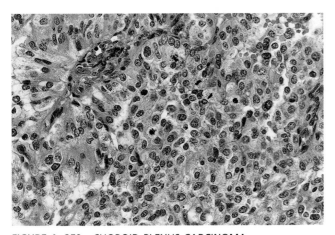

**FIGURE 4–259**   CHOROID PLEXUS CARCINOMA

Epithelial differentiation may be only focal, as seen here in the perithelial region.

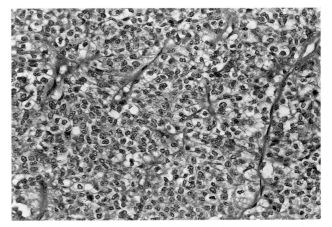

**FIGURE 4–260**   CHOROID PLEXUS CARCINOMA

Anaplastic carcinomas may resemble malignant oligodendrogliomas.

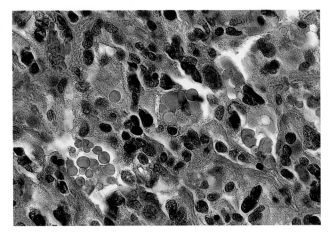

**FIGURE 4–261**   CHOROID PLEXUS CARCINOMA

Hyaline droplets are present in some pleomorphic carcinomas.

Transition from normal to neoplastic choroid plexus with variable atypia is frequently seen in both papillomas and carcinomas. Sequential biopsies showing increasing atypia and anaplasia are exceptional.[20, 35]

**Cytologic Features.** Papillary tissue fragments are readily apparent in well-differentiated tumors (Fig. 4–262). Nuclear uniformity is expected in papillomas, whereas high cellularity, cytologic atypia (nuclear pleomorphism and hyperplasia, nucleolar enlargement), mitoses, and necrosis are common features of carcinomas.

**Immunohistochemical Features.** Most choroid plexus tumors are reactive for S-100 protein and cytokeratins (Fig. 4–263). Synaptophysin has been suggested as a possible marker for choroid plexus epithelium (Fig. 4–264),[21, 25] but other laboratories have not found this useful.[34] Staining for EMA is focal at best.[9, 11, 25, 28, 35] "Ependymal differentiation" is evidenced by GFAP positivity in a minority of papillomas (see Fig. 4–256). A laminin-positive basement membrane, similar to that

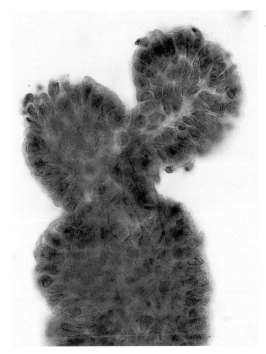

**FIGURE 4–262**   CHOROID PLEXUS PAPILLOMA—SMEAR PREPARATION

The papilloma's epithelial nature is well seen in a smear preparation.

seen in an occasional ependymoma, underlies the epithelium.[16] Although prealbumin (transthyretin) has been touted as a marker of choroid plexus and its neoplasms,[22] staining may be only focal and weak and can be present in metastatic carcinomas.[2, 5, 35] Choroid plexus carcinomas often lack uniform S-100 protein staining and occasionally show EMA reactivity. Carcinoembryonic antigen immunoreactivity is not a feature of choroid plexus tumors.

Mean MIB-1 labeling indices in papillomas and carcinomas generally are less than 10% and greater than 25%, respectively. The incidence of nuclear staining for p53 protein is said to be considerably higher in carcinomas than in papillomas.[23]

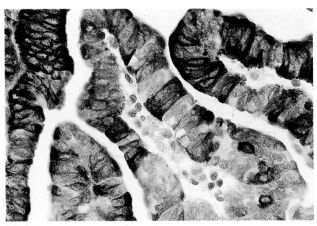

4–263

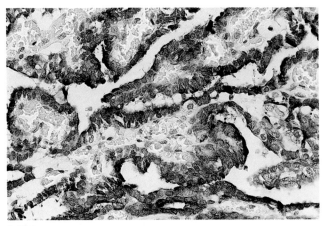

4–264

**FIGURES 4–263 AND 4–264**   CHOROID PLEXUS PAPILLOMA

Papillomas are immunoreactive for cytokeratins (Fig. 4–263) and synaptophysin (Fig. 4–264).

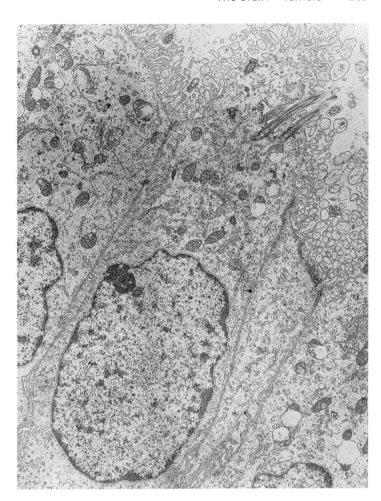

**FIGURE 4–265**    CHOROID PLEXUS PAPILLOMA

Columnar cells of choroid plexus papillomas have cilia and blunt apical microvilli. Intermediate junctions bind the apical ends of the cells.

**Ultrastructural Features.** The cells of all but the most poorly differentiated choroid plexus neoplasms exhibit apical microvilli and scattered cilia, apical junctional complexes, interdigitating lateral cell borders, a basal lamina that separates cells from underlying stroma, and fenestrated capillaries (Fig. 4–265).[12, 29, 32] Not surprisingly, cilia may exhibit the 9 + 0 microtubule config-

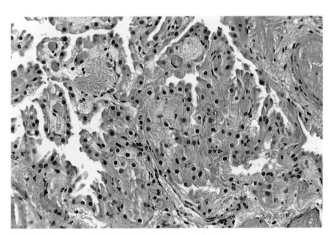

**FIGURE 4–266**    NORMAL CHOROID PLEXUS

As an artifact of tissue compression during biopsy, an apparent hypercellularity can misrepresent normal choroid plexus as papilloma. The tissue retains its normal "hobnail" appearance.

uration characteristic of neuroepithelial cells.[30] Even high-grade carcinomas often show essential epithelial features, as well as cilia and microvilli.

**Differential Diagnosis.** Although the problem is often more apparent than real, the most frequent differential diagnostic challenge is the exclusion of *normal choroid plexus* (Fig. 4–266; see also Fig. 4–499). The latter has remarkably regular, uncrowded cells with cobblestoned apices, whereas papilloma has an epithelium that is somewhat more crowded and cytologically varied. Attention to neuroradiologic studies is also helpful. The diagnosis of papilloma is difficult to defend in the absence of a contrast-enhancing intraventricular mass.

The finding of a papillary lesion within a ventricle requires exclusion of a rare *papillary ependymoma*. The distinction is rarely difficult. Cells of the ependymoma form epithelial surfaces but also intermingle with the stroma, where their fibrillar nature is readily apparent. Because many papillomas have GFAP-positive cells (see Fig. 4–256), one can challenge the distinction of choroid plexus papilloma from ependymoma. However, even papillomas that express ependymal differentiation remain phenotypically epithelial, whereas ependymomas with papillary change can generally be distinguished by their predominantly glial architecture. In the unlikely event that the distinction cannot be made in

H&E-stained tissues, immunohistochemistry can be helpful; strong staining for low-molecular-weight keratin (e.g., CAM 5.2) typifies choroid plexus tumors.

In adults, choroid plexus carcinomas are so rare that the diagnosis must be rigorously defended against the greater likelihood of *metastatic carcinoma*. Fortunately, the differential is not common. The distinction may be difficult in light of shared cytologic, ultrastructural, and immunohistochemical features. In our experience, lack of significant EMA and carcinoembryonic antigen immunoreactivity typifies choroid plexus carcinoma. It has also been suggested that immunoreactivity for synaptophysin distinguishes choroid plexus tumors.[25] BerEp4 staining is, in concept, a marker of carcinomas rather than plexus carcinomas. In the very young, the differential diagnosis of choroid plexus carcinoma must include *atypical teratoid/rhabdoid tumor*. The morphologic features of the latter, including its diverse immunophenotype, are described on pages 336 to 339.

### Diagnostic Checklist

- Is this "papilloma" just normal choroid plexus?
- Is this highly anaplastic "choroid plexus carcinoma" in an infant really an atypical teratoid tumor?

**Treatment and Prognosis.** The therapy of choroid plexus papillomas is, first and foremost, surgical resection. Nearly all patients are cured.[33, 36] The same favorable outcome is also true of some patients with carcinomas.[6, 18, 36] Even occasional recurrent carcinomas are cured by reoperation and adjuvant therapy.[15] So-called atypical choroid plexus papillomas—lesions at the cusp between papilloma and carcinoma—usually follow a benign course. Indeed, one study suggested that occasional mitoses, microscopic infiltration, and moderate atypia were not harbingers of aggressive behavior.[31] Recurrences are almost always local, although CSF seeding occurs in some carcinomas[18] and even a rare papilloma.[27] Systemic metastases are rare.[18] Not surprisingly, a tumor may be more malignant at recurrence than at the time of initial resection.[20, 35]

In view of the young age of most patients with carcinomas, radiotherapy is often initially withheld. Chemotherapy may be used, with radiotherapy reserved for a later date.[36] The need for either radio- or chemotherapy for totally resected carcinomas is debatable. This is especially true when "carcinoma" is so loosely defined as to include lesions with only moderate crowding, cytologic atypia, and mitotic activity.[33, 36]

Persistent and refractory subdural fluid accumulations are a common problem following resection of papillomas or carcinomas that present with marked ventricular dilatation.[36]

## Neuronal, Glioneuronal, and Neurocytic Tumors

### *Gangliocytoma and Ganglioglioma*

**Definition.** Neoplasms that consist entirely of large neurons (gangliocytoma) or admixtures of neurons and

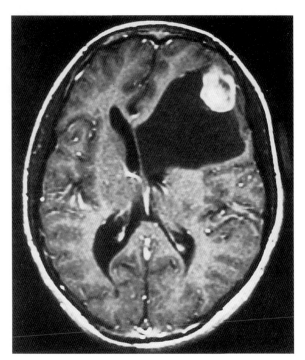

**FIGURE 4–267    GANGLIOGLIOMA**

The classic neuroimage of a ganglion cell tumor is a contrast-enhancing nodule in the wall of a cyst. This 13-year-old patient complained of pain behind the eye.

glia (ganglioglioma). Gangliocytomas are WHO grade I. Gangliogliomas may be grade I or grade II.

**General Comments.** Neoplasms with large neurons ("ganglion cells") form a diverse group of hamartomatous and neoplastic lesions. The classic ganglioglioma and gangliocytoma are described in detail later. A desmoplastic variant that occurs in the very young—desmoplastic infantile ganglioglioma—is discussed in a separate section. The rare malignant gangliogliomas are described on

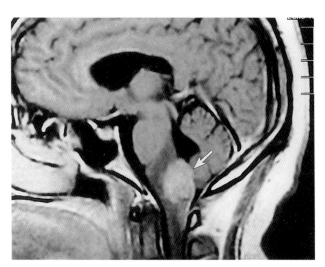

**FIGURE 4–268    GANGLIOGLIOMA**

Ganglion cell tumors occur throughout the brain and spinal cord. This ganglioglioma of the medulla (*arrow*) produced headaches and dizziness in a 29-year-old man.

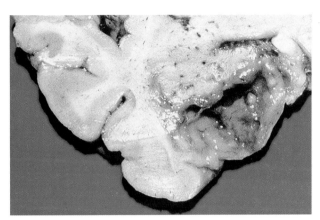

**FIGURE 4-269    GANGLIOGLIOMA**

A cyst wall nodule is common in gangliogliomas. The patient was an 18-year-old student with a lifelong history of seizures.

pages 290 to 292, and neurocytic neoplasms with ganglion cells are discussed on pages 285 and 287.

**Clinical Features.** Ganglion cell tumors occur throughout the neuraxis but favor supratentorial loci, especially the temporal lobe (see Fig. 4–269).[11] No site, including the cerebellum,[9] optic chiasm,[18] and brain stem (see Fig. 4–268),[15] is immune, not even the epiphysis.[5] Children and young adults are most often affected, but some ganglion cell tumors remain subclinical for many decades. Seizures, the most frequent presentation, may antedate surgical intervention by many years.[8, 11, 16, 23–25]

**Radiologic Features.** Although ganglion cell tumors can be either cystic (Fig. 4–267) or solid (Fig. 4–268),[3, 8, 10, 27] the cyst–mural nodule configuration is the quintessential configuration. There is little published information that draws a distinction between ganglioglioma and gangliocytoma, although contiguous extension in the subarachnoid space is more a quality of the former. This extension should not be misinterpreted as aggressive or malignant behavior.[28] Both gangliogliomas and gangliocytomas grow slowly, and either can remodel the inner table of the skull by their chronic compressive effects. CT frequently detects calcification. Table 4–7, p. 205 presents the radiologic features of well-differentiated lesions such as ganglion cell tumors.

**Macroscopic Features.** The lesions are generally well circumscribed and may sit as a mural nodule in the wall of a cyst (Fig. 4–269).

**Microscopic Features.** An important feature of many ganglion cell tumors is a compact, largely noninfiltrative pattern of growth, so that little if any infiltrated brain is seen within the lesion (Fig. 4–270). Figure 4–2 lists CNS tumors with this pattern of growth. Some ganglion cell tumors are located superficially, with their epicenter in the cortex or even subarachnoid space. Ensheathed surface vessels, a common feature of astrocytomas with a favorable prognosis, are often present in such superficial masses. Lateral extension within the subarachnoid space is not aggressive behavior; rather, it is a reassuring finding that suggests that one is dealing with a low-grade lesion such as a ganglion cell tumor, pilocytic astrocytoma, or PXA (Fig. 4–271).

The most elementary of the ganglion cell tumors—gangliocytoma—is a jumble of large neurons in a finely fibrillar, neuropil-rich stroma that is composed of tumor cell processes, that is, axons and dendrites (Figs. 4–272 and 4–273). The cellularity does not always exceed that of normal gray matter. Indeed, the lesion may even be hypocellular, because it lacks the complement of small neurons and specialized glia that populates the normal cortex. The neurons are not only disorganized and abnormally juxtaposed but also cytologically abnormal, varying in size and configuration. They often have cytoplasmic vacuolation, coarse or irregularly distributed

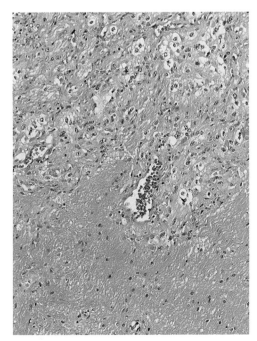

**FIGURE 4-270    GANGLIOGLIOMA**

Ganglion cell tumors are usually well demarcated.

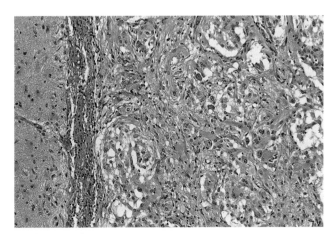

**FIGURE 4-271    GANGLIOGLIOMA**

Gangliogliomas often expand within the subarachnoid space.

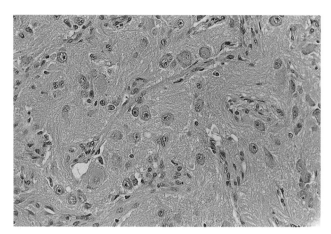

**FIGURE 4–272    GANGLIOGLIOMA**

Given their cytologic composition and architectural features, gangliogliomas often somewhat resemble disordered gray matter.

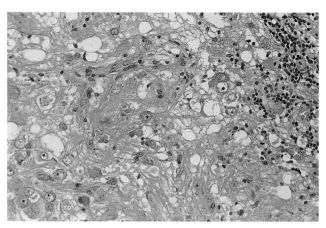

**FIGURE 4–274    GANGLIOCYTOMA**

The ganglion cells are too numerous and closely packed to represent normal neurons. The presence of perivascular lymphocytes should prompt consideration of the diagnosis of ganglion cell tumor.

Nissl substance, and nuclear abnormalities. The last may include binucleation, as well as striking variations in nuclear and nucleolar size and shape. The presence of somewhat less mature neurons ("ganglioid" cells) in transition to large cells confirms that the large, dysmorphic neurons are themselves neoplastic and not just trapped normal elements. Perivascular lymphocytes are common (Fig. 4–274).

Gangliogliomas are more complex than gangliocytomas (Figs. 4–275 to 4–278). The ganglion cell component may be dominant or subordinate and may be intimately admixed with the glial elements or spatially segregated in distinct clusters or lobules. Although the tumors have both glia and neurons, the astrocytes may be sparse, and it is often difficult to assign such cells to either neoplastic or reactive categories. Fortunately, this distinction has little prognostic significance. The division between gangliocytoma and ganglioglioma is further confounded by the occasional presence of large, pleomor-

phic cells with indeterminate histologic and immunocytologic features. The cells resemble both astrocytes and ganglion cells. The inclusive term "ganglion cell tumor" is appropriate in this setting. The glial component of most gangliogliomas is prominent. Interestingly, it can be either "fibrillary" or pilocytic.

Although no simple description of ganglion cell tumors can encompass all their architectural variations, there are several common patterns. Microcysts are common in gangliogliomas and may overshadow the aggregated or dispersed ganglion cells (see Figs. 4–275 and 4–276). Alternatively, ganglion cells may be gathered into distinct lobules with a reticulin- and collagen-rich internodular stroma (see Figs. 4–277 and 4–278).

EGBs are diagnostically important components of most ganglion cell tumors (Fig. 4–279). As seen in favorable tissue sections and in smear preparations, these

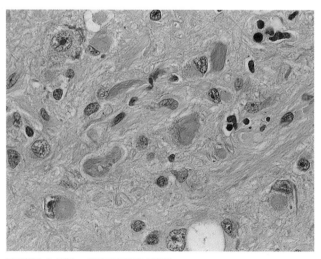

**FIGURE 4–273    GANGLIOGLIOMA**

Tumoral ganglion cells are susceptible to neurofibrillary change.

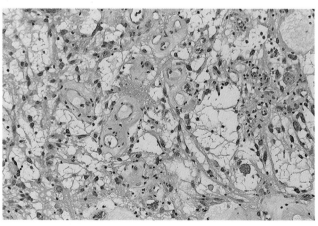

**FIGURE 4–275    GANGLIOGLIOMA**

Ganglion cell tumors with microcystic change may resemble pilocytic astrocytomas. Confirmation of the diagnosis may require immunohistochemistry. Note the eosinophilic granular body at the bottom right.

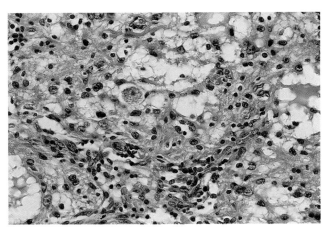

**FIGURE 4–276    GANGLIOGLIOMA**

It can be difficult to establish that ganglion cells with this degree of differentiation are part of the neoplasm, not merely trapped normal neurons. Lymphoid infiltrates are common in ganglion cell tumors.

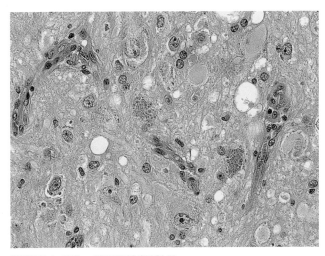

**FIGURE 4–279    GANGLIOGLIOMA**

Eosinophilic granular bodies are a common feature of ganglion cell tumors.

aggregates of small, brightly eosinophilic, hyaline droplets occupy the cytoplasm or processes of astrocytes. PAS positivity facilitates their detection. Although EGBs occur in other grade I and II lesions, such as pilocytic astrocytomas and PXAs, they are most numerous in ganglion cell tumors, especially gangliogliomas (see Table 4–8, p. 211 for CNS tumors with EGBs). They occasionally appear in high-grade infiltrating gliomas, but this is exceptional. EGBs should be taken as presumptive evidence of a well-differentiated neoplasm, particularly a relatively well-circumscribed tumor such as a pilocytic astrocytoma, PXA, or ganglion cell tumor.

Microcalcification may be prominent. Perivascular lymphocytic infiltrates are a frequent feature (see Figs. 4–274 and 4–276). A rare ganglioglioma is melanotic.[13]

Although neurons in ganglion cell tumors are interesting in their own right, some have the added appeal of

neurofibrillary change or granulovacuolar degeneration (see Fig. 4–273).[12] The former is a basophilic, faintly fibrillar blush in the cytoplasm that can be stained by any number of silver methods or, as is discussed later, by special immunohistochemical methods. Granulovacuolar degeneration, a less common feature, creates minute basophilic granules within small cytoplasmic vacuoles. These two alterations, conventionally associated with aging and Alzheimer's disease, are of no diagnostic significance but demonstrate that (1) even tumoral neurons are subject to neurodegenerative changes and (2) neurofibrillary change can occur in the absence of stainable amyloid. They appear to be somewhat more frequent in ganglion cell tumors in "older" patients—those beyond the fourth decade.[1]

Among the ganglion cell tumors, gangliocytomas in particular have been considered malformative or hamartomatous rather than neoplastic. As supportive evidence,

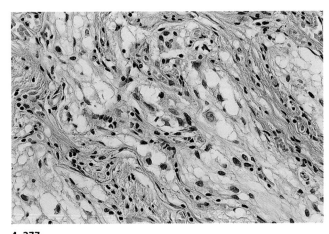

4–277

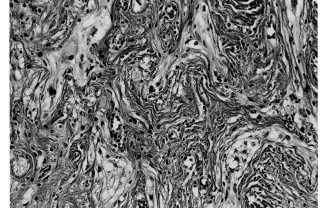

4–278

**FIGURES 4–277 AND 4–278    GANGLIOGLIOMA**

In desmoplastic lesions, islands of ganglion cell–containing neoplastic tissue (Fig. 4–277) are more readily identified after staining for connective tissue (Fig. 4–278).

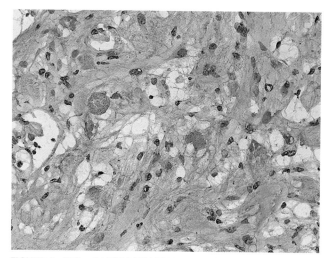

**FIGURE 4–280    GANGLIOGLIOMA—FROZEN SECTION**

The eosinophilic granular body on the left suggests the diagnosis of ganglion cell tumor or other well-differentiated discrete lesion such as pilocytic astrocytoma or pleomorphic xanthoastrocytoma. The cytologic atypia often seen in these tumors should not be misinterpreted as evidence of a high-grade neoplasm.

cortical dysplasia occurs in the cortex surrounding some ganglion cell tumors.[20]

Neuronal neoplasms composed largely of ganglion cells, "ganglioid cells," and neuroblasts (i.e., "ganglioneuroblastomas") are discussed on pages 311.

**Features in Frozen Sections.** Ganglion cells are vulnerable to freezing; they become smudged and disfigured and are easily overlooked (Fig. 4–280). Because attention is naturally drawn to the more conspicuous, pleomorphic, glial component, the diagnosis of high-grade astrocytoma is encouraged. Thus, the features of the lesion as seen in a frozen section do not always create an imperative for the diagnosis, although

pathologists should be programmed to consider the diagnosis in the presence of a radiologically discrete, enhancing, often cystic tumor, especially in a youthful patient. Fortunately, EGBs are largely unaffected by freezing and contrast nicely with the cells of this often pale-staining tumor. Perivascular lymphocytes also serve as clues.

**Cytologic Features.** Cellular processes of the glial component of gangliogliomas, whether "fibrillary" or pilocytic, produce a distinctive fibrillar background. The large neurons, with their open chromatin, prominent nucleoli, and ample amphophilic cytoplasm, are often a minority element.

**Immunohistochemical Features.** Synaptophysin is the most commonly used marker for neurons. This antibody labels the surface of ganglion cells, coating them with a granular deposit and leaving the cytoplasm only lightly stained, if at all (Fig. 4–281).[4, 19] This localization can make it difficult to assess whether the staining is bona fide or just positivity of surrounding compressed neuropil.

To complicate matters, a controversy has developed regarding the significance of surface staining for synaptophysin. It was originally envisioned as a marker of neuronal differentiation and also as an indicator of neuronal neoplasia.[19] Subsequently, however, studies of the normal CNS demonstrated similar staining of ganglion cells in spinal cord,[32] cerebellum, brain stem, basal ganglia, and hippocampus.[17, 21] Although neurons in normal cerebral cortex seemingly do not stain,[17, 21] reactivity can be induced by the presence of non-neoplastic lesions such as vascular malformations.[21] Thus, membrane pattern synaptophysin immunoreactivity per se should not be interpreted as incontrovertible evidence of neuronal neoplasia.

We usually complement staining for synaptophysin with immunostaining for chromogranin, which, when

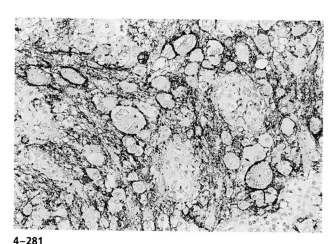

4–281

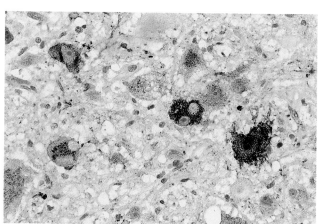

4–282

**FIGURES 4–281 AND 4–282    GANGLIOGLIOMA**

Antibodies to synaptophysin (Fig. 4–281) and chromogranin (Fig. 4–282) are useful in identifying ganglion cells.

positive, stains cytoplasm in a finely granular pattern (Fig. 4–282). Like synaptophysin, antisera to chromogranin recognize some normal neurons in surgical material, so that staining is not indicative of neoplasia. Nevertheless, cells that exhibit punctate cytoplasmic staining are clearly neuronal. Usually, only a minority of the neurons within ganglion cell tumors are immunopositive. Chromogranin preparations demonstrate these cells in a high percentage of gangliogliomas.[11]

Antibodies directed against neurofilament protein also have diagnostic application, but only when tissue is optimally fixed. The affinity is directed to the cytoplasm, particularly the neuritic processes. Anti-Hu[7] and NeuN[30] have the advantage of staining nuclei rather than cytoplasm, thus overcoming many of the interpretive limitations of synaptophysin.

Although the glial component of gangliogliomas is immunoreactive for S-100 protein and often stains intensely for GFAP (Fig. 4–283),[4] these antibodies do not always differentiate neurons from large astrocytes. Both cellular species may either lack reactivity for either antigen or, conversely, stain for both. Collagen type IV and laminin can be demonstrated, particularly in long-standing ganglion cell tumors.[14] Whether this marks the occurrence of schwannian differentiation is an unresolved issue.

A number of neurotransmitter substances, including vasoactive intestinal polypeptide, neurotensin, serotonin, somatostatin, met-enkephalin, and tyrosine hydroxylase,[6, 11, 26] have also been demonstrated in ganglion cells.[6, 11, 26] Silver stains, such as Bielschowsky's method, and immunohistochemistry for tau protein or ubiquitin confirm the occasional presence of neurofibrillary tangles. As a rule, however, H&E-stained sections alone are sufficient to identify these subtle but distinctive neuronal structures.

**Ultrastructural Features.** Electron microscopy strengthens the diagnosis of ganglioglioma if dense-core granules are abundant, because they are not found in sig-

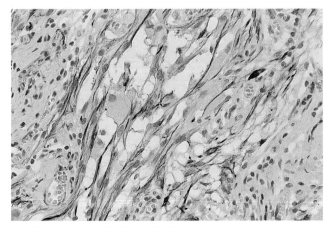

**FIGURE 4–283     GANGLIOGLIOMA**

Immunostains for glial fibrillary acidic protein highlight the glial component of gangliogliomas.

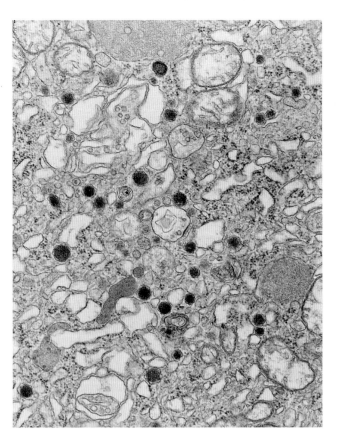

**FIGURE 4–284     GANGLIOGLIOMA**

As the ultrastructural equivalent of chromogranin immunoreactivity, neurosecretory or "dense-core" granules are a common feature of ganglion cell tumors.

nificant numbers within normal cerebral neurons (Fig. 4–284).[4, 11, 22] Although the doctrine of *res ipsa loquitur* can be invoked if microtubule-containing processes of neoplastic cells form synapses, it is often impossible to establish whether these cells are neoplastic or merely trapped normal neurons. Neurofibrillary tangles exhibit the classic architecture of paired helical filaments.[12]

**Differential Diagnosis.** One must first ask whether any lesion with large neurons is a ganglion cell tumor at all, rather than just an *infiltrating glioma with trapped normal neurons*. As the rising moon looms large when seen in reference to objects on the horizon, normal ganglion cells appear larger and more rotund when apposed to the cells of an infiltrating glioma (see Fig. 4–197). Both *diffuse astrocytoma* and *oligodendrogliomas* may thus be misinterpreted as ganglion cell tumors. The oligodendroglioma is more highly represented because of its proclivity for cortical invasion. Cytologic characteristics and spatial distribution distinguish neoplastic from normal neurons. The polarity of normal ganglion cells, seen as regimented apical dendrites that reach to the pial surface, is a helpful feature evident in favorably oriented specimens. Neoplastic ganglion cells lack this polarity. In several sites, such as in the basal ganglia, hypothalamus, central cerebellum, brain stem, and spinal cord, a less orderly distribution of normal neurons creates a problem, particularly in small specimens. Immunohistochemistry may be useful, but interpretation can be difficult because there is deep background staining in gray matter. At least in theory, there may be an absence of granular surface staining in the cerebral cortex. Importantly, neoplastic ganglion cells vary in size and shape and often keep company with smaller, less fully developed "ganglioid" forms.

If trapped normal ganglion cells are excluded, the differential diagnosis can begin by reviewing Table 4–13, which lists lesions with abnormal neurons or neuron-like cells.

The compact gangliocytoma consists largely of neurons and must be distinguished from normal brain, cortical dysplasia, cortical tuber, gray matter ectopia, and hypothalamic hamartoma. As discussed earlier, *normal brain* is distinctive for its ordered complexity. Often simpler in cytologic composition, gangliocytomas are architecturally disorganized and sometimes calcified. Their neurons are cytologically abnormal and occasionally binucleate. In both *cortical dysplasia with giant neurons* (discussed in the context of seizures in Chapter 6) and *cortical tubers*, sizable abnormal neurons lie within easily recognizable cortex and are accompanied by large, glassy, astrocyte-like cells. A rare lesion, somewhat similar to cortical dysplasia, is *focal neuronal gigantism and cerebral cortical thickening that follows brain irradiation.*[2] Like cortical dysplasia, the lesion is a symmetric, architectural alteration of cerebral cortex, not a neoplastic mass.

*Dysembryoplastic neuroepithelial tumor* is an architecturally distinctive cortical lesion characterized by patterned nodules of oligodendroglia-like cells. Large neurons are prominent. Whether these are an intrinsic component or only trapped cortical neurons may be difficult to ascertain in a given lesion, but in any case, DNT is easily misinterpreted as ganglioglioma. Unlike the neurons in ganglioglioma, the neurons in DNT show little dysmorphism and characteristically are seen "floating" or sinking in small pools of mucin. *Desmoplastic infantile ganglioglioma* is easily distinguished from ordinary ganglioglioma. This well-recognized variant is (1) restricted to the very young, (2) massive, (3) often attached to the dura, (4) cystic, and (5) remarkably desmoplastic. *Pleomorphic xanthoastrocytomas* can contain normal or even neoplastic ganglion cells, as was discussed earlier (see Fig. 4–139). *Hypothalamic hamartoma*, with its content of large neurons, is described later in a separate section.

*Neurocytic neoplasms* with *ganglion cells (ganglioneurocytoma* and *ganglioglioneurocytoma)* are discussed on pages 287 to 290. Another neuronal lesion, *dysplastic cerebellar gangliocytoma (Lhermitte-Duclos disease)*, is considered later in a separate section.

Large gemistocytes in some high-grade *diffuse astrocytomas* can resemble ganglion cells. However, based on the tissue composition and general cytologic features, their identity is usually obvious. Nuclei are more hyperchromatic and irregular than those of a normal ganglion cell. Furthermore, although some cytoplasmic basophilia may be present, discrete Nissl substance is not. Nissl substance is not a prominent feature of most neoplastic ganglion cells tumors, however, so its absence is of little diagnostic significance. Multipolar cytoplasmic processes distinguish the gemistocytic astrocyte as well.

Shared architectural features cause ganglion cell tumors to be misinterpreted as *pilocytic astrocytomas*. This is particularly true in the common microcystic pilocytic astrocytoma, in which plump, amphophilic, often multinucleated forms resemble ganglion cells. There are also occasional pilocytic astrocytomas with ganglion cell components. An immunohistochemical search for neurons is obviously appropriate in such tumors. The distinction of gangliogliomas from pilocytic astrocytomas is discussed further on page 213.

### Diagnostic Checklist

- Is this "ganglion cell tumor" really an infiltrating oligodendroglioma or astrocytoma that has trapped normal neurons?
- Is this cerebellar "ganglion cell tumor" Lhermitte-Duclos disease?

**Treatment and Prognosis.** Surgery is the principal treatment of ganglion cell tumors.[16, 23, 24, 31] It is fortunate that, in most cases, residual tissue grows slowly, if at all.[4, 8, 23, 24, 31] A finite capacity for recurrence has, however, been linked to proliferative activity.[11] Thus, the prognosis is more dependent on location than on the tumor's capacity for growth or spread. Only rarely does a ganglion cell tumor undergo malignant transformation or present with both well-differentiated and anaplastic components.[29] Such rare lesions are discussed on pages 290 to 292.

### *Desmoplastic Infantile Ganglioglioma*

**Definition.** A markedly desmoplastic variant of ganglioglioma that usually presents in the first year of life. The lesion is grade I in the WHO system.

---

**TABLE 4–13**
**Central Nervous System Tumors and Tumor-Like Lesions Potentially with Ganglion Cell Components**

Neoplasms
  Ganglion cell tumors
    Gangliocytoma
    Ganglioglioma
  Desmoplastic infantile ganglioglioma
  Dysembryoplastic neuroepithelial tumor
  Ganglioneurocytic tumors
    Extraventricular neurocytoma
    Papillary glioneuronal tumor
  Medulloblastoma
  Ganglioneuroblastoma
  Medulloepithelioma
  Pleomorphic xanthoastrocytoma
  Subependymal giant cell astrocytoma
Non-neoplastic-like lesions
  Dysplastic cerebellar gangliocytoma (Lhermitte-Duclos disease)
  Cortical dysplasia
  Cortical tuber
  Hypothalamic hamartoma

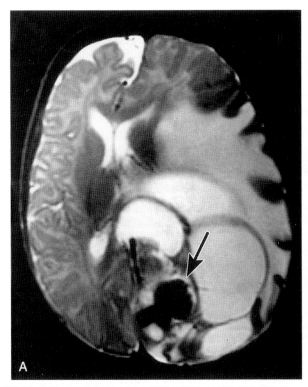
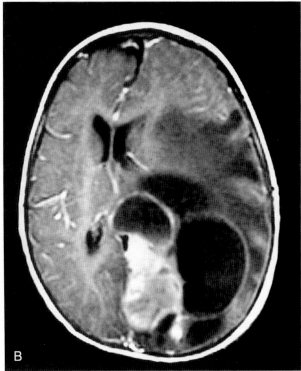

**FIGURE 4–285** DESMOPLASTIC INFANTILE GANGLIOGLIOMA

A 4-centimeter increase in head circumference over a 2-month period prompted this magnetic resonance imaging study of a 6-month-old boy. The T2-weighted (*A*) and contrast-enhanced (*B*) images illustrate the five cardinal features of desmoplastic infantile ganglioglioma: massive size, cystic architecture, superficial position, contrast enhancement, and a T2-dark desmoplastic component (*arrow*).

**Clinical Features.** Macrocephaly and signs of increased intracranial pressure are the principal expressions of this typically massive lesion.[3, 6, 11, 12]

**Radiologic Features.** Most desmoplastic infantile gangliogliomas (DIGs) appear as superficially positioned, dura-attached, contrast-enhancing masses associated with large, uni- or multiloculated cysts (Fig. 4–285).[6, 7] The desmoplastic component is dark on T2-weighted images.

**Microscopic Features.** The most prominent feature of DIG is desmoplasia that varies considerably in extent from region to region. In some areas it is so intense that it forms an almost acellular mass of collagen (Fig. 4–286). Other areas are less desmoplastic (Fig. 4–287), and elsewhere, the lesion may be free of this signature feature (Fig. 4–288). Spindled and somewhat storiform patterns are prominent. Small astrocytes with oval to elongated nuclei and pink, glassy cytoplasm are often a conspicuous feature in cellular areas.

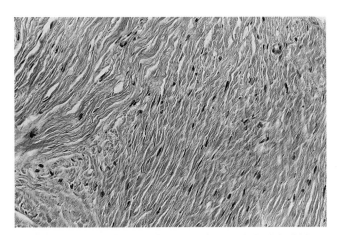

**FIGURE 4–286** DESMOPLASTIC INFANTILE GANGLIOGLIOMA

Intense desmoplasia, even if only focal, is the most distinctive feature of desmoplastic infantile gangliogliomas.

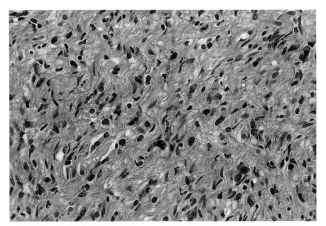

**FIGURE 4–287** DESMOPLASTIC INFANTILE GANGLIOGLIOMA

Within a given tumor, the degree of desmoplasia varies considerably from region to region. This region is considerably less sclerotic than that, from the same neoplasm, illustrated in Figure 4–286.

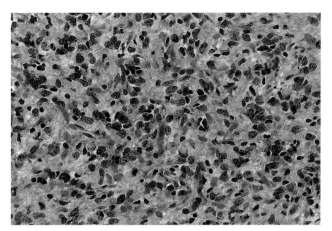

**FIGURE 4–288** DESMOPLASTIC INFANTILE GANGLIOGLIOMA

Densely cellular regions mimic either high-grade glioma or small cell embryonal tumor (primitive neuroectodermal tumor).

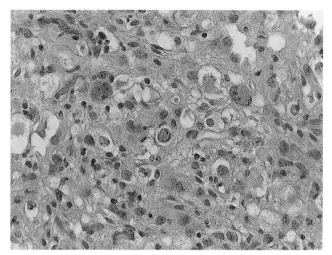

**FIGURE 4–290** DESMOPLASTIC INFANTILE GANGLIOGLIOMA

By definition, this tumor contains small ganglion-like cells, like those illustrated here. Such cells are lacking in some tumors, despite the presence of clinical, radiologic, and histopathologic features of desmoplastic infantile ganglioglioma.

The neuronal component of DIG is often difficult to recognize in H&E-stained sections (Fig. 4–289). Small, eosinophilic, and often plump, the neurons may have the conspicuous nucleolus of a ganglion cell but little cytoplasm. They can resemble astrocytes (Fig. 4–290); immunohistochemistry is then essential. In exceptional cases, there are areas of classic ganglion cell tumor with nests of large cells, microcysts, and EGBs.[8]

Some DIGs feature a highly cellular and mitotically active component resembling a high-grade glioma or a small cell embryonal tumor (primitive neuroectodermal tumor [PNET]; see Fig. 4–288). Especially disturbing are mitotically active elements that may be associated with microvascular proliferation and necrosis with pseudopalisading (Fig. 4–291). This should not be interpreted as glioblastoma multiforme, because its prognostic significance, if any, remains to be established. Some patients with these troublesome features survive for many years without tumor recurrence in the absence of any postoperative chemo- or radiotherapy.

**Immunohistochemical Features.** The extent of GFAP staining of the astrocytes hidden in the desmoplastic tissue of a DIG always comes as a surprise, even to those experienced with the entity (Fig. 4–292). Sheets of cells in which the cells have more cytoplasm are particularly immunopositive. Scattered small, pink, round cells are negative. These are cells with neuronal attributes, including cytoplasmic staining for synaptophysin (Fig. 4–293), chromogranin, neurofilament protein, and anti-Hu immunoglobulin (Fig. 4–294).[4] Synaptophysin- or chromogranin-positive neurons are often found in cellular areas in which no ganglion cells are recognizable in H&E-stained sections.

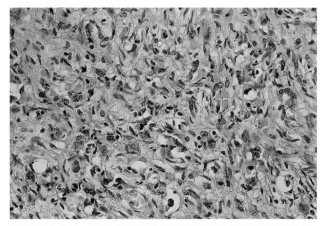

**FIGURE 4–289** DESMOPLASTIC INFANTILE GANGLIOGLIOMA

Cytologically, scattered cells of intermediate size appear ganglion like, but unequivocal neurons are often difficult to find.

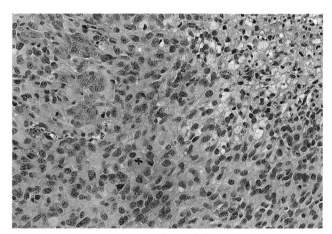

**FIGURE 4–291** DESMOPLASTIC INFANTILE GANGLIOGLIOMA

Highly cellular areas with cytologic atypia, necrosis, vascular proliferation, and brisk mitotic activity are present in some desmoplastic infantile gangliogliomas (DIGs). Remarkably, such components seem not to detract from the excellent prognosis of this tumor. In the case illustrated, the patient was treated by partial excision alone. No recurrence has been noted over a 4-year follow-up period. Elsewhere, the neoplasm showed typical features of DIG.

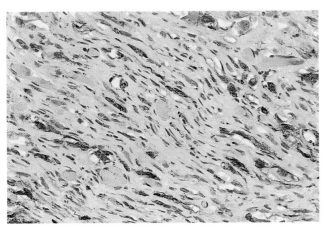

**FIGURE 4–292** DESMOPLASTIC INFANTILE GANGLIOGLIOMA

The desmoplastic regions are rich in cells that are positive for glial fibrillary acidic protein.

**Ultrastructural Features.** As expected, the astrocytes are filled with intermediate filaments. Some are partially enveloped by basement lamina. Neuronal cells have the expected organelles, including well-developed Golgi cells and rough endoplasmic reticulum, as well as processes that contain microtubules and dense-core granules, with or without accompanying clear vesicles.[11, 12] Synapses may be present in association with particularly well-differentiated neurons.

**Differential Diagnosis.** The process of differential diagnosis begins by knowing that DIGs exist, that they affect the very young, and that they have a highly characteristic radiologic profile. Without this awareness, the desmoplastic component can be mistaken for a variety of fibrous lesions such as *fibromatosis, solitary fibrous tumor,*

*gliosarcoma, fibrosarcoma,* or *fibrous histiocytoma.* Each can effectively be excluded by immunohistochemical demonstration of glial and neuronal components.

The possibility that a DIG represents a *malignant glioma*—that is, a *glioblastoma* or *gliosarcoma*—is difficult to dismiss and requires attention to radiographic and operative data. DIG is discrete, massive, cystic, and superficial, with dural attachment. The prominent, anaplastic-appearing element is particularly subject to misinterpretation. Nonetheless, reassurance can be found in the historically benign behavior of such lesions, although it is difficult to believe that these lesions are indeed not malignant—experience from past cases notwithstanding.

Not infrequently, the search for ganglion cells is fruitless in a lesion that conforms to DIG in all other aspects. This creates a quandary, because without the ganglion cells, the tumor falls into the less precise category of *desmoplastic astrocytoma of infancy.*[1, 2, 5, 9–11] Although one can debate the best nosologic niche for such tumors, we believe that they should be treated as DIGs if the clinical, neuroimaging, and morphologic features are otherwise identical, save for the truant neurons. A "see comment" addendum is appropriate.

If ganglion cells are found, one must resolve the somewhat semantic issue of whether the lesion is a DIG or a more typical *ganglion cell tumor.* This is not always possible, because features of the two entities overlap in some cases[8]; however, massive tumor size, dural attachment, remarkable desmoplasia, and very young patient age strongly favor a diagnosis of DIG.

**Treatment and Prognosis.** The treatment is surgical excision, although the size and adherence of the mass to underlying brain may preclude total removal. Patients do well, and there is little chance of recurrence, even in lesions with hypercellular foci.[3, 6]

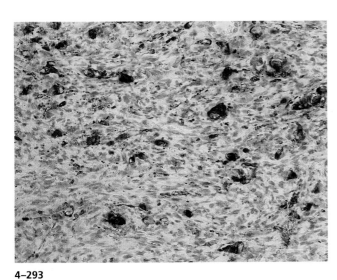

4–293

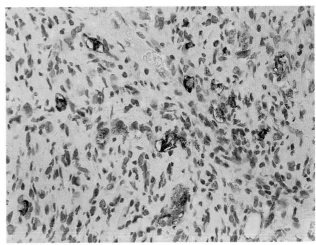

4–294

**FIGURES 4–293 AND 4–294** DESMOPLASTIC INFANTILE GANGLIOGLIOMA

Immunostaining for synaptophysin (Fig. 4–293) and chromogranin (Fig. 4–294) is useful in detecting the neuronal component. The region illustrated in Figure 4–294 is the same as in Figure 4–289.

## *Dysplastic Cerebellar Gangliocytoma (Lhermitte-Duclos Disease)*

**Definition.** A tumoral but non-neoplastic developmental abnormality of the cerebellar cortex caused primarily by massive enlargement of neurons in the internal granule cell layer.

**General Comments.** In the parlance of bird-watching, an endeavor with many similarities to surgical pathology, Lhermitte-Duclos disease is an entity not likely to be found on the "life list" of most pathologists. The lesion arises sporadically or in the setting of Cowden syndrome due to a germline mutation in the tumor suppressor gene PTEN.[4, 5, 8, 12, 14] In one series, all five patients were found to have Cowden syndrome.[13]

**Clinical Features.** Patients usually present in the second or third decade of life with cerebellar dysfunction or signs of CSF obstruction.[7]

**Radiologic Features.** The distinctive striped cerebellar mass on T2-weighted MRI scans is virtually pathognomonic (Fig. 4–295).[2, 3, 10, 14]

**Macroscopic Features.** The thickened folia produce a sometimes sizable increase in the volume of the affected hemisphere (Fig. 4–296).

**Microscopic Features.** If one is fortunate enough to have a large specimen, one can begin at the outer margin and, by moving inward, note a gradual replacement of the small neurons of the internal granular cell layer by larger neurons that attain the dimensions of small ganglion cells (Figs. 4–297 to 4–300).[1] At the lesion's center, such cells replace the internal granular cells and increase the layer's thickness several-fold. This progression from minimal to maximal involvement may be difficult to appreciate in some specimens, but abnormal neurons confined to a precise lamina are often readily apparent, even in a fragmented specimen.

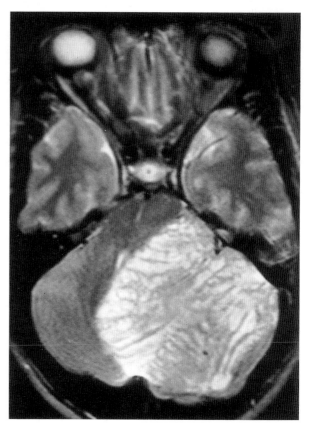

**FIGURE 4–295** DYSPLASTIC CEREBELLAR GANGLIOCYTOMA (LHERMITTE-DUCLOS DISEASE)

As seen in this T2-weighted magnetic resonance imaging scan, the lesion produces distinctive striped enlargement.

Although descriptions of Lhermitte-Duclos disease focus on alterations of the internal granular cell layer, the molecular layer is also affected. This layer, which normally exhibits little substructure, now conveys bundles of myelinated axons that fan out over the surface in an abnormal layer that stains for Luxol fast blue (Fig. 4–301).[11]

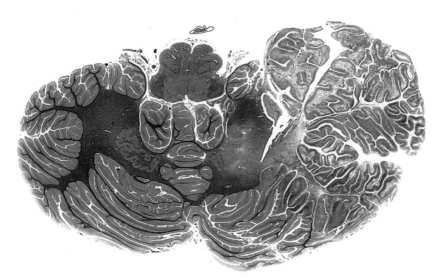

**FIGURE 4–296** DYSPLASTIC CEREBELLAR GANGLIOCYTOMA (LHERMITTE-DUCLOS DISEASE)

As seen in this whole mount histologic section, the lesion coexists in peaceful harmony with the essentially preserved anatomy of the cerebellum.

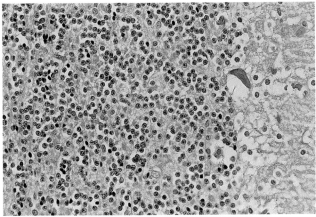
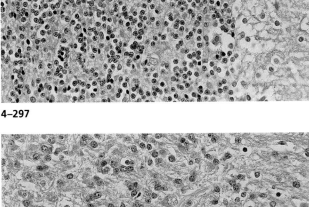

4–297

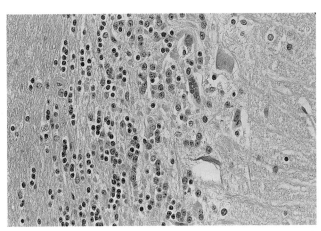

4–298

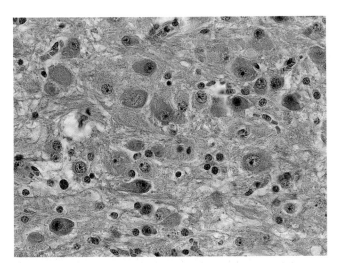

4–299

**FIGURES 4–297, 4–298, AND 4–299   DYSPLASTIC CEREBELLAR GANGLIOCYTOMA (LHERMITTE-DUCLOS DISEASE)**

Three sections from the same surgical specimen demonstrate the graduated severity of the changes occurring from the periphery to the center of the lesion. Figure 4–297 illustrates the normal cerebellar cortex with an internal granule cell layer formed of uniformly small, closely packed cells. An area of minimal involvement is seen in Figure 4–298, where some internal granule cells are replaced by neurons with larger, paler nuclei. Only a few normal internal granule cells remain in Figure 4–299.

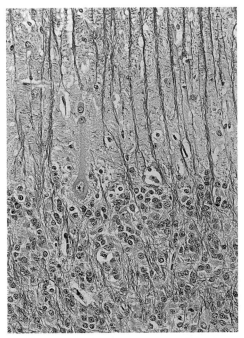

**FIGURE 4–301   DYSPLASTIC CEREBELLAR GANGLIOCYTOMA (LHERMITTE-DUCLOS DISEASE)**

In an H&E preparation also stained for myelin (H&E–Luxol fast blue), abnormal myelinated fibers extend from the internal granule cell layer (*bottom*) through the overlying molecular layer. Only a solitary Purkinje cell remains.

**FIGURE 4–300   DYSPLASTIC CEREBELLAR GANGLIOCYTOMA (LHERMITTE-DUCLOS DISEASE)**

In the fully developed lesion, small ganglion cells fully replace the internal granule cell layer.

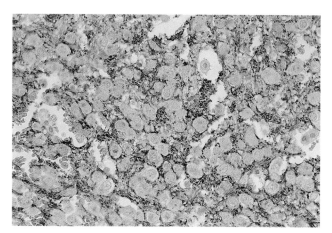

**FIGURE 4–302** DYSPLASTIC CEREBELLAR GANGLIOCYTOMA (LHERMITTE-DUCLOS DISEASE)

The abnormal small ganglion cells exhibit surface immunoreactivity for synaptophysin.

**Immunohistochemical Features.** The neurons are stained for synaptophysin (Fig. 4–302), chromogranin, and neurofibrillary protein[15]; they are negative for GFAP.

**Ultrastructural Features.** The large cells exhibit the features of neurons.[9, 11]

**Differential Diagnosis.** The lesion can be mistaken for conventional *ganglion cell tumor* when telltale radiographic features and localization of the process to the internal granular layer are not recognized (Fig. 4–303). Even without these aids, the lesion should be suspected based on neuronal monomorphism and its geographic confinement to a well-circumscribed layer. Both would be most unusual in a conventional ganglion cell neoplasm.

**Treatment and Prognosis.** Lhermitte-Duclos disease is a benign process, although a slowly growing expansion of residual tissue may necessitate subsequent resection.[6, 10]

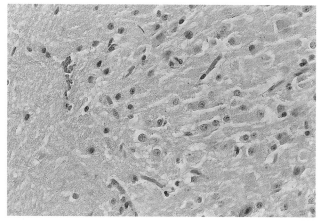

**FIGURE 4–303** DYSPLASTIC CEREBELLAR GANGLIOCYTOMA (LHERMITTE-DUCLOS DISEASE)

The diagnosis can be difficult in small fragmented specimens in which localization of the abnormal neurons to the internal granule cell layer may not be apparent.

## Dysembryoplastic Neuroepithelial Tumor

**Definition.** An intracortical multinodular mass, composed in varying parts of oligodendrocyte-like cells. The lesion is grade I in the WHO system.

**General Comments.** DNT, a relative newcomer to the WHO classification of brain tumors, was previously submerged as an entity among oligoastrocytomas and oligodendrogliomas.[4] Although the classic form of DNT is readily recognized, the diagnosis can be difficult in the face of specimens that are small, fragmented, or incomplete in their expression of classic features. Even more problematic both diagnostically and conceptually is the "nonspecific form" of DNT, discussed later. Although the lesion is classified as a neuronal or mixed glioneuronal tumor, its origin is not clear.

**Clinical Features.** Most patients present with a complaint of partial complex seizures beginning early in life, although surgery may not be performed until the second or even third decade.[3, 4, 15, 16] Most DNTs are supratentorial, with the medial or lateral temporal lobes the most common sites. Rare DNTs have been encountered in the caudate nucleus, septum pellucidum and floor of the third ventricle,[1, 2, 11] brain stem,[17] and cerebellum.[6, 10, 20] Multifocality has been reported.[11]

**Radiologic Features.** DNTs are rather well-defined, T1-dark, T2-bright lesions, often with a telltale nodular appearance (Figs. 4–304 and 4–305). The lesion's localization to the cortex may not be evident in the bulky center of the lesion, but it is often obvious peripherally, where the intracortical localization of the nodules is well seen. Erosion of the inner table is common in DNTs that are juxtaposed to the skull (see Fig. 4–305), but there is little else in the way of mass effect.[3, 4, 12, 18] The various lesions associated with skull erosion are summarized in Table 4–7, p. 205. An occasional DNT includes a narrow, uniformly and intensely enhancing ring around a dark center—a pattern that mimics that of a high-grade glioma or an abscess (see Fig. 4–304).

**Macroscopic Features.** Given their superficial location, DNTs often arise somewhat above the brain surface, with blister-like elevations that correspond to macronodules (Figs. 4–306 and 4–307). Compressive remodeling of the overlying skull is commonly seen (Fig. 4–308).

**Microscopic Features.** DNT is architecturally complex, and its recognition is greatly simplified when one is presented with an intact specimen that can be cut perpendicular to the cortical surface. Low-power assessment of the lesion is then most informative. The classic lesion includes two histologic elements: multiple nodules (Figs. 4–309 and 4–310) and an internodular, diffuse component. Both are variably mucin containing and therefore alcian blue positive (see Fig. 4–310).

The nodules are formed of small, uniform cells that are strongly reminiscent of oligodendrocytes (Fig. 4–311). Artifactual perinuclear halos are prominent. The

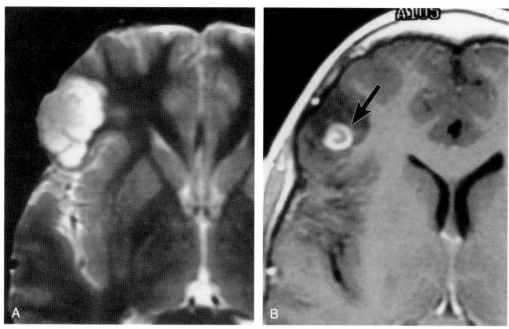

**FIGURE 4–304   DYSEMBRYOPLASTIC NEUROEPITHELIAL TUMOR**

These unique lesions have a distinctive radiologic profile. As visualized in a T2-weighted magnetic resonance imaging scan (*A*), the lesion is discrete, multinodular, intracortical, and outwardly expansile. Occasional lesions feature a well-circumscribed rim of enhancement (*arrow*), which raises concern about a possible diagnosis of malignant glioma (*B*).

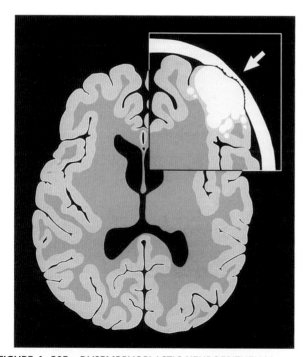

**FIGURE 4–305   DYSEMBRYOPLASTIC NEUROEPITHELIAL TUMOR**

The illustration summarizes the salient features of a dysembryoplastic neuroepithelial tumor (DNT) as seen in a fluid-attenuated inversion recovery (FLAIR) image. The small nodules, especially obvious at the periphery of the lesion, are typical of DNT. As occurs in many cases, erosion of the inner table of the skull attests to the chronicity of this lesion. (From Passe TJ, Beauchamp NJ Jr, Burger PC. Neuroimaging in the identification of low-grade and nonneoplastic CNS lesions. The Neurologist 1999;5:293–299.)

nodules are generally patternless, but they can have distinctive streaming, often in a somewhat circumferential pattern.

Between the nodules are similar oligodendrocyte-like cells that permeate the cortex (Fig. 4–312) and sometimes the subpial zone. A feature of the internodular zone is the so-called specific glioneuronal component—vertical columns of neurites traversing the cortex and sheathed by oligodendrocyte-like cells accompanied by mucin.

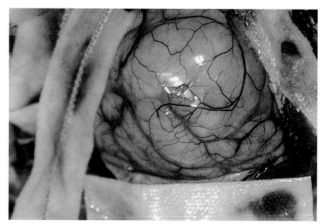

**FIGURE 4–306   DYSEMBRYOPLASTIC NEUROEPITHELIAL TUMOR**

The lobularity and outward expansion of the lesion are evident at surgery. The patient was a 15-year-old with a recent seizure. (Courtesy of Dr. Jon D. Weingart, Baltimore, MD.)

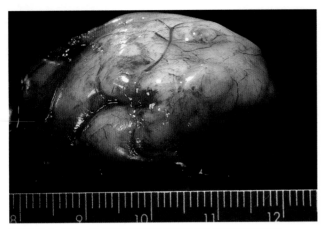

**FIGURE 4–307**    DYSEMBRYOPLASTIC NEUROEPITHELIAL TUMOR

The larger intracortical nodules are recognizable macroscopically as small nodules at the surface of an excised lesion.

A prominent, but unfortunately not specific, feature is "floating neurons," a term used to describe cortical ganglion cells sitting in individual small pools of mucin (Figs. 4–313 and 4–314). Such cells are a common in both nodular and "diffuse" areas. DNTs composed of just these structures, but no nodules, represent the lesion in its elementary, or "simple," form.

Other DNTs are more "complex" and include a variety of tissue patterns, including compact, elongated cells simulating pilocytic astrocytoma (Fig. 4–315). Nodules resembling diffuse astrocytoma, sometimes with dark, pleomorphic nuclei, are also occasionally seen (Fig. 4–316).

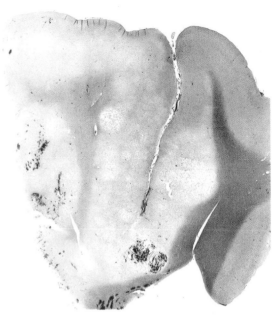

**FIGURE 4–309**    DYSEMBRYOPLASTIC NEUROEPITHELIAL TUMOR

A whole mount histologic section emphasizes the multiplicity of the intracortical nodules that typify dysembryoplastic neuroepithelial tumors.

On rare occasion, DNT and ganglioglioma are present in the same specimen.[9, 13]

Large neurons, a conspicuous feature of DNT, are found both within the lesion proper and in the adjoining brain. Whether these are merely trapped normal ganglion

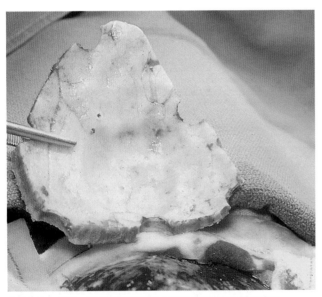

**FIGURE 4–308**    DYSEMBRYOPLASTIC NEUROEPITHELIAL TUMOR

The erosive effect of a dysembryoplastic neuroepithelial tumor on the inner table of the skull is well seen in the calvarium overlying the lesion illustrated in Figure 4–306. (Courtesy of Dr. Jon D. Weingart, Baltimore, MD.)

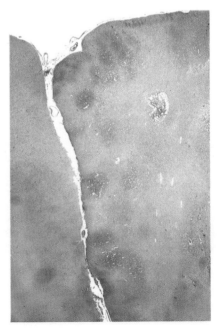

**FIGURE 4–310**    DYSEMBRYOPLASTIC NEUROEPITHELIAL TUMOR

This alcian blue stain for acid mucopolysaccharide demonstrates the typical inter- and intranodular mucin deposits.

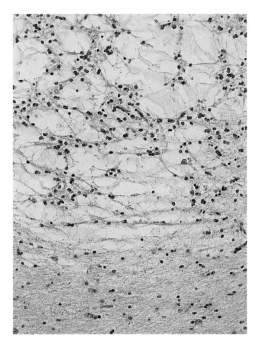

**FIGURE 4–311    DYSEMBRYOPLASTIC NEUROEPITHELIAL TUMOR**

This discrete, "patterned," intracortical nodule with abundant eosinophilic or slightly basophilic mucin content is typical of dysembryoplastic neuroepithelial tumors.

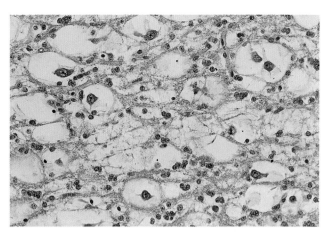

**FIGURE 4–313    DYSEMBRYOPLASTIC NEUROEPITHELIAL TUMOR**

Ganglion cells described as "floating neurons" are seen to reside in lacunae separated by cortical neuropil.

or active participants in the lesion is a matter of debate. To some observers, "cortical dysplasia"—that is, the presence of misaligned, cytologically abnormal neurons—is common in the cortex that abuts the lesion. Others find this feature less frequently. Most neurons in DNT appear to be little more than trapped cortical ganglion cells, often "floating" within the pools of mucin described earlier.

Prominent in some DNTs are arcades of glomeruloid vascular proliferation. This would raise concern about a high-grade lesion, were it not for the discordant blandness of the surrounding cells, the overall architectural features, and the radiologic findings, all of which are distinctive of DNT (Fig. 4–317). The angiogenesis is frequently circumferential about a central eosinophilic amorphous area of what is more tissue "degeneration" than necrosis. This rim of proliferating vessels corresponds to the radiologic rim of contrast enhancement seen in some examples.

Although DNT is viewed as a stable lesion, scattered mitoses are seen in some examples. A minority of DNTs are calcified.

The diagnosis of DNT, in either simple or complex form, poses a challenge. A recent attempt to expand the DNT spectrum to include a "nonspecific form" complicates this issue, and even the definition of the lesion itself.[5] Morphologically, this envisioned entity includes a heterogeneous group of histologically benign, and even malignant, lesions that are defined more on their clinical

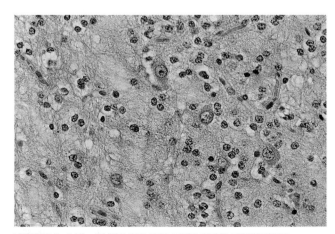

**FIGURE 4–312    DYSEMBRYOPLASTIC NEUROEPITHELIAL TUMOR**

Cells resembling oligodendrocytes diffuse through the internodular cortex. Extracellular mucopolysaccharide imparts a slight background basophilia. Tissue such as this can easily be misinterpreted as oligodendroglioma.

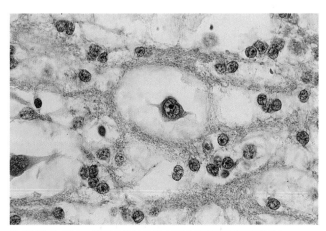

**FIGURE 4–314    DYSEMBRYOPLASTIC NEUROEPITHELIAL TUMOR**

The neurons appear to "float" in small pools of mucin.

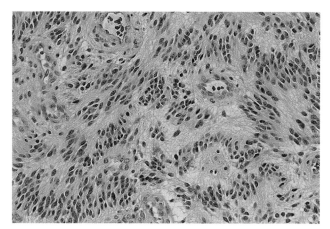

**FIGURE 4–315**    DYSEMBRYOPLASTIC NEUROEPITHELIAL TUMOR

Multiple tissue patterns can be encountered. Here, focal ribbons of elongated cells appear in a lesion that elsewhere was a typical dysembryoplastic neuroepithelial tumor.

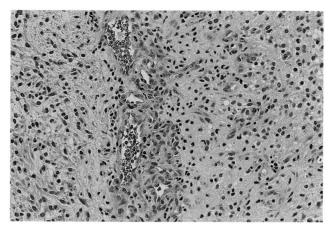

**FIGURE 4–317**    DYSEMBRYOPLASTIC NEUROEPITHELIAL TUMOR

Vascular proliferation encircling a central area of tissue degeneration may prompt concern regarding a possible diagnosis of malignant glioma. This response does not detract from the benignancy of a dysembryoplastic neuroepithelial tumor.

and radiologic features than on their histopathologic ones; it includes such lesions as pilocytic astrocytomas, astrocytomas of low or high grade, and ganglion cell tumors. As such, we do not consider it a defined pathologic entity. The common features of these lesions include (1) young age of the patient; (2) presentation with seizures; (3) intracortical location, albeit with varied neuroimaging characteristics; and (4) a favorable outcome without recurrence. Although we do not consider these histologically diverse lesions DNTs, the concept is useful in emphasizing that many seizure-producing lesions, particularly when positioned superficially and occurring in young patients, are biologically indolent and require no initial treatment beyond surgical resection.

**Immunohistochemical Features.** The small cells of DNT that resemble oligodendroglia are S-100 protein immunopositive.[3, 8] Scattered cells are positive in some

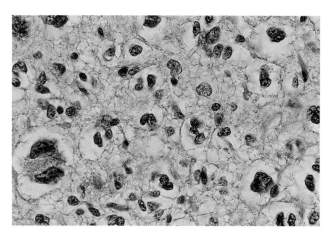

**FIGURE 4–316**    DYSEMBRYOPLASTIC NEUROEPITHELIAL TUMOR

Areas of considerable nuclear pleomorphism may suggest a diagnosis of astrocytoma.

cases for neuronal markers such as NeuN, but synaptophysin staining is largely negative.[19] Scattered cells react unpredictably with antibodies to GFAP, neurofilament protein, class III $\beta$-tubulin, or synaptophysin.[8] Naturally, astrocytic cells are GFAP positive. Synaptophysin is diffusely positive in the cortex and less so in the nodules than in the "specific glioneuronal element." One study found that the oligodendrocyte-like cells were positive for myelin oligodrocyte protein,[7] but identifying the nature of these cells has proved elusive.

The MIB-1 rate is generally less than 1% but can be higher, even reaching the ranges exhibited by lesions that enter into the differential diagnosis, such as diffuse astrocytoma and oligodendroglioma.[3, 14]

**Ultrastructural Features.** Although a few neurosecretory granules and clear vesicles—both neuronal features—can be found in some cases,[8, 11, 18] synapses are rarely encountered.[8, 11] Thus, most of the small cells are not specifically differentiated.

**Differential Diagnosis.** In most instances, the chief concern is distinguishing DNT (Fig. 4–318) from *oligodendroglioma* (see Table 4–9, p. 213). Both lesions preferentially involve the cerebral cortex; can be nodular; often possess a basophilic, mucinous matrix; and are composed predominantly of small, round cells with perinuclear halos. Distinguishing features are as follows: (1) oligodendrogliomas, to a significant extent, involve white matter, whereas DNTs are largely limited to cortex; (2) the nodules of oligodendrogliomas are generally unpatterned and of a slightly higher histologic grade than the surrounding neoplasm; (3) the nuclei of oligodendrogliomas are usually somewhat larger and slightly more varied in size and possess more open chromatin than do cells of DNTs; (4) oligodendroglioma cells within cortex are drawn to neurons as satellites, but these oligodendrocyte-neuron tête-à-têtes are largely absent in DNTs; (5) "floating" neurons, characteristic of DNTs, are less commonly

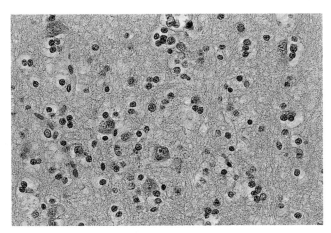

**FIGURE 4–318**  DYSEMBRYOPLASTIC NEUROEPITHELIAL TUMOR

The round, uniform nuclei of the oligodendrocyte-like cells of dysembryoplastic neuroepithelial tumor (DNT) and their perinuclear halos create a close resemblance to oligodendroglioma. "Floating neurons," though not specific, are more characteristic of DNT. Conversely, perineuronal satellitosis is considerably more prominent in oligodendroglioma.

seen in oligodendrogliomas; and (6) although not common in DNTs, vascular proliferation in such a well-differentiated lesion is more typical of DNT than of well-differentiated oligodendroglioma. In spite of this impressive list of differentiating features, DNTs and oligodendrogliomas are not always readily distinguished.

DNTs can contain overtly astrocytic tissue that resembles either *pilocytic* or *diffuse astrocytoma*. Awareness of the clinical features, coupled with a review of the neuroimaging studies, aids immeasurably in the identification of DNT, as does the finding of nodularity and large fields of very well differentiated oligodendroglia-like cells.

One occasionally encounters a lesion in a child or young adult with the overall "gestalt" of DNT, because of the mucinous background and remarkable degree of nuclear blandness and uniformity, but without the specific features of DNT. It remains unclear whether these are valid DNTs or oligodendrogliomas. We report the lesions as very well differentiated, explain the dilemma, and suggest clinical and imaging follow-up. Some such lesions will recur and require another resection. Management of the case can then be evaluated in light of the pathologic findings in the second specimen.

### Diagnostic Checklist

■ Is this DNT not really an oligodendroglioma?

**Treatment and Prognosis.** Treatment is excision, gross or subtotal, without adjuvant radio- or chemotherapy. Of the original 39 reported cases, resection was total in 22 and subtotal in 17; in no case was there clinical or radiologic evidence of subsequent progression.[4] Later series have affirmed the benign nature of DNT.[15, 18] Although tumors followed without surgery are stable in most instances,[3] slow growth has been reported in an occasional case.[12]

## Hypothalamic Hamartoma

**Definition.** A congenital, non-neoplastic mass of mature hypothalamic tissue, either in continuity with or in proximity to the hypothalamus.

**General Comments.** Hypothalamic hamartoma is an often nodular, congenital, non-neoplastic lesion that is either attached to the inferior hypothalamus or lies nearby in the suprasellar region or interpeduncular fossa (see Figs. 4–320 and 4–321).[10] Small examples are common; sizable hamartomas are rare.[4, 10] Many are incidental neuroradiologic findings that are followed for years without biopsy until the stability of the lesion obviates the need for further surveillance.

**Clinical Features.** Endocrine dysfunction, the most frequent presenting complaint, has in some cases been related to the production of hypothalamic-releasing hormones. Precocious puberty is the most common manifestation, but other endocrinologic derangements such as acromegaly are encountered.[1, 2, 5–7, 9, 10] Paroxysms of uncontrolled laughter, called "gelastic seizures," are a classic but uncommon feature.[3, 8]

**Radiologic Features.** These non–contrast-enhancing lesions have signal characteristics of normal gray matter (Fig. 4–319).[10]

**Macroscopic Features.** Of variable size, these demarcated, soft, gray lesions either dangle harmlessly from the floor of the third ventricle (Figs. 4–320 and 4–321) or lie free in the suprasellar space or interpeduncular cistern.

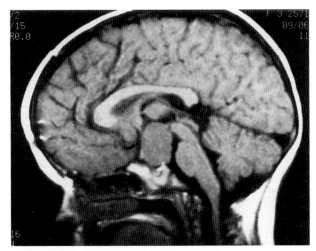

**FIGURE 4–319**  HYPOTHALAMIC HAMARTOMA

As seen in a precontrast T1-weighted magnetic resonance imaging scan, hypothalamic hamartomas show the signal characteristics of normal gray matter. This especially large lesion occurred in a 4-year-old boy.

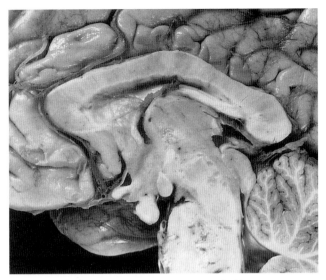

**FIGURE 4–320**   HYPOTHALAMIC HAMARTOMA

Most hypothalamic hamartomas project from the floor of the third ventricle just anterior to the pons and mamillary body. This lesion was an incidental finding in a 58-year-old man.

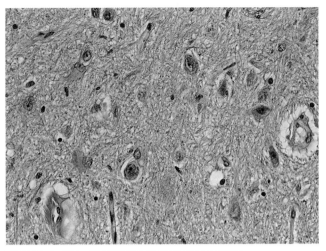

**FIGURE 4–322**   HYPOTHALAMIC HAMARTOMA

Consisting of large neurons, neuropil, and only widely scattered reactive astrocytes, the lesion may be difficult to recognize as an abnormality on histologic sections, especially when seen out of clinical and radiologic context.

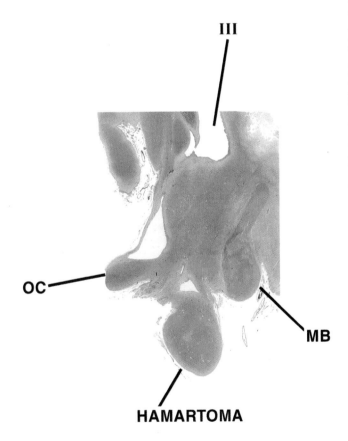

**FIGURE 4–321**   HYPOTHALAMIC HAMARTOMA

A midsagittal histologic section of the lesion depicted in Figure 4–320 illustrates the way the typical small hamartoma hangs like a pendant from the floor of the hypothalamus. III, third ventricle; MB, mamillary body; OC, optic chiasm.

**Microscopic Features.** Histologically, the hamartomas resemble normal hypothalamic tissue and consist of large, fully mature ganglion cells scattered haphazardly or loosely clustered in a delicate neuropil (Fig. 4–322).[7] A few reactive astrocytes with glassy cytoplasm and prominent processes may be present.

**Immunohistochemical Features.** The presence of hypothalamic-releasing hormones can be demonstrated in some lesions.[10]

**Ultrastructural Features.** Ultrastructurally, the bulk of the mass consists of neuropil, a fibrillar tissue composed of neuronal processes that harbor aligned microtubules. Large neurons resembling those of the hypothalamus contain large numbers of electron-dense secretory granules within their perikarya and in perivascular axonal terminals.

**Differential Diagnosis.** One's initial impression of the tissue, particularly in small, fragmented specimens, is that of *normal brain*, albeit somewhat disorganized. Indeed, the diagnosis may not be suspected unless the lesion's precise location is known. Hypothalamic hamartomas differ from *gangliocytoma* by their close similarity to normal gray matter and by the absence of neoplastic glial cells, microcysts, eosinophilic granular bodies, chronic inflammatory cells, and connective tissue. Calcification, a rather frequent feature of gangliogliomas, is uncommon in all but the largest of hamartomas. Cytologically dysmorphic neurons are also less common in hamartomas.

Also in the differential diagnosis is *neuronal metaplasia in pituitary adenoma*, a lesion discussed in Chapter 9. The distinction rests on the finding of clusters and sheets of adenoma cells admixed with neuronal tissue. Such lesions arise in the sella and are usually of macroadenomatous dimensions; as a result, their neuroimaging characteristics differ markedly from those of hypothalamic hamartomas.

**Treatment and Prognosis.** These malformative lesions are benign but may produce endocrinologic effects, such as precocious puberty with accompanying short stature. Nonsurgical treatment with gonadotropin-releasing hormone agonists may suppress precocious puberty and prevent premature maturation of bone.[8, 10]

### Central Neurocytoma

**Definition.** A well-circumscribed, intraventricular, neurocytic neoplasm that arises at or near the foramen of Monro. The lesion is grade II in the WHO system.

**General Comments.** "Neurocytes" are small but mature, round neurons that typically acquire perinuclear halos during the excision-fixation interval. An oligodendrocyte-like appearance is the diagnostically confusing result.

The neurocytic lesion under consideration is designated "central" to emphasize its deep midline position and to distinguish it from more lateralized or superficial lesions discussed later in the section on extraventricular neurocytic neoplasms. The classification of neurocytic tumors is therefore partly dependent on location. The central neurocytoma is, nevertheless, a well-defined clinicopathologic entity and the most common of the neurocytic lesions.

**Clinical Features.** Most patients, usually young adults, present with effects of CSF flow obstruction.[4, 11] Intraventricular hemorrhage brings a rare patient to attention.[18]

**Radiologic Features.** Central neurocytomas are discrete, often partly calcified masses near the foramen of

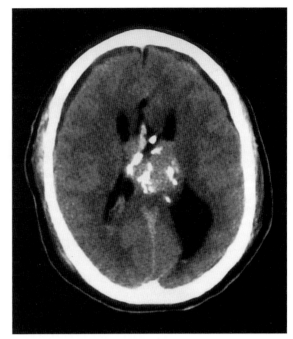

**FIGURE 4–324    CENTRAL NEUROCYTOMA**

Many central neurocytomas are calcified, which is best seen by computed tomography scanning without contrast enhancement. This patient, a 41-year-old man, relayed a 6-month history of headaches and memory loss.

Monro[5] (Figs. 4–323 and 4–324). Most are attached to the septum pellucidum and expand into one or both lateral ventricles and, less commonly, into the third ventricle. The tumors can be very large. Contrast enhancement, usually inhomogeneous, is variable in extent.

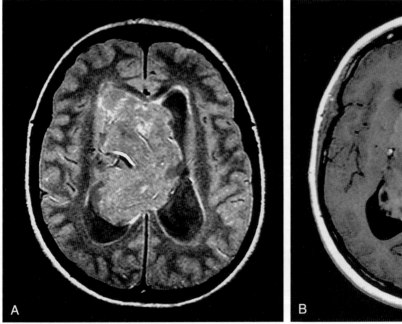

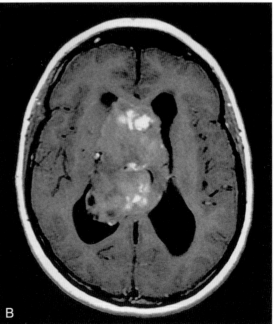

**FIGURE 4–323    CENTRAL NEUROCYTOMA**

By the time they become clinically apparent, central neurocytomas are often sizable masses that, by definition, arise within the lateral ventricles near the foramen of Monro. The lesion is well seen in a proton-density magnetic resonance imaging scan (*A*) and in a contrast-enhanced T1-weighted image (*B*). Inhomogeneous enhancement is typical (*B*). The patient, a 25-year-old woman, complained only of headaches.

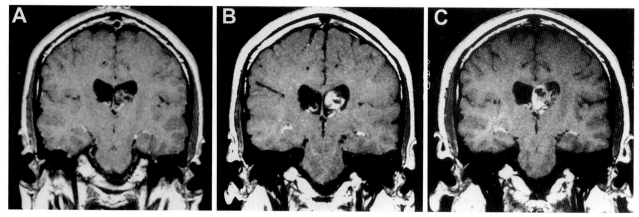

**FIGURE 4–325**   CENTRAL NEUROCYTOMA

Central neurocytomas grow slowly, as illustrated by this untreated lesion followed at 2-year intervals by magnetic resonance imaging.

Sequential scans demonstrate slow growth (Fig. 4–325). It remains to be seen whether the lesion has a distinctive proton MR spectroscopy profile.[12]

**Macroscopic Features.** The soft to gritty, tan, discrete mass may be solid or partly cystic. As a rule, little or no brain parenchyma accompanies the specimen.

**Microscopic Features.** Microscopically, a central neurocytoma has a cytologic precision that makes it one of the most gratifying entities described in this book (Figs. 4–326 to 4–328). Uniform nuclei with delicately speckled chromatin float in company or are swept individually in streams within a fine, fibrillar matrix. The cells are strikingly uniform in chromatin content and could, seemingly, be passed through a sieve without finding a single anaplastic cell. Accordingly, mitoses are rare to infrequent. "Atypical" neurocytomas, with a higher MIB-1 index and scattered mitotic figures, are discussed later in the section on grading. As in other neuronal or neuroblastic neoplasms, there are often narrow perivascular anuclear zones resembling ependymal pseudorosettes (see Fig. 4–327), as well as perinuclear halos (see Fig. 4–328). With advanced neurocytic differentiation with cell streaming, the lesion can closely resemble extensively nodular medulloblastoma. Lipofuscin and neuromelanin color a rare neurocytoma.[14]

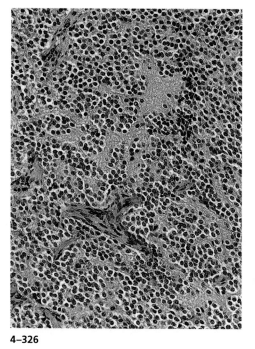

**4–326**

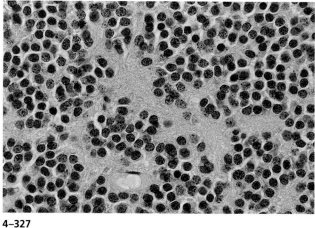

**4–327**

**FIGURES 4–326 AND 4–327**   CENTRAL NEUROCYTOMA

Central neurocytomas are densely cellular and exhibit scattered areas of neuropil, a common feature of neuronal neoplasms. The perivascular, somewhat fibrillar-appearing, zones can easily be misinterpreted as evidence of ependymoma.

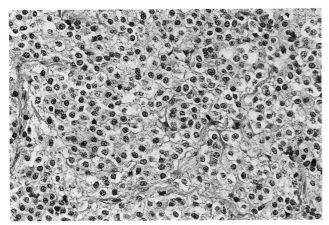

**FIGURE 4–328**  CENTRAL NEUROCYTOMA

Because of their perinuclear halos and round nuclei, neurocytomas may closely resemble oligodendrogliomas.

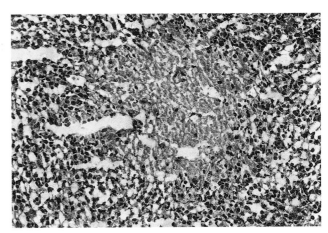

**FIGURE 4–331**  CENTRAL NEUROCYTOMA

On frozen section, fibrillar, neuropil-like regions can resemble necrosis, thus misrepresenting this indolent lesion as a malignant glioma.

Interestingly, neurocytomas, like the nodular medulloblastomas, are hesitant to take the step toward ganglion cell differentiation and produce a neoplasm with a preponderance of neuropil with variable numbers of "ganglioid" and ganglion cells. The designation "ganglioneurocytoma"[15] or "differentiated neurocytoma" can be applied.[17]

**Grading.** Most central neurocytomas are so cytologically bland and mitotically impoverished that a grade II designation is inescapable once their neurocytic nature is secured. There exists a subset, however, in which mitoses are identified easily and the MIB-1 index is increased proportionately (Figs. 4–329 and 4–330). The term "atypical neurocytoma" has been coined for these tumors, which have a significantly elevated incidence of local recurrence.[19] A MIB-1 labeling index of 2% was suggested as the break point between "typical" and "atypical" lesions. On rare occasion, an intraventricular lesion combines the features of a neurocytoma with both ganglion cells and a malignant, small cell component.[10]

**Features in Frozen Sections.** Much of the neurocytoma's histologic and cytologic distinctiveness can be effaced by the freezing process. This is particularly true for the fine fibrillarity of the background (neuropil), which lends the lesion its neuronal quality in permanent sections. The fibrillar zones can even be misinterpreted as necrosis (Fig. 4–331). Freezing also adds a degree of nuclear angulation and hyperchromatism that, in concert, can raise the possibility of "small cell malignancy."

**Cytologic Features.** The markedly uniform nuclei with their salt-and-pepper chromatin are visualized best in cytologic preparations (Fig. 4–332). The fine cell processes are inapparent, being seen only in aggregate as an amorphous background.

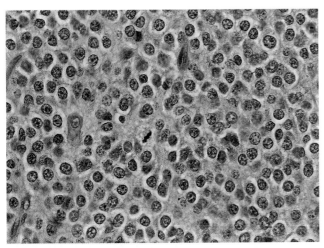

4–329

4–330

**FIGURES 4–329 AND 4–330**  ATYPICAL CENTRAL NEUROCYTOMA

Defined by increased mitotic activity (Fig. 4–329) and an elevated MIB-1 labeling index (Fig. 4–330), infrequently occurring "atypical" central neurocytomas are more likely to recur than are "typical" lesions.

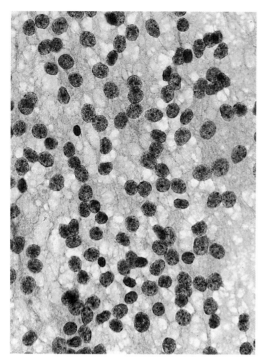

**FIGURE 4–332** CENTRAL NEUROCYTOMA

Marked nuclear uniformity and a "salt and pepper" chromatin distribution are both well seen in smear preparations.

**Immunohistochemical Features.** Antibodies to synaptophysin stain the fibrillar zones and, to a lesser extent, the perinuclear cytoplasm (Fig. 4–333). In contrast, the cells generally lack reactivity for chromogranin and neurofilament protein. Anti-Hu autoantibodies stain neurocyte nuclei.[6, 13] Indigenous reactive astrocytes reach out with their multiple, long, radiating GFAP-positive processes (Fig. 4–334).[4, 8] Some studies have shown a subpopulation of GFAP-positive neoplastic cells,[20] and glial differentiation has been substantiated in tissue culture.[9, 21] Central neurocytoma can thus be viewed as a

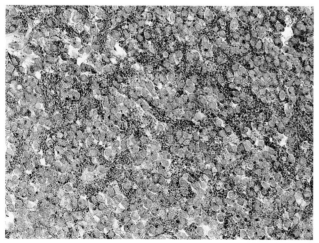

**FIGURE 4–333** CENTRAL NEUROCYTOMA

The somewhat fibrillar zones of neuropil and, to a lesser extent, the cytoplasm of individual cells are immunoreactive for synaptophysin.

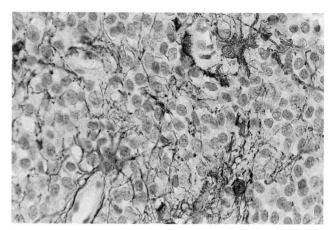

**FIGURE 4–334** CENTRAL NEUROCYTOMA

Although these lesions possess the capacity for both neuronal and glial differentiation, cells that are positive for glial fibrillary acidic protein usually represent trapped, reactive astrocytes.

mixed glioneuronal neoplasm, although one that is overwhelmingly neurocytic.

**Ultrastructural Features.** The neuronal quality of the neurocytoma is readily apparent at the ultrastructural level, where the cell processes contain microtubules and, in their terminations, both clear vesicles and dense-core granules (Fig. 4–335).[4, 7, 11] Intercellular junctions may be encountered, but well-formed synapses are rare.

**Differential Diagnosis.** In light of their cellular monomorphism and artifactual clear cytoplasm, it is not surprising that neurocytomas are often mistaken for *oligodendrogliomas* (Table 4–9, p. 213). Although the oligodendroglioma is not a discrete intraventricular mass, the two tumors can be remarkably similar histologically. Cell uniformity, finely fibrillar zones, streaming of cells, and absence of trapped or infiltrated CNS parenchyma help identify the neurocytic lesion, although these features are not always present. Immunohistochemistry for synaptophysin and neurofilament protein is therefore often a necessary adjunct. The former stains neurocytomas, whereas the latter decorates the axons that traverse oligodendrogliomas.

A neurocytoma's intraventricular location; gross characteristics; solid, noninfiltrating growth pattern; and perivascular pseudorosettes prompt consideration of *ependymoma*. Distinguishing features of the neurocytoma are its uncompromising nuclear roundness and perivascular rosettes that are less well defined than those of an ependymoma. Most importantly, the rosettes of a neurocytoma are synaptophysin positive and GFAP negative.

A lesion with neurocytic overtones, *dysembryoplastic neuroepithelial tumor*, makes a rare appearance in the third ventricle (see page 276). Both DNTs and neurocytomas are noted for nuclear uniformity and perinuclear halos. DNTs, however, are less cellular and more mucoid.

**Treatment and Prognosis.** Although permeating brain invasion is not a feature of central neurocytomas, surgical excision is not always possible because of secondary

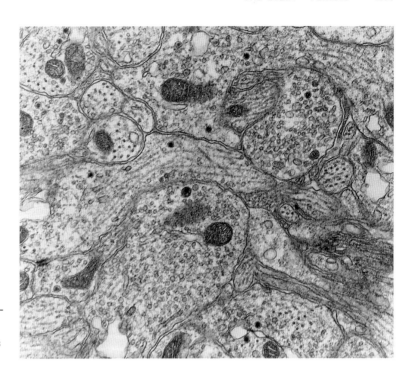

**FIGURE 4–335**   CENTRAL NEUROCYTOMA

Attesting to the neuronal nature of the lesion, cell processes contain aligned microtubules (neurotubules). Their terminations feature scattered dense-core granules and clear vesicles.

attachment to surrounding ventricular surfaces. In one series, gross total excision was possible in only 10 of 32 cases.[16] Fortunately, residual tumor grows slowly, and radiation therapy appears to be useful in controlling recurrence.[16] Some lesions may respond to chemotherapy.[1] Overall, the prognosis is excellent; the actuarial 5-year survival in one large series was 81%.[16] Craniospinal dissemination is most unusual.[3] Recurrences with an elevated MIB-1 index have been reported.[2]

### Extraventricular (Parenchymal) Neurocytic Neoplasms

**Definition.** Neurocyte-containing neuronal or glioneuronal tumors that are geographically remote from the region of the foramen of Monro.

**General Comments.** On rare occasion, neoplasms containing neurocytes arise at sites other than the region of the foramen of Monro.[5, 6, 12, 13, 18] Most are extraventricular—that is, intraparenchymal—but some are in or impinge on the ventricular system. The distinction among various classes of neurocytic tumors is less important than the need to recognize the group as a whole and not mistake its members for infiltrating gliomas, such as oligodendroglioma.

Morphologically, the lesions vary in terms of their content of neurocytes, "ganglioid cells" (small neurons with less prominent nucleoli and inconspicuous Nissl substance), ganglion cells, and, on occasion, glia. Descriptive nomenclature includes imposing and mellifluous designations such as "ganglioneurocytoma,"[14] "rosetted glioneuronal tumor,"[9, 17] "pseudopapillary neu-

rocytoma,"[10] and "papillary glioneuronal tumor."[2, 11] The last two reports describe similar if not identical lesions.

The rare lipidized cerebellar neoplasms that contain neurocyte-like cells have required such terms as "lipidized or lipomatous medulloblastoma"[3, 16] and "medullocytoma."[7] Their occurrence in adults is noteworthy. Closely related if not identical tumors have prompted the descriptive and no less imposing taxonomy "lipomatous glioneurocytoma,"[1] "neurolipocytoma,"[4] "myoneurocytoma,"[15] and "lipidized mature neuroectodermal tumor of the cerebellum with myoid differentiation."[8] Last, a rare cerebellar lesion with distinctly neurocytic qualities, but without fat, has been termed, simply, "neurocytoma."[5]

**Clinical Features.** The lesions generally favor children and young adults and manifest their presence through mass effects or by seizures.[6]

**Radiologic Features.** The tumors are sometimes large, complex, often cystic, frequently calcified, and generally discrete (Fig. 4–336).

**Microscopic Features.** Like the typical central neurocytoma, "ectopic" neurocytic neoplasms contain oligodendrocyte-like neurocytes that are either compacted into tight lobules or dispersed in a fibrillar background (Figs. 4–337 to 4–339). Although neurocytes usually predominate, this is not always the case, and some tumors are cytologically more complex, with more fibrillarity than is typical of central neurocytomas. Focal ganglion or ganglioid cells are not uncommon (Figs. 4–340 and 4–341). Calcification is frequent.

The cerebellar "medullocytoma" features sheets of round, uniform, neurocytic cells with few mitoses and a

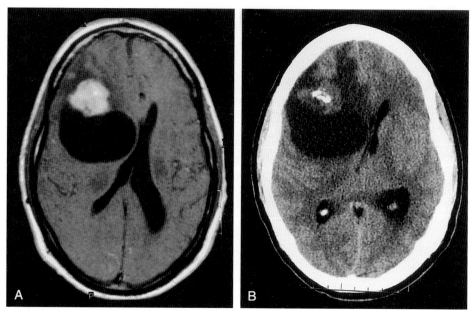

**FIGURE 4–336**    EXTRAVENTRICULAR NEUROCYTOMA

Extraventricular neurocytomas can be solid or cystic. This cystic example with a contrast-enhancing mural nodule (A) occurred in a 29-year-old man. Calcification, a common feature of neurocytomas at any site, is well seen by computed tomography (B).

low proliferation index.[7, 16] Cytologically, some closely resemble oligodendrogliomas, but the tumors are distinguished macroscopically because they are relatively discrete and noninfiltrative. Lobules of lipidized cells lie interposed among their "fat-free" compatriots. Such lesions are often "mixed" in composition, owing to the presence of an infiltrating glial component (Figs. 4–342 to 4–344).

As noted earlier, rare neurocytic lesions assume a distinctive pseudopapillary architecture, with hyalinized vessels, variable numbers of ganglion cells, and a largely perivascular zone of astrocytes (Figs. 4–345 to 4–347).

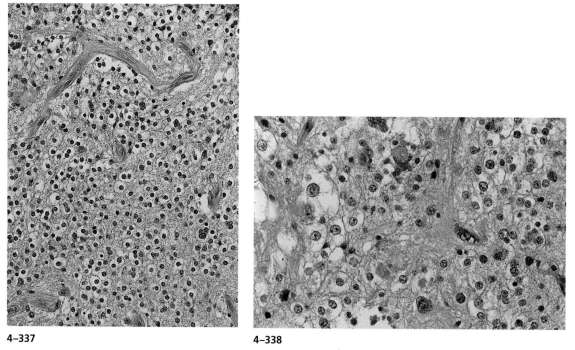

**4–337**                          **4–338**

**FIGURES 4–337 AND 4–338**    EXTRAVENTRICULAR NEUROCYTOMA

At both low (Fig. 4–337) and high (Fig. 4–338) magnification, the lesion closely resembles an oligodendroglioma. One distinguishing feature is the neurocytoma's solid, largely noninfiltrating architecture. Few normal central nervous system elements are present within the mass. In Figure 4–338, the cells have cytologic features, such as small nucleoli, that suggest ganglion cell differentiation. As is common in neuronal tumors and uncommon in oligodendrogliomas, eosinophilic granular bodies are present.

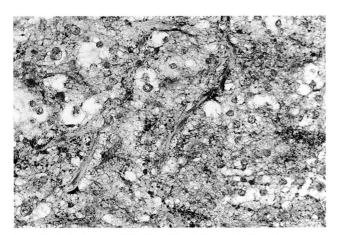

**FIGURE 4–339**   EXTRAVENTRICULAR NEUROCYTOMA

The somewhat fibrillar areas of delicate, neoplastic neuropil are immunoreactive for synaptophysin.

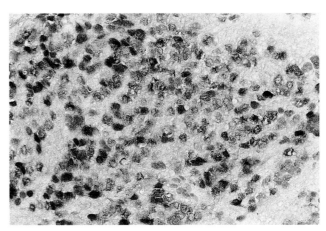

**FIGURE 4–341**   EXTRAVENTRICULAR NEUROCYTOMA

Antibodies to NeuN can be used to identify neurons. In contrast to antibodies to synaptophysin, it is the nucleus, not the cytoplasm, that is stained.

It can be debated whether these "papillary glioneuronal tumors"[2, 11] and a single example of "papillary neurocytoma"[10] are the same entity. They certainly are similar in histologic appearance and in their benign clinical course.

The most recently described entity, "rosetted glioneuronal tumor," contains an infiltrating glioma, an astrocytoma, and distinctive nodules of synaptophysin-positive neuropil (Figs. 4–348 and 4–349).[9, 17] The tumor can recur and is also discussed later in the section on malignant glioneuronal tumors.

Only rarely do neurocytic neoplasms exhibit malignant cytologic features or contain neuroblastic cells.

**Immunohistochemical Features.** The fibrillar background of neurocyte-rich areas is synaptophysin reactive, as are the surfaces of many ganglion cells (see Figs. 4–339, 4–343, and 4–347). Neurons are positive for NeuN (see Fig. 4–341). Some are also immunopositive for chromogranin. Astrocytes, either reactive or neoplastic, are GFAP positive. As with other glioneuronal lesions, it may be difficult to determine whether im-munoreactive glial cells are neoplastic or simply "stromal" elements, but the distinction appears to have little or no prognostic significance.

"Medullocytomas" are diffusely synaptophysin positive and may have a minority of GFAP-positive glia. Myocytes, striated in some cases, are reactive for appropriate muscle markers.[8, 15]

**Differential Diagnosis.** Because neurocytic neoplasms are uncommon and occur in diverse sites, they may not be considered in a differential diagnosis that restrictively focuses on *oligodendroglioma* or *mixed glioma*. Awareness of neurocytic neoplasms and their oligodendroglial mimicry minimizes the likelihood of this oversight. Review of the neuroradiologic findings is particularly appropriate in the face of any discrete lesion with oligodendroglioma-like features. Immunohistochemistry for synaptophysin resolves the issue.

It is of little importance whether one uses the term "medullocytoma" or "lipidized medulloblastoma" to designate this unique cerebellar lesion of adults, but it is of

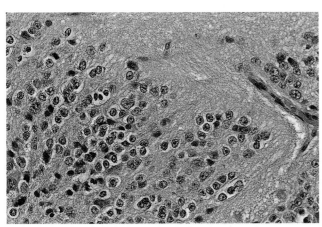

**FIGURE 4–340**   EXTRAVENTRICULAR NEUROCYTOMA

In contrast to central neurocytomas, differentiation toward ganglion cells is more common in extraventricular neurocytic neoplasms.

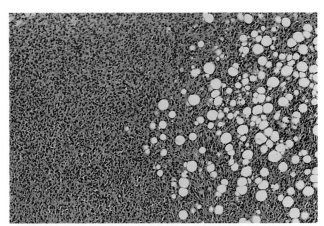

**FIGURE 4–342**   LIPIDIZED CEREBELLAR GLIONEUROCYTOMA

In these uncommon tumors, cytoplasmic accumulation of vacuoles of fat creates a superficial resemblance to adipose tissue. Lipidization is also rarely seen in central neurocytomas.

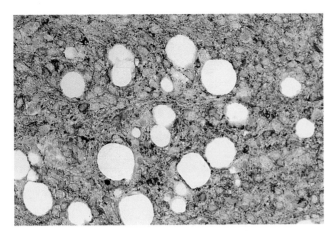

**FIGURE 4–343    LIPIDIZED CEREBELLAR GLIONEUROCYTOMA**

Immunoreactivity for synaptophysin helps define the neurocytic component.

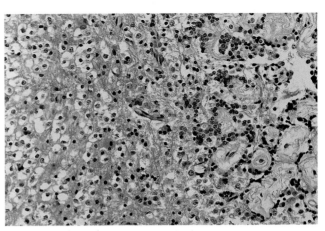

**FIGURE 4–345    PAPILLARY GLIONEURONAL TUMOR**

Small, dark glial cells that surround hyalinized vessels are associated with a neurocytic component of the neoplasm that closely resembles oligodendroglioma.

paramount importance that this cytologically bland, mitosis-poor lesion be distinguished from *medulloblastoma*.

*Medullomyoblastomas* are distinguished by their mitotic activity and malignant cytologic features.

### Diagnostic Checklist

- Is this "neurocytic" neoplasm just an infiltrating glioma, such as oligodendroglioma or mixed glioma?

**Treatment and Prognosis.** The limited recorded experience with the cerebral forms of extraventricular neurocytoma suggests that many are amenable to excision and that, in instances of subtotal resection, residual tumor behaves in a biologically indolent manner. In one series of 11 patients, most of whom were treated with neither radio- nor chemotherapy, death was attributable to the tumor in only one case.[6] Although medullocytomas can recur, cure seems possible in many cases,[7, 16] even without radiotherapy.[7]

## Malignant Neuronal and Glioneuronal Tumors

**Definition.** Neuronal or mixed glioneuronal neoplasms with malignant elements.

**General Comments.** Malignant mixed glioneuronal tumors are rare and heterogeneous lesions that must be distinguished from anaplastic astrocytomas, glioblastomas, and small cell embryonal tumors. A number of cases published in the preimmunohistochemical era are difficult to assess, because they might well have been malignant gliomas with trapped ganglion cells. Even today, using immunohistochemistry, such tumors can be difficult to identify with certainty. Their rarity has limited collective experience, and no generally accepted system of classification exists. Our simplified approach identifies four categories: (1) ganglion cell tumors with malignant glial components, (2) ganglion cell tumors with malignant neuronal components, (3) infiltrating

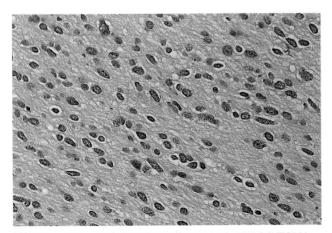

**FIGURE 4–344    LIPIDIZED CEREBELLAR GLIONEUROCYTOMA**

The glial component consists of small bipolar cells in a fibrillar background.

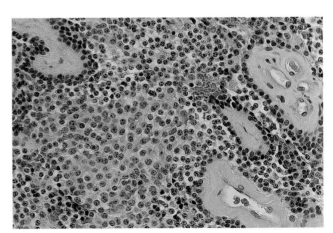

**FIGURE 4–346    PAPILLARY GLIONEURONAL TUMOR**

Sheets of neurocytic cells and palisaded, perivascular glial cells are key features of this uncommon entity.

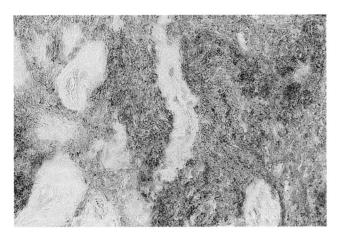

**FIGURE 4–347** PAPILLARY GLIONEURONAL TUMOR

Immunoreactivity for synaptophysin establishes the lesion's neuronal nature.

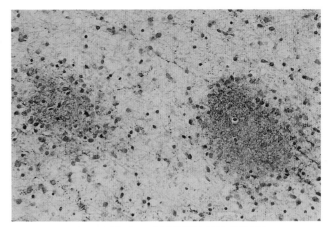

**FIGURE 4–349** ROSETTED GLIONEURONAL TUMOR

The fibrillar cores of the nodules are immunoreactive for synaptophysin. (Courtesy of Dr. Marc K. Rosenblum, New York, NY.)

gliomas with focal nodules of synaptophysin-positive neuropil, and (4) small cell neoplasms with focal neuroblastic differentiation evidenced by immunohistochemistry or electron microscopy.

**Clinical Features.** Patients of all ages are affected, but malignant tumors exhibiting ganglion cell components usually occur in children[1, 3–6, 10] or young adults.[8] In contrast, the largely undifferentiated lesions in which neuronal components are largely or exclusively immunohistochemical or ultrastructural findings usually occur in adult patients in the same age range as those with glioblastomas.

**Microscopic Features.** Patients with the most frequently occurring lesion, ganglioglioma with a malignant glial component, may have a long clinical history of seizures. Radiographic features, such as a discrete mass, often support the hypothesis that the malignant lesion arose within a preexisting low-grade lesion. Histologically, one sees both classic ganglion cell tumor and a high-grade, mitotically active, GFAP-positive glial ele-

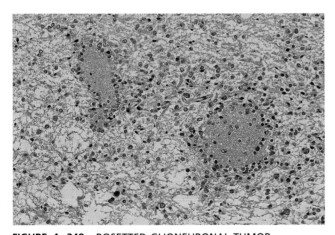

**FIGURE 4–348** ROSETTED GLIONEURONAL TUMOR

Well-circumscribed nodules, with a central neuropil-like fibrillarity, arise abruptly within the brain. (Courtesy of Dr. Marc K. Rosenblum, New York, NY.)

ment (Figs. 4–350 and 4–351).[2] In other cases, the malignant component is vimentin positive but negative for specific immunohistochemical markers. Thus, its nature remains in doubt.[1, 3, 4, 8]

The second tumor subtype has a malignant neuronal component formed of small, mitotically active, synaptophysin-positive cells in transition to larger neurons, or vice versa.[6, 10] Rare lesions are combinations of neurocytes, ganglion cells, and neuroblasts.[5] In one case, a ganglioglioma transformed biphasically to produce both malignant glia and malignant neurons.[6]

A third and rare glioneuronal lesion is one wherein distinctive, synaptophysin-positive islands of neuropil and ganglion cells occur in a lesion with all the features of an infiltrating astrocytoma. In rosetted fashion,[9] neurocytes and small ganglion cells satellite the nodules. Most commonly, the infiltrative glial component is a grade II diffuse astrocytoma. Although not malignant in the sense of anaplasia, these tumors have the potential to recur and are discussed here for that reason.

The fourth subtype, often a serendipitous finding, consists of a malignant glioma showing focal ultrastructural or immunohistochemical features of neuroblastic differentiation.[7, 10]

**Differential Diagnosis.** The principal issue in the differential diagnosis of any malignant neuronal or glioneuronal tumor is the avoidance of interpreting trapped ganglion cells in an *oligodendroglioma* or *diffuse astrocytoma* as part of the neoplasm. The section on gangliogliomas discusses this common issue.

Neoplasms in which the neuronal component is malignant must be distinguished from *high-grade gliomas* and *small cell embryonal tumors* (PNETs), including differentiating neuroblastoma or ganglioneuroblastoma. These lesions, however, consist of either solid sheets of small, undifferentiated cells or, in the latter tumor, a background of a neuropil without an accompanying glial component.

**Treatment and Prognosis.** To date, there have been so few cases that prognostication is difficult. Nonetheless, malignant gangliogliomas are aggressive and likely

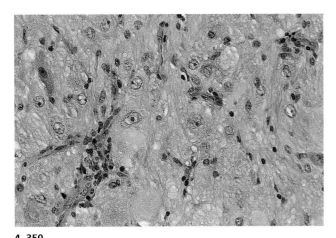

4–350

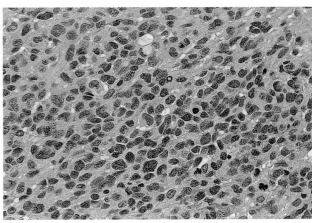

4–351

**FIGURES 4–350 AND 4–351    MALIGNANT GANGLIOGLIOMA**

Rare ganglion cell tumors combine mature ganglion cells (Fig. 4–350) with a mitotically active, cytologically malignant glioma (Fig. 4–351).

to recur. "Malignant gliomas" in which neuronal components are solely an immunohistochemical or ultrastructural feature behave like glioblastomas. The neuronal component thus has no apparent ameliorative effect on the prognosis.[10]

## Neoplasms and Non-Neoplastic Lesions of the Pineal Region

### Pineal Parenchymal Neoplasms (Pineocytoma, Pineal Parenchymal Neoplasm of Intermediate Differentiation, and Pineoblastoma)

**Definition.**  Neoplasms derived from pineocytes.

**General Comments.**  Pineal parenchymal tumors lie along a broad spectrum of differentiation, from well-differentiated lesions that are cured by simple excision to rapidly growing, disseminating tumors resistant to radio- and chemotherapy.[4, 9, 10] The WHO has partitioned this continuum into three grades: (1) pineocytoma, (2) pineal parenchymal tumor of intermediate differentiation, and (3) pineoblastoma. A less subjective approach, creating a tumor score on the basis of the mitotic count and immunostaining for neuronal markers, is discussed later in the section on treatment and prognosis.

**Clinical Features.**  Most pineocytomas occur in adults, from the third through the sixth decades. A mean age of 47 years was recorded in one study.[4, 10] Most pineoblastomas occur in childhood, but there are inevitable exceptions later in life.[2] Either neoplasm can present with symptoms that reflect obstruction to the flow of CSF or the pressure effects of the mass on adjacent structures. Rare pineoblastomas are a component of the "trilateral retinoblastoma" syndrome.[1, 18]

**Radiologic Features.**  The contrast-enhancing masses straddle in the midline, with variable infiltration of surrounding tissues that is in part proportional to tumor grade (Fig. 4–352). Some pineoblastomas have seeded CSF pathways by the time of the patient's initial presentation.

**Macroscopic Features.**  The gray, granular, relatively discrete mass fills the pineal region and compresses the subjacent aqueduct. Pineoblastomas are soft, gelatinous, and often focally necrotic.

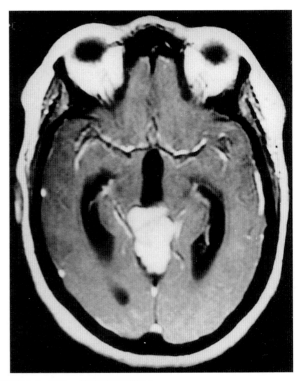

**FIGURE 4–352    PINEOCYTOMA**

Pineocytomas are well-circumscribed, contrast-enhancing masses situated in the posterior third ventricle. This lesion obstructed the flow of cerebrospinal fluid, producing headaches in a 58-year-old woman.

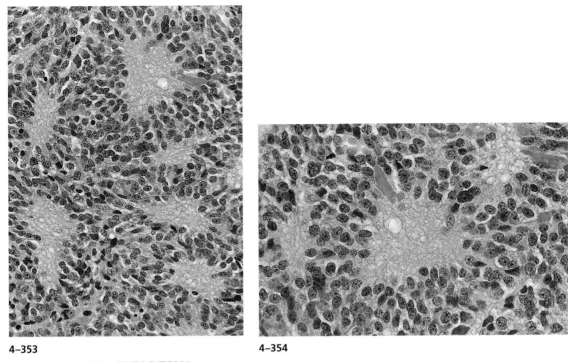

**4–353**    **4–354**

**FIGURES 4–353 AND 4–354**    PINEOCYTOMA

Large anuclear zones of neoplastic neuropil constitute the cores of pineocytomatous rosettes. As is typical, nuclei are round and regular and feature open chromatin.

**Microscopic Features.** In either diffuse or lobular forms, *pineocytomas* are formed of cells with nuclei that are larger and more open in their chromatin density than those in malignant small cell neoplasms such as pineoblastoma and medulloblastoma (Figs. 4–353 and 4–354). Mitoses are infrequent, if seen at all. There is no necrosis. Considerable nuclear polymorphism and hyperchromasia are not uncommon, but only as a form of degenerative atypia (see Fig. 4–356).[12]

The essence of a pineocytoma resides in the "pineocytomatous rosette" that is created by tumor cell processes,

which, in aggregate, form circular or slightly stellate foci of eosinophilia (Figs. 4–355 and 4–356). These interrupt a background that otherwise would be densely cellular. The structure is similar to but considerably larger than the neuroblastic, or Homer Wright, rosette seen in medulloblastomas, supratentorial embryonal tumors, and some pineoblastomas. Ganglion cells, as either solitary forms in a cellular background or large islands of neuropil, are uncommon expressions of neuronal differentiation.[6, 12, 21]

The consummate *pineoblastoma* is a classic small cell, mitotically active neoplasm (Fig. 4–357) in which necrosis

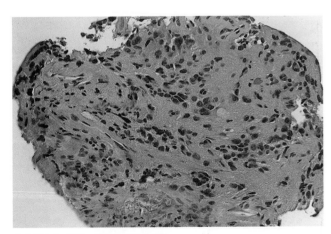

**FIGURE 4–355**    PINEOCYTOMA

The location and vascularity of the pineal region limit surgical accessibility. As a result, specimens are often quite small. Large, typical pineocytomatous rosettes are nevertheless present in this minute, somewhat distorted sample.

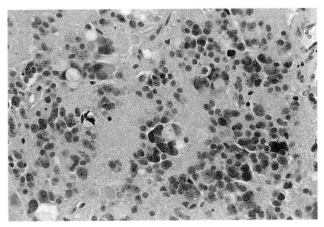

**FIGURE 4–356**    PINEOCYTOMA

In the presence of well-formed, large rosettes, nuclear pleomorphism should not be interpreted as evidence of malignancy.

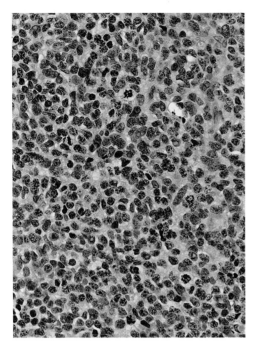

**FIGURE 4–357**    PINEOBLASTOMA

Highly cellular lesions such as this occupy the most cellular end of the pineal parenchymal tumor spectrum.

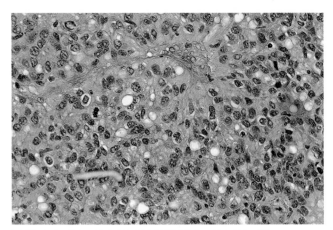

**FIGURE 4–360**    PINEAL PARENCHYMAL TUMOR OF INTERMEDIATE DIFFERENTIATION

This lesion has the large, round nuclei of pineocytoma but also features scattered mitoses. Note the lack of pineocytomatous rosettes.

and apoptosis may be prominent. Rosettes of either the Homer Wright (Fig. 4–358) or the Flexner-Wintersteiner (retinoblastoma) (Fig. 4–359) type are frequently present.[20, 25] In other examples, anaplasia is not universal, and tumor of intermediate grade is present also.

The "fleurette" is a rare, explicit form of photoreceptor differentiation in which inner and outer visual receptor segments project into a luminal rosette.[20, 24, 25] An additional form of "retinal" differentiation—pigmented epithelium—is combined with muscle differentiation in a unique neoplasm variously termed "pineal anlage tumor"[23] or "primitive pineal tumor with retinoblastomatous and retinal/ciliary epithelial differentiation."[20]

Glial differentiation, a rarity, creates cells with ample cytoplasm or GFAP-positive processes that produce background fibrillarity.[21, 24]

Although some pineal parenchymal tumors lie at one of two extremes—pineocytoma or pineoblastoma—many occupy the middle ground in terms of cellularity, differentiation, and mitotic activity. Termed "pineal parenchymal tumors of intermediate differentiation," they pose a diagnostic challenge, because their definition is not precise (Fig. 4–360). Generally, this diagnosis is appropriate in the face of a lesion without the rosettes of pineocytoma or the overt small cell appearance of pineoblastoma. Cytoplasm is discernible, mitoses are few, and necrosis is lacking.

Tumors with areas of both intermediate differentiation and pineoblastoma are considered pineoblastoma (Fig. 4–361).

Another approach to grading uses two criteria: the mitotic count, and the presence or absence of staining for neurofilament protein.[4, 10] Grade I lesions are the

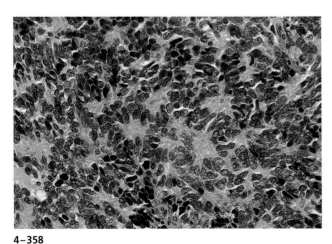

4–358

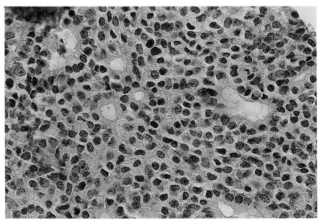

4–359

**FIGURES 4–358 AND 4–359**    PINEOBLASTOMA

Pineoblastomas can have rosettes of either the neuroblastic (Homer Wright) (Fig. 4–358) or the retinoblastic (Flexner-Wintersteiner) (Fig. 4–359) type.

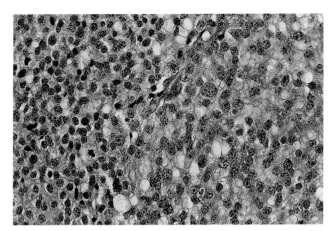

**FIGURE 4-361    COMBINED PINEOBLASTOMA AND PINEAL PARENCHYMAL TUMOR OF INTERMEDIATE DIFFERENTIATION**

This lesion contains both densely cellular pineoblastoma and neoplastic tissue in which the nuclei are larger and paler. The cells in the latter regions have more cytoplasm and are less mitotically active.

classic pineocytoma with no mitoses and strong immunopositivity for neurofilament protein. Grade II tumors have fewer than six mitoses per 10 high-power fields. Grade III tumors have either fewer than six mitoses but only +/− staining for the protein or greater than six mitoses but +/+ staining. Grade IV neoplasms have variable mitoses and only +/− staining for neurofilament protein.

**Immunohistochemical Features.** Individual tumor cells or fibrillar areas in the center of pineocytomatous or Homer Wright rosettes are positive for synaptophysin and neurofilament protein (Fig. 4–362).[3, 12] Faint immunoreactivity for tau has been noted, presumably as the equivalent of the paired helical filaments seen in some cases by electron microscopy.[5] In some cases, scattered cells are positive for retinal S-antigen.[11, 19, 20] Pineoblastomas are synaptophysin positive. Neurofilament protein is detected in accord with the degree of differentiation.[4, 10]

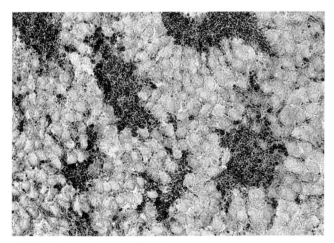

**FIGURE 4-362    PINEOCYTOMA**

The cores of pineocytomatous rosettes are immunoreactive for synaptophysin.

As is the case for the normal pineal gland, GFAP-positive processes are pervasive and should not be misinterpreted in themselves as evidence of a glioma.[19]

The MIB-1 labeling index is understandably higher in pineoblastomas than in pineocytomas (6.49% versus 0.27% in one small study).[17] In some instances, it approaches the remarkable levels seen in malignant small cell embryonal tumors (PNETs).

**Ultrastructural Features.** The cells of pineocytoma exhibit features of normal pineocytes, including dense-core vesicles, "vesicle-crowned rodlets" ("synaptic ribbons"), microtubules, and the so-called fibrous filaments.[5, 8] Paired helical filaments identical to those in Alzheimer's disease have also been observed.[5, 7] The fibrillar cores of the pineocytomatous rosettes consist of closely packed processes filled with microtubules. Their cells' club-shaped terminations contain dense-core granules.[6]

The spectrum of differentiation from pineoblastoma through pineal parenchymal tumor of intermediate differentiation to pineocytoma has correlates at the ultrastructural level. Aggressive pineoblastomas are undifferentiated lesions, whereas pineocytomas are clearly neuronal tumors with all the special features of pineocytes described earlier.[14] The cells of pineal parenchymal tumors of intermediate differentiation occupy the midportion of the spectrum; organelles, processes, and granules are less abundant than in pineocytomas.

Flexner-Wintersteiner rosettes are accepted as evidence of retinoblastomatous differentiation; their cilia possess the 9 + 0 configuration normally observed in photoreceptors.

**Differential Diagnosis.** Distinguishing pineocytoma from normal pineal parenchyma and from parenchyma incorporated in the wall of a pineal cyst is the principal issue in the differential diagnosis of pineocytoma.

The *normal pineal gland* has deceived generations of pathologists who, while examining surgical or autopsy specimens, have mistaken this peculiar tissue for a neoplasm. The normal gland varies considerably both during embryonic development and during its evolution thereafter.[15, 16] In the adult, it is a compact tissue composed of cells with meager amounts of cytoplasm and sizable, pale nuclei that differ cytologically from those of ordinary neurons and glia (Fig. 4–363). The avid immunoreactivity of the normal gland for synaptophysin helps confirm only its neuronal nature, not the diagnosis of pineal parenchymal tumor (Fig. 4–364). Reactivity for neurofilament protein highlights the orderly arrangement of processes and their terminal expansions at the vascular interface, a feature far better seen in normal tissue than in pineocytomas. The MIB-1 labeling index of normal parenchymal cells is typically 0. Importantly, the normal gland lacks the tumor's signature feature: the pineocytomatous rosette. Immunostaining for GFAP highlights the gland's lobularity (Fig. 4–365).

The normal pineal parenchyma amalgamated to the wall of a *pineal cyst* has a relatively discrete interface with the gliotic cyst wall. The latter usually contains granular bodies and/or Rosenthal fibers, as well as iron deposited in scattered histiocytes. Attention to

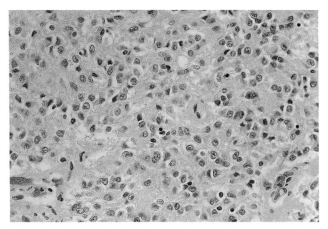

**FIGURE 4–363    NORMAL PINEAL GLAND**

The cellularity and seeming lack of specific architectural features of this normal pineal gland combine to simulate a neoplasm. The telltale lobularity of normal pineal tissue is not always apparent in small specimens.

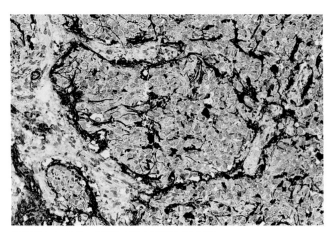

**FIGURE 4–365    NORMAL PINEAL GLAND**

Staining for glial fibrillary acidic protein emphasizes the gland's lobularity.

neuroimaging generally settles the issue. The pineal cyst is discussed separately in a later section.

The differential diagnosis of pineoblastoma invariably embraces the possibility of *medulloblastoma*. The issue is usually resolved on the basis of anatomic location. Histologically, the two can be separated to a certain extent, because pineoblastomas lack "pale islands" or a reticulin-rich (desmoplastic) stroma, and medulloblastomas rarely contain Flexner-Wintersteiner rosettes.

### Diagnostic Checklist

■ Is this "pineocytoma" nothing more than normal gland, for example, around a pineal cyst?

**Treatment and Prognosis.** Pineocytoma is essentially a benign tumor. Long survivals and even cures are expected.[13, 22] In one series,[22] the 5-year survival rate was 86%. Although radiotherapy is administered frequently, its value is unclear.[13]

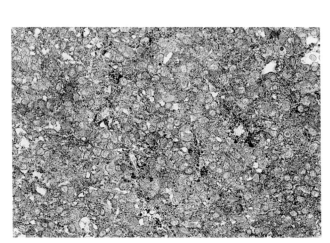

**FIGURE 4–364    NORMAL PINEAL GLAND**

The normal gland is immunoreactive for synaptophysin.

The prognosis for patients with pineoblastomas is generally poor, with few patients surviving longer than 2 years.[13, 22] The percentage of survivors is in part related to the extent of tumor resection. In one small series of adults, five patients with positive staging died of disease, whereas an equal number with negative staging were alive without progression after a median of 26 months.[2]

Using the grading system described earlier in the section on microscopic features, significant differences were apparent in the survival and disease-free survival among the four groups, with progressively poorer outcomes as the grade increased.[4, 10] All patients with grade I tumors were alive at the time of the publication, whereas all those with grade IV lesions had succumbed by 4 years. The survival experiences for patients with grade II and III neoplasms were intermediate.

### Other Neoplasms in the Pineal Region

Cells in and about the pineal gland give rise to a broad spectrum of neoplasms that are novel only because of their location. Although germ cell tumors are common in this region they are described in a separate section on pages 325 to 329, because they are not restricted to this anatomic site.

Other entities include meningioma,[9, 12] hemangiopericytoma,[15, 19] cavernous hemangioma,[5, 6, 10] ganglioglioma,[8] pilocytic astrocytoma,[4] granular cell astrocytoma,[17] ependymoma, and simply "glioma."[2, 22] Chemodectoma or paraganglioma,[16] epidermoid cyst,[1, 11, 20] metastatic carcinoma,[7, 24] myeloblastoma,[23] melanotic progonoma,[13] primary malignant melanoma,[3, 14, 25] and even craniopharyngioma[18, 21] enlarge the spectrum.

### Pineal Cyst

**Definition.** A non-neoplastic intrapineal cyst.

**Clinical Features.** An unusually large pineal cyst may obstruct CSF flow or, less commonly, compress the dorsal

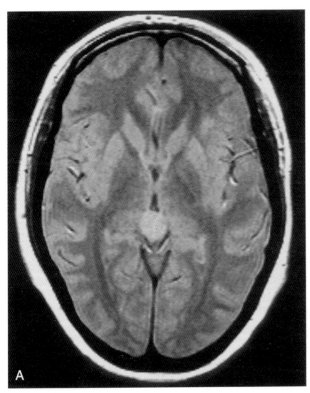 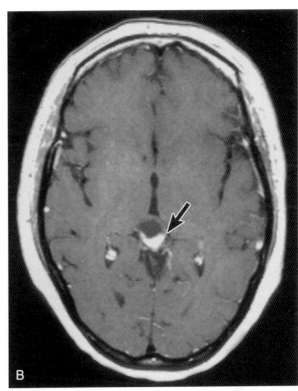

**FIGURE 4–366    PINEAL CYST**

A typical pineal cyst is illustrated in proton-density (*A*) and T1-weighted postcontrast (*B*) images. The cyst has increased signal intensity in *A*. The contrast-enhancing pineal gland is located posteriorly (*arrow*). The patient was a 40-year-old woman with headaches.

midbrain (Fig. 4–366).[2, 3, 5, 8, 9] Symptomatic patients are generally in the third through fifth decades of life.[2, 9] Most cysts, however, are discovered as incidental radiologic or autopsy findings (Fig. 4–367).[2–6, 8, 9, 11, 12] One study found 29 cysts in 672 consecutive MRI scans (4.3%).[6] A higher incidence in young women has been suggested.[2, 12]

**Radiologic Features.** Midline in location, the lesions are bright in T2-weighted images.[3, 6, 11] Contrast material, initially confined to the wall, subsequently seeps into its lumen.[7] Evidence of old hemorrhage, in the form of hemosiderin, or evidence of more recent bleed-

ing, such as a fluid-fluid level, is seen in some cases.[10] Residual pineal gland is often displaced posteroinferiorly (see Fig. 4–366).

**Macroscopic Features.** Unilocular or, less often, multilocular, the cysts have a smooth lining that may be cinnamon colored owing to hemosiderin deposition (Fig. 4–368). Ordinarily, the cyst is filled with thin, clear-to-yellow fluid.

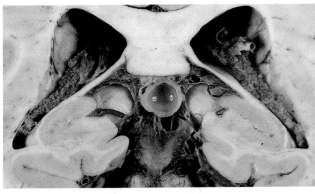

**FIGURE 4–367    PINEAL CYST**

Pineal cysts are usually incidental postmortem or neuroradiologic findings.

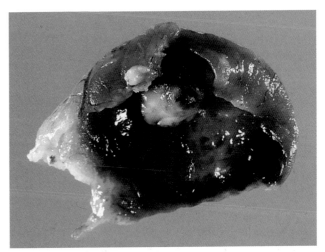

**FIGURE 4–368    PINEAL CYST**

Hemosiderin as a residue of remote hemorrhage gives many pineal cysts a rusty coloration.

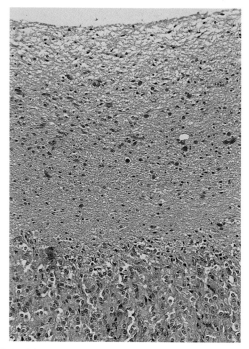

**FIGURE 4–369**   PINEAL CYST

The lumen is circumscribed by a layer of glial tissue that often contains Rosenthal fibers. In turn, this layer interfaces abruptly with the normal pineal parenchyma. Although not seen here, the entire cyst and gland are surrounded by a delicate connective tissue layer.

**Microscopic Features.** The cyst has three layers: (1) an internal zone of finely fibrillar glial tissue, (2) a lamina of pineal parenchyma, and (3) a delicate exterior layer of connective tissue (Figs. 4–369 and 4–370). The glial layer is finely fibrillar, often contains Rosenthal fibers, and frequently is hemosiderin stained. The pineal parenchyma may appear somewhat disorganized, but it is clearly confined to a lamina with a relatively abrupt demarcation from the subjacent glial cyst wall. Scalloped, basophilic concretions ("brain sand") are commonly

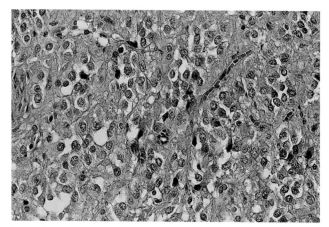

**FIGURE 4–370**   NORMAL PINEAL GLAND IN PINEAL CYST

The gland's seemingly disorganized, large polygonal cells create the impression of a neoplasm.

present. Remnants of ependyma from the posterior third ventricular wall are sometimes seen, particularly in specimens obtained post mortem.[1] As a rule, these are not apparent in the symptomatic cysts.

**Immunohistochemical Features.** The cyst wall is intensely positive for GFAP, whereas the parenchymal cells and processes of the normal gland are strongly immunoreactive for synaptophysin. Large, stellate, GFAP-positive astrocytes are a normal stromal constituent of the residual pineal gland.

**Differential Diagnosis.** The principal problem is not to confuse the cyst's parenchymal component for a *pineocytoma* (see Fig. 4–370). The latter is a solid, rosette-containing mass, whereas the normal parenchyma in the wall of a cyst is confined to a distinct lamina exterior to the glial layer. Awareness of the radiologic appearance assists in the distinction, because pineocytomas are typically solid rather than cystic. Out of this context, the normal gland, especially with the artifacts of a frozen section, may be misinterpreted as a neoplasm. The differential between pineal cyst and pineocytoma is also discussed on pages 295 to 296.

A glioma, such as a *pilocytic astrocytoma*, must be considered in view of the glial component with its Rosenthal fibers. However, pineal cyst walls are paucicellular, and they lack the biphasic, compact, microcystic architecture so typical of pilocytic astrocytomas. Hemosiderin staining is more consonant with a cyst than with an astrocytoma.

**Treatment and Prognosis.** Pineal cysts are totally benign, but occasional slow "recurrence" is possible.[2, 9]

## Small Cell Embryonal Neoplasms

### Medulloblastoma

**Definition.** A malignant, "small cell" tumor of the cerebellum.

**General Comments.** Although most medulloblastomas arise sporadically, a few appear in the setting of hereditary tumor syndromes such as Turcot's or Gorlin's (see the section on molecular and cytogenetic features). At present, the term "medulloblastoma" denotes a family of neoplasms that share clinical and pathologic features to the extent that discussion as an entity is warranted. Molecular studies, meanwhile, are dissecting these lesions into distinct subtypes, from which prognostic and therapeutic ramifications are quickly following.

Although the cytogenesis or "origin" of medulloblastomas has not been established, it has long been suspected that at least some arise from the external granular cell layer[45] or from nests of small, mitotically active cells in the posterior medullary velum[71] or cerebellar vermis.[91] There may well be more than one cell of origin; for example, nodular lesions could arise from the external granular cell layer, and "classic" medulloblastomas could stem from cells of the subventricular matrix.[49]

**Clinical Features.** Medulloblastomas usually present in the first 2 decades of life,[64, 75] declining sharply thereafter.[15, 16, 38, 42, 73] Only a rare case is congenital.[62] A slight male predominance of approximately 1.5:1 persists in many large series.[9, 43, 66, 75] Cerebellar symptoms, such as truncal ataxia (from midline tumors) and appendicular ataxia (from hemispheric lesions), often coexist with signs and symptoms of CSF flow obstruction.

**Radiologic Features.** Medulloblastomas appear as rather discrete, contrast-enhancing masses (Fig. 4–371). A remarkably botryoid and sometimes cystic architecture characterizes a subset of extremely nodular lesions that occur in the very young (Fig. 4–372).[31] Medulloblastomas in adults may be more likely than childhood lesions to be hemispheric and appear extra-axial.[4]

**Macroscopic Features.** Most medulloblastomas originate in the vermis, where they evolve into relatively discrete, soft, gray-pink masses. Some are stippled with small necrotic foci, but extensive necrosis is rare. Firmness parallels the extent of desmoplasia. Medulloblastomas of the cerebellar hemispheres are thought to occur most often in older patients and are more often discrete tumors of the nodular desmoplastic type (Fig. 4–373).[16, 17]

**Microscopic Features.** Although medulloblastomas are composed primarily of monotonous small cells, there is considerable inter- and intratumoral variation in their

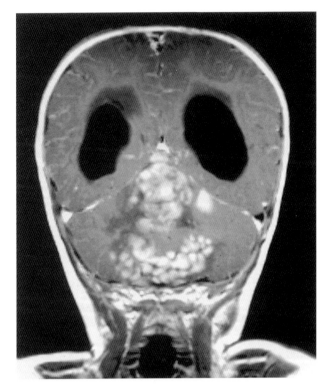

**FIGURES 4–372  MEDULLOBLASTOMA**

Multiple grape-like, contrast-enhancing nodules constitute the extensively nodular medulloblastoma that is generally seen in the first year of life. (Courtesy of Dr. F. Di Paola, Treviso, Italy.)

histologic patterns and immunohistochemical features. Medulloblastoma "variants" containing striated muscle ("medullomyoblastoma") and melanin-producing cells ("melanotic medulloblastoma") are described later in a separate section.

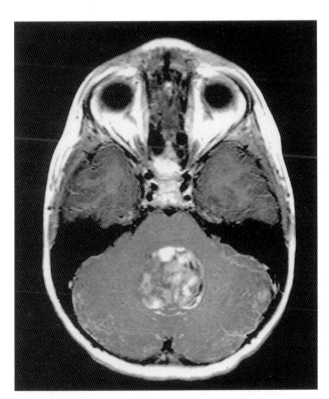

**FIGURE 4–371  MEDULLOBLASTOMA**

Medulloblastomas are generally well-circumscribed masses that, when large, enhance inhomogeneously. (Courtesy of Dr. James W. Langston, Memphis, TN.)

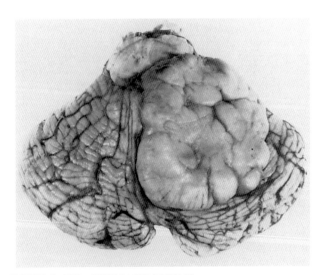

**FIGURE 4–373  MEDULLOBLASTOMA**

Nodular/desmoplastic medulloblastomas are well circumscribed and are likely to be laterally situated in a cerebellar hemisphere. (Courtesy of Professor A. Allegranza, Milan, Italy.)

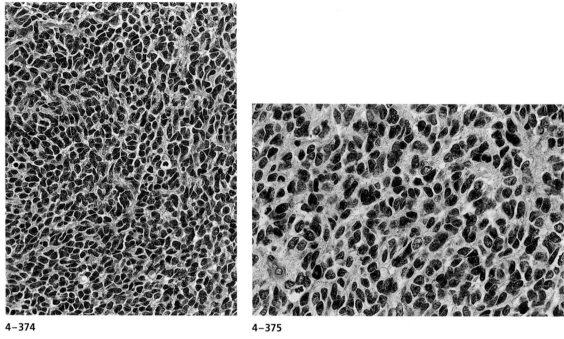

4-374                           4-375

**FIGURES 4–374 AND 4–375**   MEDULLOBLASTOMA

The "classic" medulloblastoma is composed of monomorphous sheets of small undifferentiated cells.

Based on the features in H&E-stained sections, we present five basic histologic-cytologic patterns or categories. Because cytologic differentiation rather closely parallels immunoreactivity for neuronal and glial markers, comments regarding immunophenotype are included here as well as in the section on immunohistochemical features.

*"Undifferentiated" or classic medulloblastoma:* This lesion is characterized by patternless sheets of small cells without any of the architectural features of the other variants described later (Figs. 4–374 and 4–375). Quotation marks are used advisedly around the term "undifferentiated," because electron microscopy and antibodies to synaptophysin provide evidence of neuronal differentiation in most cases. Cytologically, the cells vary considerably in nuclear shape and cytoplasmic configuration. Some cells are monomorphous and cytologically bland, to the extent that can be expected of a small cell malignant neoplasm. Other lesions are more worrisome because of nuclear irregularity and coarser chromatin. At the extreme, this group merges with the "large cell/anaplastic" category discussed later. Geographic zones of necrosis, with or without "pseudopalisading," are occasionally present. Mitotic figures range from scant to abundant. Apoptosis can be prominent.[77, 80]

*Nodular/desmoplastic medulloblastoma:* The term "desmoplastic" has been used as a generic designation for collagen-rich tumors, but also as a metaphor for medulloblastomas with prominent nodules, or "pale islands," set in reticulin-rich interlobular tumor tissue (Figs. 4–376 and 4–377).[24, 46, 48] Apoptosis is often more prominent in the intranodular areas (Fig. 4–378). In some markedly desmoplastic lesions, the tumor cells are compressed into slender columns by the deposition of collagen in a manner reminiscent of scirrhous carcinoma of the breast (Fig. 4–379). Such lesions can be nodular or anodular.

In its fullest expression, the nodular/desmoplastic pattern imparts a superficial resemblance to a lymph

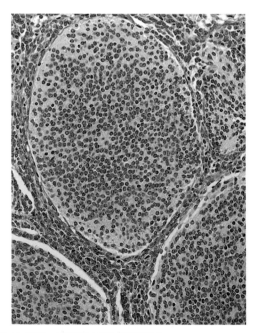

**FIGURE 4–376**   MEDULLOBLASTOMA

Rarefied nodules of reduced cellularity are found in about one third of medulloblastomas.

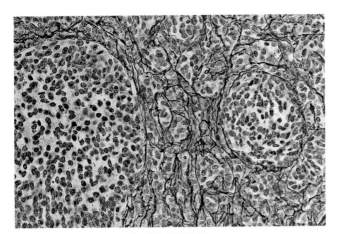

**FIGURES 4–377**   MEDULLOBLASTOMA

Reticulin is abundant in internodular regions, as illustrated here in a nodular/desmoplastic medulloblastoma from a patient with Gorlin's syndrome.

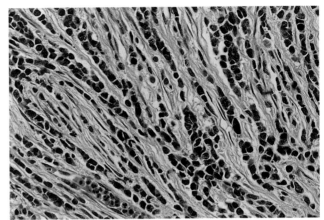

**FIGURE 4–379**   MEDULLOBLASTOMA

Desmoplasia as might be seen in a scirrhous carcinoma is a striking finding in some nodular/desmoplastic medulloblastomas.

node, with mantles of dark cells surrounding pale islands resembling germinal centers. Completing the analogy, reticulin fibers permeate the compact cellular zones but spare the "follicles" (see Fig. 4–377). In most instances, the nodules are conspicuous at low magnification, but in others, they are only appreciated at higher magnification as small, round reductions in nuclear density. As a rule, the more nodular the lesion, the more cytologically uniform are its cells. In some instances, the latter resemble neurocytes, being monotonous, perfectly spherical, and prone to the formation of oligodendrocyte-like perinuclear halos. Cellular streaming and apoptosis are common in this setting.

There are usually significant differences in the degree of cytologic atypia and mitotic rate between inter- and intranodular regions. Not only is the nuclear chromatin coarser (Fig. 4–380), but the cells are more proliferative in the internodular tissue.[47, 77] The MIB-1

indices are usually higher as well (Fig. 4–381). The nuclei at the edge of the nodules may be somewhat larger and have more prominent nucleoli, features suggestive of early ganglion cell differentiation. A fibrillar anuclear zone is also often present at the periphery of the pale islands. Flow cytofluorometry shows near diploidy, as opposed to a more varied DNA content in the "classic," non-nodular lesions.[29]

Less than 5% of medulloblastomas are so advanced in nodularity and differentiation toward cytologically bland neurocytes that little, if any, extranodular tissue is present (Figs. 4–382 and 4–383).[25, 31] The term "cerebellar neuroblastoma" has been used for these distinctive lesions,[68] but more recently they have been designated "medulloblastomas with extensive nodularity."[31] The intranodular cells, with their remarkably uniform and essentially mitosis-free nuclei, drift in a finely fibrillar background. Large, highly fibrillar, synaptophysin-positive

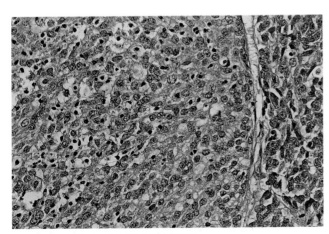

**FIGURE 4–378**   MEDULLOBLASTOMA

Apoptosis in this nodular/desmoplastic lesion is more prominent within the nodules than in the internodular areas.

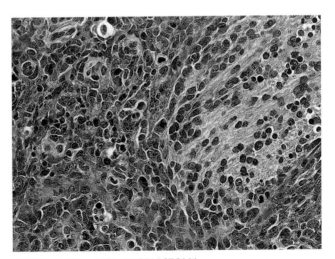

**FIGURE 4–380**   MEDULLOBLASTOMA

In this nodular/desmoplastic tumor, cytologic atypia and mitotic activity are generally more prominent in internodular regions. Cytologic atypia is especially prominent in this case.

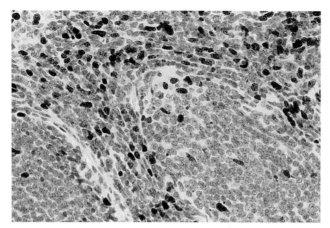

**FIGURE 4–381    MEDULLOBLASTOMA**

In accord with the cytologic features, the staining index for the cell cycling marker MIB-1 is higher in internodular regions.

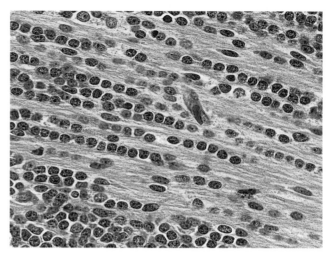

**FIGURE 4–383    MEDULLOBLASTOMA**

In extensively nodular medulloblastomas, neurocytes stream in a finely fibrillar tissue composed of aligned tumor cell processes.

areas of small ganglion cells may be present, if not at the time of the initial operation, then on subsequent resection.[28, 31] These highly nodular lesions, more neurocytic than neuroblastic, represent the extreme end of the spectrum of nodularity and differentiation. Their favorable prognosis is discussed in the section on treatment and prognosis.

The possible relationship between nodularity and mutations in the *PTCH* gene is discussed later in the section on molecular and cytogenetic features.

*Medulloblastoma with neuroblastic or neuronal differentiation:* The most common histologic expression of neuroblastic differentiation is the Homer Wright rosette, which is assembled by cells surrounding a small, circular to stellate zone of fibrillarity (Fig. 4–384). Stacked up and sectioned longitudinally, the formations appear as opposed columns of nuclei. In many medulloblastomas, neuroblastic rosettes are abortive or not fully expressed,

and one can only suspect the neuroblastic nature of the tumors in H&E-stained sections. Overtly neuroblastic lesions with well-formed Homer Wright rosettes often have perivascular pseudorosettes similar to those in ependymomas (see Fig. 4–400). Another patterned orientation of cells is found in some medulloblastomas that involve the molecular layer. Linear columns of cells stripe the molecular layer as the cells appear to orient to processes of Bergmann's glia as the latter extend to and from the foliar surface (Fig. 4–385). CNS neoplasms with ribboning or palisading are listed in Table 4–11, p. 226.

Less often, a medulloblastoma realizes a full potential for neuronal differentiation in the form of large neurons (Fig. 4–386). These appear as mature ganglion cells or as "adolescent" ganglioid cells that are intermediate in development between neuroblasts and ganglion cells. Their identification as neoplastic, rather than merely trapped, is greatly simplified if these transitional

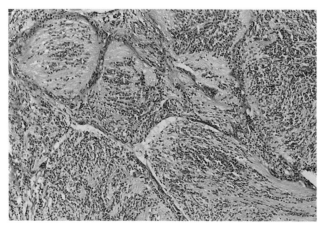

**FIGURE 4–382    MEDULLOBLASTOMA**

The rare subset of extensively nodular medulloblastomas has little or no internodular tissue. Figure 4–372 shows the radiologic appearance of this rare variant.

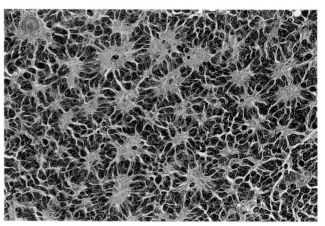

**FIGURE 4–384    MEDULLOBLASTOMA**

Homer Wright rosettes are a histologic expression of neuroblastic differentiation in a minority of medulloblastomas.

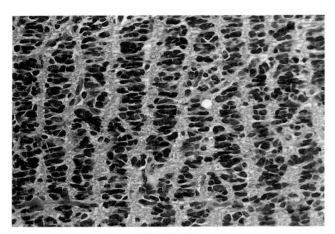

**FIGURE 4–385** MEDULLOBLASTOMA

Columns of cells in the molecular layer are sometimes prominent.

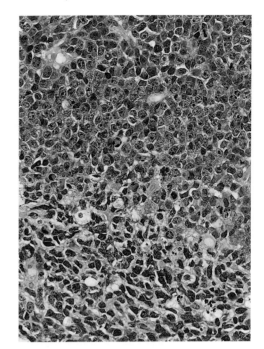

**FIGURE 4–387** MEDULLOBLASTOMA

Some medulloblastomas show marked cytologic atypia, as well as the distinctive "large cell" pattern. The "anaplastic" tissue at the bottom of the illustration appears to transform abruptly into a nodule of "large cell" medulloblastoma at the top.

cell forms are present or if the cells sit in a fibrillar neuropil background of their own creation. Widely separated, mature ganglion cells are more difficult to distinguish from preexisting normal neurons, particularly because normal neurons severed from their normal neuroanatomic surroundings frequently display nuclear and architectural abnormalities. This does not include binucleation. Attention to architectural features may also be of help. Neoplastic ganglion cells often lie jumbled in nodules and lack both the laminar architecture of the Purkinje cell layer and the uniform cellularity of deep cerebellar nuclei.

A rare cerebellar neoplasm designated "cerebellar ganglioneuroblastoma" shows extensive differentiation toward immature and mature neurons.[23] The clustered neurons are smaller than ganglion cells but possess nuclei that are larger than those of the neuroblasts. Such lesions are also intensely synaptophysin positive.

*"Large cell/anaplastic" medulloblastoma:* The designation "large cell" refers to an uncommon medulloblastoma composed of sheets and lobules of distinctive, round cells with prominent nucleoli (Figs. 4–387 and 4–388).[9, 30] "Large cell" and closely related "anaplastic" lesions represent about 4% of medulloblastomas (Fig. 4–389).[9, 30] The sheets or lobules of these round, large cells often arise in a background of "anaplastic," or markedly atypical, neoplastic tissue. In the latter, nuclei are irregular, and atypia is marked, but the roundness and prominent nucleoli of the large cell tissue are lacking.

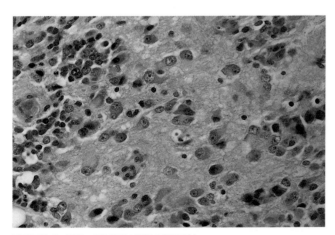

**FIGURE 4–386** MEDULLOBLASTOMA

Differentiation to ganglion cells is an uncommon feature of medulloblastoma.

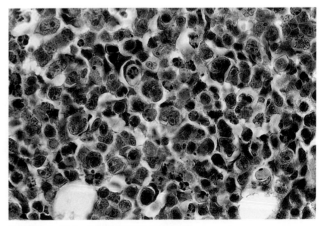

**FIGURE 4–388** MEDULLOBLASTOMA

Cells with large, round nuclei containing prominent nucleoli define the so-called large cell medulloblastoma. Frequent mitoses, conspicuous apoptosis, and cell "wrapping" are common in this aggressive tumor subtype.

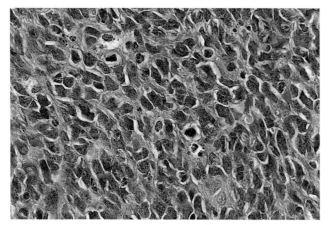

**FIGURE 4–389**   ANAPLASTIC MEDULLOBLASTOMA

Some medulloblastomas have the degree of nuclear atypia and pleomorphism seen in anaplastic carcinomas.

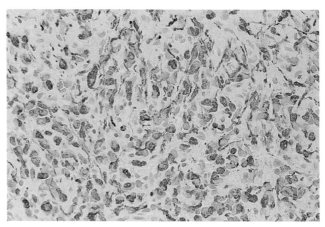

**FIGURE 4–391**   MEDULLOBLASTOMA

Immunoreactivity for glial fibrillary acidic protein in the lesion depicted in Figure 4–390 confirms the impression that the eosinophilic, highly fibrillar tissue is glial, not neuronal.

The countervailing forces of apoptosis and mitotic activity are evident in these lesions. Unfortunately, the latter prevails in this highly aggressive variant. In addition to the presence of scattered apoptotic cells, there are large regions of what resemble confluent areas of fragmented apoptotic cells. Engulfment of apoptotic fragments by neighboring viable cells is also common (see Fig. 4–388).

*Medulloblastoma with glial differentiation:* The frequency with which glial differentiation occurs in medulloblastomas has been an issue of considerable controversy because identifying it can be difficult, even by immunohistochemical methods. The facade of glial differentiation can be imparted by several factors, including trapped normal brain tissue and the delicate eosinophilic neuropil of neuroblastic lesions. Bona fide glial differentiation may be obvious in H&E sections (Figs. 4–390 and 4–391), but more often it is evident only in immunohistochemical preparations or at the ultrastructural level. Only in excep-

tional cases is it readily apparent as aggregates of cells with conspicuous eosinophilic cytoplasm, as well as processes that are immunoreactive for GFAP. The immunohistochemical expressions of glial differentiation are discussed in the section on immunohistochemical features. More frequently, glial differentiation takes the form of clustered tumor cells with short and often bipolar, GFAP-positive processes. GFAP-positive cells are usually limited to the nodules in these "nodular/desmoplastic" lesions, but in some cases they occur diffusely throughout the internodular tissue (see Fig. 4–396).

In a significant proportion of medulloblastomas, it may not be possible to distinguish reactive from neoplastic GFAP-positive cells, even when carefully focusing through the section to exclude apposition of the cytoplasm of reactive astrocytes to the nucleus of a neoplastic cell. This problem is magnified at the periphery of a lesion and around vessels, where tumor cells are intimately associated with elongated processes of reactive astrocytes.

Ependymal differentiation is rumored to occur in medulloblastomas, but its occurrence must be rare, because it is difficult to find a convincing illustration of this phenomenon.

Myoid differentiation, "medullomyocytoma," and melanin production are discussed on pages 309 to 310. Well-differentiated cerebellar neoplasms composed of lipid-containing neurocytes that resemble adipocytes are discussed on pages 287 to 288.

**Cytologic Features.** Although all are "small round cell tumors," medulloblastomas vary considerably in the degree of cytologic atypia, ranging from cells that are small and dark but uniform and scarce in mitoses to those that are overtly atypical and mitotically active (Figs. 4–392 and 4–393).

**Immunohistochemical Features.** In most medulloblastomas, individual cells are synaptophysin immunopositive, but the affinity is most pronounced in fibrillar

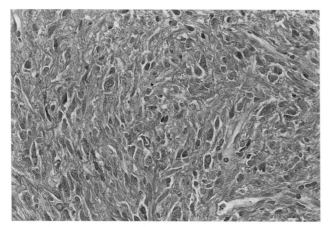

**FIGURE 4–390**   MEDULLOBLASTOMA

Glial differentiation to the degree illustrated here is unusual in medulloblastomas.

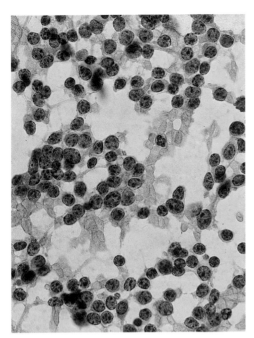

**FIGURE 4–392    MEDULLOBLASTOMA**

In a smear preparation, classic medulloblastoma consists of small, dark cells that, despite their hyperchromasia, are not notably pleomorphic.

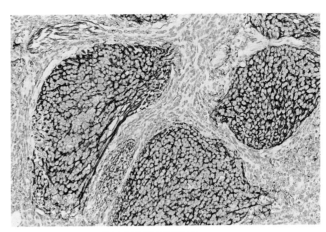

**FIGURE 4–394    MEDULLOBLASTOMA**

Nodules or "pale islands" in nodular/desmoplastic medulloblastomas are immunoreactive for synaptophysin.

zones—that is, the centers of Homer Wright rosettes, perivascular pseudorosettes, and the fibrillar areas in pale islands (Fig. 4–394).[18, 33, 82] Both large ganglion cells and some small cells may show neurofilament protein immunoreactivity. Anti-Hu is variably positive in the nuclei of small cells, but its utility as a dependable

marker for small cell neuronal tumors such as medulloblastomas has not been established.[35, 58] "Large cell medulloblastomas" are positive for synaptophysin and neurofilament protein.[9, 30] Immunoreactivity for retinal S-antigen and rhodopsin defines photoreceptor differentiation in some medulloblastomas.[20, 21, 44, 53, 55]

The significance of GFAP staining in medulloblastomas is controversial. Most tumors contain immunopositive cells that are presumably reactive in nature because they are stellate, perivascular, and evenly spaced (Fig. 4–395).[19, 60] There are tumors, however, in which unequivocal positivity is present within the scant cytoplasm of small neoplastic cells or in areas where neoplastic cells and their processes are so numerous as to create a densely fibrillar background (see Figs. 4–390 and 4–391).[33, 57] Radiating GFAP-positive cells are often prominent in the pale islands of nodular/desmoplastic medulloblastomas as large, stellate cells with nuclei that often sit at the periphery of the nodules.[33, 40, 46, 48] Less

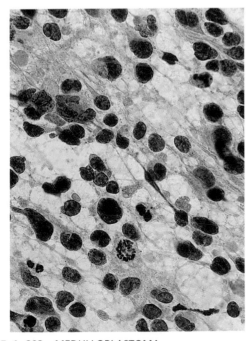

**FIGURE 4–393    MEDULLOBLASTOMA**

Cytologic atypia of the "anaplastic" variant of medulloblastoma is well seen in smear preparations.

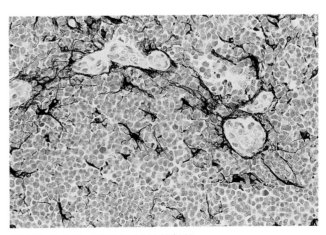

**FIGURE 4–395    MEDULLOBLASTOMA**

Many medulloblastomas feature a substantial number of glial fibrillary acidic protein–positive, reactive astrocytes. Such cells are generally concentrated in perivascular regions.

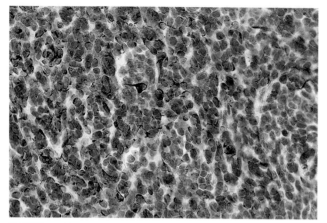

**FIGURE 4–396** MEDULLOBLASTOMA

Internodular cells in the nodular/desmoplastic tumor variant can be diffusely immunoreactive for glial fibrillary acidic protein.

frequently, small tumor cells in the internodular tissue are focally or diffusely positive (Fig. 4–396).

**Ultrastructural Features.** Processes that contain aligned microtubules, and sometimes neurosecretory granules, are the cardinal expressions of neuroblastic differentiation in medulloblastomas, especially those with advanced nodule formation (Fig. 4–397).[84] Even less common than neurosecretory granules, which may be hard to find, are signs of more advanced neuronal differ-

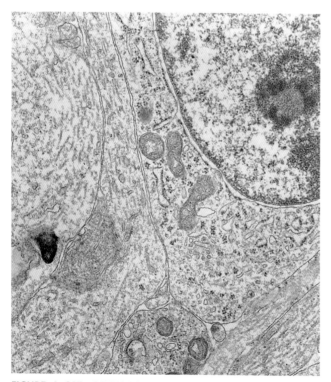

**FIGURE 4–397** MEDULLOBLASTOMA

At the ultrastructural level, the finding of cell processes filled with microtubules denotes neuroblastic differentiation.

entiation, such as clear vesicles or synapses. Glial differentiation is more difficult to document because processes containing intermediate filaments may simply represent reactive gliosis.

**Molecular and Cytogenetic Features.** Medulloblastomas occur in the setting of two inherited tumor syndromes—Turcot's and Gorlin's. It has been estimated that about 1% to 2% of all medulloblastomas arise in Gorlin's syndrome.[27] The extent to which these, or related, genetic abnormalities are responsible for sporadic medulloblastomas is unclear, but some "sporadic" medulloblastomas do appear to result from mutations or deletions in the genes that are deficient or have increased activity in these syndromes.

Turcot's syndrome has two distinct components.[36] The first reflects germline mutations in the adenomatous polyposis coli (*APC*) gene, with colonic polyposis and medulloblastoma the duplex expressions. The second component, caused by abnormalities in DNA mismatch repair, is not associated with medulloblastoma but rather nonpolyposis colon cancer and associated brain tumors, usually malignant gliomas.

Sporadic medulloblastomas have been found to show mutations in the *APC* gene itself,[41] as well as in one whose product interacts with *APC*—β-*catenin*.[26, 93] Preliminary data suggest that about 5% to 10% of sporadic medulloblastomas have dominant, "activating" mutations in this latter gene.

Gorlin's syndrome, the "nevoid basal cell carcinoma syndrome," combines a multiplicity of cutaneous lesions (basal cell carcinomas, epidermoid cysts) with ovarian fibromas. Medulloblastomas, nodular in histologic appearance, occur in some cases.[78] Of the "sporadic" medulloblastomas arising outside of Gorlin's or Turcot's syndrome, a small percentage have mutations in the *PTCH* gene, that is, in the "sonic hedgehog" signaling pathway.[70, 93]

There is evidence that some "desmoplastic" medulloblastomas are due to inactivation of the tumor suppressor *PTCH* gene.[70, 72] Loss of heterozygosity in the region of this gene at 9q has been found in sporadic medulloblastomas of the nodular type,[78] and specific mutations in the gene itself have been noted in a percentage of sporadic medulloblastomas unassociated with Gorlin's syndrome.[70, 72, 93] In one study, such a mutation was found in 3 of 11 sporadic "desmoplastic" medulloblastomas but in none of 57 conventional, "nondesmoplastic" lesions.[70] Another study did not find such a clear relationship between "desmoplastic" medulloblastomas and *PTCH* mutations.[72]

The most common cytogenetic abnormality associated with medulloblastoma is a chromosomal aberration in which all or most of one short arm of chromosome 17 is lost and replaced by a duplicated version of the long arm. This "isochromosome 17q" occurs in about 40% of all tumors (Fig. 4–398).[7, 8, 74, 81] Its relationship, if any, to mutations of the β-*catenin* gene or in genes of the sonic hedgehog pathway is unclear.

Amplification of *c-myc* and *N-myc* has been found among medulloblastomas, with a frequency that varies considerably from series to series.[1, 9, 30, 39, 74, 76] The 40%

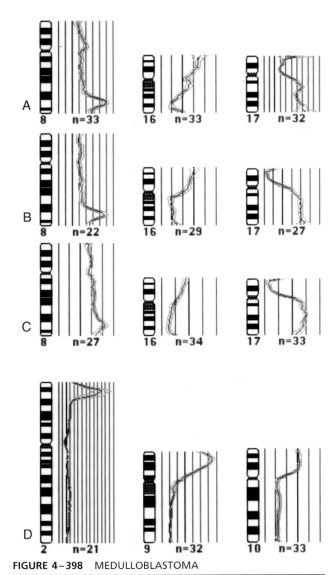

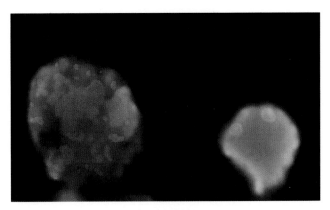

**FIGURE 4–399** MEDULLOBLASTOMA

This fluorescence in situ hybridization (FISH) preparation performed on a "large cell," or "anaplastic," medulloblastoma demonstrates a tumor cell with the normal two signals for *c-myc* (*right*), in contrast to a cell with multiple signals indicative of *c-myc* amplification (*left*). The patient with this neoplasm died within 2 years of diagnosis.

**FIGURE 4–398** MEDULLOBLASTOMA

Findings consistent with isochromosome 17q, as illustrated in tumors *A*, *B*, and *C*, is a common feature of medulloblastomas. These same three large cell medulloblastomas show high-level gain in the region of chromosome 8q24, a finding consistent with amplification of *c-myc*. A gain in the region of chromosome 2p24 in tumor *D* is consistent with amplification of *N-myc*. Either amplification is prognostically unfavorable. (From Burger PC, Kepner JL, Perlman EJ, et al. "Large cell/anaplastic" medulloblastoma: A Pediatric Oncology Group Study. J Neuropathol Exp Neurol 2000; 59:857–865.)

substantially more fibrillar and overall less cellular than a medulloblastoma and has more, and better developed, perivascular pseudorosettes. Importantly, the perivascular rosettes in medulloblastoma are synaptophysin, rather than GFAP, immunopositive.

As a common cerebellar neoplasm of childhood, *pilocytic astrocytoma* can be a suspect preoperatively, although this glioma is usually cystic, whereas medulloblastomas are almost always solid. Histologically, the pilocytic lesion lacks the cellularity of medulloblastoma and, typically, has a biphasic architecture and extensive GFAP positivity.

Some medulloblastomas are so infiltrative as to suggest a *high-grade infiltrating astrocytoma*. As a rule, however, gliomas are more fibrillar and pleomorphic than medulloblastomas. However, the distinction may be difficult and require resolution by immunohistochemistry or ultrastructural examination.

Although rare, *atypical teratoid/rhabdoid tumor* (AT/RT) is an appropriate consideration, particularly in patients younger than 2 years of age, and even more so

incidence of *c-myc* amplification in one series[76] is considerably higher than that found in others and may reflect selection bias among referral cases. Large cell/anaplastic lesions appear to have a high incidence of *c-myc* and, in some cases, *N-myc* amplification (Figs. 4–398 and 4–399).[1, 9, 30, 89]

**Differential Diagnosis.** From a clinical, radiologic, and operative perspective, *ependymoma* often heads the differential diagnosis. There are histologic similarities in these two entities, as ependymomas are often highly cellular, and medulloblastomas with Homer Wright rosettes frequently have a form of perivascular pseudorosette (Fig. 4–400). Generally, however, an ependymoma is

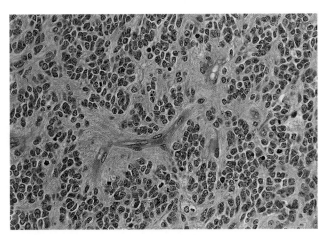

**FIGURE 4–400** MEDULLOBLASTOMA

Perivascular fibrillar zones may resemble those of ependymoma.

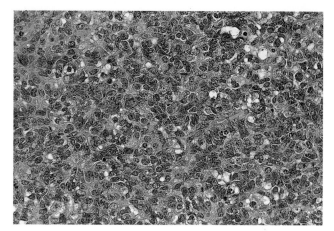

**FIGURE 4–401    ATYPICAL TERATOID/RHABDOID TUMOR**

Their shared degree of nuclear pleomorphism can make it difficult to distinguish atypical teratoid/rhabdoid tumors from medulloblastomas of the large cell or anaplastic type.

in those younger than 1 year old (Fig. 4–401). Recognition of AT/RT is easy if the diagnosis is considered and the lesion contains the classic large cells with paranuclear filamentous inclusions. A greater challenge is posed by AT/RTs with prominent small cell components and, conversely, by medulloblastomas of the large cell or anaplastic variety. The distinction often rests on the AT/RT's variation in histologic and cytologic features and immunophenotype. Large cell medulloblastomas frequently contain monomorphous sheets and lobules of round, synaptophysin-positive cells. Thus, adequate tissue sampling and application of the immunostains, discussed on pages 336 to 339, generally suffice in unmasking AT/RT. Molecular methods can be used to assess a possible loss and mutation in the *INI1* gene that are associated with AT/RT (see Fig. 4–488).[11]

The rare cerebellar *neurocytic lesions with lipidization* are discussed on pages 287 to 288.

The occurrence of a cerebellar small cell tumor in an adult invariably prompts concern about the possibility of *metastatic carcinoma*. This is less of a diagnostic problem if the lesion has nodules or pale islands, because these synaptophysin-containing and, to a lesser extent, often GFAP-positive nodules are not features of metastases. Immunoreactivity for synaptophysin is seen in medulloblastomas, especially in the nodules, but is also present in many small cell carcinomas. Combined positivity for cytokeratins and EMA, however, is limited to carcinomas. The utility of using antibodies to thyroid transcription factor 1 in the identification of metastatic lung cancer is discussed on page 349. CT of the chest may be prudent in ambiguous cases.

### Diagnostic Checklist

- Is this "medulloblastoma" a cellular ependymoma?
- Is this "medulloblastoma" in an infant really atypical teratoid/rhabdoid tumor?

**Treatment and Prognosis.** An overall long-term, disease-free survival of 50% to 60% is now possible.

Recurrences, usually local, generally obey Collin's law, which is based on the premise that embryonal tumors originate in the neonatal period. By this dictum, a postoperative "disease-free" interval of, or beyond, the patient's age at diagnosis plus the gestational period of 9 months should represent cure. There are, of course, exceptions.[10]

Long-term follow-up has disclosed an unfortunate incidence of late recurrence, sometimes delayed for 10 years or more after diagnosis.[59] In addition, some patients who had been freed of medulloblastoma succumbed to malignant glioma. The latter could represent a radiation-induced neoplasm,[51, 59, 63, 67] or perhaps a late emergence of a glial component of the original lesion.[59] A meningioma, or occasionally a schwannoma, can appear as a late radiation-induced neoplasm.

**Clinical and Radiologic Prognostic Factors.** Prognostically, the extent of resection and the stage of the neoplasm are singularly important.[64] The odds of survival drop significantly in the face of a subtotal resection[14, 52, 64, 79, 85] or when CSF dissemination is evident at the time of diagnosis.[61, 64, 69]

Generally, recurrence is local in the cerebellum, but the potential for dissemination through CSF is well recognized. Furthermore, medulloblastoma is one of the few primary intracranial neoplasms that is prone to late systemic metastasis, particularly to bone (Figs. 4–402 and 4–403).[2, 12, 50, 87] Ventriculoperitoneal shunting precedes some, but not all, of these metastatic events.[6] Large cell/anaplastic medulloblastomas appear more prone to extraneural spread.[9]

Only rarely does a medulloblastoma differentiate to form mature neurons. This may occur during local regrowth or at metastatic sites and is usually a feature of very nodular lesions.[2, 22, 28, 31, 56, 90]

**Histologic and Immunohistochemical Prognostic Features.** The morphologic heterogeneity of medulloblastomas invites conjecture regarding the prognostic significance of individual histologic or molecular features. Surprisingly little agreement has been reached,

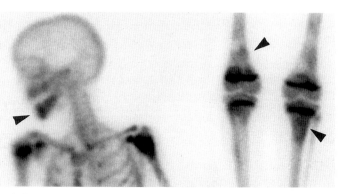

**FIGURE 4–402    MEDULLOBLASTOMA METASTATIC TO BONE**

Medulloblastomas, notably those of the large cell or anaplastic type, may metastasize to bone. The mandible and lower extremities were targeted in this 10-year-old boy, 1 year after the diagnosis of anaplastic medulloblastoma.

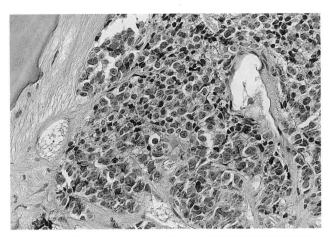

**FIGURE 4–403**    MEDULLOBLASTOMA METASTATIC TO BONE

Large cell or anaplastic medulloblastomas are particularly prone to systemic spread.

despite many detailed studies. At present, therapeutic stratification is based on the extent of resection and the tumor's stage, not on histologic or genetic subclassification. This will surely change. The significance of a tumor's level of TrkC expression is discussed later.

Whereas some reports indicate that the conventional indices of malignancy (e.g., necrosis, mitotic activity, pleomorphism, extent of vascular proliferation) are predictors of aggressive behavior,[52, 86] one investigation of adult patients did not confirm this observation.[42] Another study of pediatric cases suggested that the tumors could be graded on the basis of nuclear size and the degree of cytologic atypia.[25] Four grades were used, with significant differences in outcome between the combined none/slight versus moderate/severe categories. Apoptosis has been proffered as a favorable prognostic feature,[37] but also as a negative factor.[54]

Two histologic patterns may be predictive of biologic behavior, one favorable and the other not. A limited study suggested that patients in the first several years of life with extensively nodular lesions may do well, despite the withholding of radiotherapy because of the patients' ages.[31] Whether nodular tumors in general are better behaved than "classic," non-nodular medulloblastomas is unclear, although some series indicate that this may be the case.[5, 14, 17, 79, 85] It comes as no surprise that yet another study found patients with "desmoplastic" lesions to fare less well.[66] Few large cell/anaplastic medulloblastomas have been studied, but preliminary indications suggest an extremely aggressive nature and a high incidence of local recurrence, cerebrospinal spread, and even systemic metastases.[9, 30]

Several reports focused on cellular differentiation as a prognostic factor. One suggested that patients with neoplasms with differentiation (e.g., glial), defined by features evident in H&E-stained sections, fared less well than those with undifferentiated tumors.[65] Another investigation concluded just the opposite.[13] Whereas one study found that GFAP staining of tumor cells was prognostically favorable,[32] another suggested that glial staining of clumps and sheets of cells rather than of isolated cells confers a significantly worse prognosis.[44] Two additional studies completed the range of possibilities by concluding that differentiation has no effect on survival.[42, 86] A similar discordance has been found in studies of apoptosis, with higher levels being associated with both superior[37] and inferior outcomes.[54]

Typically, the cells of a medulloblastoma exhibit high, but variable, proliferation indices. The relationship to prognosis, if any, remains to be established. Three studies using flow cytometry suggested that aneuploidy is a favorable prognostic factor.[79, 88, 92]

The prognostic significance of molecular and cytogenetic factors remains to be established, but there is clear evidence that patients whose lesions show *c-myc* and *N-myc* amplification or overexpression[1] do considerably less well.[39, 76] This may be true in the case of large cell and anaplastic lesions.[9, 30] According to one study, isochromosome 17q, or loss of heterozygosity of chromosome 17p, is prognostically unfavorable,[3] although a subsequent study refuted this suggestion.[7] As previously noted, a high rate of apoptosis has been reported to be a favorable prognostic factor.[37]

Two studies identified elevated expression of the neurotrophin receptor TrkC as a favorable prognostic factor.[34, 83] This may be explained, in part, by the fact that nodular lesions are strongly stained for TrkC.[24]

## Medullomyoblastoma and Melanotic Medulloblastoma

**Definition.** Medulloblastoma-like neoplasms with muscle or melanocytic differentiation.

**General Comments.** As cellular cerebellar tumors, these two lesions are usually considered medulloblastoma variants. The presence of keratinizing epithelium, glands, cartilage, and smooth muscle in exceptional cases[4, 11] has prompted the alternative conclusion that some are teratomas.[4] Whether specific molecular characteristics relate these lesions to classic medulloblastomas remains to be seen, but investigation of a solitary case failed to demonstrate a common, but by no means universal, feature of medulloblastomas: isochromosome 17q.[1] Because some small cell malignant cerebellar neoplasms contain both rhabdomyoblasts and melanin,[10] it is also unclear just how distinct these two rare tumors are from each other. In the broad "PNET concept," the tumors are PNETs with muscle or melanocytic differentiation.

## Medullomyoblastoma

**Clinical Features.** Of these two medulloblastoma variants, the medullomyoblastoma is more common. Almost all patients with this lesion, generally males, have presented before the age of 7 years.[1, 4, 5, 11, 13, 15] Only rarely are adults affected.[11, 12]

**Microscopic Features.** In its "pure form," medullomyoblastoma is a biphasic tumor with a small cell, undifferentiated element and a loose-textured, collagen-rich tissue that contains myoblasts or myocytes. In some

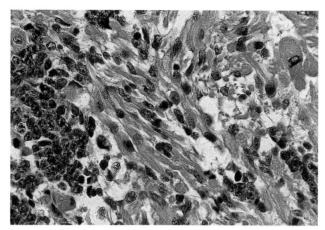

**FIGURE 4-404    MEDULLOMYOBLASTOMA**

Myoblasts, some striated, adorn this otherwise densely cellular, small cell neoplasm.

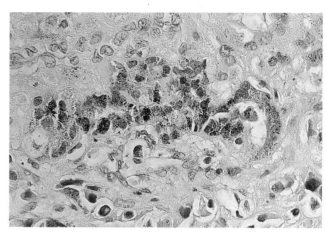

**FIGURE 4-405    MELANOTIC MEDULLOBLASTOMA**

Small tubules with melanin pigment are encountered in a small percentage of medulloblastomas.

lesions, myoblasts intermingle freely with the undifferentiated cells. Myoblastic cells assume either the classic striated "strap cell" configuration or the less readily recognized globular, or "blast," form (Fig. 4-404). At low magnification, the former may be misinterpreted as blood vessels or bundles of elongated astrocytes. On occasion, medullomyoblastomas become a veritable potpourri, garnished with areas resembling oligodendroglioma, astrocytoma, or ganglion cells in a background neuropil.[8]

**Immunohistochemical Features.** Understandably, the myoid cells are positive for actin and desmin.

**Cytologic Features.** The eosinophilic "blast" or "strap" cells are well seen in cytologic preparations.

**Ultrastructural Features.** Thick and thin filaments, Z-bands, and occasionally all the accoutrements of mature skeletal muscle are evident.[1, 12, 14, 15]

**Treatment and Prognosis.** Although it has been suggested that medullomyoblastomas are especially aggressive,[11] the limited collective experience with such tumors provides little basis to judge the behavior of these lesions vis-à-vis conventional medulloblastomas.

### Melanotic Medulloblastoma

**Clinical Features.** The lesion has appeared in children.

**Microscopic Features.** The histologic organization of pigmented cells in the so-called melanotic medulloblastoma varies from case to case. Some contain tubules or vague papillae of melanotic cells (Fig. 4-405),[2, 7, 17] whereas in other tumors, individual "melanocytes" are dispersed randomly among the small cells.[3, 9, 10] Melanosomes and premelanosomes are readily detected by electron microscopy.[3, 6, 9] True intracranial examples of melanotic neuroectodermal tumor of infancy (mela-

notic progonoma) appear clinicopathologically distinct from melanotic medulloblastoma.[16]

**Ultrastructural Features.** The pigment is melanin, not lipofuscin. Melanosomes are present.[3, 6, 9]

**Treatment and Prognosis.** There are too few data to reach conclusions about biologic behavior. Both local recurrence and CSF pathway seeding have occurred.[2, 6, 7, 9, 10, 17]

### Medulloepithelioma

**Definition.** A highly malignant (WHO grade IV) embryonal tumor with gland-like epithelial structures, often with associated divergent differentiation.

**General Comments.** Conceptually, the rare medulloepithelioma recapitulates the embryonic medullary epithelium and retains the potential for divergent glioneuronal, and even mesenchymal, differentiation.[5]

**Clinical Features.** Most patients with this rare tumor have been children younger than 3 years old; only an occasional adult has been affected.[7]

**Radiologic Features.** The lesion can arise throughout the brain, including the cerebellum, brain stem, and distal spinal cord. Many are deep-seated and lie in close proximity to the ventricular system. Although reported cases are few, and little is known of their imaging characteristics, they may show little if any contrast enhancement.[7]

**Microscopic Features.** The cardinal features of medulloepithelioma are often elongated glands and canals composed of cytologically malignant, mitotically active epithelium (Fig. 4-406) (see Table 4-11, p. 226). Externally, the epithelium rests on a basement membrane; internally, it is covered by a thin layer of amorphous material. Both are PAS positive. As expected, the outer layer is immunoreactive for type IV collagen (Fig. 4-407).

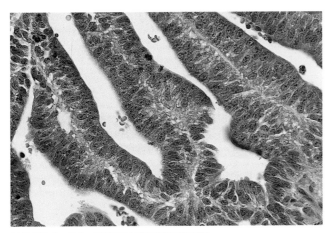

**FIGURE 4–406** MEDULLOEPITHELIOMA

Extended epithelial surfaces, an abluminal basement membrane, marked cytologic atypia, and frequent mitotic figures define the epithelium of this rare entity.

The nuclei have coarse chromatin. The rather numerous mitoses are typically situated in luminal poles of the cells. All combinations of ependymoblastic, ependymal, astrocytic, oligodendroglial, neuroblastic, and neuronal differentiation may be seen.[1, 3, 4, 7, 9] Some medulloepitheliomas even feature cartilage, bone, or rhabdomyoblasts.[1] Only a rare lesion contains melanosomes.[10]

**Immunohistochemical Features.** Reactivity for vimentin is common.[3, 6, 7] Focal staining for GFAP and neurofilament protein can also be present[3, 6, 7] and is expected in the face of glioneuronal differentiation. EMA positivity has been reported on the surface of the epithelial cells.[2] Staining for nestin, a feature of the primitive neural tube, is concentrated in the basal layer.[6] Most of the neoplastic cells are nonreactive for synaptophysin.[2]

**Ultrastructural Features.** The epithelial cells lack specialized surface features but are joined laterally by promi-

nent "intermediate junctions"[8] and rest on a basement membrane as well as a narrow zone of collagen fibrils.[8]

**Treatment and Prognosis.** There are too few cases to draw conclusions regarding biologic behavior, much less appropriate treatment. Local recurrence and cerebrospinal spread are the rule[7]; a few long-term survivals have been reported following gross total resection.[7]

## Neuroblastoma and Ganglioneuroblastoma

**Definition.** Small cell, embryonal, "primitive" neoplasms composed exclusively of neuroblasts ("neuroblastoma") or of neuroblasts and ganglion cells ("ganglioneuroblastoma").

**General Comments.** As defined before the immunohistochemical era, the criteria for neuroblastic differentiation in CNS tumors included positive metallic impregnation for neurofibrils, a fibrillar background resembling neuropil, and the classic neuroblastic (Homer Wright) rosettes. The last are recognized readily but are usually not numerous. Neuroblastic lesions defined by immunohistochemistry for neuronal markers only (i.e., without such rosettes) are discussed, arbitrarily, in the section on largely undifferentiated embryonal tumors.

**Clinical Features.** Most CNS neuroblastomas occur before the age of 2 years, although older children and even adults are affected occasionally.[2–4]

**Microscopic Features.** Histologically, typical CNS neuroblastomas are lobular, highly cellular, and often relatively discrete. Varying quantities of connective tissue may be present, and its quantitative contribution has been used to apportion these tumors into "classic," "transitional," and "desmoplastic" variants.[4]

Cerebral neuroblastomas may provide only meager histologic evidence of their neuroblastic nature. Definitive features include a process-rich, fibrillary neuropil and Homer Wright rosettes (Fig. 4–408); ganglioid or ganglion cells; immunoreactivity for neuronal markers;

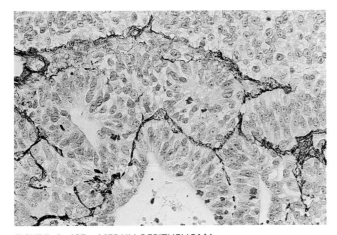

**FIGURE 4–407** MEDULLOEPITHELIOMA

The epithelium rests on a basement membrane that is immunoreactive for collagen type IV.

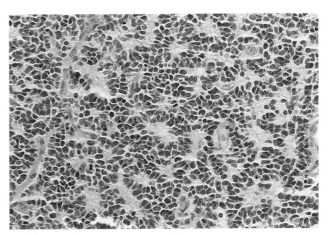

**FIGURE 4–408** CEREBRAL NEUROBLASTOMA

Neuroblastic or Homer Wright rosettes are a hallmark expression of neuroblastic differentiation.

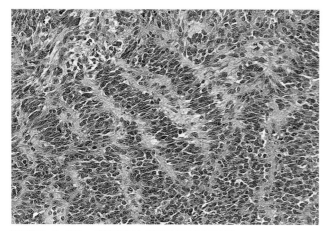

**FIGURE 4–409**    CEREBRAL NEUROBLASTOMA

Palisading or ribboning is a feature of some cerebral neuroblastomas.

and ultrastructural findings of neuronal differentiation (see later). Cellular palisades are present in some cases (Fig. 4–409).[6] Neoplasms with ribboning or palisading are summarized in Table 4–11, p. 226.

The presence of a fibrillary background in H&E-stained sections is diagnostically supportive but not diagnostic. Homer Wright rosettes are definitive evidence. The presence of cellular streaming, as occurs in nodular medulloblastomas, and the finding of ganglioid or ganglion cells provide strong evidence for the diagnosis. Convincing demonstration of neurofibrils requires immunohistochemical or ultrastructural studies.

**Immunohistochemical Features.** Ganglioid and ganglion cells are immunoreactive for neurofilament protein. Fibrillar regions, including the cores of rosettes, stain for synaptophysin. Class III $\beta$-tubulin and various neurotransmitter substances are often demonstrated as well. The same is true of labeling with anti-Hu, which circulates in the paraneoplastic syndromes.[5]

**Ultrastructural Features.** Electron microscopic studies document the presence of cytoplasmic intermediate filaments, microtubules, dense-core granules, and synaptic vesicles in cell terminations.[6] Intercellular junctions that resemble synapses are rarities (Fig. 4–410).[1]

**Differential Diagnosis.** The differential diagnosis is broad, but it must exclude other embryonal tumors with rosettes or epithelial surfaces. Homer Wright rosettes lack a lumen, unlike those of ependymoblastoma, retinoblastoma, or medulloepithelioma. Neuroblastic tumors, defined by immunohistochemical findings alone, must be differentiated from malignant gliomas (see page 314).

**Treatment and Prognosis.** A satisfactory understanding of the biologic behavior of cerebral neuroblastoma awaits further experience. Local recurrence is the rule, and cerebrospinal dissemination is a recognized complication. One series reported a "favorable" 5-year survival rate of 30%.[2] Albeit in a single case, a more favorable outcome has been reported.[7]

### Ependymoblastoma

**Definition.** A small cell, "embryonal," CNS neoplasm with "ependymoblastic rosettes."

**General Comments.** Although the term "ependymoblastoma" has been applied to anaplastic ependymoma, we use it here in a strict sense to denote a distinct, rare entity.

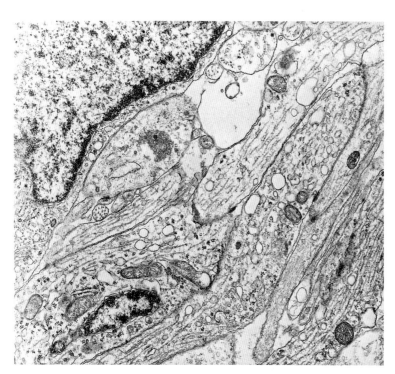

**FIGURE 4–410**    CEREBRAL NEUROBLASTOMA

Neuroblastic differentiation is expressed ultrastructurally by the formation of microtubule-containing processes.

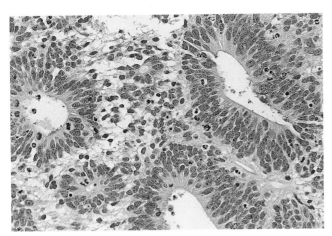

**FIGURE 4–411** EPENDYMOBLASTOMA

Large, round or slit-like, mitotically active true rosettes, in a background of small cells, are the essential features of this rare lesion.

The important distinction from anaplastic ependymoma is discussed later in the section on differential diagnosis.

**Clinical Features.** This histologically distinctive neoplasm occurs most often in childhood[4, 5] and is occasionally congenital.[3] Adults are rarely affected.[4]

**Microscopic Features.** The defining features of this markedly cellular lesion are true rosettes and canals that are composed of multilayered, markedly atypical, and mitotically active cells. These pseudostratified "ependymoblastic rosettes" encircle a distinct lumen bounded by terminal bars. They are distinguished readily from the perivascular pseudorosettes of ependymoma. The latter consist of perithelial cytoplasmic extensions originating from a surrounding cuff of tumor cells. They are also generally distinct from the "true ependymal rosette" because of their cytologic atypia and pseudostratification. Ependymoblastomatous rosettes are similar to Flexner-Wintersteiner, or "retinoblastomatous," rosettes, although they are larger and often more elliptic (Fig. 4–411). Not surprisingly, ependymoblastomatous tissue may be seen in embryonal tumors with divergent differentiation. For example, they are commonly seen in medulloepithelioma and in the "embryonal tumor with abundant neuropil and true rosettes."

**Immunohistochemical Features.** There is limited information about this lesion's immunohistochemical profile. The rosettes are positive for vimentin but negative for GFAP.[1]

**Ultrastructural Features.** As in ependymomas, the apices of the cells are joined by long junctional complexes.[1, 2]

**Differential Diagnosis.** This distinctive embryonal tumor is recognized readily as "ependymal," but its distinction from *anaplastic ependymoma* is more problematic. In contrast with the latter, the "blastoma" is more cellular and consists of fields of undifferentiated or "primitive"

cells devoid of both fibrillary processes and perivascular pseudorosettes. Most importantly, well-differentiated, true rosettes arise abruptly from a highly cellular background of "primitive" small cells. As ependymomas sink into anaplasia, they are scarcely able to form perivascular pseudorosettes, much less well-formed true rosettes or canals. As with other small cell "embryonal" or "primitive" tumors, microvascular hyperplasia, a common feature of anaplastic ependymomas, is absent or scant.

An additional lesion with lumen-containing (i.e., true) rosettes, *embryonal tumor with abundant neuropil and true rosettes*, is discussed later.

**Treatment and Prognosis.** Ependymoblastomas are aggressive tumors. Although survival statistics are scanty, one series of seven patients reported four deaths within a year of diagnosis[4]; the median survival time was 12 months or less. One patient in this study survived 9 years after initial surgery and the simple resection of multiple recurrences. Widespread cerebrospinal dissemination is recognized.[3, 4]

### Embryonal Tumor with Abundant Neuropil and True Rosettes

**General Comments.** One of the more "common" of the patterned embryonal tumors, this still rare neoplasm combines features of ependymoblastoma and neuroblastoma.[1] Whether it represents an entity distinct from either is unclear. Similar lesions have been reported as neuroblastoma[3] and ependymoblastoma.[2] It is presented here because of its distinctive features.

**Clinical Features.** Patients are young. Both supra- and infratentorial sites have been affected.

**Microscopic Features.** The lesion is distinctive for its biphasic composition of densely cellular regions and highly fibrillar areas of "neoplastic neuropil" (Fig. 4–412). True rosettes, often mitotically active and multilayered, can adorn either region but are more numerous and ap-

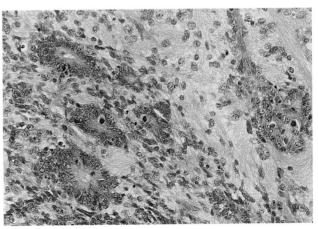

**FIGURE 4–412** EMBRYONAL TUMOR WITH ABUNDANT NEUROPIL AND TRUE ROSETTES

True rosettes occasionally appear abruptly in a paucicellular, neuropil-like background.

pear unexpectedly in the fibrillar areas, where they arise abruptly. They lack the open neural tube–like surfaces and canals of medulloepithelioma but are similar to those in ependymoblastoma. Other rosettes closely resemble the Flexner-Wintersteiner type, as seen in retinoblastoma.

**Immunohistochemical Features.** The fibrillar areas are reactive for synaptophysin. The rosettes are GFAP negative, but small foci of GFAP immunoreactive glial cells may be found in the solid areas in some cases.

**Ultrastructural Features.** The "neuropil" is composed of elongated processes containing microtubules. Zonulae adherens confederate cells in the rosettes.[1]

**Treatment and Prognosis.** The lesions are no less aggressive than the other embryonal tumors described earlier.[1]

### Retinoblastoma

Intracranial retinoblastomas are either a direct extension of an ocular lesion or a primary lesion arising in the pineal or suprasellar region as part of the "trilateral retinoblastoma" complex. The latter are found in patients with bilateral retinoblastomas and a germline mutation in the retinoblastoma gene, or in individuals with only a unilateral lesion but a family history of retinoblastoma.[4] The intracranial tumors are relatively well defined, contrast enhancing, and often calcified.[1, 3, 5] Histologically, they are densely cellular and frequently contain Flexner-Wintersteiner rosettes. The latter present precisely formed, circular lumens highlighted by a circumferential zone of terminal bars and apical protuberances (photoreceptor differentiation).

Primary intracranial retinoblastomas are aggressive and are almost invariably fatal.[1, 2] Patients with germline mutations in the retinoblastoma gene are also at risk for the development of sarcomas, especially in prior irradiation fields.

### Embryonal Tumors with Muscle Differentiation

Extracerebellar small cell neoplasms with muscle differentiation pose a special nosologic problem, as they can be considered either (1) small cell embryonal tumors with mesenchymal differentiation, analogous to medullomyoblastoma, or (2) myosarcomas.[2, 3] Immunoreactivity of the tumor for synaptophysin or GFAP establishes its neuroectodermal origin and justifies the diagnosis of an embryonal tumor rather than sarcoma.[1]

### Largely Undifferentiated Embryonal Tumors

This is a heterogeneous aggregate of small cell neoplasms that focally, if at all, differentiate or create specific histologic features. Most are supratentorial,[2] but intrapontine examples have been described.[1] Immunohistochemistry is almost obligatory for the diagnosis. Unlike most malignant gliomas, these lesions exhibit a diffuse, dense cellularity with little nuclear pleomorphism. There is little fibrillar background. Microvascular proliferation and necrosis with pseudopalisading are usually absent. The distinction from malignant glioma can be difficult, but it has significant consequences. Small cell embryonal tumors, or PNETs, are treated with radiation to the entire neuraxis if the patient's age permits, whereas only the brain is targeted in patients with malignant gliomas.

If immunoreactivity for synaptophysin is noted within tumor cells, the diagnosis of an embryonal tumor with neuroblastic differentiation is reasonably assured.[1, 4] Admittedly, one can debate the semantic issue of whether the lesion is a "neuroblastoma" without rosettes or a "small cell embryonal tumor" with neuroblastic differentiation. As is true of most neuronal and neuroblastic tumors, large, GFAP-positive, reactive astrocytes may project their long processes between the immunonegative tumor cells.

Other small cell embryonal tumors that are undifferentiated at the histologic level demonstrate clearly defined, and in some cases surprisingly extensive, GFAP reactivity (Figs. 4–413 and 4–414).[1, 3, 4] The differential diagnosis of a glioma then becomes an issue, with therapeutic and prognostic implications. As previously noted, embryonal tumors are generally more monomorphous and microcellular than are malignant gliomas. Furthermore, GFAP positivity is more uniform, featuring only a narrow circumferential rim of cytoplasmic positivity.

Rare small cell lesions exhibit both neuronal and glial differentiation. In our opinion, such tumors with divergent differentiation fulfill the essential criteria for PNET and justify the use of this diagnosis.

### Miscellaneous Embryonal Tumors

An occasional intracranial small cell tumor of childhood resembles the so-called peripheral form of PNET by immunoreactivity for 013 (HBA-71 or CD99), which recognizes a product of the MIC2 gene.[3]

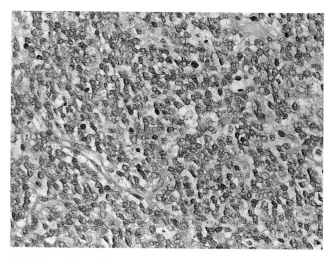

**FIGURE 4–413** EMBRYONAL TUMOR WITH GLIAL DIFFERENTIATION

Such lesions may have only the smallest amount of eosinophilic cytoplasm to suggest glial differentiation.

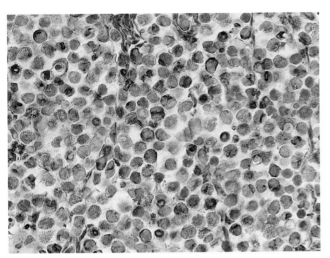

**FIGURE 4–414** EMBRYONAL TUMOR WITH GLIAL DIFFERENTIATION

A rim of cytoplasm immunopositive for glial fibrillary acidic protein is evidence of glial differentiation in this rare tumor.

Prophylactic radiotherapy, most commonly for acute lymphoblastic leukemia, has been implicated in the development of a distinctive small cell neoplasm with rosettes and palisades, as well as variable glial and neuronal differentiation.[2]

The monotony of rare small cell tumors is interrupted by adipose tissue and smooth muscle.[5] Divergent differentiation has been described in a PNET associated with von Hippel-Lindau disease.[1]

Germline mutations of p53 underlie the occurrence of rare embryonal tumors.[4]

### Primitive Polar Spongioblastoma

Figuratively and literally, this rare neoplasm is the "zebra" of the embryonal tumor group. Its stripes,

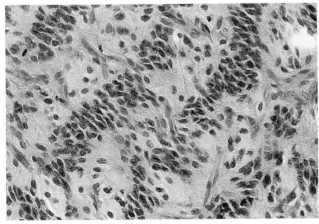

**FIGURE 4–415** CENTRAL NERVOUS SYSTEM NEOPLASM WITH PALISADING

As is summarized in Table 4–10, ribboning or palisading occurs in a wide variety of central nervous system tumors. Whether the primitive polar spongioblastoma—the tumor most associated with this feature—actually exists as a separate entity remains a subject of debate.

formed by elongated cellular palisades, are dramatic but are perhaps not as diagnostic as was once thought (Fig. 4–415).[3, 5, 7, 8, 10] The status of the lesion as an entity has been challenged, and the tumor has been downgraded to a tissue pattern rather than a specific entity, because palisading occurs in such diverse entities as oligodendroglioma, pilocytic astrocytoma, medulloblastoma, and neuroblastoma (see Table 4–11, p. 226).[4, 6, 9] As originally depicted, the cells of primitive polar spongioblastoma rest in a delicate fibrillar matrix in which capillaries may be conspicuous. Fine bipolar processes may be GFAP positive, indicating glial differentiation.[1] Ultrastructural studies, conversely, have described cell processes containing microtubules and dense-core granules.[2, 6]

Some "polar spongioblastomas" are aggressive and capable of craniospinal metastasis.[8] This is particularly true of purely spongioblastic lesions. Others, especially those exhibiting additional tumor patterns, are more indolent, abetting the skepticism about the status of the entity.

## Sarcomas

### Fibrosarcoma

**Definition.** A discrete spindle cell neoplasm composed of anaplastic fibroblasts.

**Clinical Features.** Constituting less than 1% of all intracranial neoplasms, primary fibrosarcomas can occur at any age and location. Some are "spontaneous" (Fig. 4–416), whereas others are late sequelae of radiation therapy.[1–5, 7, 8] Meningeal fibrosarcomas are discussed in Chapter 2.

**Macroscopic Features.** As if to emphasize the alien character of fibroblasts in brain parenchyma, the cells segregate themselves into a firm, discrete mass. Although most are superficial, some lie below the surface within the brain parenchyma.

**Microscopic Features.** CNS fibrosarcomas vary considerably in pattern and in their degrees of malignancy. Some contain widely spaced, spindle or stellate cells with small, uniform nuclei only infrequently engaged in mitosis. Others exhibit disarrayed warps and woofs of cellular fascicles with considerable nuclear irregularity, hyperchromasia, and mitotic activity (Fig. 4–417). A "herringbone pattern" is nonetheless classic. An intercellular matrix of reticulin and collagen is regularly seen. Necrosis is encountered in highly malignant examples.

**Immunohistochemical Features.** Immunocytologic studies show reaction for vimentin but not for GFAP, S-100 protein, or EMA.

**Ultrastructural Features.** Neoplastic fibroblasts vary in their configuration, but bipolar cells are often prominent.

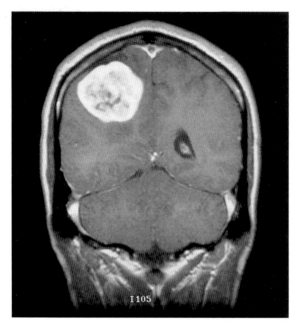

**FIGURE 4–416**  FIBROSARCOMA

Primary fibrosarcomas are discrete masses. This contrast-enhancing lesion occurred in a 34-year-old man.

Their nuclei, frequently crenated, contain coarse chromatin. Dilated cisternae of rough endoplasmic reticulum are a conspicuous feature. Although, as a rule, the cells contain few or no cytoplasmic intermediate filaments and exhibit no specialized cell junctions,[6] filaments and dense bodies are encountered beneath the cell membrane in examples with myofibroblastic features. Basement membranes are lacking.

**Differential Diagnosis.** Primary cerebral fibrosarcomas are rare, and most malignant mesenchymal-appearing neoplasms are other entities such as *malignant meningioma, solitary fibrous tumor, cellular schwannoma, gliosarcoma,* or *DIG.*

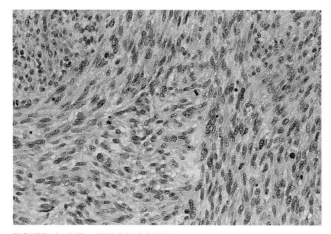

**FIGURE 4–417**  FIBROSARCOMA

Intersecting, compact fascicles produce the classic "herringbone" pattern of fibrosarcoma.

*Malignant meningioma* is the most common differential diagnostic problem, but in all but the most anaplastic meningiomas, there is evidence by history (long course, prior surgical specimen), radiology (dural tail, cranial hyperostosis), histologic examination (whorls, nuclear inclusions, psammoma bodies), electron microscopy (cytoplasmic filaments, desmosomes), or immunohistochemistry (membranous EMA staining) of the meningothelial nature of the tumor. *Gliosarcomas* are known for their more complex architecture with islands of GFAP-positive, cytologically malignant glial tissue. Before its recognition as an entity, *DIG* was often diagnosed as fibrosarcoma or gliosarcoma and treated accordingly. DIG has characteristic radiologic features (massive multicystic architecture, dural attachment). Its desmoplastic component contains GFAP-positive cells and small neurons.

**Treatment and Prognosis.** Fibrosarcomas are prone to meningeal seeding and are capable of systemic metastasis. In one study of nine patients, median survival was only 7.5 months.[5]

## Rhabdomyosarcoma

**Definition.** A malignant neoplasm with rhabdomyoblastic differentiation.

**General Comments.** Neoplasms with skeletal muscle differentiation can arise at any age, but most present during the first decade of life.[4, 7, 9, 12, 13, 16] Those that arise in the cerebellum pose a nosologic problem in the distinction from "medullomyoblastoma" (see pages 309 to 310). Indeed, it is not always clear how to classify rhabdomyocyte-containing neoplasms, especially those in childhood and adolescence, because small cell embryonal tumors (PNETs) can express muscle differentiation (see page 314). The essential nature of many such neoplasms remains unclear, as a number of cases were published before the immunohistochemical era. Supratentorial myoblastic tumors occurring in adults are, nosologically, less problematic.[1, 3, 8, 10, 11, 14, 15]

Leptomeningeal rests of striated muscle cells are a potential source for primary CNS muscle tumors,[2, 6] especially those of the leptomeninges.[7, 15]

**Microscopic Features.** Most rhabdomyosarcomas are small cell tumors, with skeletal muscle differentiation often visible in H&E-stained sections as globular ("blast") or elongated ("strap") cells (Fig. 4–418). Fibrillarity is readily evident in the former, but cross-striations are generally confined to the latter.

**Immunohistochemical Features.** Reactivity for muscle-specific markers is expected (Fig. 4–419).

**Ultrastructural Features.** Rhabdomyoblasts contain thick and thin filaments, as well as considerable glycogen.[3, 5, 9, 12, 15, 17] On occasion, Z-bands contribute to the development of remarkably well-formed sarcomeres.

**Differential Diagnosis.** In a child, the differential diagnosis often centers on a *small cell embryonal tumor,* or

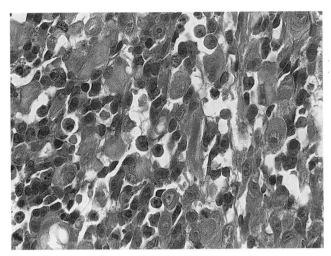

**FIGURE 4–418**   RHABDOMYOSARCOMA

Mixtures of rhabdomyoblasts and striated "strap" cells make up this rhabdomyosarcoma in the parietal lobe of a 3-year-old.

*PNET.* In concept, immunoreactivity for synaptophysin or other neural markers and/or for GFAP would place the lesion in the latter category.

**Treatment and Prognosis.** Given its rarity, the behavior of CNS rhabdomyosarcoma is not fully defined. Malignant behavior, inferred from the histologic appearance, is confirmed by the fact that only a rare patient survives beyond 2 years.[11, 16]

### Other Primary Sarcomas

Unusual forms of primary cerebral sarcomas include angiosarcoma,[3, 12, 18, 22, 25, 35] malignant fibrous histiocytoma,[11, 14, 21, 25, 28, 30, 32] hemangioendothelioma,[23] hemangiopericytoma,[1] leiomyosarcoma,[6, 8, 9, 19, 20, 25] liposar-

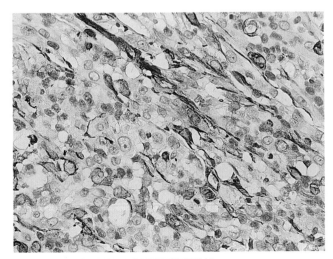

**FIGURE 4–419**   RHABDOMYOSARCOMA

As expected, the lesion in Figure 4–418 is immunoreactive for muscle-specific actin.

coma,[17, 31] chondrosarcoma,[2, 7, 13, 15, 25] mesenchymal chondrosarcoma,[25, 26] myxochondrosarcoma,[29] osteosarcoma,[5, 10, 24, 27, 33] and Ewing's sarcoma.[34]

Primary CNS leiomyosarcomas have been associated with AIDS and, on the basis of in situ hybridization studies, are known to contain the Epstein-Barr virus genome.[6, 8, 9, 19] These lesions are discussed in Chapter 2. Radiotherapy has preceded some cases of malignant fibrous histiocytoma,[11, 14, 21, 28, 30] fibrosarcoma,[4] and osteosarcoma.[16, 33]

## Lymphomas and Hematopoietic Neoplasms

### Primary Central Nervous System Lymphoma

**Definition.** A malignant primary CNS neoplasm composed of B, or less commonly T, lymphocytes.

**General Comments.** The incidence of "sporadic" primary central nervous system lymphoma (PCNSL) appeared to increase substantially over the past several decades, particularly in patients older than 60.[11, 13, 23, 41] Nonetheless, the lesion is still uncommon, and we have not perceived a notable increase in the number of PCNSL specimens over the past 10 years. A similar conclusion was reached by a population-based study in Canada.[19]

PCNSLs resemble their systemic counterparts, but with a greater incidence of high-grade lesions of the large cell type, mostly of the B-cell lineage.[17, 28, 31] T-cell lesions,[8, 14] Burkitt's lymphoma,[26] and the rare large cell anaplastic (Ki-1) types[16, 20, 29] have been reported. Two notable exceptions are both nodular variants of Hodgkin's disease—occasional reports of primary intracranial Hodgkin's disease notwithstanding.[1, 9, 10]

**Clinical Features.** Although PCNSLs occur in the setting of immunodeficiency, especially AIDS, they also arise de novo in previously healthy individuals, usually those beyond the age of 60 years. Symptoms are referable to elevated intracranial pressure and the local, destructive effects of the neoplasm. The distribution of primary lymphoma in the CNS is proportional to tissue volume; in decreasing order of incidence, the lesions affect the cerebrum, cerebellum, and brain stem. Ocular involvement may antedate intracranial disease.[8, 14, 16] Epstein-Barr virus has been implicated in the genesis of some "sporadic" and most AIDS-associated cerebral lymphomas.[2, 3, 5, 6, 8, 11, 13–15, 19, 22, 23]

"Intravascular lymphomatosis," a systemic lesion secondarily involving the CNS, is described later in a separate section.

PCNSLs are usually approached stereotactically (see Figs. 5–9 to 5–11), but even this low-risk procedure may be associated with significant morbidity in AIDS patients.[39]

**Radiologic Features.** In patients without AIDS, PCNSLs are "homogeneously" contrast enhancing and

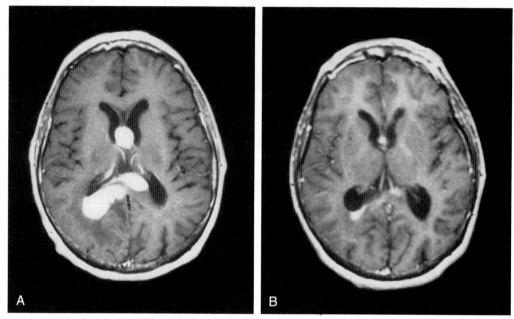

**FIGURE 4–420** PRIMARY CENTRAL NERVOUS SYSTEM LYMPHOMA

Magnetic resonance imaging scans before (A) and after (B) steroid therapy reveal the marked involution that this neoplasm can undergo in just 2 weeks. As is typical of primary central nervous system lymphoma, the multicentric process demonstrates homogeneous enhancement, giving it a solid appearance.

thus lack the dark, necrotic center so typical of glioblastoma (Fig. 4–420; see also Fig. 5–9).[24, 36] Multicentricity is common. Particularly suggestive of lymphoma are symmetric, bilateral, and subependymal foci of involvement. Some lymphomas bridge the corpus callosum and assume the "butterfly" configuration of a glioblastoma. Many abut the ventricular system.

In the setting of AIDS, PCNSLs are often centrally necrotic and appear as "ring-enhancing" lesions (Fig. 4–421). They are frequently multifocal.[34]

Cerebral lymphomas often respond dramatically, albeit transiently, to corticosteroids, generating the terms "ghost-cell tumor" or "disappearing tumor" for such lesions (see Fig. 4–420).[18] The term "sentinel lesion" has

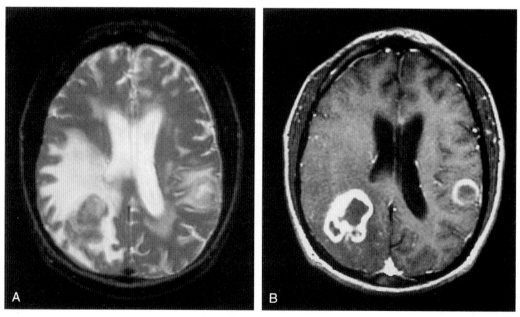

**FIGURE 4–421** PRIMARY CENTRAL NERVOUS SYSTEM LYMPHOMA

As seen in T2-weighted (A) and contrast-enhanced (B) magnetic resonance imaging scans, the multiplicity of lesions and inhomogeneous pattern of enhancement, characterized by a peripheral ring or rim pattern, are typical of AIDS-associated lymphoma. The patient was a 36-year-old HIV-positive man with a 2-day history of severe frontal headache.

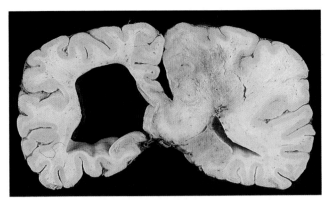

**FIGURE 4–422**  PRIMARY CENTRAL NERVOUS SYSTEM LYMPHOMA

Untreated primary central nervous system lymphoma is a granular mass. This example involves the corpus callosum. The patient was a 56-year-old man who presented with headache, right-sided weakness, and sensory loss. He died before therapy could be instituted.

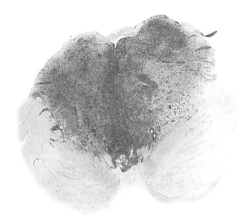

**FIGURE 4–423**  PRIMARY CENTRAL NERVOUS SYSTEM LYMPHOMA

This whole mount histologic section of the midbrain stained for cresyl fast violet illustrates the concentration of neoplastic cells around blood vessels, a typical feature of this tumor.

been applied to the initial lesion that manifests this response, as well as heralds the disease.[2] Radiologically, the duration of the response is measured in weeks to months, but in some cases, it is prolonged for years.

**Macroscopic Features.** PCNSLs form either well-circumscribed masses or ill-defined infiltrates within relatively intact brain parenchyma. Most are gray and granular (Fig. 4–422). Cerebral lymphomas are typically more deep-seated and less circumscribed than are metastatic carcinomas.

**Microscopic Features.** At low magnification, the lesion may have solid sheets of cells (Figs. 4–423 to 4–425), but in large areas it is often patchy, with solid sheets of cells and perivascular cuffs blending into less cellular zones of infiltration (Fig. 4–426). Individually, the cells are larger and rounder than those of most glioblastomas. Nucleoli are more prominent. Necrosis and, especially, apoptosis are often prominent. The latter is especially prominent after steroid therapy (see Figs. 4–431 to 4–433). An accompanying infiltrate of small reactive lymphocytes sometimes dominates the picture (Figs. 4–427 and 4–428).

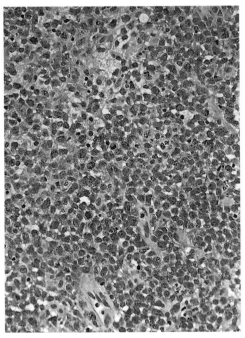

4–424

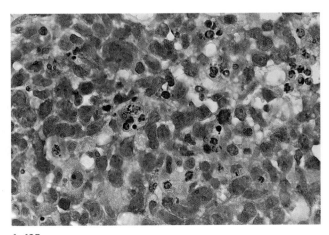

4–425

**FIGURES 4–424 AND 4–425**  PRIMARY CENTRAL NERVOUS SYSTEM LYMPHOMA

Sheets of markedly atypical, round, large cells are a classic feature. Apoptosis is often prominent.

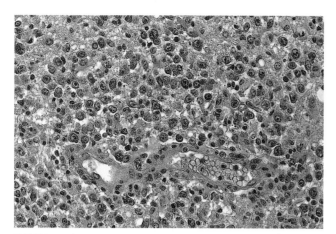

**FIGURE 4–426**   PRIMARY CENTRAL NERVOUS SYSTEM LYMPHOMA

The lesions are often looser in their growth pattern than the sheet-like pattern illustrated in Figures 4–424 and 4–425.

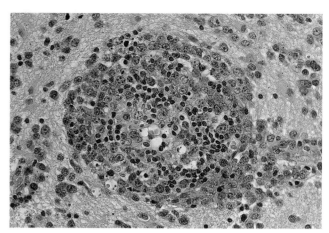

**FIGURE 4–429**   PRIMARY CENTRAL NERVOUS SYSTEM LYMPHOMA

The affinity of tumor cells for blood vessels is the most distinctive architectural feature of primary central nervous system lymphoma.

PCNSLs are typically angiocentric and angioinvasive (Figs. 4–427 and 4–429). This is evident even in the homogeneously cellular areas but is seen most readily in zones of infiltration, where cellular cuffs of neoplastic cells surround vessels. The cells laminate beneath the endothelium, insinuate themselves within the media and adventitia, and permeate the perithelial region. Simulating the annual growth rings of a tree are circumferential bands of reticulin that form laminae within and around vessel walls (Fig. 4–430).[1] In some instances, reticulin fibers are seen to arborize within the involved parenchyma.

**Effects of Prior Corticosteroid Therapy.** PCNSLs are often sensitive, sometimes exquisitely so, to corticosteroids used to control cerebral edema. Early in the post-treatment phase, there is pronounced apoptosis

(Fig. 4–431). Later, a sea of macrophages may remain (Figs. 4–432 and 4–433).

**Features in Needle Biopsy Specimens.** The diagnosis of PCNSL is usually made by stereotactic biopsy, without a subsequent attempt at resection. The cores of tissue have the features described earlier, but because of the limited sampling, the characteristic angiocentricity may be inconspicuous. Even in its absence, the diagnosis is usually possible on the basis of the cytologic features.

**Features in Frozen Sections.** The freezing process often produces considerable cellular distortion, degrading the classic appearance of lymphoma to that of a nonspecific neoplasm, which invites the diagnosis of malignant glioma (Fig. 4–434; see also Fig. 5–11). Nevertheless, the angiocentricity and angioinvasiveness are

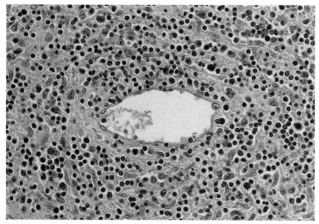

4–427

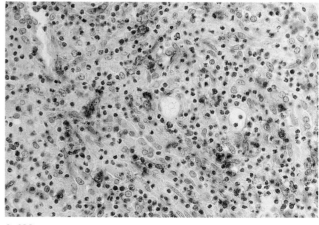

4–428

**FIGURES 4–427 AND 4–428**   PRIMARY CENTRAL NERVOUS SYSTEM LYMPHOMA

The large, atypical cells may be difficult to identify in the inflammatory infiltrate in an H&E stained section (Fig. 4–427) but may be apparent after staining for lymphoid markers, such as CD20 (Fig. 4–428).

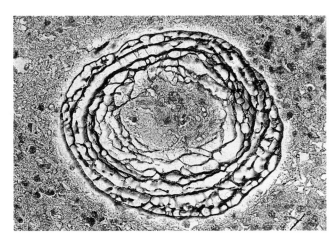

**FIGURE 4–430**    PRIMARY CENTRAL NERVOUS SYSTEM
LYMPHOMA

The angioinvasiveness of the lesion is evident from the tumor cells
locked between reticulin fibers within vessel walls.

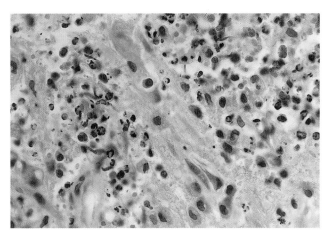

**FIGURE 4–431**    PRIMARY CENTRAL NERVOUS SYSTEM
LYMPHOMA FOLLOWING CORTICOSTEROID TREATMENT

Some primary central nervous system lymphomas respond to corticosteroid treatment by massive apoptosis. This patient had been treated
just 24 hours earlier to control cerebral edema.

retained, and if the diagnosis is considered, the significance of the round nuclei and prominent nucleoli will
be recognized. The extent of apoptosis often exceeds
that in most glioblastomas.

**Cytologic Features.** Dispersed for viewing in smear
preparations, the cells display their cytoplasmic borders,
large nuclei, coarse chromatin, and prominent nucleoli
(Fig. 4–435; see also Fig. 5–10). Apoptosis is common.
Cells of lymphomas lack the cohesiveness and nuclear
molding of metastatic carcinoma, and also the processes
that create the fibrillar background of glioblastoma.

**Immunohistochemical Features.** Most CNS lymphomas are monotypic for kappa or lambda immunoglobulin light chains and are positive for other

B-cell markers as well[38, 40] (Fig. 4–436). T-cell lymphomas are uncommon.[32] The small reactive lymphocytes
that invade most lymphomas are predominantly T cells;
these are so numerous that they overshadow the tumor
cells in some cases ("T-cell–rich B-cell lymphoma") (see
Fig. 4–427). The MIB-1 indices are high—often in the
50% range (Fig. 4–437). Immunohistochemistry or in
situ hybridization can be used to identify Epstein-Barr
virus in lymphoproliferative states associated with immunosuppression (Fig. 4–438).[25, 27, 30, 35, 37, 42]

**Ultrastructural Features.** Lacking the junctional complexes and surface specializations of carcinoma, as well
as the intermediate filaments characteristic of glioblastoma, lymphomas are the ultrastructural "have-nots"
among intracranial tumors.[22]

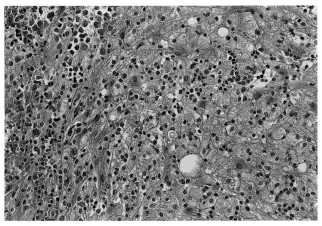

4–432

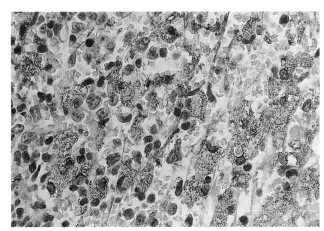

4–433

**FIGURES 4–432 AND 4–433**    PRIMARY CENTRAL NERVOUS SYSTEM LYMPHOMA FOLLOWING CORTICOSTEROID TREATMENT

Macrophage-rich lesions in the elderly should raise one's suspicion of steroid-treated malignant lymphoma. In this case, only a few residual neoplastic cells are present at the top left of the illustration (Fig. 4–432). Immunohistochemistry with the macrophage marker HAM-56 stains the phagocytes but not the neoplastic lymphoid cells (Fig. 4–433).

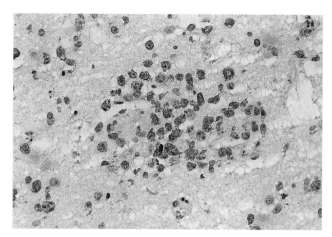

**FIGURE 4–434    PRIMARY CENTRAL NERVOUS SYSTEM LYMPHOMA—FROZEN SECTION**

In frozen sections, this tumor closely resembles an infiltrating glioma. An angiocentric cluster of cells provides a clue to the diagnosis.

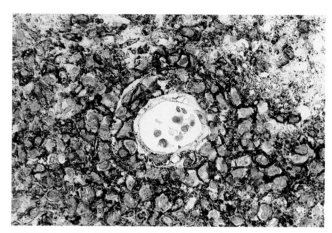

**FIGURE 4–436    PRIMARY CENTRAL NERVOUS SYSTEM LYMPHOMA**

Both the angioinvasiveness and the B-cell phenotype of typical primary central nervous system lymphoma are evident in this AIDS-associated lymphoma stained for CD20.

**Differential Diagnosis.** In a nonimmunosuppressed patient, the diagnosis of PCNSL is often suspected because of the patient's age and the radiologic features. Histologically, the diagnosis is immediately restricted to malignancy, or to an inflammatory or demyelinating lesion if there has been prior steroid therapy.

Among neoplasms, *anaplastic astrocytoma* and *glioblastoma multiforme* are of principal concern, particularly in view of the patient's age. The infiltrating edge of a lymphoma can closely mimic a high-grade glioma.

In general, *malignant gliomas* are distinguished from lymphomas by their greater degree of tissue infiltration and more marked variation in nuclear size and shape, but there is an overlap between some malignant gliomas, such as oligodendroglioma, and the infiltrating portion of PCNSL (Figs. 4–439 and 4–440). Despite their overt malignancy, PCNSLs lack microvascular proliferation and necrosis with pseudopalisading (see Table 4–6, p. 188). Malignant gliomas are often more "small cell" in composition than are PCNSLs. Furthermore, although glioma cells typically relate to vessels, they do not permeate their walls. Gliomas may contain reticulin, but it is abundant only in the face of meningeal, particularly dural, infiltration or when the tumor undergoes sarcomatous metaplasia (e.g., gliosarcoma).

*Anaplastic carcinomas* may mimic cerebral lymphomas cytologically, but with the exception of the

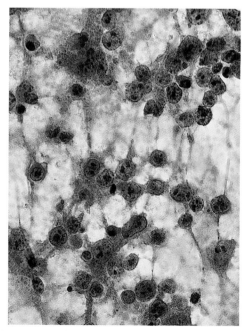

**FIGURE 4–435    PRIMARY CENTRAL NERVOUS SYSTEM LYMPHOMA**

Individually dispersed cells showing no tendency to form tissue fragments or cell processes are key cytologic features. Nucleoli are prominent.

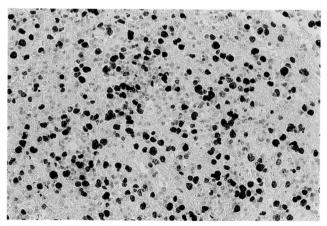

**FIGURE 4–437    PRIMARY CENTRAL NERVOUS SYSTEM LYMPHOMA**

Other than metastases, the MIB-1 index of primary central nervous system lymphomas is considerably higher than that of other central nervous system tumors.

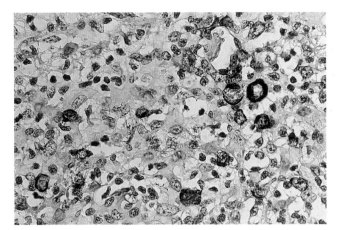

**FIGURE 4–438**   POST-TRANSPLANT LYMPHOPROLIFERATIVE SYNDROME

Immunohistochemistry for Epstein-Barr virus is positive in a high proportion of lymphoproliferative disorders occurring in the setting of immunosuppression.

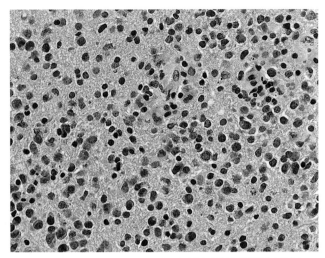

**FIGURE 4–440**   PRIMARY CENTRAL NERVOUS SYSTEM LYMPHOMA RESEMBLING INFILTRATING GLIOMA

In areas of diffuse infiltration lacking angiocentricity, lymphoma can closely mimic infiltrating glioma.

periphery of small cell carcinoma, they are not infiltrative lesions that overrun brain parenchyma. Histologically, the cells of a carcinoma are cohesive, lack both angioinvasion and the reticulin deposition of PCNSL, and cytologically show nuclear molding. Metastases are often divided by collagenous septa. In smear preparations, neoplastic epithelial cells are often cohesive and smear as tissue fragments rather than as individual cells.

One of the more common differential diagnostic problems is posed by a macrophage-rich lesion in an elderly patient. Although vascular disease with *infarction* or *demyelinating disease* immediately enters the differential diagnosis, consideration must be given to the possibility of a lymphoma treated preoperatively with steroids, as discussed earlier.[15] This scenario, especially when there are radiologic features typical of PCNSL

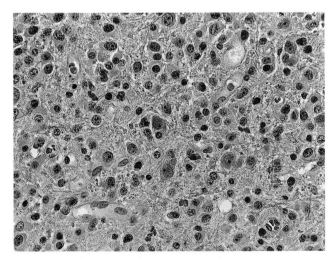

**FIGURE 4–439**   INFILTRATING GLIOMA RESEMBLING PRIMARY CENTRAL NERVOUS SYSTEM LYMPHOMA

Cytologic atypia and prominence of nucleoli in a malignant oligodendroglioma produce a resemblance to lymphoma.

before treatment, is highly suspicious for lymphoma. A repeat biopsy after discontinuation of the steroids may be needed to resolve the issue.

In the setting of immunosuppression, there is a broad spectrum of brain lesions that can be characterized, at least in part, without resort to a biopsy.[3, 39] *Toxoplasmosis* titers and a healthy index of suspicion often prompt empiric treatment of this opportunistic infection. Nevertheless, a tissue diagnosis is required in some cases. In uncomplicated cases, trophozoites are readily evident in the Giemsa- or H&E-stained section, whereas in the setting of AIDS, the organisms are distributed singly and are best seen after immunostaining.

*Progressive multifocal leukoencephalopathy* differs in almost every way from PCNSL. Lesions of the latter are usually nonenhancing and exert minimal mass effect. The histologic differences are also great. Only a few, cytologically bland lymphocytes are available to respond.

**Treatment and Prognosis.** Although the course of cerebral lymphomas varies considerably, most patients succumb within $1\frac{1}{2}$ years.[4, 7, 12, 15, 17, 21, 33] Survival in the AIDS population is especially poor. Radiotherapy, if feasible, extends the interval in some patients with AIDS,[7] but survival is often less than 3 months.[15, 18, 20]

Only a small minority of PCNSLs "peripheralize" or spread to systemic sites.[9] Even in cases in which no extraneural involvement was discernible during life, minute, incidental deposits may be found at autopsy in such organs as the testis.

### Intravascular Lymphomatosis

**Definition.** A systemic, largely intravascular lymphoma, often with prominent involvement of the CNS.

**Clinical Features.** Affected patients present with a variety of focal and nonfocal CNS manifestations, including the consequences of occlusive vascular disease,

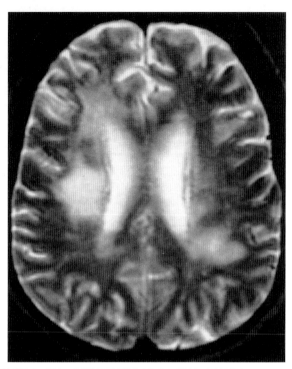

**FIGURE 4–441** INTRAVASCULAR LYMPHOMATOSIS

Multiple ill-defined patches of T2 hyperintensity were noted in the cerebral hemispheres of this 68-year-old woman experiencing a rapid decline in mental status. The histologic features of the biopsy specimen are illustrated in Figure 4–442.

subacute encephalopathy (dementia), spinal cord or nerve root symptoms, and cranial neuropathies.[1–6, 8, 9] Although affected children have been reported, the disease usually appears in the seventh decade of life.[5] The skin (rash) and endocrine glands (adrenal insufficiency) are frequently involved.

In light of the often confusing neurologic picture and the absence of a radiologic mass lesion, the disease may not be diagnosed until after death.[4, 8]

**Radiologic Features.** The range of radiologic appearances includes infarct-like areas; meningeal lesions; and multiple, diffusely distributed, T2-hyperintense foci (Fig. 4–441).[9, 10]

**Microscopic Features.** Large, malignant lymphoid cells occlude and distend small arteries, veins, and capillaries but extend little if at all into the surrounding parenchyma (Fig. 4–442).

**Immunohistochemical Features.** Almost all lesions react with markers for B cells[2, 4, 5]; a T-cell phenotype is rare.[7]

**Treatment and Prognosis.** The disease runs its fatal course in less than a year.[8]

### Lymphomatoid Granulomatosis

This unusual entity is generally viewed as a T-cell malignant lymphoma or an atypical lymphoid proliferation in evolution to lymphoma.[2, 5] CNS involvement can occur either in association with classic pulmonary disease[7] or in isolation.[2, 4–6] Intracranial lesions may be solitary or multifocal.[3, 5] They have been reported in AIDS patients.[1]

Microscopically, lymphomatoid granulomatosis is a polymorphous combination of atypical T lymphocytes, plasmacytoid lymphocytes, and macrophages. The infiltrate is angiocentric, invasive, and associated with necrosis that is often pronounced. Epstein-Barr virus genome is demonstrable in some cases.[2]

Given definitional problems, limited experience with the entity, and the frequently overriding effects of systemic disease, it is difficult to generalize about the prognosis in patients in whom CNS involvement is exclusive or predominant. Survival is typically 2 years.[5]

### Microglioma

The existence of this entity has been difficult to establish, given its rarity and the need for immunohistochemical markers. As one swallow heralds spring, one case may introduce this lesion.[1] The neoplasm was remarkably diffuse throughout the brain and spinal cord and even extended into intracranial and intraspinal nerve roots. The elongated cells of this reported case cytologically resembled the microglia and reacted for CD68 (KP1), as well as the microglial marker *Ricinus communis* agglutinin-120.

## Germ Cell Neoplasms

Intracranial germ cell neoplasms occur throughout the brain but favor the pineal and suprasellar regions,

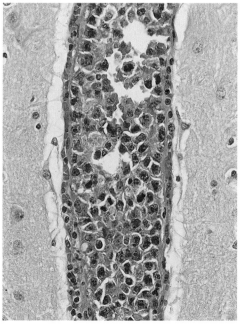

**FIGURE 4–442** INTRAVASCULAR LYMPHOMATOSIS

Markedly atypical lymphoid cells crowd the lumen of a cortical vessel in the case illustrated in Figure 4–441.

sometimes synchronously. It might be inferred from the names of authors cited in the references that the incidence of these tumors is heightened in Japan. An elevated incidence has been noted in patients with Down syndrome.[5]

The first, and larger, category of germ cell lesions—the germinoma—corresponds to seminoma of the testis and dysgerminoma of the ovary. The second, and numerically smaller, group encompasses three subgroups derived conceptually from totipotential germ cells: teratomas, yolk sac tumors, and choriocarcinomas.

The pineal germ cell tumors are more common in males and usually present during the first 3 decades of life, with the symptoms of aqueductal compression or distortion of the quadrigeminal plate. The usual signs and symptoms thus include headaches, papilledema, mental changes, and gaze palsies. Precocious puberty is a classic, but less common, presenting complaint.

## Germinoma

**Clinical Features.** Germinomas typically present in the pineal or suprasellar region, sometimes synchronously. They occasionally appear in other sites, especially the basal ganglia.

Germinomas in the suprasellar area occur either as a solitary process or, in about half the cases, in association with a pineal region lesion (Fig. 4–443). The triad of diabetes insipidus, loss of visual acuity, and hypopituitarism is typically produced by suprasellar tumors. Diabetes insipidus, as a presenting symptom in a young patient, is strongly suggestive of a germ cell tumor, because other similarly situated neoplasms, such as pilocytic astrocytoma and craniopharyngioma, produce this endocrine deficit only late in the course or after surgery. In contrast with other neoplasms of the pineal region,

germinomas are more equally divided with respect to gender.

An occasional germinoma arises at a distance from the midline, notably in the basal ganglia,[10, 18, 20, 21, 25, 42] cerebellum,[43] or midbrain.[26]

**Radiologic Features.** Germinomas are contrast-enhancing masses (see Fig. 4–443) that, owing to their content of collagen, may be dark in T2-weighted images. Initially, or at the time of recurrence, the lesion may have disseminated along the ventricular walls.

**Macroscopic Features.** Their collagen content makes these lesions tough and difficult to resect.

**Microscopic Features.** Typical germinomas consist of sheets, lobules, and nests of large, round neoplastic cells interspersed with lymphocytes and traversed by fibrous septa (Figs. 4–444 and 4–445). The ratio of neoplastic to inflammatory and stromal tissue varies from case to case. It is high in some lesions, but so low in others that the diagnosis becomes difficult, if not impossible. The nuclei of the tumor cells possess open chromatin and prominent nucleoli varying from round to bar shaped. The cytoplasm is often pale and artifactually vacuolated. Being glycogen rich, it is PAS positive and diastase labile. At the base of the brain, the tumor more often abuts the surface of the brain, but it can infiltrate superficially in the manner of a glioma (Fig. 4–446). The gliosis induced often features "reactive atypia" that also may simulate astrocytoma.

Noncaseating granulomatous inflammation replete with multinucleated giant cells accompanies some germinomas and occasionally overshadows the tumor. This can pose a diagnostic problem, especially in minute specimens that may consist entirely of fibroinflammatory tissue.[23] Neoplastic cells, even if present, may be

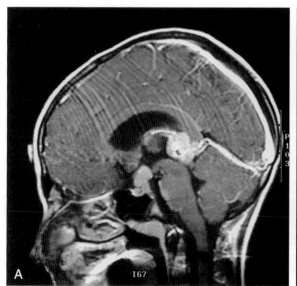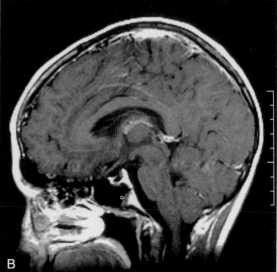

**FIGURE 4–443**   GERMINOMA

Although most germinomas are unifocal, some make a synchronous appearance in suprasellar and pineal regions, as in this 17-year-old boy who presented with diabetes insipidus (A). Neither mass was apparent on a magnetic resonance imaging scan 9 months after radiotherapy (B), illustrating germinomas' radiosensitivity.

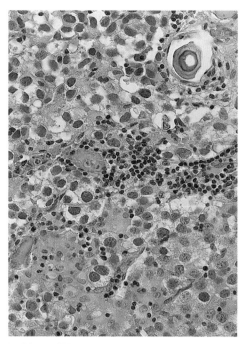

**FIGURE 4–444    GERMINOMA**

Lobules of cells with clear cytoplasm, round nuclei, and, in this instance, well-defined cell borders are typical of germinoma. A lymphoid infiltrate is frequently present. A residual pineal calcospherite ("brain sand") sits at the top right of the illustration.

pyknotic, contracted, and difficult to identify. The tumor cells are particularly susceptible to crush artifact, and it is not uncommon to seek in vain for even one intact neoplastic cell. PAS stains aid in the search.

**Features in Frozen Sections.** The tumor cell nuclei are often condensed and distorted in either the frozen section itself or in permanent sections prepared from frozen tissue (Fig. 4–447).

**Cytologic Features.** The contrast between the large malignant cells and the small benign lymphocytes is well seen in smear preparations (Fig. 4–448).

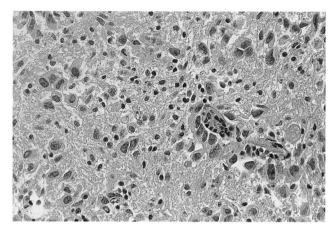

**FIGURE 4–446    GERMINOMA**

Particularly at the base of the brain, germinomas may infiltrate surrounding tissues, thus mimicking malignant gliomas.

**Immunohistochemical Features.** The surface of the neoplastic cells react for placental alkaline phosphatase (Fig. 4–449),[4, 11, 40] but this may be difficult to visualize when only isolated cells are present or in a small specimen that is distorted by prior freezing or crush artifact. Crisper and more reliable staining appears to be possible with antibodies to c-kit (Fig. 4–450).[15] Although immunohistochemistry is usually not required in larger specimens with classic histologic features, it is useful in excluding alternative diagnoses and facilitating the detection of other germ cell components.

Isolated mono- and/or multinucleate (syncytio-trophoblastic) giant cells positive for chorionic gonadotropin frequent some germinomas. Their presence has no prognostic significance, and they are not a harbinger of choriocarcinoma,[4, 45] although it has been questioned whether they are associated with a greater rate of recurrence.[2, 45] This suggestion correlates with a report of a greater risk of recurrence in the face of increased CSF levels of human chorionic gonadotropin.[12]

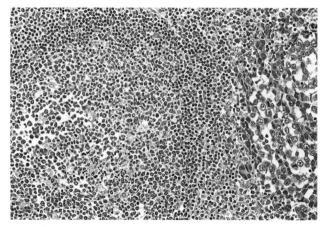

**FIGURE 4–445    GERMINOMA**

Much of the lesion may be inflammatory, sometimes with a granulomatous component.

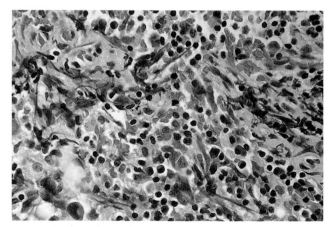

**FIGURE 4–447    GERMINOMA**

The cells may be crushed or smeared beyond recognition, particularly in small specimens.

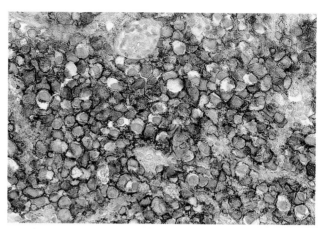

**FIGURE 4–450    GERMINOMA**

Antibodies to *c-kit* produce crisp membrane staining.

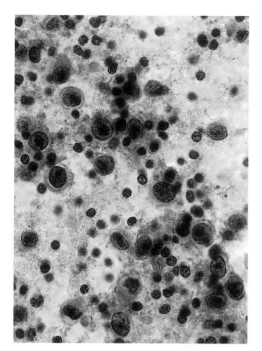

**FIGURE 4–448    GERMINOMA**

Cytologic features of germinomas include discreteness; large, round nuclei with prominent nucleoli; and, in some cases, cytoplasmic vacuolation. Reactive lymphocytes are present in variable numbers.

**Treatment and Prognosis.** The anatomic relations in the pineal region and at the base of the brain often preclude total excision of germ cell tumors. Thus, it is fortunate that germinomas are sufficiently radio- and chemosensitive to permit cure in a high percentage of cases. In one study, the 5-year survival rate was 80%.[38] In another, the 5- and 10-year survival rates were 93% and 81%, respectively.[27] In yet another, a 5-year survival of 96% was recorded.[36] Although germinomas rarely metastasize outside the CNS,[9, 16, 32] they are free to seed the craniospinal meninges or the abdominal cavity after placement of a ventriculoperitoneal shunt.[34] In some

germinomas, an initially undetected malignant germ cell component becomes apparent later in the form of a local recurrence or distant metastasis.[32]

## Other Germ Cell Neoplasms

Although other germ cell tumors frequent the same sites as germinomas, they are more likely to arise in the pineal than the suprasellar region.

The *immature teratoma*, the most common nongerminomatous tumor, is a caricature of the embryo, being composed of tissues with a distinctive embryonic or fetal appearance (Fig. 4–451). Neuroepithelial elements (glial cells of varying type, neurons, choroid plexus), muscle, and cartilage are common constituents. *Mature teratomas*, formed of "adult" tissue, are rare. The distinction between "fetal" and "adult" types is arbitrary in some instances. "Maturation" of an immature teratoma in the interval between operations is an uncommon event.[39] Radiologically, teratomas present a complex architecture; many are multicystic.[7] Immunoreactivities of the various constituent tissues are those of corresponding normal

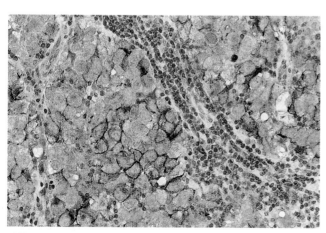

**FIGURE 4–449    GERMINOMA**

Antibodies to placental alkaline phosphatase stain the surface of the neoplastic cells.

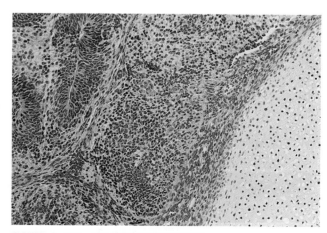

**FIGURE 4–451    IMMATURE TERATOMA**

Although deranged in structure, the lesion has many histologic features of the fetus.

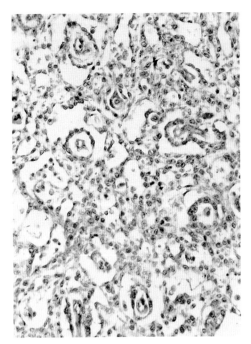

**FIGURE 4–452   YOLK SAC TUMOR**

Among hallmarks of the yolk sac tumor are "endodermal sinuses" (Schiller-Duval) that resemble structures in the rat placenta. They are formed as small blood vessels covered by epithelium project into epithelium-lined channels.

tissues and of teratomas occurring elsewhere in the body.[4, 11]

On occasion, extrapineal teratomas are congenital and present as massive lobulated, cystic lesions that virtually fill the cranial cavity.[28, 30, 31]

The capacity to mirror the pluripotentiality of germ cells is only partially expressed in most lesions but finds close to full expression in the exquisitely rare and remarkable intraventricular "fetus in fetu."[1, 48]

In rare instances, immature teratomas show transition to carcinomas and sarcomas of varying types.[6]

Although a *yolk sac tumor* may constitute a minor element in another germ cell tumor, when it is the predominant or exclusive pattern, the designation "yolk sac tumor" (or "endodermal sinus tumor") is appropriate.[4, 8, 14, 19, 29, 43, 46, 47, 49] Conceptually, this neoplasm is derived from endoderm and contains "endodermal sinuses" or Schiller-Duval bodies (Fig. 4–452). These are small glomeruloid structures formed of an epithelium-lined space invaginated by a vascular pedicle. Other patterns of yolk sac tumors include complex arrangements of perivascular endodermal cells, glands, thin-walled microscopic spaces, and loose-textured or patternless sheets (Fig. 4–453). Brightly eosinophilic, PAS-positive, diastase-resistant proteinaceous globules are a typical feature of yolk sac tumors and either occur within tumor cells or lie free within stroma. Such globules are accumulations of alpha-fetoprotein. Elevated levels of this protein in the serum or CSF are highly suggestive of the diagnosis. Immunoreactivity of the tumor for alpha-fetoprotein is expected (Fig. 4–454).[4, 11]

*Embryonal carcinoma* consists of anaplastic, cuboidal to columnar cells disposed in sheets and cords (Fig. 4–455).[33, 44, 46] Occasionally seen are embryoid bodies representing early differentiation toward embryonic (teratoid) or extraembryonic (yolk sac or placental) tissue. Embryonal carcinoma associated with teratoma, usually of the immature type, is loosely termed "teratocarcinoma." In ostensibly pure teratomas, small foci of prognostically significant embryonal carcinoma may be present. This underscores the need for a representative biopsy and thorough examination of the specimen. Embryonal carcinomas are immunoreactive for CD30.[24]

Trophoblastic differentiation in germ cell tumors may be confined to the simple presence of gonadotropin-positive syncytiotrophoblasts or may consist of fully developed bilaminar arrangements of syncytiotrophoblasts and cytotrophoblasts (i.e., *choriocarcinoma*). Neoplasms composed exclusively of human chorionic gonadotropin–positive choriocarcinoma are very rare.[3, 4, 17, 22, 41]

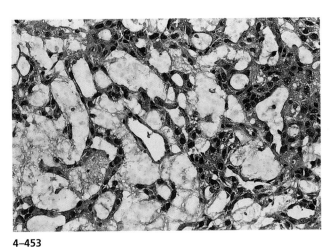
4–453

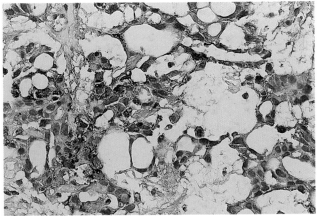
4–454

**FIGURES 4–453 AND 4–454   YOLK SAC TUMOR**

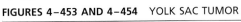
Anastomosing thin cores of cells are common in this germ cell subtype (Fig. 4–453). Positive immunostaining for alpha-fetoprotein is diagnostic (Fig. 4–454).

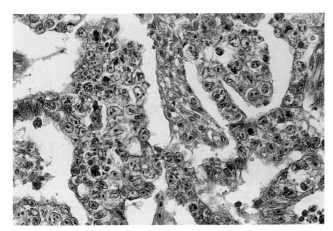

**FIGURE 4–455**  EMBRYONAL CARCINOMA

Ribbons composed of large, full-bodied, malignant epithelial cells with round nuclei, open chromatin, and macronucleoli are typical of embryonal carcinoma.

**Treatment and Prognosis.** If the mass is resectable, patients with mature or immature teratomas—especially those with the mature type—have a favorable outlook. In one study, the 5-year survival rates of patients with mature and immature teratomas were 86% and 67%, respectively.[37] In another series, the 5-year survival rate for patients with immature teratomas was also 67%.[36] In yet another series, the 10-year survival rate for patients with mature teratomas was 93%.[27] The outlook for patients with other nongerminomatous lesions is considerably less sanguine.[27, 33, 35, 37, 38] Both local recurrence and craniospinal dissemination become more likely, although systemic metastases are infrequent. One report recorded favorable results when alpha-fetoprotein–producing lesions were treated with radio- and chemotherapy.[13]

## Hemangioblastoma

**Definition.** A richly vascular neoplasm with stromal cells of uncertain histogenesis.

**General Comments.** Hemangioblastoma appeals to surgeons because of its curability, to pathologists because of its distinctive anatomy, to geneticists because of its association with phakomatosis, and to internists because of the elaboration of erythropoietin.[21, 47, 56, 57] Erythropoietin has been demonstrated within the encysted fluid, and plethora, a feature in approximately 10% of cases, resolves following resection.[27, 47, 56] Occasional intratumoral foci of erythropoiesis are yet another expression of local erythropoietin production, as are possibly granules within stromal cells.[23] Mast cells, common in hemangioblastomas,[52] are immunoreactive for erythropoietin and could play a role in angiogenesis.[16]

**Clinical Features.** Hemangioblastomas present mainly during the third through fifth decades and preferentially affect men. Examples in children are rare.[12, 39, 51] Most hemangioblastomas originate in the cerebellum, generally in a hemisphere. Although the medulla is an uncommon

site, hemangioblastoma warrants a pathologist's consideration when faced with an exophytic lesion in this region in an adult.[14, 29, 40]

Occasional hemangioblastomas are supratentorial,[9, 11, 46] such as within a ventricle[20] or on an optic nerve[28, 42, 48]; in the sella turcica[49]; or in the leptomeninges. Those in the meninges are discussed in Chapter 2. A rare example arises in peripheral nerve.[15]

Hemangioblastomas can be solitary or multifocal and may be associated with a retinal counterpart or any of a number of extra-CNS components of the von Hippel-Lindau syndrome. The latter includes renal cell carcinoma, visceral cysts (especially of kidney or pancreas), papillary cystadenoma of the epididymis or mesosalpinx, aggressive papillary middle ear tumor ("endolymphatic sac tumor"; see Fig. 1–78), and adrenal (pheochromocytoma) or extra-adrenal paraganglioma.[19, 25, 32, 36, 43, 44] Analogous to other familial multisystem disorders, the complex is variable in its expression, which includes consummate multiorgan involvement, an isolated hemangioblastoma in the setting of a positive family history, and an isolated "sporadic" tumor with a negative family history.

As enlarging posterior fossa masses, hemangioblastomas impede the flow of CSF and induce headache, vomiting, and papilledema. Tonsillar herniation with medullary compression may lead to sudden and unexpected death (see Fig. 4–458). Although hemangioblastomas are highly vascular and bleed freely when incised, spontaneous symptomatic hemorrhage is unusual.[33, 55]

**Radiologic Features.** Although some hemangioblastomas are solid, the classic architecture is a cyst with a contrast-enhancing mural nodule (Fig. 4–456).[19] Dark

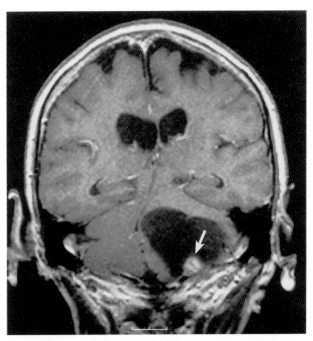

**FIGURE 4–456**  HEMANGIOBLASTOMA

Cerebellar hemangioblastoma is often a nodule (*arrow*) lying in the wall of a cyst. This example occurred in a 59-year-old woman with a 6-month history of dizziness.

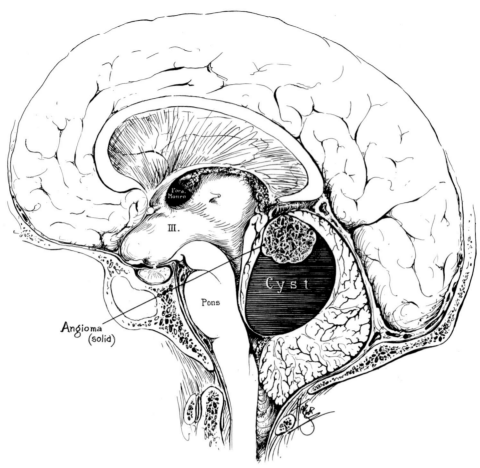

**FIGURE 4–457**    HEMANGIOBLASTOMA

A depiction by the medical illustrator Dorcas Padget captures the discreteness of the lesion and its common presentation as a mural nodule. Note the historical designation "angioma." (From Dandy WE. The Brain. New York: Harper and Row, 1969.)

"flow voids" in the large feeding and draining vessels attest to the lesion's vascularity.

**Macroscopic Features.** Much like the eccentrically positioned ovum in a graafian follicle, many hemangioblastomas are small nodules in the wall of a cyst (Figs. 4–457 to 4–459). The liquor is characteristically yellow to brown, whereas the neoplasm is red and/or yellow, reflecting its variable vascularity and lipid content (see Fig. 4–459). In properly oriented microsections, the characteristic leptomeningeal abutment is readily evident.

**Microscopic Features.** Unlike infiltrating gliomas, hemangioblastomas are relatively discrete. Nonetheless, peripheral capillaries, as well as nests and small lobules of neoplastic cells, may creep short distances into the surrounding parenchyma. Reactive astrocytes are present around, and sometimes even deep within, the substance of the tumor, a reflection of its growth by "creeping substitution" of brain tissue. In some cases, as described later in the section on immunohistochemical features, tumor cells appear GFAP positive. Exceptional tumors seemingly combine features of hemangioblastoma and glioma[2]; the nature of such "angiogliomas" is unsettled (see the section on differential diagnosis).

At low magnification, the lesion is a highly vascular mass with prominent large, often thin-walled vessels (Fig. 4–460). The cellularity is variable. Some hemangioblastomas are architecturally loose (see Fig. 4–460),

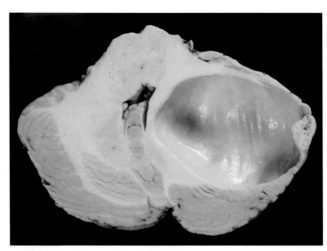

**FIGURE 4–458**    HEMANGIOBLASTOMA

The dimensions of the cyst can dwarf those of the nodule.

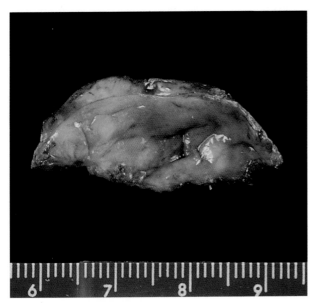

**FIGURE 4–459    HEMANGIOBLASTOMA**

Abundant lipid within the stromal cells turns some hemangioblastomas from red to yellow.

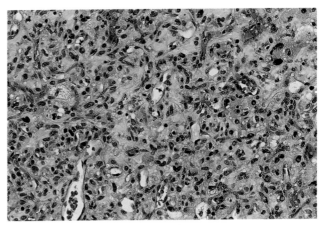

**FIGURE 4–461    HEMANGIOBLASTOMA**

Some hemangioblastomas are compact and cellular.

whereas others are more crowded and compact (Fig. 4–461). At high magnification, it is apparent that hemangioblastomas are formed of two principal components: vascular elements and interstitial, or "stromal," cells. The varied ratios of these two elements, the caliber of the vascular channels (predominantly capillaries), and the degree of lipidization of stromal cells contribute to the histologic heterogeneity of hemangioblastomas.

These constituents are often so intermingled that the capillary elements and stromal cells are distinguished only by their relation to the few intraluminal erythrocytes. When vascular channels are patulous or congested, endothelial cells are easily recognized by their flattened configuration and peripheral position. Stromal cells are discerned primarily by their prominent, variably lipidized cytoplasm (Figs. 4–462 to 4–464)[16, 18] and, to a lesser extent, by their nuclear pleomorphism and hyperchromasia (Fig. 4–465). Stromal cells may also contain moderate quantities of glycogen, a feature shared with renal cell carcinoma, the principal alternative in the differential diagnosis. Cytoplasmic hyaline droplets, at best a focal finding, are seen in a minority of cases (Fig. 4–466). PAS positive, they appear to represent large lysosomes. Foci of extramedullary hematopoiesis are not uncommon.[59]

Although an intricate network of reticulin separates the vascular compartment from stromal cells (Fig. 4–467), it is often difficult to distinguish these two cell

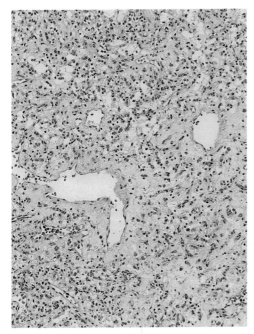

**FIGURE 4–460    HEMANGIOBLASTOMA**

Variations in cell density are common in hemangioblastomas. Large vessels are usually prominent.

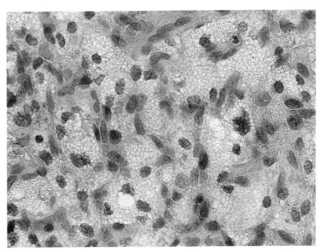

**FIGURE 4–462    HEMANGIOBLASTOMA**

Microvacuoles fill the cytoplasm of the stromal cells in this lipid-rich lesion.

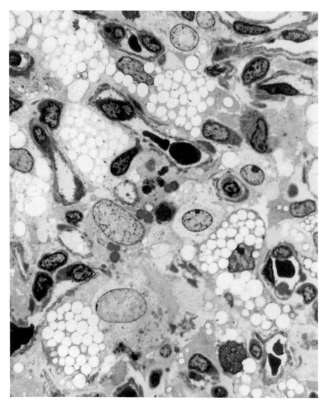

**FIGURE 4–463** HEMANGIOBLASTOMA

The extravascular position, pale nuclei, and cytoplasmic lipid of the stromal cells are illustrated in this semithin plastic-embedded section.

types when the vascular and stromal cells are densely intermingled. When stromal cells are sufficiently aggregated or engorged with lipid, however, they are readily identified (see Fig. 4–462). The dominant capillaries are delicate, whereas larger vessels are often thickened by the deposition of mature collagen. Some hemangioblastomas are extensively sclerotic (Fig. 4–468). Mast cells are common (Fig. 4–469).[16, 18, 52] CNS tumors likely to contain mast cells are listed in Table 4–10, p. 222.

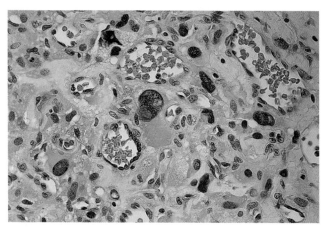

**FIGURE 4–465** HEMANGIOBLASTOMA

The nuclei of stromal cells can be large, hyperchromatic, and pleomorphic.

Hemangioblastomas occasionally play host to metastatic carcinoma.[3, 6]

**Features in Frozen Sections.** The key to the recognition of hemangioblastoma is an awareness of the entity and its distinctive radiologic and histologic features. If the possibility of hemangioblastoma is not considered, the diagnosis of glioma may be forthcoming. The dualistic cell composition frequently cannot be resolved in frozen tissues, because the cytoplasm of stromal cells is often artifactually distorted to resemble glial processes (Fig. 4–470). The presence of nuclear pleomorphism and hyperchromasia in the stromal cells lends credence to the diagnosis of malignant glioma. A malignant glioma is, however, an unlikely entity in the face of a discrete, contrast-enhancing nodule in the wall of a cerebellar cyst. The presence of abundant fat (see Fig. 4–464) supports the diagnosis of hemangioblastoma.

**Cytologic Features.** Unlike the two principal lesions in the differential diagnosis (i.e., glioma and metastatic

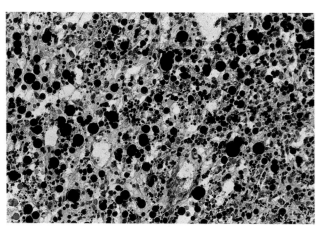

**FIGURE 4–464** HEMANGIOBLASTOMA

The lipid content of the stromal cells is readily demonstrated with fat stains such as oil red O.

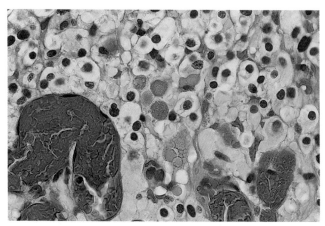

**FIGURE 4–466** HEMANGIOBLASTOMA

Intracytoplasmic eosinophilic droplets are seen in a minority of hemangioblastomas. The epithelioid quality of the stromal cells in this lesion can be misinterpreted as evidence of metastatic carcinoma.

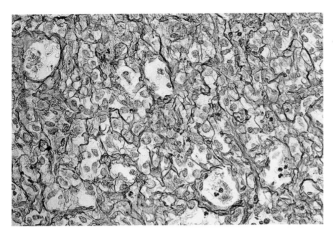

**FIGURE 4–467**   HEMANGIOBLASTOMA

Reticulin circumscribes nests of stromal cells.

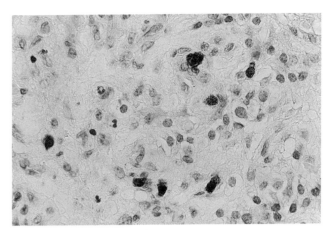

**FIGURE 4–469**   HEMANGIOBLASTOMA

As seen in a Giemsa preparation, mast cells are common in hemangioblastomas.

renal cell carcinoma), hemangioblastoma tissue resists disaggregation into individual cells (Fig. 4–471).[5] Smear preparations yield only cohesive clumps of cells entangled in capillaries, although at the edges, one may visualize stromal cells with nuclear hyperchromasia and sometimes pronounced pleomorphism. Lipid droplets can be seen if aqueous staining procedures are applied.

**Immunohistochemical Features.** Multitudes of morphologic studies and liters of antisera for immunohistochemistry have failed to resolve the nagging question of the histogenesis of hemangioblastoma. The non-neoplastic endothelial and pericytic components are obviously vascular (Fig. 4–472), but the identity of the stromal element has resisted elucidation. The torch was passed from electron microscopy to immunohistochemistry, with largely the same result—negative evidence. Although some stromal cells do stain positively for GFAP and S-100 protein, these results should be interpreted with caution, because reactive astrocytes may be numerous within the substance of hemangioblastomas.[22, 34, 53] Antisera for factor VIII/von Willebrand's factor have almost uniformly failed to stain the stromal cells.[13, 22, 35, 41]

Unfortunately, the most consistently positive staining has been to a notoriously nonspecific enzyme—neuron-specific enolase (Fig. 4–473).[10] Nevertheless, this result has raised the possibility of a neuronal origin for the stromal cells, although only a minority of stromal cells stain for a more specific neuronal marker, anti-Hu.[58] Two reports suggest a neuroendocrine derivation based on the stromal cells' content of neuropeptides.[1, 24] Electron-dense cytoplasmic granules were noted in one report.[24] Fibrohistiocytic differentiation was championed on the basis of immunoreactivity for factor XIIIa.[41]

**Ultrastructural Features.** The stromal cells are large, often lipid filled, and without specific differentiating features. They lie outside the vessel, beyond the pericyte (Fig. 4–474).[17]

**Molecular and Cytogenetic Features.** In accord with the rich vascularity of this "angioblastic" lesion, vascular endothelial growth factor is upregulated in the stromal cells, presumably as a result of mutations in the von Hippel-Lindau (*VHL*) gene.[50] Erythropoietin may also be negatively regulated by the *VHL* gene.[30] However,

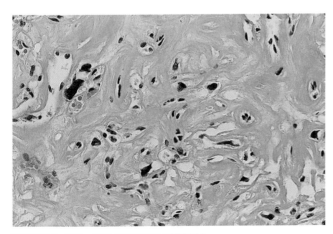

**FIGURE 4–468**   HEMANGIOBLASTOMA

Some lesions are extensively sclerotic.

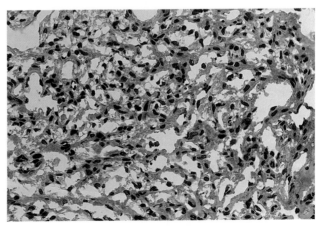

**FIGURE 4–470**   HEMANGIOBLASTOMA—FROZEN SECTION

The nuclear distortion produced by the freezing process creates a resemblance to glioma.

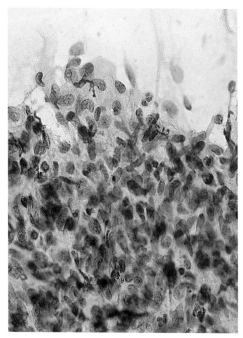

**FIGURE 4–471** HEMANGIOBLASTOMA—SMEAR PREPARATION

In contrast to most other lesions in the differential diagnosis, such as metastatic carcinoma, hemangioblastomas resist a dispersion into single cells in smear preparations. Their hyperchromatic nuclei are well visualized only at the edges of tissue fragments.

mutations or deletions in the *VHL* gene have been found in a minority of sporadic hemangioblastomas.[31] The contributions of other mechanisms for gene inactivation, such as methylation, remain unclear.[45, 54] By molecular criteria (i.e., retention of heterozygosity at the *VHL* locus), the vasculature is considered only a supportive element and not a part of the neoplasm per se.[31] The lesion is therefore neither "hemangio" nor "blastoma."

**Differential Diagnosis.** The differential diagnosis at the time of frozen section focuses on two entities—

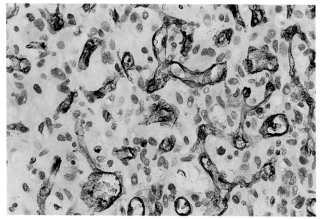

**FIGURE 4–472** HEMANGIOBLASTOMA

In spite of the tumor's name, it is only the vessels, not the stromal cells, that are immunoreactive for vascular markers such as CD31.

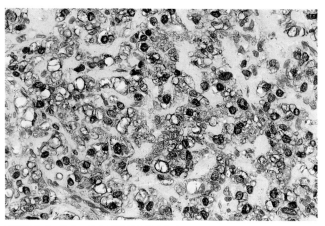

**FIGURE 4–473** HEMANGIOBLASTOMA

Stromal cells are immunoreactive for neuron-specific enolase, a finding of unknown significance.

hemangioblastoma and *malignant glioma*. The distinction is based on the largely noninfiltrative character of the hemangioblastoma, the absence of mitoses, and the presence of fat droplets.

The differential diagnosis is compounded when a neoplasm resembling a hemangioblastoma stains positively for GFAP (Figs. 4–475 and 4–476). In most cases, the positive elements are scattered reactive astrocytes near the edge of the lesion or stromal cells that can be dismissed as those that have phagocytized GFAP.[8] Other tumors, fortunately uncommon, contain or abut GFAP-positive tissue with histologic features of a glioma. The term "angioglioma" has been applied to these latter lesions.[2] We generally assign the diagnosis of hemangioblastoma if typical hemangioblastoma is found elsewhere in the specimen.

There may be striking histologic similarities between the cellular variant of hemangioblastoma and *metastatic renal cell carcinoma* (Fig. 4–477; see also Fig. 4–466). Both neoplasms are discrete, highly vascular, often lobular, composed of lipid-rich cells, and sometimes associated with erythropoietin production and erythrocytosis. The odds favor hemangioblastoma in the absence of a known renal primary tumor, although the presence of renal cell carcinoma in some cases of von Hippel-Lindau syndrome adds another dimension to the problem. Metastases of renal cell carcinoma to hemangioblastoma in the setting of von Hippel-Lindau syndrome have been reported.[3] In contrast to renal cell carcinomas, hemangioblastomas contain less glycogen. There is also a lower MIB-1 index in hemangioblastomas.[4] Renal cell carcinomas, but not hemangioblastomas, are immunoreactive for EMA.[22, 37] Negative radiologic studies of the kidneys are reassuring in doubtful cases.

A major pitfall is created by the exuberant gliosis that regularly occurs in the wall of the cyst around such lesions as *pilocytic astrocytoma*. The presence of Rosenthal fibers, which abound in these zones of reactive tissue, accompanied by a proliferation of glia, can suggest pilocytic astrocytoma. However, the latter lesion is generally a neoplasm of the young and usually has a distinctive biphasic architecture that includes loose tissue with

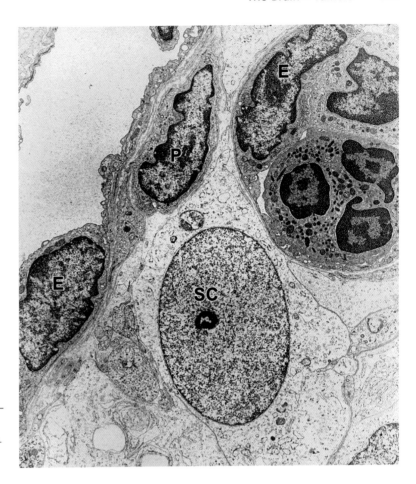

**FIGURE 4–474**   HEMANGIOBLASTOMA

The extravascular position of stromal cells is best seen by electron microscopy. A stromal cell (SC), with its large nucleus and electron-lucent cytoplasm, lies external to a capillary, with its electron-dense endothelial cells (E) and pericyte (P).

microcystic change. It lacks the marked vascularity of hemangioblastoma.

**Treatment and Prognosis.** The prognosis after removal of a hemangioblastoma is very favorable, although recurrences are possible if excision is incomplete. A new primary lesion may develop in von Hippel-Lindau syndrome, in which multiple hemangioblastomas are common, and ultimately may produce blindness as a consequence of multiple retinal neoplasms.[7, 25, 26] Dissemination along CSF pathways has been reported but is so rare as to be a pathologic curiosity.[38]

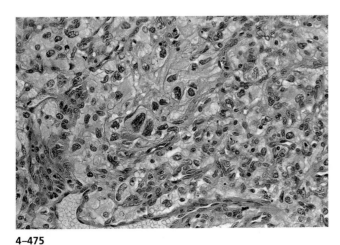

4–475

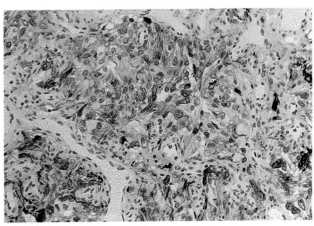

4–476

**FIGURES 4–475 AND 4–476**   GFAP-POSITIVE LESION RESEMBLING HEMANGIOBLASTOMA

Occasional cerebellar neoplasms with lobularity and a content of "stromal" cells (Fig. 4–475) are extensively immunoreactive for glial fibrillary acidic protein (Fig. 4–476). The nosologic position of such lesions relative to classic hemangioblastomas is unclear.

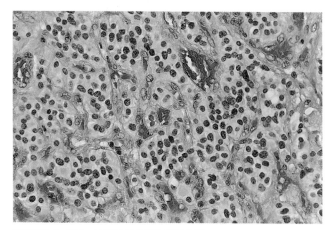

**FIGURE 4–477**    HEMANGIOBLASTOMA

Acini-like clusters of stromal cells can create a resemblance to metastatic carcinoma.

## Atypical Teratoid/Rhabdoid Tumor

**Definition.** A highly malignant neoplasm composed entirely, or in part, of distinctive large or rhabdoid cells that exhibit a diverse immunophenotype.

**General Comments.** There are multiple reports of primary CNS rhabdoid tumors with large cells, reniform nuclei, prominent nucleoli, and eccentric cytoplasmic masses of intermediate filaments.[3, 7, 8, 10] Members of what appears to be the same tumor family are more varied and less rhabdoid in appearance. Given an often broad immunophenotype representing all three germ layers, the term "atypical teratoid tumor" was suggested but was superseded by the diagnosis of atypical teratoid/rhabdoid tumor (AT/RT).[14] The simpler term "rhabdoid tumor" is now in wide use.

**Clinical Features.** Favoring males at a ratio of 3:2, AT/RTs generally present in the first 2 years of life.[6, 14] They are rare in adults.[10] With the exception of a rare intraspinal example,[6, 14] the lesions are intracranial with approximately two thirds in the posterior fossa. Synchronous occurrence of renal rhabdoid tumors and intracranial neoplasms has been described. The latter may be a small cell neoplasm, such as medulloblastoma or pineoblastoma,[4, 11] but the possibilities include rhabdoid tumors.

**Radiologic Features.** The lesions are bulky, contrast enhancing, sometimes cystic, and hemorrhagic (Fig. 4–478).[8] They are more likely to be necrotic than are the common differential diagnostic lesions—medulloblastomas. Although examples in the posterior fossa are often intracerebellar, others have their epicenter in an extracerebellar locus such as the cerebellopontine angle or brain stem. Contrast-enhancing ependymal or subarachnoid metastases are apparent at the time of presentation in some cases.

**Microscopic Features.** The histologic spectrum of AT/RT is broad, encompassing lesions that are exclu-

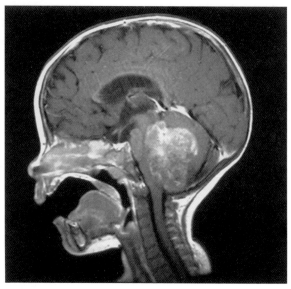

**FIGURE 4–478**    ATYPICAL TERATOID/RHABDOID TUMOR

Although atypical teratoid tumors occur throughout the central nervous system, most arise in the posterior fossa. As in this 9-month-old boy, they are usually large.

sively rhabdoid to those that are largely "small cell" in composition. Most are architecturally complex and feature a population of large cells, either rhabdoid or simply "pale" cells. These, in combination with smaller elements, give the lesion a somewhat loose, "jumbled" architecture that differs from the more compact, densely cellular composition of medulloblastoma (Fig. 4–479). In spite of the designation, the large cells are often not especially rhabdoid. The large cells possess reniform

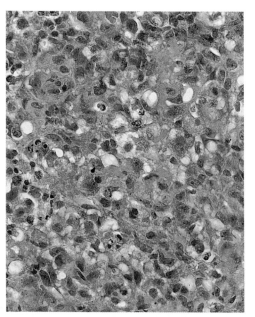

**FIGURE 4–479**    ATYPICAL TERATOID/RHABDOID TUMOR

Although the lesion has many histologic variations, the neoplasm usually has a somewhat jumbled architecture. The cells have large nuclei and prominent nucleoli, but an overt "rhabdoid" phenotype is not always prominent.

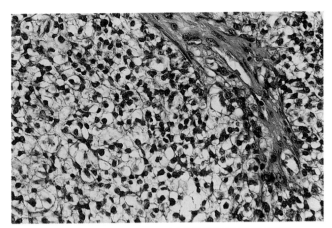

**FIGURE 4-480    ATYPICAL TERATOID/RHABDOID TUMOR**

Artifactual tumor cell vacuolization is a common finding.

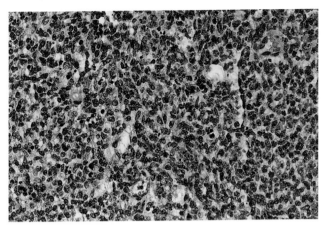

**FIGURE 4-482    ATYPICAL TERATOID/RHABDOID TUMOR**

Densely cellular areas mimic small cell embryonal tumors such as medulloblastoma.

nuclei and ample eosinophilic cytoplasm, occasionally with artifactual vacuolation (Fig. 4–480). Compact and fascicular in arrangement, small spindle cells punctuate some lesions (Fig. 4–481). Other, largely small cell examples closely resemble medulloblastoma (Fig. 4–482; see also Fig. 4–401).

Uncommonly, the cells form cords in a basophilic, mucoid matrix and thus resemble the trabecular pattern of renal rhabdoid tumors (Fig. 4–483).[15] Flexner-Wintersteiner rosettes are expressed in a small percentage of cases. Epithelial differentiation is uncommon and, if present, is confined to a few small, gland-like spaces (Fig. 4–484). Necrosis, often with dystrophic calcification, is common. A collagenous stroma is prominent in some cases. Trapped choroid plexus is common in cerebellar examples.

**Cytologic Features.** The classic large cells, often rather bland in appearance, are well seen in smear preparations, as are overtly rhabdoid cells with conspicuous nucleoli and prominent spherical cytoplasmic inclusions (Fig. 4–485). When only the spindle-shaped or small cells are represented, the diagnosis can only be suspected.

**Immunohistochemical Features.** The immunophenotype of AT/RT is broad, as the large, pale cells display a remarkable range of immunoreactivity, characteristically with clusters of immunopositive cells abutting those that are nonreactive. Surface staining for EMA is common (Fig. 4–486). Also frequent is reactivity for GFAP (Fig. 4–487) and cytokeratins.[1, 6, 8, 14] Immunopositivity for actin, neurofilament protein, and, occasionally, chromogranin is less frequent. Small cells in fascicles are often actin positive. Vimentin reactivity is universal. Staining for insulin-like growth factor II, insulin-like growth factor receptor type 1, and cathepsin has also been described.[12]

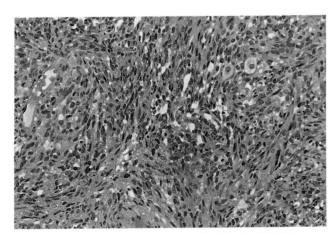

**FIGURE 4-481    ATYPICAL TERATOID/RHABDOID TUMOR**

A fascicular architecture lends a "mesenchymal" quality to some lesions.

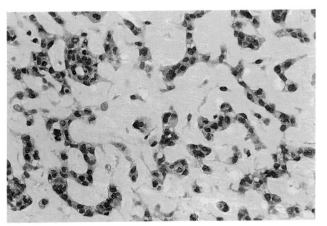

**FIGURE 4-483    ATYPICAL TERATOID/RHABDOID TUMOR**

Cords of cells in mucoid matrix are distinctive features of some lesions.

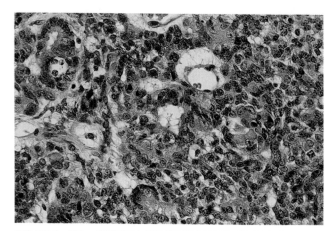

**FIGURE 4–484**    ATYPICAL TERATOID/RHABDOID TUMOR

Crude epithelial surfaces and glands are infrequent expressions of epithelial differentiation. In atypical teratoid/rhabdoid tumors, differentiation is more often an immunohistochemical than a histologic finding.

**Ultrastructural Features.** The rhabdoid component exhibits the expected cytoplasmic masses of tightly compacted, whorled intermediate filaments.[1, 3, 7, 14]

**Molecular and Cytogenetic Features.** Loss of all or part of chromosome 22 is observed in the vast majority of AT/RTs (Fig. 4–488).[2] Deletions and mutation have been found in the same gene, *INI1*, on chromosome 22q11.2, which appear to be central to the development of renal and extrarenal rhabdoid tumors. Rare germline abnormalities in this gene have also been described in both tumors.[2]

**Differential Diagnosis.** The frequent location of AT/RT in the posterior fossa raises the issue of *medulloblastoma*, of either "conventional" or "large cell" type (see Figs. 4–387 and 4–388). The large cell variant is of principal concern, but some AT/RTs are almost exclusively "small cell" (see Fig. 4–482). The distinction

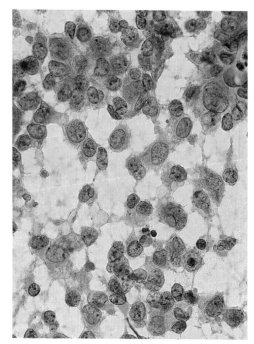

**FIGURE 4–485**    ATYPICAL TERATOID/RHABDOID TUMOR—SMEAR PREPARATION

The lesion's large nuclei with macronucleoli are especially evident in smear preparations.

between the two lies in the presence of the large, pale cells of AT/RT, whether generalized or only focal, and in the variations in histology and immunotype. Immunoreactivity for EMA, the most common reactant in AT/RT, serves as a convenient screening tool. Fluorescence in situ hybridization, for loss of chromosome 22 or the *INI1* gene, is a molecular method to distinguish these two cellular neoplasms.[5] Further distinctions between AT/RT and medulloblastoma are discussed on pages 307 to 308.

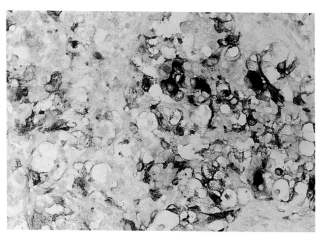

4–486

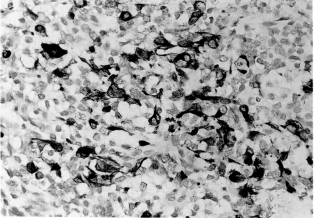

4–487

**FIGURES 4–486 AND 4–487**    ATYPICAL TERATOID/RHABDOID TUMOR

The immunophenotype of atypical teratoid/rhabdoid tumors is broad. As illustrated here, it includes reactivity for epithelial membrane antigen (Fig. 4–486) and glial fibrillary acidic protein (Fig. 4–487).

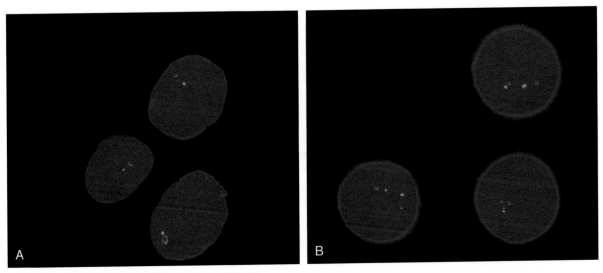

**FIGURE 4–488**    ATYPICAL TERATOID/RHABDOID TUMOR

Cells of atypical teratoid/rhabdoid tumors often lose some or all of chromosome 22. One *INI1* gene (red probe) is lost at chromosome 22q11.2, and the Ewing's sarcoma gene (green probe) is lost at 22q12 (*A*). Normal cells (*B*) have the expected two signals with each probe. (Courtesy of Dr. Jaclyn Biegel, Philadelphia, PA.)

Variants of AT/RT with overtly rhabdoid qualities can resemble *gemistocytic astrocytoma* as judged by cytoplasmic features and GFAP positivity. Unlike the astrocytoma, however, AT/RT is not highly infiltrative, and its immunophenotype, including positivity for such "nonglial" markers as EMA, is distinctive. High-grade *choroid plexus carcinoma* (Fig. 4–489) also enters into the differential diagnosis, because AT/RTs often have an epithelioid appearance; however, choroid plexus carcinomas are usually supratentorial, and most AT/RTs are infratentorial. Immunohistochemistry becomes decisive, with choroid plexus lesions being largely EMA negative but cytokeratin positive.

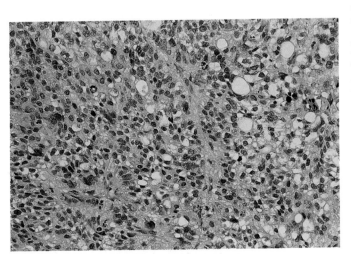

**FIGURE 4–489**    CHOROID PLEXUS CARCINOMA

High-grade choroid plexus tumors can closely resemble atypical teratoid/rhabdoid tumors (AT/RTs). The carcinoma, however, is far more likely to exhibit epithelial differentiation, while the AT/RT has a broad range of immunoreactivities for epithelial, glial, neuronal, and mesenchymal markers.

**Treatment and Prognosis.** Because of their large size and attachment to surrounding structures, gross total resection is seldom possible. Radiotherapy is generally withheld initially because of the young age of the patients. Survival times are brief—6 months to 1 year—despite aggressive chemotherapy.[6, 14] Early local recurrence and neuraxis dissemination are common. Whether a rhabdomyosarcoma-directed regimen is beneficial remains to be seen.[9, 13]

# Tumors of Intracranial Peripheral Nerves

## Schwannoma and Malignant Peripheral Nerve Sheath Tumors

**Definition.** Benign neoplasms derived from Schwann cells (schwannomas) and malignant, variously differentiated tumors of the intracranial peripheral nerves (malignant peripheral nerve sheath tumors [MPNSTs]).

**General Comments.** Like their intraspinal counterparts, intracranial schwannomas ("neurilemmomas") show a predilection for sensory nerves. Highly favored is the vestibuloacoustic (Figs. 4–490 and 4–491), followed distantly by the fifth cranial nerve[6, 58] and even more remotely by other cranial nerves.[5, 15–17, 30, 38, 39, 44, 47, 51] The "acoustic" schwannoma or "neurinoma" actually originates within the vestibular division of the eighth nerve near the zone of transition between the CNS and the peripheral nervous system (PNS). The former is myelinated by oligodendrocytes, the latter by Schwann cells.[50] With respect to the eighth nerve, this PNS-CNS interface is situated 8 to 10 mm from the pial surface of the pons, just within the internal auditory meatus. The term "vestibular schwannoma" is gradually replacing the

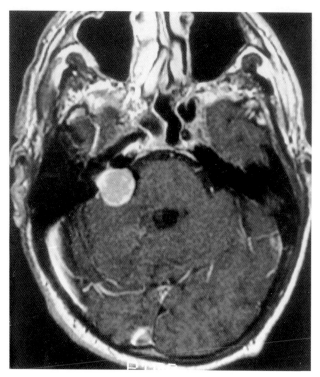

**FIGURE 4–490** VESTIBULAR SCHWANNOMA

The typical vestibular schwannoma is a contrast-enhancing mass that extends centrally from its origin in the internal auditory meatus to the cerebellopontine angle. Hearing loss in this 72-year-old man brought this lesion to medical attention.

common but anatomically incorrect designation "acoustic schwannoma."

Rare schwannomas arise within brain parenchyma,[12] including cerebrum,[2, 10, 14, 20, 21, 25, 37, 42, 49] fourth ventricle,[23, 41, 55] cerebellum,[45] and brain stem.[1, 8, 40] Presumably, the lesions take origin from small perivascular nerves. Uncommon subfrontal schwannomas[43] presumptively arise from the vestigial nervus terminalis ("cranial nerve zero") that courses in this region.[18] Perivascular extension of intraparenchymal schwannomas has been observed.[2] An intraventricular schwannoma has been reported as well.[25] Like meningiomas, a rare intracranial schwannoma plays host to metastatic carcinoma.[28, 57]

MPNSTs most often affect the fifth, or trigeminal, nerve,[4, 26, 29, 31, 32, 53] but the eighth can be affected as well.[22, 27, 36]

**Clinical Features.** With respect to schwannomas, the incidence curve plateaus from the third through the sixth decades. Bilateral examples involving the eighth cranial nerve are a frequent and almost pathognomonic manifestation of neurofibromatosis 2 (NF2; "central neurofibromatosis"), a condition that is genetically distinct from NF1 ("peripheral neurofibromatosis") and in which peripheral nerve sheath tumors, including spinal examples, predominate.[33] Multiple meningiomas and spinal ependymomas are also expressions of NF2. Schwannosis, a disorder genetically distinct from NF2, also includes intracranial schwannomas. Concurrence of meningioma and schwannoma in the cerebellopontine angle creates a mixed "collision" tumor.[19, 48]

**Radiologic Features.** Vestibular schwannomas originate within the internal auditory canal and are often "intracanalicular" at the time of presentation. The tumors enlarge or "flare" the internal auditory meatus, with larger lesions mushrooming into the intracranial compartment (see Fig. 4–490). Still further growth results in compression of the pons, cerebellum, and adjacent cranial nerves. Schwannomas can grow bidirectionally and approach the inner ear. As in schwannomas elsewhere, cystic change is not uncommon in larger examples.[52, 54]

In contrast with schwannomas, MPNSTs are aggressive and often invade bone or brain.

**Macroscopic Features.** The typical "acoustic" schwannoma is a lobulated mass, with the parent nerve stretched across the surface (see Fig. 4–491). With regard to the eighth nerve, the intracanalicular portion may be identified as a conical stalk that protrudes from the lateral aspect of the mass. Intrinsically tan in color, the tumor may be flecked by yellow foci of xanthomatous change. Consistency varies from soft to firm. The lesion may be cystic. The cellular variant of schwannoma (see later) is more homogeneously tan and lacks yellow xanthomatous change. MPNSTs are often focally necrotic.

**Microscopic Features.** Histopathologic features of Schwann cell tumors and MPNSTs are discussed in detail in Chapter 11 and in the Armed Forces Institute of Pathology's *Tumors of the Peripheral Nervous System*.[46] Intracranial examples are usually the prototypical schwannoma, with both Antoni A and Antoni B tissues (Fig. 4–492).

"Cellular schwannomas" are an uncommon variant in this location; most arise at a spinal level.[8, 13, 24] Decidedly cellular, they typically lack Antoni B tissue and show

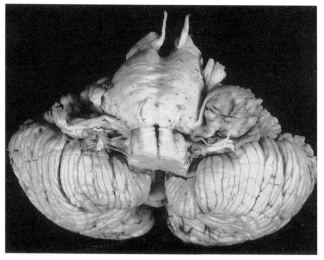

**FIGURE 4–491** VESTIBULAR SCHWANNOMA

The origin of most intracranial schwannomas of the eighth cranial nerve places them in the cerebellopontine angle, as with this incidental finding in a 65-year-old woman. The eighth nerve can be seen on the nipple-like apical portion of the neoplasm. The latter had expanded the internal auditory meatus.

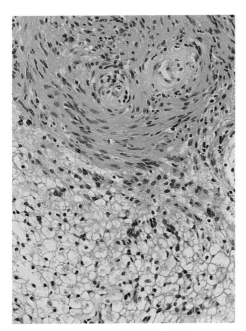

**FIGURE 4-492    VESTIBULAR SCHWANNOMA**

The prototypical lesion has both compact (Antoni A) and loose (Antoni B) components.

variable mitotic activity. Occasional tumors exhibit subcapsular, patchy, chromic inflammation. The pathologic features distinguishing cellular schwannoma from MPNST are discussed in detail in Chapter 12. Although "melanotic" schwannoma variants on the eighth cranial nerve have been described,[11, 35] the pigment is more often lipofuscin than true melanin. Nevertheless, some melanotic, psammomatous lesions are part of the Carney complex.[7] Only rare intracranial schwannomas are epithelioid.[3]

**Cytologic Features.** The cohesive tissues of a schwannoma resist disaggregation into individual cells, even when forcefully challenged during "smear" or "squash" preparation. Nonetheless, tissue can be sufficiently attenuated to visualize the elongated cells with their characteristic, "shillelagh-shaped" nuclei (Fig. 4-493). Degenerative nuclear atypia and nuclear-cytoplasmic pseudoinclusions are often seen. The cytologic features of a cellular schwannoma are indistinguishable from those of a conventional schwannoma.

**Immunohistochemical Features.** Conventional schwannomas are uniformly immunoreactive for S-100 protein. Reactivity in MPNSTs is often lacking or is a focal feature. Only low-grade and epithelial MPNSTs show uniform reactivity. Many schwannomas are reactive for Leu 7.[34] Staining for laminin and collagen IV is uniform and membranous. Cellular schwannomas share the same immunoprofile as conventional lesions.

**Ultrastructural Features.** Schwannomas feature spindle, bipolar cells with aligned and tangled processes. A single or duplicated layer of pericellular basement membrane separates the cells, which lack highly specialized intercellular junctions.[9] Striated clumps of "long spacing

collagen" are present in many conventional schwannomas but in only a small minority of cellular schwannomas.

**Differential Diagnosis.** Although the differential diagnosis of a cerebellopontine angle mass includes a host of lesions, in practice, it quickly narrows to schwannoma and *meningioma*. Schwannomas and many meningiomas are rich in collagen and may share xanthoma cells, cellular elongation, and even palisading in some cases. Psammoma bodies and tight whorls are distinctive features of meningioma. In frozen sections, the schwannoma's loose Antoni B tissue, fascicular Antoni A regions, and absence of tight whorls and psammoma bodies are helpful diagnostic features. Poorly formed whorls may be seen in NF2-associated schwannomas, whereas psammoma bodies adorn the highly distinctive "psammomatous" variant. Reticulin is abundant and distinctly pericellular in schwannomas. Staining for S-100 protein, although typical of schwannomas, is not a reliable criterion. Approximately 20% of meningiomas and 85% of fibrous variants show immunoreactivity for this protein, albeit less universally and less intensely than schwannomas do.[56] Laminin or collagen IV staining, a uniform feature of schwannomas, is not a finding in meningiomas. Last, meningiomas are reactive for EMA, whereas schwannomas are reactive only infrequently, and then without the membranous pattern of staining.[56]

**Treatment and Prognosis.** Schwannomas are variably treated in accord with the clinical circumstances. Some are followed without intervention, most are resected, and a few are treated by radiosurgery. Subtotally resected conventional schwannomas recur infrequently (3% in the Mayo Clinic experience), compared with

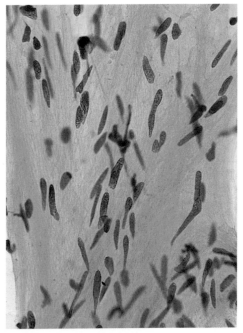

**FIGURE 4-493    VESTIBULAR SCHWANNOMA**

Although schwannomas are resistant to aggregation into single cells in smear preparations, the typical long, terminally expanded nuclei are evident in rarefied areas.

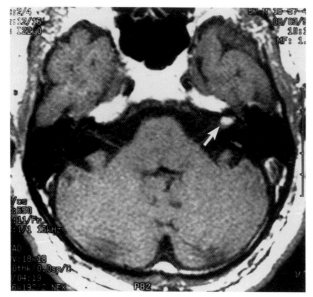

**FIGURE 4–494** LIPOMA OF THE EIGHTH CRANIAL NERVE

Intrinsically bright in a precontrast T1-weighted image, the lesion (*arrow*) resides within the auditory canal.

about 30% for cellular schwannomas.[8] Intracranial MPNSTs are aggressive, unresponsive to adjuvant treatment, and almost uniformly fatal.

### Other Tumors of Intracranial Peripheral Nerves

Small masses of fat and/or striated or smooth muscle can reside within the eighth cranial nerve. Of these, the "lipoma of the eighth cranial nerve" or "lipoma of the internal auditory canal" is most frequent. This benign lesion, which presents in adults, is variously expressed as hearing loss, tinnitus, and vertigo.[9, 11] Radiologically, it is distinguished from intracanalicular schwannoma by the bright signal that is characteristic of adipose tissue on precontrast T1-weighted MRI scans (Fig. 4–494).[4] Histologically, this distinctive lesion shows a peaceful coexistence of peripheral nerve, ganglion cells, and mature adipose tissue[10] (Fig. 4–495).

In other lesions of the eighth or other cranial nerves, striated or smooth muscle occurs alone or in association with adipose tissue. Various terms have been applied to these confederations, including "choristoma" for the smooth muscle variety,[6] "rhabdomyoma" for the striated muscle variant,[5, 13, 14] and "ectomesenchymal hamartoma" for mixed myoid-adipose lesions.[1, 12]

Other Schwann cell lesions are rarely encountered in the intracranial space. These include granular cell tumor[2, 3, 8] and neurothekeoma,[7] a lesion lacking specific features of nerve sheath differentiation.

## Benign Cystic Lesions

### Colloid Cyst

**Definition.** A benign, unilocular, mucin-containing epithelial cyst in the anterior third ventricle near the foramen of Monro.

**General Comments.** Colloid cysts have engendered speculation regarding their histogenesis. Ependyma, choroid plexus, neuroepithelium, paraphysis, and diencephalic remnants in the roof of the third ventricle have all been proffered as progenitors. Although it is natural to consider the lesion a variant of ependymal cyst, immunohistochemical and ultrastructural features speak convincingly for an endodermal derivation.[3, 5, 6, 9] Colloid cysts are, by this analysis, conjoined with enterogenous (see pages 92 to 93) and Rathke's cleft cysts (see pages 47 to 48).

**Clinical Features.** Wedged between the columns of the fornix and attached to the third ventricular roof and choroid plexus, the lesion is positioned precisely to impede CSF flow, although in some instances, the lesion is so slowly growing, if not stable, that CSF flow is not altered.[15] Chronic headaches are a common presenting complaint; sudden impaction, such as a ball valve phenomenon in the foramen of Monro, can produce abrupt "drop attacks" and even coma or death. Colloid cysts usually present in adults[11] and only rarely in children.[8]

**Radiologic Features.** Colloid cysts are imaged as spherical, well-circumscribed, nonenhancing discrete masses in the anterior third ventricle (Fig. 4–496). Although their signal characteristics vary, a central dark area of decreased signal intensity on T2-weighted images is apparent in some cases.[10]

**Macroscopic Features.** In situ, the tense, glistening cysts range in diameter from one to several centimeters and are filled with a viscid, murky substance (Figs. 4–497 and 4–498). The specimen presented to the pathologist is often only a wrinkled, gutted membrane with cautery effect.

**Microscopic Features.** The thin wall is formed of a delicate outer fibrous capsule and an inner lining of epithelium. The former consists of fibrous connective tissue of low cellularity; the latter is a simple layer of mucin-producing or ciliated epithelial cells that may be

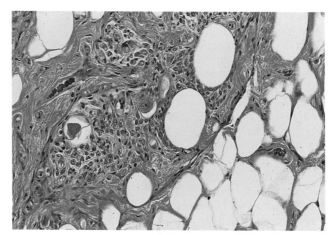

**FIGURE 4–495** LIPOMA OF THE EIGHTH CRANIAL NERVE

The lesion is a mixture of myelinated nerve fibers, ganglion cells, and adipose tissue (H&E–Luxol fast blue).

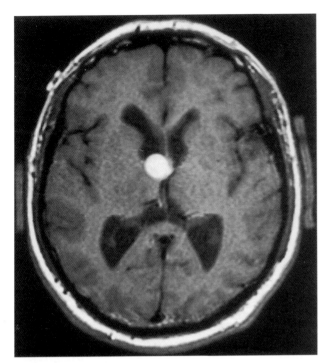

**FIGURE 4–496**   COLLOID CYST

As in this 56-year-old man with a 3-month history of headache, most colloid cysts are intrinsically bright in precontrast T1-weighted images.

pseudostratified (Figs. 4–499 and 4–500). Colloid cysts enlarge by the continuous discharge of intracellular, PAS-positive mucin, as well as by desquamation of cells that may be preserved as ghosts in the amorphous cyst contents. Some cysts contain eosinophilic filamentous masses that resemble colonies of *Actinomyces* (Fig. 4–501). Histochemical and ultrastructural studies have

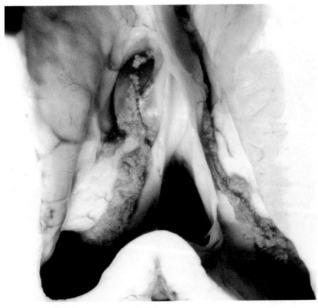

**FIGURE 4–497**   COLLOID CYST

The mechanical effects of the colloid cyst, as viewed from above, include elevation of the fornix, occlusion of the foramen of Monro, and deflection of the choroid plexus.

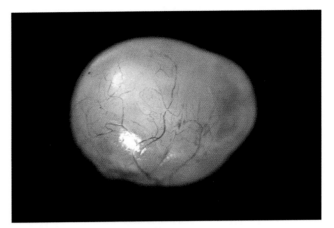

**FIGURE 4–498**   COLLOID CYST

Removed intact, a colloid cyst is discrete, translucent, and mucin filled. This lesion was removed from a 24-year-old man who presented emergently with a severe right-sided headache. He relayed an episode of "blacking out" 1 year earlier. At surgery, the lesion obstructed the right foramen of Monro. (Courtesy of Dr. Tarik Tihan, Baltimore, MD.)

excluded an infectious nature of these arresting structures and point instead to an origin from altered nucleoprotein and phospholipid.[16]

A xanthogranulomatous reaction occasionally supervenes in colloid cysts, largely replacing the epithelium in some cases. Other xanthomatous lesions in this anatomic region have no apparent epithelium. The nature of these lesions is not clear.[1, 13, 17]

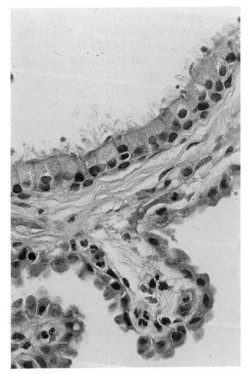

**FIGURE 4–499**   COLLOID CYST

Unless modified by compression atrophy or degenerative change, the cyst epithelium is well differentiated, ciliated, and often mucus producing. Given its anatomic location, fragments of choroid plexus frequently adhere to the cyst, as seen at the bottom of the illustration.

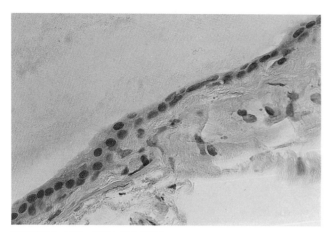

**FIGURE 4–500**    COLLOID CYST

An atrophic, simple epithelium without cilia is a frequent consequence of the lesion's intraluminal pressure.

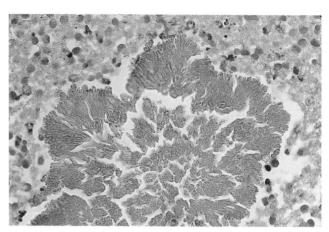

**FIGURE 4–501**    COLLOID CYST

Masses of degenerated nucleoprotein and phospholipid add interest to the cyst contents and should not be misinterpreted as infectious organisms.

**Immunohistochemical Features.** The cells are variably reactive for EMA and cytokeratins. Clara cell–specific antibodies can be used to detect the uncommon neuroendocrine cells.[6, 9]

**Ultrastructural Features.** Scanning and transmission electron microscopy disclose both nonciliated cells, some of which are mucus producing, and ciliated cells with a 9 + 2 microtubule configuration[3, 5, 7, 8] (Figs. 4–502 to 4–504). Cytoplasmic tonofilaments and well-formed desmosomes underscore the epithelial nature of the lesion. Least common are neuroendocrine cells with neurosecretory granules.[3, 5] Less differentiated, subepithelial basilar cells are also observed. It is claimed that the exterior of the cyst is covered focally by a thin layer of glia that is not appreciated readily by light microscopy.[5]

**Differential Diagnosis.** Few entities enter into the differential diagnosis. Out of context of the radiologic and operative findings, the possibility of *choroid plexus papilloma* may arise, because fragments of choroid plexus are often attached to the cyst (see Fig. 4–499). The plexus epithelium may even be the predominant tissue in the specimen. The epithelial cells of the choroid plexus are distinctively cobblestoned and lack both ciliation and mucin production.

Lesions similar to colloid cyst occur elsewhere in the ventricular system and, rarely, within the brain parenchyma, but there has been justified reluctance to include these under the designation "colloid cyst." Such generalization would diminish the individuality of the third ventricle cyst, with its characteristic location, and would detract from existing concepts about its

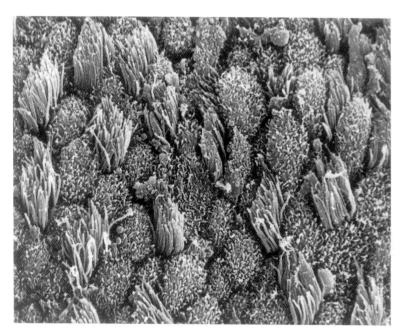

**FIGURE 4–502**    COLLOID CYST

Like tentacles of anemones, cilia wave to and fro in the cyst contents. Many of the cells are covered by microvilli rather than cilia. (Courtesy of Dr. Richard W. Leach, Oklahoma City, OK.)

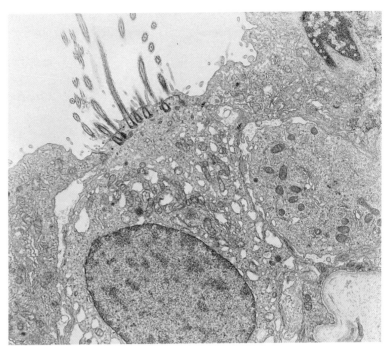

**4–503**

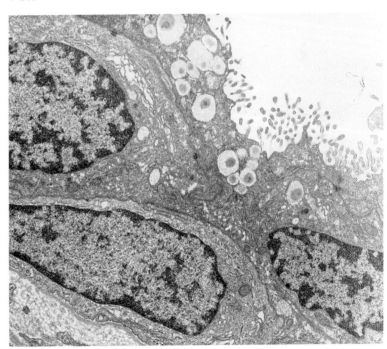

**FIGURES 4–503 AND 4–504**   COLLOID CYST

The two most distinctive cell types in the colloid cyst are
those that have cilia (Fig. 4–503) and those that secrete
mucus (Fig. 4–504).

**4–504**

histogenesis. *Ependymal cysts* and *choroid plexus cysts*
are discussed later.

Colloid cysts with advanced xanthogranulomatous
change must be distinguished from *craniopharyngiomas*
and the third ventricular or sellar *"xanthogranuloma"
without detectable epithelium* (see page 488)

**Treatment and Prognosis.** Extraction of the lesion
from the foramen of Monro restores CSF flow and
decompresses the ventricles. Although a craniotomy with

removal of the entire cyst has been the treatment of
choice, endoscopic removal is sometimes performed.[4]
Aspiration of the cyst is also possible, although this
leaves open the possibility that the lesion will re-form
and denies the pathologist the opportunity to study an
interesting lesion.[11, 12] Total excision is curative.[2, 11, 12]
Malignant degeneration has not been reported. Thus,
although surgery is generally recommended for symptomatic lesions, one study of adults noted that
in asymptomatic patients, the rate of symptomatic

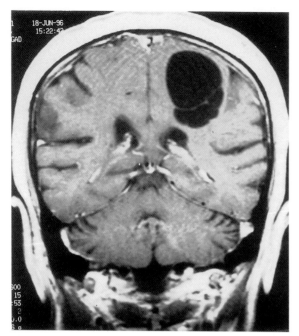

**FIGURE 4–505    EPENDYMAL CYST**

This large paraventricular cyst produced progressive right hemiparesis over a 1-year period in a 75-year-old woman.

progression was very low, and observation alone may be appropriate in some cases.[14]

### Ependymal Cyst

Variously termed "ependymal" or "glioependymal" cysts,[1–6] these fluid-filled spaces are lined by columnar, often ciliated epithelium (Figs. 4–505 and 4–506). They can lie within a ventricle[1, 6] or within the brain, where they directly abut the parenchyma with no more than a zone of intervening fibrillar glial tissue. There is no fibrous capsule. These cysts consist of ependyma, and

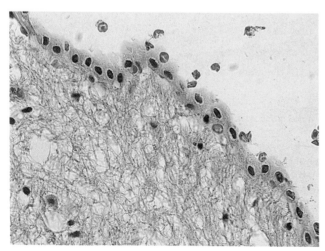

**FIGURE 4–506    EPENDYMAL CYST**

Ependymal cysts have a simple columnar or cuboidal lining.

their immunotype (S-100 protein and sometimes GFAP positive, and keratin negative) further distinguishes them from the endodermal ("enterogenous") cyst described on pages 92 to 93.

### Choroid Plexus Cyst

Cysts of the choroid plexus are rare and unlikely to appear as surgical specimens. A low cuboidal epithelium is expected.[1–4]

### Other Cysts

Because of their usual location in the leptomeninges, epidermoid and dermoid cysts, arachnoid cysts, and endodermal ("enterogenous") cysts are discussed in Chapter 2. Pineal cysts are considered on pages 296 to 298. The discussion of Rathke's cleft cysts can be found in Chapter 9, pages 484 to 485.

## METASTATIC NEOPLASMS

**General Comments.** Physicians are well acquainted with the propensity of blood-borne neoplastic cells to reach the brain, to lodge, to grow, and to kill. Surgical pathologists are regularly presented with specimens from (1) patients with unrecognized primary tumors, (2) patients with a history of systemic neoplasia but with findings that suggest a primary intracranial process, and (3) patients with CNS metastases in whom resection is expected to prolong life.

The most common tumors to metastasize to brain originate in the lung,[24, 52, 71] breast,[9, 52, 72] skin (malignant melanoma),[11, 13, 58, 61, 78] kidney,[55] and gastrointestinal tract. Their respective contributions to all CNS metastases are 35%, 20%, 10%, 10%, and 5%. Although rare, choriocarcinoma disseminates to the brain with a particularly high frequency.[3, 34] Renal cell carcinoma is curiously prone to late dissemination.[2, 56, 64] As a rule, tumors of the gastrointestinal tract show little affinity for the CNS. The rarity of metastases from such sites as bronchial carcinoid,[50] esophagus,[23] islet cells of the pancreas,[59] prostate,[21, 30, 41, 46, 68] ovary,[16, 66] thymus,[42] urinary bladder,[17, 74] and urachus[69] is sufficient to prompt case reports.

Although sarcomas of soft tissue and bone are infrequently encountered as brain metastases, their incidence may increase with prolongation of life by chemotherapy.[19, 25] Among others, metastases from alveolar soft part sarcoma,[8, 54, 60] chondrosarcoma,[25] cystosarcoma phyllodes,[32] Ewing's sarcoma[8, 80] fibrosarcoma,[14, 15, 62] hemangioendotheliosarcoma,[51] Kaposi's sarcoma,[26] leiomyosarcoma,[8, 10, 20, 25, 31, 60] liposarcoma,[40, 53] malignant cardiac myxoma,[70] malignant fibrous histiocytoma,[8, 45, 60] myxofibrosarcoma,[19] osteosarcoma,[5, 8, 19, 60] and rhabdomyosarcoma[19, 38, 65] have been recorded.

Whereas non-Hodgkin's lymphoma may undergo CNS spread, this is most unusual with Hodgkin's disease,[29, 35, 57] which is generally limited to the meninges.

**Clinical Features.** These expanding neoplasms, usually combined with marked peritumoral edema, produce headaches, seizures, motor deficits, and mental changes. Sudden expansion due to tumoral hemorrhage is prone to occur in melanoma, choriocarcinoma, and, as a consequence of its prevalence, carcinoma of the lung.[44, 52] Adenoid cystic carcinomas may undergo hematogenous CNS spread[36] but are more prone to track along divisions of the fifth cranial nerve to reach the cavernous sinus or the base of the brain (see Figs. 1–82 and 1–83).[1, 27] Understandably, pain is the most common symptom.

Patients with secondary malignant lymphomas may present with CNS symptoms at the time systemic involvement is recognized, during relapse, or during progression of the systemic disease.[57] Because the lesion is almost always meningeal, the diagnosis is typically established by CSF cytology.[29, 35, 57, 79]

**Radiologic Features.** As a rule, metastases are spherical, contrast-enhancing masses, sometimes with dark, necrotic centers (Fig. 4–507). The vast majority are situated in gray matter, usually near the gray-white junction. Thus, masses in deep white matter or the corpus callosum are unlikely to be metastases. In the absence of prior steroid treatment, there is often a sizable corona of peritumoral edema. It, and the symptoms it produces, can respond dramatically to steroids. Calcification is a very uncommon feature of metastasis.[33, 67] Highly pigmented, nonhemorrhagic melanomas can be recognized by their characteristic hyperintensity or whiteness on nonenhanced T1-weighted MRI scans, as well as by

their iso- or hypointensity relative to cerebral cortex on T2-weighted images.[4] Conversely, some adenocarcinomas are hypointense and dark on T2-weighted images.[12]

Unusual metastases diffusely colonize the subependymal region,[73] target the choroid plexus[39] or the pineal gland,[75] or, in the setting of meningeal disease, diffusely involve the brain without creating a defined mass.[43, 63] A collision between metastatic carcinoma and glioblastoma is a rarity.[22]

Metastatic neoplasms adhere to certain basic principles when they involve the brain: (1) the lesions almost always occupy gray matter, with an epicenter often near the gray-white junction; (2) the brain supplied by the middle cerebral artery is preferentially involved; (3) there is overrepresentation of metastases in arterial border zones, particularly in the parietal lobes at the confluence of the middle, anterior, and posterior cerebral arteries[18]; (4) there appears to be a heightened incidence of involvement of the posterior fossa in metastases from the gastrointestinal tract, bladder, and uterus[18, 37, 52]; (5) the brain stem is only rarely involved[30, 76]; and (6) metastases from primary lesions showing a predilection for brain, such as melanoma, are usually multiple, whereas those from such primary sites as the kidney and gastrointestinal tract are more often solitary.[52] Although most metastases are intraparenchymal, diffuse subependymal involvement has been reported.[73]

**Macroscopic Features.** The discrete nature of most metastases is accentuated by the firmness of the lesion

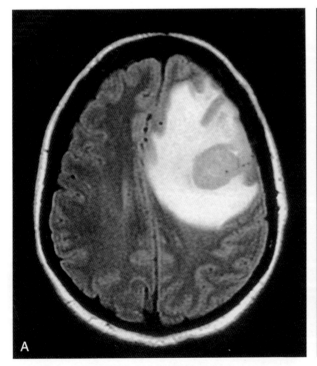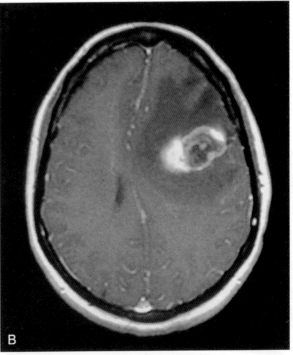

**FIGURE 4–507    METASTATIC CARCINOMA**

A contrast-enhancing solid or ring-like lesion with abundant edema is typical of metastases. This lesion is shown in fluid-attenuated inversion recovery (FLAIR) (A) and contrast-enhanced T1-weighted (B) images. The patient, a 42-year-old woman with a history of breast cancer, presented with a 1-week history of severe headache.

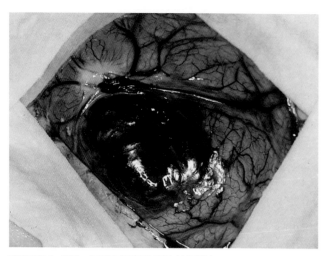

**FIGURE 4–508**    METASTATIC MELANOMA

Metastases are discrete and often superficial. This black lesion had its origin in the choroid of the eye. (Courtesy of Dr. Henry Brem, Baltimore, MD.)

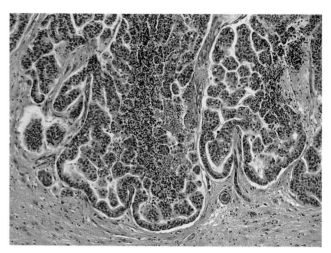

**FIGURE 4–510**    METASTATIC CARCINOMA

This moderately differentiated adenocarcinoma exhibits the typical pushing, rather than infiltrating, border of most metastatic neoplasms.

and the softness of the surrounding edematous brain (Figs. 4–508 and 4–509). Individually, the neoplastic cells are soft and, when sufficiently aggregated, produce a fleshy mass. The tumor is often firm due to the ingrowth of fibrous tissue, but it may be focally softened by necrosis, mucus production, or hemorrhage. The last is often a prominent feature of melanoma and choriocarcinoma. Melanin deposition lends a smoky gray or black coloration (see Fig. 4–508).

**Microscopic Features.** Metastases are noted for their discrete nature, fibrous tissue septa, and frequent perivascular lymphocytic infiltrates (Figs. 4–510 and 4–511). The generality of discreteness is occasionally violated by small cell carcinomas of the lung, melanomas (Fig. 4–512), and lymphomas, all of which may be diffusely infiltrative. Extensive perivascular infiltrates characterize the "encephalitic form" associated with

leptomeningeal tumor infiltrates.[43, 63] Necrosis, often prominent, is notable in many cases for its abrupt interface with viable tissue, often along a border that is isometric from the blood vessels (Fig. 4–513).

Carcinoma of the lung may be squamous, glandular, or undifferentiated; the large cell variant of the last type is the most common (Fig. 4–514). The lung is the most common source of adenocarcinoma presenting with a known primary lesion.[49] Metastatic carcinoma of the breast often mimics the parent lesion by reproduction of small ducts, cord, nest, and even cellular columns (Fig. 4–515). Adenocarcinoma of the gastrointestinal tract usually exhibits the features of intestinal epithelium (Fig. 4–516). Metastatic carcinoma of the kidney is typified by an abundance of clear cytoplasm and uniform, round nuclei with prominent nucleoli (Fig. 4–517). The cells are disposed in sheets, papillae, tubules, and lobules. Microvascular proliferation may be

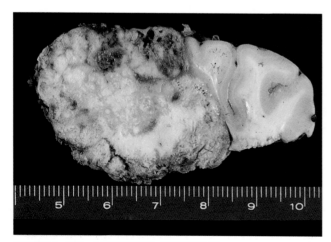

**FIGURE 4–509**    METASTATIC CARCINOMA

Metastases are often fleshy, largely necrotic, and discrete.

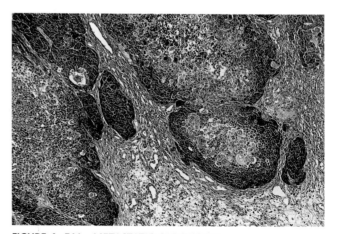

**FIGURE 4–511**    METASTATIC CARCINOMA

As seen here in a Masson trichrome–stained section, connective tissue septa often separate lobules of tumor cells.

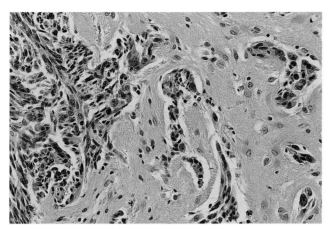

**FIGURE 4–512    METASTATIC MELANOMA**

As in this melanoma, some metastases extend along vessels, producing a lesion that is more infiltrative than a typical carcinoma metastasis.

prominent. The lobular pattern most closely resembles hemangioblastoma.

The unpredictable histologic variability of melanoma prompts one to always consider it when confronted by an undifferentiated, amelanotic lesion. The spectrum extends from round cells with generous cytoplasm to fasciculated, spindle forms (Figs. 4–518 and 4–519). Melanin may dust or distend neoplastic cells, or it may be concentrated within macrophages (melanophages). Melanin must be distinguished from hemosiderin, an easy histochemical distinction. Melanomas are often hemorrhagic, and the neoplasm may be difficult to find (Figs. 4–520 and 4–521).

**Features in Frozen Sections.** Anaplasia, connective tissue septa, and necrosis are usually apparent. Tissue taken from the edge of the lesion has added value because it commonly shows the sharp demarcation of a metastasis from brain parenchyma (Fig. 4–522).

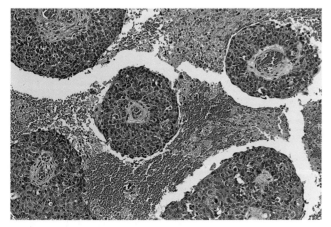

**FIGURE 4–513    METASTATIC CARCINOMA**

A uniform cuff of viable tumor surrounding vessels is a common feature of metastases.

**Cytologic Features.** Non–small cell metastases are known for cells with discrete cell borders and large, round nuclei (Fig. 4–523). Nucleoli are often prominent in adenocarcinomas and melanomas.

**Immunohistochemical Features.** Most metastatic carcinomas are reactive for cytokeratins (Figs. 4–524 and 4–525) and EMA. Antibodies to thyroid transcription factor 1 can be useful in identifying metastatic lung cancer, as is discussed in the section on differential diagnosis (Fig. 4–526). Melanomas are positive for S-100 protein, HMB-45, Melan-A (Fig. 4–527), and tyrosine hydroxylase. A subset is reportedly cytokeratin positive.[6, 48, 81] Antibodies to such tissue-specific antibodies as thyroglobulin (Figs. 4–528 and 4–529), prostate-specific antigen, and calcitonin can be used to identify uncommon metastases from these organs. Polyclonal carcinoembryonic antigen can be used to identify the canaliculi in hepatocellular carcinoma (Figs. 4–530 and 4–531). HepPar antibodies can also be used to identify metastases from a primary liver tumor.[77] The use of antibodies BEREP4 and HEA 125 to distinguish choroid plexus carcinoma and metastatic carcinoma is discussed in the section on differential diagnosis.

**Ultrastructural Features.** Squamous cell lesions are identified by their prominent desmosomes with attached tonofilaments; adenocarcinomas are recognized by their inter- or intracellular acini containing microvilli bounded by junctional complexes.[49]

**Differential Diagnosis.** The differential diagnosis of a metastatic lesion must always include the possibility of malignant glioma, PCNSL, and, in the cerebellum, hemangioblastoma and medulloblastoma.

*Anaplastic oligodendroglioma* may be macroscopically discrete and composed of compactly arranged polygonal cells that may superficially simulate carcinoma. This glioma is identified by monotony, halos, calcification, parenchymal infiltration, general absence of collagen, a distinctive "chicken wire" vasculature, and, in some instances, microvascular hypertrophy or hyperplasia. In addition, most anaplastic oligodendrogliomas contain GFAP-positive cells. In metastatic neoplasms, particularly renal cell carcinoma or melanoma, a spindle cell composition may simulate a high-grade glioma.

As a rule, certain features aid in the distinction between secondary and primary neoplasms of the CNS. Metastases retain a cohesive quality as they enlarge and thus remain demarcated from the host tissue. This feature contrasts with the infiltrative nature of most *glioblastomas* and malignant oligodendrogliomas, both of which show at least some intermingling of neoplastic cells with brain parenchyma. This underscores the value of sampling the margins of a lesion at the time of frozen section.

The neoplastic cells of metastatic carcinoma reveal their epithelial nature by their round or polygonal shape, distinct cellular borders, and lack of processes. Although the amount of fibrous tissue is variable in metastatic lesions, it generally exceeds that in most gliomas. The rapid growth of metastatic cancers produces demands

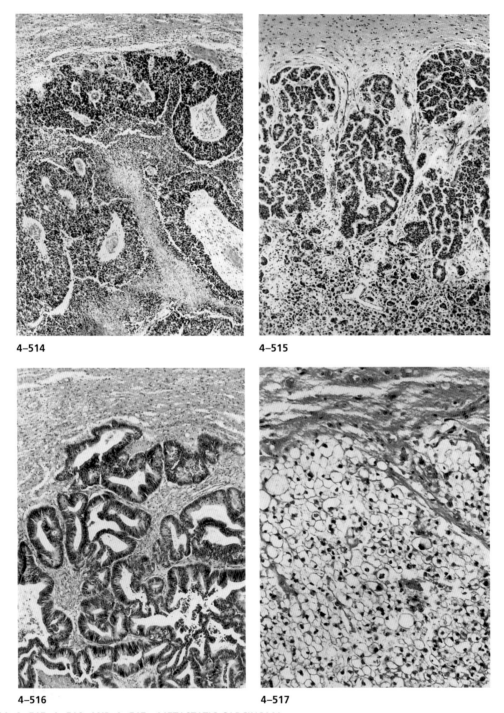

4–514

4–515

4–516

4–517

**FIGURES 4–514, 4–515, 4–516, AND 4–517**    METASTATIC CARCINOMA

These four lesions demonstrate the infiltrative yet discrete character of carcinoma metastatic to brain tissue. Each faithfully recapitulated the appearance of its primary lesion in lung (Fig. 4–514), breast (Fig. 4–515), colon (Fig. 4–516), and kidney (Fig. 4–517).

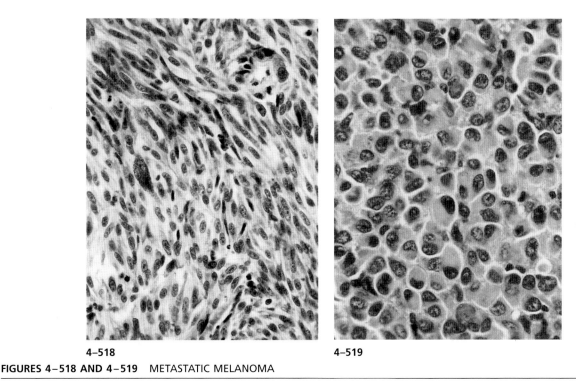

**4–518**    **4–519**

**FIGURES 4–518 AND 4–519**    METASTATIC MELANOMA

The chameleon-like nature of malignant melanoma is depicted in these two illustrations. One lesion consists of polyhedral and round cells (Fig. 4–518), and the other consists of cells that are spindle shaped (Fig. 4–519).

for sustenance that the vasculature cannot provide. Gradations of ischemia cause necrosis at a distance from the vessels, permitting only cuffs of viable cells to remain (see Fig. 4–513). Necrosis in *glioblastomas* is more random in distribution, more serpentine in configuration, more inclusive of vascular walls, and accentuated by peripheral pseudopalisading. Table 4–6, p. 188 summarizes the features of necrosis in CNS lesions.

Vascular proliferation may be encountered in metastatic carcinomas, particularly renal cell lesions, but

is usually restricted to the immediate environs of the tumor and rarely attains the degree of microvascular exuberance present in glioblastomas. Among *glioblastomas*, the small cell, "epithelioid," and "adenoid" variants most closely mimic undifferentiated carcinoma. Conversely, degenerative changes in a metastasis may simulate glioblastoma.

Histologically, *primary cerebral lymphoma*, particularly the common large cell form, can mimic metastatic carcinoma, but it is generally an anatomic or radiologic

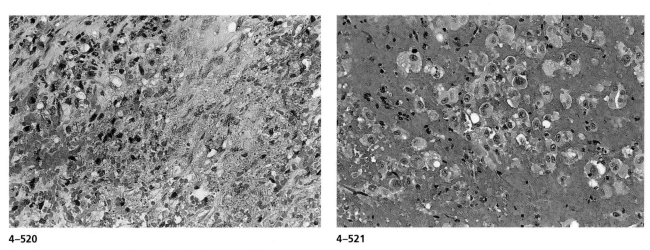

**4–520**    **4–521**

**FIGURES 4–520 AND 4–521**    METASTATIC MELANOMA

Extensive recent and old hemorrhage is a common feature of metastatic melanoma (Fig. 4–520). Neoplastic cells were only focally encountered within the hemorrhage (Fig. 4–521).

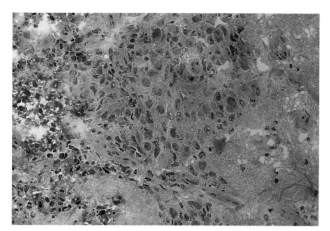

**FIGURE 4–522    METASTATIC CARCINOMA—FROZEN SECTION**

Given cytologic variation, the metastatic nature of some neoplasms may be difficult to establish at frozen section. However, their sharp borders with surrounding brain bring this diagnosis to the fore. Large nuclei with prominent nucleoli are also typical of metastases.

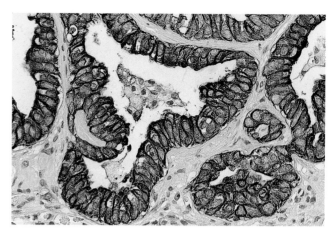

**FIGURE 4–524    METASTATIC CARCINOMA FROM THE LUNG**

Immunoreactivity for cytokeratins (AE1/AE3) is expected in such an overtly epithelial neoplasm as this adenocarcinoma.

misfit, because it mainly affects white matter, often in the periventricular region or corpus callosum. The characteristic infiltration of reticulin in vessel walls, with its target-like deposition, also distinguishes lymphomas from epithelial neoplasms. Immunopositivity for B- and rarely T-cell markers, as well as monotypism for immunoglobulin light and heavy chains, is a defining feature of lymphoma.

Aside from rare cases of *anaplastic large cell lymphoma* reactive for EMA, lack of epithelial markers aids the distinction from carcinoma.

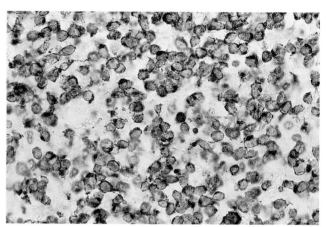

**FIGURE 4–525    METASTATIC SMALL CELL CARCINOMA FROM THE LUNG**

Immunoreactivity for cytokeratins (AE1/AE3) establishes the epithelial nature of this otherwise undifferentiated lesion.

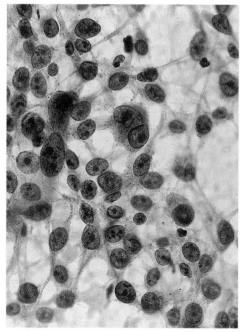

**FIGURE 4–523    METASTATIC MELANOMA—SMEAR PREPARATION**

Cells of most metastatic neoplasms are known for their sharply defined cell borders and large, round nuclei. Prominence of nucleoli is particularly noticeable in melanomas.

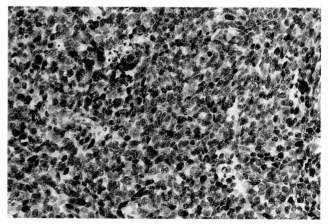

**FIGURE 4–526    METASTATIC SMALL CELL CARCINOMA FROM THE LUNG**

Nuclear staining for thyroid transcription factor-1 is present in a high percentage of pulmonary carcinomas.

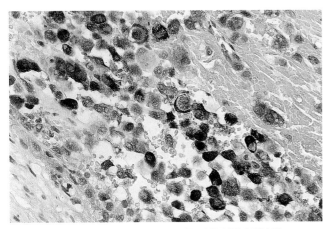

**FIGURE 4–527   METASTATIC MALIGNANT MELANOMA**

Most melanomas are immunoreactive for Melan A, as is the same neoplasm illustrated here and in Figure 4–521.

In the cerebellum, small cell carcinomas can be difficult to distinguish from *medulloblastoma*. At the H&E level, clues to the diagnosis include considerable necrosis and DNA impregnation of vessels (Azzopardi's phenomenon). Although small cell carcinomas can be synaptophysin immunopositive, clear-cut paranuclear staining for cytokeratins and surface reactivity for EMA simplify the problem, although one study noted a small percentage of medulloblastomas that were EMA or cytokeratin positive.[47] The same report recorded the presence of thyroid transcription factor 1 in a high percentage of metastatic lung cancers but in none of the medulloblastomas (see Fig. 4–526). A few cases are ambiguous and cannot be assigned clearly to either category. Even in the face of a negative CT or MRI scan of the chest, small cell carcinoma cannot be excluded in all cases.

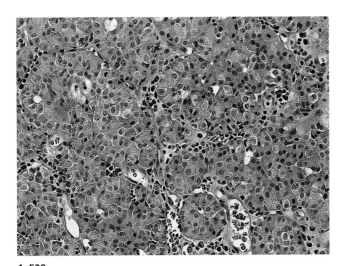

4–528

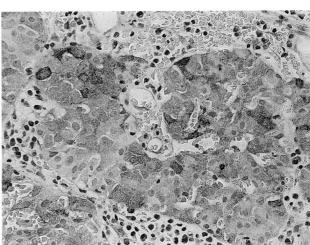

4–529

**FIGURES 4–528 AND 4–529   METASTATIC CARCINOMA FROM THE THYROID**

Immunohistochemistry is useful in defining the origin of unusual lesions such as this thyroid carcinoma immunopositive for thyroglobulin. A subsequent thyroidectomy confirmed the diagnosis.

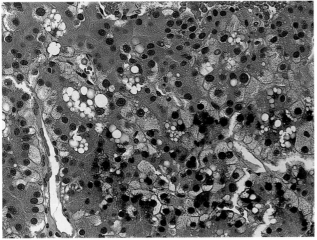

4–530

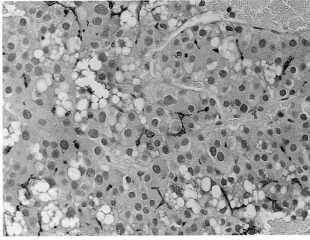

4–531

**FIGURES 4–530 AND 4–531   METASTATIC HEPATOCELLULAR CARCINOMA**

Polyclonal antibodies to carcinoembryonic antigen stain the intercellular canaliculi.

The differential of metastatic clear cell carcinoma versus *hemangioblastoma*, based largely on the reaction for EMA, is discussed on page 334.

Metastatic papillary adenocarcinoma may need to be distinguished from *choroid plexus carcinoma*, although the latter usually occurs in the first few years of life. Choroid plexus tumors are unlikely to have the strong staining for EMA seen in metastatic lesions. Staining for BEREP4 and HEA 125 can be used, because they stain almost all metastatic carcinomas and only a small minority of choroid plexus tumors.[28]

**Treatment and Prognosis.** The postsurgical treatment of patients with metastatic disease involves radiotherapy and, in some cases, chemotherapy. The duration of survival has been variously cited and obviously depends on such factors as type, site, and number of intracranial metastases; extent of the primary disease; and the presence or absence of other systemic metastases. Most patients with metastatic carcinoma or melanoma,[7, 52] as well as sarcoma,[8] survive less than 1 year.

# REFERENCES

### Diffuse Astrocytoma, Anaplastic Astrocytoma, and Glioblastoma Multiforme

1. Agosti RM, Leuthold M, Gullick WJ, et al. Expression of the epidermal growth factor receptor in astrocytic tumours is specifically associated with glioblastoma multiforme. Virchows Arch A Pathol Anat Histopathol 1992;420:321–325.
2. Albers GW, Hoyt WF, Forno LS, Shratter LA. Treatment response in malignant optic glioma of adulthood. Neurology 1988;38:1071–1074.
3. Albert FK, Forsting M, Sartor K, et al. Early postoperative magnetic resonance imaging after resection of malignant glioma: objective evaluation of residual tumor and its influence on regrowth and prognosis. Neurosurgery 1994;34:45–61.
4. Aldape K, Simmons ML, Takahashi M, et al. EGFR overexpression is prognostic in a subset of patients with glioblastoma defined by age and p53 status. J Neuropathol Exp Neurol 2000; 59:422.
5. Barnard RO, Geddes JF. The incidence of multifocal cerebral gliomas: a histologic study of large hemisphere sections. Cancer 1987;60:1519–1531.
6. Berger MS, Deliganis AV, Dobbins J, Keles GE. The effect of extent of resection on recurrence in patients with low grade cerebral hemisphere gliomas. Cancer 1994;74:1784–1791.
7. Biernat W, Tohma Y, Yonekawa Y, et al. Alterations of cell cycle regulatory genes in primary (de novo) and secondary glioblastomas. Acta Neuropathol (Berl) 1997;94:303–309.
8. Biernat W, Kleihues P, Yonekawa Y, Ohgaki H. Amplification and overexpression of MDM2 in primary (de novo) glioblastomas. J Neuropathol Exp Neurol 1997;56:180–185.
9. Bowers DC, Georgiades C, Aronson LJ, et al. Tectal gliomas: natural history of an indolent lesion in pediatric patients. Pediatr Neurosurg 2000;32:24–29.
10. Brat DJ, James CD, Jedlicka AE, et al. Molecular genetic alterations in radiation-induced astrocytomas. Am J Pathol 1999; 154:1431–1438.
11. Brat DJ, PC B. Cerebral pilocytic astrocytoma: distinction from infiltrating fibrillary astrocytomas. Pathol Case Rev 1998;3:290–295.
12. Brooks WH, Marksbery WR, Gupta GD, Roszman TL. Relationship of lymphocyte invasion and survival of brain tumor patients. Ann Neurol 1978;4:219–224.
13. Burger P, Pearl D, Aldape K, et al. Small cell architecture—a histological equivalent of EGFR amplification in glioblastoma multiforme? J Neuropathol Exp Neurol, 2001;60:1099–1104.
14. Burger PC. Pathology of brain stem astrocytomas. Pediatr Neurosurg 1996;24:35–40.
15. Burger PC, Cohen KJ, Rosenblum MK, Tihan T. Pathology of diencephalic astrocytomas. Pediatr Neurosurg 2000;32:214–219.
16. Burger PC, Dubois PJ, Schold SC, et al. Computerized tomographic and pathologic studies of the untreated, quiescent, and recurrent glioblastoma multiforme. J Neurosurg 1983;58:159–169.
17. Burger PC, Heinz ER, Shibata T, Kleihues P. Topographic anatomy and CT correlations in the untreated glioblastoma multiforme. J Neurosurg 1988;68:698–704.
18. Burger PC, Kleihues P. Cytologic composition of the untreated glioblastoma with implications for evaluation of needle biopsies. Cancer 1989;63:2014–2023.
19. Burger PC, Mahaley MS Jr, Dudka L, Vogel FS. The morphologic effects of radiation administered therapeutically for intracranial gliomas: a postmortem study of 25 cases. Cancer 1979;44:1256–1272.
20. Burger PC, Vogel FS, Green SB, Strike TA. Glioblastoma multiforme and anaplastic astrocytoma: pathologic criteria and prognostic implications. Cancer 1985;56:1106–1111.
21. Burger PC, Vollmer RT. Histologic factors of prognostic significance in the glioblastoma multiforme. Cancer 1980;46:1179–1186.
22. Campbell JW, Pollack IF, Martinez AJ, Schultz B. High-grade astrocytomas in children: radiologically complete resection is associated with an excellent long-term prognosis. Neurosurgery 1996;38:258–264.
23. Chamberlain MC, Silver P, Levin VA. Poorly differentiated gliomas of the cerebellum: a study of 18 patients. Cancer 1990;65:337–340.
24. Chan AS, Leung SY, Wong MP, et al. Expression of vascular endothelial growth factor and its receptors in the anaplastic progression of astrocytoma, oligodendroglioma, and ependymoma. Am J Surg Pathol 1998;22:816–826.
25. Chandler KL, Prados MD, Malec M, Wilson CB. Long-term survival in patients with glioblastoma multiforme. Neurosurgery 1993;32:716–720.
26. Chang S, Prados MD. Identical twins with Ollier's disease and intracranial gliomas: case report. Neurosurgery 1994;34:903–906.
27. Cheng Y, Ng HK, Zhang SF, et al. Genetic alterations in pediatric high-grade astrocytomas. Hum Pathol 1999;30:1284–1290.
28. Coons SW, Johnson PC. Regional heterogeneity in the proliferation activity of human gliomas as measured by the Ki-67 labeling index. J Neuropathol Exp Neurol 1993;52:609–618.
29. Coons SW, Pearl DK. Mitosis identification in diffuse gliomas: implications for tumor grading. Cancer 1998;82:1550–1555.
30. Cosgrove M, Fitzgibbons PL, Sherrod A, et al. Intermediate filament expression in astrocytic neoplasms. Am J Surg Pathol 1989;13:141–145.
31. Daumas-Duport C, Scheithauer BW, Kelly PJ. A histologic and cytologic method for the spatial definition of gliomas. Mayo Clin Proc 1987;62:435–449.
32. Daumas-Duport C, Scheithauer BW, O'Fallon J, Kelly P. Grading of astrocytomas: a simple and reproducible method. Cancer 1988;62:2152–2165.
33. Dropcho EJ, Soong S-J. The prognostic impact of prior low grade histology in patients with anaplastic gliomas: a case-control study. Neurology 1996;47:684–690.
34. Fisher PG, Breiter SN, Carson BS, et al. A clinicopathologic reappraisal of brain stem tumor classification: identification of pilocytic astrocytoma and fibrillary astrocytoma as distinct entities. Cancer 2000;89:1569–1576.
35. Forsting M, Albert FK, Kunze S, et al. Extirpation of glioblastomas: MR and CT follow-up of residual tumor and regrowth patterns. AJNR 1993;14:77–87.
36. Frappaz D, Ricci AC, Kohler R, et al. Diffuse brain stem tumor in an adolescent with multiple enchondromatosis (Ollier's disease). Childs Nerv Syst 1999;15:222–225.
37. Frederick L, Wang XY, Eley G, James CD. Diversity and frequency of epidermal growth factor receptor mutations in human glioblastomas. Cancer Res 2000;60:1383–1387.
38. Fujisawa H, Reis RM, Nakamura M, et al. Loss of heterozygosity on chromosome 10 is more extensive in primary (de novo) than in secondary glioblastomas. Lab Invest 2000;80:65–72.
39. Gajjar A, Sanford RA, Heideman R, et al. Low-grade astrocytoma: a decade of experience at St. Jude Children's Research Hospital. J Clin Oncol 1997;15:2792–2799.

40. Gamis AS, Egelhoff J, Roloson G, et al. Diffuse bony metastases at presentation in a child with glioblastoma multiforme: a case report. Cancer 1990;66:180–184.

41. Giangaspero F, Burger PC. Correlations between cytologic composition and biologic behavior in the glioblastoma multiforme: a postmortem study of 50 cases. Cancer 1983;52:2320–2333.

42. Giannini C, Scheithauer BW, Burger PC, et al. Cellular proliferation in pilocytic and diffuse astrocytomas. J Neuropathol Exp Neurol 1999;58:46–53.

43. Grabb PA, Albright AL, Pang D. Dissemination of supratentorial malignant gliomas via the cerebrospinal fluid in children. Neurosurgery 1992;30:64–71.

44. Haddad SF, Moore SA, Schelper RL, Goeken JA. Vascular smooth muscle hyperplasia underlies the formation of glomeruloid vascular structures of glioblastoma multiforme. J Neuropathol Exp Neurol 1992;51:488–492.

45. Hamilton SR, Liu B, Parsons RE, et al. The molecular basis of Turcot's syndrome. N Engl J Med 1995;332:839–847.

46. Hayashi Y, Ueki K, Waha A, et al. Association of EGFR gene amplification and CDKN2 (p16/MTS1) gene deletion in glioblastoma multiforme. Brain Pathol 1997;7:871–875.

47. Hayostek CJ, Shaw EG, Scheithauer BW, et al. Astrocytomas of the cerebellum. Cancer 1993;72:856–869.

48. Heros DO, Renkens K, Kasdon DL, Adelman LS. Patterns of recurrence in glioma patients after interstitial irradiation and chemotherapy: report of three cases. Neurosurgery 1988;22: 474–478.

49. Hofman S, Heeg M, Klein JP, Krikke AP. Simultaneous occurrence of a supra- and an infratentorial glioma in a patient with Ollier's disease: more evidence for non-mesodermal tumor predisposition in multiple enchondromatosis. Skeletal Radiol 1998;27:688–691.

50. Horiuchi T, Osawa M, Itoh N, et al. Extradural extension of glioblastoma multiforme into the oral cavity: case report. Surg Neurol 1996;46:42–46.

51. Hoyt WF, Meshel LG, Lessell S, et al. Malignant optic glioma of adulthood. Brain 1973;96:121–132.

52. Hsu DW, Louis DN, Efird JT, Hedley-Whyte T. Use of MIB-1 (Ki-67) immunoreactivity in differentiating grade II and grade III gliomas. J Neuropathol Exp Neurol 1997;56:857–865.

53. Huang MC, Kubo O, Tajika Y, Takakura K. A clinico-immunohistochemical study of giant cell glioblastoma. Noshuyo Byori 1996;13:11–16.

54. Ino Y, Zlatescu MC, Sasaki H, et al. Long survival and therapeutic responses in patients with histologically disparate high-grade gliomas demonstrating 1p loss. J Neurosurg 2000; 92:983–990.

55. Johnson PC, Drazkowski JF, Rossman KL, Coons SW. Cause of death in glioblastoma multiforme. J Neuropathol Exp Neurol 1993;52:289.

56. Keles GE, Anderson B, Berger MS. The effect of extent of resection on time to tumor progression and survival in patients with glioblastoma multiforme of the cerebral hemisphere. Surg Neurol 1999;52:371–379.

57. Kepes JJ, Fulling KH, Garcia JH. The clinical significance of "adenoid" formations of neoplastic astrocytes, imitating metastatic carcinoma, in gliosarcomas: a review of five cases. Clin Neuropathol 1982;1:139–150.

58. Kepes JJ, Rubinstein LJ, Chiang H. The role of astrocytes in the formation of cartilage in gliomas: an immunohistochemical study of four cases. Am J Pathol 1984;117:471–483.

59. Kim TS, Halliday AL, Hedley-Whyte T, Convery K. Correlates of survival and the Daumas-Duport grading system for astrocytomas. J Neurosurg 1991;74:27–37.

60. Kleihues P, Ohgaki H. Primary and secondary glioblastomas: from concept to clinical diagnosis. Neuro-Oncology 1999;1:44–51.

61. Kleihues P, Cavenee WK (eds). World Health Organization Classification of Tumours: Pathology and Genetics of Tumours of the Nervous System. Lyon, France: IARC Press, 2000.

62. Klein R, Molenkamp G, Sorensen N, Roggendorf W. Favorable outcome of giant cell glioblastoma in a child: report of an 11-year survival period. Childs Nerv Syst 1998;14:288–291.

63. Kosel S, Scheithauer BW, Graeber MB. Genotype-phenotype correlation in gemistocytic astrocytomas. Neurosurgery 2001;48:187–193; discussion 93–94.

64. Kros JM, Stefanko SZ, de Jong AAW, et al. Ultrastructural and immunohistochemical segregation of gemistocytic subsets. Hum Pathol 1991;22:33–40.

65. Krouwer HGJ, Prados MD. Infiltrative astrocytomas of the thalamus. J Neurosurg 1995;82:548–557.

66. Kulkarni AV, Becker LE, Jay V, et al. Primary cerebellar glioblastomas multiforme in children: report of four cases. J Neurosurg 1999;90:546–550.

67. Kuroiwa T, Numaguchi Y, Rothman MI, et al. Posterior fossa glioblastoma multiforme: MR findings. AJNR 1995;16:583–589.

68. Kyritsis AP, Bondy ML, Xiao M, et al. Germline p53 gene mutations in subsets of glioma patients. J Natl Cancer Inst 1994; 86:344–349.

69. Kyritsis AP, Levin VA, Yung WKA, Leeds NE. Imaging patterns of multifocal gliomas. Eur J Radiol 1993;16:163–170.

70. Lampl Y, Eshel Y, Gilad R, Sarova-Pinchas I. Glioblastoma multiforme with bone metastases and cauda equina syndrome. J Neurooncol 1990;8:167–172.

71. Landolfi JC, Thaler HT, DeAngelis LM. Adult brainstem gliomas. Neurology 1998;51:1136–1139.

72. Lang FF, Miller DC, Koslow M, Newcomb EW. Pathways leading to glioblastoma multiforme: a molecular analysis of genetic alterations in 65 astrocytic tumors. J Neurosurg 1994;81:427–436.

73. Leighton C, Fisher B, Bauman G, et al. Supratentorial low-grade glioma in adults: an analysis of prognostic factors and timing of radiation. J Clin Oncol 1997;15:1294–1301.

74. Levine SA, McKeever PE, Greenberg HS. Primary cerebellar glioblastoma multiforme. J Neurooncol 1987;5:231–236.

75. Louis DN, Rubio MP, Correa KM, et al. Molecular genetics of pediatric brain stem gliomas: application of PCR techniques to small and archival brain tumor specimens. J Neuropathol Exp Neurol 1993;52:507–515.

76. Lynch HT, McComb RD, Osborn NK, et al. Predominance of brain tumors in an extended Li-Fraumeni (SBLA) kindred, including a case of Sturge-Weber syndrome. Cancer 2000;88: 433–439.

77. Margetts JC, Kalyan-Raman UP. Giant-celled glioblastoma of brain: a clinico-pathological and radiological study of ten cases (including immunohistochemistry and ultrastructure). Cancer 1989;63:524–531.

78. Mattson RH, Peterson EW. Glioblastoma multiforme of the optic nerve: report of a case. JAMA 1966;196:119–120.

79. McCormack BM, Miller DC, Budzilovich GN, et al. Treatment and survival of low-grade astrocytoma in adults—1977–1988. Neurosurgery 1992;31:636–642.

80. McKeever PE, Strawderman MS, Yamini B, et al. MIB-1 proliferation index predicts survival among patients with grade II astrocytoma. J Neuropathol Exp Neurol 1998;57:931–936.

81. Mellon CD, Carter JE, Owen DB. Ollier's disease and Maffucci's syndrome: distinct entities or a continuum. Case report: enchondromatosis complicated by an intracranial glioma. J Neurol 1988; 235:376–378.

82. Meyer-Puttlitz B, Hayashi Y, Waha A, et al. Molecular genetic analysis of giant cell glioblastomas. Am J Pathol 1997;151: 853–857.

83. Millar WS, Tartaglino LM, Sergott RC, et al. MR of malignant optic glioma of adulthood. AJNR 1995;16:1673–1676.

84. Montine TJ, Vandersteenhoven JJ, Aguzzi A, et al. Prognostic significance of Ki-67 proliferation index in supratentorial fibrillary astrocytic neoplasms. Neurosurgery 1994;34:674–679.

85. Morita M, Rosenblum MK, Bilsky MH, et al. Long term survivors of glioblastoma multiforme: clinical and molecular characteristics. J Neurooncol 1996;27:259–266.

86. Mørk SJ, Rubinstein LJ, Kepes JJ. Patterns of epithelial metaplasia in malignant gliomas. I. Papillary formations mimicking medulloepithelioma. J Neuropathol Exp Neurol 1988;47:93–100.

87. Mørk SJ, Rubinstein LJ, Kepes JJ, et al. Patterns of epithelial metaplasia in malignant gliomas. II. Squamous differentiation of epithelial-like formations in gliosarcomas and glioblastomas. J Neuropathol Exp Neurol 1988;47:101–118.

88. Moulignier A, Mikol J, Pialoux G, et al. Cerebral glial tumors and human immunodeficiency virus-1 infection: more than a coincidental association. Cancer 1994;74:686–692.

89. Müller MB, Schmidt MC, Schmidt O, et al. Molecular genetic analysis as a tool for evaluating stereotactic biopsies of glioma specimens. J Neuropathol Exp Neurol 1999;58:40–45.

90. Myers T, Egelhoff J, Myers M. Glioblastoma multiforme presenting as osteoblastic metastatic disease: case report and review of the literature. AJNR 1990;11:802–803.

91. Nakamura M, Yang F, Fujisawa H, et al. Loss of heterozygosity on chromosome 19 in secondary glioblastomas. J Neuropathol Exp Neurol 2000;59:539–543.

92. Newcomb EW, Cohen H, Lee SR, et al. Survival of patients with glioblastoma multiforme is not influenced by altered expression of p16, p53, EGFR, MDM2 or Bcl-2 genes. Brain Pathol 1998;8:655–667.

93. Newton HB, Rosenblum MK, Walker RW. Extraneural metastases of infratentorial glioblastoma multiforme to the peritoneal cavity. Cancer 1992;69:2149–2153.

94. Ng HK, Lo STH. Cytokeratin immunoreactivity in gliomas. Histopathology 1989;14:359–368.

95. Nicolato A, Gerosa MA, Fina P, et al. Prognostic factors in low-grade supratentorial astrocytomas: a uni-multivariate statistical analysis in 76 surgically treated adult patients. Surg Neurol 1995; 44:208–223.

96. Nishizaki T, Ozaki S, Harada K, et al. Investigation of genetic alterations associated with the grade of astrocytic tumor by comparative genomic hybridization. Genes Chromosomes Cancer 1998;21:340–346.

97. Ohgaki H, Watanabe K, Peraud A, et al. A case history of glioma progression. Acta Neuropathol (Berl) 1999;97:525–532.

98. Olson JJ, James CD, Krisht A, et al. Analysis of epidermal growth factor receptor gene amplification and alteration in stereotactic biopsies of brain tumors. Neurosurgery 1995;36:740–746.

99. Onda K, Tanaka R, Takahashi H, et al. Cerebral glioblastoma with cerebrospinal fluid dissemination: a clinicopathological study of 14 cases examined by complete autopsy. Neurosurgery 1989; 25:533–540.

100. Ono Y, Tamiya T, Ichikawa T, et al. Malignant astrocytomas with homozygous CDKN2/p16 gene deletions have higher Ki-67 proliferation indices. J Neuropathol Exp Neurol 1996;55:1026–1031.

101. Palma L, di Lorenzo N, Guidetti B. Lymphocytic infiltrates in primary glioblastomas and recidivous gliomas: incidence, fate, and relevance to prognosis in 228 operated cases. J Neurosurg 1978; 49:854–861.

102. Parekh H, Sharma RR, Prabhu SS, et al. Multifocal giant cell glioblastoma: case report. Surg Neurol 1993;40:151–154.

103. Park CC, Hartmann C, Folkerth R, et al. Systemic metastasis in glioblastoma may represent the emergence of neoplastic subclones. J Neuropathol Exp Neurol 2000;59:1044–1050.

104. Peraud A, Watanabe K, Plate KH, et al. p53 Mutations versus EGF receptor expression in giant cell glioblastomas. J Neuropathol Exp Neurol 1997;56:1236–1241.

105. Peraud A, Watanabe K, Schwechheimer K, et al. Genetic profile of the giant cell glioblastoma. Lab Invest 1999;79:123–129.

106. Perry A, Anderl K, Borell TJ, et al. Detection of p16, RB, CDK4, and p53 gene deletion and amplification by fluorescence in situ hybridization in 96 gliomas. Am J Clin Pathol 1999;112:801–809.

107. Perry A, Jenkins RB, O'Fallon JR, et al. Clinicopathologic study of 85 similarly treated patients with anaplastic astrocytic tumors: an analysis of DNA content (ploidy), cellular proliferation, and p53 expression. Cancer 1999;86:672–683.

108. Piepmeier J, Christopher S, Spencer D, et al. Variations in the natural history and survival of patients with supratentorial low-grade astrocytomas. Neurosurgery 1996;38:872–879.

109. Pollack IF, Claassen D, Al-Shboul Q, et al. Low-grade gliomas of the cerebral hemispheres in children: an analysis of 71 cases. J Neurosurg 1995;82:536–547.

110. Raghavan R, Steart PV, Weller RO. Cell proliferation patterns in the diagnosis of astrocytomas, anaplastic astrocytomas and glioblastoma multiforme: a Ki-67 study. Neuropathol Appl Neurobiol 1990;16:123–133.

111. Rappaport ZH, Loven D, Ben-Aharon U. Radiation-induced cerebellar glioblastoma multiforme subsequent to treatment of an astrocytoma of the cervical spinal cord. Neurosurgery 1991; 29:606–608.

112. Rawlings UE, Bullard DB, Burger PC, Friedman AH. A case of Ollier's disease associated with two intracranial gliomas. Neurosurgery 1987;21:400–403.

113. Reardon DX, Gajjar A, Sanford RA, et al. Bithalamic involvement predicts poor outcome among children with thalamic glial tumors. Pediatr Neurosurg 1998;29:29–35.

114. Reifenberger J, Ring GU, Gies U, et al. Analysis of p53 mutation and epidermal growth factor receptor amplification in recurrent gliomas with malignant progression. J Neuropathol Exp Neurol 1996;55:822–831.

115. Reis RM, Herva R, Brandner S, et al. Second primary glioblastoma. J Neuropathol Exp Neurol 2001;60:208–215.

116. Ritter AM, Sawaya R, Hess KR, et al. Prognostic significance of bromodeoxyuridine labeling in primary and recurrent glioblastoma multiforme. Neurosurgery 1994;35:192–198; discussion 8.

117. Roggendorf W, Strupp S, Paulus W. Distribution and characterization of microglia/macrophages in human brain tumors. Acta Neuropathol (Berl) 1996;92:288–293.

118. Rosenblum MK, Erlandson RA, Budzilovich GN. The lipid rich epithelioid glioblastoma. Am J Surg Pathol 1991;15:925–934.

119. Rossi ML, Hughes JT, Esiri MM, et al. Immunohistochemical study of mononuclear cell infiltrate in malignant gliomas. Acta Neuropathol (Berl) 1987;74:269–277.

120. Salvati M, Artico M, Caruso R, et al. A report on radiation-induced gliomas. Cancer 1991;67:392–397.

121. Scheithauer BW, Bruner JM. The ultrastructural spectrum of astrocytic neoplasms. Ultrastruct Pathol 1987;11:535–581.

122. Scherer H. Cerebral astrocytomas and their derivatives. Am J Cancer 1940;40:159–198.

123. Schlegel J, Merdes A, Stumm G, et al. Amplification of the epidermal-growth-factor-receptor gene correlates with different growth behavior in human glioblastoma. Int J Cancer 1994; 56:72–77.

124. Schwaninger M, Patt S, Henningsen P, Schmidt D. Spinal canal metastases: a late complication of glioblastoma. J Neurooncol 1992;12:93–98.

125. Scott JN, Rewcastle NB, Brasher PM, et al. Which glioblastoma multiforme patient will become a long-term survivor? A population-based study. Ann Neurol 1999;46:183–188.

126. Shuangshoti S, Kasantikul V, Suwanwela N. Spontaneous penetration of dura mater and bone by glioblastoma multiforme. J Surg Oncol 1987;36:36–44.

127. Silbergeld DL, Rostomily RC, Alvord EC Jr. The cause of death in patients with glioblastoma is multifactoral: clinical factors and autopsy findings in 117 cases of supratentorial glioblastoma in adults. J Neurooncol 1991;10:179–185.

128. Simmons NE, Laws ER Jr. Glioma occurrence after sellar irradiation: case report and review. Neurosurgery 1998;42:172–178.

129. Sung T, Miller DC, Hayes RL, et al. Preferential inactivation of the p53 tumor suppressor pathway and lack of EGFR amplification distinguish de novo high grade pediatric astrocytomas from de novo adult astrocytomas. Brain Pathol 2000;10:249–259.

130. Tachibana O, Lampe J, Kleihues P, Ohgaki H. Preferential expression of Fas/APO1 (CD95) and apoptotic cell death in perinecrotic cells of glioblastoma multiforme. Acta Neuropathol (Berl) 1996;92:431–434.

131. Takeuchi J, Barnard RO. Perivascular lymphocytic cuffing in astrocytomas. Acta Neuropathol (Berl) 1976;35:265–271.

132. Tohma Y, Gratas C, Biernat W, et al. PTEN (MMAC1) mutations are frequent in primary glioblastomas (de novo) but not in secondary glioblastomas. J Neuropathol Exp Neurol 1998;57:684–689.

133. Tohma Y, Gratas C, Van Meir EG, et al. Necrogenesis and Fas/APO-1 (CD95) expression in primary (de novo) and secondary glioblastomas. J Neuropathol Exp Neurol 1998;57: 239–245.

134. Torp SH, Helseth E, Dalen A, Unsgaard G. Relationships between Ki-67 labeling index, amplification of the epidermal growth factor receptor gene, and prognosis in human glioblastomas. Acta Neurochir (Wien) 1992;117:182–186.

135. Uyttebroeck A, Legius E, Brock P, et al. Consecutive glioblastoma and B cell non-Hodgkin's lymphoma in a young child with von Recklinghausen's neurofibromatosis. Med Pediatr Oncol 1995;24:46–49.

136. van Nielen KM, de Jong BM. A case of Ollier's disease associated with two intracerebral low-grade gliomas. Clin Neurol Neurosurg 1999;101:106–110.

137. Vertosick FT Jr, Selker RG. Brain stem and spinal metastases of supratentorial glioblastoma multiforme: a clinical series. Neurosurgery 1990;27:516–522.

138. Vertosick FT Jr, Selker RG, Arena VC. Survival of patients with well-differentiated astrocytomas diagnosed in the era of computed tomography. Neurosurgery 1991;28:496–501.

139. von Deimling A, Louis DN, von Ammon K, et al. Association of epidermal growth factor receptor gene amplification with loss of chromosome 10 in human glioblastoma multiforme. J Neurosurg 1992;77:295–301.

140. von Deimling A, von Ammon K, Schoenfeld D, et al. Subsets of glioblastoma multiforme defined by molecular genetic analysis. Brain Pathol 1993;3:19–26.

141. von Deimling A, Fimmers R, Schmidt MC, et al. Comprehensive allelotype and genetic analysis of 466 human nervous system tumors. J Neuropathol Exp Neurol 2000;59:544–558.

142. Wakimoto H, Aoyagi M, Nakayama T, et al. Prognostic significance of Ki-67 labeling indices obtained using MIB-1 monoclonal antibody in patients with supratentorial astrocytomas. Cancer 1996;77:373–380.

143. Walker MD, Alexander E Jr, Hunt WE, et al. Evaluation of BCNU and/or radiotherapy in the treatment of anaplastic gliomas. J Neurosurg 1978;49:333–343.

144. Watanabe K, Tachibana O, Sato K, et al. Overexpression of the EGF receptor and p53 mutations are mutually exclusive in the evolution of primary and secondary glioblastomas. Brain Pathol 1996;6:217–224.

145. Watanabe K, Tachibana O, Yonekawa Y, et al. Role of gemistocytes in astrocytoma progression. Lab Invest 1997;76:277–284.

146. Wesseling P, Schlingemann RO, Rietveld FJR, et al. Early and extensive contribution of pericytes/vascular smooth muscle cells to microvascular proliferation in glioblastoma multiforme: an immuno-light and immuno-electron microscopic study. J Neuropathol Exp Neurol 1995;54:304–310.

147. Winger MJ, Macdonald DR, Cairncross JG. Supratentorial anaplastic gliomas in adults. J Neurosurg 1989;71:487–493.

148. Wood JR, Green SB, Shapiro WR. The prognostic importance of tumor size in malignant gliomas: a computed tomographic scan study by the Brain Tumor Cooperative Group. J Clin Oncol 1988;6:338–343.

149. Yanagawa Y, Miyazawa T, Ishihara S, et al. Pontine glioma with osteoblastic skeletal metastases in a child. Surg Neurol 1996;46:481–484.

150. Yaziji H, Massarani-Wafai R, Gujrati M, et al. Role of p53 immunohistochemistry in differentiating reactive gliosis from malignant astrocytic lesions. Am J Surg Pathol 1996;20:1086–1090.

## Gliosarcoma

1. Barnard RO, Bradford R, Scott T, Thomas DGT. Gliomyosarcoma: report of a case of rhabdomyosarcoma arising in a malignant glioma. Acta Neuropathol (Berl) 1986;69:23–27.

2. Biernat W, Aguzzi A, Sure U, et al. Identical mutations of the p53 tumor suppressor gene in the gliomatous and the sarcomatous components of gliosarcomas suggest a common origin from glial cells. J Neuropathol Exp Neurol 1995;54:651–656.

3. Boerman RH, Anderl K, Herath J, et al. The glial and mesenchymal elements of gliosarcomas share similar genetic alterations. J Neuropathol Exp Neurol 1996;55:973–981.

4. Haddad SF, Moore SA, Schelper RL, Goeken JA. Smooth muscle can comprise the sarcomatous component of gliosarcomas. J Neuropathol Exp Neurol 1992;51:493–498.

5. Hayashi K, Ohara N, Jeon HJ, et al. Gliosarcoma with features of chondroblastic osteosarcoma. Cancer 1993;72:850–855.

6. Jones H, Steart PV, Weller RO. Spindle-cell glioblastoma or gliosarcoma? Neuropathol Appl Neurobiol 1991;17:177–187.

7. Kepes JJ, Fulling KH, Garcia JH. The clinical significance of "adenoid" formations of neoplastic astrocytes, imitating metastatic carcinoma in gliosarcomas: a review of five cases. Clin Neuropathol 1982;1:139–150.

8. McComb RD, Jones TR, Pizzo SV, Bigner DD. Immunohistochemical detection of factor VIII/von Willebrand factor in hyperplastic endothelial cells in glioblastoma multiforme and mixed glioma-sarcoma. J Neuropathol Exp Neurol 1982;41: 479–489.

9. Meis JM, Martz KL, Nelson JS. Mixed glioblastoma multiforme and sarcoma: a clinicopathologic study of 26 radiation therapy oncology group cases. Cancer 1991;67:2342–2349.

10. Mørk SJ, Rubinstein LJ, Kepes JJ, et al. Problems of epithelial metaplasia in malignant gliomas. II. Squamous differentiation of epithelial-like formations in gliosarcomas and glioblastomas. J Neuropathol Exp Neurol 1988;47:101–118.

11. Paulus W, Jellinger K. Mixed glioblastoma and malignant mesenchymoma, a variety of gliosarcoma. Histopathology 1993;22:277–279.

12. Perry JR, Ang LC, Bilbao JM, Muller PJ. Clinicopathologic features of primary and postirradiation cerebral gliosarcoma. Cancer 1995;75:2910–2918.

13. Shintaku M, Miyaji K, Adachi Y. Gliosarcoma with angiosarcomatous features: a case report. Brain Tumor Pathol 1998;15:101–105.

14. Sreenan JJ, Prayson RA. Gliosarcoma: a study of 13 tumors, including p53 and CD34 immunohistochemistry. Arch Pathol Lab Med 1997;121:129–133.

## Granular Cell Astrocytoma of the Cerebrum

1. Albuquerque L, Pimentel J, Costa A, Cristina L. Cerebral granular cell tumors: report of a case and a note on their nature and expected behavior. Acta Neuropathol (Berl) 1992;84:680–685.

2. Dickson DW, Suzuki KI, Kanner R, et al. Cerebral granular cell tumor: immunohistochemical and electron microscopic study. J Neuropathol Exp Neurol 1986;45:304–314.

3. Geddes JF, Thom M, Robinson SFD, Révész T. Granular cell change in astrocytic tumors. Am J Surg Pathol 1996;20:55–63.

4. Kornfield M. Granular cell glioblastoma: a malignant granular cell neoplasm of astrocytic origin. J Neuropathol Exp Neurol 1986;45:447–462.

5. Markesbery WR, Duffy PE, Cowen D. Granular cell tumors of the central nervous system. J Neuropathol Exp Neurol 1973;32:92–109.

6. Medina-Flores R, Scheithauer BW, Burger PC, Brat DJ. Granular cell astrocytomas: clinicopathologic features. Mod Pathol 2000;1145:195A.

## Gliomatosis Cerebri

1. Artigas J, Cervos-Navarro J, Iglesias JR, Ebhardt G. Gliomatosis cerebri, clinical and histological findings. Clin Neuropathol 1985;4:135–148.

2. Balko GM, Blisard KS, Samaha FJ. Oligodendroglial gliomatosis cerebri. Hum Pathol 1992;23:706–707.

3. Cervos-Navarro J, Artigas J, Iglesias J. The fine structure of gliomatosis cerebri. Virchows Arch A 1987;411:93–98.

4. Cozad SC, Townsend P, Morantz RA, et al. Gliomatosis cerebri: results with radiation therapy. Cancer 1996;78:1789–1793.

5. del Carpio-O'Donovan R, Korah I, Salazar A, Melançon D. Gliomatosis cerebri. Radiology 1996;198:831–835.

6. Felsberg GJ, Silver SA, Brown MT, Tien RD. Radiologic-pathologic correlation: gliomatosis cerebri. AJNR 1994;15:1745–1753.

7. Gottesman M, Laufer H, Patel M. Gliomatosis cerebri: a case report. Clin Neuropathol 1991;10:303–305.

8. Hulette CM. Microglioma, a histiocytic neoplasm of the central nervous system. Mod Pathol 1996;9:316–319.

9. Kim DG, Yang HJ, Park IA, et al. Gliomatosis cerebri: clinical features, treatment, and prognosis. Acta Neurochir (Wien) 1998;140:755–762.

10. Malamud N, Wise BL, Jones OW. Gliomatosis cerebri. J Neurosurg 1952;9:409–417.

11. Rogers LR, Weinstein MA, Estes ML, et al. Diffuse bilateral cerebral astrocytomas with atypical neuroimaging studies. J Neurosurg 1994;81:817–821.

12. Scheinker IM, Evans JP. Diffuse cerebral glioblastosis. J Neuropathol Exp Neurosurg 1943;2:178–189.

13. Simonati A, Vio M, Iannucci AM, et al. Gliomatosis cerebri diffusa: a case report. Acta Neuropathol (Berl) 1981;54:311–314.

## Protoplasmic Astrocytoma

1. Prayson RA. Protoplasmic astrocytoma: a clinicopathologic study of 16 tumors. Am J Clin Pathol 1995;103:705–709.

## Pilocytic Astrocytoma

1. Abdollahzadeh M, Hoffman HJ, Blazer SI, et al. Benign cerebellar astrocytoma in childhood: experience at the Hospital for Sick Children 1980–1992. Childs Nerv Syst 1994;10:380–383.

2. Bowers DC, Georgiades C, Aronson LJ, et al. Tectal Gliomas: Natural History of an Indolent Lesion in Pediatric Patients. Pediatr Neurosurg 32:24–29, 2000.

3. Boydston WR, Sanford RA, Muhlbauer MS, et al. Gliomas of the tectum and periaqueductal region of the mesencephalon. Pediatr Neurosurg 1991;17:234–238.

4. Brat DJ, Burger PC. Cerebral pilocytic astrocytoma: distinction from infiltrating fibrillary astrocytomas. Pathol Case Rev 1998;3:290–295.

5. Burger PC. Pathology of brain stem astrocytomas. Pediatr Neurosurg 1996;28:245–256.

6. Burger PC, Breiter SN, Fisher PG. Pilocytic and fibrillary astrocytomas of the brain stem—a comparative clinical, radiological, and pathological study. J Neurosurg Exp Neurol 1996;55:640.

7. Burger PC, Scheithauer BW, Lee RR, O'Neill BP. An interdisciplinary approach to avoid the overtreatment of patients with central nervous system lesions. Cancer 1997;80:2040–2046.

8. Clark GB, Henry JM, McKeever PE. Cerebral pilocytic astrocytoma. Cancer 1985;56:1128–1133.

9. Coakley KJ, Huston J, Scheithauer BW, et al. Pilocytic astrocytomas: well-demarcated magnetic resonance appearance despite frequent infiltration histologically. Mayo Clin Proc 1995;70:747–751.

10. Cottingham SL, Boesel CP, Yates AJ. Pilocytic astrocytoma in infants: a distinctive histological pattern. J Neurosurg Exp Neurol 1996;55:654.

11. Cummings TJ, Provenzale JM, Hunter SB, et al. Gliomas of the optic nerve: histological, immunohistochemical (MIB-1 and p53), and MRI analysis. Acta Neuropathol (Berl) 2000;99:563–570.

12. Cushing H. Experiences with the cerebellar astrocytomas. Surg Gynecol Obstet 1931;102:129–204.

13. Dirven CMF, Mooij JJA, Molenaar WM. Cerebellar pilocytic astrocytoma: a treatment protocol based upon analysis of 73 cases and a review of the literature. Childs Nerv Syst 1997;13:17–23.

14. Fisher PG, Breiter SN, Carson BS, et al. A clinicopathologic reappraisal of brainstem tumor classification: identification of pilocytic astrocytoma and fibrillary astrocytoma as distinct entities. Cancer 2000;89:1569–1576.

15. Forsyth PA, Shaw EG, Scheithauer BW, et al. Supratentorial pilocytic astrocytomas: a clinicopathologic, prognostic, and flow cytometric study of 51 patients. Cancer 1993;72:1335–1342.

16. Gajjar A, Bhargava R, Jenkins JJ, et al. Low-grade astrocytoma with neuraxis dissemination at diagnosis. J Neurosurg 1995;83:67–71.

17. Giannini C, Scheithauer BW, Burger PC, et al. Cellular proliferation in pilocytic and diffuse astrocytomas. J Neuropathol Exp Neurol 1999;58:46–53.

18. Goldman JE, Corbin E. Rosenthal fibers contain ubiquitinated αB-crystallin. Am J Pathol 1991;139:933–938.

19. Haapasalo H, Sallinen S, Sallinen P, et al. Clinicopathological correlation of cell proliferation, apoptosis and p53 in cerebellar pilocytic astrocytomas. Neuropathol Appl Neurobiol 1999;25: 134–142.

20. Hayostek CJ, Shaw EG, Scheithauer BW, et al. Astrocytomas of the cerebellum: a comparative clinicopathologic study of pilocytic and diffuse astrocytomas. Cancer 1993;72:856–869.

21. Ito S, Hoshino T, Shibuya M, et al. Proliferative characteristics of juvenile pilocytic astrocytomas determined by bromodeoxyuridine labeling. Neurosurgery 1992;31:413–419.

22. Katsetos CD, Krishna L. Lobar pilocytic astrocytomas of the cerebral hemispheres. I. Diagnosis and nosology. Clin Neuropathol 1994;13:295–305.

23. Katsetos CD, Krishna L, Friedberg E, et al. Lobar pilocytic astrocytomas of the cerebral hemispheres. II. Pathobiology—morphogenesis of the eosinophilic granular bodies. Clin Neuropathol 1994;13:306–314.

24. Khatib ZA, Heideman RL, Kovnar EH, et al. Predominance of pilocytic histology in dorsally exophytic brain stem tumors. Pediatr Neurosurg 1994;20:2–10.

25. Lach B, Sikorska M, Rippstein P, et al. Immunoelectron microscopy of Rosenthal fibers. Acta Neuropathol (Berl) 1991;81:503–509.

26. Lang FF, Miller DC, Pisharody S, et al. High frequency of p53 protein accumulation without p53 gene mutation in human juvenile pilocytic, low grade and anaplastic astrocytomas. Oncogene 1994;9:949–954.

27. Lee Y-Y, Van Tassel P, Bruner JM, et al. Juvenile pilocytic astrocytomas: CT and MR characteristics. AJNR 1989;10:363–370.

28. Leisti E-L, Pyhtinen J, Poyhonen M. Spontaneous decrease of a pilocytic astrocytoma in neurofibromatosis type 1. AJNR 1996;17:1691–1694.

29. Listernick R, Louis DN, Packer RJ, Gutmann DH. Optic pathway gliomas in children with neurofibromatosis 1: consensus statement from the NF1 Optic Pathway Glioma Task Force. Ann Neurol 1997;41:143–149.

30. Mamelak AN, Prados MD, Obana WG, et al. Treatment options and prognosis for multicentric juvenile pilocytic astrocytoma. J Neurosurg 1994;81:24–30.

31. McGirr SJ, Kelly PJ, Scheithauer BW. Stereotactic resection of juvenile pilocytic astrocytomas of the thalamus and basal ganglia. Neurosurgery 1987;20:447–452.

32. Morikawa M, Tamaki N, Kokunai T, et al. Cerebellar pilocytic astrocytoma with leptomeningeal dissemination: case report. Surg Neurol 1997;48:49–52.

33. Murayama S, Bouldin TW, Suzuki K. Immunocytochemical and ultrastructural studies of eosinophilic granular bodies in astrocytic tumors. Acta Neuropathol (Berl) 1992;83:408–414.

34. Nishio S, Takeshita I, Fukui M, et al. Anaplastic evolution of childhood optico-hypothalamic pilocytic astrocytoma: report of an autopsy case. Clin Neuropathol 1988;7:254–258.

35. Pagni CA, Giordana MT, Canavero S. Benign recurrence of a pilocytic cerebellar astrocytoma 36 years after radical removal: case report. Neurosurgery 1991;28:606–609.

36. Palma L, Guidetti B. Cystic pilocytic astrocytomas of the cerebral hemispheres: surgical experience with 51 cases and long-term results. J Neurosurg 1985;62:811–815.

37. Parsa CF, Hoyt CS, Lesser RL, et al. Spontaneous regression of optic gliomas: 13 cases documented by serial neuroimaging. Arch Ophthalmol 2001;119:516–529.

38. Perilongo G, Carollo C, Salviati L, et al. Diencephalic syndrome and disseminated juvenile pilocytic astrocytomas of the hypothalamic-optic chiasm region. Cancer 1997;80:142–146.

39. Platten M, Giordano MJ, Dirven CMF, et al. Up-regulation of specific NF1 gene transcripts in sporadic pilocytic astrocytomas. Am J Pathol 1996;149:621–627.

40. Pollack IF, Claassen D, Al-Shboul Q, et al. Low-grade gliomas of the cerebral hemispheres in children: an analysis of 71 cases. J Neurosurg 1995;82:536–547.

41. Pollack IF, Pang D, Albright AL. The long-term outcome in children with late-onset aqueductal stenosis resulting from benign intrinsic tectal tumors. J Neurosurg 1994;80:681–688.

42. Scheithauer BW, Bruner JM. The ultrastructural spectrum of astrocytic neoplasms. Ultrastruct Pathol 1987;11:535–581.

43. Schiffer D, Cravioto H, Giordana MT, et al. Is polar spongioblastoma a tumor entity? J Neurosurg 1993;78:587–591.

44. Schwartz AM, Ghatak NR. Malignant transformation of benign cerebellar astrocytoma. Cancer 1990;65:333–336.

45. Stern J, Jakobiec FA, Housepian EM. The architecture of optic nerve gliomas with and without neurofibromatosis. Arch Ophthalmol 1980;98:505–511.

46. Takeuchi H, Kabuto M, Sato K, Kubota T. Chiasmal gliomas with spontaneous regression: proliferation and apoptosis. Childs Nerv Syst 1997;13:229–233.

47. Tihan T, Burger PC. A variant of "pilocytic astrocytoma"—a possible distinct clinicopathological entity with a less favorable outcome. J Neuropathol Exp Neurol 1999;58:1061–1068.

48. Tomlinson FH, Scheithauer BW, Hayostek CJ, et al. The significance of atypia and histologic malignancy in pilocytic astrocytoma of the cerebellum: a clinicopathologic and flow cytometric study. J Child Neurol 1994;9:301–310.

49. Ushio Y, Arita N, Yoshimime T, et al. Malignant recurrence of childhood cerebellar astrocytoma: case report. Neurosurgery 1987;21:251–255.

50. Versari P, Talamonti G, D'Aliberti G, et al. Leptomeningeal dissemination of juvenile pilocytic astrocytoma: case report. Surg Neurol 1994;41:318–321.

51. Vogel H, Dauser R, Powell S. Biphasic pilocytic ganglion cell tumor of the cerebellum. J Neuropathol Exp Neurol 1999;58:539.

52. von Deimling A, Louis DN, Menon AG, et al. Deletions on the long arm of chromosome 17 in pilocytic astrocytoma. Acta Neuropathol (Berl) 1993;86:81–85.

## Pleomorphic Xanthoastrocytoma

1. Burger PC, Nelson JS, Boyko OB. Diagnostic synergy in radiology and surgical neuropathology: neuroimaging techniques and general interpretive guidelines. Arch Pathol Lab Med 1998;122:609–619.

2. Burger PC, Nelson JS, Boyko OB. Diagnostic synergy in radiology and surgical neuropathology: radiographic findings of specific pathologic entities. Arch Pathol Lab Med 1998;122:620–632.

3. Burger PC, Scheithauer BW, Lee RR, O'Neill BP. An interdisciplinary approach to avoid the overtreatment of patients with central nervous system lesions. Cancer 1997;80:2040–2046.

4. Furuta A, Takehashi H, Ikuta F, et al. Temporal lobe tumor demonstrating ganglioglioma and pleomorphic xanthoastrocytoma components. J Neurosurg 1992;77:143–147.

5. Giannini C, Scheithauer BW, Burger PC, et al. Pleomorphic xanthoastrocytoma: what do we really know about it? Cancer 1999;85:2033–2045.

6. Haga S, Morioka T, Nishio S, Fukui M. Multicentric pleomorphic xanthoastrocytomas: case report. Neurosurgery 1996;38:1242–1245.

7. Kanzawa T, Takahashi H, Hayano M, et al. Melanotic cerebral astrocytoma: case report and literature review. Acta Neuropathol (Berl) 1997;93:200–204.

8. Kepes JJ. Pleomorphic xanthoastrocytoma: the birth of a diagnosis and a concept. Brain Pathol 1993;3:269–274.

9. Kepes JJ, Rubinstein LJ, Ansbacher L, Schreiber DJ. Histopathological features of recurrent pleomorphic xanthoastrocytomas: further corroboration of the glial nature of this neoplasm. Acta Neuropathol (Berl) 1989;78:585–593.

10. Kepes JJ, Rubinstein LJ, Eng LF. Pleomorphic xanthoastrocytoma: a distinctive meningocerebral glioma of young subjects with relatively favorable prognosis. A study of 12 cases. Cancer 1979;44:1839–1852.

11. Kros JM, Vecht CJ, Stefanko SZ. The pleomorphic xanthoastrocytoma and its differential diagnosis: a study of five cases. Hum Pathol 1991;22:1128–1135.

12. Levy RA, Allen R, McKeever P. Pleomorphic xanthoastrocytoma presenting with massive intracranial hemorrhage. AJNR 1996;17:154–156.

13. Lipper MH, Eberhard DA, Phillips CD, et al. Pleomorphic xanthoastrocytoma, a distinctive astroglial tumor: neuroradiologic and pathologic features. AJNR 1993;14:1397–1404.

14. Macaulay RJ, Jay V, Hoffman HJ, Becker LE. Increased mitotic activity as a negative prognostic indicator in pleomorphic xanthoastrocytoma: case report. J Neurosurg 1993;79:761–768.

15. Pahapill PA, Ramsay DA, Phil D, Del Maestro RF. Pleomorphic xanthoastrocytoma: case report and analysis of the literature concerning the efficacy of resection and the significance of necrosis. Neurosurgery 1996;38:822–829.

16. Perry A, Giannini C, Scheithauer BW, et al. Composite pleomorphic xanthoastrocytoma and ganglioglioma: report of four cases and review of the literature. Am J Surg Pathol 1997;21:763–771.

17. Powell SZ, Yachnis AT, Rorke LB, et al. Divergent differentiation in pleomorphic xanthoastrocytoma: evidence for a neuronal element and possible relationship to ganglion cell tumors. Am J Surg Pathol 1996;20:80–85.

18. Prayson RA, Morris HH III. Anaplastic pleomorphic xanthoastrocytoma. Arch Pathol Lab Med 1998;122:1082–1086.

19. Tonn JC, Paulus W, Warmuth-Metz M, et al. Pleomorphic xanthoastrocytoma: report of six cases with special consideration of diagnostic and therapeutic pitfalls. Surg Neurol 1997;47:162–169.

20. Wasdahl DA, Scheithauer BW, Andrews BT, Jeffrey RA Jr. Cerebellar pleomorphic xanthoastrocytoma: case report. Neurosurgery 1994;35:947–951.

21. Weldon-Linne CM, Victor TA, Groothuis DR, Vick NA. Pleomorphic xanthoastrocytoma: ultrastructural and immunohistochemical study of a case with a rapidly fatal outcome following surgery. Cancer 1983;52:2055–2063.

22. Yoshino MT, Lucio R. Pleomorphic xanthoastrocytoma. AJNR 1992;13:1330–1332.

23. Zarate JO, Sampaolesi R. Pleomorphic xanthoastrocytoma of the retina. Am J Surg Pathol 1999;23:79–81.

## Subependymal Giant Cell Astrocytoma

1. Altermatt HJ, Scheithauer BW. Cytomorphology of subependymal giant cell astrocytoma. Acta Cytol 1992;36:171–175.

2. Brown JM. Sclerosis and meningeal astrocytoma. Med J Aust 1975;1:811–814.

3. Chou TM, Chou SM. Tuberous sclerosis in the premature infant: a report of a case with immunohistochemistry on the CNS. Clin Neuropathol 1989;8:45–52.

4. Gyure KA, Prayson RA. Subependymal giant cell astrocytoma: a clinicopathologic study with HMB45 and MIB-1 immunohistochemical analysis. Mod Pathol 1997;10:313–317.

5. Hirose T, Scheithauer BW, Lopes MBS, et al. Tuber and subependymal giant cell astrocytoma associated with tuberous sclerosis: an immunohistochemical, ultrastructural, and immunoelectron microscopic study. Acta Neuropathol (Berl) 1995;90:387–399.

6. Padmalatha C, Harruff RC, Ganick D, Hafez GR. Glioblastoma multiforme with tuberous sclerosis. Arch Pathol Lab Med 1980;104: 649–650.

7. Shepherd CW, Scheithauer BW, Gomez MR, et al. Subependymal giant cell astrocytoma: a clinical, pathological, and flow cytometric study. Neurosurgery 1991;28:864–868.

8. Shepherd CW, Houser OW, Gomez MR. MR findings in tuberous sclerosis complex and correlation with seizure development and mental impairment. AJNR 1995;16:149–155.

9. Short MP, Richardson EP Jr, Haines JL, Kwiatkowski DJ. Clinical, neuropathological and genetic aspects of the tuberous sclerosis complex. Brain Pathol 1995;5:173–179.

10. Sinson G, Sutton LN, Yachnis AT, et al. Subependymal giant cell astrocytomas in children. Pediatr Neurosurg 1994;20:233–239.

11. Smirniotopoulos JG, Murphy FM. The phakomatoses. AJNR 1992;13:725–746.

12. Torres OA, Roach ES, Delgado MR, et al. Early diagnosis of subependymal giant cell astrocytoma in patients with tuberous sclerosis. J Child Neurol 1998;13:173–177.

13. Wolf HK, Roos D, Blümcke I, et al. Perilesional neurochemical changes in focal epilepsies. Acta Neuropathol (Berl) 1996; 91: 376–384.

## Oligodendroglioma and Mixed Glioma (Oligoastrocytoma)

1. Arseni C, Horvath L, Carp N, et al. Spinal dissemination following operation on cerebral oligodendroglioma. Acta Neurochir (Wien) 1977;37:125–137.

2. Barnard RO. The development of malignancy in oligodendrogliomas. J Pathol Bacteriol 1968;96:113–123.

3. Bigner SH, Rasheed BKA, Wiltshire R, McLendon RE. Morphologic and molecular genetic aspects of oligodendroglial neoplasms. Neuro-Oncology 1999;1:52–60.

4. Burger PC, Minn AY, Smith JS, et al. Losses of chromosomal arms 1p and 19q in the diagnosis of oligodendroglioma. A study of paraffin-embedded sections. Mod Pathol 2001;14:842–853.

5. Burger PC, Rawlings CE, Cox EB, et al. Clinicopathologic correlations in the oligodendroglioma. Cancer 1987;59:1345–1352.

6. Cairncross JG, Macdonald DR, Ramsay DA. Aggressive oligodendroglioma: a chemosensitive tumor. Neurosurgery 1992;31:78–82.

7. Cairncross JG, Ueki K, Zlatescu MC, et al. Specific genetic predictors of chemotherapeutic response and survival in patients with anaplastic oligodendrogliomas. J Natl Cancer Inst 1998; 90: 1473–1479.

8. Coons SW, Johnson PC, Pearl DK. The prognostic significance of Ki-67 labeling indices for oligodendrogliomas. Neurosurgery 1997;41:878–885.

9. Daumas-Duport C, Tucker M-L, Kolles H, et al. Oligodendrogliomas. Part II. A new grading system based on morphological and imaging criteria. J Neurooncol 1997;34:61–78.

10. Daumas-Duport C, Varlet P, Tucker M-L, et al. Oligodendrogliomas. Part I. Patterns of growth, histological diagnosis, clinical and imaging correlations: a study of 153 cases. J Neurooncol 1997;34:37–59.

11. Dehghani F, Schachenmayr W, Laun A, Korf H-W. Prognostic implication of histopathological, immunohistochemical and clinical features of oligodendrogliomas: a study of 89 cases. Acta Neuropathol (Berl) 1998;95:493–504.

12. Feigin I, Ransohoff J, Lieberman A. Sarcoma arising in oligodendrogliomas of the brain. J Neuropathol Exp Neurol 1976;35: 679–684.

13. Giannini C, Scheithauer BW, Mork S, et al. Oligodendrogliomas: reproducibility of grading parameters. J Neuropathol Exp Neurol 1999;58:536.

14. Giannini C, Weaver A, Scheithauer BW, et al. Histologic prognostic parameters in oligodendroglioma. J Neuropathol Exp Neurol 2000;59:443.

15. Gultekin SH, Dalmau J, Graus Y, et al. Anti-Hu immunolabeling as an index of neuronal differentiation in human brain tumors. Am J Surg Pathol 1998;22:195–200.

16. Hart MN, Peitito CK, Earle KM. Mixed gliomas. Cancer 1974; 33:134–140.

17. Heegaard S, Sommer HM, Broholm H, Broendstrup O. Proliferating cell nuclear antigen and Ki-67 immunohistochemistry

of oligodendrogliomas with special reference to prognosis. Cancer 1995;76:1809–1813.

18. Herpers JHM, Budka H. Glial fibrillary acidic protein (GFAP) in oligodendroglial tumors: gliofibrillary oligodendroglioma and transitional oligoastrocytoma as subtypes of oligodendroglioma. Acta Neuropathol (Berl) 1984;64:265–272.

19. Huang C-I, Chiou W-H, Ho DM. Oligodendroglioma occurring after radiation therapy for pituitary adenoma. J Neurol Neurosurg Psychiatry 1987;50:1619–1624.

20. James TGI, Pagel W. Oligodendroglioma with extracranial metastases. Br J Surg 1951;39:56–65.

21. Jellinger K, Minauf M, Salzer-Kuntschik M. Oligodendroglioma with extraneural metastases. J Neurol Neurosurg Psychiatry 1969; 32:249–253.

22. Kleihues P, Cavenee WK (eds). Pathology and Genetics of Tumours of the Nervous System. Lyon: IARC Press, 2000.

23. Koeppen AH, Cassidy RJ. Oligodendroglioma of the medulla oblongata in a neonate. Arch Neurol 1981;38:520–523.

24. Kraus JA, Koopmann J, Kaskel P, et al. Shared allelic losses on chromosomes 1p and 19q suggest a common origin of oligodendroglioma and oligoastrocytoma. J Neuropathol Exp Neurol 1995; 54:91–95.

25. Kros JM, de Jong AAW, van der Kwast TH. Ultrastructural characterization of transitional cells in oligodendrogliomas. J Neuropathol Exp Neurol 1992;51:186–193.

26. Kros JM, Hop WCJ, Godschalk JJCJ, Krishnadath KK. Prognostic value of the proliferation-related antigen Ki-67 in oligodendrogliomas. Cancer 1996;78:1107–1113.

27. Kros JM, Pieterman H, van Eden CG, Avezaat CJJ. Oligodendroglioma: the Rotterdam-Dijkzigt experience. Neurosurgery 1994;34:959–966.

28. Kros JM, Stefanko SZ, de Jong AAW, et al. Ultrastructural and immunohistochemical segregation of gemistocytic subsets. Hum Pathol 1991;22:33–40.

29. Kros JM, Troost D, van Eden CG, et al. Oligodendroglioma: a comparison of two grading systems. Cancer 1988;61:2251–2259.

30. Kros JM, van Eden CG, Stefanko SZ, et al. Prognostic implications of glial fibrillary acidic protein containing cell types in oligodendrogliomas. Cancer 1990;66:1204–1212.

31. Lee Y-Y, van Tassel P. Intracranial oligodendrogliomas: imaging findings in 35 untreated cases. AJNR 1989;10:119–127.

32. Ludwig CL, Smith MT, Godfrey AD, Armbrustmacher VW. A clinicopathological study of 323 patients with oligodendrogliomas. Ann Neurol 1986;19:15–21.

33. Maintz D, Fiedler K, Koopmann J, et al. Molecular genetic evidence for subtypes of oligoastrocytomas. J Neuropathol Exp Neurol 1997;56:1098–1104.

34. Mason WP, Krol GS, DeAngelis LM. Low-grade oligodendroglioma responds to chemotherapy. Neurology 1996;46: 203–207.

35. Min KW, Scheithauer BW. Oligodendroglioma: the ultrastructural spectrum. Ultrastruct Pathol 1994;18:47–60.

36. Mørk SJ, Halvorsen TB, Lindegaard K-F, Eide GE. Oligodendroglioma: histologic evaluation and prognosis. J Neuropathol Exp Neurol 1986;45:65–78.

37. Natelson SE, Dyer ML, Harp DL. Delayed CSF seeding of benign oligodendroglioma. South Med J 1992;85:1011–1012.

38. Nazek M, Mandybur TI, Kashiwagi S. Oligodendroglial proliferative abnormality associated with arteriovenous malformation: report of three cases with review of the literature. Neurosurgery 1998;23:781–785.

39. Ng H-K, Hardy CW, Tse CCH. Immunohistochemical and ultrastructural studies of oligodendrogliomas revealed features of neuronal differentiation. Int J Surg Pathol 1994;2:47–56.

40. Packer RJ, Sutton LN, Rorke LB, et al. Oligodendroglioma of the posterior fossa in childhood. Cancer 1985;56:195–199.

41. Paleologos NA, Cairncross JG. Treatment of oligodendroglioma: an update. Neuro-Oncology 1999;1:61–68.

42. Radner H, Kleinert R, Vennigerholz F, Denk H. Case report: peculiar changes in Rosenthal fibres in an atypical astrocytoma. Neuropathol Appl Neurobiol 1990;16:171–177.

43. Razack N, Baumgartner J, Bruner J. Pediatric oligodendrogliomas. Pediatr Neurosurg 1998;28:121–129.

44. Reifenberger J, Reifenberger G, Liu L, et al. Molecular genetic analysis of oligodendroglial tumors shows preferential allelic deletions on 19q and 1p. Am J Pathol 1994;145:1175–1190.

45. Reis-Filho JS, Faoro LN, Carrilho C, et al. Evaluation of cell proliferation, epidermal growth factor receptor, and bcl-2 immunoexpres-sion as prognostic factors for patients with World Health Organization grade 2 oligodendroglioma. Cancer 2000;88: 862–869.

46. Ritland SR, Ganju V, Jenkins RB. Region-specific loss of heterozygosity on chromosome 19 is related to the morphologic type of human glioma. Genes Chromosomes Cancer 1995;12:277–282.

47. Robertson DM, Vogel FS. Concentric lamination of glial processes in oligodendrogliomas. J Cell Biol 1962;15:313–334.

48. Schwechheimer K, Gass P, Berlet HH. Expression of oligodendroglia and Schwann cell markers in human nervous system tumors: an immunomorphological study and Western blot analysis. Acta Neuropathol 1992;83:283–291.

49. Shaw EG, Scheithauer BW, O'Fallon JR, et al. Oligodendrogliomas: the Mayo Clinic experience. J Neurosurg 1992; 76:428–434.

50. Smith JS, Alderete B, Minn Y, et al. Localization of common deletion regions on 1p and 19q in human gliomas and their association with histological subtype. Oncogene 1999;18:4144–4152.

51. Smith JS, Perry A, Borell TJ, et al. Alterations of chromosome arms 1p and 19q as predictors of survival in oligodendrogliomas, astrocytomas, and mixed oligoastrocytomas. J Clin Oncol 2000;18:636–645.

52. Smith MT, Ludwig CL, Godfrey AD, Armbrustmacher VW. Grading of oligodendrogliomas. Cancer 1983;52:2107–2114.

53. Sofietti R, Ruda R, Bradac GB, Schiffer D. PCV chemotherapy for recurrent oligodendrogliomas and oligoastrocytomas. Neurosurgery 1998;43:1066–1073.

54. Tice H, Barnes PD, Goumnerova L, et al. Pediatric and adolescent oligodendrogliomas. AJNR 1993;14:1293–1300.

55. von Deimling A, Louis DN, von Ammon K, et al. Evidence for a tumor suppressor gene on chromosome 19q associated with human astrocytomas, oligodendrogliomas and mixed gliomas. Cancer Res 1992;52:4277–4279.

56. von Deimling A, Fimmers R, Schmidt MC, et al. Comprehensive allelotype and genetic analysis of 466 human nervous system tumors. J Neuropathol Exp Neurol 2000;59:544–558.

57. Wharton SB, Hamilton FA, Chant WK, et al. Proliferation and cell death in oligodendrogliomas. Neuropathol Appl Neurobiol 1998;24:21–28.

58. Wolf HK, Buslei RIB, Wiestler OD, Pietsch T. Neural antigens in oligodendrogliomas and dysembryoplastic neuroepithelial tumors. Acta Neuropathol (Berl) 1997;94:436–443.

## Ependymoma

1. Afra D, Müller W, Slowik F, et al. Supratentorial lobar ependymomas: reports on the grading and survival periods in 80 cases, including 46 recurrences. Acta Neurochir (Wien) 1983;69: 243–251.

2. Bouffet E, Perilongo G, Canete A, Massimino M. Intracranial ependymomas in children: a critical review of prognostic factors and a plea for cooperation. Med Pediatr Oncol 1998;30:319–331.

3. Brown DF, Chason DP, Schwartz LF, et al. Supratentorial giant cell ependymoma: a case report. Mod Pathol 1998;11:398–403.

4. Brown WD, Tavaré CJ, Sobel EL, Gilles FH. The applicability of Collins' law to childhood brain tumors and its usefulness as a predictor of survival. Neurosurgery 1995;36:1093–1096.

5. Comi AM, Backstrom JW, Burger PC, et al. Clinical and neuroradiologic findings in infants with intracranial ependymomas. Pediatr Neurol 1998;18:23–29.

6. Doglioni C, Bontempini L, Iuzzolino P, et al. Ependymoma of the mediastinum. Arch Pathol Lab Med 1988;112:194–196.

7. Figarell-Branger D, Gambarelli D, Dollo C, et al. Infratentorial ependymomas of childhood: correlation between histological features, immunohistochemical phenotype, silver nucleolar organizer region staining value and post-operative survival in 16 cases. Acta Neuropathol (Berl) 1991;82:208–216.

8. Friede RL, Pollack A. The cytogenetic basis for classifying ependymomas. J Neuropathol Exp Neurol 1978;37:103–118.

9. Gerszten PC, Pollack IF, Martinez AJ, et al. Intracranial ependymomas of childhood: lack of correlation of histopathology and clinical outcome. Pathol Res Pract 1996;192:515–522.

10. Guerrieri C, Jarlsfelt I. Ependymoma of the ovary: a case report with immunohistochemical, ultrastructural, and DNA cytometric findings, as well as histogenetic considerations. Am J Surg Pathol 1993;17:623–632.

11. Hirato J, Nakazato Y, Iijima M, et al. An unusual variant of ependymoma with extensive tumor cell vacuolization. Acta Neuropathol (Berl) 1997;92:310–316.

12. Ho KL, Caccamo DV, Garcia JH. Intracytoplasmic lumina in ependymomas: an ultrastructural study. Ultrastruct Pathol 1994; 18:371–380.
13. Kaneko Y, Takeshita I, Matsushima T, et al. Immunohistochemical study of ependymal neoplasms: histological subtypes and glial and epithelial characteristics. Virchows Arch A Pathol Anat 1990;417:97–103.
14. Kawano N, Ohba Y, Nagashima K. Eosinophilic inclusions in ependymoma represent microlumina: a light and electron microscopic study. Acta Neuropathol (Berl) 2000;99:214–218.
15. Kovalic JJ, Flaris N, Grigsby PW, et al. Intracranial ependymoma long term outcome, patterns of failure. J Neurooncol 1993;15: 125–131.
16. Marchevsky AM. Lung tumors derived from ectopic tissues. Semin Diagn Pathol 1995;12:172–184.
17. Min K-W, Scheithauer BW. Clear cell ependymoma: a mimic of oligodendroglioma: clinicopathologic and ultrastructural considerations. Am J Surg Pathol 1997;21:820–826.
18. Molina OM, Colina JL, Luzardo GD, et al. Extraventricular cerebral anaplastic ependymomas. Surg Neurol 1999;51:630–635.
19. Nawano N, Yada K, Yagishita S. Clear cell ependymoma: a histological variant with diagnostic implications. Virchows Arch A Pathol Anat 1989;415:467–472.
20. Nazar GB, Hoffman HJ, Becker LE, et al. Infratentorial ependymomas in childhood: prognostic factors and treatment. J Neurosurg 1990;72:408–417.
21. Newton HB, Henson J, Walker RW. Extraneural metastases in ependymoma. J Neurooncol 1992;14:135–142.
22. Ng H-K. Cytologic features of ependymomas in smear preparations. Acta Cytol 1994;38:331–334.
23. Nobles E, Lee R, Kircher T. Mediastinal ependymoma. Hum Pathol 1991;22:94–96.
24. Pollack IF, Gerszten PC, Martinez AJ, et al. Intracranial ependymomas of childhood: long-term outcome and prognostic factors. Neurosurgery 1995;37:655–667.
25. Rezai AR, Woo HH, Lee M, et al. Disseminated ependymomas of the central nervous system. J Neurosurg 1996;85:618–624.
26. Robertson PL, Zeltzer PM, Boyett JM, et al. Survival and prognostic factors following radiation therapy and chemotherapy for ependymomas in children: a report of the Children's Cancer Group. J Neurosurg 1998;88:695–703.
27. Rosenblum MK, Erlandson RA, Aleksic SN, Budzilovich GN. Melanotic ependymoma and subependymoma. Am J Surg Pathol 1990;14:729–736.
28. Ruchoux MM, Kepes JJ, Dhellemmes P, et al. Lipomatous differentiation in ependymomas: a report of three cases and comparison with similar changes reported in other central nervous system neoplasms of neuroectodermal origin. Am J Surg Pathol 1998; 22: 338–346.
29. Rushing EJ, Brown DF, Hladik CL, et al. Correlation of bcl-2, p53, and MIB-1 expression with ependymoma grade and subtype. Mod Pathol 1998;11:464–470.
30. Schiffer D, Chiò A, Giordana MT, et al. Histologic prognostic factors in ependymoma. Childs Nerv Syst 1991;7:177–182.
31. Schwartz TH, Kim S, Glick RS, et al. Supratentorial ependymomas in adult patients. Neurosurgery 1999;44:721–731.
32. Shaw EG, Evans RG, Scheithauer BW, et al. Postoperative radiotherapy of intracranial ependymoma in pediatric and adult patients. Int J Radiat Oncol Biol Phys 1987;13:1457–1462.
33. Shuman RM, Alvord EC Jr, Leech RW. The biology of childhood ependymomas. Arch Neurol 1975;32:731–739.
34. Spoto GP, Press GA, Hesselink JR, Murray S. Intracranial ependymoma and subependymoma: MR manifestations. AJNR 1990;154:83–91.
35. Uematsu Y, Rojas-Corona RR, Llena JF, Hirano A. Distribution of epithelial membrane antigen in normal and neoplastic human ependyma. Acta Neuropathol (Berl) 1989;78:325–328.

## Subependymoma

1. Azzarelli B, Rekate HL, Roessmann U. Subependymoma: a case report with ultrastructural study. Acta Neuropathol (Berl) 1977; 40:279–282.
2. Changaris DG, Powers JM, Perot PL Jr, et al. Subependymoma presenting as subarachnoid hemorrhage: case report. J Neurosurg 1981;55:643–645.
3. Cheng TM, Coffey RJ, Gelber BR, Scheithauer BW. Simul-
taneous presentation of symptomatic subependymomas in siblings: case reports and review. Neurosurgery 1993;33:145–150.
4. Chiechi MV, Smirniotopoulos JG, Jones RV. Intracranial subependymomas: CT and MR imaging features in 24 cases. AJR 1995;165:1245–1250.
5. Fu Y-S, Chen ATL, Kay S, Young HF. Is subependymoma (subependymal glomerate astrocytoma) an astrocytoma or ependymoma? A comparative ultrastructural and tissue culture study. Cancer 1974;34:1992–2008.
6. Gandolfi A, Brizzi RE, Tedeschi F, et al. Symptomatic subependymoma of the fourth ventricle: case report. J Neurosurg 1981;55:841–844.
7. Hoeffel C, Boukobza M, Polivka M, et al. MR manifestations of subependymomas. AJNR 1995;16:2121–2129.
8. Kondziolka D, Bilbao JM. Mixed ependymoma-astrocytoma (subependymoma?) of the cerebral cortex. Acta Neuropathol (Berl) 1988;76:633–637.
9. Lombardi D, Scheithauer BW, Meyer FB, et al. Symptomatic subependymoma: a clinicopathological and flow cytometric study. J Neurosurg 1991;75:583–588.
10. Louis DN, Hedley-Whyte ET, Martuza RL. Case report: sarcomatous proliferation of the vasculature in subependymoma. Acta Neuropathol (Berl) 1989;78:332–335.
11. Maiuri F, Gangemi M, Iaconetta G, et al. Symptomatic subependymomas of the lateral ventricles: report of eight cases. Clin Neurol Neurosurg 1997;99:17–22.
12. Nishio S, Fujiwara S, Tashima T, et al. Tumors of the lateral ventricular wall, especially the septum pellucidum: clinical presentation and variations in pathological features. Neurosurgery 1990;27:224–230.
13. Prayson RA, Suh JH. Subependymomas: clinicopathologic study of 14 tumors, including comparative MIB-1 immunohistochemical analysis with other ependymal neoplasms. Arch Pathol Lab Med 1999;123:306–309 (see comments).
14. Rea GL, Akerson RD, Rockswold GL, Smith SA. Subependymoma in a 2½-year-old boy: case report. J Neurosurg 1983; 59: 1088–1091.
15. Rosenblum MK, Erlandson RA, Aleksic SN, Budzilovich GN. Melanotic ependymoma and subependymoma. Am J Surg Pathol 1990;14:729–736.
16. Scheithauer BW. Symptomatic subependymoma: report of 21 cases with review of the literature. J Neurosurg 1978;49:689–696.
17. Tomlinson FH, Scheithauer BW, Kelly PJ, Gorbes GS. Subependymoma with rhabdomyosarcomatous differentiation: report of a case and literature review. Neurosurgery 1991;28:761–768.
18. Yamasaki T, Kikuchi H, Higashi T, et al. Two surgically cured cases of subependymoma with emphasis on magnetic resonance imaging. Surg Neurol 1990;33:329–335.

## Astroblastoma

1. Baka JJ, Patel SC, Roebuck JR, Hearshen DO. Predominantly extraaxial astroblastoma: imaging and proton MR spectroscopy features. AJNR 1993;14:946–950.
2. Bonnin JM, Rubinstein LJ. Astroblastomas: a pathological study of 23 tumors, with a postoperative follow-up in 13 patients. Neurosurgery 1989;25:6–13.
3. Brat DJ, Hirose Y, Cohen KJ, et al. Astroblastoma: clinicopathologic features and chromosomal abnormalities defined by comparative genomic hybridization. Brain Pathol 2000;10:342–352.
4. Budka H. Non-glial specificities of immunohistochemistry for the glial fibrillary acidic protein (GFAP). Acta Neuropathol (Berl) 1986;72:43–54.
5. Cabello A, Madero S, Castresana A, Diaz-Lobato R. Astroblastoma: electron microscopy and immunohistochemical findings: case report. Surg Neurol 1991;35:116–121.
6. Husain AN, Leestma JE. Cerebral astroblastoma: immunohistochemical and ultrastructural features. J Neurosurg 1986;64: 657–661.
7. Jay V, Edwards V, Squire J, Rutka J. Astroblastoma: report of a case with ultrastructural, cell kinetic, and cytogenetic analysis. Pediatr Pathol 1993;13:323–332.
8. Pizer BL, Moss T, Oakhill A, et al. Congenital astroblastoma: an immunohistochemical study. Case report. J Neurosurg 1995;83: 550–555.
9. Rubinstein LJ, Herman MM. The astroblastoma and its possible cytogenic relationship to the tanycyte: an electron microscopic,

immunohistochemical, tissue- and organ-culture study. Acta Neuropathol (Berl) 1989;78:472–483.

10. Thiessen B, Finlay J, Kulkarni R, Rosenblum MK. Astroblastoma: does histology predict biologic behavior? J Neurooncol 1998; 40:59–65.

### Chordoid Glioma of the Third Ventricle

1. Brat DJ, Scheithauer BW, Staugaitis SM, et al. Third ventricular chordoid glioma: a distinct clinicopathologic entity. J Neuropathol Exp Neurol 1998;57:283–290.
2. Cenacchi G, Roncaroli F, Cerasoli S, et al. Chordoid neoplasm of the third ventricle: an ultrastructural study of three cases with a histogenetic hypothesis. Am J Surg Pathol 2001;25:401–405.
3. Pomper MG, Passe TJ, Burger PC, et al. Chordoid glioma: a neoplasm unique to the hypothalamus and anterior third ventricle. AJNR 2001;22:464–469.
4. Relfenberger G, Weber T, Weber RG, et al. Chordoid glioma of the third ventricle: immunohistochemical and molecular genetic characterization of a novel tumor entity. Brain Pathol 1999; 9:617–626.
5. Ricoy JR, Lobato RD, Baez B, et al. Suprasellar chordoid glioma. Acta Neuropathol (Berl) 2000;99:699–703.

### Choroid Plexus Papilloma and Carcinoma

1. Ajir F, Chanbusarakum K, Bolles JC. Acinar choroid plexus adenoma of the fourth ventricle. Surg Neurol 1982;17:290–292.
2. Albrecht S, Rouah E, Becker LE, Bruner J. Transthyretin immunoreactivity in choroid plexus neoplasms and brain metastases. Mod Pathol 1991;4:610–614.
3. Anderson DR, Falcone S, Bruce JH, et al. Radiologic-pathologic correlation: congenital choroid plexus papillomas. AJNR 1995; 16:2072–2076.
4. Andreini L, Doglioni C, Giangaspero F. Tubular adenoma of choroid plexus: a case report. Clin Neuropathol 1991;10: 137–140.
5. Ang LC, Taylor AR, Bergin D, Kaufmann JCE. An immunohistochemical study of papillary tumors in the central nervous system. Cancer 1990;65:2712–2719.
6. Berger C, Thiesse P, Lellouch-Tubiana A, et al. Choroid plexus carcinomas in childhood: clinical features and prognostic factors. Neurosurgery 1998;42:470–475.
7. Body G, Darnis E, Pourcelot D, et al. Choroid plexus tumors: antenatal diagnosis and follow-up. J Clin Ultrasound 1990;18: 575–578.
8. Buetow PC, Smirniotopoulos JG, Done S. Congenital brain tumors: a review of 45 cases. AJR 1990;155:587–593.
9. Coffin CM, Wick MR, Braun JT, Dehner LP. Choroid plexus neoplasms: clinicopathologic and immunohistochemical studies. Am J Surg Pathol 1986;10:394–404.
10. Costa JM, Ley L, Claramunt E, Lafuente J. Choroid plexus papillomas of the III ventricle in infants: report of three cases. Childs Nerv Syst 1997;13:244–249.
11. Cruz-Sanchez FF, Rossi ML, Hughes JT, et al. Choroid plexus papillomas: an immunohistological study of 16 cases. Histopathology 1989;15:61–69.
12. Dohrmann GJ, Bucy PC. Human choroid plexus: a light and electron microscopic study. J Neurosurg 1970;33:506–516.
13. Doran SE, Blaivas M, Dauser RC. Bone formation within a choroid plexus papilloma. Pediatr Neurosurg 1995;23:216–218.
14. Duckett S, Osterholm J, Schaefer D, et al. Ossified mucin-secreting choroid plexus adenoma: case report. Neurosurgery 1991; 29:130–132.
15. Duffner PK, Kun LE, Burger PC, et al. Postoperative chemotherapy and delayed radiation in infants and very young children with choroid plexus carcinomas. Pediatr Neurosurg 1995;22:189–196.
16. Furness PN, Lowe J, Tarrant GS. Subepithelial basement membrane deposition and intermediate filament expression in choroid plexus neoplasms and ependymomas. Histopathology 1990;16: 251–255.
17. Garber JE, Burke EM, Lavally BL, et al. Choroid plexus tumors in the breast cancer–sarcoma syndrome. Cancer 1990;66: 2658–2660.
18. Geerts Y, Gabreëls F, Lippens R, et al. Choroid plexus carcinoma: a report of two cases and review of the literature. Neuropediatrics 1996;27:143–148.
19. Gudeman SK, Sullivan HG, Rosner MJ, Becker DP. Surgical removal of bilateral papillomas of the choroid plexus of the lateral ventricles with resolution of hydrocephalus: case report. J Neurosurg 1979;50:677–681.
20. Gullotta F, de Melo AS. Das Karzinom des Plexus choroideus. Klinische, lichtmikroskopische und elektronenoptische Untersuchungen. Neurochirurgia 1979;22:1–9.
21. Gyure KA, Morrison AL. Expression of neuronal neuroendocrine markers in choroid plexus tumors. J Neuropathol Exp Neurol 2000;59:420.
22. Herbert J, Cavallaro T, Dwork AJ. A marker for primary choroid plexus neoplasms. Am J Pathol 1990;136:1317–1325.
23. Jay V, Ho M, Chan F, Malkin D. p53 Expression in choroid plexus neoplasms: an immunohistochemical study. Arch Pathol Lab Med 1996;120:1061–1065.
24. Ken JG, Sobel DF, Copeland B, et al. Choroid plexus papillomas of the foramen of Luschka: MR appearance. AJNR 1991;12: 1201–1203.
25. Kepes JJ, Collins J. Choroid plexus epithelium (normal and neoplastic) expresses synaptophysin: a potentially useful aid in differentiating carcinoma of the choroid plexus from metastatic papillary carcinomas. J Neuropathol Exp Neurol 1999;58:398–401.
26. Lana-Peixoto MA, Lagos J, Silbert SW. Primary pigmented carcinoma of the choroid plexus: a light and electron microscopic study. J Neurosurg 1977;47:442–450.
27. Leblanc R, Bekhor S, Melanson D, Carpenter S. Diffuse craniospinal seeding from a benign fourth ventricle choroid plexus papilloma: case report. J Neurosurg 1998;88:757–760.
28. Mannoji H, Becker LE. Ependymal and choroid plexus tumors. Cancer 1988;61:1377–1385.
29. Matsushima T. Choroid plexus papillomas and human choroid plexus: a light and electron microscopic study. J Neurosurg 1983;59:1054–1062.
30. McComb RD, Burger PC. Choroid plexus carcinoma: report of a case with immunohistochemical and ultrastructural observations. Cancer 1983;51:470–475.
31. McGirr SJ, Ebersold MJ, Scheithauer BW, et al. Choroid plexus papillomas: long-term follow-up results in a surgically treated series. J Neurosurg 1988;69:843–849.
32. Navas JJ, Battifora H. Choroid plexus papilloma: light and electron microscopic study of three cases. Acta Neuropathol (Berl) 1978;44:235–239.
33. Packer RJ, Perilongo G, Johnson D, et al. Choroid plexus carcinoma of childhood. Cancer 1992;69:580–585.
34. Paulus W, Brandner S. Synaptophysin in choroid plexus epithelial cells: no useful aid in differential diagnosis (Letter). J Neuropathol Exp Neurol 1999;58:1111–1112.
35. Paulus W, Jänisch W. Clinicopathologic correlations in epithelial choroid plexus neoplasms: a study of 52 cases. Acta Neuropathol (Berl) 1990;80:635–641.
36. Pencalet P, Sainte-Rose C, Lellouch-Tubiana A, et al. Papillomas and carcinomas of the choroid plexus in children. J Neurosurg 1998;88:521–528.
37. Reimund EL, Sitton JE, Harkin JC. Pigmented choroid plexus papilloma. Arch Pathol Lab Med 1990;114:902–905.
38. Stefanko SZ, Vuzevski VD. Oncocytic variant of choroid plexus papilloma. Acta Neuropathol (Berl) 1985;66:160–162.
39. Talacchi A, de Micheli E, Lombardo C, et al. Choroid plexus papilloma of the cerebellopontine angle: a twelve patient series. Surg Neurol 1999;51:621–629.
40. Tomita T, Naidich TP. Successful resection of choroid plexus papillomas diagnosed at birth: report of two cases. Neurosurgery 1987;20:774–779.
41. Tomlinson FA, Scheithauer BW, Hammack JE, et al. Choroid plexus neoplasia: a correlative clinical and pathologic study. J Neuropathol Exp Neurol 1995;54:423.
42. Trifiletti RR, Incorpora G, Polizzi A, et al. Aicardi syndrome with multiple tumors: a case report with literature review. Brain Dev 1995;17:283–285.
43. Vital A, Bringuier P-B, Huang H, et al. Astrocytomas and choroid plexus tumors in two families with identical p53 germline mutations. J Neuropathol Exp Neurol 1998;57:1061–1069.
44. Watanabe K, Ando Y, Iwanaga H, et al. Choroid plexus papilloma containing melanin pigment. Clin Neuropathol 1995;14:159–161.
45. Yuasa H, Tokito S, Tokunaga M. Primary carcinoma of the

choroid plexus in Li-Fraumeni syndrome: case report. Neurosurgery 1993;32:131–134.

## Gangliocytoma and Ganglioglioma

1. Brat DJ, Gearing M, Goldthwaite PT, et al. Tau-associated neuropathology in ganglion cell tumours increases with patient age but appears unrelated to ApoE genotype. Neuropathol Appl Neurobiol 2001;27:197–205.
2. Caccamo D, Herman MM, Urich H, Rubinstein LJ. Focal neuronal gigantism and cerebral cortical thickening after therapeutic irradiation of the central nervous system. Arch Pathol Lab Med 1989;113:880–885.
3. Castillo M, Davis PC, Takei Y, Hoffman JC Jr. Intracranial ganglioglioma: MR, CT, and clinical findings in 18 patients. AJNR 1990;11:109–114.
4. Diepholder HM, Schwechheimer K, Mohadjer M, et al. A clinicopathologic and immunomorphologic study of 13 cases of ganglioglioma. Cancer 1991;68:2192–2201.
5. Faillot T, Sichez J-P, Capelle L, et al. Ganglioglioma of the pineal region: case report and review of the literature. Surg Neurol 1998;49:104–108.
6. Giangaspero F, Burger PC, Budwit DA, et al. Regulatory peptides in neuronal neoplasms of the central nervous system. Clin Neuropathol 1985;4:111–115.
7. Gultekin SH, Dalmau J, Graus Y, et al. Anti-Hu immunolabeling as an index of neuronal differentiation in human brain tumors: a study of 112 central neuroepithelial neoplasms. Am J Surg Pathol 1998;22:195–200.
8. Haddad SF, Moore SA, Menezes AH, VanGilder JC. Ganglioglioma: 13 years of experience. Neurosurgery 1992;31: 171–178.
9. Handa J, Yamagami T, Furuta M. An adult patient with cerebellar ganglioglioma. J Neurooncol 1994;18:183–189.
10. Hashimoto M, Fujimoto K, Shinoda S, Masuzawa T. Magnetic resonance imaging of ganglion cell tumours. Neuroradiology 1993;35:181–184.
11. Hirose T, Scheithauer BW, Lopes MB, et al. Ganglioglioma: an ultrastructural and immunohistochemical study. Cancer 1997;79:989–1003.
12. Hori A, Weiss R, Schaake T. Ganglioglioma containing osseous tissue and neurofibrillary tangles. Arch Pathol Lab Med 1988;112:653–655.
13. Hunt SJ, Johnson PC. Melanotic ganglioglioma of the pineal region. Acta Neuropathol (Berl) 1989;79:222–225.
14. Jaffey PB, Mundt AJ, Baunoch DA, et al. The clinical significance of extracellular matrix in gangliogliomas. J Neuropathol Exp Neurol 1996;55:1246–1252.
15. Karamitopoulou E, Perentes E, Probst A, Wegmann W. Ganglioglioma of the brain stem: neurological dysfunction of 16-year duration. Clin Neuropathol 1995;14:162–168.
16. Khajavi K, Comair YG, Prayson RA, et al. Childhood ganglioglioma and medically intractable epilepsy: a clinicopathological study of 15 patients and a review of the literature. Pediatr Neurosurg 1995;22:181–188.
17. Lindboe CF, Hansen HB. Epiperikaryal synaptophysin reactivity in the normal human central nervous system. Clin Neuropathol 1998;17:237–240.
18. Liu GT, Galetta SL, Rorke LB, et al. Gangliogliomas involving the optic chiasm. Neurology 1996;46:1669–1673.
19. Miller DC, Koslow M, Budzilovich GN, Burstein DE. Synaptophysin: a sensitive and specific marker for ganglion cells in central nervous system neoplasms. Hum Pathol 1990;21:271–276.
20. Prayson RA, Khajava K, Comair YG. Cortical architectural abnormalities and MIB1 immunoreactivity in gangliogliomas: a study of 60 patients with intracranial tumors. J Neuropathol Exp Neurol 1995;54:513–520.
21. Quinn B. Synaptophysin staining in normal brain: importance for diagnosis of ganglioglioma. Am J Surg Pathol 1998;22:550–556.
22. Rubinstein LJ, Herman MM. A light- and electron-microscopic study of a temporal-lobe ganglioglioma. J Neurol Sci 1972;16:27–48.
23. Scheithauer BW, Gay D, Kispert B, et al. Ganglioglioma: a clinicopathologic, radiologic, and immunocytologic study of 31 surgically treated cases diagnosed over a 40-year period. Pathol Res Pract, in press.
24. Silver JM, Rawlings CE III, Rossitch E Jr, et al. Ganglioglioma: a clinical study with long-term follow-up. Surg Neurol 1991;35:261–266.
25. Smith NM, Carli MM, Hanieh A, et al. Gangliogliomas in childhood. Childs Nerv Syst 1992;8:258–262.
26. Takahashi H, Wakabayashi K, Kawai K, et al. Neuroendocrine markers in central nervous system neuronal tumors (gangliocytoma and ganglioglioma). Acta Neuropathol (Berl) 1989;77: 237–243.
27. Tampieri D, Moumdjian R, Melanson D, Ethier R. Intracerebral gangliogliomas in patients with partial complex seizures: CT and MR imaging findings. AJNR 1991;12:749–755.
28. Tien RD, Tuori SL, Pulkingham N, Burger PC. Ganglioglioma with leptomeningeal and subarachnoid spread: results of CT, MR and PET imaging. AJR 1992;159:391–393.
29. Tihan T, Brat DJ, Goldthwaite PT, Burger PC. Glioneuronal tumors with malignant histological features. J Neuropathol Exp Neurol 1999;58:509.
30. Wolf HK, Buslei R, Schmidt-Kastner R, et al. NeuN: a useful neuronal marker for diagnostic histopathology. J Histochem Cytochem 1996;44:1167–1171.
31. Zentner J, Wolf HK, Ostertun B, et al. Gangliogliomas: clinical, radiological, and histopathological findings in 51 patients. J Neurol Neurosurg Psychiatry 1994;57:1497–1502.
32. Zhang PJ, Rosenblum MK. Synaptophysin expression in the human spinal cord: diagnostic implications of an immunohistochemical study. Am J Surg Pathol 1996;20:273–276.

## Desmoplastic Infantile Ganglioglioma

1. Aydin F, Ghatak NR, Salvant J, Muizelaar P. Desmoplastic cerebral astrocytoma of infancy. Acta Neuropathol (Berl) 1993;86:666–670.
2. de Chadarévian J-P, Pattisapu JV, Faerber EN. Desmoplastic cerebral astrocytoma of infancy. Cancer 1990;66:173–179.
3. Duffner PK, Burger PC, Cohen ME, et al. Desmoplastic infantile gangliogliomas: an approach to therapy. Neurosurgery 1994;34:583–589.
4. Gultekin SH, Dalmau J, Graus Y, et al. Anti-Hu immunolabeling as an index of neuronal differentiation in human brain tumors. Am J Surg Pathol 1998;22:195–200.
5. Louis DN, von Deimling A, Dickersin RG, et al. Desmoplastic cerebral astrocytomas of infancy: a histopathologic, immunohistochemical, ultrastructural, and molecular genetic study. Hum Pathol 1992;23:1402–1409.
6. Mallucci C, Lellouch-Tubiana A, Salazar C, et al. The management of desmoplastic neuroepithelial tumours in childhood. Childs Nerv Syst 2000;16:8–14.
7. Martin DS, Levy B, Awwad EE, Pittman T. Desmoplastic infantile ganglioglioma: CT and MR features. AJNR 1991;12:1195–1197.
8. Parisi JE, Scheithauer BW, Priest JR, et al. Desmoplastic infantile ganglioglioma (DIG): a form of ganglioglioma. J Neuropathol Exp Neurol 1992;51:365.
9. Paulus W, Scholte W, Perentes E, et al. Desmoplastic supratentorial neuroepithelial tumours of infancy. Histopathology 1992;21: 43–49.
10. Taratuto AL, Monges J, Lylyk P, Leiguarda R. Superficial cerebral astrocytoma attached to dura: report of six cases in infants. Cancer 1984;54:2505–2512.
11. VandenBerg SR. Desmoplastic infantile ganglioglioma and desmoplastic cerebral astrocytoma of infancy. Brain Pathol 1993;3:275–281.
12. VandenBerg SR, May EE, Rubinstein LR, et al. Desmoplastic supratentorial neuroepithelial tumors of infancy with divergent differentiation potential ("desmoplastic infantile gangliogliomas"): report on 11 cases of a distinctive embryonal tumor with favorable prognosis. J Neurosurg 1987;66:58–71.

## Dysplastic Cerebellar Gangliocytoma (Lhermitte-Duclos Disease)

1. Ambler M, Pogacar S, Sidman R. Lhermitte-Duclos disease (granule cell hypertrophy of the cerebellum): pathological analysis of the first familial cases. J Neuropathol Exp Neurol 1969;28:622–647.
2. Ashley DG, Zee C-S, Chandrasoma PT, Segall HD. Case report. Lhermitte-Duclos disease: CT and MR findings. J Comput Assist Tomogr 1990;14:984–987.

3. Carter JE, Merren MD, Swann KW. Preoperative diagnosis of Lhermitte-Duclos disease by magnetic resonance imaging. J Neurosurg 1989;70:135–137.

4. Koch R, Scholz M, Nelen MR, et al. Lhermitte-Duclos disease as a component of Cowden's syndrome. J Neurosurg 1999;90:776–779.

5. Lindboe CF, Helseth E, Myhr G. Lhermitte-Duclos disease and giant meningioma as manifestations of Cowden's disease. Clin Neuropathol 1995;14:327–330.

6. Marano SR, Johnson PC, Spetzler RF. Recurrent Lhermitte-Duclos disease in a child: case report. J Neurosurg 1988;69:599–603.

7. Milbouw G, Born JD, Martin D, et al. Clinical and radiological aspects of dysplastic gangliocytoma (Lhermitte-Duclos disease): a report of two cases with review of the literature. Neurosurgery 1988;22:124–128.

8. Padberg PW, Schot JDL, Vielvoye GJ, et al. Lhermitte-Duclos disease and Cowden disease: a single phakomatosis. Ann Neurol 1991;29:517–523.

9. Pritchett PS, King TI. Dysplastic gangliocytoma of the cerebellum—an ultrastructural study. Acta Neuropathol (Berl) 1978;42:1–5.

10. Reeder RF, Saunders RL, Roberts DW, et al. Magnetic resonance imaging in the diagnosis and treatment of Lhermitte-Duclos disease (dysplastic gangliocytoma of the cerebellum). Neurosurgery 1988;23:240–245.

11. Reznik M, Schoenen J. Lhermitte-Duclos disease. Acta Neuropathol (Berl) 1983;59:88–94.

12. Rimbau J, Isamat F. Dysplastic gangliocytoma of the cerebellum (Lhermitte-Duclos disease) and its relation to the multiple hamartoma syndrome (Cowden disease). J Neurooncol 1994;18:191–198.

13. Robinson S, Cohen AR. Cowden disease and Lhermitte-Duclos disease: characterization of a new phakomatosis. Neurosurgery 2000;46:371–383.

14. Williams DW III, Elster AD, Ginsberg LE, Stanton C. Recurrent Lhermitte-Duclos disease: report of two cases and association with Cowden's disease. AJNR 1992;13:287–290.

15. Yachnis AT, Trojanowski JQ, Memmo M, Schlaepfer WW. Expression of neurofilament proteins in the hypertrophic granule cells of Lhermitte-Duclos disease: an explanation for the mass effect and the myelination of parallel fibers in the disease state. J Neuropathol Exp Neurol 1988;47:206–216.

## Dysembryoplastic Neuroepithelial Tumor

1. Baisden BL, Brat DJ, Melhem ER, et al. Dysembryoplastic neuroepithelial tumor–like neoplasm of the septum pellucidum: a lesion often misdiagnosed as glioma: report of 10 cases. Am J Surg Pathol 2001;25:494–499.

2. Cervera-Pierot P, Varlet P, Chodkiewicz J-P, Daumas-Duport C. Dysembryoplastic neuroepithelial tumors located in the caudate nucleus area: report of four cases. Neurosurgery 1997;40:1065–1070.

3. Daumas-Duport C. Dysembryoplastic neuroepithelial tumours. Brain Pathol 1993;3:283–295.

4. Daumas-Duport C, Scheithauer BW, Chodkiewicz J-P, et al. Dysembryoplastic neuroepithelial tumor: a surgically curable tumor of young patients with intractable partial seizures. Report of thirty-nine cases. Neurosurgery 1988;23:545–556.

5. Daumas-Duport C, Varlet P, Bacha S, et al. Dysembryoplastic neuroepithelial tumors: nonspecific histological forms—a study of 40 cases. J Neurooncol 1999;41:267–280.

6. Fujimoto K, Ohnishi H, Tsujimoto M, et al. Dysembryoplastic neuroepithelial tumor of the cerebellum and brainstem: case report. J Neurosurg 2000;93:487–489.

7. Gyure KA, Sandberg GD, Prayson RA, et al. Dysembryoplastic neuroepithelial tumor: an immunohistochemical study with myelin oligodendrocyte glycoprotein. Arch Pathol Lab Med 2000;124:123–126.

8. Hirose T, Scheithauer BW, Lopes MBS, VandenBerg SR. Dysembryoplastic neuroepithelial tumor (DNT): an immunohistochemical and ultrastructural study. J Neuropathol Exp Neurol 1994;53:184–195.

9. Hirose T, Scheithauer BW. Mixed dysembryoplastic neuroepithelial tumor and ganglioglioma. Acta Neuropathol (Berl) 1998;95:649–654.

10. Kuchelmeister K, Demirel T, Schlörer E, et al. Dysembryoplastic neuroepithelial tumour of the cerebellum. Acta Neuropathol (Berl) 1995;89:385–390.

11. Leung SY, Gwi E, Ng HK, Yam KY. Dysembryoplastic neuroepithelial tumor. Am J Surg Pathol 1994;18:604–614.

12. Ostertun B, Wolf HK, Campos MG, et al. Dysembryoplastic neuroepithelial tumors: MR and CT evaluation. AJNR 1996;17:419–430.

13. Prayson RA. Composite ganglioglioma and dysembryoplastic neuroepithelial tumor. Arch Pathol Lab Med 1999;123:247–250.

14. Prayson RA, Morris HH, Estes ML, Comair YG. Dysembryoplastic neuroepithelial tumor: a clinicopathologic and immunohistochemical study of 11 tumors including MIB1 immunoreactivity. Clin Neuropathol 1996;15:47–53.

15. Raymond AA, Halpin SFS, Alsangari N, et al. Dysembryoplastic neuroepithelial tumor: features in 16 patients. Brain 1994;117:461–475.

16. Scully RE, Mark EJ, McNeely WF, et al. Dysembryoplastic neuroepithelial tumors: case records of the Massachusetts General Hospital. Case 14-1997. N Engl J Med 1997;336:1373–1379.

17. Shimada A, Chin SS, Goldman JE, et al. Dysembryoplastic neuroepithelial tumor occurring within the midbrain. J Neuropathol Exp Neurol 1996;55:623.

18. Taratuto AL, Pomata H, Sevlever G, et al. Dysembryoplastic neuroepithelial tumor: morphological, immunocytochemical, and deoxyribonucleic acid analysis in a pediatric series. Neurosurgery 1995;36:474–481.

19. Wolf HK, Buslei R, Blümcke I, et al. Neural antigens in oligodendrogliomas and dysembryoplastic neuroepithelial tumors. Acta Neuropathol (Berl) 1997;94:436–443.

20. Yasha TC, Mohanty A, Radhesh S, et al. Infratentorial dysembryoplastic neuroepithelial tumor (DNT) associated with Arnold-Chiari malformation. Clin Neuropathol 1998;17:305–310.

## Hypothalamic Hamartoma

1. Alvarez-Garijo JA, Albiach VJ, Vila MM, et al. Precocious puberty and hypothalamic hamartoma with total recovery after surgical treatment: case report. J Neurosurg 1983;58:583–585.

2. Curnes JT, Oakes WJ, Burger PC, Boyko OB. Hamartomas of the tuber cinereum: CT and MR imaging. AJNR 1991;12:309–314.

3. Fukuda M, Kameyama S, Wachi M, Tanaka R. Stereotaxy for hypothalamic hamartoma with intractable gelastic seizures: technical case report. Neurosurgery 1999;44:1347–1350.

4. Guibaud L, Rode V, Sainte-Pierre G, et al. Giant hypothalamic hamartoma: an unusual neonatal tumor. Pediatr Radiol 1995;25:17–18.

5. Price RA, Lee PA, Albright AL, et al. Treatment of sexual precocity by removal of a luteinizing hormone–releasing hormone secreting hamartoma. JAMA 1984;251:2247–2249.

6. Sato M, Ushio Y, Arita N, Mogami H. Hypothalamic hamartoma—report of two cases. Neurosurgery 1985;16:198–206.

7. Sherwin RP, Grassi JE, Sommers SC. Hamartomatous malformation of the posterolateral hypothalamus. Lab Invest 1962;11:89–97.

8. Stewart L, Steinbok P, Daaboul J. Role of surgical resection in the treatment of hypothalamic hamartomas causing precocious puberty: report of six cases. J Neurosurg 1998;88:340–345.

9. Takeuchi J, Handa H, Miki Y, et al. Precocious puberty due to a hypothalamic hamartoma. Surg Neurol 1979;11:456–460.

10. Valdueza JM, Cristante L, Dammann O, et al. Hypothalamic hamartomas: with special reference to gelastic epilepsy and surgery. Neurosurgery 1994;34:949–958.

## Central Neurocytoma

1. Brandes AA, Amista P, Gardiman M, et al. Chemotherapy in patients with recurrent and progressive central neurocytoma. Cancer 2000;88:169–174.

2. Christov C, Adle-Biassette H, Le Guerinel C. Recurrent central neurocytoma with marked increase in MIB-1 labelling index. Br J Neurosurg 1999;13:496–499.

3. Eng DY, DeMonte F, Ginsberg L, et al. Craniospinal dissemination of central neurocytoma: report of two cases. J Neurosurg 1997;86:547–552.

4. Figarella-Branger D, Pellissier JF, Daumas-Duport C, et al. Central neurocytomas: critical evaluation of a small-cell neuronal tumor. Am J Surg Pathol 1992;16:97–109.

5. Goergen SK, Gonzales MF, McLean CA. Intraventricular neuro-cytoma: radiologic features and review of the literature. Radiology 1992;182:787–792.
6. Gultekin SH, Dalmau J, Graus Y, et al. Anti-Hu immunolabeling as an index of neuronal differentiation in human brain tumors: a study of 112 central neuroepithelial neoplasms. Am J Surg Pathol 1998;22:195–200.
7. Hassoun J, Gambarelli D, Grisoli F, et al. Central neurocytoma: an electron-microscopic study of two cases. Acta Neuropathol (Berl) 1982;56:151–156.
8. Hessler RB, Lopes MBS, Frankfurter A, et al. Cytoskeletal immunohistochemistry of central neurocytomas. Am J Surg Pathol 1992;16:1031–1038.
9. Ishiuchi S, Tamura M. Central neurocytoma: an immunohisto-chemical, ultrastructural and cell culture study. Acta Neuropathol (Berl) 1997;94:425–435.
10. Jay V, Edwards V, Hoving E, et al. Central neurocytoma: morpho-logical, flow cytometric, polymerase chain reaction, fluorescence in situ hybridization, and karyotypic analyses. J Neurosurg 1999;90:348–354.
11. Kim DG, Chi JG, Park SH, et al. Intraventricular neurocytoma: clinicopathological analysis of seven cases. J Neurosurg 1992;76:759–765.
12. Kim DG, Choe WJ, Chang KH, et al. In vivo proton magnetic resonance spectroscopy of central neurocytomas. Neurosurgery 2000;46:329–333; discussion 33–34.
13. Laeng RH, Scheithauer BW, Altermatt HJ. Anti-neuronal nuclear autoantibodies, types 1 and 2: their utility in the study of tumors of the nervous system. Acta Neuropathol (Berl) 1998;96:329–339.
14. Ng TH, Wong AY, Boadle R, Compton JS. Pigmented central neurocytoma: case report and literature review. Am J Surg Pathol 1999;23:1136–1140.
15. Nishio S, Takeshita I, Fukui M. Primary cerebral ganglioneurocy-toma in an adult. Cancer 1990;66:358–362.
16. Schild SE, Scheithauer BW, Haddock MG, et al. Central neuro-cytomas. Cancer 1997;79:790–795.
17. Schweitzer JB, Davies KG. Differentiating central neurocytoma: case report. J Neurosurg 1997;86:543–546.
18. Smoker WRK, Townsend JJ, Reichman MV. Neurocytoma accom-panied by intraventricular hemorrhage: case report and literature review. AJNR 1991;12:765–770.
19. Söylemezoglu F, Scheithauer BW, Esteve J, Kleihues P. Atypical central neurocytoma. J Neuropathol Exp Neurol 1997;56:551–556.
20. von Deimling A, Janzer R, Kleihues P, Wiestler OD. Patterns of differentiation in central neurocytoma: an immunohistochemical study of eleven biopsies. Acta Neuropathol (Berl) 1990;79:473–479.
21. Westphal M, Stavrou D, Nausch H, et al. Human neurocytoma cells in culture show characteristics of astroglial differentiation. J Neurosci Res 1994;38:698–704.

## Extraventricular (Parenchymal) Neurocytic Neoplasms

1. Alleyne CH Jr, Hunter S, Olson JJ, Barrow DL. Lipomatous glioneurocytoma of the posterior fossa with divergent differentia-tion: case report. Neurosurgery 1998;42:639–643.
2. Bouvier-Labit C, Daniel L, Dufour H, et al. Papillary glioneu-ronal tumour: clinicopathological and biochemical study of one case with 7-year follow up. Acta Neuropathol (Berl) 2000;99:321–326.
3. Chimelli L, Hahn MD, Budka H. Lipomatous differentiation in a medulloblastoma. Acta Neuropathol (Berl) 1991;81:471–473.
4. Ellison DW, Zygmunt SC, Weller RO. Case report: neurocy-toma/lipoma (neurolipocytoma) of the cerebellum. Neuropathol Appl Neurobiol 1993;19:95–98.
5. Enam SA, Rosenblum ML, Ho K-L. Neurocytoma in the cere-bellum: case report. J Neurosurg 1997;87:100–102.
6. Giangaspero F, Cenacchi G, Losi L, et al. Extraventricular neo-plasms with neurocytoma features: a clinicopathological study of 11 cases. Am J Surg Pathol 1997;21:206–212.
7. Giangaspero F, Cenacchi G, Roncaroli F, et al. Medullocytoma (lipidized medulloblastoma): a cerebellar neoplasm of adults with favorable prognosis. Am J Surg Pathol 1996;20:656–664.
8. González-Cámpora R, Wellert RO. Lipidized mature neuroecto-dermal tumour of the cerebellum with myoid differentiation. Neuropathol Appl Neurobiol 1998;24:397–402.

9. Gultekin SH, Teo JGC, Rosenblum MK. Rosetted glioneuronal tumors of the cerebrum. J Neuropathol Exp Neurol 1999;58:510.
10. Kim DH, Suh Y-L. Pseudopapillary neurocytoma of temporal lobe with glial differentiation. Acta Neuropathol (Berl) 1997;94:187–191.
11. Komori T, Scheithauer BW, Anthony DC, et al. Papillary glione-uronal tumor: a new variant of mixed neuronal-glial neoplasm. Am J Surg Pathol 1998;22:1171–1183.
12. Louis DN, Swearingen B, Linggood RM, et al. Central nervous system neurocytoma and neuroblastoma in adults—report of eight cases. J Neurooncol 1990;9:231–238.
13. Miller DC, Kim R, Zagzag D. Neurocytomas: non-classical sites and mixed elements. J Neuropathol Exp Neurol 1992;51:364.
14. Nishio S, Takeshita I, Fukui M. Primary cerebral ganglioneurocy-toma in an adult. Cancer 1990;66:358–362.
15. Pal L, Santosh V, Gayathri N, et al. Neurocytoma/rhabdomyoma (myoneurocytoma) of the cerebellum. Acta Neuropathol (Berl) 1998;95:318–323.
16. Söylemezoglu F, Soffer D, Onol B, et al. Lipomatous medul-loblastoma in adults: a distinct clinicopathological entity. Am J Surg Pathol 1996;20:413–418.
17. Teo JC, Gultekin SH, Bilsky M, et al. A distinctive glioneuronal tumor of the adult cerebrum with neuropil-like (including roset-ting) islands: report from a case. Am J Surg Pathol 1999;23:502–510.
18. Warmuth-Metz M, Klein R, Sorensen N, Solymosi L. Central neurocytoma of the fourth ventricle: case report. J Neurosurg 1999;91:506–509.

## Malignant Neuronal and Glioneuronal Tumors

1. Campos MG, Zentner J, Ostertun B, et al. Anaplastic ganglio-glioma: case report and review of the literature. Neurol Res 1994;16:317–320.
2. Dash RC, Provenzale JM, McComb RD, et al. Malignant supra-tentorial ganglioglioma (ganglion cell–giant cell glioblastoma). Arch Pathol Lab Med 1999;123:342–345.
3. Hall WA, Yunis EJ, Albright AL. Anaplastic ganglioglioma in an infant: case report and review of the literature. Neurosurgery 1986;19:1016–1020.
4. Hirose T, Kannuki S, Nishida K, et al. Anaplastic ganglioglioma of the brain stem demonstrating active neurosecretory features of neoplastic neuronal cells. Acta Neuropathol (Berl) 1992;83:365–370.
5. Jay V, Edwards V, Hoving E, et al. Central neurocytoma: morpho-logical, flow cytometric, polymerase chain reaction, fluorescence in situ hybridization, and karyotypic analyses: case report. J Neurosurg 1999;90:348–354.
6. Jay V, Squire J, Becker LE, Humphreys R. Malignant transforma-tion in a ganglioglioma with anaplastic neuronal and astrocytic components. Cancer 1994;73:2862–2868.
7. McLendon RE, Bentley RC, Parisi JE, et al. Malignant supraten-torial glial-neuronal neoplasms: report of two cases and review of the literature. Arch Pathol Lab Med 1997;121:485–492.
8. Sasaki A, Hirato J, Nakazato Y, et al. Recurrent anaplastic gan-glioglioma: pathological characterization of tumor cells. J Neurosurg 1996;84:1055–1059.
9. Teo JGC, Gultekin SH, Bilsky M, et al. A distinctive glioneuronal tu-mor of the adult cerebrum with neuropil-like (inclusing "rosetted") islands: report of 4 cases. Am J Surg Pathol 1999;23: 502–510.
10. Tihan T, Brat TJ, Goldthwaite PT, Burger PC. Glioneuronal tu-mors with malignant histological features. J Neuropathol Exp Neurol 1999;58:509.

## Primary Pineal Parenchymal Neoplasms (Pineocytoma, Pineal Parenchymal Neoplasm of Intermediate Differentiation, and Pineoblastoma)

1. Bagley LJ, Hurst RW, Zimmerman RA, et al. Imaging in the trilat-eral retinoblastoma syndrome. Neuroradiology 1996;38: 166–170.
2. Chang SM, Lillis-Hearne PK, Larson DA, et al. Pineoblastoma in adults. Neurosurgery 1995;37:383–391.
3. Collins VP. Pineocytoma with neuronal differentiation demon-strated immunocytochemically: a case report. Acta Pathol Microbiol Immunol Scand [A] 1987;95:113–117.
4. Fauchon F, Jouvet A, Paquis P, et al. Parenchymal pineal tumors: a clinicopathological study of 76 cases. Int J Radiat Oncol Biol Phys 2000;46:959–968.

5. Fèvre-Montange M, Jouvet A, Privat K, et al. Immunohisto-chemical, ultrastructural, biochemical and in vitro studies of a pineocytoma. Acta Neuropathol (Berl) 1998;95:532–539.
6. Fukushima T, Tomonaga M, Sawada T, Iwasaki H. Pineocytoma with neuronal differentiation: case report. Neurol Med Chir (Tokyo) 1990;30:63–68.
7. Hassoun J, Devictor B, Gambarelli D, et al. Paired twisted filaments: a new ultrastructural marker of human pinealomas. Acta Neuropathol (Berl) 1984;65:163–165.
8. Hassoun J, Gambarelli D, Peragut JC, Toga M. Specific ultrastructural markers of human pinealomas: a study of four cases. Acta Neuropathol (Berl) 1983;62:31–40.
9. Herrick MK, Rubinstein LJ. The cytological differentiating potential of pineal parenchymal neoplasms (true neoplasms): clinicopathological study of 28 tumors. Brain 1979;102:289–320.
10. Jouvet A, Saint-Pierre G, Fauchon F, et al. Pineal parenchymal tumors: a correlation of histological features with prognosis in 66 cases. Brain Pathol 2000;10:49–60.
11. Korf HW, Klein DC, Zigler JS, et al. S-antigen-like immunoreactivity in a human pineocytoma. Acta Neuropathol (Berl) 1986; 69:165–167.
12. Kuchelmeister K, von Borcke IM, Klein H, et al. Pleomorphic pineocytoma with extensive neuronal differentiation: report of two cases. Acta Neuropathol (Berl) 1994;88:448–453.
13. Mena H, Rushing EJ, Ribas JL, et al. Tumors of pineal parenchymal cells: a correlation of histological features, including nucleolar organizer regions, with survival in 35 cases. Hum Pathol 1995; 26:20–30.
14. Min KW, Scheithauer BW, Bauserman SC. Pineal parenchymal tumors: an ultrastructural study with prognostic implications. Ultrastruct Pathol 1994;18:69–85.
15. Min KW, Seo IS, Song J. Postnatal evolution of the human pineal gland: an immunohistochemical study. Lab Invest 1987;57: 724–728.
16. Moller M. The ultrastructure of the human fetal pineal gland. I. Cell types and blood vessels. Cell Tissue Res 1974;152:13–30.
17. Numoto RT. Pineal parenchymal tumors: cell differentiation and prognosis. J Cancer Res Clin Oncol 1994;120:683–690.
18. Paulino AC. Trilateral retinoblastoma: is the location of the intracranial tumor important? Cancer 1999;86:135–141.
19. Perentes E, Rubinstein LJ, Herman MM, Donoso LA. S-antigen immunoreactivity in human pineal glands and pineal parenchymal tumors: a monoclonal antibody study. Acta Neuropathol (Berl) 1986;71:224–227.
20. Raisanen J, Vogel H, Horoupian DS. Primitive pineal tumor with retinoblastomatous and retinal/ciliary epithelial differentiation: an immunohistochemical study. J Neurooncol 1990;9:165–170.
21. Rubinstein LJ, Ozazaki H. Gangliogliomatous differentiation in a pineocytoma. J Pathol 1970;102:27–32.
22. Schild SE, Scheithauer BW, Haddock MG, et al. Histologically confirmed pineal tumors and other germ cell tumors of the brain. Cancer 1996;78:2564–2571.
23. Schmidbauer M, Budka H, Pilz P. Neuroepithelial and ectomesenchymal differentiation in a primitive pineal tumor ("pineal anlage tumor"). Clin Neuropathol 1989;8:7–10.
24. Sobel RA, Trice JE, Nielsen SL, Ellis WG. Pineoblastoma with ganglionic and glial differentiation: report of two cases. Acta Neuropathol (Berl) 1981;55:243–246.
25. Stefanko SZ, Manschot WA. Pinealoblastoma with retinoblastomatous differentiation. Brain 1979;102:321–332.

## Other Neoplasms in the Pineal Region

1. Braga FM, Magalhaes FW. Epidermoid tumor of the pineal region. Surg Neurol 1987;27:370–372.
2. Cho BK, Wang KC, Nam DH, et al. Pineal tumors: experience with 48 cases over 10 years. Childs Nerv Syst 1998;14:53–58.
3. Czirjak S, Vitanovic D, Slowik F, Magyar A. Primary meningeal melanocytoma of the pineal region: case report. J Neurosurg 2000;92:461–465.
4. DeGirolami U, Armbrustmacher VW. Juvenile pilocytic astrocytoma of the pineal region: report of a case. Cancer 1982; 50:1185–1188.
5. Donati P, Maiuri F, Gangemi M, et al. Cavernous angioma of the pineal region. J Neurosurg Sci 1992;36:155–160.
6. Fukui M, Matsuoka S, Hasuo K, et al. Cavernous hemangioma in the pineal region. Surg Neurol 1983;20:209–215.

7. Halpert B, Erikson EE, Fields WS. Intracranial involvement from carcinoma of the lung. Arch Pathol 1960;69:93–103.
8. Hunt SJ, Johnson PC. Melanotic ganglioglioma of the pineal region. Acta Neuropathol (Berl) 1989;79:222–225.
9. Konovalov AN, Spallone A, Pitzkhelauri DI. Meningioma of the pineal region: a surgical series of 10 cases. J Neurosurg 1996; 85: 586–590.
10. Lombardi D, Scheithauer BW, Villani RM, et al. Cavernous haemangioma of the pineal region. Acta Neurochir (Wien) 1996; 138:678–683.
11. MacKay CI, Baeesa SS, Ventureyra EC. Epidermoid cysts of the pineal region. Childs Nerv Syst 1999;15:170–178.
12. Madawi AA, Crockard HA, Stevens JM. Pineal region meningioma without dural attachment. Br J Neurosurg 1996;10: 305–307.
13. Rickert CH, Probst-Cousin S, Blasius S, Gullotta F. Melanotic progonoma of the brain: a case report and review. Childs Nerv Syst 1998;14:389–393.
14. Rubino GJ, King WA, Quinn B, et al. Primary pineal melanoma: case report. Neurosurgery 1993;33:511–515.
15. Sell JJ, Hart BL, Rael JR. Hemangiopericytoma: a rare pineal mass. Neuroradiology 1996;38:782–784.
16. Smith WT, Hughes B, Ermocilla R. Chemodectoma of the pineal region, with observations on the pineal body and chemoreceptor tissues. J Pathol Bacteriol 1966;92:69–76.
17. Snipes GJ, Horoupian DS, Shuer LM, Silverberg GD. Pleomorphic granular cell astrocytoma of the pineal gland. Cancer 1992;70:2159–2165.
18. Solarski A, Panke ES, Panke TW. Craniopharyngioma in the pineal gland. Arch Pathol Lab Med 1978;102:490–491.
19. Stone JL, Cybulski GR, Rhee HL, Bailey OT. Excision of a large pineal region hemangiopericytoma (angioblastic meningioma, hemangiopericytoma type). Surg Neurol 1983;19:181–189.
20. Talacchi A, Sala F, Alessandrini F, et al. Assessment and surgical management of posterior fossa epidermoid tumors: report of 28 cases. Neurosurgery 1998;42:242–251.
21. Usanov EI, Hatomkin DM, Nikulina TA, Gorban NA. Craniopharyngioma of the pineal region. Childs Nerv Syst 1999;15:4–7.
22. Vaquero J, Ramiro J, Martinez R. Glioblastoma multiforme of the pineal region. J Neurosurg Sci 1990;34:149–150.
23. Voessing R, Berthold F, Richard K-E, et al. Primary myeloblastoma of the pineal region. Clin Neuropathol 1992;11:11–15.
24. Weber P, Shepard KV, Vijayakumar S. Case report: metastases to pineal gland. Cancer 1989;63:164–165.
25. Yamane K, Shima T, Okada Y, et al. Primary pineal melanoma with long-term survival: case report. Surg Neurol 1994;42: 433–437.

## Pineal Cyst

1. Cooper ERA. The human pineal gland and pineal cysts. J Anat 1932;67:28–46.
2. Fain JS, Tomlinson FH, Scheithauer BW, et al. Symptomatic glial cysts of the pineal gland. J Neurosurg 1994;80:454–460.
3. Fleege MA, Miller GM, Fletcher GP, et al. Benign glial cysts of the pineal gland: unusual imaging characteristics with histological correlation. AJNR 1994;15:161–166.
4. Hasegawa A, Ohtsubo K, Mori W. Pineal gland in old age: quantitative and qualitative morphological study of 168 human autopsy cases. Brain Res 1987;409:343–349.
5. Klein P, Rubinstein LJ. Benign symptomatic glial cysts of the pineal gland: a report of seven cases and review of the literature. J Neurol Neurosurg Psychiatry 1989;52:991–995.
6. Mamourian AC, Towfighi J. Pineal cysts: MR imaging. AJNR 1986;7:1081–1086.
7. Mamourian AC, Yarnell T. Enhancement of pineal cysts on MR images. AJNR 1991;12:773–774.
8. Maurer PK, Ecklund J, Parisi JE, Ondra S. Symptomatic pineal cyst: case report. Neurosurgery 1990;27:451–454.
9. Mena H, Armonda RA, Ribas JL, et al. Nonneoplastic pineal cysts: a clinicopathologic study of twenty-one cases. Ann Diagn Pathol 1997;1:11–18.
10. Osborn RE, Deen HG, Kerber CW, Glass RF. A case of hemorrhagic pineal cyst: MR/CT correlation. Neuroradiology 1989; 31:187–189.
11. Sandhu JS, McLaughlin JR, Gomez CR. Characteristics of incidental pineal cysts on magnetic resonance imaging. Neurosurgery 1989;25:636–640.

12. Sawamura Y, Ikeda J, Ozawa M, et al. Magnetic resonance images reveal a high incidence of asymptomatic pineal cysts in young women. Neurosurgery 1995;37:11–16.

## Medulloblastoma

1. Aldosari N, Bigner SH, Burger PC, et al. Genetic analysis by FISH on paraffin sections of medulloblastoma. Arch Pathol Lab Med, in press.
2. Alwasiak J, Mirecka B, Wozniak L, Liberski PP. Neuroblastic differentiation of metastases of medulloblastoma to extracranial lymph node: an ultrastructural study. Ultrastruct Pathol 1991;15:647–654.
3. Batra SK, McLendon RE, Koos JS, et al. Prognostic implications of chromosome p17 deletions in human medulloblastomas. J Neurooncol 1995;24:39–45.
4. Becker RL, Becker AD, Sobel DF. Adult medulloblastoma: review of 13 cases with emphasis on MRI. Neuroradiology 1995;37:104–108.
5. Belza MG, Donaldson SS, Steinberg GK, et al. Medulloblastoma: freedom from relapse longer than 8 years—a therapeutic cure? J Neurosurg 1991;75:575–582.
6. Berger MS, Baumeister B, Geyer JR, et al. The risks of metastases from shunting in children with primary central nervous system tumors. J Neurosurg 1991;74:872–877.
7. Biegel JA, Janss AJ, Raffel C, et al. Prognostic significance of chromosome 17p deletions in childhood primitive neuroectodermal tumors (medulloblastomas) of the central nervous system. Clin Cancer Res 1997;3:473–478.
8. Biegel JA, Rorke LB, Janss AJ, et al. Isochromosome 17q demonstrated by interphase fluorescence in situ hybridization in primitive neuroectodermal tumors of the central nervous system. Genes Chromosomes Cancer 1995;14:85–96.
9. Brown HG, Kepner JL, Perlman EJ, et al. "Large cell/anaplastic" medulloblastomas: a pediatric oncology group study. J Neuropathol Exp Neurol 2000;59:857–865.
10. Brown WD, Tavaré CJ, Sobel EL, Gilles FH. The applicability of Collins' law to childhood brain tumors and its usefulness as a predictor of survival. Neurosurgery 1995;36:1093–1096.
11. Bruch LA, Hill DA, Cai DX, et al. A role for fluorescence in situ hybridization detection of chromosome 22q dosage in distinguishing atypical teratoid/rhabdoid tumors from medulloblastoma/central primitive neuroectodermal tumors. Hum Pathol 2001;32:156–162.
12. Campbell AN, Chan HSL, Becker LE, et al. Extracranial metastases in childhood primary intracranial tumors. Cancer 1984;53:974–981.
13. Caputy AJ, McCullough DC, Manz HJ, et al. A review of the factors influencing the prognosis of medulloblastoma: the importance of cell differentiation. J Neurosurg 1987;66:80–87.
14. Cervoni L, Cantore G. Medulloblastoma in pediatric age: a single-institution review of prognostic factors. Childs Nerv Syst 1995;11:80–85.
15. Cervoni L, Maleci A, Salvati M, et al. Medulloblastoma in late adults: report of two cases and critical review of the literature. J Neurooncol 1994;19:169–173.
16. Chan AW, Tarbell NJ, Black PM, et al. Adult medulloblastoma: prognostic factors and patterns of relapse. Neurosurgery 2000;47:623–631; discussion 31–32.
17. Chatty EM, Earle KM. Medulloblastoma: a report of 201 cases with emphasis on the relationship of histologic variants to survival. Cancer 1971;28:977–983.
18. Coffin CM, Braun JT, Wick MR, Dehner LP. A clinicopathologic and immunohistochemical analysis of 53 cases of medulloblastoma with emphasis on synaptophysin expression. Mod Pathol 1990;3:164–170.
19. Coffin CM, Mukai K, Dehner LP. Glial differentiation in medulloblastomas. Am J Surg Pathol 1983;7:555–565.
20. Cruz-Sanchez FF, Rossi ML, Hughes JT, Moss TH. Differentiation in embryonal neuroepithelial tumors of the central nervous system. Cancer 1991;67:965–976.
21. Czerwionka M, Korf H-W, Hoffmann O, et al. Differentiation in medulloblastomas: correlation between the immunocytochemical demonstration of photoreceptor markers (S-antigen, rod-opsin) and the survival rate in 66 patients. Acta Neuropathol (Berl) 1989;78:629–636.
22. De Chadarévian J-P, Montes JL, O'Gorman AM, Freeman CR.

Maturation of cerebellar neuroblastoma into ganglioneuroma with melanosis: a histologic, immunocytochemical, and ultrastructural study. Cancer 1987;59:69–76.
23. Durity FA, Dolman CL, Moyes PD. Ganglioneuroblastoma of the cerebellum: case report. J Neurosurg 1968;28:270–273.
24. Eberhart CG, Kaufman W, Burger PC. Apoptosis, neuronal maturation, and neurotropin signaling within medulloblastoma nodules. J Neuropathol Exp Neurol 2001;60:462–469.
25. Eberhart CG, Kepner JL, Goldthwaite PT, et al. Histopathologic grading of medulloblastomas: a pediatric oncology group study. Cancer, in press.
26. Eberhart CG, Tihan T, Burger PC. Nuclear localization and mutation of beta-catenin in medulloblastomas. J Neuropathol Exp Neurol 2000;59:333–337.
27. Evans DGR, Farndon PA, Burnell LD, et al. The incidence of Gorlin syndrome in 173 consecutive cases of medulloblastoma. Br J Cancer 1991;64:959–961.
28. Geyer JR, Schofield D, Berger M, Milstein J. Differentiation of a primitive neuroectodermal tumor into a benign ganglioglioma. J Neurooncol 1992;14:237–241.
29. Giangaspero F, Chieco P, Ceccarelli C, et al. "Desmoplastic" versus "classic" medulloblastoma: comparison of DNA content, histopathology and differentiation. Virchows Arch A Pathol Anat 1991;418:207–214.
30. Giangaspero F, Rigobello L, Badiali M, et al. Large-cell medulloblastomas. Am J Surg Pathol 1992;16:687–693.
31. Giangaspero F, Perilongo G, Fondelli MP, et al. Medulloblastoma with extensive nodularity: a variant with favorable prognosis. J Neurosurg 1999;91:971–977.
32. Goldberg-Stern H, Gadoth N, Stern S, et al. The prognostic significance of glial fibrillary acidic protein staining in medulloblastoma. Cancer 1991;68:568–573.
33. Gould VE, Jansson DS, Molenaar WM, et al. Primitive neuroectodermal tumors of the central nervous system: patterns of expression of neuroendocrine markers, and all classes of intermediate filament proteins. Lab Invest 1990;62:498–509.
34. Grotzer MA, Janss AJ, Fung K, et al. TrkC expression predicts good clinical outcome in primitive neuroectodermal brain tumors. J Clin Oncol 2000;18:1027–1035.
35. Gultekin SH, Dalmau J, Graus Y, et al. Anti-Hu immunolabeling as an index of neuronal differentiation in human brain tumors. Am J Surg Pathol 1998;22:195–200.
36. Hamilton SR, Liu B, Parsons RE, et al. The molecular basis of Turcot's syndrome. N Engl J Med 1995;332:839–847.
37. Haslam RH, Lamborn KR, Becker LE, Isreal MA. Tumor cell apoptosis present at diagnosis may predict treatment outcome for patients with medulloblastoma. J Pediatr Hematol Oncol 1998; 20:520–527.
38. Hazuka MB, DeBiose DA, Henderson RH, Kinzie JJ. Survival results in adult patients treated for medulloblastoma. Cancer 1992;69:2143–2148.
39. Herms J, Neidt I, Luscher B, et al. C-myc expression in medulloblastoma and its prognostic value. Int J Cancer (Pred Oncol) 2000;89:395–402.
40. Herpers MJHM, Budka H. Primitive neuroectodermal tumors including the medulloblastoma: glial differentiation signaled by immunoreactivity for GFAP is restricted to the pure desmoplastic medulloblastoma ("arachnoidal sarcoma of the cerebellum"). Clin Neuropathol 1985;4:12–18.
41. Huang H, Mahler-Araujo BM, Sankila A, et al. APC mutations in sporadic medulloblastomas. Am J Pathol 2000;156:433–437.
42. Hubbard JL, Scheithauer BW, Kispert DB, et al. Adult cerebellar medulloblastomas: the pathological, radiographic, and clinical disease spectrum. J Neurosurg 1989;70:536–544.
43. Hughes EN, Shillito J, Sallan SE, et al. Medulloblastoma at the Joint Center for Radiation Therapy between 1968 and 1984: the influence of radiation dose on the patterns of failure and survival. Cancer 1988;61:1992–1998.
44. Janss AJ, Yachnis AT, Silber JH, et al. Glial differentiation predicts poor clinical outcome in primitive neuroectodermal brain tumors. Ann Neurol 1996;39:481–489.
45. Kadin ME, Rubinstein LJ, Nelson JS. Neonatal cerebellar medulloblastoma originating from the fetal external granular layer. J Neuropathol Exp Neurol 1970;29:583–600.
46. Katsetos CD, Herman MM, Frankfurter A, et al. Cerebellar desmoplastic medulloblastomas. Arch Pathol Lab Med 1989; 113:1019–1029.

47. Katsetos CD, Krishna L, Frankfurter A, et al. A cytomorphological scheme of differentiating neuronal phenotypes in cerebellar medulloblastomas based on immunolocalization of class III β-tubulin isotype (βIII) and proliferating cell nuclear antigen (PCNA)/cyclin. Clin Neuropathol 1995;14:72–80.

48. Katsetos CD, Liu HM, Zacks SI. Immunohistochemical and ultrastructural observations on Homer Wright (neuroblastic) rosettes and the "pale islands" of human cerebellar medulloblastomas. Hum Pathol 1988;19:1219–1227.

49. Katsetos CD, Burger PC. Medulloblastoma. Semin Diagn Pathol 1994;11:85–97.

50. Kleinman GM, Hochberg FH, Richardson EP. Systemic metastases from medulloblastoma: report of two cases and review of the literature. Cancer 1981;48:2296–2309.

51. Klériga E, Sher JH, Nallainathan S-K, et al. Development of cerebellar malignant astrocytoma at site of a medulloblastoma treated 11 years earlier: case report. J Neurosurg 1978;49: 445–449.

52. Kopelson G, Linggood RM, Kleinman GM. Medulloblastoma: the identification of prognostic subgroups and implications for multimodality management. Cancer 1983;51:312–319.

53. Korf H-W, Czerwionka M, Reiner J, et al. Immunocytochemical evidence of molecular photoreceptor markers in cerebellar medulloblastomas. Cancer 1987;60:1763–1766.

54. Korshunov A, Golanov A, Ozerov S, Sycheva R. Prognostic value of tumor-associated antigens immunoreactivity and apoptosis in medulloblastomas: an analysis of 73 cases. Brain Tumor Pathol 1999;16:37–44.

55. Kramm CM, Korf H-W, Czerwionka M, et al. Photoreceptor differentiation in cerebellar medulloblastoma: evidence for a functional photopigment and authentic S-antigen (arrestin). Acta Neuropathol (Berl) 1991;81:296–302.

56. Kudo M, Shimizu M, Akutsu Y, et al. Ganglioglial differentiation in medulloblastoma. Acta Pathol Jpn 1990;40:50–56.

57. Kumanishi T, Washiyama K, Watabe K, Sekiguchi K. Glial fibrillary acidic protein in medulloblastomas. Acta Neuropathol (Berl) 1985;67:1–5.

58. Laeng RH, Scheithauer BW, Altermatt HJ. Anti-neuronal nuclear autoantibodies, types 1 and 2: their utility in the study of tumors of the nervous system. Acta Neuropathol (Berl) 1998;96:329–339.

59. Lefkowitz IB, Packer RJ, Ryan SG, et al. Late recurrence of primitive neuroectodermal tumor/medulloblastoma. Cancer 1988; 62:826–830.

60. Mannoji H, Takeshita I, Fukui M, et al. Glial fibrillary acidic protein in medulloblastoma. Acta Neuropathol (Berl) 1981;55:63–69.

61. Miralbell R, Bieri S, Huguenin P, et al. Prognostic value of cerebrospinal fluid cytology in pediatric medulloblastoma: Swiss pediatric oncology group. Ann Oncol 1999;10:239–241.

62. Mitchell D, Rojiani AM, Richards D, et al. Congenital CNS primitive neuroectodermal tumor: case report and review of the literature. Pediatr Pathol Lab Med 1995;15:949–956.

63. Osumi AK, McLendon RE, Tien RD, et al. Well differentiated astrocytoma occurring nine years after radiation therapy for medulloblastoma. Clin Neuropathol 1994;13:281–285.

64. Packer RJ, Cogen P, Vezina G, Rorke LB. Medulloblastoma: clinical and biologic aspects. Neuro-Oncology 1999;1:232–250.

65. Packer RJ, Sutton LN, Rorke LB, et al. Prognostic importance of cellular differentiation in medulloblastoma of childhood. J Neurosurg 1984;61:296–301.

66. Park TS, Hoffman HJ, Hendrick EB, et al. Medulloblastoma: clinical presentation and management: experience at the Hospital for Sick Children, Toronto, 1950–1980. J Neurosurg 1983;58: 543–552.

67. Pearl GS, Mirra SS, Miles ML. Glioblastoma multiforme occurring 13 years after treatment of a medulloblastoma. Neurosurgery 1980;6:546–551.

68. Pearl GS, Takei Y. Cerebellar "neuroblastoma": nosology as it relates to medulloblastoma. Cancer 1981;47:772–779.

69. Perek D, Perek-Polnik M, Drogosiewicz M, et al. Risk factors of recurrence in 157 MB/PNET patients treated in one institution. Childs Nerv Syst 1998;14:582–586.

70. Pietsch T, Waha A, Kock A, et al. Medulloblastomas of the desmoplastic variant carry mutations of the human homologue of Drosophila patched. Cancer Res 1997;57:2085–2088.

71. Raaf J, Kernohan JW. Relation of abnormal collections of cells in posterior medullary velum of cerebellum to origin of medulloblastoma. Arch Neurol 1994;52:163–169.

72. Raffel C, Jenkins RB, Frederick L, et al. Sporadic medulloblastomas contain PTCH mutations. Cancer Res 1997;57:842–845.

73. Ramsay DA, Bonnin J, MacDonald DR, Assis L. Medulloblastomas in late middle age and the elderly: report of 2 cases. Clin Neuropathol 1995;14:337–342.

74. Reardon DA, Michalkiewicz E, Boyett JM, et al. Extensive genomic abnormalities in childhood medulloblastoma by comparative genomic hybridization. Cancer Res 1997;57:4042–4047.

75. Roberts RO, Lynch CF, Jones MP, Hart MN. Medulloblastoma: a population-based study of 532 cases. J Neuropathol Exp Neurol 1991;50:134–144.

76. Scheurlen WB, Schwabe GC, Joos S, et al. Molecular analysis of childhood primitive neuroectodermal tumors defines markers associated with poor outcome. J Clin Oncol 1998;16:2478–2485.

77. Schiffer D, Cavalla P, Chio A, et al. Tumor cell proliferation and apoptosis in medulloblastoma. Acta Neuropathol (Berl) 1994; 87:362–370.

78. Schofield D, West DC, Anthony DC, et al. Correlation of loss of heterozygosity at chromosome 9q with histological subtype in medulloblastomas. Am J Pathol 1995;146:472–480.

79. Schofield DE, Yunis EJ, Geyer JR, et al. DNA content and other prognostic features in childhood medulloblastoma: proposal of a scoring system. Cancer 1992;69:1307–1314.

80. Schubert TEO, Cervos-Navarro J. The histopathological and clinical relevance of apoptotic cell death in medulloblastomas. J Neuropathol Exp Neurol 1998;57:10–15.

81. Schütz BR, Scheurlen W, Krauss J, et al. Mapping of chromosomal gains and losses in primitive neuroectodermal tumors by comparative genomic hybridization. Genes Chromosomes Cancer 1996;16:196–203.

82. Schwechheimer K, Wiedenmann B, Franke WW. Synaptophysin: a reliable marker for medulloblastomas. Virchows Arch A 1987; 411:53–59.

83. Segal RA, Goumnerova LC, Kwon YK, et al. Expression of the neurotrophin receptor TrkC is linked to a favorable outcome in medulloblastoma. Proc Natl Acad Sci U S A 1994;91:12867–12871.

84. Shin W-Y, Laufer H, Lee Y-C, et al. Fine structure of a cerebellar neuroblastoma. Acta Neuropathol (Berl) 1978;42:11–13.

85. Sure U, Berghorn WJ, Bertalanffy H, et al. Staging, scoring and grading medulloblastoma. Acta Neurochir (Wien) 1995;132: 59–65.

86. Taomoto K, Tomita T, Raimondi AJ, Leestma JE. Medulloblastomas in childhood: histological factors influencing patients' outcome. Childs Nerv Syst 1987;3:354–360.

87. Tarbell NJ, Loeffler JS, Silver B, et al. The change in patterns of relapse in medulloblastoma. Cancer 1991;68:1600–1604.

88. Tomita T, Yasue M, Engelhard HH, et al. Flow cytometric DNA analysis of medulloblastoma: prognostic implication of aneuploidy. Cancer 1988;61:744–749.

89. Tomlinson FH, Jenkins RB, Scheithauer BW, et al. Aggressive medulloblastoma with high-level N-myc amplification. Mayo Clin Proc 1994;69:359–365.

90. Warzok R, Jaenisch W, Lang G. Morphology and biology of cerebellar neuroblastomas. J Neurooncol 1983;1:373–379.

91. Yachnis AT, Rorke LB, Trojanowski JQ. Cerebellar dysplasias in humans: development and possible relationship to glial and primitive neuroectodermal tumors of the cerebellar vermis. J Neuropathol Exp Neurol 1994;53:61–71.

92. Yasue M, Tomita T, Engelhard H, et al. Prognostic importance of DNA ploidy in medulloblastoma of childhood. J Neurosurg 1989; 70:385–391.

93. Zurawel RH, Allen C, Chiappa S, et al. Analysis of PTCH/SMO/SHH pathway genes in medulloblastoma. Genes Chromosomes Cancer 2000;27:44–51.

### Medullomyoblastoma and Melanotic Medulloblastoma

1. Bergmann M, Pietsch T, Herms J, et al. Medullomyoblastoma: a histological, immunohistochemical, ultrastructural and molecular genetic study. Acta Neuropathol (Berl) 1998;95:205–212.

2. Best PV. A medulloblastoma-like tumour with melanin formation. J Pathol 1973;110:109–111.

3. Boesel CP, Suhan JP, Sayers MP. Melanotic medulloblastoma: report of a case with ultrastructural findings. J Neuropathol Exp Neurol 1978;37:531–543.

4. Chowdhury C, Roy S, Mahapatra AK, Bhatia R. Medullomyoblastoma. Cancer 1985;55:1495–1500.

5. Dickson DW, Hart MN, Menezes A, Cancilla PA. Medulloblastoma with glial and rhabdomyoblastic differentiation. J Neuropathol Exp Neurol 1983;42:639–647.
6. Dolman CL. Melanotic medulloblastoma: a case report with immunohistochemical and ultrastructural examination. Acta Neuropathol (Berl) 1988;76:528–531.
7. Fowler M, Simpson DA. A malignant melanin-forming tumour of the cerebellum. J Pathol Bacteriol 1962;84:307–311.
8. Höll T, Kleihues P, Yasargil MG, Wiestler OD. Cerebellar medullomyoblastoma with advanced neuronal differentiation and hamartomatous component. Acta Neuropathol (Berl) 1991;82:408–413.
9. Jimenez CL, Carpenter BF, Robb IA. Melanotic cerebellar tumor. Ultrastruct Pathol 1987;11:751–759.
10. Kalimo H, Päljarvi L, Ekfors T, Pelliniemi LJ. Pigmented primitive neuroectodermal tumor with multipotential differentiation in cerebellum (pigmented medullomyoblastoma). Pediatr Neurosci 1987;13:188–195.
11. Mahapatra AK, Sinha AK, Sharma MC. Medullomyoblastoma: a rare cerebellar tumour in children. Childs Nerv Syst 1998;14:312–316.
12. Rao C, Friedlander ME, Klein E, et al. Medullomyoblastoma in an adult. Cancer 1990;65:157–163.
13. Schiffer D, Giordana MT, Pezotta S, et al. Medullomyoblastoma: report of two cases. Childs Nerv Syst 1992;8:268–272.
14. Smith TW, Davidson RI. Medullomyoblastoma: a histologic, immunohistochemical, and ultrastructural study. Cancer 1984;54:323–332.
15. Stahlberger R, Friede RL. Fine structure of myomedulloblastoma. Acta Neuropathol (Berl) 1977;37:43–48.
16. Stowens D, Lin T-HL. Melanotic progonoma of the brain. Hum Pathol 1974;5:105–113.
17. Sung JH, Mastri AR, Segal EL. Melanotic medulloblastoma of the cerebellum. J Neuropathol Exp Neurol 1973;32:437–445.

## Medulloepithelioma

1. Auer RN, Becker LE. Cerebral medulloepithelioma with bone, cartilage, and striated muscle: light microscopic and immunohistochemical study. J Neuropathol Exp Neurol 1983;42:256–267.
2. Best PV. Posterior fossa medulloepithelioma: report of a case. J Neurol Sci 1974;22:511–518.
3. Caccamo DV, Herman MM, Rubinstein LJ. An immunohistochemical study of the primitive and maturing elements of human cerebral medulloepitheliomas. Acta Neuropathol (Berl) 1989;79:248–254.
4. Deck JHN. Cerebral medulloepithelioma with maturation into ependymal cells and ganglion cells. J Neuropathol Exp Neurol 1969;28:442–454.
5. Karch SB, Urich H. Medulloepithelioma: definition of an entity. J Neuropathol Exp Neurol 1972;31:27–53.
6. Khoddami M, Becker LE. Immunohistochemistry of medulloepithelioma and neural tube. Pediatr Pathol Lab Med 1997;17:913–925.
7. Molloy PT, Yachnis AT, Rorke LB, et al. Central nervous system medulloepithelioma: a series of eight cases including two arising in the pons. J Neurosurg 1996;84:430–436.
8. Pollak A, Friede RL. Fine structure of medulloepithelioma. J Neuropathol Exp Neurol 1977;36:712–725.
9. Scheithauer BW, Rubinstein LJ. Cerebral medulloepithelioma: report of a case with multiple divergent neuroepithelial differentiation. Childs Brain 1979;5:62–71.
10. Sharma MC, Mahapatra AK, Gaikwad S, et al. Pigmented medulloepithelioma: report of a case and review of the literature. Childs Nerv Syst 1998;14:74–78.

## Neuroblastoma and Ganglioneuroblastoma

1. Azzarelli B, Richards DE, Anton AH, Roessmann U. Central neuroblastoma: electron microscope observations and catecholamine determinations. J Neuropathol Exp Neurol 1977;36:384–397.
2. Bennett JP Jr, Rubinstein LJ. The biological behavior of primary cerebral neuroblastoma: a reappraisal of the clinical course in a series of 70 cases. Ann Neurol 1984;16:21–27.
3. Berger MS, Edwards MSB, Wara WM, et al. Primary cerebral neuroblastoma: long-term follow-up review and therapeutic guidelines. J Neurosurg 1983;59:418–423.

4. Horten BC, Rubinstein LJ. Primary cerebral neuroblastoma: a clinicopathological study of 35 cases. Brain 1976;99:735–756.
5. Laeng RH, Scheithauer BW, Altermatt HJ. Anti-neuronal nuclear autoantibodies, types 1 and 2: their utility in the study of tumors of the nervous system. Acta Neuropathol (Berl) 1998;96:329–339.
6. Ojeda VJ, Spagnelo DV, Vaughn RJ. Palisades in primary central neuroblastoma simulating so-called polar spongioblastoma: a light and electron microscopical study of an adult case. Am J Surg Pathol 1987;11:316–322.
7. Torres LF, Grant N, Harding BN, Scaravilli F. Intracerebral neuroblastoma: report of a case with neuronal maturation and long survival. Acta Neuropathol (Berl) 1985;68:110–114.

## Ependymoblastoma

1. Cruz-Sanchez FF, Haustein J, Rossi ML, et al. Ependymoblastoma: a histological, immunohistological and ultrastructural study of five cases. Histopathology 1988;12:17–27.
2. Langford LA. The ultrastructure of the ependymoblastoma. Acta Neuropathol (Berl) 1986;71:136–141.
3. Lorentzen M, Hägerstrand I. Congenital ependymoblastoma. Acta Neuropathol (Berl) 1980;49:71–74.
4. Mørk SJ, Rubinstein LJ. Ependymoblastoma: a reappraisal of a rare embryonal tumor. Cancer 1985;55:1536–1542.
5. Rubinstein LJ. The definition of the ependymoblastoma. Arch Pathol 1970;90:35–45.

## Embryonal Tumor with Abundant Neuropil and True Rosettes

1. Eberhart CG, Brat DJ, Cohen K, Burger PC. Pediatric neuroblastic brain tumors containing abundant neuropil and true rosettes. Pediatr Dev Pathol 2000;3:346–352.
2. Queiroz LS, de Faria JL, Cruz JN. An ependymoblastoma of the pons. J Pathol 1975;115:207–212.
3. Yagishita S, Itoh Y, Chiba Y, Yuda K. Cerebral neuroblastoma. J Pathol Anat Histol 1978;381:1–11.

## Retinoblastoma

1. Amoaku WMK, Willshaw HE, Parkes SE, et al. Trilateral retinoblastoma: a report of five patients. Cancer 1996;78:858–863.
2. Bader JL, Meadows AT, Zimmerman LE, et al. Bilateral retinoblastoma with ectopic intracranial retinoblastoma: trilateral retinoblastoma. Cancer Genet Cytogenet 1982;5:203–213.
3. Bagley LJ, Hurst RW, Zimmerman RA, et al. Imaging in the trilateral retinoblastoma syndrome. Neuroradiology 1996;38:166–170.
4. Paulino AC. Trilateral retinoblastoma: is the location of the intracranial tumor important? Cancer 1999;86:135–141.
5. Provenzale JM, Weber AL, Klintworth GK, McLendon RE. Radiologic-pathologic correlation: bilateral retinoblastoma with coexistent pinealoblastoma (trilateral retinoblastoma). AJNR 1995;16:157–165.

## Embryonal Tumors with Muscle Differentiation

1. Abenoza P, Wick MR. Primitive cerebral neuroectodermal tumor with rhabdomyoblastic differentiation. Ultrastruct Pathol 1986;10:347–354.
2. Caputo V, Repetti ML, Grimoldi N, et al. Cerebral rhabdomyosarcoma with rhabdoid tumor-like features. J Neurooncol 1997;32:81–86.
3. Celli P, Cervoni L, Maraglino C. Primary rhabdomyosarcoma of the brain: observations on a case with clinical and radiological evidence of cure. J Neurooncol 1998;36:259–267.

## Largely Undifferentiated Embryonal Tumors

1. Behnke J, Mursch K, Brück W, et al. Intra-axial endophytic primitive neuroectodermal tumors in the pons: clinical, radiological, and immunohistochemical aspects in four children. Childs Nerv Syst 1996;12:125–129.
2. Dirks PB, Harris L, Hoffman HJ, et al. Supratentorial primitive neuroectodermal tumors in children. J Neurooncol 1996;29:75–84.
3. Gaffney CC, Sloane JP, Bradley NJ, Bloom HJG. Primitive neuroectodermal tumours of the cerebrum: pathology and treatment. J Neurooncol 1985;3:23–33.
4. Grant JW, Steart PV, Gallagher PJ. Primitive neuroectodermal tumors of the cerebrum: a histological and immunohistochemical study of 10 cases. Clin Neuropathol 1988;7:228–233.

## Miscellaneous Embryonal Tumors

1. Becker R, Bauer BL, Mennel HD, Plate KH. Cerebellar primitive neuroectodermal tumor with multipotent differentiation in a family with von Hippel-Lindau disease: case report. Clin Neuropathol 1993;12:107–111.
2. Brüstle O, Ohgaki H, Schmitt HP, et al. Primitive neuroectodermal tumors after prophylactic central nervous system irradiation in children. Cancer 1992;69:2385–2392.
3. Katayama Y, Kimura S, Watanabe T, et al. Peripheral-type primitive neuroectodermal tumor arising in the tentorium: case report. J Neurosurg 1999;90:141–144.
4. Reifenberger J, Janssen G, Weber RG, et al. Primitive neuroectodermal tumors of the cerebral hemispheres in two siblings with TP53 germline mutation. J Neuropathol Exp Neurol 1998;57:179–187.
5. Selassie L, Rigotti R, Kepes JJ, Towfighi J. Adipose tissue and smooth muscle in a primitive neuroectodermal tumor of cerebrum. Acta Neuropathol (Berl) 1994;87:217–222.

## Primitive Polar Spongioblastoma

1. Bignami A, Adelman LS, Perides G, Dahl D. Glial hyaluronate-binding protein in polar spongioblastoma. J Neuropathol Exp Neurol 1989;48:187–196.
2. de Chadarévian J-P, Guyda HJ, Hollenberg RD. Hypothalamic polar spongioblastoma associated with the diencephalic syndrome: ultrastructural demonstration of a neuro-endocrine organization. Virchows Arch [A] 1989;402:465–474.
3. Jansen GH, Troost D, Dingemans KP. Polar spongioblastoma: an immunohistochemical and electron microscopical study. Acta Neuropathol (Berl) 1990;81:228–231.
4. Langford LA, Camel MH. Palisading pattern in cerebral neuroblastoma mimicking the primitive polar spongioblastoma: an ultrastructural study. Acta Neuropathol (Berl) 1987;73:153–159.
5. Ng H, Path MRC, Tang NLS, Poon WS. Polar spongioblastoma with cerebrospinal fluid metastases. Surg Neurol 1994;41:137–142.
6. Ojeda VJ, Spagnolo DV, Vaughan RJ. Palisades in primary cerebral neuroblastoma simulating so-called polar spongioblastoma: a light and electron microscopical study of an adult case. Am J Surg Pathol 1987;11:316–322.
7. Rubinstein LJ. Cytogenesis and differentiation in primitive central neuropathologic tumors. J Neuropathol Exp Neurol 1972;31:7–26.
8. Rubinstein LJ. Discussion on polar spongioblastomas. Acta Neurochir (Wien) 1964;10(Suppl):126–140.
9. Schiffer D, Cravioto H, Giordana T, et al. Is polar spongioblastoma a tumor entity? J Neurosurg 1993;78:587–591.
10. Schochet SS, Violett TW Jr, Nelson J, et al. Polar spongioblastoma of the cervical spinal cord: case report. Clin Neuropathol 1984;3:225–227.

## Fibrosarcoma

1. Aung TH, Tse CH. Bifrontal meningeal fibrosarcoma in a patient with metastases to the liver, kidneys and suprarenal glands. Aust N Z J Surg 1993;63:746–748.
2. Aydin F, Ghatak NR, Leshner RT. Possible radiation-induced dural fibrosarcoma with an unusually short latent period: case report. Neurosurgery 1995;36:591–595.
3. Chang SM, Barker FG II, Larson DA, et al. Sarcomas subsequent to cranial irradiation. Neurosurgery 1995;36:685–690.
4. Coppeto JR, Roberts M. Fibrosarcoma after proton-beam pituitary ablation. Arch Neurol 1979;36:380–381.
5. Gasper LE, Mackenzie IRA, Gilbert JJ, et al. Primary cerebral fibrosarcomas: clinicopathologic study and review of the literature. Cancer 1993;72:3277–3281.
6. Mena H, Garcia JH. Primary brain sarcomas: light and electron microscope features. Cancer 1978;42:1298–1307.
7. Paulus W, Slovik F, Jellinger K. Primary intracranial sarcomas: histopathological features in 19 cases. Histopathology 1991;18:395–402.
8. Schrantz JL, Araoz CA. Radiation induced meningeal fibrosarcoma. Arch Pathol 1972;93:26–31.

## Rhabdomyosarcoma

1. de Faria JL. Rhabdomyosarcoma of cerebellum. Arch Pathol 1957;63:234–238.
2. Fix SE, Nelson J, Schochet SS Jr. Focal leptomeningeal rhabdomyomatosis of the posterior fossa. Arch Pathol Lab Med 1989;113:872–873.
3. Hayashi K, Ohtsuki Y, Ikehara I, et al. Primary rhabdomyosarcoma combined with chronic paragonimiasis in the cerebrum: a necropsy case and review of the literature. Acta Neuropathol (Berl) 1986;72:170–177.
4. Herva R, Serlo W, Laitinen J, Becker LE. Intraventricular rhabdomyosarcoma after resection of hyperplastic choroid plexus. Acta Neuropathol (Berl) 1996;92:213–216.
5. Hinton DR, Halliday WC. Primary rhabdomyosarcoma of the cerebellum—a light, electron microscope, and immunohistochemical study. J Neuropathol Exp Neurol 1984;43:439–449.
6. Hoffman SF, Rorke LB. On finding striated muscle in the brain. J Neurol Neurosurg Psychiatry 1971;34:761–764.
7. Korinthenberg R, Edel G, Palm D, et al. Primary rhabdomyosarcoma of the leptomeninx: clinical, neuroradiological and pathological aspects. Clin Neurol Neurosurg 1984;86:301–305.
8. Leedham PW. Primary cerebral rhabdomyosarcoma and the problem of medullomyoblastoma. J Neurol Neurosurg Psychiatry 1972;35:551–559.
9. Masuzawa T, Shimabukuro H, Kamoshita S, Sato F. The ultrastructure of primary cerebral rhabdomyosarcoma. Acta Neuropathol (Berl) 1982;56:307–310.
10. Min K-W, Gyorkey F, Halpert B. Primary rhabdomyosarcoma of the cerebrum. Cancer 1975;35:1405–1411.
11. Namba K, Aschenbrener C, Nikpour M, VanGilder JC. Primary rhabdomyosarcoma of the tentorium with peculiar angiographic findings. Surg Neurol 1979;11:39–43.
12. Olson JJ, Menezes AH, Godersky JC, et al. Primary intracranial rhabdomyosarcoma. Neurosurgery 1985;17:25–34.
13. Paulus W, Slowik F, Jellinger K. Primary intracranial sarcomas: histopathological features in 19 cases. Histopathology 1991;18:395–402.
14. Shuangshoti S, Phonprasert C. Primary intracranial rhabdomyosarcoma producing proptosis. J Neurol Neurosurg Psychiatry 1976;39:531–535.
15. Smith M, Armbrustmacher VW, Violett TW. Diffuse meningeal rhabdomyosarcoma. Cancer 1981;47:2081–2086.
16. Taratuto AL, Molina HA, Diez B, et al. Primary rhabdomyosarcoma of brain and cerebellum. Report of four cases in infants: an immunohistochemical study. Acta Neuropathol (Berl) 1985;66:98–104.
17. Yagishita S, Itoh Y, Chiba Y, Fujino H. Primary rhabdomyosarcoma of the cerebrum: an ultrastructural study. Acta Neuropathol (Berl) 1979;45:111–115.

## Other Primary Sarcomas

1. Abrahams JM, Forman MS, Lavi E, et al. Hemangiopericytoma of the third ventricle. J Neurosurg 1999;90:359–362.
2. Adegbite ABO, McQueen JD, Paine KWE, Rozdilsky B. Primary intracranial chondrosarcoma: a report of two cases. Neurosurgery 1985;17:490–493.
3. Antoniadis C, Selviaridis P, Zaramboukas T, Fountzilas G. Primary angiosarcoma of the brain: case report. Neurosurgery 1996;38:583–586.
4. Aydin F, Ghatak NR, Leshner RT. Possible radiation-induced dural fibrosarcoma with an unusually short latent period: case report. Neurosurgery 1995;36:591–594.
5. Bauman GS, Wara WM, Ciricillo SF, et al. Primary intracerebral osteosarcoma: a case report. J Neurooncol 1997;32:209–213.
6. Bejjani GK, Stopak B, Schwartz A, Santi R. Primary dural leiomyosarcoma in a patient infected with human immunodeficiency virus: case report. Neurosurgery 1999;44:199–202.
7. Bernstein M, Perrin RG, Platts ME, Simpson WJ. Radiation-induced cerebellar chondrosarcoma: case report. J Neurosurg 1984;61:174–177.
8. Blumenthal DT, Raizer JJ, Rosenblum MK, et al. Primary intracranial neoplasms in patients with HIV. Neurology 1999;52:1648–1651.
9. Brown HG, Burger PC, Olivi A, et al. Intracranial leiomyosarcoma in a patient with AIDS. Neuroradiology 1999;41:35–39.
10. Cannon TC, Bane BL, Kistler D, et al. Primary intracerebellar osteosarcoma arising within an epidermoid cyst. Arch Pathol Lab Med 1998;122:737–739.
11. Chang SM, Barker FG II, Larson DA, et al. Sarcomas subsequent to cranial irradiation. Neurosurgery 1995;36:685–690.

12. Charman HP, Lowenstein DH, Cho KG, et al. Primary cerebral angiosarcoma: case report. J Neurosurg 1988;68:806–810.

13. Cybulski GR, Russell EJ, D'Angelo CM, Bailey OT. Falcine chondrosarcoma: case report and literature review. Neurosurgery 1985;16:412–415.

14. Gonzalez-Vitale JC, Slavin RE, McQueen JD. Radiation-induced intracranial malignant fibrous histiocytoma. Cancer 1976; 37: 2960–2963.

15. Hassounah M, Al-Mefty O, Akhtar M, et al. Primary cranial and intracranial chondrosarcoma: a survey. Acta Neurochir (Wien) 1985;78:123–132.

16. Koot RW, Tan WF, Dreissen JJ, et al. Irradiation induced osteosarcoma in the posterior cranial fossa six years after surgery and radiation for medulloblastoma. J Neurol Neurosurg Psychiatry 1996;61:429–430.

17. Kothandaram P. Dural liposarcoma associated with subdural hematoma: case report. J Neurosurg 1970;33:85–87.

18. Kuratsu J-I, Seto H, Kochi M, et al. Metastatic angiosarcoma of the brain. Surg Neurol 1991;35:305–309.

19. Litofsky NS, Pihan G, Corvi F, Smith TW. Intracranial leiomyosarcoma: a neuro-oncological consequence of acquired immunodeficiency syndrome. J Neurooncol 1998;40:179–183.

20. Louis DN, Richardson EP Jr, Dickersin GR, et al. Primary intracranial leiomyosarcoma: case report. J Neurosurg 1989;71: 279–282.

21. Martinez-Salazar A, Supler M, Rojiani AM. Primary intracerebral malignant fibrous histiocytoma: immunohistochemical findings and etiopathogenetic considerations. Mod Pathol 1997;10: 149–154.

22. Mena H, Ribas JL, Enzinger FM, Parisi JE. Primary angiosarcoma of the central nervous system. J Neurosurg 1991;75:73–76.

23. Nora FE, Scheithauer BW. Primary epithelioid hemangioendothelioma of the brain. Am J Surg Pathol 1996;20:707–714.

24. Ohara N, Hayashi K, Shinohara C, et al. Primary osteosarcoma of the cerebrum with immunohistochemical and ultrastructural studies: report of a case. Acta Neuropathol (Berl) 1994;88:384–388.

25. Paulus W, Slowick F, Jellinger K. Primary intracranial sarcomas: histopathological features of 19 cases. Histopathology 1991; 18:395–402.

26. Raskind R, Grant S. Primary mesenchymal chondrosarcoma of the cerebrum: report of a case. J Neurosurg 1966;24:676–678.

27. Reznick M, Lenelle J. Primary intracerebral osteosarcoma. Cancer 1991;68:793–797.

28. Roosen N, Cras P, Paquier P, Martin JJ. Primary thalamic malignant fibrous histiocytoma of the dominant hemisphere causing severe neuropsychological symptoms. Clin Neuropathol 1989;8: 16–21.

29. Scott RM, Dickersin GR, Wolpert SM, Twitchell T. Myxochondrosarcoma of the fourth ventricle: case report. J Neurosurg 1976;44:386–389.

30. Scully RE (ed). Case records of the Massachusetts General Hospital: case 26-1988. N Engl J Med 1988;318:1742–1750.

31. Sima A, Kindblom LG, Pelletteiri L. Liposarcoma of the meninges: a case report. Acta Pathol Microbiol Scand 1976;84: 306–310.

32. Sima AAF, Ross RT, Hoag G, et al. Malignant intracranial fibrous histiocytomas: histologic, ultrastructural and immunohistochemical studies of two cases. Can J Neurol Sci 1986;13:138–145.

33. Smith MM, Thompson JE, Castillo M. Radiation-induced cerebral osteogenic sarcoma. AJR 1996;167:1067.

34. Stechschulte SU, Kepes JJ, Holladay FP, McKittrick RJ. Primary meningeal extraosseous Ewing's sarcoma: case report. Neurosurgery 1994;35:143–147.

35. Suzuki Y, Yoshida YK, Shirane R, et al. Congenital primary cerebral angiosarcoma: case report. J Neurosurg 2000;92:466–468.

## Primary Central Nervous System Lymphoma

1. Aho R, Ekfors T, Haltia M, Kalimo H. Pathogenesis of primary central nervous system lymphoma: invasion of malignant lymphoid cells into and within the brain parenchyme. Acta Neuropathol (Berl) 1993;86:71–76.

2. Alderson L, Fetell MR, Sisti M, et al. Sentinel lesions of primary CNS lymphoma. J Neurol Neurosurg Psychiatry 1996;60: 102–105.

3. Antinori A, Ammassari A, De Luca A, et al. Diagnosis of AIDS-related focal brain lesions: a decision-making analysis based on clinical and neuroradiologic characteristics combined with polymerase chain reaction assays in CSF. Neurology 1997;48:687–694.

4. Ashby MA, Barber PC, Holmes AE, et al. Primary intracranial Hodgkin's disease. Am J Surg Pathol 1988;12:294–299.

5. Auperin I, Mikolt J, Oksenhendler E, et al. Primary central nervous system malignant non-Hodgkin's lymphomas from HIV-infected and non-infected patients: expression of cellular surface proteins and Epstein-Barr viral markers. Neuropathol Appl Neurobiol 1994;20:243–252.

6. Bashir RM, Hochberg FH, Wei MX. Epstein-Barr virus and brain lymphomas. J Neurooncol 1995;24:195–206.

7. Baumgartner JE, Rachlin JR, Beckstead JH, et al. Primary central nervous system lymphomas: natural history and response to radiation therapy in 55 patients with acquired immunodeficiency syndrome. J Neurosurg 1990;73:206–211.

8. Bednar MM, Salerni A, Flanagan ME, Pendlebury WW. Primary central nervous system T-cell lymphoma: case report. J Neurosurg 1991;74:668–672.

9. Brown MT, McClendon RE, Gockerman JP. Primary central nervous system lymphoma with systemic metastasis: case report and review. J Neurooncol 1995;23:207–221.

10. Camilleri-Broët S, Davi F, Feuillard J, et al. AIDS-related primary brain lymphomas: histopathologic and immunohistochemical study of 51 cases. Hum Pathol 1997;28:367–374.

11. Coté TR, Manns A, Hardy CR, et al. Epidemiology of brain lymphoma among people with or without acquired immunodeficiency syndrome. J Natl Cancer Inst 1996;88:675–679.

12. DeAngelis LM, Wong E, Rosenblum M, Furneaux H. Epstein-Barr virus in acquired immune deficiency syndrome (AIDS) and non-AIDS primary central nervous system lymphoma. Cancer 1992;70:1607–1611.

13. Eby NL, Grufferman S, Flannelly CM, et al. Increasing incidence of primary brain lymphoma in the US. Cancer 1988; 62: 2461–2465.

14. Ferracini R, Bergmann M, Pileri S, et al. Primary T-cell lymphoma of the central nervous system. Clin Neuropathol 1995; 14:125–129.

15. Geppert M, Ostertag CB, Seitz G, Kiessling M. Glucocorticoid therapy obscures the diagnosis of cerebral lymphoma. Acta Neuropathol (Berl) 1990;80:629–634.

16. Goldbrunner R, Warmuth-Metz M, Tonn J-C, et al. Primary Ki-1-positive T-cell lymphoma of the brain—an aggressive subtype of lymphoma: case report and review of the literature. Surg Neurol 1996;46:37–41.

17. Grant JW, Isaacson PG. Primary central nervous system lymphoma. Brain Pathol 1992;2:97–109.

18. Gray RS, Abrahams JJ, Hufnagel TJ, et al. Ghost-cell tumor of the optic chiasm: primary CNS lymphoma. J Clin Neuro-ophthalmol 1989;9:98–104.

19. Hao D, DiFrancesco LM, Brasher PM, et al. Is primary CNS lymphoma really becoming more common? A population-based study of incidence, clinicopathological features and outcomes in Alberta from 1975 to 1996. Ann Oncol 1999;10:65–70.

20. Havlioglu N, Manepalli A, Galindo L, et al. Primary Ki-1 (anaplastic large cell) lymphoma of the brain and spinal cord. Am J Clin Pathol 1995;103:496–499.

21. Hayakawa T, Takakura K, Abe H, et al. Primary central nervous system lymphoma in Japan: a retrospective, co-operative study of CNS-Lymphoma Study Group in Japan. J Neurooncol 1994;19: 197–215.

22. Hirano A. A comparison of the fine structure of malignant lymphoma and other neoplasms in the brain. Acta Neuropathol (Berl) 1975;6(Suppl):141–145.

23. Hochberg FH, Miller DC. Primary central nervous system lymphoma. J Neurosurg 1988;68:835–853.

24. Johnson BA, Fram EK, Johnson PC, Jacobowitz R. The variable MR appearance of primary lymphoma of the central nervous system: comparison of histopathologic features. AJNR 1997;18: 563–572.

25. Klein R, Müllges W, Bendszus M, et al. Primary intracerebral Hodgkin's disease: report of a case with Epstein-Barr virus association and review of the literature. Am J Surg Pathol 1999; 23:477–481.

26. Kobayashi H, Sano T, Hizawa K. Primary Burkitt-type lymphoma of the central nervous system. Acta Neuropathol (Berl) 1984;64: 12–14.

27. Krogh-Jensen M, Johansen P, D'Amore F. Primary central nervous system lymphomas in immunocompetent individuals: histology, Epstein-Barr virus genome, Ki-67 proliferation index, p53 and bcl-2 gene expression. Leuk Lymphoma 1998;30:131–142.

28. Miller DC, Hochberg FH, Harris NL, et al. Pathology with clinical correlations of primary central nervous system non-Hodgkin's lymphoma. Cancer 1994;74:1383–1397.

29. Miyazono M, Iwaki T, Tateishi J, Fukui M. Anaplastic large cell Ki-1 lymphoma in the central nervous system: report of an autopsy case. Acta Neuropathol (Berl) 1992;84:577–580.

30. Morgello S. Epstein-Barr and human immunodeficiency viruses in acquired immunodeficiency syndrome–related primary central nervous system lymphoma. Am J Pathol 1992;141:441–450.

31. Morgello S. Pathogenesis and classification of primary central nervous system lymphoma: an update. Brain Pathol 1995;5: 383–393.

32. Novak JA, Katzin WE. Primary central nervous system T-cell lymphoma with a predominant CD8 immunophenotype. Cancer 1995;75:2180–2185.

33. O'Neill BP, Wang CH, O'Fallon JR, et al. Primary central nervous system non-Hodgkin's lymphoma (PCNSL): survival and advantages with combined initial therapy? A final report of the North Central Cancer Treatment Group (NCCTG) Study 86-72-52. Int J Radiat Oncol Biol Phys 1999;43:559–563.

34. Poon T, Matoso I, Tchertkoff V, et al. CT features of primary cerebral lymphoma in AIDS and non-AIDS patients. J Comput Assist Tomogr 1989;13:6–9.

35. Raez LE, Patel P, Feun L, et al. Natural history and prognostic factors for survival in patients with acquired immune deficiency syndrom (AIDS)–related primary central nervous system lymphoma (PCNSL). Crit Rev Oncog 1998;9:199–208.

36. Roman-Goldstein SM, Goldman DL, Howieson J, et al. MR of primary CNS lymphoma in immunologically normal patients. AJNR 1992;13:1207–1213.

37. Rouah E, Rogers BB, Wilson DR, et al. Demonstration of Epstein-Barr virus in primary central nervous system lymphomas by polymerase chain reaction and in situ hybridization. Hum Pathol 1990;21:545–550.

38. Schwechheimer K, Braus DF, Schwartzkopf G, et al. Polymorphous high-grade B cell lymphoma is the predominant type of spontaneous primary cerebral malignant lymphomas: histological and immunomorphological evaluation of computed tomography–guided stereotactic brain biopsies. Am J Surg Pathol 1994;18:931–937.

39. Skolasky RL, Dal Pan GJ, Olivi A, et al. HIV-associated primary CNS lymorbidity and utility of brain biopsy. J Neurol Sci 1999; 163:32–38.

40. Tomlinson FH, Kurtin PJ, Suman VJ, et al. Primary intracerebral malignant lymphoma: a clinicopathological study of 89 patients. J Neurosurg 1995;82:558–566.

41. Werner MH, Phuphanich S, Lyman GH. The increasing incidence of malignant gliomas and primary central nervous system lymphoma in the elderly. Cancer 1995;76:1634–1642.

42. Yu GH, Montone KT, Frias-Hidvegi D, et al. Cytomorphology of primary CNS lymphoma: review of 23 cases and evidence for the role of EBV. Diagn Cytopathol 1996;14:114–120.

## Intravascular Lymphomatosis

1. Bergmann M, Terzija-Wessel U, Blasius S, et al. Intravascular lymphomatosis of the CNS: clinicopathologic study and search for expression of oncoproteins and Epstein-Barr virus. Clin Neurol Neurosurg 1994;96:236–243.

2. Clark WG, Dohan FC Jr, Moss T, Schweitzer JB. Immunocytochemical evidence of lymphocytic derivation of neoplastic cells in malignant angioendotheliomatosis. J Neurosurg 1991;74: 757–762.

3. Dubas F, Sainte-Andre JP, Pouplard-Barthelaix A, et al. Intravascular malignant lymphomatosis (so called malignant angioendotheliomatosis): a case confined to the lumbosacral spinal cord and nerve roots. Clin Neuropathol 1990;9:115–120.

4. Fredericks RK, Walker FO, Elster A, Challa V. Angiotropic intravascular large-cell lymphoma (malignant angioendotheliomatosis): report of a case and review of the literature. Surg Neurol 1991;35:218–223.

5. Glass J, Hochberg FH, Miller DC. Intravascular lymphomatosis: a systemic disease with neurologic manifestations. Cancer 1993;71:3156–3164.

6. Hamada K, Hamada T, Satoh M, et al. Two cases of neoplastic angioendotheliomatosis presenting with myelopathy. Neurology 1991;41:1139–1140.

7. Sepp N, Schuler G, Romani N, et al. "Intravascular lymphomatosis" (angioendotheliomatosis): evidence for a T-cell origin in two cases. Hum Pathol 1990;21:1051–1058.

8. Smadja D, Mas J-L, Fallet-Bianco C, et al. Intravascular lymphomatosis (neoplastic angioendotheliosis) of the central nervous system: case report and literature review. J Neurooncol 1991;11: 171–180.

9. Vieren M, Sciot R, Robberecht W. Intravascular lymphomatosis of the brain: a diagnostic problem. Clin Neurol Neurosurg 1999; 101:33–36.

10. Williams RL, Meltzer CC, Smirniotopoulos JG, et al. Cerebral MR imaging in intravascular lymphomatosis. AJNR 1998;19: 427–431.

## Lymphomatoid Granulomatosis

1. Anders KH, Latta H, Chang BS, et al. Lymphomatoid granulomatosis and malignant lymphoma of the central nervous system in the acquired immunodeficiency syndrome. Hum Pathol 1989;20:326–334.

2. Hamilton MG, Demetrick DJ, Tranmer BI, Curry B. Isolated cerebellar lymphomatoid granulomatosis progressing to malignant lymphoma. J Neurosurg 1994;80:314–320.

3. Kapila A, Gupta KL, Garcia JH. CT and MR of lymphomatoid granulomatosis of the CNS: report of four cases and review of the literature. AJNR 1988;9:1139–1143.

4. Kerr RSC, Hughes JT, Blamires T, Teddy PJ. Lymphomatoid granulomatosis apparently confined to one temporal lobe: case report. J Neurosurg 1987;67:612–615.

5. Kleinschmidt-DeMasters BK, Filley CM, Bitter MA. Central nervous system angiocentric, angiodestructive T-cell lymphoma (lymphomatoid granulomatosis). Surg Neurol 1992;37:130–137.

6. Schmidt BJ, Meagher-Villemure K, Carpio JD. Lymphomatoid granulomatosis with isolated involvement of the brain. Ann Neurol 1984;15:478–481.

7. Verity MA, Wolfson WL. Cerebral lymphomatoid granulomatosis: a report of two cases, with disseminated necrotizing leukoencephalopathy in one. Acta Neuropathol (Berl) 1976;36:117–124.

## Microglioma

1. Hulette CM. Microglioma, a histiocytic neoplasm of the central nervous system. Mod Pathol 1996;9:316–319.

## Germ Cell Neoplasms

1. Afshar F, King TT, Berry CL. Intraventricular fetus-in-fetu: case report. J Neurosurg 1982;56:845–849.

2. Akai T, Iizuka H, Kadoya S, Nojima T. Extraneural metastasis of intracranial germinoma with syncytiotrophoblastic giant cells—case report. Neurol Med Chir 1998;38:574–577.

3. Bjornsson J, Scheithauer BW, Leech RW. Primary intracranial choriocarcinoma: a case report. Clin Neuropathol 1986;5: 242–245.

4. Bjornsson J, Scheithauer BW, Okazaki H, Leech RW. Intracranial germ cell tumors: pathobiological and immunohistochemical aspects of 70 cases. J Neuropathol Exp Neurol 1985;44:32–46.

5. Chik K, Li C, Shing MM, et al. Intracranial germ cell tumors in children with and without Down syndrome. J Pediatr Hematol Oncol 1999;21:149–151.

6. Freilich RJ, Thompson SJ, Walker RW, Rosenblum MK. Adenocarcinomatous transformation of intracranial germ cell tumors. Am J Surg Pathol 1995;19:537–544.

7. Fujimaki T, Matsutani M, Funada N, et al. CT and MRI features of intracranial germ cell tumors. J Neurooncol 1994;19:217–226.

8. Fujiwara T, Honjo Y, Nagao S, et al. Primary cerebellar yolk sac tumor: case report. Surg Neurol 1994;42:121–124.

9. Gay JC, Janco RL, Lukens JN. Systemic metastases in primary intracranial germinoma: case report and literature review. Cancer 1985;55:2688–2690.

10. Higano S, Takahashi S, Ishii K, et al. Germinoma originating in the basal ganglia and thalamus: MR and CT evaluation. AJNR 1994;15:1435–1441.

11. Ho DM, Liu H-C. Primary intracranial germ cell tumor: pathologic study of 51 patients. Cancer 1992;70:1577–1584.

12. Inamura T, Nishio S, Ikezaki K, Fukui M. Human chorionic gonadotrophin in CSF, not serum, predicts outcome in germinoma. J Neurol Neurosurg Psychiatry 1999;66:654–665.

13. Itoyama Y, Kochi M, Kuratsu J-I, et al. Treatment of intracranial nongerminomatous malignant germ cell tumors producing α-fetoprotein. Neurosurgery 1995;36:459–466.
14. Iwanowski L, Kupryjanczyk J, Kuchna I, et al. Embryonal carcinoma of the pineal gland with yolk sac tumor differentiation: a case report. Folia Neuropathol 1997;35:128–132.
15. Izquierdo MA, Van der Valk P, Van Ark-Otte J, et al. Differential expression of the *c-kit* proto-oncogene in germ cell tumours. J Pathol 1995;177:253–258.
16. Jennings CD, Powell DE, Walsh JW, Mortara RH. Suprasellar germ cell tumor with extracranial metastases. Neurosurgery 1985;16:9–12.
17. Kawakami Y, Yamada O, Tabuchi K, et al. Primary intracranial choriocarcinoma. J Neurosurg 1980;53:369–374.
18. Kim DI, Yoon PH, Ryu YH, et al. MRI of germinomas arising from the basal ganglia and thalamus. Neuroradiology 1998;40:507–511.
19. Kirikae M, Arai H, Hidaka T, et al. Pineal yolk sac tumor in a 65-year-old man. Surg Neurol 1994;42:253–258.
20. Kobayashi T, Kageyama N, Kida Y, et al. Unilateral germinomas involving the basal ganglia and thalamus. J Neurosurg 1981;55:55–62.
21. Kobayashi T, Yoshida J, Kida Y. Bilateral germ cell tumors involving the basal ganglia and thalamus. Neurosurgery 1989;24:579–583.
22. Koyama S, Tsubokawa T, Katayama Y, Hirota H. Choriocarcinoma of the septum pellucidum: case report. Surg Neurol 1991;35:478–482.
23. Kraichoke S, Cosgrove M, Chandrasoma PT. Granulomatous inflammation in pineal germinoma: a cause of diagnostic failure at stereotaxic brain biopsy. Am J Surg Pathol 1988;12:655–660.
24. Latza U, Foss HD, Durkop H, et al. CD30 antigen in embryonal carcinoma and embryogenesis and release of the soluble molecule. Am J Pathol 1995;146:463–471.
25. Liu E, Robertson RL, de Plessis A, Pomeroy SL. Basal ganglia germinoma with progressive cerebral hemiatrophy. Pediatr Neurol 1999;20:312–314.
26. Matsumoto K, Tabuchi A, Tamesa N, et al. Primary intracranial germinoma involving the midbrain. Clin Neurol Neurosurg 1998;100:292–295.
27. Matsutani M, Saño K, Takakura K, et al. Primary intracranial germ cell tumors: a clinical analysis of 153 histologically verified cases. J Neurosurg 1997;86:446–455.
28. Nanda A, Schut L, Sutton LN. Congenital forms of intracranial teratoma. Childs Nerv Syst 1991;7:112–114.
29. Nishio S, Fukui M, Iwaki T, et al. Primary pineal yolk sac tumor: ultrastructural and immunohistochemical features—case report. Neurol Med Chir 1986;26:564–570.
30. Odell JM, Allen JK, Badura RJ, Weinberger E. Massive congenital intracranial teratoma: a report of two cases. Pediatr Pathol 1987;7:333–340.
31. Oi S, Tamaki N, Kondo T, et al. Massive congenital intracranial teratoma diagnosed in utero. Childs Nerv Syst 1990;6:459–461.
32. Ono N, Isobe I, Uki J, et al. Recurrence of primary intracranial germinomas after complete response with radiotherapy: recurrence patterns and therapy. Neurosurgery 1994;35:615–621.
33. Packer RJ, Sutton LN, Rorke LB, et al. Intracranial embryonal cell carcinoma. Cancer 1984;54:520–524.
34. Rickert CH, Reznik M, Lenelle J, Rinaldi P. Shunt-related abdominal metastases of cerebral teratocarcinoma: report of an unusual case and review of the literature. Neurosurgery 1998;42:1378–1383.
35. Salzman KL, Rojiani AM, Buatti J, et al. Primary intracranial germ cell tumors: clinicopathologic review of 32 cases. Pediatr Pathol Lab Med 1997;17:713–727.
36. Sawamura Y, Ikeda J, Shirato H, et al. Germ cell tumours of the central nervous system: treatment consideration based on 111 cases and their long-term clinical outcomes. Eur J Cancer 1998;34:104–110.
37. Schild SE, Haddock MG, Scheithauer BW, et al. Nongerminomatous germ cell tumors of the brain. Int J Radiat Oncol Biol Phys 1996;36:557–563.
38. Schild SE, Scheithauer BW, Haddock MG, et al. Histologically confirmed pineal tumors and other germ cell tumors of the brain. Cancer 1996;78:2564–2571.
39. Shaffrey ME, Lanzino G, Lopes MB, et al. Maturation of in-

40. Shinoda J, Miwa Y, Sakai N, et al. Immunohistochemical study of placental alkaline phosphatase in primary intracranial germ-cell tumors. J Neurosurg 1985;63:733–739.
41. Sievers EL, Berger M, Geyer JR. Long-term survival of a patient with primary sellar choriocarcinoma with pulmonary metastases: a case report. Med Pediatr Oncol 1996;26:293–295.
42. Tamaki N, Lin T, Shirataki K, et al. Germ cell tumors of the thalamus and the basal ganglia. Childs Nerv Syst 1990;6:3–7.
43. Tsukamoto H, Matsushima T, Shono S, et al. Primary yolk sac tumor of the cerebellar vermis: case report. Surg Neurol 1992;38:50–56.
44. Tsunoda S, Sasaoka Y, Sakaki T, et al. Suprasellar embryonal carcinoma which developed ten years after local radiation therapy for pineal germinoma. Surg Neurol 1993;40:146–150.
45. Uematsu Y, Tsuura Y, Miyamoto K, et al. The recurrence of primary intracranial germinomas: special reference to germinoma with STGC (syncytiotrophoblastic giant cell). J Neurooncol 1992;13:247–256.
46. Ushio Y, Kochi M, Kuratsu J, et al. Preliminary observations for a new treatment in children with primary intracranial yolk sac tumor or embryonal carcinoma: report of five cases. J Neurosurg 1999;90:133–137.
47. Wilson ER, Takei Y, Bikoff WT, et al. Abdominal metastases of primary intracranial yolk sac tumors through ventriculoperitoneal shunts: report of three cases. Neurosurgery 1979;5:356–364.
48. Yang S-T, Leow S-W. Intracranial fetus-in-fetu: CT diagnosis. AJNR 1992;13:1326–1329.
49. Yoshiki T, Itoh T, Shirai T, et al. Primary intracranial yolk sac tumor: immunofluorescent demonstration of alpha-fetoprotein synthesis. Cancer 1976;37:2343–2348.

## Hemangioblastoma

1. Becker I, Paulus W, Roggendorf W. Histogenesis of stromal cells in cerebellar hemangioblastomas: an immunohistochemical study. Am J Clin Pathol 1989;134:271–275.
2. Bonnin JM, Peña CE, Rubinstein LJ. Mixed capillary hemangioblastoma and glioma: a redefinition of the "angioglioma." J Neuropathol Exp Neurol 1983;42:504–516.
3. Bret P, Streichenberger N, Guyotat J. Metastasis of renal carcinoma to a cerebellar hemangioblastoma in a patient with von Hippel-Lindau disease: a case report. Br J Neurosurg 1999;13:413–416.
4. Brown DF, Gazdar AF, White CL III, et al. Human telomerase RNA expression and MIB-1 (Ki-67) proliferation index distinguish hemangioblastomas from metastatic renal cell carcinomas. J Neuropathol Exp Neurol 1997;56:1349–1355.
5. Commins DL, Hinton DR. Cytologic features of hemangioblastoma: comparison with meningioma, anaplastic astrocytoma and renal cell carcinoma. Acta Cytol 1998;42:1104–1110.
6. Crockard HA, Barnard RO, Isaacson PG. Metastasis of carcinoma to hemangioblastoma cerebelli: case report. Neurosurgery 1988;23:382–384.
7. de la Monte S, Horowitz SA. Hemangioblastomas: clinical and histopathological factors correlated with recurrence. Neurosurgery 1989;25:695–698.
8. Deck JHN, Rubinstein LJ. Glial fibrillary acidic protein in stromal cells of some capillary hemangioblastomas: significance and possible implications of an immunoperoxidase study. Acta Neuropathol (Berl) 1981;54:173–181.
9. Faiss J, Wild G, Schroth G, et al. Multiple supratentorial hemangioblastomas following primary infratentorial manifestations. Clin Neuropathol 1991;10:21–25.
10. Feldenzer JA, McKeever PE. Selective localization of γ-enolase in stromal cells of cerebellar hemangioblastomas. Acta Neuropathol (Berl) 1987;72:281–285.
11. Ferrante L, Acqui M, Mastronardi L, Fortuna A. Supratentorial hemangioblastoma: report of a case and review of the literature. Zentralbl Neurochir 1988;49:151–161.
12. Ferrante L, Celli P, Fraioli B. Supratentorial hemangioblastomas in children: case report. Acta Neurochir (Wien) 1982;62:241–246.
13. Frank TS, Trojanowski JQ, Roberts SA, Brooks JJ. A detailed immunohistochemical analysis of cerebellar hemangioblastoma: an undifferentiated mesenchymal tumor. Mod Pathol 1989;2:638–651.

14. Fukushima T, Sakamoto S, Iwaasa M, et al. Intramedullary hemangioblastoma of the medulla oblongata: two case reports and review of the literature. Neurol Med Chir 1998;38:489–498.

15. Giannini C, Scheithauer BW, Hellbusch LC, et al. Peripheral nerve hemangioblastoma. Mod Pathol 1998;11:999–1004.

16. Ho KL. Ultrastructure of cerebellar capillary hemangioblastoma. II. Mast cells and angiogenesis. Acta Neuropathol (Berl) 1984; 64:308–318.

17. Ho KL. Ultrastructure of cerebellar capillary hemangioblastoma. IV. Pericytes and their relationship to endothelial cells. Acta Neuropathol (Berl) 1985;67:254–264.

18. Ho KL. Ultrastructure of cerebellar capillary hemangioblastoma. I. Weibel-Palade bodies and stromal cell histogenesis. J Neuropathol Exp Neurol 1984;43:592–608.

19. Ho VB, Smirniotopoulos JG, Murphy FM, Rushing EJ. Radiologic-pathologic correlation: hemangioblastoma. AJNR 1992; 13:1343–1352.

20. Ho Y-S, Plets C, Goffin J, Dom R. Hemangioblastoma of the lateral ventricle. Surg Neurol 1990;33:407–412.

21. Horton JC, Harsh GR, Fisher JW, Hoyt WF. Von Hippel-Lindau disease and erythrocytosis: radioimmunoassay of erythropoietin in cyst fluid from a brainstem hemangioblastoma. Neurology 1991; 41:753–754.

22. Hufnagel TJ, Kim JH, True LD, Maneulidis EE. Immunohistochemistry of capillary hemangioblastoma: immunoperoxidase-labeled antibody staining resolves the differential diagnosis with metastatic renal cell carcinoma, but does not explain the histogenesis of the capillary hemangioblastoma. Am J Surg Pathol 1989;13:207–216.

23. Ishwar S, Taniguchi RM, Vogel FS. Multiple supratentorial hemangioblastomas: case study and ultrastructural characteristics. J Neurosurg 1971;35:396–405.

24. Ismail SM, Jasani B, Cole G. Histogenesis of haemangioblastomas: an immunocytochemical and ultrastructural study in a case of von Hippel-Lindau syndrome. J Clin Pathol 1985;38:417–421.

25. Jeffreys R. Pathological and haematological aspects of posterior fossa haemangioblastomata. J Neurol Neurosurg Psychiatry 1975; 38:112–119.

26. Jennings AM, Smith C, Cole DR, et al. Von Hippel-Lindau disease in a large British family: clinicopathological features and recommendations for screening and follow-up. Q J Med 1998;n.s. 66:233–249.

27. Kawafuchi J-I, Shirakura T, Azuma M, et al. Hematological study on a case with cerebellar hemangioblastoma associated with erythrocytosis, with special reference to an erythropoiesis-stimulating activity present in the fluid of the cyst of tumor. Blut 1970; 20:69–75.

28. Kerr DJ, Scheithauer BW, Miller GM, et al. Hemangioblastoma of the optic nerve: case report. Neurosurgery 1995;36:573–581.

29. Kohno K, Matsui S, Nishizaki A, et al. Successful total removal of intramedullary hemangioblastoma from the medulla oblongata. Surg Neurol 1993;39:25–30.

30. Krieg M, Marti HH, Plate KH. Coexpression of erythropoietin and vascular endothelial growth factor in nervous system tumors associated with von Hippel-Lindau tumor suppressor gene loss function. Blood 1998;92:3388–3393.

31. Lee J-Y, Dong S-M, Park W-S, et al. Loss of heterozygosity and somatic mutations of the VHL tumor suppressor gene in sporadic cerebellar hemangioblastomas. Cancer Res 1998;58:504–508.

32. Maher ER, Kaelin WG Jr. Reviews in molecular medicine: von Hippel-Lindau disease. Medicine 1997;76:381–391.

33. Matsumura A, Maki Y, Munekata K, Kobayashi E. Intracerebellar hemorrhage due to cerebellar hemangioblastoma. Surg Neurol 1985;24:227–230.

34. McComb RD, Eastman PJ, Hahn FJ, Bennett DR. Cerebellar hemangioblastoma with prominent stromal astrocytosis: diagnostic and histogenetic considerations. Clin Neuropathol 1987;6: 149–154.

35. McComb RD, Jones TR, Pizzo SV, Bigner DD. Localization of factor VIII/von Willebrand factor and glial fibrillary acidic protein in the hemangioblastoma: implications for stromal cell histogenesis. Acta Neuropathol (Berl) 1982;56:207–213.

36. Melmon KL, Rosen SW. Lindau's disease: review of the literature and study of a large kindred. Am J Med 1964;36:595–617.

37. Mills SE, Ross GW, Perentes E, et al. Cerebellar hemangioblastoma: immunohistochemical distinction from metastatic renal cell carcinoma. Surg Pathol 1990;3:121–132.

38. Mohan J, Brownell B, Oppenheimer DR. Malignant spread of haemangioblastoma: report on two cases. J Neurol Neurosurg Psychiatry 1976;39:515–525.

39. Naik RT, Purohit AK, Dinakar I, Ratnakar KS. Hemangioblastoma of the IV ventricle. Childs Nerv Syst 1995;11:499–500.

40. Nakamura N, Sekino H, Taguchi Y, Fuse T. Successful total extirpation of hemangioblastoma originating in the medulla oblongata. Surg Neurol 1985;24:87–94.

41. Nemes Z. Fibrohistiocytic differentiation in capillary hemangioblastoma. Hum Pathol 1992;23:805–810.

42. Nerad JA, Kersten RC, Anderson RL. Hemangioblastoma of the optic nerve: report of a case and review of the literature. Ophthalmology 1988;95:398–402.

43. Neumann HPH, Eggert HR, Scheremet R, et al. Central nervous system lesions in the von Hippel-Lindau syndrome. J Neurol Neurosurg Psychiatry 1992;55:898–901.

44. Neumann HPH, Lips CJM, Hsia YE, Zbar B. Von Hippel-Lindau syndrome. Brain Pathol 1995;5:181–193.

45. Prowse AH, Webster AR, Richards FM, et al. Somatic inactivation of the VHL gene in von Hippel-Lindau disease tumors. Am J Hum Genet 1997;60:765–771.

46. Richmond BK, Schmidt JH III. Congenital cystic supratentorial hemangioblastoma: case report. J Neurosurg 1995;82:113–115.

47. Rosenlöf K, Fyhrquist F, Grönhagen-Riska C, et al. Erythropoietin and renin substrate in cerebellar haemangioblastoma. Acta Med Scand 1985;218:481–485.

48. Rubio A, Meyers SP, Powers JM, et al. Hemangioblastoma of the optic nerve. Hum Pathol 1994;25:1249–1251.

49. Sawin PD, Follett KA, Wen C, Laws ER Jr. Symptomatic intrasellar hemangioblastoma in a child treated with subtotal resection and adjuvant radiosurgery. J Neurosurg 1996;84:1046–1050.

50. Stratmann R, Krieg M, Haas R, Plate KH. Putative control of angiogenesis in hemangioblastomas by the von Hippel-Lindau tumor suppressor gene. J Neuropathol Exp Neurol 1997;56: 1242–1252.

51. Sutton LN, Lasner T, Hunter J, et al. Thirteen-year-old female with hemangioblastoma. Pediatr Neurosurg 1997;27:50–55.

52. Tachibana O, Yamashima T, Yamashita J. Immunohistochemical study of erythropoietin in cerebellar hemangioblastomas associated with secondary polycythemia. Neurosurgery 1991;28:24–26.

53. Tanimura A, Nakamura Y, Hachishuka H, et al. Hemangioblastoma of the central nervous system: nature of the stromal cells as studied by the immunoperoxidase technique. Hum Pathol 1984;15:866–869.

54. Tse JYM, Wong JHC, Lo K-W, et al. Molecular genetic analysis of the von Hippel-Lindau disease tumor suppressor gene in familial and sporadic cerebellar hemangioblastomas. Am J Clin Pathol 1997;107:459–466.

55. Wakai S, Inoh S, Ueda Y, Nagai M. Hemangioblastoma presenting with intraparenchymatous hemorrhage. J Neurosurg 1984; 61:956–960.

56. Waldmann TA, Levin EH, Baldwin M. The association of polycythemia with a cerebellar hemangioblastoma: the production of an erythropoiesis stimulating factor by the tumor. Am J Med 1961;31:318–324.

57. Ward AA Jr, Foltz EL, Knopp LM. "Polycythemia" associated with cerebellar hemangioblastoma. J Neurosurg 1958;13: 248–258.

58. Zagzag D, Gultekin SH, Rosenblum MK. Immunolocalization of anti-Hu and RMDO-20 in stromal cells of hemangioblastomas. J Neuropathol Exp Neurol 1999;58:566.

59. Zec N, Cera P, Towfighi J. Extramedullary hematopoiesis in cerebellar hemangioblastoma. Neurosurgery 1991;29:34–36.

## Atypical Teratoid/Rhabdoid Tumor

1. Behring B, Brück W, Goebel HH, et al. Immunohistochemistry of primary central nervous system malignant rhabdoid tumors: report of five cases and review of the literature. Acta Neuropathol (Berl) 1996;91:578–586.

2. Biegel JA, Zhou J-Y, Rorke LB, et al. Germ-line and acquired mutations of INI1 in atypical teratoid and rhabdoid tumors. Cancer Res 1999;59:74–79.

3. Biggs PJ, Garen PD, Powers JM, Garvin AJ. Malignant rhabdoid tumor of the central nervous system. Hum Pathol 1987;18: 332–337.

4. Bonnin JM, Rubinstein LJ, Palmer NF, Beckwith JB. The association of embryonal tumors originating in the kidney and in the brain: a report of seven cases. Cancer 1984;54:2137–2146.

5. Bruch LA, Hill DA, Cai DX, et al. A role for fluorescence in situ hybridization detection of chromosome 22q dosage in distinguishing atypical teratoid/rhabdoid tumors from medulloblastoma/central primitive neuroectodermal tumors. Hum Pathol 2001; 32:156–162.

6. Burger PC, Yu I-T, Tihan T, et al. Atypical teratoid/rhabdoid tumor of the central nervous system: a highly malignant tumor of infancy and childhood frequently mistaken for medulloblastoma: a Pediatric Oncology Group study. Am J Surg Pathol 1998;22: 1083–1092.

7. Chou SM, Anderson JS. Primary CNS malignant rhabdoid tumor (MRT): report of two cases and review of the literature. Clin Neuropathol 1991;10:1–10.

8. Hanna SL, Langston JW, Parham DM, Douglass EC. Primary malignant rhabdoid tumor of the brain: clinical, imaging, and pathologic findings. AJNR 1993;14:107–115.

9. Hilden JM, Watterson J, Longee DC, et al. Central nervous system atypical teratoid tumor/rhabdoid tumor: response to intensive therapy and review of the literature. J Neurooncol 1998;40: 265–275.

10. Horn M, Schlote W, Lerch KD, et al. Malignant rhabdoid tumor: primary intracranial manifestation in an adult. Acta Neuropathol (Berl) 1992;83:445–448.

11. Howat AJ, Gonzales MF, Waters KD, Campbell PE. Primitive neuroectodermal tumour of the central nervous system associated with malignant rhabdoid tumour of the kidney: report of a case. Histopathology 1986;10:643–650.

12. Ogino S, Cohen ML, Abdul-Karim FW. Atypical teratoid/rhabdoid tumor of the CNS: cytopathology and immunohistochemistry of insulin-like growth factor-II, insulin-like growth factor receptor type 1, cathepsin D, and Ki-67. Mod Pathol 1999;12: 379–385.

13. Olson TA, Bayar E, Kosnik E, et al. Successful treatment of disseminated central nervous system malignant rhabdoid tumor. J Pediatr Hematol Oncol 1995;17:71–75.

14. Rorke LB, Packer RJ, Biegel JA. Central nervous system atypical teratoid/rhabdoid tumors of infancy and childhood: definition of an entity. J Neurosurg 1996;85:56–65.

15. Weeks DA, Beckwith JB, Mierau GW, Luckey DW. Rhabdoid tumor of kidney: a report of 111 cases from the National Wilms' Tumor Study Pathology Center. Am J Surg Pathol 1989;13: 439–458.

## Schwannoma and Malignant Peripheral Nerve Sheath Tumors

1. Aryanpur J, Long DM. Schwannoma of the medulla oblongata: case report. J Neurosurg 1988;69:446–449.

2. Aur RN, Budney J, Drake CG, Ball MJ. Frontal lobe perivascular schwannoma. J Neurosurg 1982;56:154–157.

3. Benhaiem-Sigaux N, Ricolfi F, Keravel Y, Poirier J. Epithelioid schwannoma of the acoustic nerve. Clin Neuropathol 1996; 15:231–233.

4. Best PV. Malignant triton tumour in the cerebellopontine angle: report of a case. Acta Neuropathol (Berl) 1987;74:92–96.

5. Boggan JE, Rosenblum ML, Wilson CB. Neurilemmoma of the fourth cranial nerve: case report. J Neurosurg 1979;50:519–521.

6. Bunc G, Milojkovic V, Kosir G, et al. Dumb-bell hypoglossal neurinoma with intra- and extracranial paravertebral expansion. Acta Neurochir (Wien) 1998;140:1209–1210.

7. Carney JA. Psammomatous melanotic schwannoma: a distinctive, heritable tumor with special associations, including cardiac myxoma and the Cushing syndrome. Am J Surg Pathol 1990;14: 206–222.

8. Casadei GP, Scheithauer BW, Hirose T, et al. Cellular schwannoma: a clinicopathologic, DNA flow cytometric, and proliferation marker study of 70 patients. Cancer 1995;75:1109–1119.

9. Cravioto H. The ultrastructure of acoustic nerve tumors. Acta Neuropathol (Berl) 1969;12:116–140.

10. Cruz-Sanchez F, Cervos-Navarrro J, Kashihara M. Intracerebral neurinomas in a case of von Recklinghausen's disease (neurofibromatosis). Clin Neuropathol 1987;6:174–178.

11. Dastur DK, Sinh G, Pandya SK. Melanotic tumor of the acoustic nerve: case report. J Neurosurg 1967;27:166–170.

12. Demyer W. Aberrant peripheral nerve fibres in the medulla oblongata of man. J Neurol Neurosurg Psychiatry 1965;28:121–123.

13. Deruaz JP, Janzer RC, Costa J. Cellular schwannomas of the intracranial and intraspinal compartment: morphological and immunological characteristics compared with classical benign schwannomas. J Neuropathol Exp Neurol 1993;52:114–118.

14. Di Biasi C, Trasimeni G, Iannilli M, et al. Intracerebral schwannoma: CT and MR findings. AJNR 1994;15:1956–1958.

15. Dolan EJ, Tucker WS, Rotenberg D, Chui M. Intracranial hypoglossal schwannoma as an unusual cause of facial nerve palsy. J Neurosurg 1982;56:420–423.

16. Dolenc VV, Coscia S. Cystic trochlear nerve neurinoma. Br J Neurosurg 1996;10:593–597.

17. Fink LH, Early CB, Bryan RN. Glossopharyngeal schwannomas. Surg Neurol 1978;9:239–245.

18. Fuller GN, Burger PC. Nervus terminalis (cranial nerve zero) in the adult human. Clin Neuropathol 1990;9:279–283.

19. Geddes JF, Sutcliffe JC, King TT. Mixed cranial nerve tumors in neurofibromatosis type 2. Clin Neuropathol 1995;14:310–313.

20. Ghatak NR, Norwood CW, Davis CH. Intracerebral schwannoma. Surg Neurol 1975;3:45–47.

21. Gökay H, İzgi N, Barlas O, Erseven G. Supratentorial intracerebral schwannomas. Surg Neurol 1984;22:69–72.

22. Han DH, Kim DG, Chi JG, et al. Malignant triton tumor of the acoustic nerve: case report. J Neurosurg 1992;76:874–877.

23. Huang PP, Zagzag D, Benjamin V. Intracranial schwannoma presenting as a subfrontal tumor: case report. Neurosurgery 1997; 40:194–197.

24. Ishii N, Sawamura Y, Tada M, Abe H. Acoustic cellular schwannoma invading the petrous bone: case report. Neurosurgery 1996; 38:576–578.

25. Jung J-M, Shin H-J, Chi JG, et al. Malignant intraventricular schwannoma: case report. J Neurosurg 1995;82:121–124.

26. Karmody CS. Malignant schwannoma of the trigeminal nerve. Otolaryngol Head Neck Surg 1979;87:594–598.

27. Kudo M, Matsumoto M, Terao H. Malignant nerve sheath tumor of acoustic nerve. Arch Pathol Lab Med 1983;107:293–297.

28. LeBlanc RA. Metastasis of bronchogenic carcinoma to acoustic neurinoma. J Neurosurg 1974;41:614–617.

29. Levy WJ, Ansbacher L, Byer J, et al. Primary malignant nerve sheath tumor of the gasserian ganglion: a report of two cases. Neurosurgery 1983;13:572–576.

30. Lilequist B, Thulin C, Tovi D, et al. Neurinoma of the labyrinthine portion of the facial nerve: case report. J Neurosurg 1972;37:105–109.

31. Liwnicz B. Bilateral trigeminal neurofibrosarcoma. J Neurosurg 1979;50:253–256.

32. Majoie CB, Hulsmans FJ, Castelijns JA, et al. Primary nerve-sheath tumours of the trigeminal nerve: clinical and MRI findings. Neuroradiology 1999;41:100–108.

33. Martuza RL, Ojemann RG. Bilateral acoustic neuromas: clinical aspects, pathogenesis, and treatment. Neurosurgery 1982;10: 1–12.

34. Memoli VA, Brown EF, Gould VE. Glial fibrillary acidic protein (GFAP) immunoreactivity in peripheral nerve sheath tumors. Ultrastruct Pathol 1984;7:269–275.

35. Miller RT, Sarikaya H, Sos A. Melanotic schwannoma of the acoustic nerve. Arch Pathol Lab Med 1986;110:153–154.

36. Mrak RE, Flanigan S, Collins CL. Malignant acoustic schwannoma. Arch Pathol Lab Med 1994;118:557–561.

37. New PFJ. Intracerebral schwannoma. J Neurosurg 1972;36: 795–797.

38. Okada Y, Shima T, Nishida M, Okita S. Large sixth nerve neuroma involving the prepontine region: case report. Neurosurgery 1997;40:608–610.

39. Ortiz O, Reed L. Spinal accessory nerve schwannoma involving the jugular foramen. AJNR 1995;16:986–989.

40. Prakash B, Roy S, Tandon PN. Schwannoma of the brain stem. J Neurosurg 1980;53:121–123.

41. Redekop G, Elisevich K, Gilbert J. Fourth ventricular schwannoma: case report. J Neurosurg 1990;73:777–781.

42. Rodriguez-Salazar A, Carillo R, de Miguel J. Intracerebral schwannoma in a child: report of a case. Childs Brain 1984;11: 69–72.

43. Sabel LHW, Teepen JLJM. The enigmatic origin of olfactory schwannoma: case report. Clin Neurol Neurosurg 1995;97: 187–191.

44. Santoreneos S, Hanieh A, Jorgensen RE. Trochlear nerve schwannomas occurring in patients without neurofibromatosis: case report and review of the literature. Neurosurgery 1997; 41:282–287.

45. Sarkar C, Mehta VS, Roy S. Intracerebellar schwannoma: case report. J Neurosurg 1987;67:120–123.
46. Scheithauer BW, Woodruff JM, Erlandson RA. Tumors of the Peripheral Nervous System. 3rd ed. Washington, DC: Armed Forces Institute of Pathology, 1999.
47. Shen W-C, Yang D-Y, Ho WL, et al. Neurilemmoma of the oculomotor nerve presenting as an orbital mass: MR findings. AJNR 1993;14:1253–1254.
48. Sobel RA, Wang Y. Vestibular (acoustic) schwannomas: histologic features in neurofibromatosis 2 and in unilateral cases. J Neuropathol Exp Neurol 1993;52:106–113.
49. Stefanko SZ, Vuzevski VD, Mass AIR, van Vroonhoven CCJ. Intracerebral malignant schwannoma. Acta Neuropathol (Berl) 1986;71:321–325.
50. Sterkers JM, Perre J, Viala P, Foncin J. The origin of acoustic neuromas. J Otolaryngol 1987;103:427–431.
51. Suzuki F, Handa J, Todo G. Intracranial glossopharyngeal neurinomas: report of two cases with special emphasis on computed tomography and magnetic resonance imaging findings. Surg Neurol 1989;31:390–394.
52. Tali ET, Yuh WTC, Nguyen HD, et al. Cystic acoustic schwannomas: MR characteristics. AJNR 1993;14:1241–1247.
53. Tegos S, Georgouli G, Gogos C, et al. Primary malignant schwannoma involving simultaneously the right gasserian ganglion and the distal part of the right mandibular nerve: case report. J Neurosurg Sci 1997;41:293–297.
54. Tran-Dinh HD, Soo YS, O'Neil P, Chaseling R. Cystic cerebellar schwannoma: case report. Neurosurgery 1991;29:296–300.
55. Weiner HL, Zagzag R, Weinreb HJ, Ransohoff J. Schwannoma of the fourth ventricle presenting with hemifacial spasm: report of two cases. J Neurooncol 1993;15:37–43.
56. Winek RR, Scheithauer BW, Wink MR. Meningioma, meningeal hemangiopericytoma (angioblastic meningioma), peripheral hemangiopericytoma and acoustic schwannoma: a comparative immunohistochemical study. Am J Surg Pathol 1989;13:251–261.
57. Wong T, Bennington JL. Metastasis of a mammary carcinoma to an acoustic neuroma. J Neurosurg 1962;19:1088–1093.
58. Yoshida K, Kawase T. Trigeminal neurinomas extending into multiple fossae: surgical methods and review of the literature. J Neurosurg 1999;91:202–211.

## Other Tumors of Intracranial Peripheral Nerves

1. Apostolides PJ, Spetzler RF, Johnson PC. Ectomesenchymal hamartoma (benign "ectomesenchymoma") of the VIIIth nerve: case report. Neurosurgery 1995;37:1204–1207.
2. Carvalho GA, Lindeke A, Tatagiba M, et al. Cranial granular-cell tumor of the trigeminal nerve: case report. J Neurosurg 1994;81:795–798.
3. Chimelli L, Symon L, Scaravilli F. Granular cell tumor of the fifth cranial nerve: further evidence for Schwann cell origin. J Neuropathol Exp Neurol 1984;43:634–642.
4. Cohen TI, Powers SK, Williams DW III. MR appearance of intracanalicular eighth nerve lipoma. AJNR 1992;13:1188–1190.
5. Lee JI, Nam DH, Kim JS, et al. Intracranial oculomotor nerve rhabdomyoma. J Neurosurg 2000;93:715.
6. Lena G, Dufour T, Gambarelli D, et al. Choristoma of the intracranial maxillary nerve in a child: case report. J Neurosurg 1994;81:788–791.
7. Paulus W, Warmuth-Metz M, Sörensen N. Intracranial neurotheleoma (nerve-sheath myxoma): case report. J Neurosurg 1993;79:280–282.
8. Rao TV, Puri R, Reddy GNN. Intracranial trigeminal nerve granular cell myoblastoma: case report. J Neurosurg 1983;59:706–709.
9. Saunders JE, Kwartler JA, Wolf HK, et al. Lipomas of the internal auditory canal. Laryngoscope 1991;101:1031–1037.
10. Scheithauer BW, Woodruff JM, Erlandson RA. Tumors of the Peripheral Nervous System. Washington, DC: Armed Forces Institute of Pathology, 1999.
11. Singh SP, Cottingham SL, Slone W, et al. Lipomas of the internal auditory canal. Arch Pathol Lab Med 1996;120:681–683.
12. Smith MM, Thompson JE, Thomas D, et al. Choristomas of the seventh and eighth cranial nerves. AJNR 1997;18:327–330.
13. Vandewalle G, Brucher J-M, Michotte A. Intracranial facial nerve rhabdomyoma: case report. J Neurosurg 1995;83:919–922.
14. Zwick DL, Livingston K, Clapp L, et al. Intracranial trigeminal nerve rhabdomyoma/choristoma in a child: a case report and discussion of possible histogenesis. Hum Pathol 1989;20:390–392.

## Colloid Cyst

1. Hadfield MG, Ghatak NR, Wanger GP. Xanthogranulomatous colloid cyst of the third ventricle. Acta Neuropathol (Berl) 1985;66:343–346.
2. Hernesniemi J, Leivo S. Management outcome in third ventricular colloid cysts in a defined population: a series of 40 patients treated mainly by transcallosal microsurgery. Surg Neurol 1996;45:2–14.
3. Ho KL, Garcia JH. Colloid cysts of the third ventricle: ultrastructural features are compatible with endodermal derivation. Acta Neuropathol (Berl) 1992;83:605–612.
4. King WA, Ullman JS, Frazee JG, et al. Endoscopic resection of colloid cysts: surgical considerations using the rigid endoscope. Neurosurgery 1999;44:1103–1110.
5. Lach B, Scheithauer BW. Colloid cyst of the third ventricle: a comparative ultrastructural study of neuraxis cysts and choroid plexus epithelium. Ultrastruct Pathol 1992;16:331–349.
6. Lach B, Scheithauer BW, Gregor A, Wick MR. Colloid cyst of the third ventricle: a comparative immunohistochemical study of neuraxis cysts and choroid plexus epithelium. J Neurosurg 1993;78:101–111.
7. Leech RW, Freeman T, Johnson R. Colloid cyst of the third ventricle: a scanning and transmission electron microscopic study. J Neurosurg 1982;57:108–113.
8. Macaulay RJB, Felix I, Jay V, Becker LE. Histological and ultrastructural analysis of six colloid cysts in children. Acta Neuropathol (Berl) 1997;93:271–276.
9. MacKenzie IR, Gilbert JJ. Cysts of the neuraxis of endodermal origin. J Neurol Neurosurg Psychiatry 1991;54:572–575.
10. Maeder PP, Holtåns SL, Basibüyük LN, et al. Colloid cysts of the third ventricle: correlation of MR and CT findings with histology and chemical analysis. AJNR 1990;11:575–581.
11. Mathiesen T, Grane P, Lindgren L, Lindquist C. Third ventricle colloid cysts: a consecutive 12-year series. J Neurosurg 1997;86: 5–12.
12. Mathiesen T, Grane P, Lindquist C, von Holst H. High recurrence rate following aspiration of colloid cysts in the third ventricle. J Neurosurg 1993;78:748–752.
13. Paulus W, Honegger J, Keyvani K, Fahlbusch R. Xanthogranuloma of the sellar region: a clinicopathological entity different from adamantinomatous craniopharyngioma. Acta Neuropathol (Berl) 1999;97:377–382.
14. Pollock BE, Huston J III. Natural history of asymptomatic colloid cysts of the third ventricle. J Neurosurg 1999;91:364–369.
15. Pollock BE, Schreiner SA, Huston J III. A theory on the natural history of colloid cysts of the third ventricle. Neurosurgery 2000;46:1077–1081.
16. Powers JM, Dodds HM. Primary actinomycoma of the third ventricle—the colloid cyst: a histochemical and ultrastructural study. Acta Neuropathol (Berl) 1977;37:21–26.
17. Tatter SB, Ogilvy CS, Golden JA, et al. Third ventricular xanthogranulomas clinically and radiologically mimicking colloid cysts: report of two cases. J Neurosurg 1994;81:605–609.

## Ependymal Cyst

1. Boockvar JA, Shafa R, Forman MS, O'Rourke DM. Symptomatic lateral ventricular ependymal cysts: criteria for distinguishing these rare cysts from other symptomatic cysts of the ventricles: case report. Neurosurgery 2000;46:1229–1232.
2. Bouch DC, Mitchell I, Maloney AF. Ependymal lined paraventricular cerebral cysts: a report of three cases. J Neurol Neurosurg Psychiatry 1973;36:611–617.
3. Friede RL, Yasargil MG. Supratentorial intracerebral epithelial (ependymal) cysts: review, case reports, and fine structure. J Neurol Neurosurg Psychiatry 1977;40:127–137.
4. Gherardi R, Lacombe MJ, Poirer J, et al. Asymptomatic encephalic intraparenchymatous neuroepithelial cysts. Acta Neurol Pathol 1984;63:264–268.
5. Ho KL, Chason JL. A glioependymal cyst of the cerebellopontine angle: immunohistochemical and ultrastructural studies. Acta Neuropathol (Berl) 1987;74:382–388.
6. Pant B, Uozumi T, Hirohata T, et al. Endoscopic resection of intraventricular ependymal cyst presenting with psychosis. Surg Neurol 1996;46:573–576.

## Choroid Plexus Cyst

1. Giorgi C. Symptomatic cyst of the choroid plexus of the lateral ventricle. Neurosurgery 1979;5:53–56.
2. Inoue T, Kuromatsu C, Iwata Y, Matsushima T. Symptomatic choroidal epithelial cyst in the fourth ventricle. Surg Neurol 1985;24:57–62.
3. Inoue T, Matsushima T, Fukui M, et al. Choroidal epithelial cyst of the cerebral hemisphere: an immunohistochemical study. Surg Neurol 1987;28:119–122.
4. Odake G, Tenjin H, Murakami N. Cyst of the choroid plexus in the lateral ventricle: case report and review of the literature. Neurosurgery 1990;27:470–476.

## Metastatic Neoplasms

1. Alleyne CH, Bakay RAE, Costigan D, et al. Intracranial adenoid cystic carcinoma: case report and review of the literature. Surg Neurol 1996;45:265–271.
2. Ammirati M, Samii M, Skaf G, Sephernia A. Solitary brain metastasis 13 years after removal of renal adenocarcinoma. J Neurooncol 1993;15:87–90.
3. Athanassiou A, Begent RHJ, Newlands ES, et al. Central nervous system metastases of choriocarcinoma: 23 years' experience at Charing Cross Hospital. Cancer 1983;52:1728–1735.
4. Atlas SW, Grossman RI, Gomori JM, et al. MR imaging of intracranial metastatic melanoma. J Comput Assist Tomogr 1987;11:577–582.
5. Baram TZ, van Tassel P, Jaffe NA. Brain metastases in osteosarcoma: incidence, clinical and neuroradiological findings and management options. J Neurooncol 1988;6:47–52.
6. Ben-Izhak O, Stark P, Levy R, et al. Epithelial markers in malignant melanoma: a study of primary lesions and their metastases. Am J Dermatopathol 1994;16:241–246.
7. Bindal RK, Sawaya R, Leavens ME, Lee JJ. Surgical treatment of multiple brain metastases. J Neurosurg 1993;79:210–216.
8. Bindal RK, Sawaya RE, Leavens ME, et al. Sarcoma metastatic to the brain: results of surgical treatment. Neurosurgery 1994;35:185–191.
9. Boogerd W, Vos VW, Hart AAM, Baris G. Brain metastases in breast cancer: natural history, prognostic factors and outcome. J Neurooncol 1993;15:165–174.
10. Buff BJ, Schick RM, Norregaard T. Meningeal metastasis of leiomyosarcoma mimicking meningioma: CT and MR findings. J Comput Assist Tomogr 1991;15:166–167.
11. Bullard DE, Cox EB, Seigler HF. Central nervous system metastases in malignant melanoma. Neurosurgery 1981;8:26–30.
12. Carrier DA, Mawad ME, Kirkpatrick JB, Schmid MF. Metastatic adenocarcinoma to the brain: MR with pathologic correlation. AJNR 1994;15:155–159.
13. Choi KN, Withers HR, Rotman M. Intracranial metastases from melanoma: clinical features and treatment by accelerated fractionation. Cancer 1985;56:1–9.
14. Colon G, Quint DJ, Blaivas M, McGillicuddy J. Cardiac sarcoma metastatic to the brain. AJNR 1995;16:1739–1741.
15. dal Canto M, Valsamis MP. Fibrosarcoma metastatic to the brain. Arch Pathol 1973;96:108–110.
16. Dauplat J, Nieberg RK, Hacker NF. Central nervous system metastases in epithelial ovarian carcinoma. Cancer 1987;60:2559–2562.
17. Davis RP, Spigelman MK, Zappulla RA, et al. Isolated central nervous system metastasis from transitional cell carcinoma of the bladder: report of a case and review of the literature. Neurosurgery 1986;18:622–624.
18. Delattre JY, Krol G, Thaler HT, Posner JB. Distribution of brain metastases. Arch Neurol 1988;45:741–744.
19. España P, Chang P, Wiernik PH. Increased incidence of brain metastases in sarcoma patients. Cancer 1980;45:377–380.
20. Feeney JJ, Popek EJ, Bergman WC. Leiomyosarcoma metastatic to the brain: case report and literature review. Neurosurgery 1985;16:398–401.
21. Fervenza FC, Wolanskyj AP, Eklund HE, Richardson RL. Brain metastasis: an unusual complication from prostatic adenocarcinoma. Mayo Clin Proc 2000;75:79–82.
22. Franke FE, Altmannsberger M, Schachenmayr W. Metastasis of renal carcinoma colliding with glioblastoma. Carcinoma to glioma: an event only rarely detected. Acta Neuropathol (Berl) 1990;80:448–452.
23. Gabrielsen TO, Eldevik OP, Orringer MB, Marshall BL. Esophageal carcinoma metastatic to the brain: clinical value and cost-effectiveness of routine enhanced head CT before esophagectomy. AJNR 1995;16:1915–1921.
24. Galluzzi S, Payne PM. Brain metastases from primary bronchial carcinoma: a statistical study of 741 necropsies. Br J Cancer 1956;10:408–414.
25. Gercovich FG, Luna MA, Gottlieb JA. Increased incidence of cerebral metastases in sarcoma patients with prolonged survival from chemotherapy: report of cases of leiomyosarcoma and chondrosarcoma. Cancer 1975;36:1843–1851.
26. Gorin FA, Bale JF, Halks-Miller M, Schwartz RA. Kaposi's sarcoma metastatic to the CNS. Arch Neurol 1985;42:162–165.
27. Gormley WB, Sekhar LN, Wright DC, et al. Management and long-term outcome of adenoid cystic carcinoma with intracranial extension: a neurosurgical perspective. Neurosurgery 1996;38:1105–1113.
28. Gottschalk J, Jautzke G, Paulus W, et al. The use of immunomorphology to differentiate choroid plexus tumors from metastatic carcinomas. Cancer 1993;72:1343–1349.
29. Griffin JW, Thompson RW, Mitchinson MJ, et al. Lymphomatous leptomeningitis. Am J Med 1971;51:200–208.
30. Gupta A, Baidas S, Cumberlin RK. Brain stem metastasis as the only site of spread in prostate carcinoma: a case report. Cancer 1994;74:2516–2519.
31. Haykal HA, Wang A-M, Zamani A. Leiomyosarcoma metastatic to the brain: CT features and review. AJNR 1987;8:911–912.
32. Hlavin ML, Kaminski HJ, Cohen M, et al. Central nervous system complications of cystosarcoma phyllodes. Cancer 1993;72:126–130.
33. Hwang T-L, Valdivieso JG, Yang C-H, Wolin MJ. Calcified brain metastasis. Neurosurgery 1993;32:451–454.
34. Ishizuka T, Tomoda Y, Kaseki S, et al. Intracranial metastasis of choriocarcinoma: a clinicopathologic study. Cancer 1983;52:1896–1903.
35. Jellinger K, Radaszkiewicz T. Involvement of the central nervous system in malignant lymphomas. Virchows Arch A Pathol Anat Histol 1976;370:345–362.
36. Kazumoto K, Hayase N, Kurosumi M, et al. Multiple brain metastases from adenoid cystic carcinoma of the parotid gland: case report and review of the literature. Surg Neurol 1998;50: 475–479.
37. Kindt GW. The pattern of location of cerebral metastatic tumors. J Neurosurg 1964;21:54–57.
38. Kleinert R, Beham A, Rosanelli G. Alveolar rhabdomyosarcoma in a young female patient metastasizing to the brain. Acta Neuropathol (Berl) 1985;67:341–344.
39. Kohno M, Matsutani M, Sasaki T, Takakura K. Solitary metastasis to the choroid plexus of the lateral ventricle. J Neurooncol 1996;27:47–52.
40. Lu AT, Lee CO. Liposarcoma of chest wall with metastasis to the cerebrum: review of literature and report of case. Bull Los Angeles Neurol Soc 1961;26:217–224.
41. Lynes WL, Bostwick DG, Freiha FS, Stamey TA. Parenchymal brain metastases from adenocarcinoma of prostate. Urology 1986;28:280–287.
42. MacDonald J, Parker JC Jr, Brown S, et al. Cerebral metastasis from a malignant thymoma. Surg Neurol 1978;9:58–60.
43. Madow L, Alpers BJ. Encephalitic form of metastatic carcinoma. Am Arch Neurol Psych 1951;65:161–173.
44. Mandybur TI. Intracranial hemorrhage caused by metastatic tumors. Neurology 1977;27:650–655.
45. Maruki C, Suzukawa K, Kioke J, Sato K. Cardiac malignant fibrous histiocytoma metastasizing to the brain: development of multiple neoplastic cerebral aneurysms. Surg Neurol 1994;41: 40–44.
46. McCutcheon IE, Eng DY, Logothetis CJ. Brain metastasis from prostate carcinoma: antemortem recognition and outcome after treatment. Cancer 1999;86:2301–2311.
47. McKenney JK, Varma VA, Hunter SB. Distinguishing metastatic small cell carcinoma (SCC) from a primary cerebellar medulloblastoma (MB) in an adult: an immunohistochemical study of thyroid transcription factor (TTF), cytokeratin AE1/3 (AE1/3), and epithelial membrane antigen. J Neuropathol Exp Neurol 2000;59:420.
48. Miettinen M, Franssila K. Immunohistochemical spectrum of malignant melanoma: the common presence of keratins. Lab Invest 1989;6:623–628.

49. Mrak RE. Origins of adenocarcinomas presenting as intracranial metastases. Arch Pathol Lab Med 1993;117:1165–1169.

50. Nida TY, Hall WA, Glantz MJ, Clark HB. Metastatic carcinoid tumor to the orbit and brain. Neurosurgery 1992;31:949–952.

51. Nurick S, Mair WGP. Brain metastases from haemangioendothelioma of the spleen: report of a case. Acta Neuropathol (Berl) 1970;14:345–349.

52. Nussbaum ES, Djalilian HR, Cho KH, Hall WA. Brain metastases: histology, multiplicity, surgery, and survival. Cancer 1996; 78:1781–1788.

53. Paraf F, Deloche A, Scholl J-M, et al. Primary liposarcoma of the heart. Am J Cardiovasc Pathol 1990;3:175–180.

54. Perry JR, Bilbao JM. Metastatic alveolar soft part sarcoma presenting as a dural-based cerebral mass. Neurosurgery 1994;34: 168–170.

55. Postler E, Meyermann R. Brain metastasis in renal cell carcinoma: clinical data and neuropathological differential diagnoses. Anticancer Res 1999;19:1579–1581.

56. Radley MG, McDonald JV, Pilcher WH, Wilbur DC. Late solitary cerebral metastases from renal cell carcinoma: report of two cases. Surg Neurol 1993;39:230–234.

57. Recht L, Straus DJ, Cirrincione C, et al. Central nervous system metastases from non-Hodgkin's lymphoma: treatment and prophylaxis. Am J Med 1988;84:425–435.

58. Retsas S, Gershuny AR. Central nervous system involvement in malignant melanoma. Cancer 1988;61:1926–1934.

59. Sabo RA, Kalyanan-Raman UP. Multiple intracerebral metastases from an islet cell carcinoma of the pancreas: case report. Neurosurgery 1995;37:326–328.

60. Salvati M, Cervoni L, Caruso R, et al. Sarcoma metastatic to the brain: a series of 15 cases. Surg Neurol 1998;49:441–444.

61. Sampson JH, Carter JH Jr, Friedman AH, Seigler HF. Demographics, prognosis, and therapy in 702 patients with brain metastases from malignant melanoma. J Neurosurg 1998;88: 11–20.

62. Saris S, Vavoulis G, Linder J, Friedman A. Fibrosarcoma of the heart metastatic to the brain. Neurosurgery 1983;13:327–329.

63. Scully RE, Mark EJ, McNeely WF, McNeely BU. Case records of the Massachusetts General Hospital: case 28-1992. N Engl J Med 1992;327:107–116.

64. Seaman EK, Ross S, Sawczuk IS. High incidence of asymptomatic brain lesions in metastatic renal cell carcinoma. J Neurooncol 1995;23:253–256.

65. Shimada H, Newton WA Jr, Soule EH, et al. Pathology of fatal rhabdomyosarcoma: report from Intergroup Rhabdomyosarcoma Study (IRS-I and IRS-II). Cancer 1987;59:459–465.

66. Stein M, Steiner M, Klein B, et al. Involvement of the central nervous system by ovarian carcinoma. Cancer 1986;58: 2066–2069.

67. Tashiro Y, Kondo A, Aoyama I, et al. Calcified metastatic brain tumor. Neurosurgery 1990;26:1065–1070.

68. Taylor HG, Lefkowitz M, Skoog SJ, et al. Intracranial metastases in prostate cancer. Cancer 1984;53:2728–2730.

69. Tewari MK, Khosla VK, Sharma BS, et al. Brain metastasis from urachal carcinoma: case report. Surg Neurol 1994;42:340–342.

70. Todo T, Usui M, Nagashima K. Cerebral metastasis of malignant cardiac myxoma. Surg Neurol 1992;37:374–379.

71. Trillet V, Catajar J-F, Croisile B, et al. Cerebral metastases as first symptom of bronchogenic carcinoma. Cancer 1991;68:2935–2940.

72. Tsukada Y, Fouad A, Pickren JW, Lane WW. Central nervous system metastasis from breast carcinoma: autopsy study. Cancer 1983;52:2349–2354.

73. Vannier A, Gray F, Gherardi R, et al. Diffuse subependymal periventricular metastases: report of three cases. Cancer 1986;58: 2720–2725.

74. Vinchon M, Ruchoux MM, Seuer JP, et al. Solitary brain metastasis as only recurrence of a carcinoma of the bladder. Clin Neuropathol 1994;13:338–340.

75. Weber P, Shepard KV, Vijayakumar S. Metastases to pineal gland. Cancer 1989;63:164–165.

76. Weiss HD, Richardson EP Jr. Solitary brainstem metastasis. Neurology 1978;28:562–566.

77. Wennerberg AE, Nalesnik MA, Coleman WB. Hepatocyte paraffin 1: a monoclonal antibody that reacts with hepatocytes and can be used for differential diagnosis of hepatic tumors. Am J Pathol 1993;143:1050–1054.

78. Wronsky MAE. Surgical treatment of brain metastases from melanoma: a retrospective study. J Neurosurg 2000;93:9–18.

79. Young RC, Howser DM, Anderson T, et al. Central nervous system complications of non-Hodgkin's lymphoma: the potential role for prophylactic therapy. Am J Med 1979;66:435–443.

80. Yu L, Craver R, Baliga M, et al. Isolated CNS involvement in Ewing's sarcoma. Med Pediatr Oncol 1990;18:354–358.

81. Zarbo RJ, Gown AM, Nagle RB, et al. Anomalous cytokeratin expression in malignant melanoma: one- and two-dimensional Western blot analysis and immunohistochemical survey of 100 melanomas. Mod Pathol 1990;3:494–501.

# The Brain: Stereotactically Directed Needle Biopsy

5

The application of stereotactic methods to specific entities is discussed throughout this book. The present chapter is intended only as a general guide for specimen preparation and interpretation. Many of the recommendations presented here are equally applicable to the study of larger specimens obtained by craniotomy. For a more in-depth discussion, the reader is referred to several articles regarding specimen preparation and analysis[3, 9, 17, 26] and the historical development of the technique.[16]

## INDICATIONS

Stereotactic biopsies are not always justified by strict criteria but are undertaken in many instances on the basis of convenience, financial considerations, or the fact that some lesions, such as primary central nervous system lymphomas, are more safely sampled by this technique than by an open approach. The procedure is also used in cases in which patients are too ill to undergo a craniotomy. In some instances, the biopsy is the definitive procedure; in others it is only a preliminary sampling done in the anticipation of a later open or stereotactic procedure after the histologic nature of a lesion has been clarified. Although the procedure is employed generally for morphologic studies, procuring material for culture of microorganisms and obtaining it for molecular biologic purposes are other potential roles.[19, 21]

The advantages of the stereotactic biopsy method include safety, reduced hospital stay, and the ability to sample a predetermined target point with great precision. Optimally, the yield of diagnostic tissue exceeds 90%.[11, 22] Disadvantages include the size and frequent fragmentation of the specimen. Nonetheless, small but representative samples from a definable target point are often preferable to larger, but less representative, tissues obtained freehand by open craniotomy.

Complications of stereotactically directed biopsy are uncommon and are variably reported to occur in 0.5% to 4% of cases.[1, 2, 11, 12, 20] The lower figure represents our own experience. Hemorrhage, the principal concern, is more likely when the instrument penetrates periventricular or particularly vascular deep gray matter, for example, thalamus and basal ganglia. Clinically occult hemorrhages are not uncommonly found by postbiopsy computed tomographic (CT) scanning.[17]

Obviously, sampling becomes an issue with stereotactic biopsies. This is particularly true in infiltrative gliomas. In one systematic study of the accuracy of stereotactic biopsy versus that obtained by open resection of lesions, an average of six stereotactic biopsies per patient allowed accurate grading in 98% of cases. When the mean number of biopsies was only four, tumor grade was underestimated in 25% of cases.[8]

## TARGET SELECTION

Any area of the brain, including the brain stem, can be safely reached. Nonetheless, most sampled lesions are supratentorial, deep seated, and intrinsic. Cerebellar or brain stem lesions, usually infiltrating astrocytomas, are less often subjected to biopsy (Figs. 5–1 to 5–3). Infiltrating gliomas (astrocytomas and oligodendrogliomas) (Figs. 5–1 to 5–8),[9] primary central nervous system lymphomas (Figs. 5–9 to 5–11),[18, 21] and inflammatory lesions are common targets (Figs. 5–12 and 5–13).[14] Even vascular lesions are sometimes approached (Figs. 5–14 to 5–17). On the other hand, discrete and potentially resectable masses, such as ganglion cell tumors, pilocytic astrocytomas, pleomorphic xanthoastrocytomas, astroblastoma, ependymoma, and hemangioblastomas, are usually

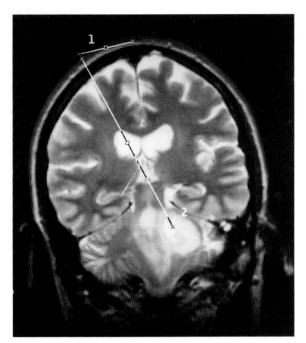

**FIGURE 5–1** ANAPLASTIC ASTROCYTOMA OF THE BRAIN STEM AND CEREBELLUM

A 49-year-old man presented with a 2½-year history of progressive weakness followed by sensory and motor cranial nerve deficits. The deep-seated lesion was approached stereotactically.

approached by craniotomy with the goal of excision or decompression. The wide variety of processes amenable to stereotactic biopsy is well illustrated by lesions occurring in the population with acquired immunodeficiency syndrome (AIDS).[7, 13–15] In contrast, extra-axial lesions such as meningiomas are approached by open procedures with the intent of excision, not with the purely diagnostic aim of stereotactic biopsy.

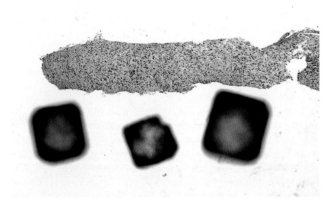

**FIGURE 5–2** ANAPLASTIC ASTROCYTOMA OF THE BRAIN STEM AND CEREBELLUM

Grains of table salt placed on the slide emphasize the size of this small, but adequate, tissue core obtained from the lesion illustrated in Figure 5–1. Although specimen size was not a limiting factor in this case, it can complicate the diagnosis of a paucicellular, well-differentiated glioma as illustrated in Figures 5–29 to 5–31.

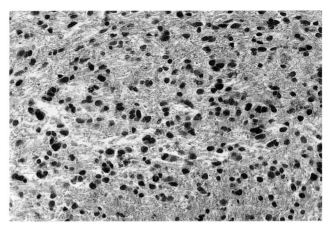

**FIGURE 5–3** ANAPLASTIC ASTROCYTOMA OF THE BRAIN STEM AND CEREBELLUM

Higher magnification of the lesion in Figure 5–2 shows the typical features of a grade III astrocytoma.

The hardware and software systems utilized in stereotactic procedures vary considerably from one institution to another, but classical methods begin by identifying reference points created by a frame attached to the skull. Newer techniques use small fiducial markers attached to the skull that obviate the cumbersome superstructure of a frame.[10] One or more target points most likely to yield diagnostic tissue are identified by either CT or magnetic resonance imaging (MRI). If present, an area of enhancement is generally chosen. As discussed later in the section Correlation of Clinical, Radiologic, and Pathologic Data, it is essential that radiographic images guide the interpretation of pathologic findings. Such questions as "Does the biopsy explain the imaging abnormality?" and "Does this apparently low-grade lesion actually have the radiologic features of a high-grade lesion?" must be answered.

The stereotactic system is based on three dimensions and generates X (left-right), Y (anterior-posterior), and Z (superior-inferior) coordinates. The computer directs the appropriate settings on the gantry that is attached to the frame. The sampling device is advanced to the prescribed depth and accepts the tissue drawn into its aperture by the suction from an attached syringe. The caliber and configuration of the device vary from those of a fine needle to the substantial core obtained by stout trocars with cutting sideports (Figs. 5–18 and 5–19). By preference of the surgeon, one or more specimens may be obtained at a given target point. A trocar may be rotated "around the clock," stopping periodically to obtain additional samples. The surgeon may then wait for the results of the pathologic study or proceed immediately to a different target point along the same trajectory. Sampling at a new target point may be necessary if the cores from the initial point do not contain diagnostic tissue. Depending on the nature of the sampling device and the nature of the lesion, specimens

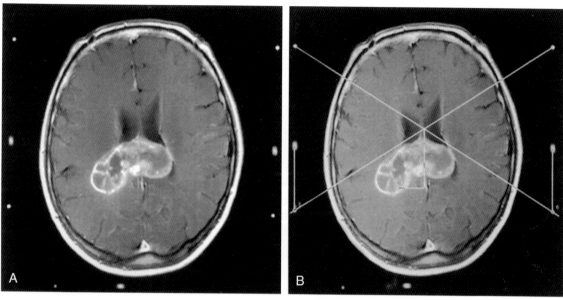

**FIGURE 5–4**   GLIOBLASTOMA MULTIFORME

As seen in reference to the stereotactic frame, this deep-seated "butterfly" lesion of the corpus callosum exhibits the peripheral rim of contrast enhancement so typical of glioblastoma (A). The coordinates identified by the surgeon triangulated a point on the contrast-enhancing rim where diagnostic tissue is most likely to be found. This 56-year-old woman had presented emergently with headaches and changes in mental status. (Courtesy of Dr. Alessandro Olivi, Baltimore, MD.)

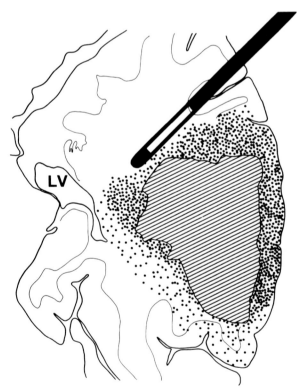

**FIGURE 5–5**   GLIOBLASTOMA MULTIFORME

Although glioblastoma is an infiltrative neoplasm, its densely cellular rim can be sharply defined. While very close to the diagrammed temporal lobe lesion seen in the horizontal plane, this needle is about to obtain tissue that is either normal or so marginally hypercellular as to be nondiagnostic. Referring to neuroimages at the time of intraoperative tissue analysis would quickly identify a problem of tissue sampling. LV, lateral ventricle.

range from minute fragments to sizable (1 cm long, 0.2 cm wide) intact tissue cores (Fig. 5–19). Occasionally, only blood gushes out, or pus pours forth in the case of an abscess.

The accuracy of the technique is impressive, both in theory and usually in practice,[19] but pathologists are familiar with "stereotactic misses," even of large lesions.[22] As discussed later, active participation by the

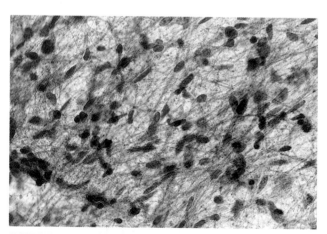

**FIGURE 5–6**   GLIOBLASTOMA MULTIFORME

In a smear preparation of the lesion illustrated in Figure 5–4, the tissue fragment can be seen to be composed of aggregated cells whose processes form a background. The small, somewhat elongated, rather bland nuclei are common in glioblastomas.

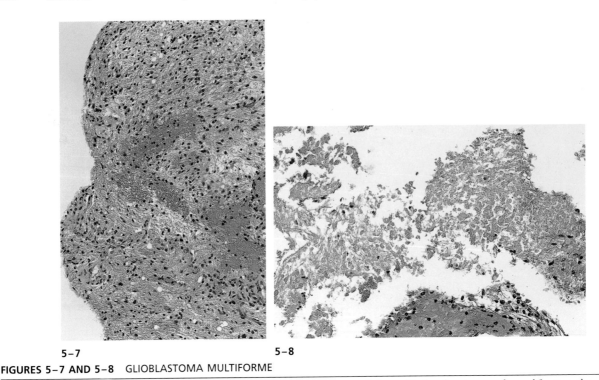

5-7                              5-8

**FIGURES 5-7 AND 5-8**   GLIOBLASTOMA MULTIFORME

Although the tissue removed from the patient illustrated in Figure 5–4 was hypercellular and had early microvascular proliferation, the abnormalities seen were less than expected on the basis of radiologic features (Fig. 5–7). The presence of necrosis elsewhere in the specimen helped secure the diagnosis of glioblastoma (Fig. 5–8).

pathologist goes a long way toward preventing this unfortunate outcome.

## SPECIMEN PREPARATION

Assessment of a specimen begins as consultation with the surgeon, ideally in the operating room, to review goals of the procedure and determine the amount of tissue to be provided. If the specimen is limited, a smear preparation from a portion of it may have to suffice. More options are open if multiple cores are available, and the use of smears as well as frozen sections can be entertained. Although the relative merits of frozen sections and cytologic preparations can be debated,[13] as can the use of any tissue at all for frozen section, most laboratories perform both. Either can ensure that adequate and representative tissue has been obtained and can often establish a definitive diagnosis. In the usual setting in which multiple tissue cores are available, it is our practice to divide the specimen into portions for (1) a smear preparation, (2) a frozen section and permanent specimens prepared therefrom, and (3) permanent sections of unfrozen tissue. Tissue for electron microscopy and molecular-cytogenetic studies can be set aside as well. Only under most unusual circumstances should all tissue be used for frozen sections.

In regard to cytologic preparations, some lesions are so cellular and stroma poor that sufficient numbers of cells can be harvested by merely pressing a slide against the specimen. Although such lesions as lymphomas, macrophage-rich processes such as demyelination, pituitary adenomas, meningiomas, and some metastatic carcinomas are adequately sampled by such touch preparations, most tumors yield either no cells or tissue that is confined to unsightly hypercellular mounds. For these, we clearly prefer smear preparations because this more forceful method achieves uniform cell dispersion. A minute (1 to 2 mm) portion of tissue is separated from a core, placed between two slides, and compressed until the nail beds turn white. The slides are then drawn slowly apart to minimize artifactual cell elongation and then immersed immediately in fixative to avoid drying (Fig. 5–20). We find 95% alcohol the ideal fixative because subsequent staining with hematoxylin and eosin (H&E) or hemalum-phloxine[9] yields crisp nuclear and cytoplasmic details that are entirely comparable to those seen in routinely stained tissue sections. In the tradition of fine-needle aspirations at other body sites, some pathologists use dried smears stained with such stains such as Diff-Quik. Our clear preference is for H&E.

Preparation of the tissue cores for frozen and permanent histologic sections must be done in such a way as to neither waste tissue nor introduce unnecessary artifacts. Whatever their fate in the frozen section suite, the integrity of these precious specimens must be ensured. For example, the cores should be transported from the operating room on a moist, smooth-surfaced carrier—not on cotton pledgets or gauze, to

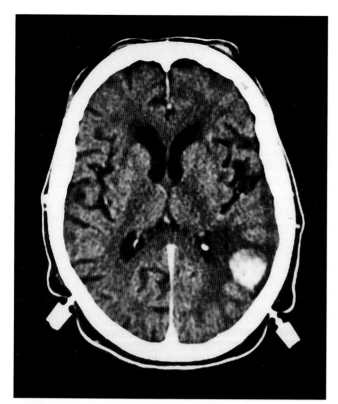

**FIGURE 5–9    PRIMARY CENTRAL NERVOUS SYSTEM LYMPHOMA**

Primary lymphomas of the brain are often approached stereotactically, as in this case of an 82-year-old woman. In immunocompetent patients the diagnosis is suggested by a homogeneous pattern of enhancement, that is, the one illustrated here, where the enhancing area is uninterrupted by nonenhancing regions. In the setting of immunocompromise, however, enhancement is usually inhomogeneous because of the presence of a dark-appearing, usually central, zone of necrosis. The gyral atrophy and ventricular enlargement are consistent with the patient's age.

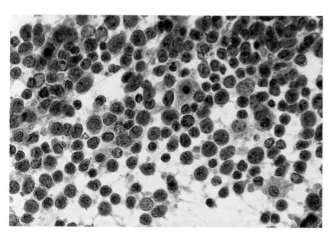

**FIGURE 5–10    PRIMARY CENTRAL NERVOUS SYSTEM LYMPHOMA**

Smear preparations are invaluable in identifying CNS lymphomas. The cells are dispersed and lack the cohesion typical of metastatic carcinoma or the meshwork of fibrillar processes seen in most glioblastomas. The cytologic profile, including nuclear roundness or indentation, as well as prominence of single or multiple nucleoli, is also typical.

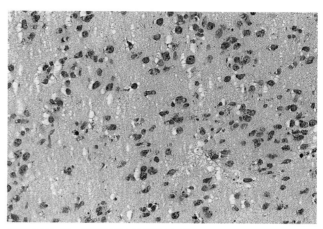

**FIGURE 5–11    PRIMARY CENTRAL NERVOUS SYSTEM LYMPHOMA**

A frozen section of the needle biopsy specimen from the lesion illustrated in Figure 5–9 illustrates the diffuse or infiltrative quality of this tumor. Whereas some cells show cytologic features typical of lymphoma, such as large round nuclei, others are angulated. Out of radiologic and cytologic (smear preparation) context, this lesion could be misinterpreted as a glioma.

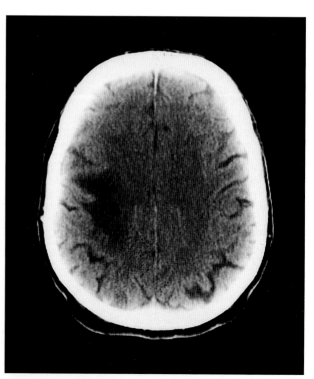

**FIGURE 5–12    PROGRESSIVE MULTIFOCAL LEUKOENCEPHALOPATHY**

In an immunocompromised patient, a nonenhancing white matter lesion with little mass effect is highly suggestive of progressive multifocal leukoencephalopathy (PML).

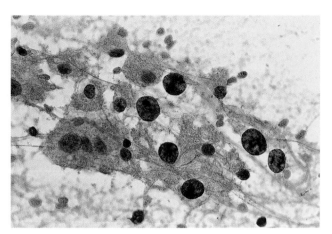

**FIGURE 5-13** PROGRESSIVE MULTIFOCAL LEUKOENCEPHALOPATHY

These large hyperchromatic cells in a smear preparation could be misinterpreted as those of a glioma. In the setting of AIDS, however, they are highly suggestive of oligodendroglia infected by papovavirus.

which tissue adheres to form an inseparable amalgam. The freeze-thaw sequence of frozen section preparation is the ultimate in "tissue abuse."

## SPECIMEN ANALYSIS

Using smears and frozen sections, as desired, one can often arrive at a specific intraoperative pathologic diagnosis.

Nonetheless, one must avoid freezing valuable tissue after the surgeon's principal questions have been answered. Using the smears alone, it is usually simple to identify basic lesions, such as metastatic carcinoma, lymphoma, and patently malignant gliomas. Precise grading of gliomas is not always possible and, for that matter, often not necessary. In the case of a glioblastoma with typical imaging characteristics, that is, a rim or ring pattern of contrast enhancement, the finding of a clearly malignant glioma may suffice. Additional cores can be assessed in the unusual circumstance that a strict diagnosis of glioblastoma is required. Aside from establishing the adequacy of a specimen, one can often narrow the differential diagnosis and finger the principal suspect. Review of radiographic images and a discussion with the surgeon are instrumental in judging how far to proceed with additional smears or frozen sections. It may be necessary to emphasize to the surgeon the need for tissue beyond that used for smear and/or frozen section preparation. Lastly, the pathologist must always be ready to admit that pathologic findings are negative or note that they are inconsistent with clinical-radiologic data.

As discussed throughout this book, cytologic preparations quickly provide information regarding the identity of a lesion, the wait being shorter than that for a frozen section. Smears are generally informative about general architecture, cell relations, presence or absence of cellular processes, and degree of cytologic atypia or malignancy. They are particularly useful in identifying gliomas, especially astrocytomas of any grade, in which processes and their content of fibrils are easily seen

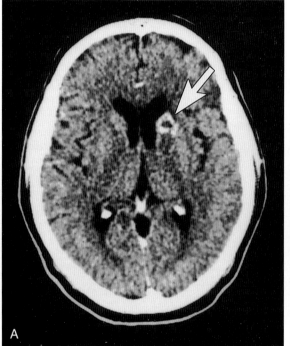

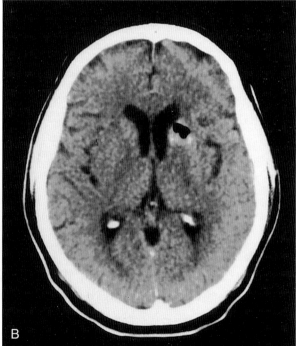

**FIGURE 5-14** INFARCT

Not all ring or rim enhancing processes are glioblastomas. This deep-seated lesion produced transient right-sided weakness in a 67-year-old man. As seen with the patient in the stereotactic frame (*A*), the contrast-enhancing lesion (*arrow*) occupies the caudate nucleus and adjacent internal capsule. Confirming the precision of the procedure, a postoperative scan found the dark MR signal of air at the biopsy site (*B*).

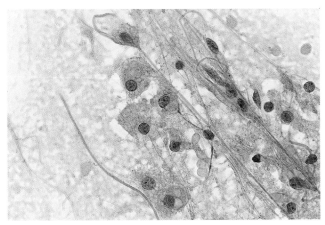

**FIGURE 5–15**  INFARCT

Emphasizing the value of smear preparation, macrophages with their discrete cell borders, foamy cytoplasm, and uniform nuclei provide important clues to the nature of the lesion in Figure 5–14.

(Fig. 5–6). Lastly, gliosis, with its radial arrangement of tapering processes emanating circumferentially from cells with benign nuclei, is readily recognized on smear preparations (Fig. 5–21). Neoplastic cells from a grade II astrocytoma are cytologically more atypical and have fewer processes (Fig. 5–22).

Several caveats are in order regarding the interpretation of cytologic preparations. The first relates to potential overinterpretation of normal white matter as hypercellular and therefore potentially neoplastic (Fig. 5–23). Smears augment the apparent cellularity of neoplasms as well; a lesion that appears markedly cellular in a smear may be surprisingly paucicellular in histologic sections. While so distinctive histologically, cortical neurons lose much of their cytologic uniqueness in smears and appear as generic, large, somewhat hyperchromatic cells, stripped of their cytoplasm so as to appear as neoplastic elements (Fig. 5–24). Smears of cerebellum are even more deceptive because the cells of the densely populated internal granule layer are easily mistaken for a small cell neoplasm, particularly medulloblastoma or metastatic carcinoma (Fig. 5–25). This is doubly true on frozen section, where their smaller size, remarkable uniformity, and lack of atypia are obscured. The encounter with a Purkinje cell is a welcome indicator of the correct diagnosis—normal cerebellar cortex. Lastly, one must be careful not to interpret nonspecifically thickened vessels as evidence of microvascular hyperplasia, a classical feature of high-grade gliomas.

Prior freezing of tissue introduces both nuclear hyperchromasia and pleomorphism that can compromise an accurate diagnosis on permanent sections. This effect is best exemplified by oligodendrogliomas, where tissues that were previously frozen and then processed for permanent sections acquire cytologic features of an astrocytoma (Figs. 5–26 and 5–27). During preparation of a burr hole, microscopic fragments of bone are created that often contaminate the tissue core. Although the larger fragments have a lamellar architecture of the haversian system, they lack the geode-like concentric lamella of calcospherites (Fig. 5–28).

## CORRELATION OF CLINICAL, RADIOLOGIC, AND PATHOLOGIC FINDINGS

Even under the best of circumstances, stereotactic biopsies sometimes fail to yield diagnostic tissue. The likelihood of this unfortunate outcome is minimized by comparing radiographic and pathologic findings as the intraoperative examination proceeds. With imaging findings

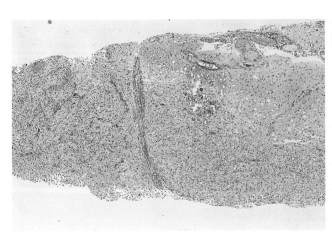

5–16                          5–17

**FIGURES 5–16 AND 5–17**  INFARCT

The core of tissue from the lesion in Figure 5–14 consists of a mass of macrophages, not of tumor cells.

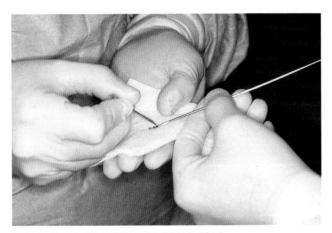

**FIGURE 5–18    TROCAR WITH TISSUE CORE**

A large-bore needle with a cutting side port obtains "large" cylinders of tissue.

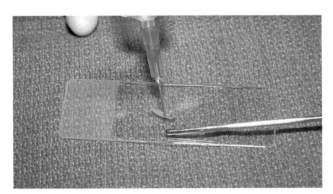

**FIGURE 5–19    DISSECTION OF TISSUE CORE**

A small portion of the tissue core can be removed for smear preparation, microbiologic studies, electron microscopy, or molecular analyses.

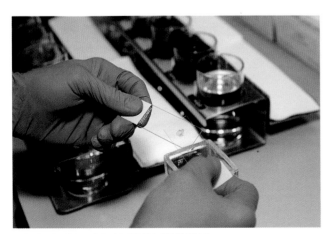

**FIGURE 5–20    PREPARATION OF SMEAR**

We prefer the smear technique by which tissue is first firmly compressed and then slowly drawn between two slides. Immediate fixation in alcohol precedes H&E staining.

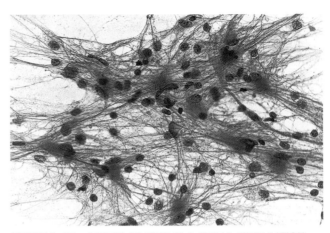

**FIGURE 5–21    GLIOSIS AS SEEN IN A SMEAR PREPARATION**

The lush corona of processes surrounding reactive astrocytes is well seen in this smear of a demyelinating disease plaque.

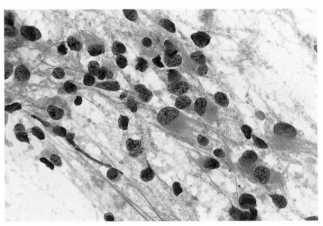

**FIGURE 5–22    SMEAR OF AN ASTROCYTOMA**

In contrast to reactive astrocytes, neoplastic astrocytes generally have more nuclear abnormalities and a lesser amount of cytoplasm.

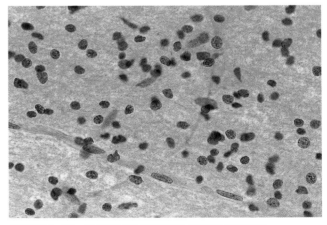

**FIGURE 5–23    SMEAR OF NORMAL WHITE MATTER**

Although there is no cytologic atypia, apparent hypercellularity in thick smears can suggest a glioma.

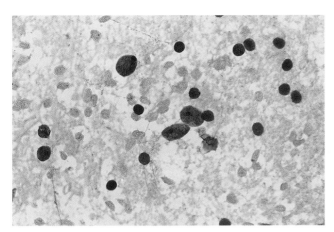

**FIGURE 5–24**   SMEAR OF NORMAL CORTICAL GRAY MATTER

Stripped of their cytoplasm, normal ganglion cells with their often prominent nucleoli can be misinterpreted as neoplastic cells in smear preparations.

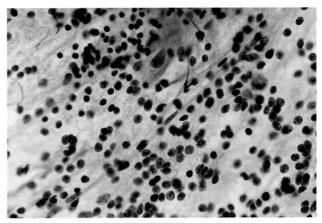

**FIGURE 5–25**   SMEAR OF NORMAL CEREBELLUM

The densely populated small neurons of the internal granule cell layer can be misinterpreted as those of a small cell neoplasm such as medulloblastoma. Such cells have perfectly round nuclei and central distinct nucleoli and lack the greater cytologic variation of a neoplasm. The admixture of Purkinje cells also alerts the pathologist to the nature of the tissue.

in hand, one can generally determine whether a pathologic diagnosis agrees with radiographic features of lesions at the target point(s). Needless to say, the adequacy of a specimen should be determined before, not after, the biopsy procedure is terminated.

Contrast enhancement is a common feature of lesions that include both neoplastic (both low and high grade) and non-neoplastic entities. Metastatic carcinoma, lymphoma, and high-grade gliomas are all enhancing, but so are cerebral infarcts, abscesses, and demyelinating disease, at least in some phase of their evolution. Because all these lesions exhibit obvious histologic abnormalities, the finding of only minimal histologic deviation from normal indicates a serious

problem in tissue sampling in the presence of a contrast-enhancing lesion. Marginally abnormal tissue with only a hint of hypercellularity is thus prima facie evidence of a stereotactic miss if on CT or MRI the lesion is contrast enhancing.

Nonenhancing lesions largely include low-grade infiltrating gliomas, mainly oligodendroglioma and fibrillary astrocytoma. Most focal inflammatory processes are contrast enhancing, progressive multifocal leukoencephalopathy (PML) being a notable exception (Fig. 5–12).

Radiographic images are occasionally stereotypic and alert the pathologist to certain diagnostic possibilities. This is especially true of several low-grade,

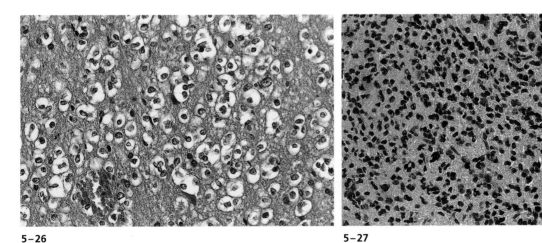

5–26                                                                5–27

**FIGURES 5–26 AND 5–27**   EFFECT OF PRIOR FREEZING ON OLIGODENDROGLIOMA

The classical features of oligodendroglioma are seen in tissue processed for permanent sections without prior freezing (Fig. 5–26). A permanent section of tissue from the same specimen, previously subjected to frozen section, shows artifactual nuclear condensation and angulation that suggest the diagnosis of astrocytoma (Fig. 5–27). Distinguishing between these two gliomas in previously frozen tissue can be difficult if not impossible. Only under most unusual circumstances should a specimen be entirely subjected to frozen section.

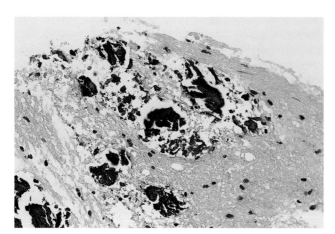

**FIGURE 5–28** BONE DUST

Contaminating fragments of bone incident to preparation of the burr hole should not be interpreted as pathologic calcification.

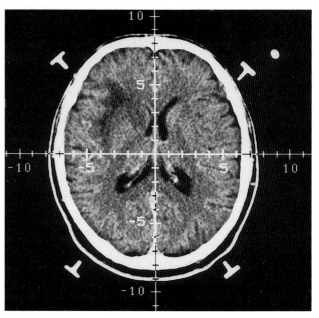

**FIGURE 5–29** RULE OUT INFILTRATING GLIOMA

This nonenhancing lesion in a 54-year-old man was approached stereotactically with the assumption that the deep-seated, nonenhancing abnormality was a grade II astrocytoma or oligodendroglioma.

localized tumors. For example, a cyst lesion containing a mural nodule suggests ganglion cell tumor, pleomorphic xanthoastrocytoma, or pilocytic astrocytoma.[3-6] Densely calcified, discrete lesions with little surrounding cerebral edema are also likely to be low grade or even hamartomatous. Members of the two major architectural categories of brain tumors, infiltrating and localized, are summarized in Figure 4–2, page 165. Radiologic features of low-grade brain tumors are given in Table 4–7, page 205.

There are times that, with a non–contrast-enhancing lesion, histologic findings do not live up to the expectations of the surgeon and consist of either normal brain or tissue that, while abnormal, is much less impressive than the radiographic images would suggest. In many cases, however, the tissue is indeed representative. Paucicellular, low-grade infiltrating gliomas, either relatively localized or remarkably diffuse (gliomatosis), can create an imposing degree of whiteness in T2-weighted or fluid-attenuated inversion recovery (FLAIR) MR images, despite only minimal abnormality in frozen or even permanent sections (Figs. 5–29 to 5–31). Only with a dialogue between pathologist and neurosurgeon can these issues be resolved and a degree of tissue sampling achieved that fulfills everyone's expectations. The position of the needle tract or the presence of air can determine the site of biopsy in postoperative neuroimages (see Fig. 5–14).

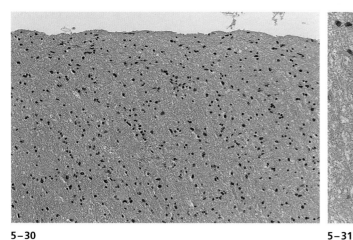

5–30

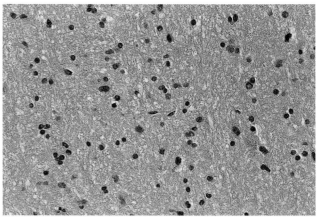

5–31

**FIGURES 5–30 AND 5–31** RULE OUT INFILTRATING GLIOMA

Well-differentiated, paucicellular gliomas can be difficult to evaluate in small specimens, even when processed optimally. This tissue core from the lesion illustrated in Figure 5–29, which was generous by stereotactic standards, has only minimal degrees of hypercellularity and nuclear pleomorphism. Experienced consultants differed as to whether there were sufficient criteria for the diagnosis of a glioma.

# COMMUNICATION

Pathologists are sometimes hesitant to commit themselves during the intraoperative phase of tissue examination and qualify diagnoses with such modifiers as "probably is," "highly suggestive of," "I think this," or "consistent with." Although these equivocations are not inappropriate if intended to convey a degree of uncertainty that is explained to the surgeon, they are often interpreted as "diagnostic of," especially if the diagnosis confirms the clinical impression. Although the pathologist may feel that these reservations are exculpatory if the permanent sections do not bear out the intraoperative diagnosis, the surgeon may feel differently. It is essential that the pathologist's level of certainty be communicated explicitly before the procedure is terminated. Recording this opinion in writing forestalls ambiguity. The surgeon should be forthcoming about clinical and radiologic findings and the amount of additional tissue that will be obtained. Details of the clinical history are crucial, as is a statement regarding the likelihood of additional tissue. Without a clear understanding, the pathologist may freeze all the specimen, leaving no artifact-free tissue for permanent sections.

# REFERENCES

1. Apuzzo MLJ, Chandrasoma PT, Cohen D, et al. Computed imaging stereotaxy: experience and perspective related to 500 procedures applied to brain masses. Neurosurgery 1987;20:930–937.
2. Bernstein M, Parrent AG. Complications of CT-guided stereotactic biopsy of intra-axial brain lesions. J Neurosurg 1994;81:165–168.
3. Burger PC, Nelson JS. Stereotactic brain biopsies. Specimen preparation and evaluation. Arch Pathol Lab Med 1997;121:477–480.
4. Burger PC, Nelson JS, Boyko OB. Diagnostic synergy in radiology and surgical neuropathology. Neuroimaging techniques and general interpretation guidelines. Arch Pathol Lab Med 1998;122:609–619.
5. Burger PC, Nelson JS, Boyko OB. Diagnostic synergy in radiology and surgical neuropathology. Radiographic findings of specific pathologic entities. Arch Pathol Lab Med 1998;122:620–632.
6. Burger PC, Scheithauer BW, Roland RL, et al. An interdisciplinary approach to avoid the overtreatment of patients with central nervous system lesions. Cancer 1997;80:2040–2046.
7. Ciricillo SF, Rosenblum ML. AIDS and the neurosurgeon–an update. Adv Tech Stand Neurosurg 1994;21:155–182.
8. Daumas-Duport C. Histological grading of gliomas. Curr Opin Neurol Neurosurg 1992;5:924–931.
9. Daumas-Duport C, Scheithauer BW, Kelly PJ. A histologic and cytologic method for the spatial definition of gliomas. Mayo Clin Proc 1987;62:435–449.
10. Fountas KN, Kapsalaki EZ, Smisson HF, et al. Results and complications for the use of a frameless stereotactic microscope navigator system. Stereotact Funct Neurosurg 1998;71:76–82.
11. Fritsch MJ, Leber MJ, Gossett L, et al. Stereotactic biopsy of intracranial brain lesions. High diagnostic yield without increased complications: 65 consecutive biopsies and early postoperative CT scans. Stereotact Funct Neurosurg 1998;71:36–42.
12. Hall WA. The safety and efficacy of stereotactic biopsy for intracranial lesions. Cancer 1998;82:1749–1755.
13. Hayden R, Cajulis RS, Frias-Hidvegi D, et al. Intraoperative diagnostic techniques for stereotactic brain biopsy: cytology versus frozen-section histopathology. Stereotact Funct Neurosurg 1995;65:187–193.
14. Hirschfeld A, Pellegrin K, Rawanduzy A. Stereotactic brain biopsies in AIDS patients: superior diagnostic yield with side-cutting needle than with cup forceps. Stereotact Funct Neurosurg 1994;63:150–153.
15. Holloway RG, Mushlin AI. Intracranial mass lesions in acquired immunodeficiency syndrome: using decision analysis to determine the effectiveness of stereotactic brain biopsy. Neurology 1996;46:1010–1015.
16. Kelly P. Stereotactic surgery: what is past is prologue. Neurosurgery 2000;46:16–27.
17. Kulkarni AV, Guha A, Lozano A, et al. Incidence of silent hemorrhage and delayed deterioration after stereotactic brain biopsy. J Neurosurg 1998;89:31–35.
18. O'Neill BP, Kelly PJ, Earle JD, et al. Computer-assisted stereotaxic biopsy for the diagnosis of primary central nervous system lymphoma. Neurology 1987;37:1160–1164.
19. Revesz T, Scaravilli F, Coutinho L, et al. Reliability of histologic diagnosis including grading in gliomas biopsied by image-guided stereotactic technique. Brain 1993;116:781–793.
20. Sawin PD, Hitchon PW, Follett KA, et al. Computed imaging–assisted stereotactic brain biopsy. A risk analysis of 225 consecutive cases. Surg Neurol 1998;49:640–649.
21. Sherman ME, Erozan YS, Mann RB, et al. Stereotactic brain biopsy in the diagnosis of malignant lymphoma. Am J Clin Pathol 1991;95:878–883.
22. Soo TM, Bernstein M, Provias J, et al. Failed stereotactic biopsy in a series of 518 cases. Stereotact Funct Neurosurg 1996;64:183–196.

# THE BRAIN: SURGERY FOR SEIZURES

**6**

Seizures are initiated by a wide variety of cerebral hemispheric lesions. Some are malignant neoplasms for which the seizures are only the initial expression of a soon-to-be-fatal disease. Others are chronic, not life threatening, and without an underlying morphologic correlate. Many lesions fall between these two extremes. Most entities that are approached surgically are found among the neoplasms and vascular lesions discussed in Chapters 4 and 7, respectively. These entities need little description here. There are, nevertheless, certain neoplastic and non-neoplastic entities so regularly associated with chronic seizures as to deserve additional or exclusive attention in this chapter.

The goals of surgery vary as dictated by the nature and location of the lesion. The intent in some cases is a curative removal of radiologically evident tumor or malformative focus. In others, that is, "seizure surgery," the goal is a palliative attempt to reduce seizure frequency by the resection of an epileptogenic focus in the absence of a defined lesion other than hippocampal sclerosis in some cases. Although chronic seizure-inciting foci occur throughout the cerebral hemispheres,[1] most occur in the temporal lobe. A lesion, albeit minor in some cases, is found in some specimens; extratemporal specimens are often histologically normal.[1]

Neuroradiologic studies are essential in the clinical evaluation of a patient with seizures. Thus, it is helpful for the pathologist to consider the approach to seizure-producing lesions in the context of these images (Table 6–1).[2] Although the resulting algorithm accommodates any seizure-producing lesion, it is intended for application to surgical specimens from patients with seizures that are chronic, arbitrarily defined as two or more years in duration.

## NEOPLASMS AND NON-NEOPLASTIC MASS LESIONS

Irritant neoplasms in the cerebral cortex are more likely to produce seizures than are deep-seated lesions in white matter, wherein myelin "insulation" impedes the propagation of electrical outbursts. Neoplasms that produce seizures thus usually arise in, or invade, the cortex. Those of subcortical gray matter (basal ganglia and thalamus), cerebellum, or brain stem do not generally initiate convulsive events. Seizures can be precipitated by extra-axial neoplasms, such as meningiomas, but this is much less frequent than with the intrinsic lesions discussed herein. Generally, patients with neoplasms that cause epilepsy do not have coincidental malformative lesions, but the two can coexist. Whether this association is by chance or related to a common pathogenesis is not clear.[12]

Almost any neoplasm that affects the cerebral cortex can incite seizures, but some are disproportionately represented. Almost by definition, chronic seizures reflect a well-differentiated lesion, that is, of World

**TABLE 6-1**
**Categorization of Epileptogenic Lesions by Radiologic Findings**

**Radiologic Abnormality Present**

Focal lesion
  Neoplasm
  Hippocampal (mesial) sclerosis
  Cortical dysplasia or microdysgenesis
  Vascular lesion
  Encephalomalacia
  Inflammatory lesion
  Hypothalamic hamartoma
  Meningioangiomatosis
Diffuse lesion
  Neoplasm
  Rasmussen's encephalitis
  Sturge-Weber angiomatosis
  Hemimegalencephaly

**No Radiologic Abnormality Present**

Focal or mild cortical dysplasia or microdysgenesis
Focal inflammation
No histologic abnormality

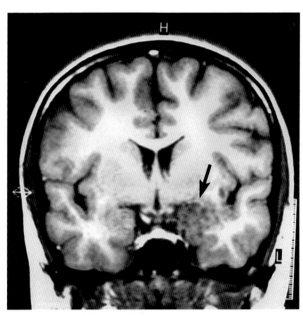

**FIGURE 6-1** DYSEMBRYOPLASTIC NEUROEPITHELIAL TUMOR (DNT)

As is typical, this DNT (arrow) has a distinctive "bubbly" quality in a precontrast T1-weighted image. The lesion in the medical temporal lobe produced seizures in a 20-year-old woman.

Health Organization grade I or II.[4] Deep-seated, high-grade tumors such as primary central nervous system lymphomas are unlikely to produce seizures, certainly not ones of long duration. Intracortical metastases are occasionally epileptogenic but obviously run an acute course.

Magnetic resonance (MR) imaging detects a wide range of seizure-producing neoplasms, sometimes at an early stage. Some of the long-standing examples appear discrete and often contrast enhancing. Others, for example, well-differentiated infiltrating astrocytomas and oligodendrogliomas, are ill defined and non–contrast enhancing. Macroscopically discrete neoplasms include ganglion cell tumors, pleomorphic xanthoastrocytoma, astroblastoma, and cortically based pilocytic astrocytomas (see Fig. 4–2). Skull erosion, common in many of these entities and also in dysembryoplastic neuroepithelial tumor, is always an alert to the possibility of a slowly growing lesion.[1–3, 10]

Particularly in patients with oligodendrogliomas, seizures may have been present for years, and there may be little if any mass effect or neurologic abnormality other than the seizures. The chronicity of the seizures has its correlate in the very well-differentiated nature of the lesion and an explanation in the oligodendroglioma's affinity for the cerebral cortex. Some oligodendrogliomas are entirely intracortical and are then difficult to distinguish from a dysembryoplastic neuroepithelial tumor (DNT), particularly in small specimens.

The DNT is a now a well-recognized, if not always easy to diagnose, entity for which seizures, and seizures alone, are the clinical manifestation.[5–9, 11, 13, 15–17] Children and young adults are typically affected. The entity and its sometimes difficult differential from oligo-

dendroglioma are discussed in Chapter 4 on pages 239 and 280. Fortunately, the lesion often presents a distinctive neuroradiologic profile, as a usually rather discrete, "bubbly" intracortical mass in precontrast T1-weighted images (Fig. 6–1). An intense intratumoral ring of enhancement appears in a minority of cases. The similarity of the lesion to oligodendroglioma (Fig. 6–2) is discussed in Chapter 4 on pages 239 and 280.

A non-neoplastic intracortical mass that appears exclusively with seizures is meningioangiomatosis.[14] This uncommon lesion is discussed in Chapter 2 on pages 99 to 101.

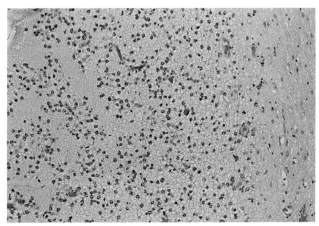

**FIGURE 6-2** DYSEMBRYOPLASTIC NEUROEPITHELIAL TUMOR

Well-defined nodules of oligodendroglioma-like cells are classical features. Out of context, the lesion can be readily misinterpreted as oligodendroglioma.

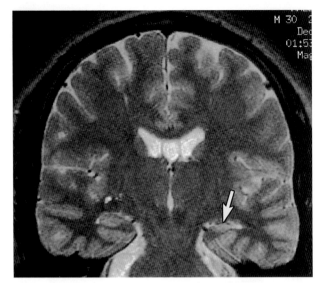

**FIGURE 6-3** HIPPOCAMPAL ("MESIAL") SCLEROSIS

As seen in a T2-weighted image, the affected hippocampus (arrow) is atrophic in comparison with its counterpart on the opposite side. The patient, a 30-year-old man, had a history of partial complex seizures from childhood.

## NON-NEOPLASTIC LESIONS

## Hippocampal ("Mesial") Sclerosis

**Definition.** A seizure-associated neuronal loss with gliosis in the hippocampus and adjacent structures.

**General Comments.** For reasons still debated, the hippocampus is frequently altered by a combined neuronal dropout and gliosis. The term "mesial sclerosis" is widely employed. "Hippocampal sclerosis" and "Ammon's horn sclerosis" are alternative designations. Similar changes in the amygdala often coexist with hippocampal sclerosis, or they can appear as isolated changes.[18] Understanding the concept and histopathology of the lesion is essential to the pathologic study of a temporal lobe specimen obtained at the time of seizure surgery.

**Radiologic Features.** Radiographically, mesial sclerosis appears as an ill-defined area of increased (white) signal in T2-weighted images, with loss of distinction between gray and white matter.[16] The hippocampus is atrophic in some cases (Fig. 6-3). With rare exceptions, the lesion is lateralized to the temporal lobe from which the seizures emanate[9] and may be accompanied by atrophy of surrounding tissues with enlargement of the adjacent temporal horn of the lateral ventricle.[9, 11, 14]

**Microscopic Features.** Recognition of mesial sclerosis depends upon an understanding of the normal anatomy of the hippocampus, and a specimen sectioned in the coronal plane. Histologically, this complicated anatomic formation can be simplified by viewing it as a spiral of pyramidal neurons inserting at one end into a V-shaped formation of small neurons known as the dentate gyrus (Fig. 6-4).[8] The "V" is composed of so-called granular neurons. From the dentate gyrus, the pyramidal cells sweep in a seahorse configuration, known as Ammon's horn, that disappears as a distinct lamina in the subiculum and presubiculum on the medial aspect of the temporal lobe. The spiral is divided into four zones on the basis of cytoarchitectural features—CA1 through CA4. "CA" is an acronym for cornu ammonis. CA4, or the end folium, is the segment that is tucked into the dentate gyrus, whereas CA1 is farthest removed from the V and lies adjacent to the temporal horn of the lateral ventricle. CA1 is also known as Sommer's sector.

Fortunately, the diagnosis of mesial sclerosis does not require expertise in the architectonic details of this anatomically complex region. The specimen is often

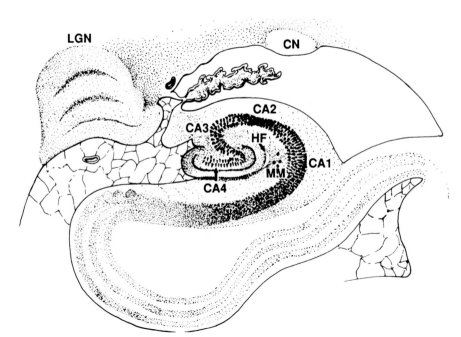

**FIGURE 6-4** NORMAL ANATOMY OF THE HIPPOCAMPAL REGION

The segment of Ammon's horn designated CA1 or Sommer's sector is preferentially involved in hippocampal, or "mesial," sclerosis. LGN, lateral geniculate nucleus; CN, tail of the caudate nucleus; HF, hippocampal fissure. MM indicates a region prone to incidental microcalcifications in older patients. (From Fuller GN, Burger PC. Central nervous system. In Sternberg SS [ed]. Histology for Pathologists. 2nd ed. Philadelphia: Lippincott Raven, 1997.)

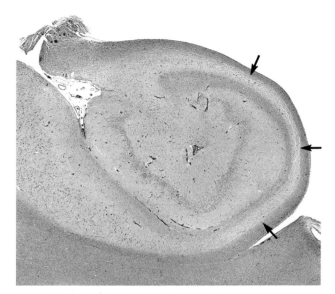

**FIGURE 6–5**  HIPPOCAMPAL ("MESIAL") SCLEROSIS

Thinning of the CA1 segment of Ammon's horn (arrows) is the cardinal feature of hippocampal sclerosis. As is sometimes the case, the process also affects CA2.

submitted as "hippocampus" or simply "medial temporal lobe." In an en bloc removal, the bulge of the hippocampus is readily evident as a landmark that facilitates coronal sectioning. Microsections taken in other planes can be extremely confusing. In a specimen properly oriented, the density of neurons in the affected areas can be contrasted with that in the less vulnerable sectors. In small specimens without proper orientation, and when almost all pyramidal neurons are lost, it can be difficult to identify any abnormality. In such cases, staining for myelin and glial fibrillary acidic protein (GFAP) may help define the laminations and facilitate identification of the abnormality. Neuronal loss is generally most prominent in, if not restricted to, CA1 (Figs. 6–5 to 6–9). However, on occasion, CA4 bears the brunt, whereas in other instances the entirety of Ammon's horn is involved.[1, 6, 7, 13] When the pyramidal cell loss is severe, adjacent granular cells in the dentate gyrus may be depopulated, disorganized, or seemingly dispersed in gliotic parenchyma (Fig. 6–10).[1, 13, 15] Synaptophysin staining is proportionally reduced.[12] Corpora amylacea are often numerically increased (Fig. 6–11).[4, 5]

The chronic astrogliosis that characterizes mesial sclerosis is usually only a fine background fibrillarity containing bland nuclei of astrocytes and a few remaining neurons (Fig. 6–7). Occasionally, the gliosis is more active, that is, the classical gemistocytic variety (Fig. 6–10).

In addition to the hippocampal specimen, temporal lobectomies often provide a portion of tissue labeled "lateral temporal lobe" that consists largely of cerebral cortex and underlying white matter. Herein, as in the hippocampus, one may find a malformative or dysplastic lesion discussed later under Cortical Dysplasia, but often there is nothing to be seen. How often changes are encountered depends on the presence or absence of radi-

ographic visualization of a lesion, other than mesial sclerosis, the size of the specimen, the experience and persistence of the observer, and his or her threshold for accepting minor variations in cytoarchitectonics as bona fide abnormalities. In one series, cortical dysplasia was noted in 5 of 27 patients with mesial sclerosis.[17] Care should be taken to distinguish artifacts created by electroencephalography electrodes from meningeal inflammatory lesions (see Fig. 6–28).

**Differential Diagnosis.** The differential diagnosis of mesial sclerosis lies between *normal brain* on the one hand and an *infiltrating, well-differentiated glioma* on the other. The distinction from normal brain has already been discussed. The possibility of a glial neoplasm should be approached with great caution and an awareness that mesial sclerosis is associated only uncommonly with a glioma.[10] The distinction is usually straightforward; the former features neither an increase in cellularity nor significant cytologic atypia. Thus, in the presence of classical radiographic evidence of mesial sclerosis with atrophy, a diagnosis of glioma is largely untenable. This is not to say that oligodendrogliomas and astrocytomas cannot occur in this region and mimic the radiologic signal changes, but there is no atrophy.

**Treatment and Prognosis.** The significance of Ammon's horn sclerosis has long been the subject of debate. The uncertainty centers upon whether the lesion is the result of, the cause of, or the result and then the cause of seizure activity. Although current thinking favors an ultimate causal role that justifies hippocampal resection, the issue continues to be discussed.[1, 3, 15] Fortunately, one need not enter this contentious arena to assess a specimen adequately. The presence of mesial sclerosis in a surgical specimen is a favorable prognostic sign relative to the future frequency of seizures.[2, 9]

## Malformative Lesions

Under the rubrics cortical dysplasia, microdysgenesis, hamartia, hamartoma, and neuronal migration disorder are a variety of non-neoplastic developmental faux pas of varying extent and clinical importance. Some are massive hemispheric, or even bihemispheric, malformations of profound clinical importance; others are microscopic discoveries encountered in patients with or without seizures. Some focal lesions are visible in radiographic studies. Although attempts have been made to order these varied lesions along a continuum so as to relate them to the timing of embryogenetic insults,[18, 19] the following discussion divides the spectrum on the basis of histologic criteria.

### Cortical Dysplasia with Giant Neurons (Focal Cortical Dysplasia)

This distinctive entity occurs throughout the cerebrum and is a cause of chronic seizures in both children and adults.[5, 6, 8, 9, 11, 18, 19, 23, 25, 29, 31, 33, 36, 37] Typically, the duration of seizures is prolonged.[29] As visualized radiologically,

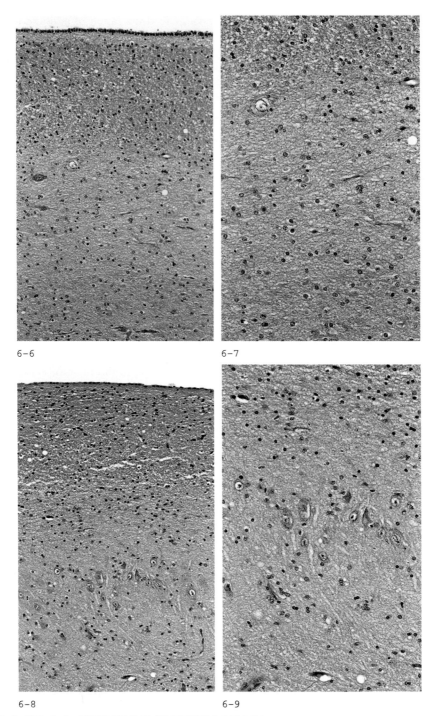

6-6

6-7

6-8

6-9

**FIGURES 6-6, 6-7, 6-8, AND 6-9    HIPPOCAMPAL ("MESIAL") SCLEROSIS**

The loss of pyramidal cell neurons leaves only a narrow, neuron-poor (or even neuron-free) lamina showing no other significant histologic abnormality. In this field, only a single neuron survives (Figs. 6-6 and 6-7). The abnormality in Figures 6-6 and 6-7 is best appreciated by comparing these findings with those in a less affected sector in the same specimen (Figs. 6-8 and 6-9).

focal cortical dysplasia thickens the cortex and blurs the underlying gray-white demarcation. An abnormal, bright T2 signal may be seen in the subjacent white matter (Fig. 6-12).[21, 22, 28, 31] As a more diffuse form of the disease, the same abnormality is encountered in some examples of hemimegalencephaly, a lesion discussed on page 398 (see Figs. 6-20 and 6-21). Some examples of

cortical dysplasia may not be large enough to be recognized by the naked eye. Macroscopically, the process effaces the normal cortical laminar architecture and blurs the gray-white junction (Fig. 6-13), but it can be a very focal finding difficult to detect at low magnification, particularly in palely stained hematoxylin and eosin (H&E) sections.

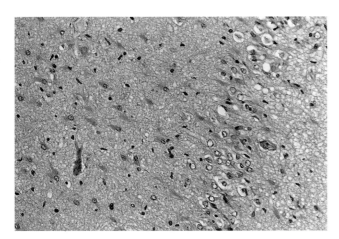

**FIGURE 6–10** HIPPOCAMPAL ("MESIAL") SCLEROSIS

In some cases, gliosis is more "active" or "gemistocytic" in appearance, featuring hypertrophic astrocytes with glassy cytoplasm and coarse processes. The molecular layer, at the right of the illustration, is somewhat depopulated and disorganized.

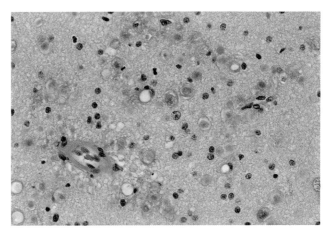

**FIGURE 6–11** HIPPOCAMPAL ("MESIAL") SCLEROSIS

Corpora amylacea may be abundant in sclerotic areas.

Cytologically, focal cortical dysplasia is characterized by extremely large cells, some clearly neuronal and others obviously astrocytic, intermingled with renegades that cannot be assigned readily to either category (Figs. 6–14 and 6–15).[2, 8, 11, 18, 19, 28, 29] Prominent among the latter are especially large cells with "ballooned" glassy cytoplasm.[6] GFAP-positive astrocytes may be prominent in the first or most superficial, cortical lamina, whereas others are unpredictably and unevenly distributed throughout the remaining cortex and subcortical white matter. The white matter is characteristically hypomyeli-

nated, may contain the large cells (Fig. 6–16), appears pale in myelin-stained sections, and is correspondingly bright in T2-weighted or FLAIR MR images.[15] A linear, often perivascular, tracking of these large cells from white to gray matter suggests that the process is, at least in part, a disorder of cellular migration.

Identifying the large cells is elementary when they are numerous but requires exacting microscopic review when they are not. Abnormal clustering of cells and lack of polarization of apical dendrites to the cortical surface are helpful index features of abnormality. Size per se can

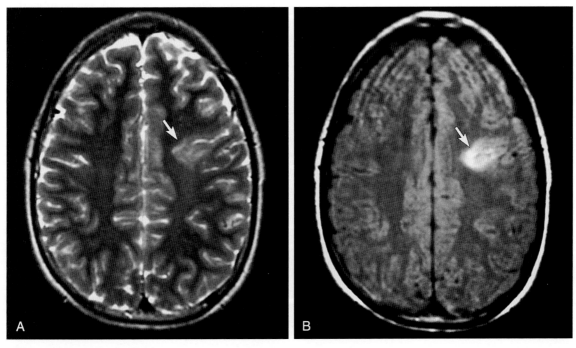

**FIGURE 6–12** CORTICAL DYSPLASIA

Radiologically, focal cortical dysplasia may appear as an abnormal sector of the cerebral cortex, as seen in A in a T2-weighted image (arrow). As seen in a FLAIR image, abnormal signal in the hypomyelinated white matter (arrow) may be present in some cases (B). The patient was an 11-year-old boy with focal right-sided seizures. (Courtesy of Dr. Tom Milligan, Corpus Christi, TX.)

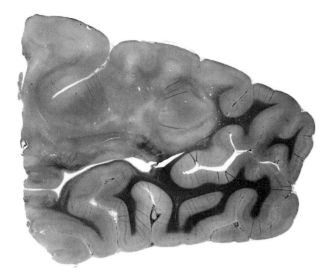

**FIGURE 6–13    CORTICAL DYSPLASIA**

As is evident in a section stained for myelin (H&E–Luxol fast blue), focal cortical dysplasia thickens the cortex and effaces the normally sharp gray-white junction.

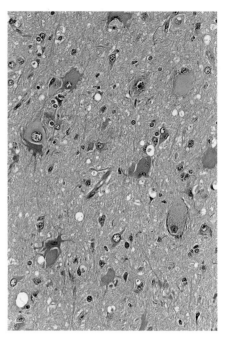

**FIGURE 6–15    CORTICAL DYSPLASIA**

Abnormally large, sometimes "giant" neurons as well as large glassy astrocytes are the principal components of this process.

be diagnostic because neurons comparable in size to giant motor neurons of Betz would be abnormal in the temporal lobe.

As neuronal-astrocytic hybrids, these large glassy cells and the lesions themselves resemble cortical tubers. Nonetheless, one study found contrasting features. The balloon cells in hemimegalencephaly were negative immunohistochemically for tuberin, the tuberous sclerosis 2 gene product, and were always negative for GFAP.[1] Efforts to find molecular abnormalities of the two tuberous

sclerosis genes in the sporadic cortical dysplasia have been unrewarding.[35]

## Microscopic Malformative Lesions (Microdysgenesis)

The term *microdysgenesis* has been applied to a diverse group of radiologically subthreshold findings. Their significance is difficult to determine in a given case because the same "lesions" are occasionally found in patients without seizures, and more than one variant may be found in a single specimen from a patient with seizures. Although their presence may satisfy the

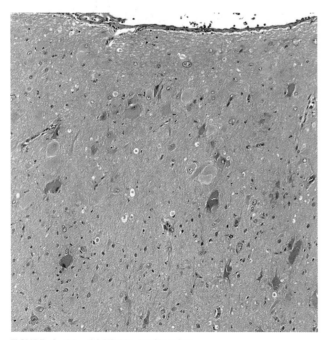

**FIGURE 6–14    CORTICAL DYSPLASIA**

The process in this case spans the cortical ribbon. Note the large cells.

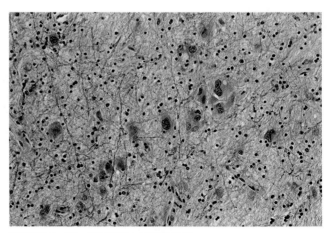

**FIGURE 6–16    CORTICAL DYSPLASIA**

In the specimen illustrated in Figure 6–13, large, cytologically abnormal cells lie ectopically within subcortical white matter.

pathologist's desire to identify an abnormality, the findings may be unrelated to seizure activity in a given case.[12] One study compared the microscopic findings in a series of surgical specimens from patients with temporal lobe epilepsy with those of control brains acquired at autopsy.[12] Although most of the changes described in the following were found in both groups, four features were statistically more frequent in specimens from the patients with epilepsy. These were (1) clustering of neurons in the cortex, (2) perivascular clustering of oligodendroglia, (3) increased numbers of heterotopic neurons in the white matter, and (4) glioneuronal hamartias.

**Neuron-Oligodendroglial Foci.** Clusters of small cells with haloed nuclei resembling those of oligodendroglia are occasionally encountered in surgical specimens from the temporal lobe. Mature ganglion cells are often interspersed between the small cells (Fig. 6–17).[33, 34, 36, 38, 39] The term *glioneuronal hamartia* has been employed for these microscopic findings. In other cases, small clusters of abnormal neurons without accompanying glia are microscopic findings (Fig. 6–18).

**Isolated Neurons in the White Matter.** Scattered heterotopic neurons in white matter are a common finding, particularly in specimens from the temporal lobe.[7, 10, 12, 17–19, 25, 27, 38] Some of these ectopic cells are merely deep cortical neurons that appear displaced as a consequence of plane of section. Yet others, by a process of triangulation, can clearly be accepted as indeed out of

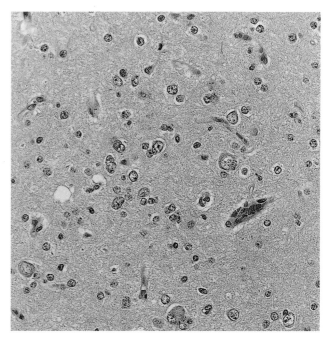

**FIGURE 6–18** MICRODYSGENESIS

Microscopic clusters of abnormal cortical neurons are findings in some specimens removed for seizure control.

place. The significance of this radiologically invisible finding is difficult to assess in any given patient.[7, 12, 17, 27] Albeit generally in lesser numbers, such neurons can be present in the white matter of neurologically normal patients.

**Oligodendroglial Hyperplasia.** During the examination of an occasional surgical specimen, one is struck occasionally by a seeming hyperplasia of small uniform cells with the cytologic features of oligodendroglia (Fig. 6–19).[2, 3, 12] There are no neuroradiologic correlates; the

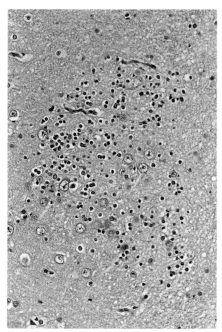

**FIGURE 6–17** MICRODYSGENESIS

Small clusters of oligodendrocyte-like cells associated with large neurons are occasionally encountered in specimens obtained at the time of "seizure surgery." Such foci are more common in specimens from patients with seizures but are occasionally encountered in nonepileptic patients. The significance of these cells is unknown.

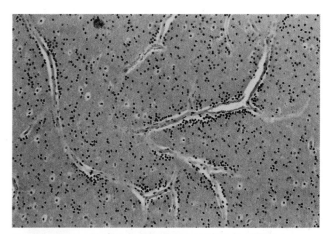

**FIGURE 6–19** OLIGODENDROGLIAL "HYPERPLASIA"

Apparent hypercellularity of the white matter and deep cortical laminae is occasionally encountered in tissues removed for seizure control. These well-differentiated cells, which closely resemble oligodendrocytes, are distributed along vessels as well as about neurons ("satellitosis"). The significance of this "lesion" is unclear because it is occasionally encountered in patients without epilepsy.

"affected" white matter is normally myelinated and free of gliosis. A form of perineuronal satellitosis may also be created in deep cortical layers. Equally arresting is the orderly lamination of such cells around blood vessels, sometimes in layers that are two to three cells deep. Although this appearance is sometimes considered a form of microdysgenesis, it is seen in some "control brains"[12] or in association with lesions other than those that produce seizures. There is no evidence that oligodendroglial hyperplasia is neoplastic or even preneoplastic.

**Other Malformative Lesions.** Ectopic neurons in the most superficial cortical layer, clustering of neurons, remnants of the subpial granular cell layer, and glioneuronal hamartomas at the brain surface are other microscopic malformations.[10, 12, 13, 18, 19, 24] Glial hamartomatous lesions, sometimes in association with other forms of cortical dysplasia, may also be encountered.[32]

### Hemimegalencephaly

Although this macroscopic lesion usually lies outside the purview of the surgical pathologist, it can prompt a massive surgical resection of the affected hemisphere to control seizures (Figs. 6–20 and 6–21). A wide variety of malformative, dysgenetic, and anomalous lesions can be encountered in such specimens.[4, 16, 20, 22, 26] These include (1) a diffuse form of the focal cortical dysplasia already described[26] and (2) multiple congenital aberrations such as polymicrogyria, pachygyria, and heterotopias as well as the so-called double cortex.[21] These gross abnormalities are apparent neuroradiologically.

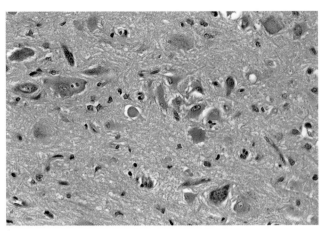

**FIGURE 6–21**   HEMIMEGALENCEPHALY

The cortex of the surgical specimen of Figure 6–20 contained large neurons and "glassy" astrocytes similar to those seen in the case of focal cortical dysplasia illustrated in Figures 6–14 and 6–15.

### Hypothalamic Hamartoma

With the neuroradiographic signal characteristics of gray matter, this usually small, globular anomaly projects from the undersurface of the hypothalamus. Whereas many are clinically silent and are discovered incidentally, if at all, some come to attention because of seizures or endocrine dysfunction (precocious puberty). As a rule, the seizures are neither absence (petit mal) nor convulsive events but rather outbursts of raucous laughter known as gelastic seizures.[15, 30] The clinical and pathologic features of hypothalamic hamartoma are discussed on pages 281 to 283.

## Vascular Lesions

### Vascular Malformations

Although seizures may be instigated by either *arteriovenous malformations* or *cavernous angiomas*, the latter predominate in specimens resected for chronic epilepsy.[2, 4, 5] As discussed in detail in Chapter 7 on pages 403 to 405, the oft-calcified cavernoma has a distinctive radiologic appearance. As a result, the informed pathologist anticipates the diagnosis. In a futile attempt to find a legitimate lesion in a seizure specimen, one should not grasp at artifactually compacted normal leptomeningeal vessels that are common in surgical specimens from the brain (see Fig. 7–13).

### Encephalomalacia

Although cerebral infarcts rarely induce seizures, occasional foci of chronic encephalomalacia do appear culpable (Figs. 6–22 to 6–24).[6] These lesions may be attributed to ischemia in some cases and to trauma in others. The abnormality consists largely of tissue rarefaction associated with residual macrophages and gliosis—both nonspecific evidence of the original insult. A history of surgery in the area, of birth injury,[3] or of the prior placement of electrodes provides an alternative explanation.

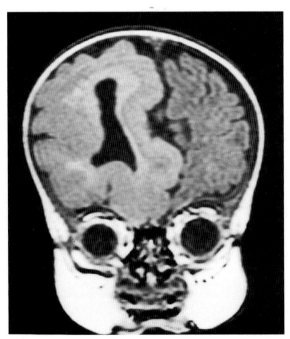

**FIGURE 6–20**   HEMIMEGALENCEPHALY

The right cerebral hemisphere of this 12-month-old girl was markedly enlarged because of diffuse gyral thickening. A hemispherectomy was successful in relieving the patient's intractable seizures.

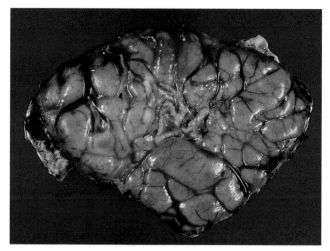

**FIGURE 6–22    INFARCT**

The surgical specimen of this 11-year-old boy with a history of cerebral palsy and seizures contains a central area of gyral atrophy consistent with a remote infarct.

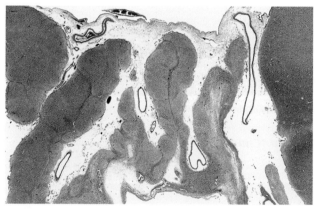

**FIGURE 6–23    INFARCT**

A remote event, presumably ischemia, produced the gyral atrophy seen in the center of the specimen of Figure 6–22.

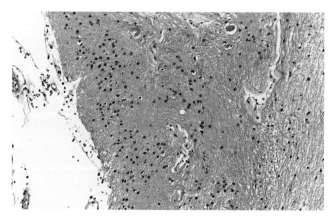

**FIGURE 6–24    INFARCT**

At this late date, no specific histological changes remain, only atrophy, gliosis, and neuronal depopulation.

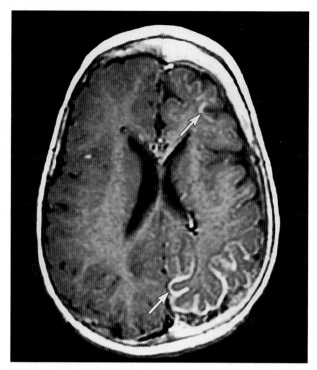

**FIGURE 6–25    STURGE-WEBER DISEASE**

Leptomeningeal angiomatosis is apparent as a thin band of contrast enhancement in the subarachnoid space (arrows). The patient was a 16-month-old girl with a seizure disorder from the age of 3 months. A near-total hemispherectomy was effective in seizure control. (Courtesy of Dr. Elias Melhem, Baltimore, MD.)

## Sturge-Weber Angiomatosis

This rare syndrome complex includes a massive increase in the number of small leptomeningeal vessels and calcification of underlying gyri. These intracranial lesions are associated with an ipsilateral, facial port-wine stain in the distribution of the trigeminal nerve. The choroid plexus may be hypertrophied, and abnormal retinal vessels may be associated with glaucoma. Seizures, diminished mental acuity, and hemiparesis are the variable clinical expressions. When viewed in section, the calcifications produce a classical "tram track" image on computed tomography scans. A diffuse, contrast-enhancing angiomatosis is seen by MR imaging[1] or angiography (Fig. 6–25).

A surgeon may be recruited to control the seizures by the removal of the offending epileptogenic cortex, of which an impressive amount may be excised.[6–9] Sturge-Weber angiomatosis is therefore one of the few justifications for hemispherectomy.

Histologically, the subarachnoid space is packed with small vein-like vessels (Fig. 6–26) Laminated, scalloped concretions are strewn throughout the underlying cortex. Gliosis and neuronal depletion are common in chronic lesions. Subpial (Chaslin's) gliosis may be prominent (Fig. 6–27; see Fig. 6–26). Sturge-Weber disease is also discussed in Chapter 7 on pages 407 to 408.

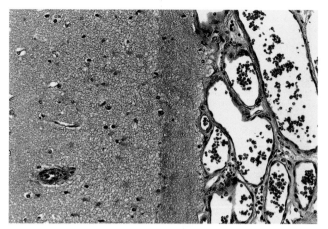

**FIGURE 6–26**    STURGE-WEBER DISEASE AND SUBPIAL (CHASLIN'S) GLIOSIS

Numerous thin-walled vessels fill the subarachnoid space. An eosinophilic, paucicellular band of gliosis (Chaslin's gliosis) effaces the superficial, subpial cortex immediately beneath the malformation.

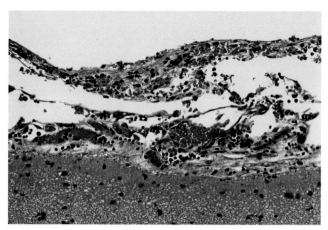

**FIGURE 6–28**    REACTIVE CHANGES SECONDARY TO GRID PLACEMENT

Leptomeningeal lymphocytes and reactive changes in meningovascular elements in this case are the consequence of surface electrode placement and are not evidence of preexisting disease.

## Reactive and Inflammatory Lesions

### Rasmussen's Encephalitis

Rasmussen's encephalitis, a rare cause of intractable epilepsy, is discussed in Chapter 3 on pages 148 to 149.

### Other Inflammatory Lesions

Probably the most common form of chronic inflammation encountered in tissues removed surgically for seizures is initiated by electrodes of either the superficial (surface) or penetrating (depth) type. The former incites acute and chronic leptomeningitis (Fig. 6–28), whereas the latter leaves a macrophage-rich tract and a few scattered lymphocytes. Obviously, neither tissue response should be considered a disease process.

The significance of focal, or even extensive, inflammation outside this rare setting is not always clear. Small aggregates of lymphocytes or microglia (glial nodule) may be seen in specimens from patients with seizures who have not undergone prior electrode placement. Also, inflammatory lesions similar to but without the hemiatrophy of the latter may be seen. The etiology is usually unclear, although a viral or rickettsial infection is often suspected. Past episodes of meningitis are incriminated in some cases.[1]

### Subpial (Chaslin's) Gliosis

This is a finely fibrillar, brightly eosinophilic, and intensely GFAP-positive change in the subpial layer (see Figs. 6–26 and 6–27). Although seen in many patients with seizures, it is not specific and its role in the latter is not clear.

## REFERENCES

**Introduction**

1. Frater JL, Prayson RA, Morris IH, et al. Surgical pathologic findings of extratemporal-based intractable epilepsy: a study of 133 consecutive resections. Arch Pathol Lab Med 2000;124:545–549.
2. Kuznicky RI, Barkovich AJ. Pathogenesis and pathology of focal malformations of cortical development and epilepsy. J Clin Neurophysiol 1996;13:468–480.

**Neoplasms and Non-Neoplastic Masses**

1. Burger PC, Scheithauer BW, Lee RR, et al. An interdisciplinary approach to avoid the overtreatment of patients with central nervous system lesions. Cancer 1997;80:2040–2046.
2. Burger PC, Nelson JS, Boyko OB. Diagnostic synergy in radiology and surgical neuropathology: neuroimaging techniques and general interpretive guidelines. Arch Pathol Lab Med 1998;122: 609–619.
3. Burger PC, Nelson JS, Boyko OB. Diagnostic synergy in radiology and surgical neuropathology: radiographic findings of specific pathologic entities. Arch Pathol Lab Med 1998; 122:620–632.
4. Frater JL, Prayson RA, Morris IH, et al. Surgical pathologic findings of extratemporal-based intractable epilepsy: a study of 133 consecutive resections. Arch Pathol Lab Med 2000; 124:545–549.
5. Fried I, Kim JH, Spencer DD. Limbic and neocortical gliomas

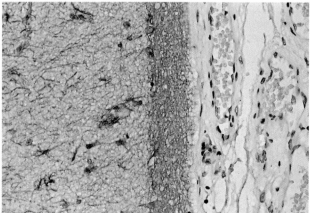

**FIGURE 6–27**    STURGE-WEBER DISEASE AND SUBPIAL (CHASLIN'S) GLIOSIS

The affected lamina is intensely immunopositive for GFAP.

associated with intractable seizures: a distinct clinicopathological group. Neurosurgery 1994;34:815–824.

6. Khajavi K, Comair YG, Prayson RA, et al. Childhood ganglioglioma and medically intractable epilepsy. A clinicopathological study of 15 patients and a review of the literature. Pediatr Neurosurg 1995;22:181–188.

7. Kirkpatrick PJ, Honavar M, Janota I, et al. Control of temporal lobe epilepsy following en bloc resection of low-grade tumors. J Neurosurg 1993;78:19–25.

8. Montes JL, Rosenblatt B, Farmer J-P, et al. Lesionectomy of MRI detected lesions in children with epilepsy. Pediatr Neurosurg 1995;22:167–173.

9. Morris HH, Estes ML, Gilmore R, et al. Chronic intractable epilepsy as the only symptom of primary brain tumor. Epilepsia 1993;34:1038–1043.

10. Passe TJ, Beauchamp BN, Burger PC. Neuroimaging in the identification of low-grade and nonneoplastic CNS lesions. Neurologist 1999;5:293–299.

11. Plate KH, Wieser H-G, Yasargil MG, et al. Neuropathological findings in 224 patients with temporal lobe epilepsy. Acta Neuropathol (Berl) 1993;86:433–438.

12. Prayson RA, Estes ML, Morris HH. Coexistence of neoplasia and cortical dysplasia in patients presenting with seizures. Epilepsia 1993;34:609–615.

13. Tampieri D, Moumdjian R, Melanson D, et al. Intracerebral gangliogliomas in patients with partial complex seizures: CT and MR imaging findings. AJNR 1991;12:749–755.

14. Wiebe S, Munoz DG, Smith S, et al. Meningioangiomatosis. A comprehensive analysis of clinical and laboratory features. Brain 1999;122:709–726.

15. Wolf HK, Campos MG, Zentner J, et al. Surgical pathology of temporal lobe epilepsy. Experience with 216 cases. J Neuropathol Exp Neurol 1993;52:499–506.

16. Wolf HK, Wellmer J, Muller MB, et al. Glioneuronal malformative lesions and dysembryoplastic neuroepithelial tumors in patients with chronic pharmacoresistant epilepsies. J Neuropathol Exp Neurol 1995;54:245–254.

17. Wolf HK, Zentner J, Hufnagel A, et al. Surgical pathology of chronic epileptic seizure disorders: experience with 63 specimens from extratemporal corticectomies, lobectomies and functional hemispherectomies. Acta Neuropathol (Berl) 1993;86:466–472.

## Hippocampal ("Mesial") Sclerosis

1. Armstrong DD. The neuropathology of temporal lobe epilepsy. J Neuropathol Exp Neurol 1993;52:433–443.

2. Bronen RA, Cheung G, Charles JT, et al. Imaging findings in hippocampal sclerosis: correlation with pathology. AJNR 1991;12:933–940.

3. Cendes F, Andermann F, Gloor P, et al. Atrophy of mesial structures in patients with temporal lobe epilepsy: cause or consequence of repeated seizures? Ann Neurol 1993;34:795–801.

4. Chung MH, Horoupian DS. Corpora amylacea: a marker for mesial temporal sclerosis. J Neuropathol Exp Neurol 1996;55: 403–408.

5. Erdamar S, Zhu ZQ, Hamilton WJ, et al. Corpora amylacea and heat shock protein 27 in Ammon's horn sclerosis. J Neuropathol Exp Neurol 2000;59:698–706.

6. Falconer MA, Serafetinides EA, Corsellis JAN. Etiology and pathogenesis of temporal lobe epilepsy. Arch Neurol 1964;10: 233–248.

7. Fried I, Kim JH, Spencer DD. Hippocampal pathology in patients with intractable seizures and temporal lobe masses. J Neurosurg 1992;76:735–740.

8. Fuller GN, Burger PC. Central nervous system. In Sternberg SS (ed). Histology for Pathologists. 2nd ed. Philadelphia: Lippincott-Raven, 1997, pp 243–282.

9. Heinz R, Ferris N, Lee EK, et al. MR and positron emission tomography in the diagnosis of surgically correctable temporal lobe epilepsy. AJNR 1994;15:1341–1348.

10. Kim JH, Guimaraes PO, Shen MY, et al. Hippocampal neuronal density in temporal lobe epilepsy with and without gliomas. Acta Neuropathol (Berl) 1989;80:41–45.

11. Kim JH, Tien RD, Felsberg GJ, et al. Fast spin-echo MR in hippocampal sclerosis: correlation with pathology and surgery. AJNR 1995;16:627–636.

12. Looney MR, Dohan FC Jr, Davies KG, et al. Synaptophysin immunoreactivity in temporal lobe epilepsy–associated hippocampal sclerosis. Acta Neuropathol (Berl) 1999;98:179–185.

13. Margerison JH, Corsellis JAN. Epilepsy and the temporal lobes. A clinical, electroencephalographic and neuropathological study of the brain in epilepsy, with particular reference to the temporal lobes. Brain 1966;89:499–580.

14. Mark LP, Daniels DL, Naidich TP, et al. Hippocampal anatomy and pathologic alterations on conventional MR images. AJNR 1993;14:1237–1240.

15. Mathern GW, Kuhlman PA, Mendoza D, et al. Human fascia dentata anatomy and hippocampal neuron densities differ depending on the epileptic syndrome and age at first seizure. J Neuropathol Exp Neurol 1997;56:199–212.

16. Meiners LC, van Gils A, Jansen GH, et al. Temporal lobe epilepsy: the various MR appearances of histologically proven mesial temporal sclerosis. AJNR 1994;15:1547–1555.

17. Prayson RA, Reith JD, Najm IM. Mesial temporal sclerosis. A clinicopathologic study of 27 patients, including 5 with coexistent cortical dysplasia. Arch Pathol Lab Med 1996;120:532–536.

18. Zentner J, Wolf HK, Helmstaedter C, et al. Clinical relevance of amygdala sclerosis in temporal lobe epilepsy. J Neurosurg 1999;91:59–67.

## Malformative Lesions

1. Arai Y, Edwards V, Becker LE. A comparison of cell phenotypes in hemimegalencephaly and tuberous sclerosis. Acta Neuropathol (Berl) 1999;98:407–413.

2. Armstrong DD. The neuropathology of temporal lobe epilepsy. J Neuropathol Exp Neurol 1993;52:433–443.

3. Armstrong DL, Grossman RG, Zhu ZQ, et al. Changes in glial cells in temporal lobes of patients treated for intractable complex partial seizures. J Neuropath Exp Neurol 1988;49:328.

4. Barkovich AJ, Chuang SH. Unilateral megalencephaly: correlation of MR imaging and pathologic characteristics. AJNR 1990;11:523–531.

5. Cotter D, Honavar M, Lovestone S, et al. Disturbance of Notch-1 and Wnt signalling proteins in neuroglial balloon cells and abnormal large neurons in focal cortical dysplasia in human cortex. Acta Neuropathol (Berl) 1999;98:465–472.

6. De Rosa MJ, Farrell MA, Burke MM, et al. An assessment of the proliferative potential of 'balloon cells' in focal cortical resections performed in childhood epilepsy. Neuropathol Appl Neurobiol 1992;18:566–574.

7. Emery JA, Roper SN, Rojiani AM. White matter neuronal heterotopia in temporal lobe epilepsy: a morphometric and immunohistochemical study. J Neuropathol Exp Neurol 1997;56: 1276–1282.

8. Farrell MA, DeRosa MJ, Curran JG, et al. Neuropathologic findings in cortical resections (including hemispherectomies) performed for the treatment of intractable childhood epilepsy. Acta Neuropathol (Berl) 1992;83:246–259.

9. Frater JL, Prayson RA, Morris IH, et al. Surgical pathologic findings of extratemporal-based intractable epilepsy: a study of 133 consecutive resections. Arch Pathol Lab Med 2000;124:545–549.

10. Hardiman O, Burke T, Phillips J, et al. Microdysgenesis in resected temporal neocortex: incidence and clinical significance in focal epilepsy. Neurology 1988;38:1041–1047.

11. Jay V, Becker LE, Otsubo H, et al. Pathology of temporal lobectomy for refractory seizures in children. Review of 20 cases including some unique malformative lesions. J Neurosurg 1993;79: 53–61.

12. Kasper BS, Stefan H, Buchfelder M, et al. Temporal lobe microdysgenesis in epilepsy versus control brains. J Neuropathol Exp Neurol 1999;58:22–28.

13. Kaufman WE, Galaburda AM. Cerebrocortical microdysgenesis in neurologically normal subjects: a histopathologic study. Neurology 1989;39:238–244.

14. Kuzniecky R, Garcia J, Faught E, et al. Cortical dysplasia in temporal lobe epilepsy: magnetic resonance imaging correlations. Ann Neurol 1991;29:293–298.

15. Kuzniecky R, Guthrie B, Mountz J, et al. Intrinsic epileptogenesis of hypothalamic hamartomas in gelastic epilepsy. Ann Neurol 1997;42:60–67.

16. Manz HJ, Phillips TM, Rowden G, et al. Unilateral megalencephaly, cerebral cortical dysplasia, neuronal hypertrophy, and heterotopia: cytomorphometric, fluorometric cytochemical, and biochemical analyses. Acta Neuropathol (Berl) 1979;45:97–103.

17. Meencke HJ, Janz D. The significance of microdysgenesis in primary generalized epilepsy: an answer to the considerations of Lyon and Gastaut. Epilepsia 1985;26:368–371.

18. Mischel PS, Nguyen LP, Vinters HV. Cerebral cortical dysplasia associated with pediatric epilepsy. Review of neuropathologic features and proposal for a grading system. J Neuropathol Exp Neurol 1995;54:137–153.

19. Mischel PS, Vinters HV. Neuropathology. Neurosurg Clin North Am 1995;6:565–579.

20. Osborn RE, Byrd SE, Naidich TP, et al. MR imaging of neuronal migrational disorders. AJNR 1988;9:1101–1106.

21. Palmini A, Andermann F, Aicardi J, et al. Diffuse cortical dysplasia, or the 'double cortex' syndrome: the clinical and epileptic spectrum in 10 patients. Neurology 1991;41:1656–1662.

22. Palmini A, Andermann F, Olivier A, et al. Focal neuronal migration disorders and intractable partial epilepsy: a study of 30 patients. Ann Neurol 1991;30:741–749.

23. Plate KH, Wieser H-G, Yasargil MG, et al. Neuropathological findings in 224 patients with temporal lobe epilepsy. Acta Neuropathol (Berl) 1993;86:433–438.

24. Prayson RA, Estes ML. Cortical dysplasia: a histopathologic study of 52 cases of partial lobectomy in patients with epilepsy. Hum Pathol 1995;26:493–500.

25. Raymond AA, Fish DR, Sisodiya SM, et al. Abnormalities of gyration, heterotopias, tuberous sclerosis, focal cortical dysplasia, microdysgenesis, dysembryoplastic neuroepithelial tumour and dysgenesis of the archicortex in epilepsy. Clinical, EEG and neuroimaging features in 100 adult patients. Brain 1995;118:629–660.

26. Robain O, Floquet CH, Heldt N, et al. Hemimegalencephaly: a clinicopathological study of four cases. Neuropathol Appl Neurobiol 1988;14:125–135.

27. Rojiani AM, Emery JA, Anderson KJ, et al. Distribution of heterotopic neurons in normal hemispheric white matter: a morphometric analysis. J Neuropathol Exp Neurol 1996;55:178–183.

28. Scully RE (ed). Case records of the Massachusetts General Hospital. Case 7-1996. N Engl J Med 1996;334:586–592.

29. Taylor DC, Falconer MA. Focal dysplasia of the cerebral cortex in epilepsy. J Neurol Neurosurg Psychiatry 1971;34:369–387.

30. Valdueza JM, Cristante L, Dammann O, et al. Hypothalamic hamartomas: with special reference to gelastic epilepsy and surgery. Neurosurgery 1994;34:949–958.

31. Vital A, Marchal C, Loiseau H, et al. Glial and neuronoglial malformative lesions associated with medically intractable epilepsy. Acta Neuropathol (Berl) 1994;87:196–201.

32. Volk EE, Prayson RA. Hamartomas in the setting of chronic epilepsy: a clinicopathologic study of 13 cases. Hum Pathol 1997;28:227–232.

33. Wolf HK, Birkholz T, Wellmer J, et al. Neurochemical profile of glioneuronal lesions from patients with pharmacoresistant focal epilepsies. J Neuropathol Exp Neurol 1995;54:689–697.

34. Wolf HK, Campos MG, Zentner J, et al. Surgical pathology of temporal lobe epilepsy. Experience with 216 cases. J Neuropathol Exp Neurol 1993;52:499–506.

35. Wolf HK, Normann S, Green AJ, et al. Tuberous sclerosis–like lesions in epileptogenic human neocortex lack allelic loss at the TSC1 and TSC2 regions. Acta Neuropathol (Berl) 1997;93:93–96.

36. Wolf HK, Wellmer J, Muller MB, et al. Glioneuronal malformative lesions and dysembryoplastic neuroepithelial tumors in patients with chronic pharmacoresistant epilepsies. J Neuropathol Exp Neurol 1995;54:245–254.

37. Wolf HK, Wiestler OD. Surgical pathology of chronic epileptic seizure disorders. Brain Pathol 1993;3:371–380.

38. Wolf HK, Zentner J, Hufnagel A, et al. Surgical pathology of chronic epileptic seizure disorders: experience with 63 specimens from extratemporal corticectomies, lobectomies and functional hemispherectomies. Acta Neuropathol (Berl) 1993;86:466–472.

39. Yachnis AT, Owell SZ, Olmsted JJ, et al. Distinct neurodevelopmental patterns of Bcl-2 and Bcl-x expression are altered in glioneuronal hamartias of the human temporal lobe. J Neuropathol Exp Neurol 1997;56:186–198.

**Vascular Lesions**

1. Benedikt RA, Brown DC, Walker R, et al. Sturge-Weber syndrome: cranial MR imaging with Gd-DTPA. AJNR 1993;14: 409–415.

2. Buckingham MJ, Crone KR, Ball WS, et al. Management of cerebral cavernous angiomas in children presenting with seizures. Childs Nerv Syst 1989;5:347–349.

3. Davies KG, Maxwell RE, French LA. Hemispherectomy for intractable seizures: long-term results in 17 patients followed for up to 38 years. J Neurosurg 1993;78:733–740.

4. Dodick DW, Cascino GD, Meyer FB. Vascular malformations and intractable epilepsy: outcome after surgical treatment. Mayo Clin Proc 1994;69:741–745.

5. Edgar R, Baldwin M. Vascular malformations associated with temporal lobe epilepsy. J Neurosurg 1960;17:638–656.

6. Frater JL, Prayson RA, Morris IH, et al. Surgical pathologic findings of extratemporal-based intractable epilepsy: a study of 133 consecutive resections. Arch Pathol Lab Med 2000;124:545–549.

7. Hoffman HJ, Hendrick EB, Dennis M, et al. Hemispherectomy for Sturge-Weber syndrome. Childs Brain 1979;5:233–248.

8. Ito M, Sato K, Ohnuki A, et al. Sturge-Weber disease: operative indications and surgical results. Brain Dev 1990;12:473–477.

9. Ogunmekan AO, Hwang PA, Hoffman HJ. Sturge-Weber-Dimitri disease: role of hemispherectomy in prognosis. Can J Neurol Sci 1989;16:78–80.

**Reactive and Inflammatory Lesions**

1. Davies KG, Hermann BP, Dohan FC Jr, et al. Intractable epilepsy due to meningitis: results of surgery and pathological findings. Br J Neurosurg 1996;10:567–570.

# THE BRAIN: VASCULAR DISEASE

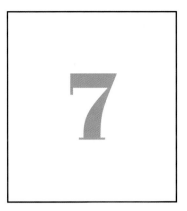

## VASCULAR MALFORMATIONS
    Capillary Telangiectasis
    Venous Angioma
    Cavernous Angioma
    Arteriovenous Malformation
    Vascular Malformations in Dysgenetic
      Syndromes
## VASCULITIS AND VASCULOPATHY
    Temporal (Giant Cell) Arteritis
    Granulomatous Angiitis
    Amyloid (Congophilic) Angiopathy
## CEREBRAL INFARCT
## SUBDURAL HEMATOMA
## REFERENCES

Most cerebrovascular disorders are diagnosed and treated without recourse to surgery. However, when they arise as mass lesions or epileptogenic foci, some ultimately come to the attention of the surgical pathologist.

## VASCULAR MALFORMATIONS

Vascular malformations have been classified on the basis of (1) the caliber, configuration, and histologic composition of the component vessels; (2) the continuity with the normal cerebral vasculature; and (3) the quantitative interrelationship between vessels and intervening parenchyma.[4, 26] Relationships among and apparent transitions between specific lesions within this group are the subjects of ongoing discussion. This is particularly true in regard to a possible relationship between telangiectasis and cavernous angioma. Selected references are provided for the reader interested in pursuing this nosologic nightmare.[4, 12, 52, 64, 70] Although the following discussion presents the vascular malformations as specific entities, sharp morphologic distinctions are not always possible, especially in small specimens.

## Capillary Telangiectasis

This, the most innocent lesion of the group, appears to persist throughout the life of the host and is encountered most often as an incidental neuroradiologic or postmortem finding. Angiographically, it is a nebulous blush, often within the pons.[5] Contrast enhancement is seen by magnetic resonance (MR) imaging.[32] Only a rare lesion is symptomatic.[16, 61]

Telangiectases are aggregates of thin-walled, ectatic vessels resembling dilated capillaries. Their aneurysmal dilatations are seen best in injection studies.[6] Microscopically, the vessels are individually dispersed throughout a region of parenchyma that is unaltered by gliosis or hemosiderin deposits.

## Venous Angioma

Lesions on the venous limb of the cerebral circulation appear as loose or compact conglomerates. Loosely organized examples are little more than varicosities. These bleed only rarely and are generally incidental MR findings.[9, 37, 41, 45, 53] A cavernous angioma hovers nearby in some cases.[69]

## Cavernous Angioma

**Definition.** A compact mass of malformed vessels.

**Clinical Features.** The cavernous angioma or "cavernoma" is a well-defined clinicopathologic entity that is approached surgically in an attempt to control seizures and to eliminate the possibility of future hemorrhage.[4, 39, 44, 64] Cavernomas are usually seen clinically in adults, although, given their malformative nature, they can appear in children as well.[20, 39, 57]

**Radiologic Features.** The typical lesion consists of a small, discrete nidus surrounded by a rim of hemosiderin-stained brain parenchyma. The ferruginous penumbra is

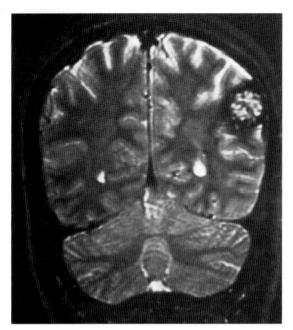

**FIGURE 7–1    CAVERNOUS ANGIOMA**

This MR image of a 27-year-old man with a 9-year history of seizures is almost diagnostic of a cavernous angioma. The compact mass of vessels is surrounded by a dark halo of decreased signal produced by the iron in hemosiderin. (Courtesy of Dr. John T. Curnes, Durham, NC.)

obvious on MR imaging and, in concert with vascular profiles, is virtually diagnostic (Fig. 7–1).[39, 48] Viewed in cross section, the closely packed vessels have a so-called popcorn appearance, at least to the radiologist. Chronic lesions are often calcified. A neighboring venous angioma may be evident in some cases[1, 43, 69]; an associated telangiectasis may be seen in others.[31, 64]

Cavernous angiomas occur throughout the central nervous system and meninges. The reader is referred to the references for accounts of examples involving specific sites: meninges,[8, 33, 40, 56, 66] hypothalamus (mammillary bodies),[35] thalamus,[62] basal ganglia,[62] pineal region,[23] brain stem,[13, 62, 67] cerebellum,[24] cerebellopontine angle,[8] ventricular system,[8, 11, 28, 50, 60] and cavernous sinus.[34, 58] Dural lesions are discussed in Chapter 2 on page 79

Angiographically, cavernomas do not shunt blood from arterial to venous limbs. In the presence of such diversion, the surgeon assumes the presence of an arteriovenous malformation (AVM) and is skeptical about the diagnosis of cavernous malformation. The noncommittal diagnosis of "vascular malformation" can be utilized to avoid this conflict and appease diagnostic uncertainty.

Although many cavernous angiomas remain clinically silent, seizures, focal neurologic deficits, or signs of increased intracranial pressure may herald their presence.[3, 10, 14, 39, 44, 59] Female patients are more likely to present with the complications of hemorrhage and neurologic deficits, whereas men are more likely to present with seizures.[1, 39, 44] Hemorrhages are usually smaller and less life threatening than those from AVMs. Cavernous angiomas in the brain stem may be responsible for progressive deficits.[61, 67]

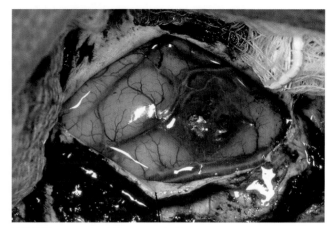

**FIGURE 7–2    CAVERNOUS ANGIOMA**

The discrete quality of the lesion is readily apparent in this operative view of a temporal lobe lesion. Courtesy of Dr. William. E. Krauss, Rochester, MN.

A familial predilection for cavernous angiomas is noted in some cases, particularly among Spanish-American individuals of Mexican descent.[29, 44, 51, 71] Multiple lesions may occur in such genetically susceptible individuals as well as in families with an as yet undefined genetic abnormality.[29] Multiple lesions may occur in the absence of a family history. Although linkage studies have focused attention upon chromosome 7q as the likely locus of a gene responsible in some familial cases, this genomic domain is exculpated in others.[19, 22] One study found a point mutation in the *KRIT1* gene in this region in four Hispanic-American families.[72] Radiation therapy appears responsible in the genesis of multiple cavernoma-like lesions that share histologic features with telangiectases.[17, 49]

**Macroscopic Features.** The lesion is a compact mass of interwoven vessels (Figs. 7–2 and 7–3). Any brain attached to the lesion is likely to be hemosiderin stained.

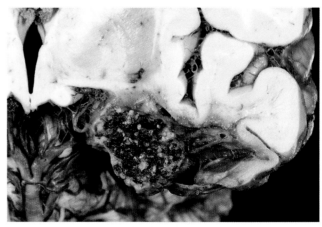

**FIGURE 7–3    CAVERNOUS ANGIOMA**

As illustrated by this lesion in the leptomeninges of a 64-year-old patient with a 43-year history of seizures, a cavernous angioma is a well-circumscribed mass of vessels.

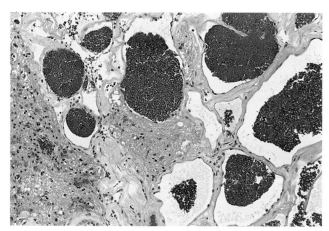

**FIGURE 7–4    CAVERNOUS ANGIOMA**

A calcified right frontal lobe mass was detected by computed tomography in a 31-year-old woman with an 18-year history of seizures. The lesion, which did not fill during angiography, was excised as a discrete mass without apparent feeding or draining vessels.

**Microscopic Features.** In contrast to the telangiectasis, cavernous angiomas are composed of featureless, hyalinized vascular channels. These are variably disposed but usually form a compact mass of back-to-back vessels with little if any interposed brain parenchyma (Fig. 7–4). In other cases, brain parenchyma is interposed between the channels.[64] Thick, amuscular vessels are frequently calcified (Fig. 7–5) and sometimes even ossified. Lumens are often occluded by thrombi that may show evidence of recanalization. The surrounding gliotic tissue bears the stain of hemosiderin.

**Treatment and Prognosis.** The prognosis after excision is excellent. The incidence of hemorrhage from unexcised examples has been estimated to be approximately 1% per lesion per year[39, 54, 55] or 0.25% per person (lesion) per year.[14] Factors predisposing to this risk include female gender, pregnancy, familial or multiple form of the disease, previous irradiation, prior hemorrhage, and an associated venous malformation.[3, 30, 44, 48, 54, 55] The

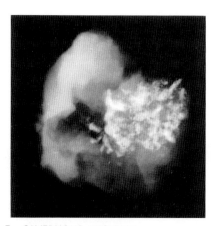

**FIGURE 7–5    CAVERNOUS ANGIOMA**

"Cavernomas" are compact masses of vessels with little intervening parenchyma. Note the hemosiderin that is commonly present in the brain immediately surrounding the lesion.

occasional association between a cavernoma and astrocytoma may be fortuitous.[2]

## Arteriovenous Malformation

**Definition.** A vascular malformation with arteriovenous shunting.

**General Comments.** AVMs may germinate anywhere in the embryonic brain or spinal cord, but most originate above the tentorium, where their roots extend over the hemispheric surfaces and dig deep into the underlying cortical soil. In some instances, a vascular fistula lies outside the brain within the dura.[42, 65, 68] The most plausible explanation for the pathogenesis of AVMs incriminates congenital absence of the regional capillary bed. This theory is in agreement with in vivo and in vitro arteriographic studies that clearly demonstrate arteriovenous shunting, and it is further substantiated by the histologic absence of capillary communications between arterial and venous channels. Shunting elevates intraluminal venous pressure and produces ectasia and muscularization so that hybrid vessels with both venous and arterial characteristics are created. Altered by time and pressure gradients, the lesion thereafter contains large vessels with shunt-related changes in addition to the original malformation per se.

**Clinical Features.** The lesion enlarges insidiously, generally becoming symptomatic during the second to fifth decades of life. Hemorrhage, headaches, seizures, and focal neurologic deficits are common.[7] In infants and children, the effluent may be sufficient to dilate the great vein of Galen and produce cardiac failure.

Vascular malformations occurring in dysgenetic syndromes are described in a separate section on pages 407 to 408.

**Radiologic Features.** Vascular profiles and dark flow voids are readily evident on MR imaging, and the excised lesion is sent to the pathology laboratory with little uncertainty regarding the diagnosis. Almost by definition, arteriovenous shunting is apparent angiographically (Figs. 7–6 and 7–7).

**Macroscopic Findings.** Cushing and Bailey[15] aptly characterized the angry, tangled mass of vessels that grossly constitute arteriovenous malformations as a "snarl." Its cortical surface is covered by thickened, sometimes hemosiderin-stained, leptomeninges (Figs. 7–8 to 7–10) through which the vascular channels appear at surgery as blue veins, red pulsatile arteries, and vessels of indeterminate parentage with laminar or turbulent streams of blue or red. Unfortunately for the pathologist, these kinetic qualities are lost when the lesion is uprooted from the vascular bed that gives it life. Nonetheless, some semblance of vitality can be recaptured by the injection of contrast material, which floods both feeder and draining vessels to swell the body of the malformation.[25, 27] The wormy mass often extends deep into the cerebrum. If its apex approaches a ventricle, the

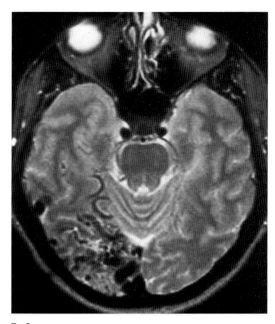
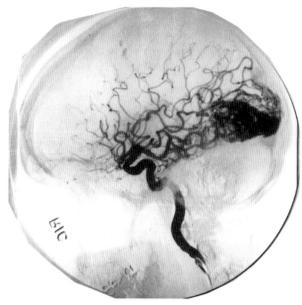

7–6                                                          7–7

**FIGURES 7–6 AND 7–7    ARTERIOVENOUS MALFORMATION**

Serpiginous profiles of abnormal vessels with dark lumens (flow voids) are typical of arteriovenous malformations (Fig. 7–6). Arteriovenous shunting seen during angiography (Fig. 7–7) established the diagnosis in this 40-year-old woman with headaches.

outflow may discharge into the deep cerebral veins. Vascular or interstitial calcification imparts grittiness to some specimens.

**Microscopic Features.** Microscopic diversity characterizes the vessels of this blunder of angiogenesis.[25, 26, 38] Some vessels have the thin, amuscular walls of veins, whereas others have the media and the elastic laminae of arteries. Still others are structural hybrids (Figs. 7–11 and 7–12). Although interposed parenchyma is often gliotic and hemosiderin stained, some lesions show surprisingly little of either alteration. At the core, or nidus, of the lesion, vessels lie densely packed with only scant intervening parenchyma. Elsewhere, brain parenchyma

fills the interstices between vascular profiles. Crescents of mural calcification outline the contours of some vessels, and granules and pebbles of mineral lie strewn in surrounding brain tissue. Although usually not sufficiently dense to be visualized in clinical radiographs, calcifications are often seen in radiographs of the excised specimen.

In an attempt to reduce their vascularity to aid in excision, some AVMs are embolized therapeutically with any of a number of occlusive or thrombogenic substances. The foreign material and secondary giant cell reactions can be seen in surgical specimens.[18] Partially occluded AVMs may recanalize.[21] Previously irradiated lesions are often fibrotic.[63]

**Differential Diagnosis.** The histologic composition of an AVM generally permits confident recognition. One should not misconstrue *small clusters of normally structured arteries* in the subarachnoid space that become artifactually compacted during surgical excision of the brain or meninges (Fig. 7–13). The diagnosis in this setting would come as a surprise to the surgeon because only rarely are arteriovenous lesions unanticipated or incidental findings. Hypercellularity by oligodendroglia, as occurs on occasion in the environs of an AVM, should not be misinterpreted as *glioma, particularly oligodendroglioma*.[46] Nonetheless, gliomas of varying types have been reported in association with the vascular malformations.[2] A cited reference discusses in detail these vessel-rich gliomas (angiogliomas) and glioma-like tissue responses.[36]

**FIGURE 7–8    ARTERIOVENOUS MALFORMATION**

This occipital lesion demonstrates the classical large vessels that feed and drain the compact central mass of an arteriovenous anomaly.

**Treatment and Prognosis.** The prognosis of patients with untreated AVMs is contingent upon the unpre-

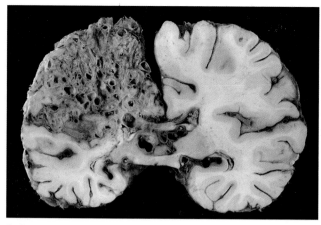

7–9

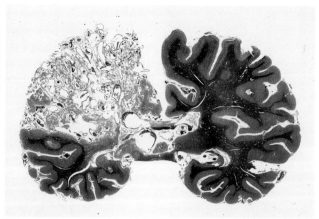

7–10

**FIGURES 7–9 AND 7–10**    ARTERIOVENOUS MALFORMATION

As seen macroscopically (Fig. 7–9) and in a whole mount histologic section (Fig. 7–10), arteriovenous malformations can be large and may involve large areas of the brain.

dictable occurrence of hemorrhage, an event estimated to occur at the rate of 2% to 4% per patient year.[7, 47] Complete excision precludes this eventuality, whereas partial resection leaves the patient at continued jeopardy. Embolization is effective temporarily in reducing vasculature. The sclerosing effects of radiotherapy are finding increased usage.

## Vascular Malformations in Dysgenetic Syndromes

**Sturge-Weber Disease.** In its full expression, this uncommon entity combines vascular malformations of the face, eye, and brain with glaucoma, cerebral atrophy, mental retardation, and seizures.[8, 13, 15, 19] The entity is also discussed in regard to epilepsy in Chapter 6 on pages 399. Extensive resections, including hemispherectomy, may be undertaken to control seizures.[2, 8, 11]

The classical vascular abnormalities include a cutaneous vascular malformation or nevus in the distribution of the trigeminal nerve, a similar abnormality in the choroid, and a carpet of small vessels in the leptomeninges ipsilateral to the facial abnormality (Fig. 7–14). The latter is seen well in contrast-enhanced MR imaging studies, as are other vascular abnormalities such as vessels in an enlarged choroid plexus.[3–6, 18, 19] Ocular

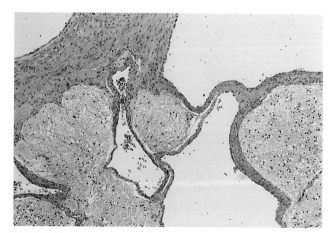

**FIGURE 7–11**    ARTERIOVENOUS MALFORMATION

Irregularity in size, shape, and degree of muscularization characterize the vessels of an arteriovenous malformation.

**FIGURE 7–12**    ARTERIOVENOUS MALFORMATION

Brain parenchyma is frequently found sequestered between the vascular channels.

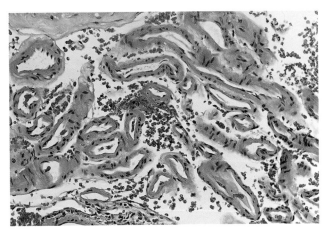

**FIGURE 7–13    LEPTOMENINGEAL VESSELS SIMULATING ARTERIOVENOUS MALFORMATION**

Artifactually compacted normal leptomeningeal vessels should not be misinterpreted as a vascular malformation. They are normally and uniformly muscularized.

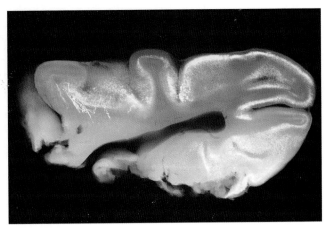

**FIGURE 7–15    STURGE-WEBER DISEASE**

As seen in a radiograph of a surgical specimen, cortical calcifications produce an undulating band of radiodensity. (Courtesy of Dr. Douglas C. Anthony, Boston, MA.)

lesions can also be visualized by MR imaging.[7] The laminar, intracortical calcifications are well seen by computed tomography of the brain or radiographs of the specimen (Fig. 7–15).

Histologically, the redundant leptomeningeal vessels consist of closely packed veins (Fig. 7–16). Layering of calcospherites in the subjacent cortex is the basis of so-called tram-track calcifications that follow gyral contours. The cerebellum may also be affected.[4, 19, 21] Parenchymal loss with gliosis attends some cases.

**Wyburn-Mason Syndrome.** AVMs of the midbrain and ipsilateral eye (retina) combine with a facial vascular nevus to form this rare oculocerebral syndrome complex.[12, 17, 20]

**Hereditary Hemorrhagic Telangiectasia (Rendu-Osler-Weber Syndrome).** Although the visceral components of this vasomalformative syndrome are the classical components of this disease, symptomatic in-

tracranial AVMs, sometimes multiple, are occasionally seen as well.[1, 9, 10, 14, 16]

# VASCULITIS AND VASCULOPATHY

## Temporal (Giant Cell) Arteritis

**Definition.** An inflammatory process of unknown etiology that affects predominantly branches of the external carotid artery system.

**General Comments.** The temporal, ophthalmic, and posterior ciliary arteries are primarily affected in this common condition.[6, 10, 13, 14, 16, 26] In unusual cases, intracranial vessels are affected as well[13] and histologically analogous lesions have been described in the aorta and intracranial vessels.[16] Vertebral arteries are susceptible; their involvement, albeit uncommon, may result in spinal cord infarction as well as basilar artery thrombosis.[8]

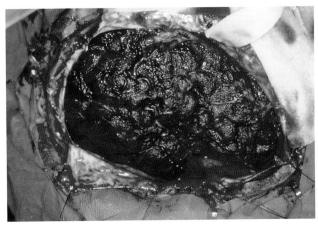

**FIGURE 7–14    STURGE-WEBER DISEASE**

A lush carpet of leptomeningeal vessels covers the surface of the brain. (Courtesy of Dr. Harold J. Hoffman, Toronto, Canada.)

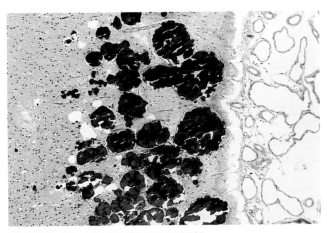

**FIGURE 7–16    STURGE-WEBER DISEASE**

Vessels with venous features fill the subarachnoid space; the characteristic calcifications occur in superficial cortex.

Selective involvement of the internal elastic membrane, as well as the specific T-cell composition of the inflammatory response, has focused attention on an immunologic pathogenetic mechanism.[22] Arterial deposition of immunoglobulin and complement, although a regular finding, provides only circumstantial evidence. Inflammatory cytokines have been incriminated, but an inciting antigen has yet to be identified.[25] One imaginative hypothesis indicts actinic radiation in the pathogenesis of giant cell arteritis.[11, 18] Not surprisingly, the etiology of temporal arteritis has eluded electron microscopists.[22, 23]

**Clinical Features.** Temporal arteritis is uncommon before the seventh decade of life and occurs at a higher incidence in women.[7, 10, 13–16] It rarely affects blacks.[27] Specific signs and symptoms are referable to involvement of a regional artery: headaches and scalp tenderness to the temporal artery, jaw claudication to the facial artery, and visual loss to the ophthalmic and posterior ciliary vessels. The disorder is often a component of polymyalgia rheumatica syndrome, with its fever, weight loss, malaise, myalgias, arthralgias, and an increased erythrocyte sedimentation rate. Pathologic changes in temporal arteritis can be visualized in some cases by ultrasonography.[21]

Biopsy of an asymptomatic and palpably normal temporal artery may show the typical changes of giant cell arteritis. Because, conversely, a negative biopsy does not exclude the disease and patients with classical signs and symptoms may be effectively treated with corticosteroids, the need for biopsy has been debated.[2, 9]

**Macroscopic Features.** The involved artery may be thickened and nodular (Fig. 7–17). More commonly,

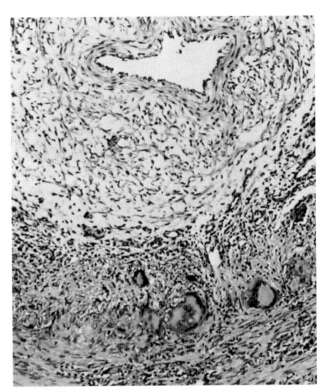

**FIGURE 7–18    GIANT CELL (TEMPORAL) ARTERITIS**

A 56-year-old woman experienced headaches for 2 weeks prior to the onset of loss of visual acuity. A temporal artery shows vascularization and marked thickening of the intima with heavy inflammation and giant cell formation in the media. Characteristically, the giant cells are aligned along the internal elastic lamina, where they surround and engulf fragments of elastica. As often seen, the latter show decreased affinity for elastic stains.

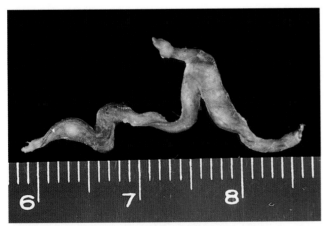

**FIGURE 7–17    GIANT CELL (TEMPORAL) ARTERITIS**

A 75-year-old woman presented with the polymyalgia rheumatica syndrome and an erythrocyte sedimentation rate (ESR) of 86 mm/hr. Aside from a single adventitial focus of lymphocytes, the left temporal artery was histologically unremarkable. Steroid therapy reduced the symptoms and ESR, but the latter rose abruptly when the glucocorticoid dose was reduced. A biopsy of the right temporal artery was then performed and this thickened nodular segment was excised. Microscopically, it showed typical features of giant cell (temporal) arteritis.

however, it is normal by sight and touch. If a frozen section is requested to ensure a diagnostic biopsy, it is expeditious to focus upon a nodular segment. Because temporal cell arteritis is characteristically segmental, the entire surgical specimen should be transected at close intervals and examined histologically in step sections.[5, 12]

**Microscopic Features.** Inflammatory cells are generally present within the media and to a lesser extent in the adventitia or intima. In some cases, adventitial involvement predominates. As a rule, lymphocytes and plasma cells are most numerous but may be joined by eosinophils and polymorphonuclear leukocytes. The intima is usually thickened by fibrous tissue and may be vascularized (Fig. 7–18). A granular eosinophilic zone equated with fibrinoid necrosis is not uncommon (Fig. 7–19).[15, 20] Mucoid degeneration of the intima is frequent.

Multinucleated giant cells are the hallmark of temporal arteritis, although their presence is not obligatory.[3] Typically, they congregate along the internal elastic membrane at the interface between the media and intima (see Fig. 7–18). Lesser numbers are attracted to the external elastic membrane. Varying in number from few to many, giant cells may be inconspicuous as they conform to the undulations of the disrupted elastica

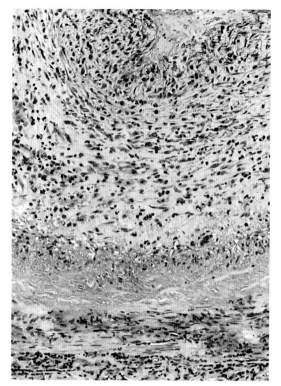

**FIGURE 7–19** GIANT CELL (TEMPORAL) ARTERITIS

A granular, eosinophilic, circumferential zone of necrosis may border the internal elastic membrane.

(Fig. 7–20). Fragments of membrane may be engulfed by giant cells and lose their affinity for elastic stains.

Healed temporal arteritis is characterized by medial fibrosis, fragmentation of the internal elastic lamina, and vascularization of the arterial wall (Fig. 7–21).[1, 13] Vessels with such features are usually encountered after corticosteroid treatment,[2, 21] but there is not always a close correlation between the activity of the clinical disease and its histologic expressions. Their distinction from the degenerative changes of aging and arteriosclerosis may not always be possible[1, 4, 13, 14, 19] Calcification of the internal elastic membrane is of no diagnostic significance, as it is a common finding in elderly patients (Fig. 7–22).

**Differential Diagnosis.** Generally, the histologic features of temporal arteritis are diagnostic. The occasional absence of giant cells in the presence of an otherwise typical temporal arteritis raises the question of a *non–giant cell variant*. One can accept the lack of giant cells in the typical clinical setting, albeit with hesitance in use of the term giant cell arteritis. The finding of prominent mucin deposition in the intima in the absence of arteritis has prompted the suggestion that there exists an early intimal phase of the disease process.[4,14] In the absence of mural inflammation, we are reluctant to make the diagnosis of temporal arteritis but feel obliged to bring this observation to attention because clinicians are inclined to treat such patients if the sedimentation rate is elevated.

Whereas the presence of frank, transmural necrosis should prompt consideration of *polyarteritis*, necrosis in

giant cell arteritis is generally limited to the vicinity of the elastica.[4, 13, 14]

**Treatment and Prognosis.** Temporal arteritis is generally a self-limited disorder that typically resolves within 1 year. Excision of the affected artery may relieve symptoms but does not modify the effects of the process at other sites. Steroid therapy generally aborts the disease and prevents visual loss. The risk of blindness, a common justification for steroid therapy for polymyalgia rheumatica and temporal arteritis, has not been defined with precision.[24] Giant cell arteritis is rarely fatal.[17]

## Granulomatous Angiitis

**Definition.** A granulomatous angiitis affecting intracranial vessels.

**General Comments.** The nosology of granulomatous angiitis is beset with the same ambiguities as are the classifications of other vasculitides.[17] Nonetheless, it represents a distinct clinicopathologic entity when it occurs sporadically in a previously normal individual. Although the suggestion has been made that it is but an intracranial variant of giant cell or temporal arteritis, the two

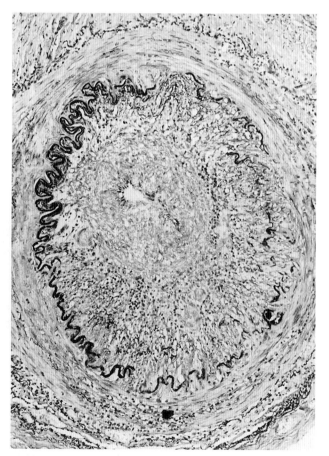

**FIGURE 7–20** GIANT CELL (TEMPORAL) ARTERITIS

Fragmentation of the internal elastic membrane is characteristic of giant cell (temporal) arteritis.

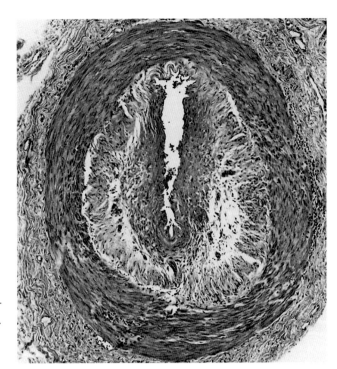

**FIGURE 7–21    GIANT CELL (TEMPORAL) ARTERITIS**

The healed phase of giant cell arteritis is illustrated in this vessel in which the now thickened, vascularized intima is no longer inflamed. Only a few adventitial lymphocytes remain. This patient with polymyalgia rheumatica syndrome had been treated with corticosteroids.

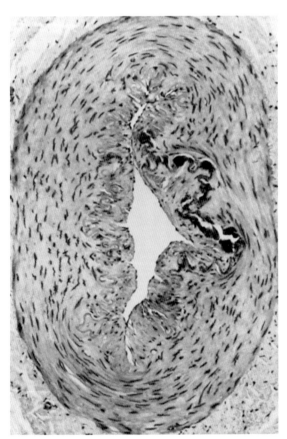

**FIGURE 7–22    TEMPORAL ARTERY CALCIFICATION IN A PATIENT WITHOUT GIANT CELL (TEMPORAL) ARTERITIS**

Calcification along the internal elastic membrane is a common nonspecific finding in the temporal arteries of elderly patients.

entities have a number of important distinguishing features. These include (1) predominance of epithelioid histiocytes in granulomatous angiitis, (2) involvement of veins, (3) occurrence in adults younger than those typically affected by temporal arteritis, (4) a higher incidence in men than women, and (5) occurrence outside the polymyalgia rheumatica syndrome. It remains to be established whether the rare examples of granulomatous vasculitis that occur in the setting of Hodgkin's disease and herpes zoster are the same disorder as the sporadic disease.

In any setting, biopsy may be necessary to confirm the diagnosis.[3]

**Clinical Features.** Segmental in distribution, granulomatous angiitis constricts and occludes intracranial arteries with resultant infarction[2, 4, 5, 9–13, 17, 19] and sometimes hemorrhage.[4] Extracranial disease is uncommon.[11] One analysis of its clinical presentations, in biopsy-proven cases, emphasized "diffuse" or "encephalopathic" symptoms rather than the focal manifestations of ischemia expected of vaso-occlusive disease.[19] Headache was the most common presenting symptom in yet another series.[5] In any case, a subacute or chronic course can cause diagnostic confusion. Occasional cases affect the spinal cord.[8, 16, 18, 20]

Granulomatous angiitis generally occurs during or beyond the fifth decade of life. Men are more often targeted.[19] Although Hodgkin's disease appears to be a predisposing factor in some cases,[8, 22] the etiology of the disorder is obscure.[11]

**Radiologic Features.** The presumptive diagnosis is often suggested by angiography, when the larger intracranial vessels cast beaded shadows (Fig. 7–23).[2, 5, 7, 12, 15] The diagnosis remains presumptive because these

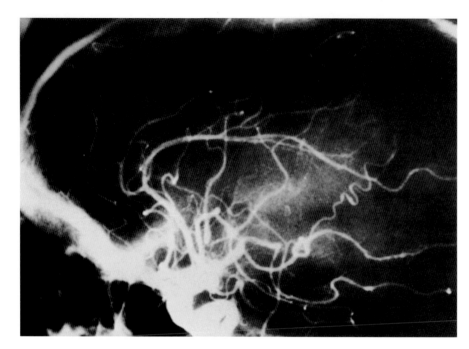

**FIGURE 7–23**   GRANULOMATOUS
ANGIITIS

Angiographically, granulomatous angiitis
appears as "beading" of cerebral vessels.
Affected branches of the middle cerebral
artery are evident at the lower right of the
illustration. The patient was a 43-year-old
man with a 1-year history of headache,
weakness, and unilateral sensory loss.

angiographic changes are not always found and, when they are present, they are not specific. Infarcts or lesions mimicking glioma may also be seen.[7] In the absence of histologic confirmation, the differential diagnosis is broad,[7, 17] and the need for a tissue diagnosis has been emphasized.[5, 11, 12, 17, 21]

**Microscopic Features.** Granulomatous angiitis is predominantly an arterial process, but veins are not immune. Leptomeningeal vessels are particularly vulnerable. Because the lesions contain mixtures of epithelioid histiocytes, lymphocytes, and giant cells, the term *granulomatous* is appropriate (Fig. 7–24). Epithelioid histiocytes can predominate.[2, 9–11, 13] Distributed segmentally along vessels, individual discrete granulomas affect mainly the adventitia.

Uncommonly, both granulomatous inflammation and amyloid affect the same vessels (see Fig. 7–29).[1, 6, 14] It is not clear whether this is a chance occurrence, a granulomatous response to amyloid, or a deposition of amyloid in granulomatous angiitis. One study concluded that, for therapeutic purposes, such cases should be considered as granulomatous angiitis.[6]

**Treatment and Prognosis.** Granulomatous angiitis is effectively treated with corticosteroids.[4, 5, 12, 15, 23]

## Amyloid (Congophilic) Angiopathy

**Definition.** An idiopathic deposition of amyloid in leptomeningeal and cortical vessels.

**General Comments.** The possibility of amyloid, or congophilic, angiopathy adds a welcomed element of expectation to the often unrewarding examination of specimens of intracerebral hemorrhage. The entity, familiar

to clinicians and radiologists alike, is not well known to pathologists.

**Clinical Features.** This form of angiopathy is a disorder of the elderly in whom amyloid normally accumulates within small- and medium-sized vessels of the

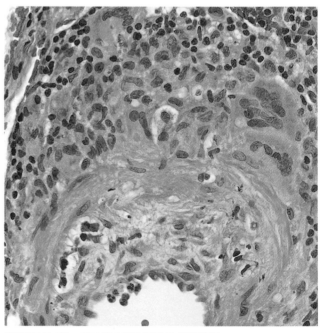

**FIGURE 7–24    GRANULOMATOUS ANGIITIS**

As seen in this biopsy specimen from a 59-year-old woman with a 1-week history of personality change and headache, granulomatous angiitis is most prominent in vessels of the leptomeninges and superficial cortex. The inflammatory infiltrate is composed of epithelioid cells, giant cells, and lymphocytes. The patient's disordered personality responded dramatically to corticosteroids.

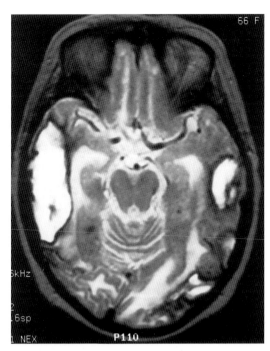

**FIGURE 7-25**   AMYLOID (CONGOPHILIC) ANGIOPATHY

Multiple hemorrhages and/or infarcts are common in the advanced stages of amyloid angiopathy. The T2-bright hemorrhages noted here are surrounded by dark rims of hemosiderin-rich tissue. The patient, a 66-year-old woman, had acquired multiple neurologic deficits over an 18-month period.

cerebral cortex and leptomeninges.[23] The process is independent of systemic amyloidosis and becomes clinically relevant only when amyloid deposition is marked.

Amyloid angiopathy should be considered when hemorrhage and/or infarction occurs in a patient 60 years or older. It is a disease of the leptomeningeal and cortical vasculature and is not to be found in the white matter, although the parenchyma of the latter is abnormal radiologically in some cases, as discussed subsequently.

As a consequence of its rather restricted distribution, the cerebral hemorrhages are typically superficial in location, in contrast to the deep-seated hemorrhages that occur in hypertension (Fig. 7-25).[2, 4, 6, 9-12, 17, 21, 22, 26] Infarction is less common. Occasional patients develop focal white matter changes including edema and gliosis that may be independent of hemorrhage and infarction.[1, 5, 8, 13, 19] Dementia, a prominent feature in some,[7] is usually attributable to a concurrent neurodegenerative disease (see later).

**Radiologic Features.** Hemorrhages and infarcts of various ages are common (see Fig. 7-25).

**Microscopic Features.** The amyloid deposits are visible in hematoxylin and eosin–stained preparations as the waxy eosinophilic material familiar to all pathologists (Fig. 7-26). The amyloid is applied to the outer vessel wall. Any doubt about the authenticity of the deposit is resolved by Congo red staining (Fig. 7-27) and microscopy with polarized light (Fig. 7-28). Affected vessels may show structural redundancies, descriptively referred to as glomeruli, double-barreled lumens, microaneurysms, and telangiectases.[14] A granulomatous reaction to the amyloid is occasionally seen (Fig. 7-29).[3, 6, 20] This association is discussed further in this chapter under Granulomatous Angiitis on pages 410 to 412. Fibrinoid necrosis may be seen and is associated with the apolipoprotein E ε2 allele.[16]

A puzzling issue is the relation between congophilic angiopathy with intracerebral hemorrhage and senile dementia of Alzheimer's type (SDAT).[15, 22, 24, 25] Several

**FIGURES 7-26 AND 7-27**   AMYLOID (CONGOPHILIC) ANGIOPATHY

Amyloid thickens the walls of vessels, as seen in a section first stained for H&E (Fig. 7-26) and then later Congo red (Fig. 7-27). The affected vessels are restricted to the subarachnoid space and cortex; those of the white matter are spared.

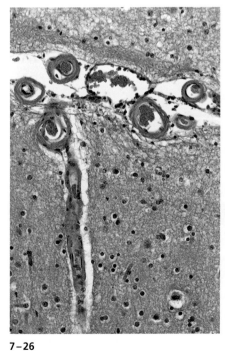

7-26

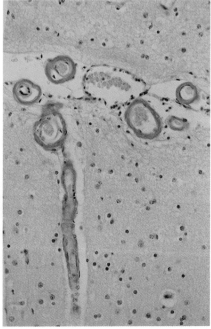

7-27

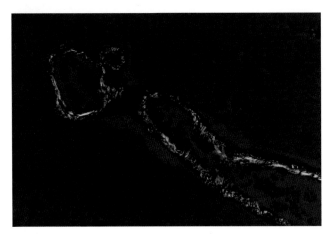

**FIGURE 7–28    AMYLOID (CONGOPHILIC) ANGIOPATHY**

"Apple green" birefringence with polarized light establishes the diagnosis, as would staining for beta amyloid.

observations hint at a relationship: (1) amyloid deposition is frequent in Alzheimer's disease, wherein it occurs in the center of neuritic or "senile" plaques as well as within blood vessel walls; (2) dementia may precede cerebral hemorrhage in the setting of congophilic angiopathy; and (3) senile plaques are often numerous in congophilic angiopathy and are accompanied by neurofibrillary tangle formation.[2, 10, 18] When prominent, perivascular plaques give the visual impression that the amyloid incited the plaques.

No doubt, some of the dementia associated with congophilic angiopathy in the elderly can be attributed to coincidence rather than to any shared pathogenesis with Alzheimer's disease. Furthermore, patients with congophilic angiopathy are not unfailingly demented, nor do postmortem studies invariably demonstrate histologic evidence of senile dementia. The histologic features of Alzheimer's disease and SDAT are discussed on pages 427 to 430.

**Treatment and Prognosis.** There is no treatment for amyloid angiopathy. Patients are susceptible to repeated hemorrhagic and/or ischemic events.

## CEREBRAL INFARCT

**General Comments.** With rare exceptions, cerebral infarcts are distinguished clinically and radiologically from other mass lesions,[2] and only a rare impostor is deceptive enough to convince clinicians that a biopsy is appropriate. A progressive clinical course and a worrisome mass on MR or computed tomography are the usual justifications for surgery. The possibility of a neoplasm seems even more compelling when the patient is young. A rare form of multi-infarct dementia, with subcortical infarcts and diffuse white matter degeneration, cerebral autosomal dominant arteriopathy with subcortical infarcts and leukoencephalopathy (CADASIL), is discussed in Chapter 8 on page 434.

**Radiologic Features.** Large cerebral hemispheric infarcts classically have a wedge shape, a vascular distribution, and, often, gyriform enhancement (Figs. 7–30 to 7–32). When seen in the coronal plane, small lesions in the basal ganglia may exhibit a telltale linear profile along the course of a lenticulostriate artery. When viewed axially, the zone of contrast enhancement in the latter lesions is more or less ring shaped and thus can simulate that of a glioblastoma.

**Macroscopic Features.** Acute infarcts are swollen and soft. Thrombosed veins are evident in some cases (Fig. 7–33).

**Microscopic Features.** After approximately 24 hours, infarcted brain is expansile, edematous, and sometimes hemorrhagic. Microscopic alterations become diagnostic

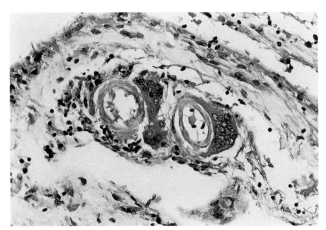

**FIGURE 7–29    AMYLOID (CONGOPHILIC) ANGIOPATHY WITH GRANULOMATOUS INFLAMMATION**

Amyloid angiopathy and granulomatous inflammation can coexist.

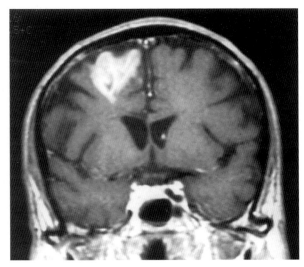

**FIGURE 7–30    CEREBRAL INFARCT**

Mass effect and a rim or ring configuration of contrast enhancement create a likeness to high-grade glioma. Progressive neurologic deficit prompted a craniotomy in this 61-year-old man.

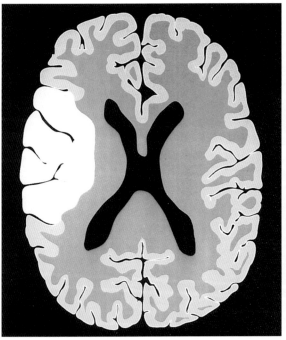

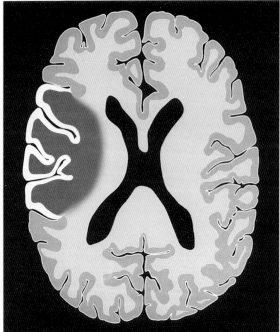

7-31                                          7-32

**FIGURES 7-31 AND 7-32    CEREBRAL INFARCT**

Cerebral infarcts appear as wedge-shaped T2-bright areas that conform to a vascular distribution (Fig. 7-31). A peripheral rim of contrast enhancement, particularly in the cerebral cortex, is also a common feature (Fig. 7-32). (From Passe TJ, Beauchamp NJ Jr, Burger PC. Neuroimaging in the identification of low grade and non-neoplastic CNS lesions. Neurologist 1999;5:293-299.)

when neuronal cytoplasm is hypereosinophilic and the nuclei are karyolytic. Referred to as "red" or "red-dead" neurons, these distinctive eosinophilic cells are reliable evidence of recent cell death (Fig. 7-34).[1] Red-dead neurons are to be distinguished from dark normal neurons undergoing autolysis after biopsy or resection. The latter become densely hyperchromatic, rather than dissolving through progressively paler stages of eosinophilia. Although ischemia is the prototypical mechanism underlying the formation of red or red-dead neurons, other

processes such as herpes simplex infection produce identical changes.

Early in the evolution of an infarct, capillary endothelial cells and pericytes enlarge and, to some extent, multiply. This hypertrophy of microvascular cells superficially resembles the vascular hyperplasia of malignant gliomas (Fig. 7-35). Focal acute inflammatory cell infiltrates appear, and clear, astrocytic processes surrounding the microvasculature and neurons become prominent. After several days, monocytes emigrate from the blood

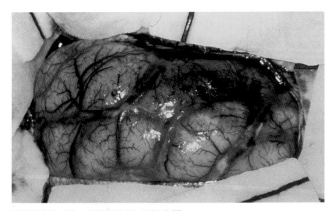

**FIGURE 7-33    CEREBRAL INFARCT**

The recent onset of headaches in a 32-year-old woman and the presence on imaging of an expansile mass with ring enhancement prompted surgery for what was presumed to be a malignant glioma. At the time of craniotomy, the lesion was a soft expansile infarct related to venous thrombi. The latter are seen at the lower portion of the illustration.

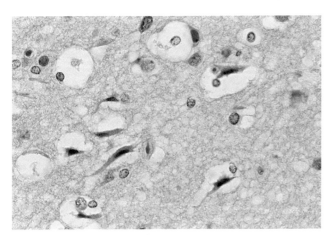

**FIGURE 7-34    CEREBRAL INFARCT**

Brightly eosinophilic cytoplasm and pale karyolytic nuclei are the principal features of red neurons, the pathognomonic feature of recent neuronal death. Few, if any, macrophages are present at this early stage of infarction.

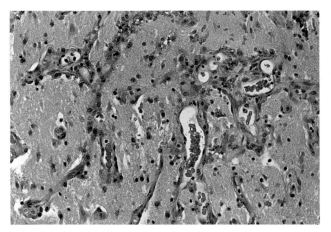

**FIGURE 7–35**   CEREBRAL INFARCT

Hypertrophy and, to a lesser extent, hyperplasia of microvascular cells in a recent infarct should not be misconstrued as the vascular proliferation of a glioma. Note the red neurons.

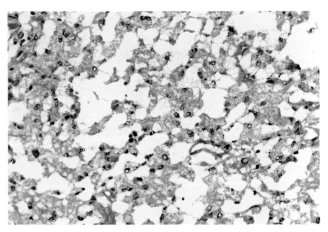

**FIGURE 7–37**   CEREBRAL INFARCT

The specific histologic features of macrophages can be obscured in frozen sections. As a result, the lesion can be misinterpreted as a glioma.

stream to assume their long-awaited destiny as foamy macrophages or "gitter cells." Over subsequent days or weeks, these full-bodied scavengers come to predominate as they gorge themselves on necrotic cell debris (Fig. 7–36). The resultant hypercellularity and vascular prominence can, in concert, create the histologic appearance of a glioma.

Having cleared a cavity, or "cyst," traversed by a web-like network of residual blood vessels, most of the macrophages eventually return to the vessels and hence the blood stream. In contrast to the response in other organs, fibrosis plays little role in the resolution of a cerebral infarct. At this juncture, the lesion is still of in-

terest to neurologists but has lost its fascination for neurosurgeons.

**Features in Frozen Sections.** The hypercellular lesions can be misinterpreted as a neoplasm in light of the distortion inherent in the freezing process (Fig. 7–37). Nevertheless, the outlines of macrophages are usually discernible here, and even more so in an accompanying cytologic preparation.

**Cytologic Features.** The histiocytes are recognized with great assurance because of their discrete cell borders, granular contents, and round bland nuclei (Fig. 7–38).

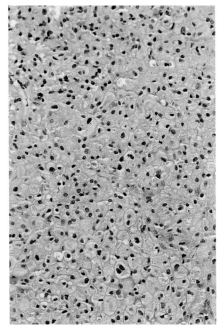

**FIGURE 7–36**   CEREBRAL INFARCT

The cellularity of a macrophage-rich infarct can prompt consideration of a glioma. The distinct cell borders and bland nuclei are, however, features of macrophages, not of malignant glia.

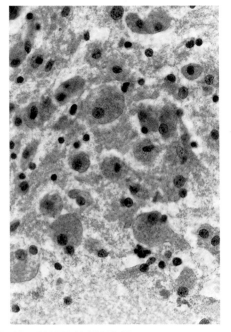

**FIGURE 7–38**   CEREBRAL INFARCT

Cytologic preparations are ideally suited to identify the specific features of macrophages, that is, discrete cell borders, granular cytoplasm, and "benign" nuclei.

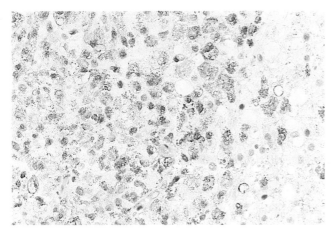

**FIGURE 7–39**   CEREBRAL INFARCT

Macrophages are readily identified by their immunoreactivity with such antibodies as KP-1, lysozyme, or, as in this case, HAM-56.

**Immunohistochemical Features.** Immunohistochemical studies are strongly recommended when a tissue sample has even the slightest suggestion of a macrophage infiltrate. Macrophage markers such as HAM-56 or CD68 (KP-1 or PGM-1) are of particular utility (Fig. 7–39).

**Differential Diagnosis.** Rarely do the diagnosis and therapy of cerebral infarcts intentionally involve surgery, and the pathologist receives a lesion for which a neoplasm is the principal, or only, suspected entity. The pathologist must guard against uncritical confirmation of the clinical diagnosis, usually *malignant glioma*. Macrophages, the critical feature, are identified by their cytologic characteristics and their tendency to accumulate about vessels (see Table 4–6, page 188).

Determining the cause of an infarct is possible in some cases when *amyloid angiopathy*, or a clearly antecedent thrombosis, is found. *Venous thrombosis* is sometimes the cause. The etiology is not apparent in many cases from either clinical or angiographic analysis or microscopic study.

## SUBDURAL HEMATOMA

**Definition.** A hematoma in the potential space between the arachnoid and the dura.

**General Comments.** A subdural hematoma is formed when venous, or rarely arterial, blood dissects between the dura and the leptomeninges. Although the hematoma occupies the "subdural space," there is normally no such anatomic compartment. The latter is only a potential space; the arachnoid and dura are conjoined, albeit tenuously, by intercellular junctions.[10, 17]

Subdural hematomas occur most frequently over and between the convexities of the cerebral hemispheres (Fig. 7–40).[4, 6] The posterior fossa is less often involved.[5, 23] Traditionally, subdural hematomas have been classified as acute, subacute, or chronic on the

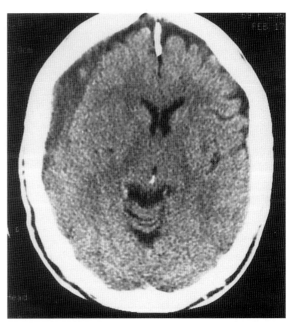

**FIGURE 7–40**   SUBDURAL HEMATOMA

A computed tomographic scan discloses the mass effect of a subdural hematoma. Its chronicity is apparent in the isodensity to the brain. Acute hemorrhages are white. (Courtesy of Dr. Martin G. Pomper, Baltimore, MD.)

basis of the interval between the traumatic episode and the onset of neurologic symptoms.

Most chronic lesions that generate surgical specimens are attributed to tearing of "bridging" veins that pass from the cortical surface to the superior sagittal sinus.[21] Other potential sources of hemorrhage, particularly in acute lesions, include torn anomalous arteries that pass between the dura and the arachnoid, ruptured parenchymal vessels at the sites of cortical lacerations, and arachnoidal arteries and veins avulsed in a meningeal tear.

It is assumed that the rupture of vessels responsible for a subdural hematoma results from a shearing force whose magnitude varies from case to case. Whereas a major traumatic incident is well documented for some patients with an acute lesion, a history of trauma may be difficult or impossible to elicit from some patients with chronic hematomas. The ability of the cerebral veins to withstand even minor trauma is compromised by anticoagulant therapy,[23] thrombocytopenia,[2] carcinoma metastatic to the dura,[2] long-term hemodialysis,[13] cerebral atrophy, and shunting procedures that acutely reduce the size of the cerebrum. Both atrophy and shunting exert traction upon the superior cortical veins and compromise their capacity to elongate or resist shearing forces.

**Clinical Features.** Patients with acute subdural hematomas usually have a history of major cranial trauma within 2 to 3 days before the onset of clinical signs and symptoms of increased intracranial pressure. Immediate surgical evacuation is the treatment of choice. If not removed, the lesion enters the chronic phase 2 to 3 weeks thereafter. Mental changes or focal

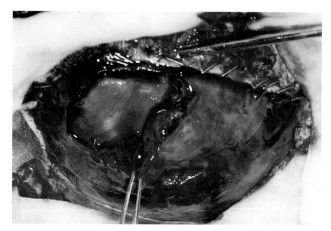

**FIGURE 7–41    SUBDURAL HEMATOMA**

Surgical retraction of the hematoma exposes the thin inner membrane that directly overlies the arachnoid.

neurologic deficits may become apparent; this is particularly true in the elderly. In many instances, the apparent absence of increased intracranial pressure belies the presence of an expanding intracranial mass.[4, 6]

**Macroscopic and Microscopic Features.** Persistence of blood in the subdural space incites a tissue reaction that organizes and resorbs the hematoma. In the process, "membranes" are formed. Although simple drainage, rather than membrane removal, is generally accepted treatment,[14] the membranes may be submitted for pathologic examination (Figs. 7–41 and 7–42).[7, 8] Currently, many patients are treated without surgery.

Most of the organization and resorptive activity in a persistent hematoma take place on its outer or dural aspect, where proliferating fibroblasts and capillaries permeate the clot to a uniform depth of several millimeters. Given its surprisingly abrupt interface with the remaining hematoma, this lamina of granulation tissue is termed the outer membrane (Fig. 7–43). The development of this layer proceeds at a relatively predictable rate, thus being useful for dating the hematoma.[7, 8] Interestingly, one study has suggested that the collagen-producing cells are not fibroblastic[16] but rather reactive meningeal cells ("dural border cells") that normally populate the dural-arachnoid interface.[7, 8, 22] Some of the

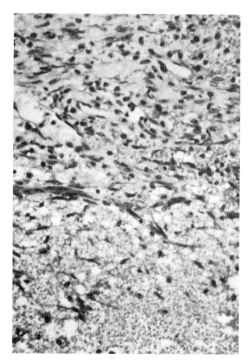

**FIGURE 7–43    SUBDURAL HEMATOMA**

The outer membrane consists of granulation tissue formed of fibroblasts and capillaries that have migrated and grown into the hematoma.

spindle cells appear to be myofibroblasts.[11] Small aggregates of small dark erythropoietic cells may also be encountered within the granulation tissue of the outer membrane (Fig. 7–44).[18] Truly surprising are the large numbers of eosinophils, with resultant Charcot-Leyden crystals, that converge on some hematomas (Fig. 7–45).[9]

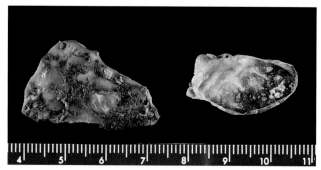

**FIGURE 7–42    SUBDURAL HEMATOMA**

The thick rubbery outer membrane (left) contrasts with the delicate transparent inner membrane (right).

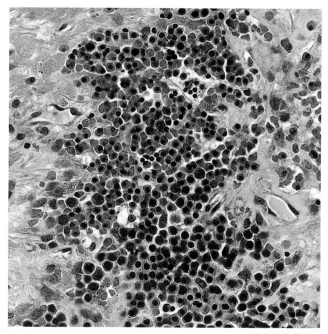

**FIGURE 7–44    SUBDURAL HEMATOMA**

Foci of extramedullary hematopoiesis are not uncommon in the outer membrane of chronic subdural hematomas.

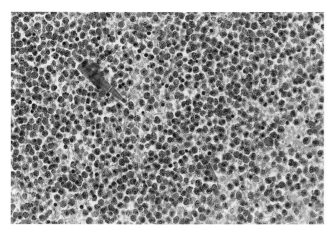

**FIGURE 7–45    SUBDURAL HEMATOMA**

On occasion, large numbers of eosinophils congregate in chronic subdural hematomas. Note the Charcot-Leyden crystals.

Concurrent with maturation of the outer membranes, a delicate layer of reactive tissue also develops on the inner or arachnoidal aspect. The origin of its constituent cells remains in doubt, but presumably they represent either dural fibroblasts or the dural border cells just described[22] that have migrated inward from the circumferential edge of the hematoma. In either case, the inner membrane is devoid of capillaries so conspicuous in the outer membrane (Fig. 7–46). The formation of the inner membrane is a tardy, less dynamic process; only after 10 days to 2 weeks does a fibrocollagenous sheet become visible to the naked eye. It then chronicles the hematoma as it thickens predictably with age, but it never achieves the opaque rubbery state of the outer membrane.[7, 8]

An important property of subdural hematomas is their capacity for expansion. It is this quality, rather than the size of the initial hemorrhage, that brings many chronic lesions to medical attention. Enlargement has been attributed either to osmotic absorption of fluid drawn from the cerebrospinal fluid compartment across the inner membrane or to rebleeding from the delicate capillaries of the outer membrane. The latter appears to be the more likely mechanism, given the finding of fresh hemorrhage adjacent to the outer membrane in many otherwise chronic subdural hematomas. Rebleeding has also been observed in experimental animals, although in this setting significant expansion of the lesion is debated.[3, 19] Some hematomas resolve completely, whereas others may undergo extensive calcification or even ossification.[1, 12, 15, 20]

# REFERENCES

**Vascular Malformations**

1. Abdulrauf SI, Kaynar MY, Awad IA. A comparison of the clinical profile of cavernous malformations with and without associated venous malformations. Neurosurgery 1999;44:41–46.
2. Acciarri N, Padovani R, Giulioni M, et al. Cerebral astrocytoma and cavernous angioma: a case report. Br J Neurosurg 1994;8:607–610.
3. Aiba T, Tanaka R, Koike T, et al. Natural history of intracranial cavernous malformations. J Neurosurg 1995;83:56–59.
4. Awad IA, Robinson JR Jr, Mohanty S, et al. Mixed vascular malformations of the brain: clinical and pathogenetic considerations. Neurosurgery 1993;33:179–188.
5. Barr RM, Dillon WP, Wilson CB. Slow-flow vascular malformations of the pons: capillary telangiectasias? AJNR 1996;17:71–78.
6. Blackwood W. Two cases of benign cerebral telangiectasis. J Pathol 1941;52:209–212.
7. Brown RD Jr, Wiebers DO, Forbes G, et al. The natural history of unruptured intracranial arteriovenous malformations. J Neurosurg 1988;68:352–357.
8. Brunori A, Chiappetta F. Cystic extra-axial cavernoma of the cerebellopontine angle. Surg Neurol 1996;46:475–476.
9. Cabanes J, Blasco R, Garcia M, et al. Cerebral venous angiomas. Surg Neurol 1979;11:385–389.
10. Casazza M, Broggi G, Franzini A, et al. Supratentorial cavernous angiomas and epileptic seizures: preoperative course and postoperative outcome. Neurosurgery 1996;39:26–34.
11. Chadduck WM, Binet EF, Farrell FW Jr. Intraventricular cavernous hemangioma: report of three cases and review of the literature. Neurosurgery 1985;16:189–197.
12. Challa VR, Moody DM, Brown WR. Vascular malformations of the central nervous system. J Neuropathol Exp Neurol 1995;54:609–621.
13. Chandra PS, Manjari T, Chandramouli BA, et al. Cavernous-venous malformation of brain stem—report of a case and review of literature. Surg Neurol 1999;52:280–285.
14. Curling OD Jr, Kelly DL Jr, Elster AD, et al. An analysis of the natural history of cavernous angiomas. J Neurosurg 1991;75:702–708.
15. Cushing H, Bailey P. Tumors Arising from the Blood Vessels of the Brain: Angiomatous Malformations and Hemangioblastomas. Springfield, IL: Charles C Thomas, 1928.
16. Farrell DF, Forno LS. Symptomatic capillary telangiectasis of the brainstem without hemorrhage. Report of an unusual case. Neurology 1970;20:341–346.
17. Gaensler EH, Dillon WP, Edwards MS, et al. Radiation-induced telangiectasia in the brain simulates cryptic vascular malformations at MR imaging. Radiology 1994;193:629–636.
18. Germano IM, Davis RL, Wilson CB, et al. Histopathological follow-up study of 66 cerebral arteriovenous malformations after therapeutic embolization with polyvinyl alcohol. J Neurosurg 1992;76:607–614.
19. Gil-Nagel A, Dubovsky J, Wilcox KJ, et al. Familial cerebral cavernous angioma: a gene localized to a 15-cM interval on chromosome 7q. Ann Neurol 1996;39:807–810.
20. Giulioni M, Acciarri N, Padovani R, et al. Surgical management of cavernous angiomas in children. Surg Neurol 1994;42:194–199.

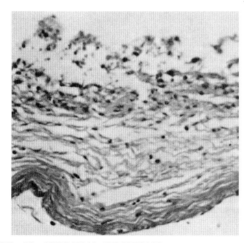

**FIGURE 7–46    SUBDURAL HEMATOMA**

The inner membrane of a subdural hematoma is a delicate, paucicellular lamina of loose fibrous tissue. In this illustration, the membrane underlies erythrocytes of the hematoma.

21. Gruber A, Mazal PR, Bavinzski G, et al. Repermeation of partially embolized cerebral arteriovenous malformations: a clinical, radiologic, and histologic study. AJNR 1996;17:1323–1331.

22. Günel M, Awad IA, Finberg K, et al. Genetic heterogeneity of inherited cerebral cavernous malformation. Neurosurgery 1996; 38:1265–1271.

23. Hubschman O, Kasoff S, Doniger D. Cavernous haemangioma in the pineal region. Surg Neurol 1976;6:349–351.

24. Ishikawa S, Kuwabara S, Fukuma A, et al. Cavernous angioma of the cerebellum—case report. Neurol Med Chir (Tokyo) 1989;29:35–39.

25. Isoda K, Fukuda H, Takamura N, et al. Arteriovenous malformation of the brain—histological study and micrometric measurement of abnormal vessels. Acta Pathol Jpn 1981;31:883–893.

26. Jellinger K. Vascular malformations of the central nervous system: a morphological overview. Neurosurg Rev 1986;9:177–216.

27. Kaplan HA, Aronson SM, Browder EJ. Vascular malformations of the brain. J Neurosurg 1961;18:630–635.

28. Katayama Y, Tsubokawa T, Maeda T, et al. Surgical management of cavernous malformations of the third ventricle. J Neurosurg 1994;80:64–72.

29. Kattapong VJ, Hart BL, Davis LE. Familial cerebral cavernous angiomas: clinical and radiologic studies. Neurology 1995;45: 492–497.

30. Kondziolka D, Lunsford LD, Kestle JRW. The natural history of cerebral cavernous malformations. J Neurosurg 1995;83:820–824.

31. Lee C, Pennington MA, Kenney CM III. MR evaluation of developmental venous anomalies: medullary venous anatomy of venous angiomas. AJNR 1996;17:61–70.

32. Lee R, Becher MW, Benson ML, et al. Brain capillary telangiectasia: MR imaging appearance and clinicohistopathologic findings. Radiology 1997;205:797–805.

33. Lewis AI, Tew JM Jr, Payner TD, et al. Dural cavernous angiomas outside the middle cranial fossa: a report of two cases. Neurosurgery 1994;35:498–504.

34. Linskey ME, Sekhar LN. Cavernous sinus hemangiomas: a series, a review, and an hypothesis. Neurosurgery 1992;30:101–108.

35. Loesch DV, Gilman S, Del Dotto J, et al. Cavernous malformation of the mammillary bodies: neuropsychological implications. J Neurosurg 1995;83:354–358.

36. Lombardi D, Scheithauer BW, Piepgras D, et al. "Angioglioma" and the arteriovenous malformation–glioma association. J Neurosurg 1991;75:589–596.

37. Malik GM, Morgan JK, Boulos RS, et al. Venous angiomas: an underestimated cause of intracranial hemorrhage. Surg Neurol 1988;30:350–358.

38. Mandybur TI, Nazek M. Cerebral arteriovenous malformations. Arch Pathol Lab Med 1990;114:970–973.

39. Maraire JN, Awad IA. Intracranial cavernous malformations: lesion behavior and management strategies. Neurosurgery 1995;37: 591–605.

40. McCormick WF, Boulter TR. Vascular malformations ("angiomas") of the dura mater. J Neurosurg 1966;25:309–311.

41. McLaughlin MR, Kondziolka D, Flickinger JC, et al. The prospective natural history of cerebral venous malformations. Neurosurgery 1998;43:195–201.

42. Mironov A. Classification of spontaneous dural arteriovenous fistulas with regard to their pathogenesis. Acta Radiol 1995;36: 582–592.

43. Miyagi Y, Mannoji H, Akaboshi K, et al. Intraventricular cavernous malformation associated with medullary venous malformation. Neurosurgery 1993;32:461–464.

44. Moriarty JL, Wetzel M, Clatterbuck RE, et al. The natural history of cavernous malformations: a prospective study of 68 patients. Neurosurgery 1999;44:1166–1173.

45. Naff NJ, Wemmer J, Utkarsh J, et al. A longitudinal study of 53 patients with venous malformations: documentation of a benign natural history. Neurology [Suppl] 1996:S-369.

46. Nazek M, Mandybur TI, Kashiwagi S. Oligodendroglial proliferative abnormality associated with arteriovenous malformation: report of three cases with review of the literature. Neurosurgery 1988;23:781–785.

47. Ondra SL, Troupp H, George ED, et al. The natural history of symptomatic arteriovenous malformations of the brain: a 24-year follow-up assessment. J Neurosurg 1990;73:387–391.

48. Pozzati E, Acciarri N, Tognetti F, et al. Growth, subsequent bleeding, and de novo appearance of cerebral cavernous angiomas. Neurosurgery 1996;38:662–670.

49. Pozzati E, Giangaspero F, Marliani F, et al. Occult cerebrovascular malformations after irradiation. Neurosurgery 1996;39: 677–684.

50. Reyns N, Assaker R, Louis E, et al. Intraventricular cavernomas: three cases and review of the literature. Neurosurgery 1999;44: 648–655.

51. Rigamonti D, Hadley MN, Drayer BP, et al. Cerebral cavernous malformations. Incidence and familial occurrence. N Engl J Med 1988;319:343–347.

52. Rigamonti D, Johnson PC, Spetzler RF, et al. Cavernous malformations and capillary telangiectasia: a spectrum within a single pathological entity. Neurosurgery 1991;28:60–64.

53. Rigamonti D, Spetzler RF, Medina M, et al. Cerebral venous malformations. J Neurosurg 1990;73:560–564.

54. Robinson JR, Awad IA, Little JR. Natural history of the cavernous angioma. J Neurosurg 1991;75:709–714.

55. Robinson JR Jr, Awad IA, Magdinec M, et al. Factors predisposing to clinical disability in patients with cavernous malformations of the brain. Neurosurgery 1993;32:730–736.

56. Sathi S, Folkerth R, Madsen JR. Cavernous angioma of the posterior fossa dura mimicking a meningioma: case report and review of literature. Surg Neurol 1992;38:257–260.

57. Scott RM, Barnes P, Kupsky W, et al. Cavernous angiomas of the central nervous system in children. J Neurosurg 1992;76:38–46.

58. Shi J, Hang C, Pan Y, et al. Cavernous hemangiomas in the cavernous sinus. Neurosurgery 1999;45:1308–1314.

59. Simard JM, Garcia-Bengochea F, Ballinger WE Jr, et al. Cavernous angioma: a review of 126 collected and 12 new clinical cases. Neurosurgery 1986;18:162–172.

60. Sinson G, Zager EL, Grossman RI, et al. Cavernous malformations of the third ventricle. Neurosurgery 1995;37:37–42.

61. Stahr SM, Johnson KP, Malamud N. The clinical and pathological spectrum of brain stem vascular malformations: long-term course simulates multiple sclerosis. Arch Neurol 1980;37:25–29.

62. Steinberg GK, Chang SD, Gewirtz RJ, et al. Microsurgical resection of brainstem, thalamic, and basal ganglia angiographically occult vascular malformations. Neurosurgery 2000;46:260–271.

63. Szeifert GT, Kemeny AA, Timperley WR, et al. The potential role of myofibroblasts in the obliteration of arteriovenous malformations after radiosurgery. Neurosurgery 1997;40:61–66.

64. Tomlinson FH, Houser OW, Scheithauer BW, et al. Angiographically occult vascular malformations: a correlative study of features on magnetic resonance imaging and histological examination. Neurosurgery 1994;34:792–800.

65. Versari PP, D'Aliberti G, Talamonti G, et al. Progressive myelopathy caused by intracranial dural arteriovenous fistula: report of two cases and review of the literature. Neurosurgery 1993;33: 914–919.

66. Vogler R, Castillo M. Dural cavernous angioma: MR features. AJNR 1995;16:773–775.

67. Vrethem M, Thuomas K-A, Hillman J. Cavernous angioma of the brain stem mimicking multiple sclerosis (Letter). N Engl J Med 1997;336:875–876.

68. Willinsky RA, Lasjaunias P, Terbrugge K, et al. Multiple cerebral arteriovenous malformations (AVMs); review of our experience from 203 patients with cerebral vascular lesions. Neuroradiology 1990;32:207–210.

69. Wilms G, Bleus E, Demaerel P, et al. Simultaneous occurrence of developmental venous anomalies and cavernous angiomas. AJNR 1994;15:1247–1254.

70. Wilson CB. Cryptic vascular malformations. Clin Neurosurg 1992;38:49–84.

71. Zabramski JM, Wascher TM, Spetzler RF, et al. The natural history of familial cavernous malformations: results of an ongoing study. J Neurosurg 1994;80:422–432.

72. Zhang J CR, Rigamonti D, Dietz HC. Mutations in *KRIT1* in familial cerebral cavernous malformations. Neurosurgery 2000;46: 1272–1279.

### Vascular Malformations in Dysgenetic Syndromes

1. Aesch B, Lioret E, de Toffol B, et al. Multiple cerebral angiomas and Rendu-Osler-Weber disease: case report. Neurosurgery 1991;29:599–602.

2. Bebin EM, Gomez MR. Prognosis in Sturge-Weber disease: comparison of unihemispheric and bihemispheric involvement. J Child Neurol 1988;3:181–184.
3. Benedikt RA, Brown DC, Walker R, et al. Sturge-Weber syndrome: cranial MR imaging with Gd-DTPA. AJNR 1993;14: 409–415.
4. Chamberlain MC, Press GA, Hesselink JR. MR imaging and CT in three cases of Sturge-Weber syndrome: prospective comparison. AJNR 1989;10:491–496.
5. Elster AD, Chen MY. MR imaging of Sturge-Weber syndrome: role of gadopentetate dimeglumine and gradient-echo techniques. AJNR 1990;11:685–689.
6. Griffiths PD, Blaser S, Boodram MB, et al. Choroid plexus size in young children with Sturge-Weber syndrome. AJNR 1996;17:175–180.
7. Griffiths PD, Boodram MB, Blaser S, et al. Abnormal ocular enhancement in Sturge-Weber syndrome: correlation of ocular MR and CT findings with clinical and intracranial imaging findings. AJNR 1996;17:749–754.
8. Ito M, Sato K, Ohnuki A, et al. Sturge-Weber disease: operative indications and surgical results. Brain Dev 1990;12:473–477.
9. Kadoya C, Momota Y, Ikegami Y, et al. Central nervous system arteriovenous malformations with hereditary hemorrhagic telangiectasia: report of a family with three cases. Surg Neurol 1994;42:234–239.
10. Kikuchi K, Kowada M, Sasajima H. Vascular malformations of the brain in hereditary hemorrhagic telangiectasia (Rendu-Osler-Weber disease). Surg Neurol 1994;41:374–380.
11. Ogunmekan AO, Hwang PA, Hoffman HJ. Sturge-Weber-Dimitri disease: role of hemispherectomy in prognosis. Can J Neurol Sci 1989;16:78–80.
12. Patel U, Gupta SC. Wyburn-Mason syndrome. A case report and review of the literature. Neuroradiology 1990;31:544–546.
13. Peterman AF, Hayles AB, Dockerty MB, et al. Encephalotrigeminal angiomatosis (Sturge-Weber disease). JAMA 1958;167:2169–2176.
14. Putman CM, Chaloupka JC, Fulbright RK, et al. Exceptional multiplicity of cerebral arteriovenous malformations associated with hereditary telangiectasis (Osler-Weber-Rendu Syndrome). AJNR 1996;17:1733–1742.
15. Smirniotopoulos JG, Murphy FM. The phakomatoses. AJNR 1992;13:725–746.
16. Sobel D, Norman D. CNS manifestations of hereditary hemorrhagic telangiectasia. AJNR 1984;5:569–573.
17. Théron J, Newton TH, Hoyt WF. Unilateral retinocephalic vascular malformations. Neuroradiology 1974;7:185–196.
18. Vogl TJ, Stemmler J, Bergman C, et al. MR and MR angiography of Sturge-Weber syndrome. AJNR 1993;14:417–425.
19. Wasenko JJ, Rosenbloom SA, Duchesneau PM, et al. The Sturge-Weber syndrome: comparison of MR and CT characteristics. AJNR 1990;11:131–134.
20. Wyburn-Mason R. Arteriovenous aneurysm of mid-brain and retina, facial nevi and mental changes. Brain 1943;66:163–203.
21. Yeakley JW, Woodside M, Fenstermacher MJ. Bilateral neonatal Sturge-Weber-Dimitri disease: CT and MR findings. AJNR 1992;13:1179–1182.

## Temporal ("Giant Cell") Arteritis

1. Allison MC, Gallagher PJ. Temporal artery biopsy and corticosteroid treatment. Ann Rheum Dis 1984;43:416–417.
2. Allsop CJ, Gallagher PJ. Temporal artery biopsy in giant cell arteritis: a reappraisal. Am J Surg Pathol 1981;5:317–323.
3. Baldursson Ö, Steinsson K, Björnsson J, et al. Giant cell arteritis in Iceland. An epidemiologic and histopathologic analysis. Arthritis Rheum 1994;37:1007–1012.
4. Bevan AT, Dunnill MS, Harrison MJG. Clinical and biopsy findings in temporal arteritis. Ann Rheum Dis 1968;27:271–277.
5. Brownstein S, Nicolle DA, Codere F. Bilateral blindness in temporal arteritis with skip areas. Arch Ophthalmol 1983;101:388–391.
6. Crompton MR. The visual changes in temporal (giant-cell) arteritis: report of a case with autopsy findings. Brain 1959;82:377–390.
7. Fauchald P, Rygvold O, Oystese B. Temporal arteritis and polymyalgia rheumatica. Clinical and biopsy findings. Ann Intern Med 1972;77:845–852.
8. Gibb WR, Urry PA, Lees AJ. Giant cell arteritis with spinal cord infarction and basilar artery thrombosis. J Neurol Neurosurg Psychiatry 1985;48:945–948.
9. Hall S, Hunder GG. Is temporal artery biopsy prudent? Mayo Clin Proc 1984;59:793–796.
10. Huston KA, Hunder GG, Lie JT, et al. Temporal arteritis: a 25-year epidemiologic, clinical, and pathologic study. Ann Intern Med 1968;88:162–167.
11. Kinmont PDC, McCallum DI. The aetiology, pathology and course of giant-cell arteritis: the possible role of light sensitivity. Br J Dermatol 1964;77:193–202.
12. Klein RG, Campbell RJ, Hunder GG, et al. Skip lesions in temporal arteritis. Mayo Clin Proc 1976;51:504–510.
13. Lie JT. The classification and diagnosis of vasculitis in large and medium-sized blood vessels. Pathol Annu 1987;22:125–162.
14. Lie JT. Illustrated histopathologic classification criteria for selected vasculitis syndromes. American College of Rheumatology Subcommittee on Classification of Vasculitis. Arthritis Rheum 1990;33:1074–1087.
15. Mambo NC. Temporal (granulomatous) arteritis: a histopathological study of 32 cases. Histopathology 1979;3:209–221.
16. McDonnell PJ, Moore GW, Miller NR, et al. Temporal arteritis. A clinicopathologic study. Ophthalmology 1986;93:518–530.
17. Nordborg E, Bengtsson BA. Death rates and causes of death in 284 consecutive patients with giant cell arteritis confirmed by biopsy. BMJ 1989;299:549–550.
18. O'Brien JP. A concept of diffuse actinic arteritis. The role of actinic damage to elastin in 'age change' and arteritis of the temporal artery and in polymyalgia rheumatica. Br J Dermatol 1978;98:1–13.
19. Parker R, Healey LA, Wilske KR, et al. Light and electron microscopic studies of human temporal arteries with special reference to alterations related to senescence, atherosclerosis, and giant cell arteritis. Am J Pathol 1975;79:57–80.
20. Russell RWF. Giant-cell arteritis: a review of 35 cases. Q J Med 1959;28:471–489.
21. Schmidt WA, Kraft HE, Vorpahl K, et al. Color duplex ultrasonography in the diagnosis of temporal arteritis. N Engl J Med 1997;337:1336–1342.
22. Shiiki H, Shimokama T, Watanabe T. Temporal arteritis: cell composition and the possible pathogenetic role of cell-mediated immunity. Hum Pathol 1989;20:1057–1064.
23. Smith KR Jr. Electron microscopy of giant cell (temporal) arteritis. J Neurol Neurosurg Psychiatry 1969;32:348–353.
24. Turnbull J. Temporal arteritis and polymyalgia rheumatica: nosographic and nosologic considerations. Neurology 1996;46:901–906.
25. Weyand CM, Tetzlaff N, Björnsson J, et al. Disease patterns and tissue cytokine profiles in giant cell arteritis. Arthritis Rheum 1997;40:19–26.
26. Wilkinson IMS, Russell RWR. Arteries of the head and neck in giant cell arteritis: a pathological study to show the pattern of arterial involvement. Arch Neurol 1972;27:378–391.
27. Wilson JW, Topolosky MK, Hettleman BD, et al. Giant cell arteritis in a black patient. South Med J 1979;72:1221–1222.

## Granulomatous Angiitis

1. Anders KH, Wang ZZ, Kornfeld M, et al. Giant cell arteritis in association with cerebral amyloid angiopathy: immunohistochemical and molecular studies. Hum Pathol 1997;28:1237–1246.
2. Burger PC, Burch JG, Vogel FS. Granulomatous angiitis. An unusual etiology of stroke. Stroke 1977;8:29–35.
3. Chu CT, Gray L, Goldstein LB, et al. Diagnosis of intracranial vasculitis: a multi-disciplinary approach. J Neuropathol Exp Neurol 1998;57:30–38.
4. Clifford-Jones RE, Love S, Gurusinghe N. Granulomatous angiitis of the central nervous system: a case with recurrent intracerebral hemorrhage. J Neurol Neurosurg Psychiatry 1985;48:1054–1056.
5. Cupps TR, Moore PM, Fauci AS. Isolated angiitis of the central nervous system. Prospective diagnostic and therapeutic experience. Am J Med 1983;74:97–105.
6. Fountain NB, Eberhard DA. Primary angiitis of the central nervous system associated with cerebral amyloid angiopathy: report of two cases and review of the literature. Neurology 1996;46: 190–197.

7. Greenan TJ, Grossman RI, Goldberg HI. Cerebral vasculitis: MR imaging and angiographic correlation. Radiology 1992;182:65–72.
8. Inwards DJ, Piepgras DG, Lie JT, et al. Granulomatous angiitis of the spinal cord associated with Hodgkin's disease. Cancer 1991;68:1318–1322.
9. Jellinger K. Giant cell granulomatous angiitis of the central nervous system. J Neurol 1977;215:175–190.
10. Kolodny EH, Rebeiz JJ, Caviness VS Jr, et al. Granulomatous angiitis of the central nervous system. Arch Neurol 1968;19:510–524.
11. Lie JT. Primary (granulomatous) angiitis of the central nervous system: a clinicopathologic analysis of 15 new cases and a review of the literature. Hum Pathol 1992;23:164–171.
12. Moore PM. Diagnosis and management of isolated angiitis of the central nervous system. Neurology 1989;39:167–173.
13. Nurick S, Blackwood W, Mair WG. Giant cell granulomatous angiitis of the central nervous system. Brain 1972;95:133–142.
14. Probst A, Ulrich J. Amyloid angiopathy combined with granulomatous angiitis of the central nervous system: report on two patients. Clin Neuropathol 1985;4:250–259.
15. Rajjoub RK, Wood JH, Ommaya AK. Granulomatous angiitis of the brain: a successfully treated case. Neurology 1977;27:588–591.
16. Rawlinson DG, Braun CW. Granulomatous angiitis of the nervous system first seen as relapsing myelopathy. Arch Neurol 1981;38:129–131.
17. Rhodes RH, Madelaire NC, Petrelli M, et al. Primary angiitis and angiopathy of the central nervous system and their relationship to systemic giant cell arteritis. Arch Pathol Lab Med 1995;119:334–349.
18. Shoemaker EI, Lin ZS, Rae-Grant AD, et al. Primary angiitis of the central nervous system: unusual MR appearance. AJNR 1994;15:331–334.
19. Vollmer TL, Guarnaccia J, Harrington W, et al. Idiopathic granulomatous angiitis of the central nervous system. Diagnostic challenges. Arch Neurol 1993;50:925–930.
20. Yoong MF, Blumbergs PC, North JB. Primary (granulomatous) angiitis of the central nervous system with multiple aneurysms of spinal arteries. Case report. J Neurosurg 1993;79:603–607.
21. Younger DS, Hays AP, Brust JC, et al. Granulomatous angiitis of the brain. An inflammatory reaction of diverse etiology. Arch Neurol 1988;45:514–518.
22. Yuen RW, Johnson PC. Primary angiitis of the central nervous system associated with Hodgkin's disease. Arch Pathol Lab Med 1996;120:573–576.
23. Zimmerman RS, Young HF, Hadfield MG. Granulomatous angiitis of the nervous system: a case report of long-term survival. Surg Neurol 1990;33:206–212.

## Amyloid ("Congophilic") Angiopathy

1. Bogucki A, Papierz W, Szymanska R, et al. Cerebral amyloid angiopathy with attenuation of the white matter on CT scans: subcortical arteriosclerotic encephalopathy (Binswanger) in a normotensive patient. J Neurol 1988;235:435–437.
2. Cosgrove GR, Leblanc R, Meagher-Villemure K, et al. Cerebral amyloid angiopathy. Neurology 1985;35:625–631.
3. Fountain NB, Eberhard DA. Primary angiitis of the central nervous system associated with cerebral amyloid angiopathy: report of two cases and review of the literature. Neurology 1996;46:190–197.
4. Gilles C, Brucher JM, Khoubesserian P, et al. Cerebral amyloid angiopathy as a cause of multiple intracerebral hemorrhages. Neurology 1984;34:730–735.
5. Gray F, Dubas F, Rouller E, et al. Leukoencephalopathy in diffuse hemorrhagic cerebral amyloid angiopathy. Ann Neurol 1985;18:54–59.
6. Gray F, Vinters HV, LeNoan H, et al. Cerebral amyloid angiopathy and granulomatous angiitis: immunohistochemical study using antibodies of the Alzheimer A4 peptide. Hum Pathol 1990;21:1290–1293.
7. Greenberg SM, Rebeck GW, Vonsattel JPG, et al. Apolipoprotein E ε4 and cerebral hemorrhage associated with amyloid angiopathy. Ann Neurol 1995;38:254–259.
8. Greenberg SM, Vonsattel JP, Stakes JW, et al. The clinical spectrum of cerebral amyloid angiopathy: presentations without lobar hemorrhage. Neurology 1993;43:2073–2079.
9. Ishii N, Nishihara Y, Horie A. Amyloid angiopathy and lobar cerebral hemorrhage. J Neurol Neurosurg Psychiatry 1984;47:1203–1210.
10. Jellinger K. Cerebrovascular amyloidosis with cerebral hemorrhage. J Neurol 1977;214:195–206.
11. Kalyan-Raman UP, Kalyan-Raman K. Cerebral amyloid angiopathy causing intracranial hemorrhage. Ann Neurol 1984;16:321–329.
12. Leblanc R, Preul M, Robitaille Y, et al. Surgical considerations in cerebral amyloid angiopathy. Neurosurgery 1991;29:712–718.
13. Loes DJ, Biller J, Yuh WTC, et al. Leukoencephalopathy in cerebral amyloid angiopathy: MR imaging in four cases. AJNR 1990;11:485–488.
14. Mandybur TI. Cerebral amyloid angiopathy: the vascular pathology and complications. J Neuropathol Exp Neurol 1986;45:79–90.
15. Maury CPJ. Biology of disease. Molecular pathogenesis of β-amyloidosis in Alzheimer's disease and other cerebral amyloidoses. Lab Invest 1995;72:4–16.
16. McCarron MO, Nicoll JAR, Stewart J, et al. The apolipoprotein E ε2 allele and the pathological features in cerebral amyloid angiopathy-related hemorrhage. J Neuropathol Exp Neurol 1999;58:711–718.
17. Neumann MA. Combined amyloid vascular changes and argyrophilic plaques in the central nervous system. J Neuropathol Exp Neurol 1960;19:370–382.
18. Okazaki H, Reagan TJ, Campbell RJ. Clinicopathologic studies of primary cerebral amyloid angiopathy. Mayo Clin Proc 1979;54:22–31.
19. Osumi AK, Tien RD, Felsberg GJ, et al. Cerebral amyloid angiopathy presenting as a brain mass. AJNR 1995;16(4 Suppl):911–915.
20. Powers JM, Stein BM, Torres RAA. Sporadic cerebral amyloid angiopathy with giant cell reaction. Acta Neuropathol (Berl) 1990;81:95–98.
21. Roosen N, Martin J-J, de la Porte C, et al. Intracerebral hemorrhage due to cerebral amyloid angiopathy. Case report. J Neurosurg 1985;63:965–969.
22. Scully RE (ed). Case records of the Massachusetts General Hospital: case 22-1996. N Engl J Med 1996;335:189–196.
23. Tomonaga M. Cerebral amyloid angiopathy in the elderly. J Am Geriatr Soc 1981;29:151–157.
24. Vinters HV. Cerebral amyloid angiopathy. A critical review. Stroke 1987;18:311–324.
25. Vinters HV, Gilbert JJ. Cerebral amyloid angiopathy: incidence and complications in the aging brain: II. The distribution of amyloid vascular changes. Stroke 1983;14:924–928.
26. Wagle WA, Smith TW, Weiner M. Intracerebral hemorrhage caused by cerebral amyloid angiopathy: radiographic-pathologic correlation. AJNR 1984;5:171–176.

## Cerebral Infarct

1. Chuaqui R, Tapia J. Histologic assessment of the age of recent brain infarcts in man. J Neuropathol Exp Neurol 1993;52:481–489.
2. Wardlaw JM, Sellar R. A simple practical classification of cerebral infarcts on CT and its interobserver reliability. AJNR 1994;15:1933–1939.

## Subdural Hematoma

1. Afra D. Ossification of subdural hematoma: report of two cases. J Neurosurg 1961;18:393–397.
2. Ambiavagar PC, Sher J. Subdural hematoma secondary to metastatic neoplasm: report of two cases and a review of the literature. Cancer 1978;42:2015–2018.
3. Apfelbaum RI, Guthkelch AN, Shulman K. Experimental production of subdural hematomas. J Neurosurg 1974;40:336–346.
4. Cameron MM. Chronic subdural hematoma: a review of 114 cases. J Neurol Neurosurg Psychiatry 1978;41:834–839.
5. Ciembroniewicz JE. Subdural hematoma of the posterior fossa: review of the literature with addition of three cases. J Neurosurg 1965;22:465–473.
6. De Jesus PV Jr, Poser CM. Subdural hematomas: a clinicopathologic study of 100 cases. Postgrad Med 1968;44:172–177.
7. Friede RL. Incidence and distribution of neomembranes of dura mater. J Neurol Neurosurg Psychiatry 1971;34:439–446.

8. Friede RL, Schachenmayr W. The origin of subdural neomembranes: II. Fine structure of neomembranes. Am J Pathol 1978;92:69–84.
9. Golden J, Frim DM, Chapman PH, et al. Marked tissue eosinophilia within organizing chronic subdural hematoma membranes. Clin Neuropathol 1994;13:12–16.
10. Haines DE, Harkey I, Al-Mefty O. The "subdural" space: a new look at an outdated concept. Neurosurgery 1993;32:111–120.
11. Kulali A, Erel C, Ozyilmaz F, et al. Giant calcified subdural empyemas. Surg Neurol 1994;42:442–447.
12. Leonard A, Shapiro FL. Subdural hematoma in regularly hemodialyzed patients. Ann Intern Med 1975;82:650–658.
13. Markwalder T-M, Reulen J-J. Influence of neomembranous organisation, cortical expansion and subdural pressure on the postoperative course of chronic subdural hematoma—an analysis of 201 cases. Acta Neurochir 1986;79:100–106.
14. Niwa J, Nakamura T, Fujishige M, Hashi K, et al. Removal of a large asymptomatic calcified chronic subdural hematoma. Surg Neurol 1988;30:135–139.
15. Sambasivan M. An overview of chronic subdural hematoma: experience with 2300 cases. Surg Neurol 1997;47:418–422.
16. Sato S, Suzuki J. Ultrastructural observation of the capsule of chronic subdural hematoma in various clinical stages. J Neurosurg 1975;43:569–578.
17. Schachenmayr W, Friede RL. The origin of subdural neomembranes. I. Fine structure of the dura-arachnoid interface in man. Am J Pathol 1978;92:53–68.
18. Slater JP. Extramedullary hematopoiesis in a subdural hematoma: case report. J Neurosurg 1966;25:211–214.
19. Watanabe S, Shimade H, Ishii S. Production of clinical forms of chronic subdural hematoma in experimental animals. J Neurosurg 1972;37:552–561.
20. Watts C. The management of intracranial calcified subdural hematomas. Surg Neurol 1976;6:247–250.
21. Yamashima T, Friede RL. Why do bridging veins rupture into the virtual subdural space? J Neurol Neurosurg Psychiatry 1984;47:121–127.
22. Yamashima T, Yamamoto S. The origin of inner membranes in chronic subdural hematomas. Acta Neuropathol 1985;67:219–225.
23. Zenteno-Alanis GH, Covera J, Mateos JH. Subdural hematomas of the posterior fossa as a complication of anticoagulant therapy: presentation of a case. Neurology 1968;18:1133–1136.

# THE BRAIN: BIOPSY FOR DEMENTIA

**8**

In some measure, dementia tarnishes the minds of the aged but, like atherosclerosis, is often accepted as a natural consequence of advancing age. However, when dementia appears during the younger decades as an unseemly and alien occurrence, its causation may be sought, by biopsy of the brain, among the entities discussed in this chapter.

## CREUTZFELDT-JAKOB DISEASE

**General Comments.** The concatenation of events leading to our present understanding of Creutzfeldt-Jakob disease (CJD) had an unlikely beginning in the mountainous terrain of New Guinea with the scientific recognition of a related disorder, termed kuru.[14] A seminal observation was the appreciation of the correspondence between the pathologic findings in the patients with kuru and those of scrapie, a partially characterized "slow virus" infection in sheep.[17] Following this lead, the intracerebral inoculation of cerebral tissue from patients with kuru into chimpanzees produced a tissue reaction similar to that of the parent disease.[3, 4, 13] Morphologic similarities then linked human and experimental kuru to CJD and prompted the inoculation of brain tissue from patients with CJD into chimpanzees as well as other laboratory animals.[15, 16, 18, 35] The resultant spongiform

encephalopathy established the transmissibility of CJD. The similarity of natural scrapie to the encephalopathy produced in laboratory animals by the inoculation of brain tissue from patients with CJD clearly indicated a relationship between these two conditions.[18, 28, 29] Contrary to early presumptions, CJD, although transmissible, is not due to a virus. The term prion was coined to denote this heretofore unrecognized class of disease-transmitting proteins.[28, 29] Since then, there has been rapid progress in the characterization of the interactions between the abnormal prion protein and the host that produce the phenotypic variations in the human disease.[26, 27, 30, 31]

**Clinical Features.** CJD is a rapidly progressive, dementing disease with a tempo notably faster than that of Alzheimer's disease. This tempo, in concert with myoclonus and distinctive electroencephalographic changes, produces a clinical picture that, although not specific, is highly characteristic. In appropriate clinical settings, where other conditions can be excluded, the detection of elevated "14-3-3 protein" and neuron-specific enolase levels in cerebrospinal fluid may obviate the need for a brain biopsy.[1, 2, 19, 32] Radiologic features, described in the following section, may also be useful in establishing the diagnosis without resort to brain biopsy.

The symptoms of CJD vary from patient to patient. In some, extrapyramidal signs predominate as an expression of basal ganglia involvement, whereas visual impairment reflects occipital lobe disease in patients with the Heidenhain variant.[21] Most cases are sporadic; about 10% are familial.[20] Only rarely can transmission from dural grafts,[7, 22] corneal grafts,[12] or pooled human pituitary growth hormone[7, 8] be incriminated in the pathogenesis.

**Radiologic Features.** Diffusion-weighted or T2-weighted magnetic resonance imaging detects an increased (whiter) signal in affected cerebral cortex, thalamus, or basal ganglia (Fig. 8–1).[1, 11, 24, 33, 34] Diffuse cerebral hypometabolism has been noted with positron emission tomography.[25]

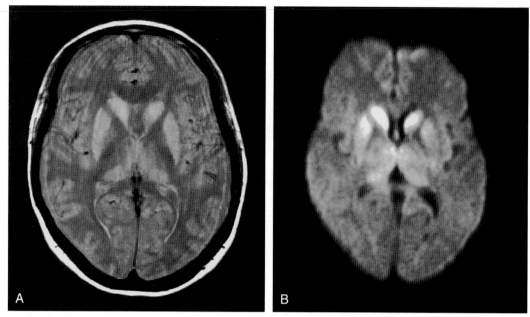

**FIGURE 8-1    CREUTZFELDT-JAKOB DISEASE**

Increased signal in the basal ganglia and thalamus in T2-weighted (*A*) and diffusion (*B*) images is typical of some cases of CJD. The patient was a 53-year-old woman with rapidly progressive dementia and ataxia. (Courtesy of Dr. Carlos Pardo, Baltimore, MD.)

**Macroscopic Features.** Although the brain of a patient with end-stage CJD may be atrophic, it is often macroscopically normal, even late in the course of the disease.

**Microscopic Features.** In its advanced form, the disease has a triad of features: spongiform change, neuronal loss, and gliosis.

Spongiform change, sometimes quite subtle, is usually the only abnormality in biopsy specimens of lesions, and its recognition is therefore essential to the histologic diagnosis (Figs. 8-2 and 8-3). Restricted to gray matter, it creates a moth-eaten appearance by its multitude of vacuoles, which are variable in size but mostly smaller than the diameter of a neuron. These are situated

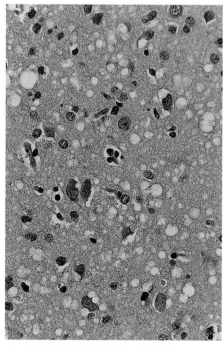

**FIGURE 8-2    CREUTZFELDT-JAKOB DISEASE**

Spongiform change may be subtle when it consists only of small circular vacuoles.

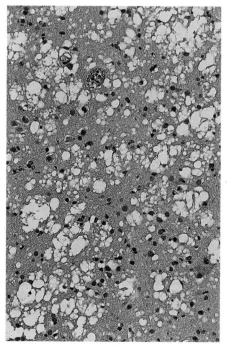

**FIGURE 8-3    CREUTZFELDT-JAKOB DISEASE**

Spongiform change is pronounced when larger and more irregular vacuoles create a moth-eaten appearance.

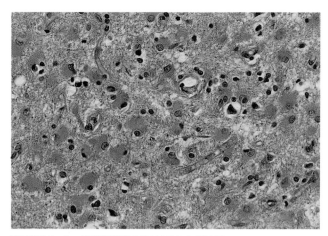

**FIGURE 8–4** CREUTZFELDT-JAKOB DISEASE

Severe neuronal depopulation and astrogliosis mark the late stage of Creutzfeldt-Jakob disease. In this field, only one shrunken neuron remains.

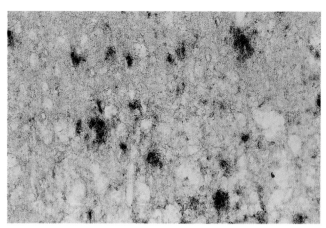

**FIGURE 8–5** CREUTZFELDT-JAKOB DISEASE

Immunohistochemistry for tau protein stains either in a diffuse or patchy manner, depending on the molecular subtype of the disease. Immunoreactivity is patchy in this case. (Courtesy of Dr. Pierluigi Gambetti, Cleveland, OH.)

principally in the neuropil, but a few reside in perikarya, where some indent the nuclei and produce a "signet ring" appearance. Generally, the size, distribution, and complexity of the vacuoles of CJD leave little doubt of their authenticity, but in some cases the changes, while suggestive, are not diagnostic. In such instances, tissue can be referred to a reference laboratory for the immunohistochemical detection of the prion protein, as discussed later. Frozen tissue can be used for Western blot analysis.

In the later stages of CJD, as usually seen only in autopsy specimens, neuronal dropout is diffuse. Residual neurons are often shrunken, distorted, and tinted with lipochrome (Fig. 8–4). Such neurons should be distinguished from the artifactually contracted, intensely pyknotic neurons often seen in biopsy specimens, particularly near the margins of excision (see Fig. 8–15). Gliosis is usually absent in biopsy specimens but can be extreme at autopsy (see Fig. 8–4).

**Immunohistochemical Features.** Immunopositivity for the prion protein may be focal and plaque-like or diffusely reactive (Fig. 8–5).[26]

**Ultrastructural Features.** The sponginess is created by vacuoles with membranous debris (Fig. 8–6).

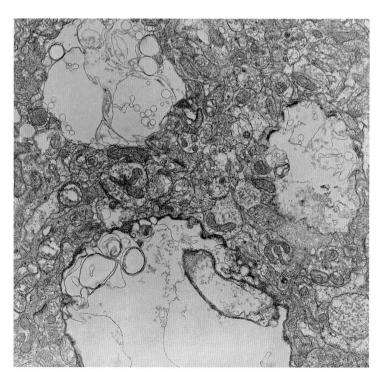

**FIGURE 8–6** CREUTZFELDT-JAKOB DISEASE

Ultrastructurally, the vacuoles of Creutzfeldt-Jakob disease contain cytoplasmic and membranous debris (×16,000).

**Precautions in Handling Tissue.** Although the chance of accidental acquisition without inoculation of tissue is very small, it cannot be dismissed, and specific guidelines have been proposed to isolate medical personnel from the "agent."[9] Devoid of nucleic acid, the latter is not an organism but an abnormally configured protein that affects and perpetuates a similar pathogenic configuration in its normal protein counterpart. Although the risk of acquiring the disease is very small, laboratory personnel are understandably distressed when they have unknowingly handled the tissue without precautions. The disease appears to be transmissible to nonhuman primates from formalin-fixed, paraffin-embedded material,[6, 8] and medical personnel have acquired the disease.[5] In any case of dementia, the likelihood of CJD should be discussed with the clinicians before proceeding with tissue preparation. Rapidly progressing dementia should alert medical personnel to the possibility of CJD.

A number of safety guidelines have been formulated. To prevent penetrating wounds, safety gloves are recommended when handling both fresh and fixed tissues. With regard to chemical decontamination of surgical specimens, it is recommended that initial fixation with formalin (24 hours) be followed by immersion in 100% formic acid for at least 1 hour. Thereafter, the specimen, is maintained in formalin until ready for processing. Instruments, gloves, and other items that have been in contact with tissue at any stage before formic acid treatment should be decontaminated by immersion in 2N sodium hydroxide (NaOH) for at least 1 hour.[9, 10] Plastic sheets conveniently serve as a working surface and can be incinerated with other discarded objects. Instruments can be decontaminated by immersion in 2N NaOH for 1 hour.

**Differential Diagnosis.** Care should be exercised when interpreting small vacuoles because they may be artifacts of fixation, for example, minute clearings about axons. Perivascular clearing is also a common autolytic change and not a component of spongiform change. The latter is not limited to perithelial regions.

Other degenerative diseases may on occasion involve spongiform change, notably some cases of *advanced Alzheimer's disease, dementia with Lewy bodies, frontotemporal dementias,* and *tauopathies.*[23]

**Treatment and Prognosis.** There is no specific treatment; most patients succumb within 6 months.

# ALZHEIMER'S DISEASE AND NEURODEGENERATIVE CHANGES OF THE ALZHEIMER TYPE

**General Comments.** Alzheimer's disease is primarily a disease of the aged, and diagnostic brain biopsies are usually reserved for younger patients, in whom dementia is statistically uncommon.[5]

**Clinical Features.** Alzheimer's disease begins with a loss of recent memory and later progresses to a loss of other cognitive domains and dissolution of personality.

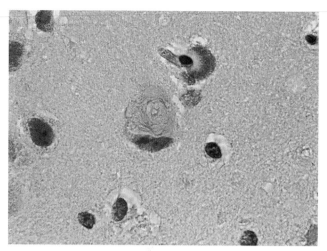

**FIGURE 8–7    ALZHEIMER'S DISEASE**

Slightly basophilic and finely fibrillar, the neurofibrillary tangle may be difficult to identify in H&E-stained sections.

**Radiologic Features.** Atrophy is minimal in the early cases that come to biopsy but typically becomes severe with the passage of time. Ventricles enlarge and hippocampi contract.

**Microscopic Features.** Two distinctive cortical alterations characterize Alzheimer's disease, namely neurofibrillary change and senile plaques. Other features are amyloid (congophilic) angiopathy and granulovacuolar degeneration. The latter is largely confined to neurons of the hippocampus and is not expected in biopsy specimens.

Neurofibrillary change is the deposition of cytoplasmic fibrillar material that usually requires special stains or immunohistochemistry for positive identification. In some cases, the alteration is apparent with the hematoxylin and eosin (H&E) stain alone, appearing as a subtle basophilic wisp, but even then is often difficult to distinguish from Nissl substance (Fig. 8–7). With silver stains the filamentous aggregates appear as tangles that cradle or envelop the nucleus and branch into neuritic processes (Fig. 8–8), assuming configurations that have been likened to flames, spirals, torches, loops, rings, triangle spools, strands, baskets, and even pretzels. Scattered argyrophilic neurites, "neuropil threads," are commonly seen in cases wherein neurofibrillary change is advanced.

Senile plaques are intriguing structures that predominate numerically over neurofibrillary tangles. Although there are transitional forms, plaques are envisioned as occurring as one of two types. The first, or neuritic plaque, is closely associated with dementia when present in large numbers. It is often detectable with H&E staining alone because it is more coarsely granular than normal cortical neuropil and often contains an eosinophilic amyloid core (Fig. 8–9). Trapped nuclei of microglia or reactive astrocytes add an element of cellularity to some plaques. With silver staining (e.g., Bielschowsky, Bodian, Holmes), the plaque is a fuzzy domain of argyrophilia that contains scattered densely argyrophilic neuronal processes (neurites). The amyloid

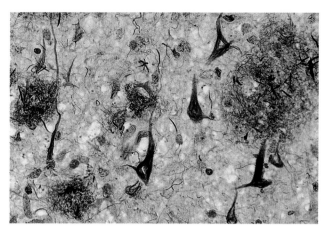

**FIGURE 8–8**   ALZHEIMER'S DISEASE

Neurofibrillary tangles, here accompanied by neuritic plaques, are well seen after silver staining.

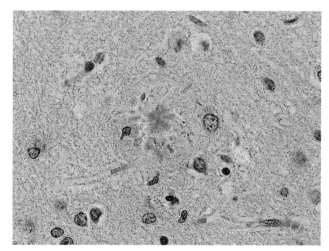

**FIGURE 8–9**   ALZHEIMER'S DISEASE

When their amyloid cores are prominent, neuritic plaques are readily visible in H&E-stained sections.

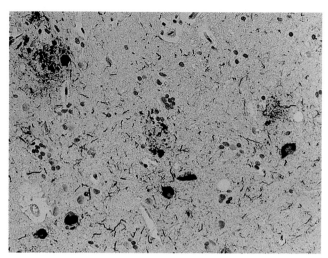

**FIGURE 8–10**   ALZHEIMER'S DISEASE

Neurofibrillary tangles and plaques are immunoreactive for phosphorylated tau protein.

lation between vascular amyloid deposition in the setting of Alzheimer's disease and the hemorrhage or infarct-associated disease amyloid angiopathy is discussed in Chapter 7 on pages 412–414.

Not infrequently, high-magnification microscopy, especially when abetted by immunohistochemistry for α-synuclein or ubiquitin, reveals small discrete intraneuronal inclusions and cortical Lewy bodies in addition to the Alzheimer's changes. These nosologically problematic mixed lesions are discussed on pages 430–431.

**Immunohistochemical Features.** Neurofibrillary tangles react with antibodies to phosphorylated tau protein (Fig. 8–10)[9, 17] and ubiquitin (Fig. 8–11).[3, 8] Neuropil threads are also tau positive. The senile plaque is a nearly circular area of positivity for Aβ amyloid. As is the case with neurofibrillary tangles, neuritic plaques can be demonstrated readily with antibodies to tau

core is evident on special histochemical stains such as periodic acid–Schiff (PAS) or thioflavin S or with immunostaining for Aβ amyloid.

The second type of plaque, the diffuse form, requires special procedures for detection, most commonly the silver stains noted before, or immunostaining for Aβ amyloid. These plaques appear as a cobweb of argyrophilia and are diffusely positive for Aβ amyloid but are devoid of an amyloid core. The "primitive" plaque is not as closely associated with dementia as is the neuritic form.

Granulovacuolar degeneration consists of multiple small intraneuronal vacuoles, each with its own central dense granule. It is infrequently present in neocortex, and its absence is of no diagnostic significance. Pyramidal cells of the hippocampal formation are principally affected.

Leptomeningeal and intracortical vessels often lose their substructure, become thickened and eosinophilic, and acquire both reactivity with antibodies to Aβ amyloid and affinity for Congo red and thioflavin S. The re-

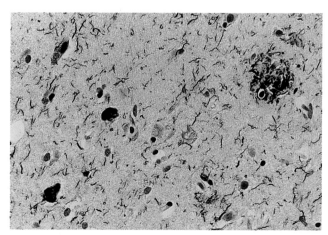

**FIGURE 8–11**   ALZHEIMER'S DISEASE

Both neurofibrillary tangles and neuritic plaques are immunoreactive for ubiquitin.

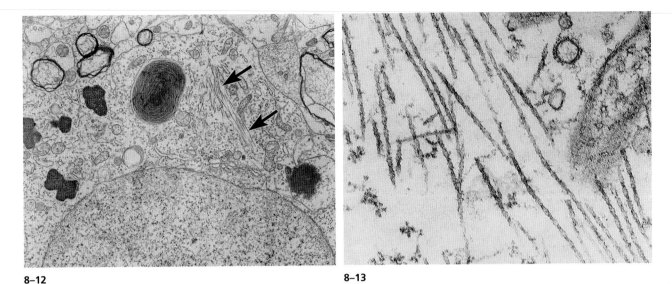

8–12                                                                   8–13

**FIGURES 8–12 AND 8–13**   ALZHEIMER'S DISEASE

Ultrastructurally, neurofibrillary change consists of cytoplasmic accumulation of filamentous material, here seen to course diagonally above the nucleus and to the right of the dark laminated myelin body (*arrows*) (Fig. 8–12, ×11,000). At higher magnification, what appear to be single threads at low magnification are paired, helically arranged filaments (Fig. 8–13, ×70,000). (From Burger PC, Vogel FS. Degenerative and demyelinating diseases. Am J Pathol 1980;99:479–520.)

protein (see Fig. 8–10) and ubiquitin (Fig. 8–11),[3] the former being more specific. Immunohistochemical features of the various inclusions encountered in brains of patients with dementia have been summarized by Lowe.[9]

**Ultrastructural Features.** At the ultrastructural level, neurofibrillary change consists of aggregates of paired helical filaments with a maximum diameter of approxi-

mately 200 Å. As a consequence of the helical structure, the pairs appear segmentally constricted along the longitudinal axes at intervals of 800 Å (Figs. 8–12 and 8–13).[14, 16] As defined by electron microscopy, neuritic plaques contain focally expanded neurites distended by degenerating mitochondria, dense bodies, and abnormal neurofibrillary material (Fig. 8–14).[6, 7] In contrast, diffuse plaques are composed largely of extracellular amyloid fibrils.[4, 18]

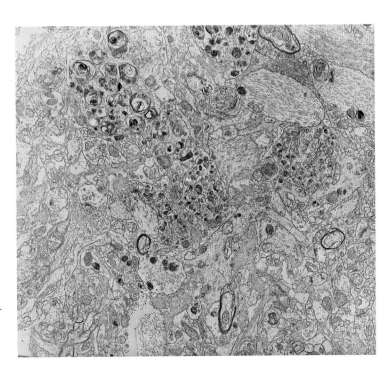

**FIGURE 8–14**   ALZHEIMER'S DISEASE

Senile plaques are composed of expanded neurites filled with degenerating organelles, dense bodies, and paired helical filaments. The last are best seen at the upper right of the illustration.

**Differential Diagnosis.** In most biopsy specimens, the principal issue is to distinguish the brain of patients with Alzheimer's disease from *normal brain*. For autopsy material, standardized criteria based largely on plaque density[10, 11] or on the distribution of neurofibrillary tangles[2] have been suggested to establish the probability of the disease. No such guidelines exist for the interpretation of biopsy material. However, in young patients, the presence in neocortex of neurofibrillary tangles in conjunction with neuritic plaques is abnormal and strongly supports the diagnosis of Alzheimer's disease.[1, 12] The presence of plaques alone, particularly of the diffuse type, does not establish the diagnosis, although a large number of the neuritic type would be highly consistent with the diagnosis.

The presence of α-synuclein–positive cortical Lewy bodies places the disease in the *dementia with Lewy bodies* category, a pathologic state discussed immediately below.

In the absence of neuritic plaques, the presence of immunohistochemically demonstrable tau protein in neurons and glia establishes the diagnosis of a tauopathy and requires exclusion of other members of this disease group.[15] This differential is discussed on pages 432–433.

In surgical specimens, one frequently encounters clusters of markedly contracted, hyperchromatic neurons, particularly at the edges of the specimen (Fig. 8–15). Such cells should not be confused with the diffusely distributed, lipochrome-laden dark neurons seen in late-stage Alzheimer's or in other degenerative disorders. It has been established experimentally that the contracted state of these cells is induced by surgical trauma.[13] They contrast sharply with neighboring neurons, which, as is typical in promptly fixed tissue, seem unduly plump when compared with the triangular shape they assume in postmortem specimens. The presence of a *storage disease* therefore should not be inferred from this rotundity.

**Treatment and Prognosis.** Regrettably, there is no cure for Alzheimer's disease, although symptomatic treatments are available. The condition is relentlessly progressive and death usually results from an intercurrent infection within a decade after the onset of symptoms.

# DEMENTIA WITH LEWY BODIES

**General Comments.** Variably referred to in the past as cortical Lewy body disease, diffuse Lewy body disease, or any of a long list of similar names, this form of dementia is second in prevalence only to Alzheimer's disease.[3, 6] A consensus on the definition of the entity, particularly in regard to mixed lesions that combine Alzheimer's features and cortical Lewy bodies, has been elusive. Because dementia with Lewy bodies almost always appears in elderly people, it is an entity that surgical pathologists must confront only rarely.[4] If only the same could be said of another mixed lesion, oligoastrocytoma.

**Clinical Features.** Patients generally present in their seventies or eighties. Those with "pure" Lewy body disease are more likely to present with parkinsonian symptoms.[2, 3, 6, 9–11]

**Macroscopic Features.** In its pure form without changes of Alzheimer's disease, dementia with Lewy bodies lacks progressive cerebral atrophy.

**Microscopic Features.** In H&E-stained sections, the typical widely distributed intraneuronal inclusions are often found only after an exacting search at high magnification (Fig. 8–16). Unlike the classical Lewy body with

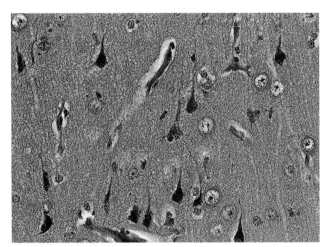

**FIGURE 8–15** NORMAL CEREBRAL CORTEX WITH TRAUMATIC NEURONAL CONDENSATION

Even minor surgical trauma of the biopsy procedure produces dark contracted neurons that should not be interpreted as evidence of disease. Note normal, unaffected, neighboring neurons promptly fixed after excision.

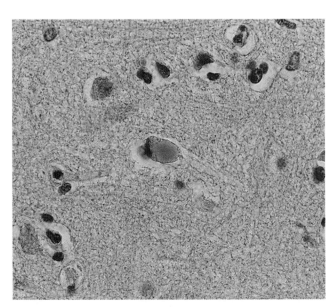

**FIGURE 8–16** DEMENTIA WITH LEWY BODIES

Cortical Lewy bodies are small, cytoplasmic, hyaline masses often difficult to identify in H&E-stained sections. In contrast to their counterparts in the substantia nigra, cortical Lewy bodies have no core.

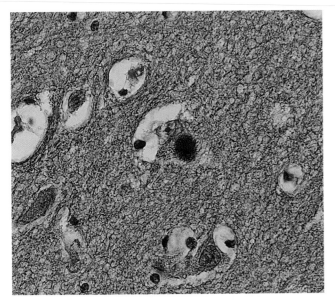

**FIGURE 8-17**   DEMENTIA WITH LEWY BODIES

Immunoreactivity for α-synuclein greatly facilitates the detection of Lewy bodies.

its targetoid profile, as it occurs in the substantia nigra in Parkinson's disease, the cortical Lewy body is a pale, structureless hyaline mass.

**Immunohistochemical Features.** The Lewy body is immunoreactive for ubiquitin, α-synuclein (Fig. 8–17), and phosphorylated neurofilament protein.[5-8]

**Ultrastructural Features.** Lewy bodies are largely fibrillar and non–membrane bound.[1, 12]

**Differential Diagnosis.** Once cortical Lewy bodies are identified, there is little differential diagnosis. Although cortical Lewy bodies resemble the Pick bodies of *Pick's disease*, the latter are immunoreactive for tau protein, whereas the Lewy body is reactive for α-synuclein. Both are ubiquitin positive.

## PICK'S DISEASE AND OTHER NON-ALZHEIMER TAUOPATHIES

**General Comments.** Only rarely is a brain biopsy utilized in the diagnosis of this rare disorder. Pick's disease is considered a form of frontotemporal dementia because of its symptoms and the severity of the changes centered in this region. It is one of the tauopathies.[2, 10, 12] Mutations in the tau gene have been reported.[10]

**Clinical Features.** The disease expresses itself in adults, often in their forties and fifties.[2] Reflecting the localization of the atrophy, personality change and language difficulties are more common in Pick's disease than in Alzheimer's disease, but memory and cognitive disturbances are less severe.[1, 3] Nonetheless, the symptoms are quite variable.[2]

**Radiologic Features.** A presumptive diagnosis is usually offered because of the characteristic distribution and degree of gyral atrophy (Fig. 8–18). This finding, in combination with clinical expressions of the disorder, establishes the diagnosis of a frontotemporal dementia.[4, 5] In Pick's disease, the anterior and orbital portions of the frontal lobe are most affected, whereas the most posterior aspect, the precentral gyrus, is usually spared. In

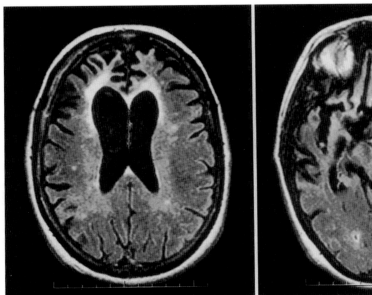
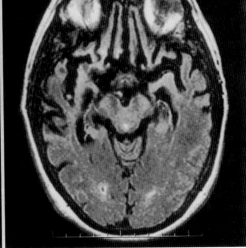

**FIGURE 8-18**   PICK'S DISEASE

Marked frontotemporal gyral atrophy is typical of Pick's disease and other frontotemporal dementias. (Courtesy of Dr. Ronald C. Peterson, Rochester, MN.)

the temporal lobe, the middle and inferior gyri are affected along their entirety, but the atrophy curiously spares the posterior one half to two thirds of the superior temporal gyrus. In late stages, convolutional atrophy becomes so severe as to resemble the cutting edge of a knife and the brain the meat of a dried walnut.

**Microscopic Features.** The hallmarks of Pick's disease are the Pick body and the balloon cell. The former is an intracytoplasmic inclusion most numerous in the small neurons of the second cortical lamina. It is scant or absent in regions of severe atrophy. Although often inconspicuous in H&E-stained sections, the Pick body forms a relatively discrete, pale eosinophilic mass (Fig. 8–19). Argyrophilia facilitates its detection. Many laboratories find immunohistochemistry for tau protein to be more user-friendly (see Fig. 8–21). It is certainly more specific.

The second index feature of Pick's disease, swelling or ballooning of the neurons, results when Nissl substance is lysed and the cytoplasm assumes a glassy, eosinophilic translucency (Fig. 8–20). This cytoplasmic expansion is most apparent in large neurons of the fifth and sixth cortical laminae. Their nuclei are often peripherally displaced and flattened against the cell membrane. Balloon cells are often scant, even in the early stages of the disease, and become less frequent in advanced cases. Ballooned neurons are also characteristic of some other tauopathies, such as corticobasilar degeneration.

**Immunohistochemical Features.** The Pick body is immunopositive for tau protein (Fig. 8–21), phosphorylated neurofilament protein, and ubiquitin.[2, 6, 8, 14] Unlike the Lewy body, it is negative for α-synuclein.

**Ultrastructural Features.** The Pick body is a non–membrane-bound mass of 100 Å filaments. Scattered paired helical filaments similar to those of Alzheimer's disease, but with a greater period of rotation, are also found.[2, 8, 11, 13]

**Differential Diagnosis.** The presence of immunohistochemically demonstrable tau protein establishes the

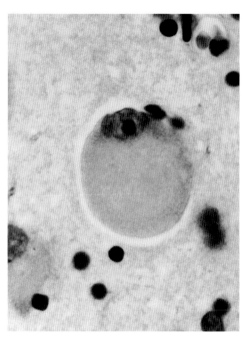

**FIGURE 8–20** PICK'S DISEASE

Balloon cells have distended, translucent cytoplasm. Peripheral displacement of the nucleus is common.

diagnosis of a tauopathy and requires exclusion of other members of this disease group. Tauopathies comprise a diverse array of entities, of which Alzheimer's disease is the dominant member.[12] All accumulate an abnormal form of tau protein. The neurofibrillary tangle of

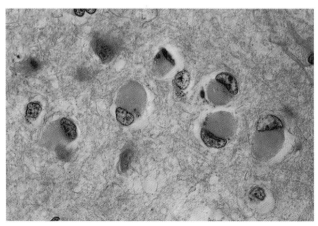

**FIGURE 8–19** PICK'S DISEASE

The intracytoplasmic Pick body is small and eosinophilic.

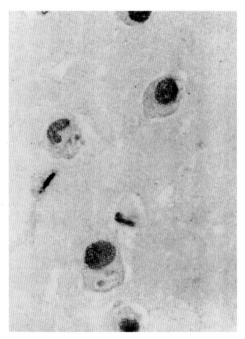

**FIGURE 8–21** PICK'S DISEASE

Pick bodies are immunoreactive for tau protein. (Courtesy of Dr. Suzanne S. Mirra, Brooklyn, NY.)

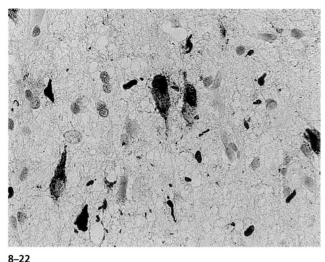

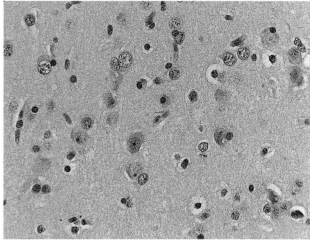

8–22                                          8–23

**FIGURES 8–22 AND 8–23     NON-PICK TAUOPATHY**

This frontal lobe biopsy specimen (Fig. 8–22) features numerous tau-positive intracytoplasmic neuronal inclusions, as well as many tau-positive deposits in neuritic processes. Note that the H&E-stained section from the same case shows only minimal changes (Fig. 8–23), emphasizing the need for immunohistochemistry. The patient was a 33-year-old woman with evolving frontotemporal dementia of 2 years' duration.

*Alzheimer's disease* is tau protein immunopositive but is finely fibrillar with H&E or silver staining. In addition, tangles often wrap about the nucleus and extend into neurites. Pick bodies are discrete globular masses.

*Non-Pick, tau-positive, frontotemporal dementias* contain less well-structured tau-immunoreactive deposits. These have neither the structure of the Pick body nor the fibrillar constitution of the neurofibrillary tangle. The brains in these tauopathies may be surprisingly normal histologically despite extensive tau deposits as detected immunohistochemically and striking atrophy as seen radiologically (Figs. 8–22 and 8–23).

Pick bodies must be distinguished from the intraneuronal inclusions of *dementia with Lewy bodies*.

Lewy bodies are reactive for α-synuclein, but not for tau protein. The immunohistochemical profile is reversed for the Pick body. Dementia with Lewy bodies is generally not as strikingly restricted to the frontotemporal cortex.

Yet other frontotemporal dementias are those with nonspecific changes such as neuronal loss, gliosis, and spongiform change as well as examples with abundant accumulation but without Pick bodies.[7, 9, 12]

**Treatment and Prognosis.** There is no treatment for these progressive diseases.

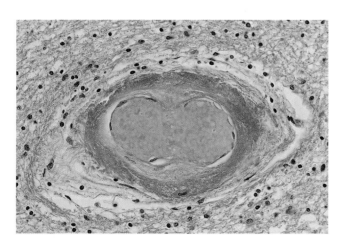

**FIGURE 8–24     CEREBRAL AUTOSOMAL DOMINANT ARTERIOPATHY WITH SUBCORTICAL INFARCTS AND LEUKOENCEPHALOPATHY (CADASIL)**

An arteriole in the white matter is altered by a fine, slightly basophilic granularity.

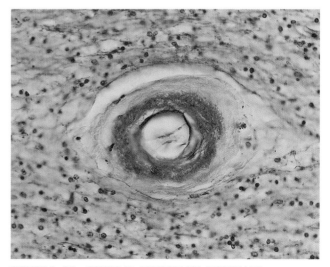

**FIGURE 8–25     CEREBRAL AUTOSOMAL DOMINANT ARTERIOPATHY WITH SUBCORTICAL INFARCTS AND LEUKOENCEPHALOPATHY (CADASIL)**

The granularity of the vessel wall is highlighted by the periodic acid–Schiff stain.

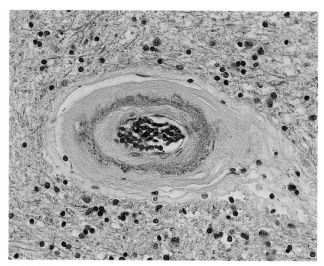

**FIGURE 8–26** CEREBRAL AUTOSOMAL DOMINANT ARTERIOPATHY WITH SUBCORTICAL INFARCTS AND LEUKOENCEPHALOPATHY (CADASIL)

A Movat stain for vessel components clearly demonstrates the finely granular material in the muscularis of this small artery.

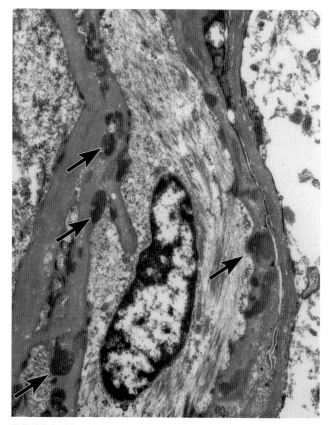

**FIGURE 8–27** CEREBRAL AUTOSOMAL DOMINANT ARTERIOPATHY WITH SUBCORTICAL INFARCTS AND LEUKOENCEPHALOPATHY (CADASIL)

Ultrastructurally, granular, electron-dense deposits (*arrows*) are intimately associated with basement membranes of myocytes in this cutaneous vessel. The deposits typically indent the cells and are often associated with underlying pinocytotic activity.

# CEREBRAL AUTOSOMAL DOMINANT ARTERIOPATHY WITH SUBCORTICAL INFARCTS AND LEUKOENCEPHALOPATHY (CADASIL)

CADASIL is an autosomal dominant vasculopathy with infarcts in the basal ganglia and deep white matter, pseudobulbar palsy, dementia, and, in some cases, migraine headaches.[1–12] Patients are typically in their forties.

Neuroradiologically, the infarcts are well seen in the basal ganglia, internal capsule, and white matter. The loss of myelin (leukoencephalopathy) results in a diffuse increase in T2 signal.

Biopsy of the brain can be employed in the diagnosis,[6, 9] but a simpler approach targets more accessible tissues, such as skin or muscle.[10, 12] The responsible lesion is a distinctive vasculopathy wherein small arteries are thickened and smudged by the deposition of eosinophilic, partially PAS-positive, material within the media (Figs. 8–24 to 8–26).[2] The elastica is duplicated and fragmented.

Ultrastructurally, a peculiar extracellular, granular and osmiophilic material is associated with vascular smooth muscle cells that themselves are often disorganized and numerically depleted (Fig. 8–27).[2, 6, 9–12]

CADASIL is a progressive disorder. Patients usually succumb within two decades.

# REFERENCES

**Creutzfeldt-Jakob Disease**

1. Bahn MM, Parchi P. Abnormal diffusion-weighted magnetic resonance images in Creutzfeldt-Jakob disease. Arch Neurol 1999;56:577–583.
2. Beaudry P, Cohen P, Brandel JP, et al. 14-3-3 protein, neuron-specific enolase, and S-100 protein in cerebrospinal fluid of patients with Creutzfeldt-Jakob disease. Dement Geriatr Cogn Disord 1999;10:40–46.
3. Beck E, Daniel PM, Alpers DM, et al. Experimental kuru in the chimpanzee: a neuropathological study. Brain 1973;96:441–462.
4. Beck E, Daniel PMD, Alpers MA, et al. Experimental "kuru" in chimpanzees: a pathological report. Lancet 1966;2:1056–1059.
5. Berger JR, David NJ. Creutzfeldt-Jakob disease in a physician: a review of the disorder in health care workers. Neurology 1993;43:205–206.
6. Brown P, Gibbs GC Jr, Gadjusek, DC. Transmission of Creutzfeldt-Jakob disease from formalin-fixed, paraffin-embedded human brain tissue. N Engl J Med 1986;315:1614–1615.
7. Brown P, Preece M, Brandel JP, et al. Iatrogenic Creutzfeldt-Jakob disease at the millennium. Neurology 2000;55:1075–1081.
8. Brown P, Preece MA, Will RG. Friendly fire in medicine: hormones, homografts, and Creutzfeldt-Jakob disease. Lancet 1992;340:24–27.
9. Budka H, Aguzzi A, Brown P, et al. Tissue handling in suspected Creutzfeldt-Jakob disease (CJD) and other human spongiform encephalopathies (prion diseases). Brain Pathol 1995;5:319–322.
10. Crain BJ. Safety guidelines for anatomic studies of possible Creutzfeldt-Jakob disease. CAP Today, January, 1996:56.
11. Demaerel P, Heiner L, Robberecht W, et al. Diffusion-weighted MRI in sporadic Creutzfeldt-Jakob disease. Neurology 1999;52:205–208.
12. Duffy P, Wolf J, Collins G, et al. Letter: Possible person-to-person transmission of Creutzfeldt-Jakob disease. N Engl J Med 1974;290:692–693.

13. Gadjusek DC, Gibbs CJ Jr, Alpers M. Experimental transmission of a kuru-like syndrome to chimpanzees. Nature 1966;209:794–796.
14. Gadjusek DC, Zigas V. Degenerative disease of the central nervous system in New Guinea: the endemic occurrence of "kuru" in the native population. N Engl J Med 1957;294:974–978.
15. Gibbs CJ, Gadjusek DC. Experimental subacute spongiform virus encephalopathies in primates and other laboratory animals. Science 1973;182:67–68.
16. Gibbs CJ, Gadjusek DC, Aher DM, et al. Creutzfeldt-Jakob disease (spongiform encephalopathy): transmission to the chimpanzee. Science 1968;161:388–389.
17. Hadlow W. Scrapie and kuru (Letter). Lancet 1959;2:289–290.
18. Hadlow W, Prusiner SB, Kennedy RC, et al. Brain tissue from person dying of Creutzfeldt-Jakob disease causes scrapie-like encephalopathy in goats. Ann Neurol 1980;8:628–632.
19. Hsich G, Kenney K, Gibbs CJ, et al. The 14-3-3 brain protein in cerebrospinal fluid as a marker for transmissible spongiform encephalopathies. N Engl J Med 1996;335:924–930.
20. Johnson RT, Gibbs CJ Jr. Creutzfeldt-Jakob disease and related transmissible spongiform encephalopathies. N Engl J Med 1998;339:1994–2004.
21. Kropp S, Schulz-Schaeffer WJ, Finkenstaedt M, et al. The Heidenhain variant of Creutzfeldt-Jakob disease. Arch Neurol 1999;56:55–61.
22. Lane KL, Brown P, Howell DN, et al. Creutzfeldt-Jakob disease in a pregnant woman with an implanted dura mater graft. Neurosurgery 1994;34:737–739.
23. Mann DM. Dementia of frontal type and dementias with subcortical gliosis. Brain Pathol 1998;8:325–338.
24. Na DL, Suh CK, Choi SH, et al. Diffusion-weighted magnetic resonance imaging in probable Creutzfeldt-Jakob disease: a clinical-anatomic correlation. Arch Neurol 1999;56:951–957.
25. Ogawa T, Inugami A, Fujita H, et al. Serial positron emission tomography with fludeoxyglucose F 18 in Creutzfeldt-Jakob disease. AJNR 1995;16:978–981.
26. Parchi P, Castellani R, Capellari S, et al. Molecular basis of phenotypic variability in sporadic Creutzfeldt-Jakob disease. Ann Neurol 1996;39:767–778.
27. Parchi P, Giese A, Capellari S, et al. Classification of sporadic Creutzfeldt-Jakob disease based on molecular and phenotypic analysis of 300 subjects. Ann Neurol 1999;46:224–233.
28. Prusiner S. Prions and neurodegenerative diseases. N Engl J Med 1987;318:1571–1581.
29. Prusiner S, DeArmond SJ. Biology of disease: prions causing nervous system degeneration. Lab Invest 1987;56:349–363.
30. Prusiner SB. The prion diseases. Brain Pathol 1998;8:499–513.
31. Prusiner SB. Prions. Proc Natl Acad Sci U S A 1998;95:13363–13383.
32. Satoh J, Kurohara K, Yukitake M, et al. The 14-3-3 protein detectable in the cerebrospinal fluid of patients with prion-unrelated neurological diseases is expressed constitutively in neurons and glial cells in culture. Eur Neurol 1999;41:216–225.
33. Schroter A, Zerr I, Henkel K, et al. Magnetic resonance imaging in the clinical diagnosis of Creutzfeldt-Jakob disease. Arch Neurol 2000;57:1751–1757.
34. Urbach H, Klisch J, Wolf HK, et al. MRI in sporadic Creutzfeldt-Jakob disease: correlation with clinical and neuropathological data. Neuroradiology 1998;40:65–70.
35. Zlotnik I, Grant DP, Dayan AD, et al. Transmission of Creutzfeldt-Jakob disease from man to squirrel monkey. Lancet 1974;2:435–438.

## Alzheimer's Disease and Neurodegenerative Changes of the Alzheimer Type

1. Arriagada PV, Growdon JH, Hedley-Whyte ET, et al. Neurofibrillary tangles but not senile plaques parallel duration and severity of Alzheimer's disease. Neurology 1992;42:631–639.
2. Braak H, Braak E. Neuropathological staging of Alzheimer-related changes. Acta Neuropathol (Berl) 1991;82:239–259.
3. Chu CT, Caruso JL, Cummings TJ, et al. Ubiquitin immunochemistry as a diagnostic aid for community pathologists evaluating patients who have dementia. Mod Pathol 2000;13:420–426.
4. Davies CA, Mann DM. Is the "preamyloid" of diffuse plaques in Alzheimer's disease really nonfibrillar? Am J Pathol 1993;143:1594–1605.
5. Hulette CM, Earl NL, Crain BJ. Evaluation of cerebral biopsies for the diagnosis of dementia. Arch Neurol 1992;49:28–31.
6. Krigman M, Feldman RG, Bensch K. Alzheimer's presenile dementia: a histochemical and electron microscopic study. Lab Invest 1965;14:381–396.
7. Lampert P. Fine structural changes of neurites in Alzheimer's disease. Acta Neuropathol Suppl 1971;5:49–53.
8. Love S, Saitoh T, Quijada S, et al. Alz-50, ubiquitin and tau immunoreactivity of neurofibrillary tangles, Pick bodies and Lewy bodies. J Neuropathol Exp Neurol 1988;47:393–405.
9. Lowe J. Establishing a pathological diagnosis in degenerative dementias. Brain Pathol 1998;8:403–406.
10. Mirra SS, Gearing M, McKeel DW Jr, et al. Interlaboratory comparison of neuropathology assessments in Alzheimer's disease: a study of the Consortium to Establish a Registry for Alzheimer's Disease (CERAD). J Neuropathol Exp Neurol 1994;53:303–315.
11. Mirra SS, Heyman A, McKeel D, et al. The Consortium to Establish a Registry for Alzheimer's Disease (CERAD). Part II. Standardization of the neuropathologic assessment of Alzheimer's disease. Neurology 1991;41:479–486.
12. Nagy Z, Esiri MM, Jobst KA, et al. Relative roles of plaques and tangles in the dementia of Alzheimer's disease: correlations using three sets of neuropathological criteria. Dementia 1995;6:21–31.
13. Queiroz LdeS, Eduardo RMdeP. Occurrence of dark neurons in living mechanically injured rat neocortex. Acta Neuropathol (Berl) 1977;38:45–48.
14. Terry R. The fine structure of neurofibrillary tangles in Alzheimer's disease. J Neuropathol Exp Neurol 1963;22:629–642.
15. Tolnay M, Probst A. Review: tau protein pathology in Alzheimer's disease and related disorders. Neuropathol Appl Neurobiol 1999;25:171–187.
16. Wisniewski H, Narang H, Terry RD. Neurofibrillary change of paired helical filaments. J Neurol Sci 1976;27:173–181.
17. Wood JG, Mirra SS, Pollock NJ, et al. Neurofibrillary tangles of Alzheimer disease share antigenic determinants with the axonal microtubule-associated protein tau (tau). Proc Natl Acad Sci U S A 1986;83:4040–4043.
18. Yamaguchi H, Nakazato Y, Hirai S, et al. Electron micrograph of diffuse plaques. Initial stage of senile plaque formation in the Alzheimer brain. Am J Pathol 1989;135:593–597.

## Dementia with Lewy Bodies

1. Arima K, Ueda K, Sunohara N, et al. Immunoelectron-microscopic demonstration of NACP/alpha-synuclein-epitopes on the filamentous component of Lewy bodies in Parkinson's disease and in dementia with Lewy bodies. Brain Res 1998;808:93–100.
2. Gearing M, Mirra SS, Hedreen JC, et al. The Consortium to Establish a Registry for Alzheimer's Disease (CERAD). Part X. Neuropathology confirmation of the clinical diagnosis of Alzheimer's disease. Neurology 1995;45:461–466.
3. Hansen L, Salmon D, Galasko D, et al. The Lewy body variant of Alzheimer's disease: a clinical and pathologic entity. Neurology 1990;40:1–8.
4. Hulette CM, Earl NL, Crain BJ. Evaluation of cerebral biopsies for the diagnosis of dementia. Arch Neurol 1992;49:28–31.
5. Hurtig HI, Trojanowski JQ, Galvin J, et al. Alpha-synuclein cortical Lewy bodies correlate with dementia in Parkinson's disease. Neurology 2000;54:1916–1921.
6. Ince PG, Perry EK, Morris CM. Dementia with Lewy bodies. A distinct non-Alzheimer dementia syndrome? Brain Pathol 1998;8:299–324.
7. Lowe J. Establishing a pathological diagnosis in degenerative dementias. Brain Pathol 1998;8:403–406.
8. Mukaetova-Ladinska EB, Hurt J, Jakes R, et al. Alpha-synuclein inclusions in Alzheimer and Lewy body diseases. J Neuropathol Exp Neurol 2000;59:408–417.
9. Papka M, Rubio A, Schiffer RB. A review of Lewy body disease, an emerging concept of cortical dementia. J Neuropsychiatry Clin Neurosci 1998;10:267–279.
10. Perry RH, Irving D, Blessed G, et al. Senile dementia of Lewy body type. A clinically and neuropathologically distinct form of

Lewy body dementia in the elderly. J Neurol Sci 1990;95: 119–139.

11. Samuel W, Galasko D, Masliah E, et al. Neocortical Lewy body counts correlate with dementia in the Lewy body variant of Alzheimer's disease. J Neuropathol Exp Neurol 1996;55:44–52.

12. Wakabayashi K, Hayashi S, Kakita A, et al. Accumulation of alpha-synuclein/NACP is a cytopathological feature common to Lewy body disease and multiple system atrophy. Acta Neuropathol (Berl) 1998;96:445–452.

## Pick's Disease

1. Binetti G, Locascio JJ, Corkin S, et al. Differences between Pick disease and Alzheimer disease in clinical appearance and rate of cognitive decline. Arch Neurol 2000;57:225–232.

2. Dickson D. Pick's disease: a modern approach. Brain Pathol 1998;8:339–354.

3. Duara R, Barker W, Luis CA. Frontotemporal dementia and Alzheimer's disease: differential diagnosis. Dement Geriatr Cogn Disord 1999;10:37–42.

4. Groen JJ, Hekster RE. Computed tomography in Pick's disease: findings in a family affected in three consecutive generations. J Comput Assist Tomogr 1982;6:907–911.

5. Knopman DS, Christensen KJ, Schut LJ, et al. The spectrum of imaging and neuropsychological findings in Pick's disease. Neurology 1989;39:362–368.

6. Lowe J. Establishing a pathological diagnosis in degenerative dementias. Brain Pathol 1998;8:403–406.

7. Mann DM. Dementia of frontal type and dementias with subcortical gliosis. Brain Pathol 1998;8:325–338.

8. Murayama S, Mori H, Ihara Y, et al. Immunocytochemical and ultrastructural studies of Pick's disease. Ann Neurol 1990;27: 394–405.

9. Neary D, Snowden JS, Mann DM. The clinical pathological correlates of lobar atrophy. Dementia 1993;4:154–159.

10. Pickering-Brown S, Baker M, Yen SH, et al. Pick's disease is associated with mutations in the tau gene. Ann Neurol 2000;48: 859–867.

11. Takauchi S, Hosomi M, Marasigan S, et al. An ultrastructural study of Pick bodies. Acta Neuropathol (Berl) 1984;64:344–348.

12. Tolnay M, Probst A. Review: tau protein pathology in Alzheimer's disease and related disorders. Neuropathol Appl Neurobiol 1999;25:171–187.

13. Towfighi J. Pick's disease. A light and electron microscopic study. Acta Neuropathol (Berl) 1972;21.

14. Ulrich J, Haugh M, Anderton BH, et al. Alzheimer dementia and Pick's disease: neurofibrillary tangles and Pick bodies are associated with identical phosphorylated neurofilament epitopes. Acta Neuropathol (Berl) 1987;73:240–246.

## Cerebral Autosomal Dominant Arteriopathy with Subcortical Infarcts and Leukoencephalopathy (CADASIL)

1. Baudrimont M, Dubas F, Joutel A, et al. Autosomal dominant leukoencephalopathy and subcortical ischemic stroke. A clinicopathological study. Stroke 1993;24:122–125.

2. Bauserman SC, Scheithauer BW. CADASIL (cerebral autosomal dominant arteriopathy with subcortical infarcts and leukoencephalopathy); ultrastructural confirmation by skin biopsy. Pathol Case Rev 1998;3:319–322.

3. Bousser MG, Tournier-Lasserve E. Summary of the proceedings of the First International Workshop on CADASIL. Paris, May 19–21, 1993. Stroke 1994;25:704–707.

4. Chabriat H, Tournier-Lasserve E, Vahedi K, et al. Autosomal dominant migraine with MRI white-matter abnormalities mapping to the CADASIL locus. Neurology 1995;45:1086–1091.

5. Chabriat H, Vahedi K, Iba-Zizen MT, et al. Clinical spectrum of CADASIL: a study of 7 families. Cerebral autosomal dominant arteriopathy with subcortical infarcts and leukoencephalopathy. Lancet 1995;346:934–939.

6. Estes ML, Chimowitz MI, Awad IA, et al. Sclerosing vasculopathy of the central nervous system in nonelderly demented patients. Arch Neurol 1991;48:631–636.

7. Joutel A, Corpechot C, Ducros A, et al. Notch3 mutations in CADASIL, a hereditary adult-onset condition causing stroke and dementia. Nature 1996;383:707–710.

8. Kalimo H, Viitanen M, Amberla K, et al. CADASIL: hereditary disease of arteries causing brain infarcts and dementia. Neuropathol Appl Neurobiol 1999;25:257–265.

9. Lammie GA, Rakshi J, Rossor MN, et al. Cerebral autosomal dominant arteriopathy with subcortical infarcts and leukoencephalopathy (CADASIL)—confirmation by cerebral biopsy in 2 cases. Clin Neuropathol 1995;14:201–206.

10. Ruchoux MM, Maurage CA. CADASIL: cerebral autosomal dominant arteriopathy with subcortical infarcts and leukoencephalopathy. J Neuropathol Exp Neurol 1997;56:947–964.

11. Ruchoux MM, Maurage CA. Endothelial changes in muscle and skin biopsies in patients with CADASIL. Neuropathol Appl Neurobiol 1997;23:60–65.

12. Ruchoux MM, Guerouaou D, Vandenhaute B, et al. Systemic vascular smooth muscle cell impairment in cerebral autosomal dominant arteriopathy with subcortical infarcts and leukoencephalopathy. Acta Neuropathol (Berl) 1995;89: 500–512.

# REGION OF THE SELLA TURCICA

**9**

The sellar region contains a diversity of skeletal, vascular, meningeal, endocrine, and central nervous system (CNS) structures, all in close approximation (Figs. 9–1 to 9–4). These tissues, and ones presumably displaced during embryogenesis, provide the substrate for numerous lesions of interest to clinicians and pathologists alike.

## NORMAL ANATOMY OF THE PITUITARY

Given the complexity of the pituitary gland and the uneven distribution of its cell types, an understanding of the normal anatomy is essential for optimal assessment of surgical specimens.

**Anterior Lobe (Adenohypophysis).** In the horizontal plane the pituitary can be conveniently divided into lateral "wings" and a midline "mucoid wedge" (Fig. 9–5).

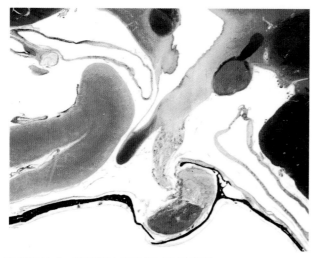

**FIGURE 9-1    NORMAL SELLAR ANATOMY**

This midsagittal histologic section emphasizes the intimate relation of normal anatomic structures in the region of the sella turcica (H&E–Luxol fast blue).

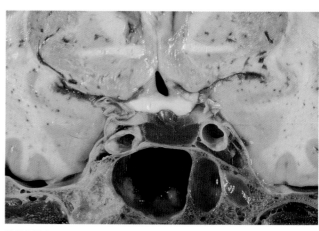

**FIGURE 9-3    NORMAL SELLAR ANATOMY**

This photograph of a coronal section at the level of the pituitary stalk and gland illustrates the intimate relationships between cavernous sinuses, sphenoid sinus, and pituitary gland. Invasive adenomas may extend laterally into one or both cavernous sinuses or inferiorly into the sphenoid sinus. Note the proximity of the optic chiasm to the pituitary.

An additional portion, the pars tuberalis, extends upward along anterolateral surface of the pituitary stalk.

Principal cell types include growth hormone (GH) cells or somatotrophs, prolactin (PRL) cells or lactotrophs, adrenocorticotropic hormone (ACTH) cells or corticotrophs, luteinizing hormone (LH) and follicle-stimulating hormone (FSH) cells or gonadotrophs, and thyroid-stimulating hormone (TSH) cells or thyrotrophs. As a rule, these various cells lie admixed within acini (Fig. 9–6). The latter are surrounded by a capillary-rich reticulin network (Fig. 9–7). The lateral wings of the

gland consist primarily of acidophilic cells that produce GH. The cellular monotony produced by their sheer number (Fig. 9–8) may mimic adenoma, particularly in frozen sections and in small or fragmented specimens. PRL cells are largely chromophobic and are concentrated in the posterior portions of the lateral wings. Basophilic periodic acid–Schiff (PAS)–positive and largely ACTH-producing cells predominate in the mucoid wedge, where nodules of these cells are a common feature (Fig. 9–9). These should not be mistaken for hyperplasia or adenoma. Particularly in adults and elderly

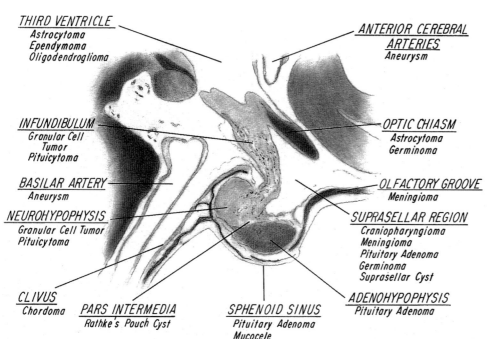

THIRD VENTRICLE
*Astrocytoma*
*Ependymoma*
*Oligodendroglioma*

ANTERIOR CEREBRAL ARTERIES
*Aneurysm*

INFUNDIBULUM
*Granular Cell Tumor*
*Pituicytoma*

OPTIC CHIASM
*Astrocytoma*
*Germinoma*

BASILAR ARTERY
*Aneurysm*

OLFACTORY GROOVE
*Meningioma*

NEUROHYPOPHYSIS
*Granular Cell Tumor*
*Pituicytoma*

SUPRASELLAR REGION
*Craniopharyngioma*
*Meningioma*
*Pituitary Adenoma*
*Germinoma*
*Suprasellar Cyst*

CLIVUS
*Chordoma*

PARS INTERMEDIA
*Rathke's Pouch Cyst*

SPHENOID SINUS
*Pituitary Adenoma*
*Mucocele*

ADENOHYPOPHYSIS
*Pituitary Adenoma*

**FIGURE 9-2    SELLAR REGION LESIONS**

Topographic distribution of lesions in the region of the sella turcica.

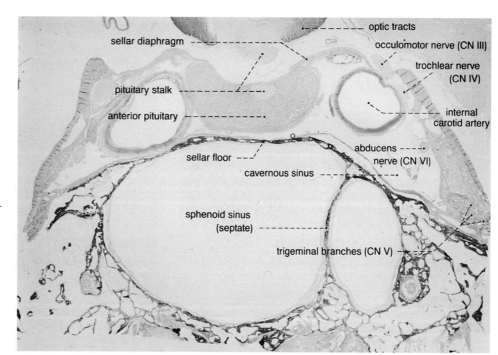

**FIGURE 9–4    NORMAL SELLAR ANATOMY**

In a coronal whole mount section, note the location of cranial nerves III, IV, and VI and branches of nerve V within the cavernous si-nuses, a relationship explaining the occurrence of cranial nerve palsy in association with invasive pituitary adenomas. This section also illustrates the proximity of the internal carotid arteries to the pituitary gland (Luxol fast blue–PAS).

people, such cells are also seen in the posterior or neural lobe, a phenomenon termed basophil invasion (Fig. 9–10). It is of no physiologic significance and must not be misinterpreted as infiltration of the neural lobe

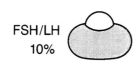

**FIGURE 9–5    DISTRIBUTION OF CELL TYPES IN THE NORMAL ADENOHYPOPHYSIS**

The various hormone-producing cells of the adenohypophysis are not uniformly distributed. The PAS-positive ACTH- and TSH-producing cells are concentrated in the midline mucoid wedge, whereas the generally chromophobic prolactin cells and the typically eosinophilic growth hormone cells are concentrated in the lateral wings. Gonadotrophs or follicle-stimulating hormone (FSH) and luteinizing hormone (LH) cells, which are diffusely distributed throughout the adenohypophysis, are depicted by stippling in the small gland at the right of the illustration. The percentages indicate the approximate proportions of these various cell types.

by an ACTH cell adenoma. Although ACTH immunoreactive, these cells are functionally distinct from other corticotrophs. For example, they do not undergo Crooke's change in the setting of cortisol excess. The presence of axons of the posterior lobe among these cells serves to distinguish basophil invasion from anterior lobe or adenoma tissue. A smaller subset of basophilic cells produces the glycoprotein hormones thyrotropin (TSH) and the gonadotropins (FSH and LH). The former are somewhat concentrated in the anterior mucoid wedge and the latter are distributed throughout the gland.

An eye-catching feature of the normal gland is squamous metaplasia in the pars tuberalis. This affects mainly the gonadotrophs and ACTH-producing cells

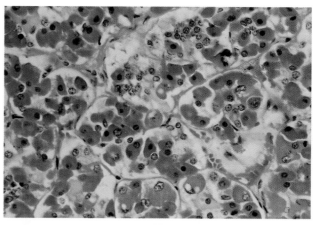

**FIGURE 9–6    NORMAL ADENOHYPOPHYSIS**

This H&E preparation shows several pituitary acini and their composition of eosinophilic, basophilic, and chromophobic cells.

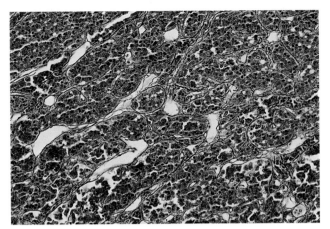

**FIGURE 9–7**   NORMAL ADENOHYPOPHYSIS

This reticulin stain highlights the capillary network that encloses the round to elongate acini of secretory cells.

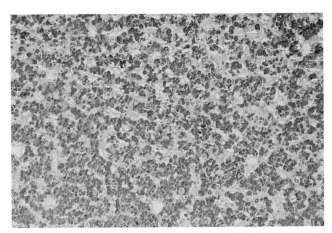

**FIGURE 9–8**   SOMATOTROPHS IN NORMAL ADENOHYPOPHYSIS

Seen after immunostaining for GH, the bulk of GH cells are densely granulated and hence strongly immunopositive. Their sheer number, particularly on H&E-stained frozen or permanent sections, lend a monotonous appearance that can mimic adenoma.

common at this site (Fig. 9–11). Also present are stellate cells not engaged in hormone production. These are analogous to sustentacular cells in some other endocrine organs and lie distributed in small number throughout the pituitary (Fig. 9–12). Lastly, salivary gland rests may be encountered near the junction of the pituitary stalk and gland (Fig. 9–13).

The general characteristics of major anterior pituitary cell types are summarized in Table 9–1.

**Posterior Lobe (Neurohypophysis).** This consists almost entirely of axonal terminations and accompanying glial cells (pituicytes) in a delicate capillary stroma (Fig. 9–14). Granular axonal expansions termed Herring bodies are a common feature and are vasopressin immunoreactive (see Fig. 9–14). Pituicytes are variably glial fibrillary acidic protein (GFAP)–positive (Fig. 9–15).

Detailed discussions of the anatomy and pathophysiology of the pituitary gland, including the posterior lobe

**TABLE 9–1**
**The Normal Anterior Pituitary: Morphological and Functional Features of Secretory Cells**

| Cell | Product | Serum Level (Males/Females) | Location | Percentage of Cells | Histochemical Staining* | Immunoperoxidase Staining |
|---|---|---|---|---|---|---|
| Somatotroph† | Growth hormone (GH); 21,000-dalton polypeptide | 0–5 ng/mL 0–10 ng/mL | Lateral wings | 50 | Acidophilic; PAS (−) | GH |
| Lactotroph† | Prolactin (PRL); 23,500-dalton polypeptide | 0–20 ng/mL 0–23 ng/mL | Resting cells— generalized; secreting cells— posterolateral wings | 15–20 | Acidophilic/PAS (−) Herlant's erythrosin and Brooke's carmoisine (+) | PRL |
| Corticotroph | Adrenocorticotropic hormone (ACTH); 4507-dalton polypeptide | <60 pg/mL | Mucoid wedge | 15–20 | Basophilic; PAS and lead hematoxylin (+) | ACTH, β-LPH, MSH, endorphin, enkephalin |
| Gonadotroph | Follicle-stimulating hormone and luteinizing hormone (FSH/LH); 35,100- and 28,260-dalton glycoproteins | <22 IU/L <20 IU/L FSH§ <4–24 IU/L <30 IU/L LH¶ | Generalized | 10 | Basophilic; PAS, lead hematoxylin, aldehyde fuchsin, and aldehyde thionine (+) | FSH and LH‡ |
| Thyrotroph | Thyrotropic hormone (TSH); 28,000-dalton glycoprotein | 0.4–6 mIU/L | Anterior mucoid wedge | ~5 | Same as for gonadotroph | TSH |

\* The tinctorial characteristics of normal pituitary cells depend on adequate cytoplasmic granule storage. If sparsely granulated, cells otherwise functional may appear nonreactive or "chromophobic."

† Rare acidophilic stem cells (presumed somatotroph and lactotroph precursor cells producing both GH and PRL) are present in the normal pituitary.

‡ Many gonadotrophs are capable of producing both FSH and LH, although immunohistochemical and ultrastructural evidence suggests that some gonadotrophs may produce only one hormone.

§ Value given for females is non-midcycle value. Midcycle, <40 IU/L, postmenopausal, 40 to 160 IU/L.

¶ Value given for females is non-midcycle value. Midcycle, 30 to 150 IU/L, postmenopausal, 30 to 120 IU/L.

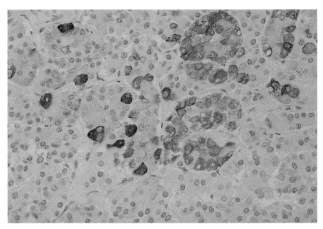

**FIGURE 9–9**  CORTICOTROPHS IN NORMAL ADENOHYPOPHYSIS

Clusters and nodules of ACTH-immunoreactive cells are a normal feature of the pituitary. Large and basophilic after H&E staining, they must not be mistaken for pathologic hyperplasia or adenoma.

and hypothalamus, are available in more comprehensive texts.[1-12]

# PITUITARY NEOPLASIA

## Adenoma—General Features

**Definition.** A benign neoplasm derived from parenchymal cells of the adenohypophysis.

**Clinical and Radiographic Features.** Evidence has confirmed their clonal origin[62] as well as the presence of various cytogenetic[122] and molecular genetic abnormalities.[15, 22, 47, 60, 65, 90]

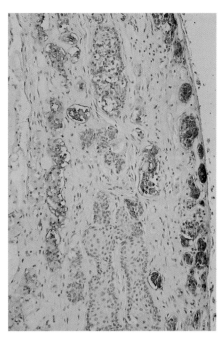

**FIGURE 9–11**  SQUAMOUS CELL NESTS IN THE INFUNDIBULUM

Nests of well-differentiated squamous epithelium form a partial bark around the trunk of the infundibulum. These foci result from metaplasia of mainly ACTH and FSH/LH cells and are usually seen in adults. Although it had been suggested that such cells represent progenitors of craniopharyngioma, this concept has been abandoned (immunostain for ACTH).

**Clinical Features.** Pituitary adenomas that exhibit endocrine activity or attain sufficient size to produce symptoms make up 10% to 20% of all intracranial neoplasms (see Table 9–1). Most are solitary, but multiple lesions are occasionally encountered.[74, 151] The bell-shaped incidence curve levels off from the third through the sixth decades. Women are more often affected. Adenomas

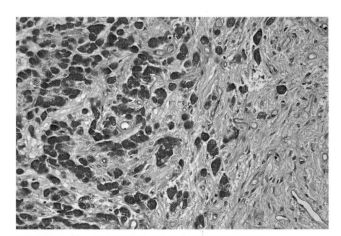

**FIGURE 9–10**  "BASOPHIL INVASION" IN NORMAL ADENOHYPOPHYSIS

With age, there is a tendency for PAS-positive, ACTH-immunoreactive cells that appear to invade the neurohypophysis. The latter is seen as the pale-staining, neuroglial tissue on the right. Dense aggregation of such ACTH cells must not be interpreted as adenoma.

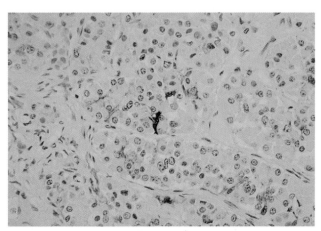

**FIGURE 9–12**  STELLATE CELLS IN THE NORMAL ADENOHYPOPHYSIS

The function of these elongated, S-100 protein–immunopositive and non–hormone-containing cells is poorly understood, but they appear to play a paracrine role in the regulation of hormone secretion and may also function as phagocytes. No tumors have been attributed to such cells.

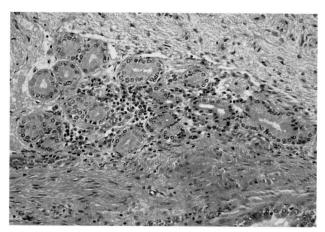

**FIGURE 9–13    SALIVARY GLAND REST OF THE PITUITARY**

Serous acini are a common finding on the superior aspect of the gland near its junction with the pituitary stalk.

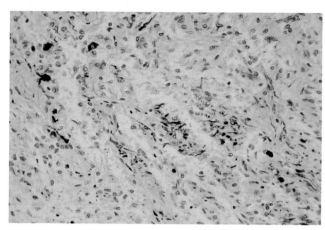

**FIGURE 9–15    POSTERIOR PITUITARY**

Pituicytes constitute the nucleated cells of the neurohypophysis. The functionally specialized astrocytes play an important role in the regulation of water metabolism. As seen here, they are variably GFAP positive.

occurring in children are usually PRL or ACTH producing.[64, 86, 101, 112] Approximately 3% of operated adenomas are associated with multiple endocrine neoplasia type I. Of these, most are macroadenomas associated with acromegaly or hyperprolactinemia.[133]

High-resolution radiographic techniques (Figs. 9–16 and 9–17) and sensitive radioimmunoassays for circulating hormones bring many adenomas to attention at the early, "microadenoma" stage. By definition, they measure less than 1 cm in diameter (Figs. 9–18 to 9–21). Symptoms referable to the mass effects of larger lesions, that is, "macroadenomas," reflect their strategic position at the crossroads of the visual and hypothalamic-hypophyseal

systems. Particularly when nonfunctioning, these large, contrast-enhancing (Figs. 9–17, 9–22, and 9–23) tumors often expand or "balloon" the sella, undergo suprasellar extension, encroach upon the cavernous sinus, and occur as lobulated masses that compress or displace cranial nerves, blood vessels, or the brain (Figs. 9–24 to 9–27). Invasive adenomas are discussed later.

Ectopic adenomas are rare.[49, 91, 138] Some arise in the sphenoid sinus or beneath the oral mucoperiosteum, where they represent neoplastic transformation of the pharyngeal pituitary.[49, 70, 91] Rare examples occur in the nasal cavity[70] or lie entirely in the suprasellar region[134] or the third ventricle.[72] The common histogenetic rela-

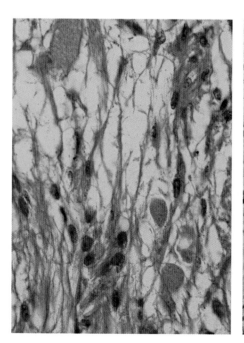

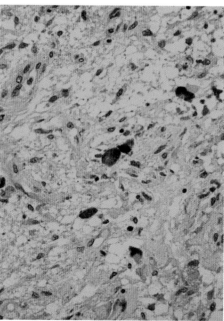

**FIGURE 9–14    POSTERIOR PITUITARY**

The neurohypophysis is composed largely of axons showing occasional swellings (Herring bodies) containing hormones (*left*), including vasopressin (*right*, immunostain) and oxytocin, as well as their respective carrier proteins. Supportive cells include specialized glia (see Fig. 9–15) and a vascular stoma.

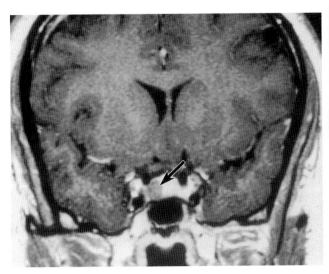

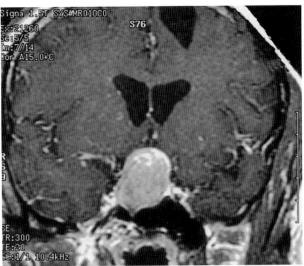

9–16                                    9–17

**FIGURES 9–16 AND 9–17**    MICROADENOMAS AND MACROADENOMAS

Microadenomas are visualized during MR contrast studies by their "delayed" enhancement relative to that of the normal gland (Fig. 9–16). They thus appear as a small darker area within the adenohypophysis (*arrow*). Macroadenomas, in contrast, are larger, rapidly enhancing masses that, as in this case, often extend above the sella (Fig. 9–17). The macroadenoma, in a 56-year-old man, produced bilateral constriction of the visual field.

tionship between Rathke's cleft cyst and pituitary adenoma has been used to explain the occurrence of occasional cystic, intrasellar masses with combined features of both.[71, 107, 108] Pituitary adenoma may even be a component of an ovarian teratoma.[110]

When carefully sought, incidental pituitary adenomas are present in nearly 25% of all autopsies[21]; the majority are either PRL producing or devoid of demonstrable hormones, that is, null cell adenomas.[100]

Pituitary apoplexy, that is, sudden enlargement of an adenoma by hemorrhage and/or infarction, occurs in 1% of adenomas. It not only worsens pituitary hypofunction but also may induce visual disturbance, even blindness because of compression of the optic chasm.[2, 13, 18, 24, 102, 148] Extensive

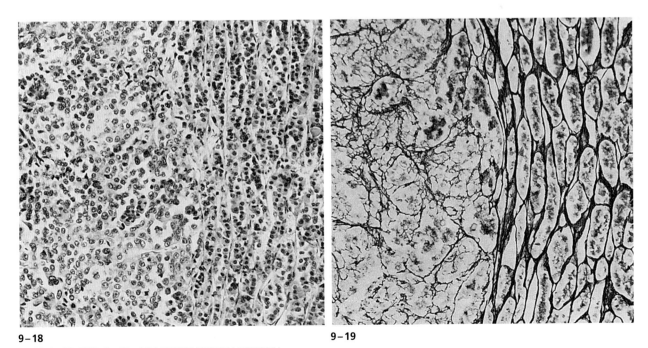

9–18                                    9–19

**FIGURES 9–18 AND 9–19**    PITUITARY MICROADENOMA

The interface between a microadenoma and adjacent compressed pituitary is usually abrupt. Note that the nuclei of the adenoma (*left*) are larger and have increased nuclear/cytoplasmic ratios as compared with cells in surrounding tissue on the right (Fig. 9–18). Reticulin precisely defines the uniform lobules of the normal gland but incompletely invests large, coarse lobules in the neoplasm (Fig. 9–19).

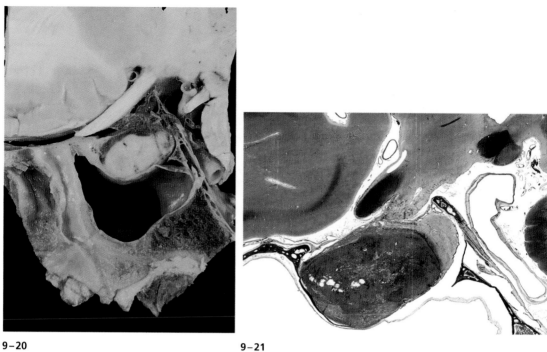

9–20                                  9–21

**FIGURES 9–20 AND 9–21    PITUITARY ADENOMA**

During work-up for acromegaly and an enlarged sella, a 60-year-old man died of coronary artery disease. Responsible for the endocrine hyperactivity, which was apparent at autopsy as visceromegaly, was the light-colored pituitary adenoma seen in the midsagittal section of the sellar region (Fig. 9–20). A whole mount histologic section stained for H&E–luxol fast blue discloses the discrete, darkly staining adenoma that erodes the sellar floor (Fig. 9–21). Note the surgical accessibility of the neoplasm via the subjacent sphenoid sinus.

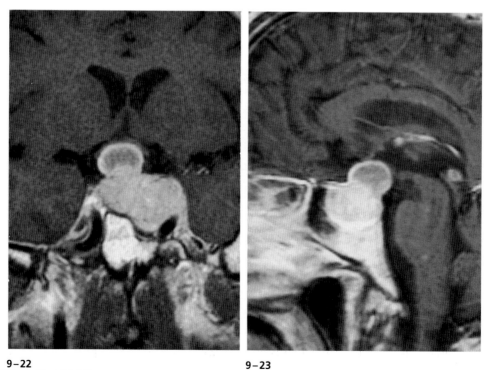

9–22                                  9–23

**FIGURES 9–22 AND 9–23    PITUITARY ADENOMA**

Macroadenomas enlarge the sella and often extend into the suprasellar region. In these coronal (Fig. 9–22) and sagittal (Fig. 9–23) T1-weighted images after gadolinium administration, the lesion is an enhancing mass that involves the cavernous sinus on the patient's left. A cystic component of the tumor extends into the suprasellar region, where the mass compresses and elevates the optic chiasm.

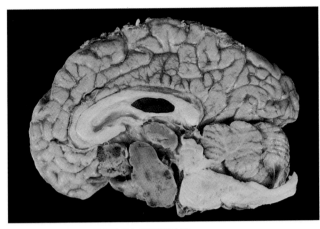

**FIGURE 9–24**    PITUITARY ADENOMA

In advanced cases, continued expansion of pituitary adenomas brings them forcefully in contact with the floor of the third ventricle to produce hydrocephalus. This particularly large adenoma was encountered in a 57-year-old woman who died of Hodgkin's disease 17 years after incomplete primary resection of an adenoma and 7 years after partial excision of its recurrence.

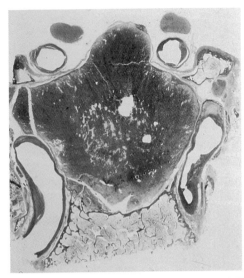

**FIGURE 9–25**    MACROADENOMA WITH CAVERNOUS SINUS EXTENSION

Seen in coronal section, this nonfunctioning adenoma shows lateral extension with indentation of the cavernous sinus. Such massive adenomas often obliterate the sella but lack frank invasiveness.

subarachnoid hemorrhage is also common (Fig. 9–28). Emergency decompression of the optic nerves and chiasm may be required. Sudden hemorrhagic necrosis occurs primarily in large nonfunctioning tumors but can affect adenomas of any size and immunotype.[18, 24] Although clinically apparent apoplexy is often a dramatic event, hemorrhagic infarction of an adenoma is far more often subclini-

cal. Approximately 10% of operated adenomas contain areas of hemorrhagic necrosis, hemosiderin deposits, granulation tissue, or cystic change.[102] On occasion, apoplexy is induced by endocrine testing. Spontaneous hemorrhagic infarction of a functioning adenoma rarely results in permanent endocrine cure.[99] Pituitary apoplexy specimens are hemorrhagic and largely, if not entirely, necrotic. On

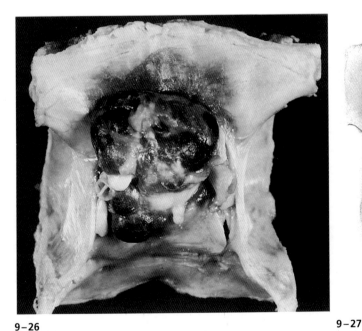

9–26

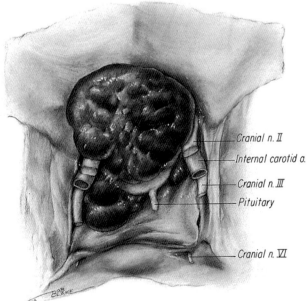

9–27

Cranial n. II
Internal carotid a.
Cranial n. III
Pituitary
Cranial n. VI

**FIGURES 9–26 AND 9–27**    PITUITARY ADENOMA

As a pituitary adenoma extends dorsally, it enters the suprasellar region, where it displaces and compresses such structures as the optic chiasm, cranial nerves, blood vessels, and infundibulum (Fig. 9–26). Headaches and bitemporal hemianopia in a 64-year-old woman prompted skull radiographs that revealed sellar enlargement produced by this lobulated pituitary macroadenoma (Fig. 9–27).

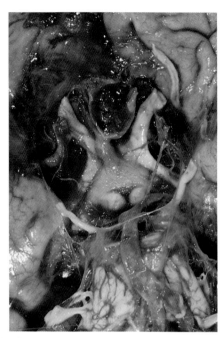

**FIGURE 9–28** PITUITARY APOPLEXY

Massive hemorrhage in a pituitary is a surgical emergency with significant mortality. Necrotic tumor and clot fill the suprasellar space and displace the optic nerves.

staining with hematoxylin and eosin (H&E), it may be difficult to identify adenoma tissue, but in most instances the tumor pattern of reticulin staining is still discernible (Fig. 9–29). Immunostaining of infarcted adenoma often yields misleading results and should not be pursued unless some viable fragments are also available for study.

**Radiologic Features.** Unless invasive of bone, pituitary adenomas appear radiographically well defined. On computed tomographic (CT) and magnetic resonance imaging (MRI) scans, contrast enhancement is temporally somewhat retarded relative to normal gland. Thus, immediately after injection of the contrast agent, the adenoma appears darker than the surrounding pituitary, the enhancement of which is immediate and avid. A radiographic classification of pituitary adenoma stage devised by Hardy[45] is based upon tumor size, the presence or absence of various extensions, and the degree to which adenomas invade surrounding structures (Fig. 9–30).

**Macroscopic Features.** Although most pituitary adenomas are solid, their consistency is often that of pudding. Cystic change with or without evidence of hemorrhage is seen in only a minority of cases. Calcification is largely, but not entirely, limited to PRL-producing adenomas; rare examples are so densely calcified as to resemble stones.[149]

**Specimen Handling.** To avoid drying or impregnation of the soft tumor into the supportive surface of gauze, specimens should be promptly submitted on a moist, smooth-surfaced material. Processing should proceed in such a way as to provide unfrozen tissue for histologic and immunohistochemical study and, if necessary, for electron microscopy.

Intraoperative confirmation of a clinical diagnosis of pituitary adenoma is frequently requested. Although the frozen section method can be used, H&E-stained smears or touch preparations are preferable (see Fig. 9–34). The preparation time is shorter, the evaluation is reliable, and smears complement permanent microsections. Furthermore, these methods conserve artifact-free tissue for paraffin embedding and for electron microscopy.

Frozen section assessment of margins is of questionable efficacy and, because of the technical artifacts that affect minute specimens, is difficult at best. If requested, it should be understood that a final assessment

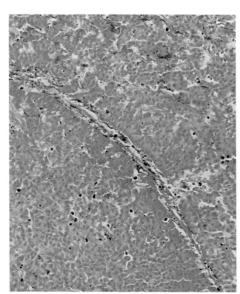

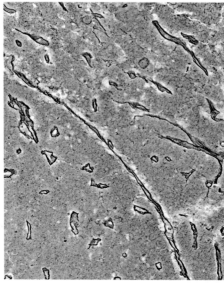

**FIGURE 9–29** PITUITARY APOPLEXY

Although the adenoma may be obscured by the infarction (*left*), the characteristic stomal pattern of the adenoma can often be identified with reticulin staining (*right*).

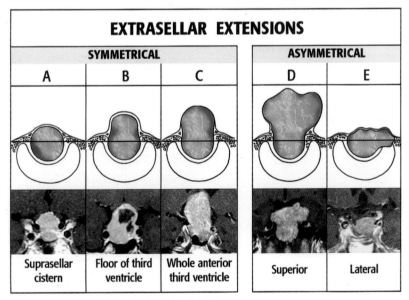

**FIGURE 9–30** RADIOLOGIC CLASSIFICATION OF PITUITARY TUMORS

This classification considers pituitary tumors to be either noninvasive (Grades I and II) or invasive (Grades III and IV) based on the MRI integrity of the bony floor of the sella or its invasion by the tumor with inferior extension. Other extrasellar tumoral extensions are superior symmetrical (A, B, and C) or asymmetrical (D), and lateral (E). They are designated by adding the proper suffix letter to the grade (e.g., Grade II B).

**Grade Ø:** Added to the above grades to designate a small tumor seen within a normal-sized gland and sella with a normal floor.

**Grade I:** Subtle localized blistering, bulging, or lowering of the floor by a tumor measuring less than 10 mm (microadenoma).

**Grade II:** Enlargement of the sella by a tumor of more than 10 mm. The cortex of the floor may be thinned, but it appears intact.

**Grade III:** Partial destruction of the floor with localized protrusion of the tumor downward into the sphenoid sinus.

**Grade IV:** Total destruction of the floor by a large tumor invading diffusely the sphenoid sinus.

**A:** Small, superior tumoral extension protruding into the suprasellar cistern.

**B:** Medium-size extension indenting the floor of the third ventricle.

**C:** Large symmetrical, superior extension filling the anterior portion of the third ventricle.

**D:** Asymmetrical superior extension sprouting anteriorly, laterally, or posteriorly.

**E:** Lateral extension into the adjacent cavernous sinus.

(From Hardy J, Vezina JL. Transsphenoidal neurosurgery of intracranial neoplasm. In Thompson RA, Green JR (eds). Advances in Neurology. New York: Raven Press, 1976, pp 261–274; Hardy J. Atlas of Transsphenoidal Microsurgery in Pituitary Tumors. New York: Igaku-Shoin Medical Publishers, 1991, p 3.)

of margins awaits the use of special stains on permanent sections of optimally fixed tissue. We have not found intraoperative reticulin stains to be of practical use.[1, 147] With regard to enhancement of immunoreactivity, both enzyme digestion and microwave treatment are applicable. Caution is advised because both methods may result in artifactual staining.

For electron microscopy, glutaraldehyde fixation is clearly optimal, but even a 1-mm fragment reserved in formalin may save the day by permitting the characterization of adenomas with an unusual immunoprofile or clinical presentation.

**Microscopic Features.** When adenomas are small in size, their location within the gland reflects the distribution of their normal cellular counterparts (Fig. 9–31). Like other endocrine tumors, they show a range of histologic appearances (Figs. 9–32 and 9–33). Some patterns are associated with specific hormonal phenotypes. We first discuss the "generic" adenoma and then continue with discussions of specific hormonal subtypes. The section concludes with an overall discussion of differential diagnosis, treatment, and prognosis.

The adenoma consists of patternless sheets of uniform cells interrupted only by a delicate capillary network. The epithelial nature of adenoma cells is most apparent in perivascular zones, where the cells often display regimentation, columnar shape, tapering processes, and polarization of nuclei. When exaggerated, this arrangement produces pseudorosettes and contributes to papilla formation. Nuclei are typically uniform, round to oval, and exhibit the delicate "salt-and-pepper" chromatin pattern so characteristic of neuroendocrine neoplasms. Cell borders are often well defined. Features best seen in touch preparations include small but distinct nucleoli and mild anisonucleosis (Fig. 9–34). Binucleation or multinucleation may be seen, but nuclear pleomorphism is rarely prominent. Unlike the cells of normal pituitary, which vary from eosinophilic to basophilic and chromophobic, those of most adenomas are uniform in their tinctorial characteristics.

With PAS and reticulin staining, adenomas lack the acinar pattern of normal pituitary tissue. The normal small, uniform acini are replaced by sheets of cells with fragmented or incomplete circumscription by reticulin. This relative lack of stroma imparts the neoplasm's typical soft texture.

**Artifacts.** A common "crush" artifact produced by the rough handling of normal and neoplastic pituitary tissue is the formation of hyperchromatic cells that mimic metastatic small cell carcinoma (Fig. 9–35). The distinction is simple, given the low MIB-1 labeling indices of normal and adenomatous tissue.[139] The effect of suction on the normal gland is the formation of unsightly empty acini (see Fig. 9–35).

**Cytologic Features.** Smear or touch preparations are of great value in differentiating pituitary adenoma from other lesions. As previously noted, adenoma cells are cytologically benign and have an endocrine chromatin pattern (Fig. 9–34). Cellular pleomorphism, binucleation, and nucleolar enlargement are only occasionally seen and mitoses are uncommon. Cytoplasmic granulation varies among the different adenoma subtypes but tends to be uniform in any one tumor. Adenoma cells detach individually rather than in cohesive tissue fragments as characterizes metastatic carcinoma.

**Immunohistochemical Features.** Adenomas are generally reactive for both synaptophysin and chromogranin. Aside from some null cell lesions, all exhibit immunohistochemical staining for one or more pituitary hormones. Hormonal immunotypes are discussed in regard to specific subtypes on the following pages. Their general, nonhormonal phenotype is the subject of several studies[61, 94, 95] (see Table 9–6).

## Adenomas of Specific Cell Type

Decades of correlative clinical, immunohistochemical, and ultrastructural study by Kovacs and Horvath[51, 77, 79] and their colleagues have resulted in the now widely accepted World Health Organization (WHO) classification of pituitary adenomas (Tables 9–2 to 9–4).[129] Numerous smaller studies by other authors support their conclusions.[39, 97, 106, 119] The classification is doubly satisfying because it is at the same time morphologic and clinically informative (see Table 9–1). For example, the benefit of

### ADENOMAS

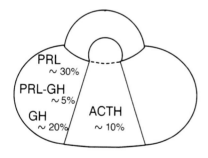

| | |
|---|---|
| Acidophil stem cell | 2% |
| ACTH (silent) | 2% |
| FSH/LH | 10% |
| TSH | 1% |
| Null cell | 20% |

**FIGURE 9–31** REGIONAL DISTRIBUTION OF PITUITARY ADENOMAS BY CELL TYPE

The ACTH-producing neoplasms are largely confined to the mucoid wedge, whereas prolactin- and growth hormone–producing adenomas usually arise in the lateral wings. Nonfunctioning tumors most of which are macroadenomas, so disrupt local anatomy that they defy precise localization (indicated by the stippled area in the small diagram at the bottom right).

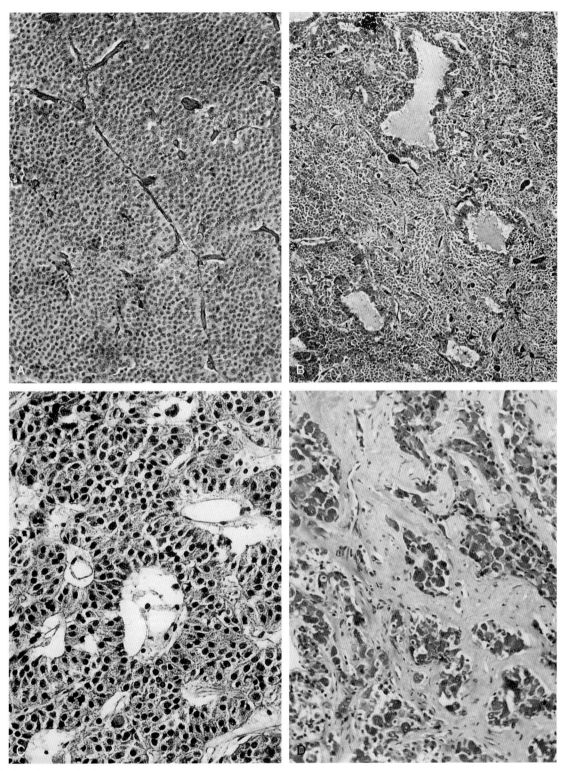

**FIGURE 9–32**    PITUITARY ADENOMA

Pituitary adenomas assume many histologic patterns. *A*, The neoplasm forms a diffuse sheet of cells creating a monotonous appearance unlike that of the normal gland, which is acinar in architecture and heterogeneous in its cytologic composition. *B*, The lesion contains small colloid-filled cysts. *C*, The pattern is one of anastomosing ribbons of cells. *D*, The lesion has a dense fibrovascular stroma, an uncommon feature, but one occasionally seen in ACTH-producing tumors.

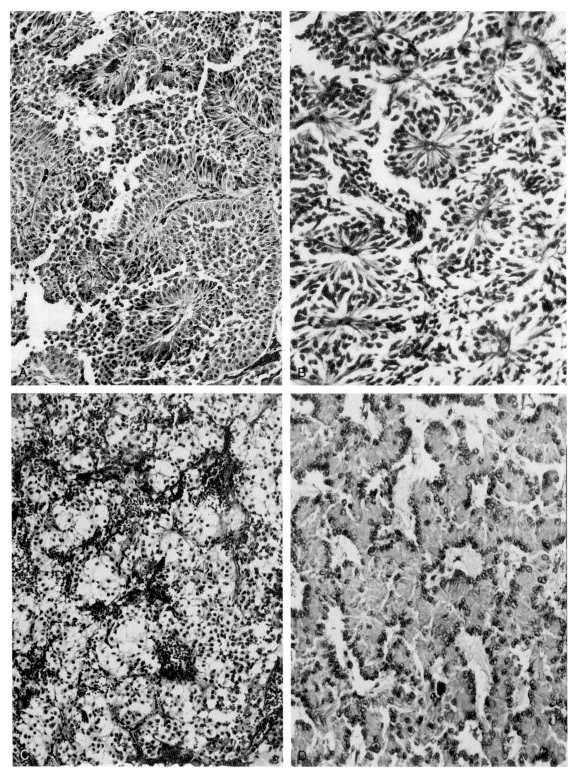

**FIGURE 9–33** PITUITARY ADENOMA

*A*, This neoplasm assumes a papillary pattern, and some cells possess long cytoplasmic processes. *B*, Cytoplasmic processes insert into blood vessels and simulate the perivascular pseudorosettes of ependymoma. *C*, Cytoplasmic clearing, an uncommon feature, mimics oligodendroglioma. *D*, Festoons, an infrequent pattern, lend a distinct neuroendocrine quality.

**FIGURE 9–34** PITUITARY ADENOMA

Compared with smears or touch preparations of normal pituitary (*left*), many cells are shed from adenomas (*right*). Adenoma nuclei possess less delicate chromatin and exhibit somewhat larger, less regular nucleoli. Pleomorphism and multinucleation, although uncommon, may be encountered, particularly in growth hormone cell adenomas. In addition, the cytoplasm of adenoma cells is tinctorially uniform. The presence of a mitotic figure in the adenoma smear (*right*) clearly indicates the neoplastic nature of the lesion.

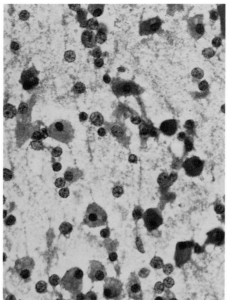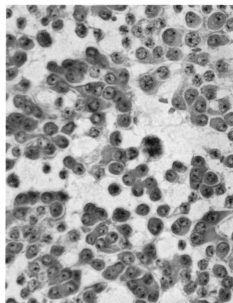

**FIGURE 9–35** HISTOLOGIC ARTIFACTS IN PITUITARY ADENOMA AND THE NORMAL PITUITARY

Adenohypophyseal cells, both adenomatous and normal, are sensitive to crush artifact. The affected cells may become so condensed and hyperchromatic as to mimic those of a small cell malignancy (*left*). Also unsightly is a suction artifact in normal pituitary tissue by which acini are evacuated and "empty" in histologic sections (*right*).

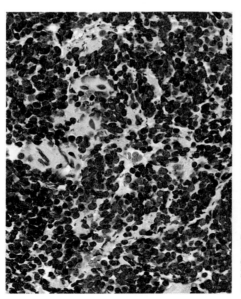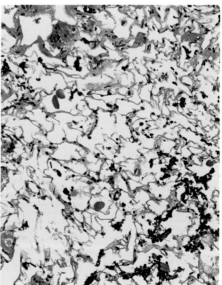

**TABLE 9–2**
**Histologic Classification of Adenohypophysial Tumors: 2000 WHO Classification**

1. Adenoma
    1.1. Typical                          8140/0
    1.2 Atypical                          8140/1
2. Carcinoma                            8010/3
3. Soft tissue tumors
    3.1. Postirradiation sarcoma
    3.2. Benign soft tissue tumors
4. Secondary tumors
5. Tumor-like lesions
    5.1. Pituitary hyperplasia
    5.2. Rathke cleft cyst
    5.3. Lymphocytic hypophysitis
    5.4. Giant cell granuloma

From Scheithauer BW, Kovacs K, Horvath E, et al. Tumors of the adenohypophysis. In Solcia E, Kloppel G, Sobin LH (eds). Histologic Typing of Endocrine Tumors. The World Health Organization. Berlin: Springer, 2000, pp. 15–29, 75–90.

**TABLE 9–3**
**Immunohistochemical Classification of Adenohypophysial Tumors: 2000 WHO Classification**

| Principal Immunoreactivity | Secondary Immunoreactivity* |
|---|---|
| A. GH | PRL, α-SU(f), TSH, FSH, LH(i) |
| B. PRL | α-SU(i) |
| C. GH and PRL | α-SU(f), TSH(i) |
| D. ACTH | LH, α-SU(i) |
| E. TSH | α-SU(f), GH, PRL(i) |
| F. FSH/LH/α-SU | PRL, GH, ACTH(i) |
| G. Plurihormonal† | |
| H. Hormone immunonegative | |

* Secondary hormone immunoreactivities are commonly observed. Although most are not clinically expressed, the hormones may be biochemically detected in blood. i, infrequent; f, frequent.

† Combinations of immunoreactivities, the most common being GH-PRL-TSH and/or α-SU. Other combinations are rare, for example, ACTH-LH, GH-ACTH, PRL-TSH.

GH, growth hormone; PRL, prolactin; ACTH, adrenocorticotropic hormone; TSH, thyroid-stimulating hormone; FSH, follicle-stimulating hormone; LH, luteinizing hormone; α-SU, alpha-subunit.

From Scheithauer BW, Kovacs K, Horvath E, et al. Tumors of the adenohypophysis. In Solcia E, Kloppel G, Sobin LH (eds). Histologic Typing of Endocrine Tumors. The World Health Organization. Berlin: Springer, 2000, pp. 15–29, 75–90.

identifying the various functional subtypes of pituitary adenoma is clear. Immunocytologic and selective ultrastructural characterization of pituitary adenomas not only correlates with clinical and endocrinologic data but also provides information regarding their aggressive potential. Despite a current deemphasis on electron microscopy in the work-up of pituitary adenomas,[4] we find it an indispensable tool in the identification of several specific adenoma types. As some of these are aggressive and relatively unresponsive to conventional therapies, their identification is of clinical importance.[55, 56, 57] The essential clinicopathologic features of the various adenoma subtypes (Table 9–5) are individually discussed in the following subsections.

**TABLE 9–4**
**Ultrastructural Classification of Adenohypophysial Tumors: 2000 WHO Classification**

| Tumor Type | Ultrastructural Variant | Frequency (%)* |
|---|---|---|
| PRL cell adenoma | Densely granulated | 10–30 |
| | Sparsely granulated | 10–20 |
| GH cell adenoma | Sparsely granulated | 10–20 |
| | Densely granulated | 1 |
| Adenomas with GH and PRL cell differentiation | Mixed GH-PRL cell adenoma | 5 |
| | Mammosomatotroph cell adenoma | 2 |
| | Acidophil stem cell adenoma | 2 |
| ACTH cell adenoma | Densely granulated | 10 |
| | Sparsely granulated | 1 |
| | Crooke cell variant | 1 |
| LH-FSH cell adenoma | Male and female type | 10 |
| TSH cell adenoma | | 1 |
| Null cell adenoma | Nononcocytic | 10 |
| | Oncocytic | 5–10 |
| Other adenomas | Silent "corticotroph" subtype 1 | 2 |
| | Silent "corticotroph" subtype 2 | 1 |
| | Silent adenoma subtype 3 | 2 |
| | Plurimorphous adenomas, e.g., GH-PRL-TSH, PRL-ACTH | 1 |
| | Unclassified | <1% |

FSH, follicle-stimulating hormone; GH, growth hormone; LH, luteinizing hormone; PRL, prolactin; TSH, thyroid-stimulating hormone.

*Frequencies vary by institution and practice mode.

Modified from Scheithauer BW, Kovacs K, Horvath E, et al. Tumors of the adenohypophysis. In Solcia E, Kloppel G, Sobin LH (eds). Histologic Typing of Endocrine Tumors. The World Health Organization. Berlin: Springer, 2000, pp. 15–29, 75–90.

## TABLE 9–5
## Clinicopathologic Features of Pituitary Adenomas

| Tumor Type | Incidence (%) | Clinical | Staining* | Hormone | Blood | Immunostaining | Gross Features Size | Invasion |
|---|---|---|---|---|---|---|---|---|
| **PRL cell adenomas** | | | | | | | | |
| Sparsely granulated | 10–30 ⎫ | Amenorrhea/ galactorrhea Impotence | C | PRL | + | + | 35% micro 65% macro | 52% overall |
| Densely granulated | 1 ⎭ | | A | PRL | + | + | | |
| **GH cell adenomas** | | | | | | | | |
| Sparsely granulated | 5–10 ⎫ | Acromegaly/ gigantism | C-A | GH | + | + | 15% macro/ 85% macro | 50% overall |
| Densely granulated | 5–10 ⎭ | | A | GH | + | + | | |
| **Adenomas with combined GH and PRL cell features** | | | | | | | | |
| Mixed GH cell–PRL cell | 5 | Acromegaly or gigantism ± hyperprolactinemia | A/C | GH/PRL | +/+ | +/+ | 25% micro/ 72% macro | 31% overall |
| Mammosomatotroph | 2 | Acromegaly ± hyperprolactinemia | A | GH/PRL | +/+ | +/+ | Features similar to mixed GH cell–PRL cell adenoma | |
| Acidophil stem cell | 2 | Hyperprolactinemia or nonfunctional Occasional acromegaly | C | GH/PRL | ±/+ | +/+ | Usually invasive macroadenomas | |
| **ACTH cell adenomas** | | | | | | | | |
| Cushing's | 10 | Hypercortisolism | B | ACTH ± β-endorphin, β-LPH, MSH | + | − | 85% micro/ 15% macro | 10% 65% |
| Crook's cell | 0.5 | Hypercortisolism nonfunctioning | B | | ± | + | 80% macro | 70% |
| Silent | 2 | Mass symptoms, hypopituitarism | B-C | Endorphins and related compounds | − | + | 100% macro | 82% |
| Nelson's | 2 | Pigmentation Mass symptoms | B-C | ACTH ± β-endorphin, β-LPH, MSH | + | + | 30% micro/ 70% macro | 17% 64% |
| **LH-FSH adenoma** | 10 | Setting of hypogonadism Functionally silent, mass effects | C-B | FSH/LH, alpha subunit | − | + (± alpha subunit) | 100% macro | 21% |
| **TSH cell adenoma** | 1 | Setting of hypo- or hyperthyroidism | C-B | TSH | + | + (± alpha subunit) | Usually macro | 75% |
| **Plurihormonal adenoma** | 10 | Usually acromegaly ± hyperprolactinemia Glycoprotein hormone production rarely expressed | C-A | Usually GH/PRL/TSH, alpha subunit. Also includes other unusual combinations. | +/±/−/± | Usually +/+/+ | 25% micro/ 75% macro | 31% 59% |
| **Null cell** | 15–20 | | | | | | | |
| Nononcocytic | 10 | Visual symptoms Hypopituitarism Headaches | C | None ± mild PRL increase due to pituitary stalk compression | − | None or minimal glycoprotein hormone or other reactivities in occasional cells | 2% micro/ 98% macro | 42% overall |
| Oncocytic | 5 | | A | | − | | | |
| **Silent subtype III** | 3 | Mass effects; mimics prolactinoma in females | C to mild A | Variable | − | Low level reactivities for various hormones | Macro (males), Micro (females) | |

* A, acidophilic; B, basophilic; C, chromophobic.

† Micro, microadenoma (≤1 cm diameter); macro, macroadenoma (≥1 cm diameter).

ACTH, adrenocorticotropic hormone; FSH, follicle-stimulating hormone; GH, growth hormone; LH, luteinizing hormone; PRL, prolactin; TSH, thyroid-stimulating hormone.

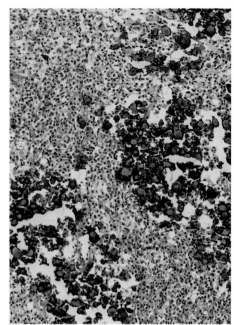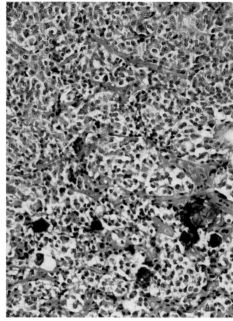

**FIGURE 9–36**    PROLACTIN CELL ADENOMA

These two chromophobic tumors typify the appearance of prolactin cell adenomas. Both exhibit calcospherite formation, occurring in approximately 10% to 20% of prolactinomas.

### Prolactin Cell Adenoma (Prolactinoma)

Prolactinomas are among the most common of pituitary adenomas and have been thoroughly characterized.[59, 129] Comprising up to 30% of all pituitary adenomas, their incidence has increased.[115] Most arise in women of reproductive age and occur with galactorrhea and/or amenorrhea.[115, 118] Because of the efficacy of dopamine agonists in the treatment of prolactinomas, their incidence in surgical series is decreasing. Fully half of pituitary adenomas incidentally encountered at autopsy are prolactinomas. Interestingly, these show no sex predilection.[100]

Clinical manifestations of prolactinoma vary with patient sex and age. Young women are exquisitely sensitive to hyperprolactinemia (amenorrhea, galactorrhea). As a result, their prolactinomas are often detected at the microadenoma stage. In postreproductive women and in men, prolactinomas are often functionally silent, coming to clinical attention only at the macroadenoma stage when hypopituitarism, symptomatic compression of the visual system, and invasion (cranial neuropathy, skull base destruction) become apparent.[17] In any case, serum PRL levels are elevated and roughly proportional to tumor size. Values above 150 ng/mL are nearly diagnostic of a PRL-producing adenoma. Elevations below this level may be nonspecific because any mass lesion, neoplastic or non-neoplastic, can produce hyperprolactinemia by compression of the pituitary stalk. Apparently, this interrupts the down-flow of dopamine, the principal PRL-inhibiting factor of the hypothalamus, with resultant release of PRL by normal lactotrophs.[84, 117, 118] In clinical parlance, any lesion causing elevations of PRL by this mechanism of "stalk section effect" is termed a "pseudoprolactinoma."[117]

In approximately 10% of cases, a diagnosis of PRL cell adenoma can be inferred from the presence of psam-momatous calcification on the H&E-stained section[89] (Fig. 9–36). When abundant, such calcification can transform the tumor into a gravel-like mass termed a "pituitary stone."[149] Calcification is rare in other forms of adenoma.[149] Far less frequent is massive amyloid deposition in the form of spherical, somewhat green bodies grossly resembling caviar[80, 82, 135] (Figs. 9–37 to 9–39). Their origin has been attributed to abnormal processing of PRL.[48] With rare exception,[12] such amyloid spheres are limited to prolactinomas. Interstitial (perivascular) and even crystalline forms of amyloid may be encountered in PRL-producing as well as in GH-producing adenomas.[82, 105]

In H&E-stained sections, most PRL cell adenomas are sparsely granulated. Such tumors appear either chro-

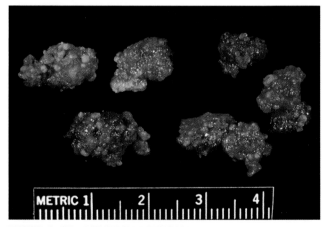

**FIGURE 9–37**    PITUITARY ADENOMA

Macroscopically resembling caviar, these multiple golden spherules of amyloid are a rare but virtually diagnostic feature of prolactin-producing adenomas.

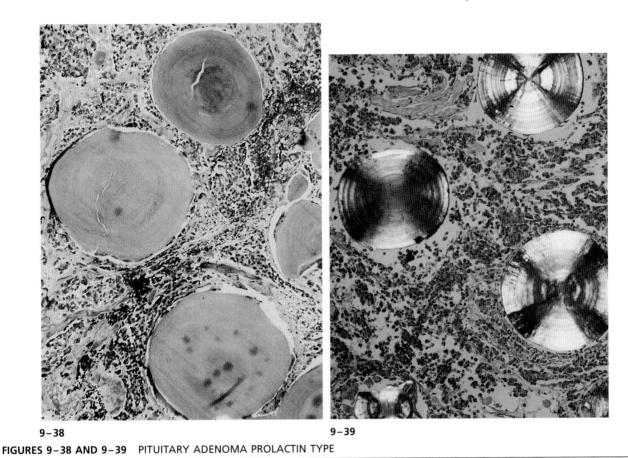

9–38                                    9–39

**FIGURES 9–38 AND 9–39**   PITUITARY ADENOMA PROLACTIN TYPE

The amyloid spheres grossly illustrated in Figure 9–37 are concentrically laminated eosinophilic bodies (Fig. 9–38) that exhibit birefringence when Congo red–stained sections are viewed with polarized light (Fig. 9–39).

mophobic (see Fig. 9–36) or somewhat basophilic because of the abundance of rough endoplasmic reticulum (Fig. 9–40). Densely granulated, acidophilic examples are rare. Immunoreactivity for PRL is typically paranuclear, a distribution corresponding to the Golgi zone[23, 46, 59] (Fig. 9–41). Ultrastructural features of diagnostic importance include abundance of rough endoplasmic reticulum and the presence of "misplaced" exocytosis, that is, extrusion of secretory granules between neoplastic cells rather than at their capillary interface (Fig. 9–42).

The prognosis for patients with prolactinomas has been related to tumor size and PRL level,[115] as well as to age and sex.[17, 115] As PRL levels rise, the likelihood of achieving a biochemical cure diminishes.[115] Whereas most microadenomas are amenable to gross total removal by the transsphenoidal route, prolactinomas are often invasive. Occasional tumors, particularly in postreproductive females and in males, are widely infiltrative of the skull base.

Bromocriptine, the most common dopamine agonist used to treat prolactinomas, has a dramatic effect on their morphology. Essentially, it produces atrophy of neoplastic cells with resultant tumor shrinkage. The "small cell" appearance induced is due to loss of cytoplasmic volume. Ultrastructurally, granules remain, but

synthetic organelles undergo involution and lysosomes accumulate. Long-term treatment often results in extensive tumoral fibrosis[8, 93, 104, 109, 143] (Fig. 9–43). Bromocriptine is not tumoricidal, and cessation of therapy results in adenoma regrowth.

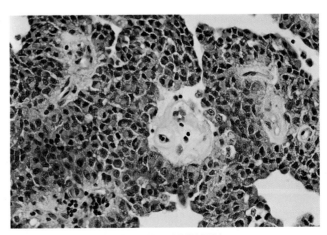

**FIGURE 9–40**   PROLACTIN CELL ADENOMA

Although most prolactin cell adenomas are chromophobic, sheer abundance of rough endoplasmic reticulum gives some a basophilic hue (H&E, ×400).

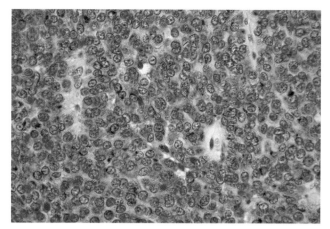

**FIGURE 9–41    PROLACTIN CELL ADENOMA**

The typical paranuclear distribution of immunoreactivity for prolactin corresponds to the Golgi region. Because of sparsity of secretory granules, the cytoplasm otherwise shows little staining.

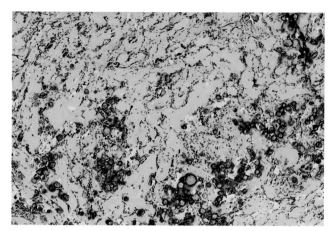

**FIGURE 9–43    BROMOCRIPTINE EFFECT UPON PROLACTIN CELL ADENOMA**

Note shrinkage of cytoplasm with resultant small cell appearance as well as stromal fibrosis. Overall, the tissue may suggest a malignancy.

## Growth Hormone Cell Adenoma

Approximately 10% to 20% of pituitary adenomas are GH producing. Significant clinicopathologic variation exists in the spectrum of these tumors.[59, 129] Virtually all are functional and associated with acromegaly or, less often,

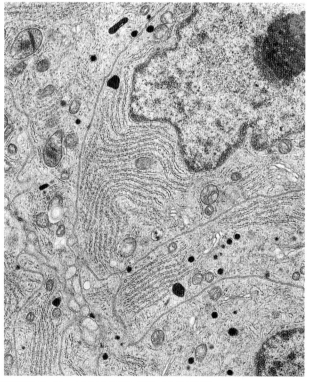

**FIGURE 9–42    PROLACTIN CELL ADENOMA**

This sparsely granulated neoplasm is a typical prolactinoma. Note the presence of well-developed rough endoplasmic reticulum and Golgi as well as sparse secretory granules, some of which are undergoing misplaced exocytosis (×8000). (Courtesy of Dr. E. Horvath, Toronto, Canada.)

gigantism.[84, 132] With equal frequency, GH cell adenomas are either densely or sparsely granulated, that is, acidophilic (Figs. 9–44 and 9–45) or chromophobic (Figs. 9–46 and 9–47). Most consist of patternless sheets of monomorphous cells. The majority of acromegaly-associated adenomas produce not only GH but also PRL, TSH, and alpha subunit. Thus, most GH-containing adenomas are actually plurihormonal.[58, 126] The various forms of plurihormonal adenomas are discussed separately in a following section. In adult patients, the secretory activity of GH-producing tumors causes acromegaly, whereas in childhood or adolescence the result is gigantism.[84, 132] Fundamental differences exist between the lesions responsible for these two disorders[154] (see Pituitary Hyperplasia, pages 472 to 473).

In the densely granulated or acidophilic variant, immunoreactivity for GH is strong and diffuse (see Fig. 7–44). It is this form of GH cell adenoma that most often coexpresses PRL and/or TSH or alpha subunit staining (see also Plurihormonal Adenomas, page 464). Ultrastructurally, the cells resemble normal GH cells and contain large numbers of secretory granules in the 300- to 600-nm range (see Fig. 7–40).[76, 93]

In contrast to the densely granulated variant, sparsely granulated or chromophobic tumors show often weak immunoreactivity for GH. Occasional examples are nearly devoid of staining. Fibrous bodies are a distinctive feature virtually diagnostic of GH-producing adenoma of the sparsely granulated type (see Fig. 9–46). These consist in large part of cytokeratin (see Fig. 9–46). Ultrastructurally, they are represented by paranuclear masses of whorled intermediate filaments[61, 76, 93] (see Fig. 9–47).

Although the clinical features and biochemical abnormalities associated with the eosinophilic and chromophobic variants of GH adenoma are similar, the latter are more aggressive. Multinucleation and nuclear pleomorphism occur more often in such adenomas, but are of no prognostic significance per se. In one large study, chromophobic lesions included no microadenomas and were considerably more invasive than their eosinophilic

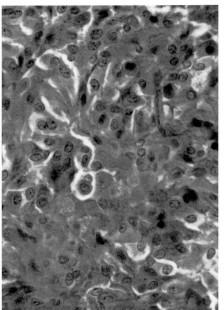
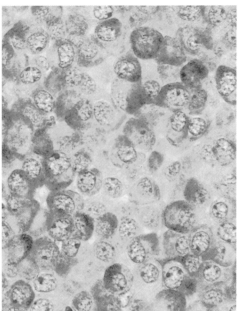

**FIGURE 9–44** DENSELY GRANULATED GROWTH HORMONE CELL ADENOMA

Approximately one half of somatotropic adenomas are strongly eosinophilic (*left*) because of their high content of cytoplasmic secretory granules. Immunoreactivity for growth hormone is uniformly strong in this variant (*right*).

counterparts.[119] This may be a manifestation of autocrine stimulation, because sparsely granulated GH cell adenomas often produce growth hormone–releasing hormone (GHRH).[140] As previously noted, interstitial amyloid deposition may be evident in GH-producing adenomas.[82, 105]

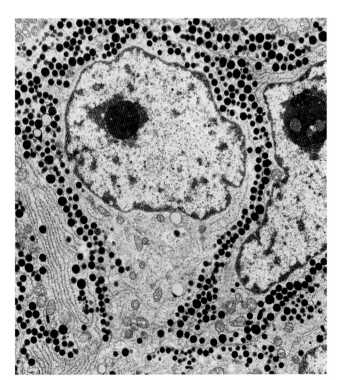

**FIGURE 9–45**   DENSELY GRANULATED GROWTH HORMONE CELL ADENOMA

In this form of growth hormone cell adenoma, the cells contain sizable secretory granules with tight-fitting membranes. No fibrous bodies, such as are seen in sparsely granulated somatotropic tumors, are identified (×5500). (Courtesy of Dr. E. Horvath, Toronto, Canada.)

## Adenomas Producing Both Growth Hormone and Prolactin

As previously noted, relatively few adenomas associated with either acromegaly or gigantism produce GH alone. An important subgroup of three adenoma types also produce PRL.[59, 129] These include (1) mixed GH cell–PRL cell adenoma, (2) mammosomatotroph cell adenoma, and (3) acidophil stem cell adenoma. With the exception of acidophil stem cell adenoma, their predominant clinical manifestation is GH excess. If expressed at all, the effects of hyperprolactinemia are minor.

**Mixed GH Cell–PRL Cell Adenomas.** This rather uncommon lesion is a true mixed tumor, being composed of two cell types, eosinophilic (densely granulated) and chromophobic (sparsely granulated) cells (Fig. 9–48), corresponding to GH cells and PRL cells[20, 59, 93, 129] (Figs. 9–49 and 9–50) Clinically, these adenomas cause acromegaly and are generally indolent in behavior. Although PRL elevation is a feature, the mere presence of hyperprolactinemia in association with a GH-producing adenoma is not hard evidence of a mixed tumor. As previously noted, it may be the result of stalk section effect. Mixed GH cell–PRL cell adenomas must be distinguished from the more "primitive" and aggressive acidophil stem cell adenoma (see later). Their separation from mammosomatotroph and plurihormonal adenomas (see below) is of less consequence.

**Mammosomatotroph Cell Adenoma.** This unusual, variably acidophilic, GH- and PRL-producing adenoma is composed of a single cell type.[29, 59, 76, 129] Its unique ultrastructural features, which include large (1000 to 1500 nm), ovoid to irregular secretory granules as well as extrusion of granules of uneven, mottled texture, are intermediate between those of GH and PRL cells. Immunostains show generalized reactivity for both hormones.

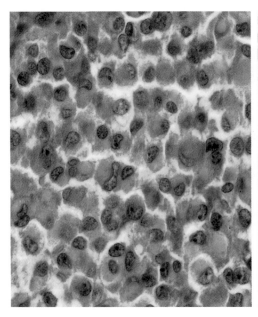

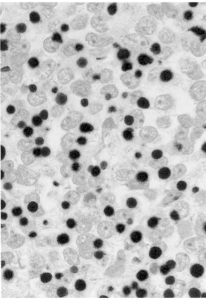

**FIGURE 9–46** SPARSELY GRANULATED GROWTH HORMONE CELL ADENOMA

In contrast to the densely granulated neoplasm illustrated in Figure 9–44, the cytoplasm in this variant is poorly granulated (*left*). In addition, careful examination reveals the presence of paranuclear eosinophilic fibrous bodies. The latter are immunoreactive for cytokeratin (*right*, CAM 5.2).

Unlike acidophil stem cell adenoma, an often invasive macroadenoma usually unassociated with GH effects, mammosomatotroph cell adenomas are clinically indolent and cause acromegaly.[29] Endocrine signs of hyperprolactinemia may also be evident. Mammosomatotroph cells have been shown to play an important role in the development of gigantism.[154]

**Acidophil Stem Cell Adenoma.** This rare form of adenoma represents about 2% of GH-producing tumors. Conceptually, it is a neoplasm of stem cells of the acidophil (GH and PRL cell) line.[55, 59, 76, 129] It may be clinically nonfunctioning, but it is more often associated with hyperprolactinemia. Unlike in prolactinomas, PRL levels are disproportionately low in comparison with tumor size. Because GH levels are often normal, signs of GH excess are uncommon. Acidophil stem cell adenomas are generally chromophobic. Careful examination of a well-fixed specimen occasionally shows cytoplasmic vacuoles corresponding to the presence of giant mitochondria

**FIGURE 9–47** SPARSELY GRANULATED GROWTH HORMONE CELL ADENOMA

The fibrous bodies of sparsely granulated growth hormone cell adenomas represent intermediate filament whorls (cytokeratin). Contrast the sparse granularity of this tumor with that of the densely granulated variant in Figure 9–45 (×5500).

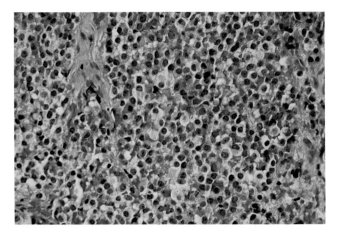

**FIGURE 9–48** MIXED GROWTH HORMONE AND PROLACTIN CELL ADENOMA

Composed of densely granulated GH cells and sparsely granulated PRL cells, this cytologically heterogenous adenoma may be mistaken for normal pituitary on a small biopsy. A reticulin stain would demonstrate loss of acinar architecture.

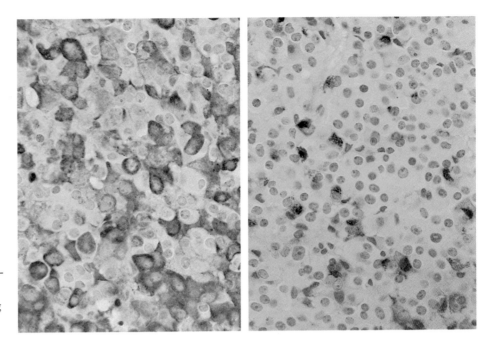

**FIGURE 9–49** MIXED GROWTH HORMONE AND PROLACTIN CELL ADENOMA

Immunostaining for GH (*left*) and PRL (*right*) is evident in separate cells. Note diffuse cytoplasmic staining of GH cells and paranuclear Golgi zone reactivity of PRL cells.

(Figs. 9–51 and 9–52), a neither constant nor specific feature. Immunoreactivity for PRL generally exceeds that for GH, but neither reaction is strong. Ultra-structurally, the less than fully differentiated cells show some features of both GH- and PRL-producing cells. Respectively, these include fibrous bodies and misplaced exocytoses.[55, 59, 129] Oncocytic change is also common. The recognition of acidophil stem cell adenomas is important because they are prone to inexorable growth and invasive behavior. Interestingly, mitotic activity is infrequent and MIB-1 labeling indices are often not high. Bromocriptine treatment for what is mistakenly presumed to be a prolactinoma is often ineffective.[55]

### ACTH Cell Adenomas

Three clinical subtypes of ACTH producing adenoma are recognized within this well-characterized

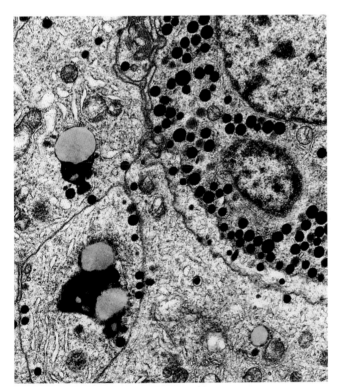

**FIGURE 9–50** MIXED GROWTH HORMONE CELL–PROLACTIN CELL ADENOMA

This uncommon adenoma is composed of two distinct cell types: densely granulated growth hormone cells (*top right*) and sparsely granulated lactotrophs (seen throughout the remainder of the microscopic field). The latter are engaged in misplaced exocytosis of secretory granules (×8400). (Courtesy of Dr. E. Horvath, Toronto, Canada.)

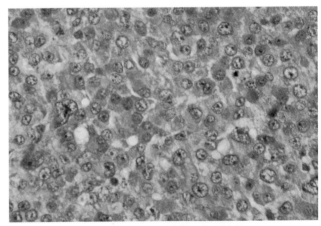

**FIGURE 9–51** ACIDOPHILIC STEM CELL ADENOMA

On routine H&E stains this rare aggressive form of growth hormone- and prolactin-producing adenoma occasionally shows paranuclear vacuoles that correspond to markedly enlarged mitochondria. The latter are best seen at the ultrastructural level.

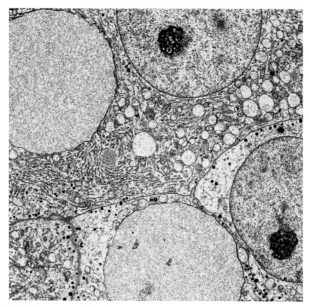

**FIGURE 9–52**   ACIDOPHILIC STEM CELL ADENOMA

The intracytoplasmic vacuoles seen by light microscopy in Figure 9–51 are recognized ultrastructurally as markedly enlarged mitochondria (×7200). Such tumors are monomorphous but typically show ultrastructural features of growth hormone (fibrous bodies) and prolactin cell differentiation (misplaced exocytosis). (Courtesy of Dr. E. Horvath, Toronto, Canada.)

family of lesions.[59, 129] They are (1) tumors underlying pituitary-based ACTH excess (Cushing's disease),[59, 86, 92, 120, 121, 124, 129, 150] (2) similar but often more aggressive adenomas in patients having previously undergone adrenalectomy (Nelson's syndrome),[124, 150] and (3) so-called silent corticotropic adenomas of subtypes I and II, which, for reasons unclear, are unassociated with biochemical or clinical evidence of cortisol excess.[52, 128]

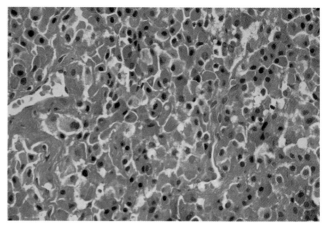

**FIGURE 9–53**   ACTH CELL ADENOMA

This functioning Cushing's disease–associated adenoma is typically amphophilic to basophilic because of its significant granule content.

**Adenomas of Cushing's Disease.** Classical basophilic adenomas of Cushing's disease are microadenomas and constitute about 10% of all pituitary adenomas.[59] Most occur in women (sex ratio 5:1) and exhibit high hormonal activity. When untreated, they may be lethal as a consequence of cortisol excess. With H&E stain, the cells of Cushing's adenomas are amphophilic to basophilic (Fig. 9–53) and are PAS-positive (Fig. 9–54). Mitoses are rare, and the MIB-1 labeling index is low. Massive spherical amyloid deposition is rarely seen.[12] ACTH immunoreactivity varies but may be strong (Fig. 9–54). Other peptides derived from pro-opiomelanocortin, the precursor of ACTH, may also be produced. These include beta-endorphin, beta LPH, CLIP, and melanocyte-stimulating hormone. Gonadotropic hormone or alpha subunit production is infrequently also seen.[10, 125]

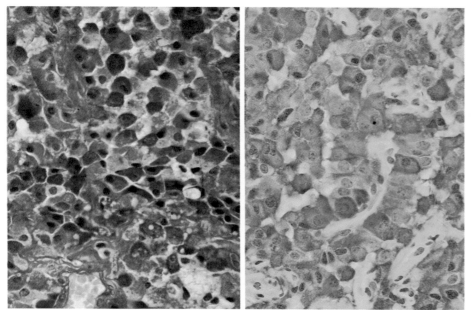

**FIGURE 9–54**   CORTICOTROPH CELL ADENOMA

Histochemical staining by the PAS method (*left*) as well as ACTH immunoreactivity (*right*) varies considerably in such tumors. Here it is variable, correlating with differing degrees of cytoplasmic granularity.

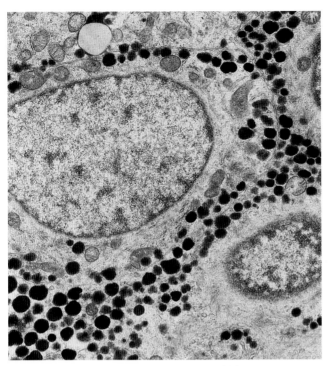

**FIGURE 9–55    CORTICOTROPH CELL ADENOMA**

This tumor from a patient with Cushing's syndrome shows the two principal characteristics of corticotroph cells: the presence of perinuclear cytokeratin microfilament bundles and somewhat pleomorphic, indented or teardrop-shaped granules of varying electron density (×8500). (Courtesy of Dr. E. Horvath, Toronto, Canada.)

At the ultrastructural level, most tumors are densely granulated and resemble normal corticotrophs containing variably electron-dense, teardrop- or heart-shaped secretory granules, as well as perinuclear bundles of intermediate filaments (cytokeratin)[59, 129] (Fig. 9–55).

The very size of these adenomas poses diagnostic problems. Because 85% are microadenomas, some as small as 2 mm, they may be undetectable by neuroradiologic methods and difficult to find at surgery. Furthermore, only a small part of the specimen may represent tumor. Thus, failure to identify an adenoma by frozen sections should prompt retrieval and processing of the contents of the suction bottle, superficial cutting of paraffin blocks in order to avoid waste, and perhaps systematic leveling of the block to ensure thorough sampling of the specimen. We also find that PAS and reticulin preparations complement ACTH immunostains in maximizing the recognition of adenoma tissue. A note of caution: because ACTH cells often lie clustered in the normal gland (see Fig. 9–9), it may be difficult to distinguish such nodules from neoplasm in small, fragmented specimens. It is here that the issue of distinguishing adenoma from pituitary hyperplasia, a rare cause of Cushing's disease, comes into play. The issue is discussed further in the Pituitary Hyperplasia section (page 472).

Crooke's hyaline change, a conspicuous finding in non-neoplastic pituitary tissue surrounding an ACTH-producing adenoma, is a response to glucocorticoid excess. It consists of massive perinuclear accumulation of keratin microfilaments in corticotrophs.[59] Doughnut-like, the pale-staining, hyaline ring of cytokeratin encircles the nucleus and centrally displaces organelles (Figs. 9–56 and 9–57). The degree of Crooke's cell formation varies from case to case; it is difficult to find in some instances and conspicuous in others. Posterior lobe basophils do not undergo this change. The suggestion that absence of Crooke's hyaline change is associated with adenoma recurrence[43] remains to be confirmed. On occasion, Crooke's change is seen in the cells of ACTH adenomas[28, 36, 59, 129] (Fig. 9–58), a finding that suggests the presence of cortisol receptors on the neoplastic cells. Such "Crooke's cell adenomas" represent about 2% of Cushing's adenomas and 4% of silent corticotroph adenomas and behave in an aggressive manner.[36] Although most occur with Cushing's disease, an occasional example is silent, manifesting as mass effects or psychiatric symptoms.[78]

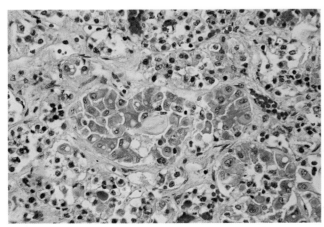
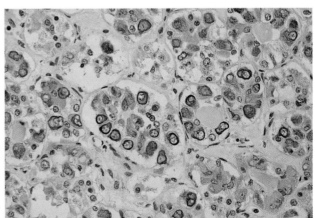

9–56                9–57

**FIGURES 9–56 AND 9–57    CROOKE'S HYALINE CHANGE**

In the setting of Cushing's syndrome, ACTH cells of the extratumoral pituitary acquire a circumnuclear band of hyalin or faintly fibrillar material termed Crooke's hyalin (Fig. 9–56). This band-like mass of cytokeratin filaments is more apparent on ACTH staining (Fig. 9–57).

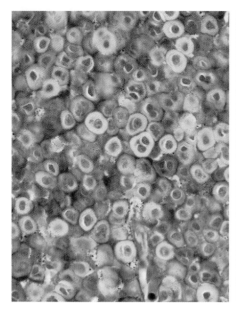
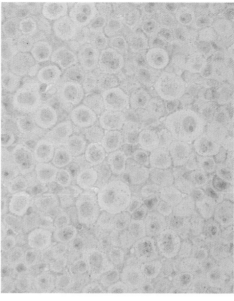

**FIGURE 9–58    CROOKE'S CELL ADENOMA**

A small minority of ACTH cell adenomas, the majority associated with Cushing's disease, exhibit Crooke's hyaline change. Such tumors are aggressive (*left*, PAS; *right*, ACTH). Note the prominent nonstaining bands of hyaline change in both preparations.

As previously noted, typical ACTH cell adenomas associated with Cushing's disease are small and nonaggressive. In the Mayo Clinic experience, the majority (85%) are microadenomas; of these only 10% are invasive and all but a few (<5%) are cured by transsphenoidal resection. Macroadenomas make up the remaining 15% and are frequently (65%) invasive. Often chromophobic and only weakly PAS positive, they have less pronounced hormonal activity than the smaller, basophilic adenomas. Not surprisingly, tumor size and invasiveness contribute significantly to persistent or recurrent Cushing's disease. In a minority of cases, failure to achieve remission is due to concurrent ACTH cell hyperplasia (see Pituitary Hyperplasia section, page 472).

**Adenomas of Nelson's Syndrome.** In the past more than at present, radiologic work-up of patients with Cushing's syndrome occasionally failed to reveal an adenoma. As a result, adrenalectomy was performed to remove what was ostensibly primary adrenocortical hyperplasia. Thereafter, no longer exposed to the inhibitory effects of circulating glucocorticoids, an undetected microadenoma was free to grow unsuppressed.[124, 146] The majority of "Nelson's adenomas" progress to become invasive macroadenomas. Approximately 20% of patients die of the local, aggressive effects of the tumor. With advances in neuroimaging, even small Cushing's adenomas are now being discovered. As a result, few patients are subjected to adrenalectomy for primary control of the disease. Nelson's syndrome is disappearing.

**Silent Corticotroph Cell Adenomas.** Approximately 10–15% of corticotroph cell adenomas are unaccompanied by elevations in ACTH or clinical evidence of Cushing's disease.[52, 59, 128, 129] Possible explanations for this phenomenon include (1) inability of the tumor to secrete ACTH, (2) secretion of an ACTH-like molecule either undetected by routine laboratory testing or lacking bioactivity, or (3) a shift to the production of pro-opiomelanocortin derivatives that share the immunoreactivity of ACTH but differ in their endocrine effects. The last is the most likely explanation.[46] The cytogenesis of silent corticotroph adenomas is unclear, but an origin in intermediate corticotrophs is likely.[53]

Unlike the adenomas of Cushing's disease, silent corticotroph adenomas attain large size and are frequently invasive,[52, 128] the figure being 82% in one large series.[128] These adenomas occur in two types that differ considerably in their degree of differentiation. Designated subtypes I and II, they range from basophilic to chromophobic, strongly to weakly PAS and ACTH positive, and densely to sparsely granulated, respectively[129] (Fig. 9–59). A Mayo Clinic study clarified the differences between tumors of types I and II.[128] They are

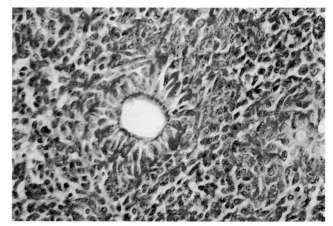

**FIGURE 9–59    SILENT CORTICOTROPH CELL ADENOMA**

A small minority of corticotropic adenomas, despite PAS positivity and immunoreactivity for pro-opiomelanocortin–derived hormones including ACTH, are clinically nonfunctioning. Such tumors are more aggressive than ordinary Cushing's adenomas (PAS).

related to gender (male/female ratio 6:1 versus 1.7:1), frequency of radiographic or gross invasion (44% versus 71%), and postoperative pituitary failure (38% versus 86%). MIB-1 proliferation indices did not differ, the mean being less than 1% in both types. Silent corticotropic tumors rarely metastasize.[128]

Once thought to be a third variant of silent corticotropic adenoma, the silent subtype III adenoma is now considered a distinct entity (see later). Such tumors may produce not only small quantities of ACTH but also a variety of other pituitary hormones.[57]

### Glycoprotein Adenomas

This group of tumors includes gonadotropic (FSH-LH) and thyrotropic (TSH) adenomas.[59, 129] Both are characterized by the production of hormones that consist of a PAS-positive carbohydrate component as well as two amino acid chains, a 92-amino-acid alpha subunit common to all glycoprotein hormones, and a longer beta subunit that underlies functional specificity. Serum elevation of alpha subunit is often seen, not only in glycoprotein adenomas but also in GH-plurihormonal and null cell adenomas.[10] Its secretion is unassociated with physiologic effects. A word of caution is in order regarding the interpretation of glycoprotein immunostains. Extensive homology in beta subunits, coupled with virtual identity of the alpha subunits, results in some tendency to cross-reactivity.

**Gonadotroph Cell Adenoma.** Representing 10% of pituitary adenomas, gonadotrophic tumors are the principal form of glycoprotein adenoma.[50, 59, 129, 145, 152] They presumably arise from LH- or FSH-secreting cells scattered throughout the normal gland. All are macroadenomas, but with an invasion rate as low as 20%.[152] As a rule, they occur in the elderly, most often in males. Endocrine hypofunction is common, as are mass effects such as headache, visual disturbance, and cranial nerve palsies. Because elevation of gonadotropic hormones is normal in aged females, the contribution of tumoral secretion is difficult to assess in this population.

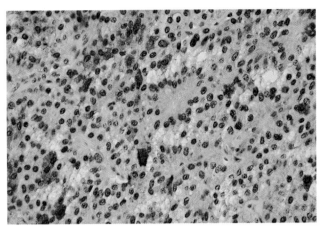

**FIGURE 9-61   GONADOTROPH CELL ADENOMA**

Immunoreactivity for FSH and/or LH is generally patchy and varies in strength (FSH).

Sparsely granulated and thus chromophobic, many show a tendency to perivascular pseudorosette formation and/or oncocytic change (Fig. 9-60). Delicate, stippled PAS positivity is commonly seen beneath the cell membrane and corresponds to the pattern of granule distribution. Staining for FSH and/or LH is highly variable and often patchy (Fig. 9-61). The same is true of alpha subunit reactivity. Chromogranin is a reliable feature of gonadotropic adenomas as well as other tumors containing glycoprotein hormone–producing cells, for example, plurihormonal GH as well as null cell adenomas.

Ultrastructurally, gonadotroph adenomas vary greatly in differentiation.[50, 59, 78, 129, 152] Only a minority of gonadotroph adenomas resemble normal gonadotrophs in being distinctly PAS positive, strongly LH or FSH immunoreactive, and endowed with medium size (up to 450 nm) secretory granules. Yet others are nearly indistinguishable from null cell adenomas. For reasons unknown, the tumors of most female patients feature a distinctive "honeycomb" Golgi complex.[50, 59, 129] In the Mayo Clinic experience, postoperative normalization of the pituitary-gonadal axis and of visual function was low (22% and 30%), but the same was true of the need for reoperation (8%).[148]

**Thyrotroph Cell Adenoma.** Thyrotropin-producing tumors are the least common (1%) of pituitary adenomas.[27, 37, 40, 59, 66, 129] The majority arise in the setting of hypothyroidism and are probably preceded by TSH cell hyperplasia,[27, 66] a subject discussed later. They occur at all ages and with no sex predilection. Only a small proportion elevate TSH levels and cause hyperthyroidism.[37, 40] The majority of thyrotroph cell adenomas (75%) are invasive macroadenomas.[130]

Histologically, thyrotropic adenomas are composed of often elongated, weakly PAS-positive cells engaged in pseudorosette formation (Fig. 9-62). The TSH reaction is variable and alpha subunit staining is commonly seen (see Fig. 9-62). Only a minority of tumors are somewhat basophilic and PAS positive. Occasional lesions are markedly sclerotic. Ultrastructurally, synthetic organelles

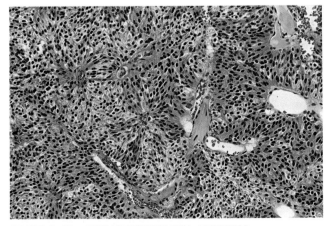

**FIGURE 9-60   GONADOTROPH CELL ADENOMA**

Perivascular pseudorosette formation and oncocytic change are common features.

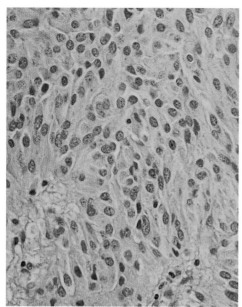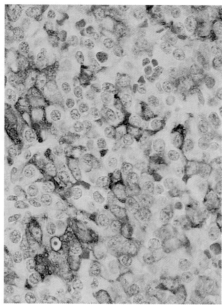

**FIGURE 9–62** THYROTROPH CELL ADENOMA

This rare form of adenoma often features elongated cells (*left*) that vary in TSH immunoreactivity (*right*).

are abundant and secretory granules are few and small (200 nm).[59, 129] Other features include sizable lysosomes and cell processes containing microtubules.

As noted earlier in the discussion of plurihormonal GH cell adenomas, TSH immunoreactivity occasionally predominates and ultrastructural studies reveal largely or only thyrotropic cells.[58, 59, 76, 126, 129]

### Plurihormonal Adenomas

Adenomas producing combinations of major hormone types, that is, amino acid (GH, PRL, ACTH) and glycoprotein (LH, FSH, TSH, alpha subunit) hormones, are termed plurihormonal.[58, 59, 126, 129] Most are associated with acromegaly. As previously noted, such plurihormonal GH-producing adenomas may show greater light microscopic and ultrastructural variation than tumors making GH alone.[58, 59, 76, 126, 129] Ultrastructurally, some consist entirely of densely granulated GH cells, whereas others also feature PRL and/or glycoprotein cells, usually thyrotrophs. Despite their frequent content of TSH, it is rarely secreted or clinically expressed. In contrast, alpha subunit levels are often increased.[10]

Plurihormonal adenomas of other immunotypes are less common. Examples include ACTH-LH-alpha subunit, LH/FSH-ACTH-β-endorphin, LH/FSH-PRL, GH-ACTH, and PRL-TSH.[26, 125, 126]

### Silent Adenoma, Subtype III

The cellular derivation of this adenoma is indeterminate. Once considered a subtype of silent corticotroph adenoma, it now occupies a distinct nosologic niche.[57, 59, 129] No sex predilection is seen. When it occurs in young women, it often mimics prolactinoma. Dopamine agonist therapy normalizes serum PRL levels through suppression of normal lactotrophs but does not affect tumor growth.[57] In men, the tumors occur as functionally silent macroadenomas. Often diffuse or lobular in pattern, this chromophobic or slightly acidophilic tumor consists of large cells with mild nuclear pleomorphism and delicate, PAS-positive granules. Minor immunopositivity for any combination of pituitary hormones may be seen. A minority of lesions are entirely immunonegative. Unlike null cell adenomas, however, they are shown ultrastructurally to be highly differentiated tumors with some resemblance to glycoprotein hormone–producing adenomas. The pleomorphic nuclei often contain conspicuous spheridia. The abundant cytoplasm is richly endowed with rough and smooth endoplasmic reticulin, often a prominent Golgi apparatus, and numerous mitochondria. Secretory granules are sparse and small (200 nm) (Fig. 9–63). Inexorable growth and a distinct tendency to invasion make it important to recognize this uncommon tumor.

### Null Cell Adenomas

Null cell adenomas constitute 15–25% of all pituitary adenomas and the majority of nonfunctioning tumors.[25, 59, 75, 129] Many are immunonegative for pituitary hormones or show only scant glycoprotein hormone or alpha subunit production.[5, 10, 14, 73, 96] Being macroadenomas, they clinically present with mass effects and hypopituitarism.

Histologically, most null cell adenomas are chromophobic (Figs. 9–64 and 9–65); a minority are oncocytic (Figs. 9–66 and 9–67). Chromophobic tumors are similar to other sparsely granulated adenomas and cannot be distinguished without the use of immunohistochemistry. Similarly, oncocytic change is not specific to null cell adenoma, being seen in acidophil stem cell, silent ACTH cell, and gonadotroph cell adenomas as well. At the ultrastructural level, null cell tumors possess little in

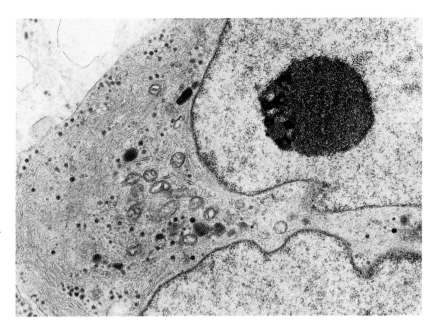

**FIGURE 9–63**   SILENT CORTICOTROPH ADENOMA, SUBTYPE III

Of unknown cellular derivation, this adenoma features nuclear pleomorphism and occasional spheridia, as well as organelle-rich cytoplasm in-cluding not only rough but also smooth endo-plas-mic reticulum. Secretory granules are sparse and small (×7700). (Courtesy of Dr. E. Horvath, Toronto, Canada.)

the way of synthetic organelles and only few small granules.[59, 75, 129] The cytogenesis of null cell adenomas is un-settled,[75] but there is evidence to suggest a relationship to the family of glycoprotein adenomas.[5, 10, 14, 73]

Like gonadotroph cell adenomas, null cell adenomas show a relatively low (40%) rate of invasion[130] and be-have in an indolent fashion.[25, 31]

### Pituitary Adenomas with Neuronal Metaplasia

On rare occasion, ganglion cells occur in pituitary adenomas. Most, but not all,[7, 35, 88, 123] are GH-producing and functional.[7, 35, 54, 76, 88, 117, 131, 144] Evidence indicates that they are not developmental malformations, a once popular notion,[7, 131] but a manifestation of neuronal metaplasia of adenoma cells.[54] In support of this concept

are (1) lack of pituitary hyperplasia that should accompany excess GHRH production, (2) immunohistochemical and ultrastructural studies demonstrating cells with transitional features, and (3) demonstrable GHRH in some GH-producing pituitary adenomas.[87, 140]

Morphologically, ganglion cells may be few or numerous and accompanied by variable amounts of

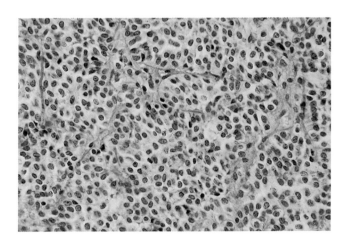

**FIGURE 9–64**   NULL CELL ADENOMA

The chromophobic variant of this nonfunctioning adenoma is virtually nonreactive for the full spectrum of pituitary hormones. At most, it shows alpha subunit or mild focal glycoprotein hormone immunoreactivity.

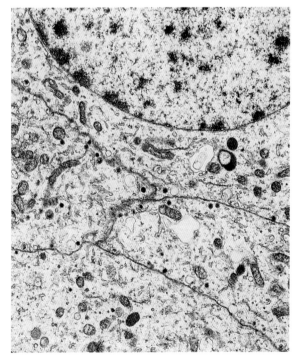

**FIGURE 9–65**   NULL CELL ADENOMA

This rather poorly differentiated tumor contains only rudimentary Golgi complexes, scattered profiles of rough endoplasmic reticulum, and a few minute scattered secretory granules (×7700). (Courtesy of Dr. E. Horvath, Toronto, Canada.)

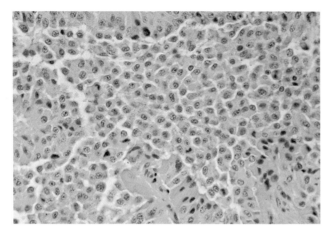

**FIGURE 9–66**   NULL CELL ADENOMA, ONCOCYTIC VARIANT

Like ordinary null cell adenomas, this lesion is largely devoid of anterior pituitary hormones. Loosely termed pituitary oncocytoma, it owes its eosinophilia and apparent granularity to the accumulation of mitochondria.

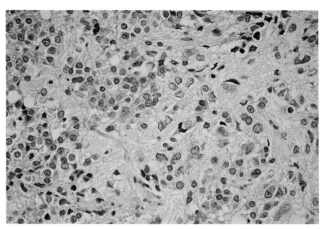

**FIGURE 9–68**   NEURONAL METAPLASIA IN PITUITARY ADENOMA

This rare lesion consists of a mixture of adenoma cells, neurons, and cells with intermediate features. Note the presence of neuropil.

neuropil (Fig. 9–68). In most cases, adenoma cells lie clustered among the neurons. Transitional cells feature ample cytoplasm and vesicular nuclei with a sizable central nucleolus. As in other ganglion cell lesions, binucleation may be observed. Fully developed neurons feature varying amounts of Nissl substance as well as processes. Neurons exhibit not only the hormone immunoprofile of the adenoma cells (Fig. 9–69), including epithelial markers (cytokeratin), but also neuronal markers (class III beta tubulin and occasionally neurofilament protein).[127] Nerve growth factor receptor has also been demonstrated in both adenoma cells and neurons.[127] Ultrastructural studies have clearly documented the transition of adenoma to ganglion cells.[54, 127] With the rare exception of one pituitary carcinoma in which the primary tumor was neuron containing,[127] the behavior of tumors showing neuronal metaplasia is benign and like that of ordinary adenomas. This was even true of one example in which the neuronal element appeared immature or "neuroblastic."[81]

## Differential Diagnosis of Pituitary Adenoma

First and foremost, the differential diagnosis of pituitary adenoma must include normal or compressed anterior pituitary tissue. The distinction is of obvious importance

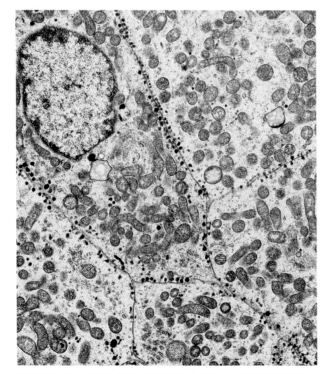

**FIGURE 9–67**   NULL CELL ADENOMA, ONCOCYTIC VARIANT

This mitochondrion-rich tumor with poorly developed synthetic organelles contains only occasional, small secretory granules (×5500). (Courtesy of Dr. E. Horvath, Toronto, Canada.)

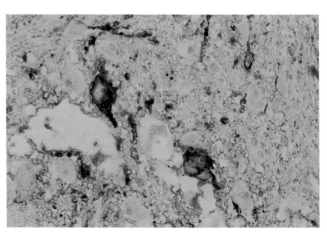

**FIGURE 9–69**   NEURONAL METAPLASIA IN PITUITARY ADENOMA

The PRL produced in this adenoma is also seen in the neurons (immunostain for PRL).

but may be difficult in the sometimes minute specimens obtained by transsphenoidal surgery. Although adenomas are characterized by cellular monotony, at high magnification even fragments of normal gland may appear monomorphous. This is particularly true of specimens from the lateral wings, where GH cells abound (see Fig. 9–8). In other portions of the gland, the usual mix of acidophilic, basophilic, and chromophobic cells is more obvious, but even this may be obscured in frozen sections. Good-quality permanent sections stained with H&E usually reveal not only cytologic variation but also the normal pattern of acini encompassed by delicate capillaries. In contrast, adenoma tissue lacks the acinar pattern. The distinction between normal tissue and adenoma is also obvious with reticulin stains on frozen[1, 147] or permanent sections (see Figs. 9–7 and 9–19). Lastly, because the nuclear/cytoplasmic ratio in adenomas may be higher than that of normal cells, sections of adenomas often look somewhat "bluer."

A number of tumors, some very rare, enter into the differential diagnosis of pituitary adenoma. These include mainly monomorphous or small cell tumors of the sellar region, such as metastatic carcinoma,[16] plasmacytoma,[11, 146] lymphoma, meningioma,[37, 133] germinoma,[33, 109] paraganglioma,[11, 153] and glomangioma.[6] Carcinoma metastatic to pituitary adenoma has been reported on more than one occasion.[103, 114] Even rare salivary gland tumors primary in the sellar region enter into the differential.[44] Although pituitary adenomas may closely resemble oligodendroglioma and ependymoma, with the exception of pituicytoma, a rare astrocytic tumor (see Miscellaneous Neoplasms later), gliomas do not enter into the differential diagnosis of adenoma. Rathke's cleft cysts occasionally mimic adenoma, but only at the neuroimaging level.[123] As a rule, the sharply defined lesions with their mucinous contents create an image that clearly suggests a cyst.

The immunohistochemical features of these various neoplasms are summarized in Table 9–6. Although electron microscopy plays a role in the subclassification of adenomas, routine histochemical and immunostains usually suffice in the differential diagnosis with nonpituitary neoplasms.

### Treatment and Prognosis

As a rule, adenomas are surgically dealt with, the goal being total resection without postoperative adjuvant therapy. Most are approached by the transsphenoidal route. Craniotomy is reserved for large lesions showing significant suprasellar extension.

Despite the frequency of pituitary adenomas, precise correlation of their pathologic features with optimal therapy and prognosis remains to be established. Biochemical cure is a measure of success with functional adenomas, but success with nonfunctional or silent adenomas is more difficult to assess. Given the slow growth of pituitary adenomas,[83] particularly of nonfunctioning tumors, recurrence may not become apparent for years.[111] As a result, long periods of follow-up are required to establish associations between pathologic factors and outcome.[41, 115] Invasive and atypical adenomas

(see later) can be expected to recur with greater frequency and rapidity. The anticipated biologic behavior of the various adenoma subtypes was discussed previously.

A number of studies have attempted to correlate DNA content with tumor behavior.[3, 30, 32] Although aneuploidy is often seen in invasive, particularly functioning adenomas, its finding is of little prognostic significance.

Cytogenetic studies have sought to identify karyotypic patterns associated with aggressive behavior. In one series, abnormalities were found more often in hormonally functioning tumors than in null cell adenomas; most involved chromosomes 1, 4, 7, and 19.[122] Despite the fact that functioning tumors are more often invasive,[130] no significant differences in karyotype have been observed between invasive and noninvasive tumors.

## Invasive Adenoma

The reported frequency with which adenomas invade surrounding tissue, not simply pituitary parenchyma (Fig. 9–70) but dura and bone (Figs. 9–71 to 9–73), varies depending upon the means of assessment. Respective radiographic, surgically apparent, and microscopic invasion rates of 10%, 35%, and 85% have been reported.[136] We consider only radiographic or operative invasion to justify the term invasive adenoma (see Figs. 9–22 and 9–23).[63, 98, 130] Obviously, dural invasion is more frequent than involvement of cavernous sinus, sphenoid bone, or nasopharynx. Such invasion may be of prognostic significance, particularly with respect to biochemical cure, that is, postoperative normalization of hormone levels in functional adenomas. No doubt, osseous or cavernous sinus involvement more substantially increases the likelihood of recurrence. Because most surgical specimens consist only of tumor and contain little or no dura or bone, pathologists generally lack the opportunity to evaluate invasion.

There is another good reason why invasion should be determined radiographically and at surgery. The frequency

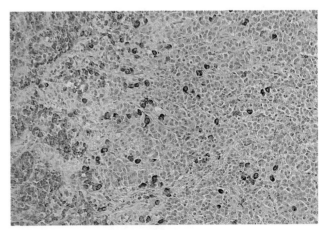

**FIGURE 9–70**  PITUITARY ADENOMA INVADING SURROUNDING ANTERIOR LOBE TISSUE

The tumor (*right*), a PRL cell adenoma, freely infiltrates among GH cells in the lateral wing of the gland. This common finding has no prognostic significance (immunostain for GH).

# TABLE 9–6
## Immunostaining in the Differential Diagnosis of Sellar and Perisellar Lesions

| Staining | Pituitary Adenoma* | Carcinoma | Melanoma | Germinoma | Meningioma | Chordoma | Olfactory Neuroblastoma | Lymphoma | Myeloma | Astrocytoma (Pituicytoma)/Oligodendroglioma/Ependymoma | Granular Cell Tumor | Paraganglioma | Schwannoma |
|---|---|---|---|---|---|---|---|---|---|---|---|---|---|
| Pituitary hormones | ± | – | – | – | – | – | – | – | – | –/–/– | – | – | – |
| Keratin | 90% | + | – | ±(10%) | 5% | + | – | – | – | –/–/– | – | – | – |
| EMA | >50% | + | – | – | + | + | – | ±§ | ± | –/–/–°° | – | – | – |
| S-100 protein | – | 10%‡ | + | – | 20% | + | ± | – | – | +/+/+ | + | +†† | + |
| CEA | – | ±† | – | – | 5% | – | – | – | – | –/–/– | ±# | – | – |
| Vimentin | – | 10%‡ | + | – | + | + | – | ±¶ | ± | +/±/+ | – | ? | + |
| Neurofilament | – | – | – | – | – | – | + | – | – | –/–/– | – | ? | – |
| GFAP | – | – | – | – | – | – | – | – | – | +/±/+ | – | +§§ | 50% |
| Leuk C Ag | – | – | – | – | – | – | – | + | – | –/–/– | – | – | – |
| Ig light chains | – | – | – | – | – | – | – | ± | + | –/–/– | – | – | – |
| Synaptophysin | + | ± | – | – | – | – | + | – | – | –/–/– | – | + | – |
| Chromogranin | 90% | ± | – | – | – | – | 70% | – | – | –/–/– | – | 95% | – |

* See Lloyd et al.[94]

† Breast and mullerian carcinomas.

‡ Carcinomas of thyroid, kidney, and adrenal, and germ cell tumors.

§ Lymphocytoplasmacytoid and pleomorphic large cell (Ki-1) lymphomas.

¶ Approximately 50% of large cell lymphomas.

°° Paranuclear but nonmembranous staining may be observed in the ependymoma.

# Cytoplasmic lysosomes may produce artifactual positivity.

†† Sustentacular and often chief cells react.

§§ Sustentacular cells may react.

EMA, epithelial membrane antigen; CEA, carcinoembryonic antigen; GFAP, glial fibrillary acidic protein; Leuk C Ag, leukocyte common antigen; Ig, immunoglobulin.

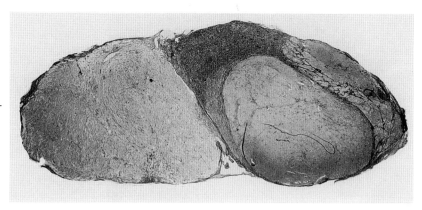

**FIGURE 9–71** PITUITARY ADENOMA WITH MICROSCOPIC DURAL INVASION

This reticulin preparation of the pituitary cut in the sagittal plane demonstrates a pale-staining, partly discrete adenoma on the right and the larger reticulin-free neurohypophysis on the left. The adenoma extends superiorly to involve the pituitary capsule. The prognostic significance of such invasion is unclear, but it is certainly less than that of osseous or grossly apparent dural invasion (reticulin, ×6).

of microscopically apparent dural invasion is high (66% in microadenomas, 87% in macroadenomas, and 94% in macroadenomas with suprasellar exten-sion).[136] As a result, its prognostic significance is questionable. In contrast, gross invasion, as determined by the surgeon, is noted in only 35% of adenomas and varies in frequency with tumor subtype[136] (Table 9–5). Roughly 50% of prolactinomas, GH cell adenomas, and plurihormonal tumors are grossly invasive, as compared with 20% of gonadotroph and 40% of null cell adenomas.[130] The rate of invasion of ACTH-producing adenomas is closely related to tumor size, being approximately 10% for microadenomas and 65% for macroadenomas. Some adenomas, particularly prolactinomas in male patients, acidophil stem cell adenomas, silent corticotroph adenomas, the tumors in Nelson's syndrome, thyrotroph adenomas, and silent subtype III adenomas, show high invasion rates.

Cytology is a poor discriminator between noninvasive and invasive adenomas and is only somewhat bettered by assessment of mitotic activity.[142] Nevertheless, mitotic activity, MIB-1 labeling indices (1.4% versus 4.9%), and frequencies of p53 protein immunoreactivity (0% versus 15%) are significantly higher in invasive adenomas.[139, 141]

Expression of the cytokine interleukin-6,[34] heat shock protein 27,[34] and type IV collagenase[69] is associated with invasiveness in pituitary adenomas, as is reduced expression of the metastasizing suppressor gene *NM-23*.[60] Preliminary studies suggest that neither metalloproteinase[67] nor cadherin expression significantly contributes to invasiveness.[68]

## Atypical Adenoma

In an effort to identify tumors likely to behave in an aggressive manner, a histologic category intermediate between ordinary or "typical" adenomas and pituitary carcinoma has been established.[79, 113, 129] The designation "atypical adenoma" denotes tumors showing increased proliferative activity, that is, more than an occasional mitosis, an MIB-1 labeling index exceeding 3%, and p53 immunoreactivity (Figs. 9–74 and 9–75).[79, 113, 129] Because combinations of these findings are clearly associated with invasion and/or recurrence, the designation "atypical" earmarks potentially more aggressive lesions. Its utility in identifying tumors capable of metastasis remains to be established in prospective studies.

## Pituitary Carcinoma

Defined as tumors showing craniospinal and/or systemic spread, pituitary carcinomas are often endocrinologically functioning tumors. Of these, most produce PRL or ACTH[32]; GH-, LH/FSH-, or TSH-producing lesions are very uncommon. Nonfunctioning carcinomas are rare.[9]

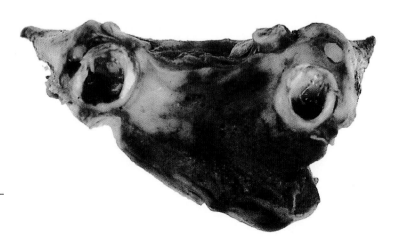

**FIGURE 9–72** INVASIVE PITUITARY ADENOMA

This tumor involved both the sphenoid sinus and the cavernous sinuses bilaterally. Note encirclement of both carotid arteries and of cranial nerves, particularly on the right.

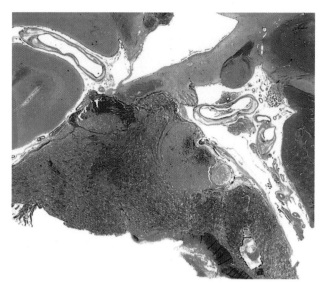

**FIGURE 9–73** INVASIVE PITUITARY ADENOMA

Multiple surgical procedures failed to arrest the growth of this neo-plasm, which, in a sagittal section of the sphenoid region, shows destruc-tion of bone. The case was associated with lethal meningitis and ven-triculitis. Despite the aggressive behavior, the histologic appearance was that of a well-differentiated pituitary adenoma with a low mitotic index.

Most carcinomas appear well differentiated, but, as with meningiomas, their histologic spectrum ranges from le-sions with little cellular atypia to ones exhibiting frank malignancy (Figs. 9–77 to 9–79). As previously discussed, some adenomas are histologically benign but widely infiltrative. Thus, as with various other endocrine neoplasms, arriving at a clear-cut and useful definition of malignancy has been problematic.[79, 113, 129] We adhere to the 2000 WHO Classification of Endocrine Tumors,[79] which restricts the designation pituitary carcinoma to the rare lesions demonstrating craniospinal (subarachnoid or parenchymal) metastases and/or metastasis to extracra-nial sites, usually lymph nodes, liver, or bone[79, 113, 129] (Fig. 9–76). Proliferative activity is not closely linked with cytologic appearance (Fig. 9–77). Most carcinomas do feature an elevated mitotic rate (see Fig. 9–77), but are not overtly malignant at the microscopic level. Al-though the presence of brisk mitotic activity suggests a higher likelihood of invasion and perhaps the eventual occurrence of metastatic spread, it is not an indicator of malignancy per se. Indeed, not all mitotically active ade-nomas pursue an aggressive course. Even tumors with very few mitoses may metastasize (Figs. 9–77 and 9–79). Although electron microscopy shows carcinomas to be less differentiated than their adenoma counter-parts,[134] the prognostic value of fine-structural features remains to be determined. Time will tell whether "ear-marking" atypical adenomas, as defined above, will be clinically useful. The goal of identifying pituitary carci-nomas before metastasis remains elusive. Its importance is underscored by the fact that once metastases become apparent, life expectancy is often less than 1 year.[113]

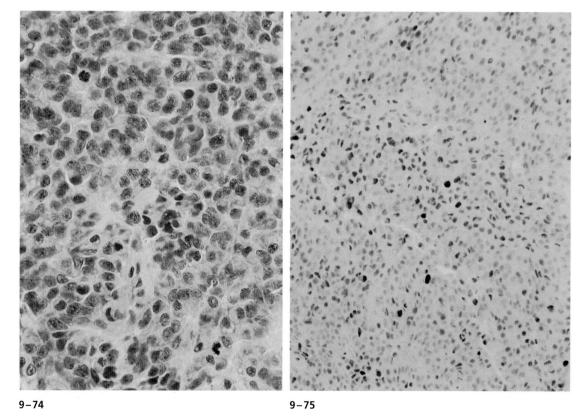

9–74                                              9–75

**FIGURES 9–74 AND 9–75** ATYPICAL PITUITARY ADENOMA

This PRL-producing tumor exhibited increased mitotic activity (Fig. 9–74), an elevated MIB-1 labeling index of 7%, and p53 immunoreactivity (Fig. 9–75). Nucleolar prominence is also a common feature of atypical adenomas.

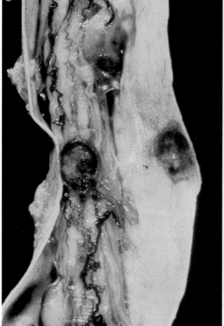
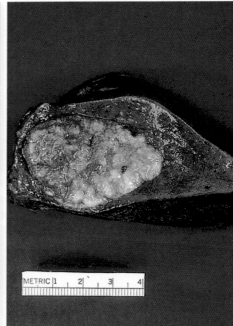

**FIGURE 9–76    PITUITARY CARCINOMA**

Craniospinal and/or systemic metastases define malignancy in adenohypophysial tumors. Seen here are spinal spread of an ACTH cell carcinoma (*left*) and hepatic metastasis of a PRL-producing tumor (*right*).

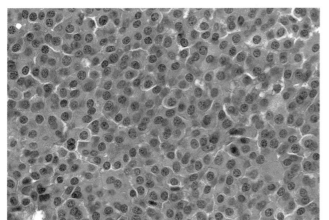

9–77

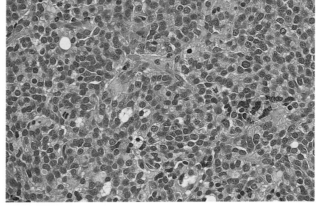

9–78

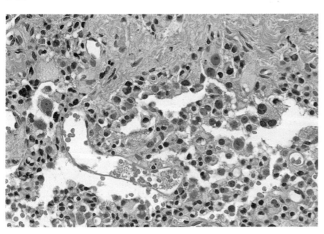

9–79

**FIGURES 9–77, 9–78, AND 9–79    PITUITARY CARCINOMA**

The histologic features of pituitary carcinomas vary considerably. Although some tumors exhibit benign features and low proliferative activity (Fig. 9–77; H&E, ×250), others show brisk mitotic activity (Fig. 9–78; H&E, ×250). Yet other tumors feature marked cytologic atypia and only occasional mitoses (Fig. 9–79; H&E, ×250). This broad spectrum is the reason that, at present, a confident diagnosis of carcinoma requires the presence of metastases.

# PITUITARY HYPERPLASIA

The concept that pituitary hyperplasia does not occur has been disproved. Clearly, it may be the basis of clinically and biochemically manifest disease.[2, 3, 5] It is difficult to diagnose, especially in small or fragmented surgical specimens, because GH, PRL, ACTH, and TSH cells are not evenly distributed in the normal pituitary. There is also substantial evidence that the condition occasionally undergoes transformation to adenoma.

Pituitary hyperplasia is a response to endocrinologic stimulation by either orthotopic or ectopic production of hypothalamic releasing hormones. The former is a normal physiologic response to end-organ failure, whereas the latter is usually associated with neuroendocrine neoplasms. Either nodular or diffuse in pattern, hyperplasia may involve one or occasionally several cell types.

The diagnosis poses a challenge and relies entirely upon routine histochemical stains and immunostains. In biopsy specimens, nodular hyperplasia is more readily diagnosed. It is characterized by marked expansion of pituitary acini, a conspicuous architectural alteration best seen with reticulin stain (Figs. 9–80 to 9–82). On the other hand, diffuse hyperplasia usually escapes detection unless a formal cell count is performed. This laborious process is not applicable to small specimens and is only rarely undertaken in intact pituitary glands.

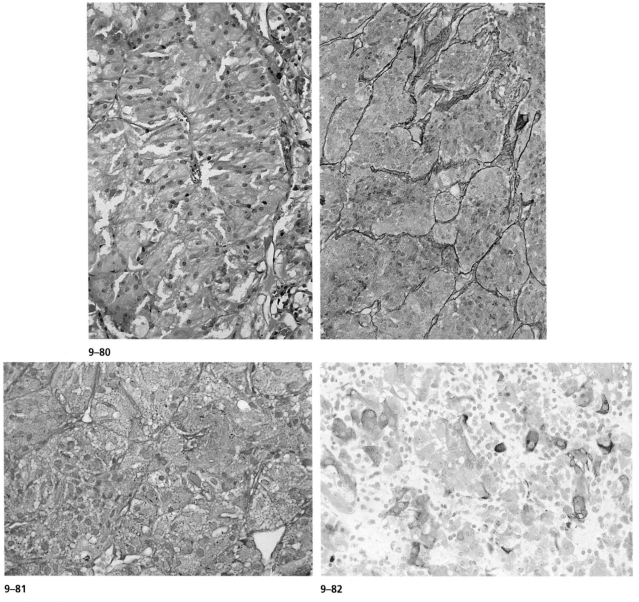

9–80

9–81                                9–82

**FIGURES 9–80, 9–81, AND 9–82**   TSH CELL HYPERPLASIA

This hypothyroid young woman presented with visual abnormalities, hyperprolactinemia, and what appeared on MRI scanning to be a macroadenoma with suprasellar extension. Although an H&E stain showed monomorphism suggestive of adenoma (Fig. 9–80, *left*), a reticulin preparation revealed expansion rather than effacement of the acinar pattern (Fig. 9–80, *right*). The diagnosis of TSH cell hyperplasia was confirmed by the finding of numerous cells with large PAS-positive lysosomes (Fig. 9–81) and abundant immunoreactivity for TSH (Fig. 9–82).

*Growth hormone cell hyperplasia* is usually of the diffuse type and occurs in association with GHRH-producing neuroendocrine tumors. Examples include pancreatic islet cell tumor, bronchial and thymic carcinoid tumor, and pheochromocytoma.[11, 12, 19] The hyperplastic cells are primarily acidophils immunoreactive for GH. Hyperplasia of GH-producing cells is not seen in the pituitary surrounding ordinary GH cell adenomas but may be an integral part of the adenomas of gigantism.[22] Adenoma formation only rarely supervenes upon hyperplasia accompanying orthotopic[131] or ectopic production of GRH.[12]

*Prolactin cell hyperplasia* is more often diffuse than nodular. It is a regular and conspicuous feature of pregnancy and lactation,[17, 18] estrogen treatment,[16] long-standing primary hypothyroidism wherein it is caused by an increase of thyrotropin-releasing hormone (TRH),[8, 15] and Cushing's disease.[2, 3, 5] Only rarely is it seen in the normal pituitary adjacent to a PRL cell adenoma. An example of PRL cell adenoma occurring in the setting of massive estrogen treatment may represent an example of hyperplasia undergoing neoplastic transformation.[6]

*Corticotroph hyperplasia,* either nodular or diffuse, may underlie the development of Cushing's disease.[21] In addition, it has been reported in patients with corticotropin-releasing hormone (CRH)–producing neuroendocrine tumors,[1, 20] in long-standing and untreated Addison's disease,[14] and in the nontumorous pituitary containing a corticotroph cell adenoma.[9] In rare instances, corticotroph hyperplasia has no apparent cause.[21] Loosely termed primary hyperplasia, it may be the result of an undisclosed hypothalamic stimulus.[21] Unquestionably, nodular corticotroph hyperplasia can transform into an adenoma.[5, 7]

*Thyrotroph hyperplasia* is regularly observed in patients with long-standing primary hypothyroidism[2, 3, 8, 15] (see Figs. 9–80 to 9–82). It may simulate adenoma clinically[2, 3, 8, 15] and is not difficult to identify on immunostained sections, wherein aggregates of often elongated TSH cells are a conspicuous feature. Cytoplasmic, PAS-positive lysosomes are also a regular feature (see Fig. 9–81). As previously noted, PRL cell hyperplasia is a common accompaniment and results from stimulation by TRH.[8, 15] Occasional TSH cell adenomas are associated with thyrotroph hyperplasia.

*Gonadotroph hyperplasia* may be seen in patients in whom primary hypogonadism has its onset at a young age, notably in Klinefelter's or Turner's syndrome. This form of hyperplasia is not well defined and awaits the establishment of morphologic criteria. Interestingly, gonadotropin hyperplasia is not a feature of the aged pituitary,[10] nor is there evidence that it precedes the development of LH or FSH cell adenomas.

# PITUICYTOMA (INFUNDIBULOMA) AND GRANULAR CELL TUMOR OF THE INFUNDIBULUM

**Definition.** Rare, well-differentiated sellar and suprasellar neoplasms apparently originating from pituicytes.

Phenotypically, pituicytomas appear astrocytic, whereas granular cell tumors do not.

**General Comments.** The infundibulum or neurohypophysis is composed of axons originating from hypothalamic neurons as well as functionally specialized astrocytes known as pituicytes,[9, 10] somewhat elongated cells reacting only moderately for GFAP (see Fig. 9–15). Eosinophilic, granular expansions of axons (Herring bodies) are also a regular feature of the normal infundibulum[1, 9] (see Fig. 9–14).

Symptomatic granular cell tumors represent large versions of the granular cell tumorlets so often an incidental postmortem finding in the infundibulum[5] (Fig. 9–83). Only occasional incidental nodules consist of nongranulated cells resembling those of symptomatic pituicytoma.[5] Both lesions may be attributable to these cells. Whether pituicytoma and granular cell tumor, either infundibular or neurohypophysial, are phenotypic variations is unclear. Nonetheless they share a number of clinical and anatomic features.

**Clinical Features.** Adults are generally affected and present with headaches and the effects of chiasmal and hypothalamic compression.[1, 2, 3, 7, 8]

**Radiologic Features.** Both pituicytoma and granular cell tumor are discrete, contrast-enhancing masses having their epicenter in the sella turcica or suprasellar space[3, 8] (Fig. 9–84).

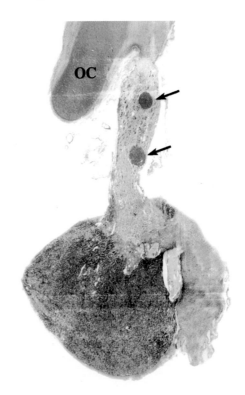

**FIGURE 9–83    GRANULAR CELL TUMORLET**

Multiple small nests of granular cells (*arrows*) are commonly encountered in the neurohypophysis and infundibulum. Their histologic appearance is identical to that of larger, symptomatic lesions. OC, optic chiasm.

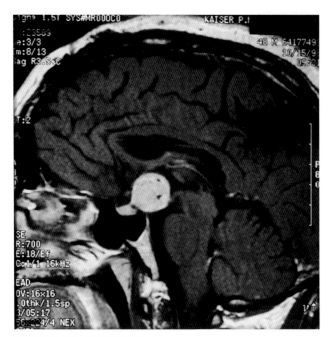

**FIGURE 9–84   PITUICYTOMA**

Circumscribed and solid in nature, the tumors enhance uniformly.

**Microscopic Features.** In their early form, granular cell tumors consist of ill-defined accumulations of such low cellularity that it would be difficult to distinguish them from normal infundibulum were it not for their distinctly granular, PAS-positive and diastase-resistant cytoplasm. More fully formed tumors are circumscribed and feature compact, polygonal to fascicular cells (Fig.

9–85). Often eccentrically placed, their nuclei contain inconspicuous nucleoli. Cytoplasm is PAS-positive (Fig. 9–85). Perivascular aggregates of lymphocytes may be seen focally.

Pituicytomas are moderately cellular lesions (see Fig. 9–86) whose cells are often somewhat fascicular in arrangement and lack cytoplasmic granulation. Their uniform, bland nuclei contain small, precisely defined nucleoli. If present at all, mitoses are rare. Although the tumor background may be somewhat fibrillar, overall the lesion is less process rich and more compact than most gliomas. Because pituicytomas are relatively solid, axons and their Herring bodies are absent.

**Immunohistochemical Features.** Both granular cell tumors and pituicytomas are S-100 protein-positive. Whereas GFAP staining is variable in pituicytoma (Fig. 9–86), it is weak or lacking in granular cell tumor.[1, 4, 6, 11]

**Ultrastructural Features.** Heterolysosomes fill the cells of granular cell tumor (Fig. 9–87). The basement membrane material occasionally surrounding cell clusters in peripheral granular cell tumor is lacking in this central variety. Pituicytoma are morphologically nondescript and, short of varying numbers of intermediate filaments, contain no specific organelles[1] (Fig. 9–88).

**Differential Diagnosis.** If the entity is considered, granular cell tumors pose little diagnostic difficulty. The differential diagnosis of pituicytoma can be more challenging and focuses on excluding normal infundibulum-neurohypophysis and pilocytic astrocytoma. The variable cellularity of normal neurohypophysis can, at its upper end, overlap that of pituicytoma. However, the normal tissue is looser in texture, features perivascular fibrillar

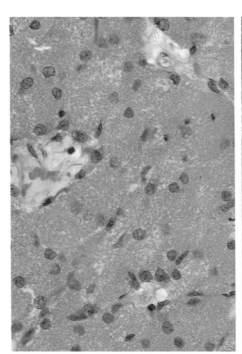

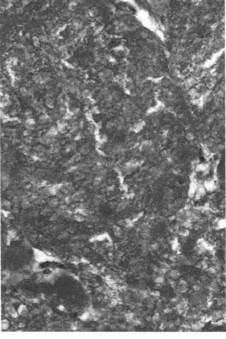

**FIGURE 9–85   SYMPTOMATIC GRANULAR CELL TUMOR**

At high magnification the nuclei are uniform and dense, and the cytoplasm exhibits distinctive granularity (*left*). The PAS positivity (*right*) is due to abundance of lysosomes.

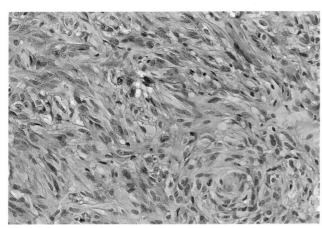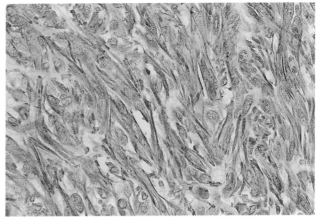

**FIGURE 9-86**    PITUICYTOMA

Architecturally solid, the tumor is composed of spindle cells arranged in interlacing fascicles or in storiform pattern (*left*). GFAP immunoreactivity varies from mild to moderate (*right*).

zones, is rich in axons, and contains occasional PAS-positive Herring bodies. Nonetheless, with very small specimens it can be difficult to arrive at a firm diagnosis. In such instances, correlation with radiologic images is essential.

Unlike pituicytomas, pilocytic astrocytomas usually occur as a sizable, hypothalamic–third ventricular mass in childhood. Furthermore, they vary in pattern from compact to microcystic as well as in cytologic features, which range from piloid to protoplasmic. Rosenthal

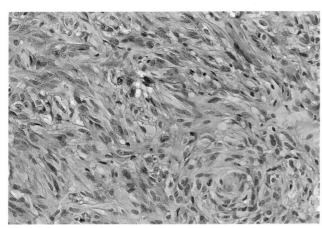

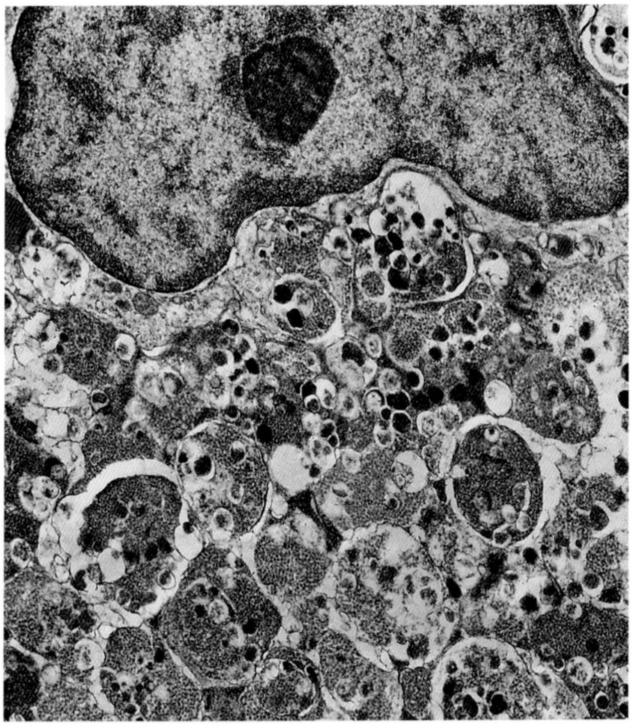

**FIGURE 9-87    GRANULAR CELL TUMOR**

The cells contain innumerable heterolysosomes, the basis for the lesions' PAS positivity (×11,000).

fibers and eosinophilic granular bodies are commonly seen.

**Treatment and Prognosis.** Although curative resection is possible in most cases of granular cell tumor and pituicytoma, recurrence after subtotal removal has been noted.[1, 8] At present, the value of adjuvant therapy is unclear.[8]

## CRANIOPHARYNGIOMAS

Constituting 2% to 5% of all intracranial neoplasms and 10% of non-neuroepithelial, intracranial tumors of childhood, craniopharyngiomas are epithelial neoplasms largely confined to the sellar or third ventricular region. Only rare examples arise elsewhere. Although some authors fail to comment upon the histologic features of adult and childhood craniopharyngiomas, in aggregate they paint an account of two clinical and radiographic variants corresponding to adamantinomatous and papillary types.[44] These are expressly different in age at presentation, clinical and radiographic features, and histologic appearance. Of the two subtypes, the classical or adamantinomatous variety is 10-fold more common and affects mainly children. In contrast, the papillary form occurs almost exclusively in adults. Each variant is discussed separately.

### Adamantinomatous Craniopharyngioma

**Definition.** An epithelial neoplasm arising in the suprasellar region and bearing a similarity to certain odontogenic tumors.

**General Comments.** The origin of the adamantinomatous craniopharyngioma has been sought in the nests of squamous cells that normally frequent the anterior

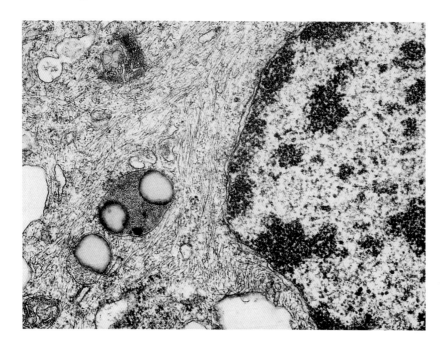

**FIGURE 9–88**   PITUICYTOMA

Ultrastructurally, the spindle cells are rich in intermediate filaments. They also possess scattered intermediate junctions as well as basement membrane at stromal interfaces.

surface of the pituitary stalk[19, 30] (see Fig. 9–11). Formerly considered remnants of the craniopharyngeal duct,[19] such cell nests are now known to result from metaplasia of adenohypophyseal cells of the pituitary stalk.[5] Although these cells represent a natural source of suprasellar squamous epithelium, their increased frequency with age is at odds with the largely juvenile incidence of craniopharyngioma.

The idea that craniopharyngiomas, either adamantinomatous or the papillary type described next, are derived from Rathke's cleft is supported by (1) the occasional capacity of the tumor cells to focally express one or more pituitary hormones,[45] chromogranin A,[51] or human chorionic gonadotropin and (2) the capacity of Rathke's cleft cyst to undergo impressive squamatization.

On the basis of the tumor's resemblance to adamantinomas of the jaw, it has been suggested that adamantinomatous craniopharyngiomas arise from embryonic rests with enamel organ potential.[8] Admittedly, there is a resemblance to adamantinoma of the jaw. Even more striking is the similarity to so-called keratinizing and calcifying odontogenic cyst[8, 21] (Fig. 9–89). Therefore, a histogenetic relationship is difficult to deny. Indeed, the eruption of teeth in rare craniopharyngiomas adds bite to the argument.[4, 26, 42]

**Clinical Features.** This distinctive neoplasm usually occurs during the first two decades of life; only a minority occur in middle-aged adults. The elderly are rarely affected.[39] Congenital examples are most unusual.[51] Despite the report of two cases in consanguineous twins,[9] there appears to be no genetic susceptibility to the development of the tumor. As a rule, this form of craniopharyngioma results in hypothalamic-pituitary axis dysfunction, visual symptoms, and hydrocephalus resulting from obstruction of cerebrospinal fluid flow. Endocrine abnormalities include growth retardation, diabetes in-

sipidus (15%), and amenorrhea. Signs of increased intracranial pressure are most often seen in pediatric patients (Fig. 9–90).

Although typically suprasellar, the tumor may undergo various extensions, including intrasellar, anterior or middle fossa, and retroclival. Approximately 5% are

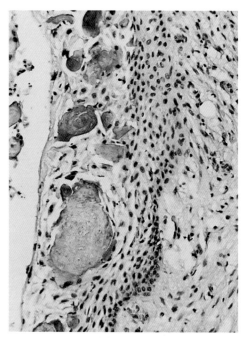

**FIGURE 9–89**   KERATINIZING AND CALCIFYING ODONTOGENIC CYST

The close resemblance of the so-called keratinizing and calcifying odontogenic cyst to the adamantinoma-like craniopharyngioma suggests a common origin of these neoplasms from cells with enamel organ potential.

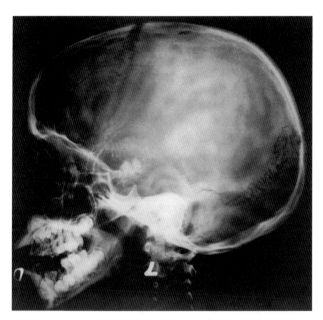

**FIGURE 9–90    ADAMANTINOMATOUS CRANIOPHARYNGIOMA**

Suprasellar calcification is an important diagnostic feature of typical craniopharyngiomas. In this instance, the patient was a 10-year-old boy with growth retardation, polyuria, polydipsia, and visual impairment. Note the "beaten copper" appearance of the skull, a reflection of increased intracranial pressure.

**Radiologic Features.** On CT or MRI (Fig. 9–91), adamantinomatous craniopharyngiomas appear as contrast-enhancing, often partly calcified, cystic, suprasellar masses.[37, 40] Most are sufficiently calcified to be visualized on plain radiographs of the skull (see Fig. 9–90).

**Macroscopic Features.** Adamantinomatous craniopharyngiomas fill the suprasellar region, exhibit a ragged interface with surrounding brain, and displace as well as adhere to adjacent vessels and cranial nerves (Figs. 9–92 to 9–94). Internally, they present a kaleidoscopic array of cysts, necrotic debris, fibrous tissue, and calcification (see Figs. 9–93 and 9–94). Particularly notable is the presence of encysted fluid that wells forth on sectioning, sparkling with minute cholesterol particles (Figs. 9–95 and 9–96). Spontaneous or operative spillage of this irritative "machinery oil" into the cerebrospinal space can produce severe chemical meningitis.[35, 41]

**Microscopic Features.** The histologic patterns of adamantinomatous craniopharyngioma include sheets, nodular whorls, intricate anastomosing trabeculae, and "clover leaves," as well as cysts lined by an attenuated epithelium (Fig. 9–97). In an orderly manner, the epithelial cells form a peripheral palisaded layer of columnar cells, loosely knit epithelium termed stellate reticulum, and an intervening layer of polygonal cells (Fig. 9–98; see Fig. 9–97). All are squamous in nature and immunoreactive for high- and low-molecular-weight keratins as well as epithelial membrane antigen (EMA).

Small or nonrepresentative specimens may consist entirely of fibrohistiocytic reaction, necrotic debris, calcification, and cholesterol clefts (see xanthogranuloma of the sellar region later). This array of features is only suggestive of the diagnosis. Instead, nodules of so-called

confined entirely to the sella. Rare craniopharyngiomas appear ectopically in the sphenoid bone,[10, 22] paranasal sinus,[2] nasopharynx,[30] cerebellopontine angle,[3] optic chiasm,[14] or pineal gland.[43] Implantation in a needle aspiration tract has also been recorded.[6, 24, 38] Malignant transformation is rare.[32]

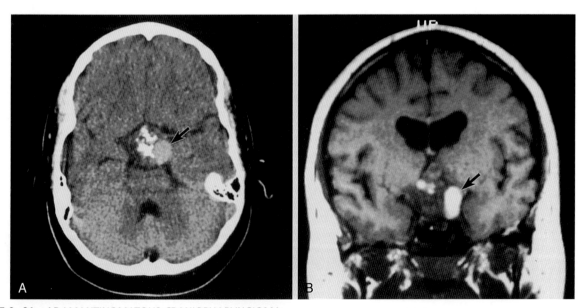

**FIGURE 9–91    ADAMANTINOMATOUS CRANIOPHARYNGIOMA**

A typical craniopharyngioma is illustrated by both CT (*A*) and MR (*B*). By CT, the cystic component (*arrow*) adjoins a densely calcified region. In a precontrast T1-weighted MR image, the cystic areas (*arrow*) appear bright because of their protein-rich contents. (Courtesy of Dr. Elias R. Melhem, Baltimore, MD.)

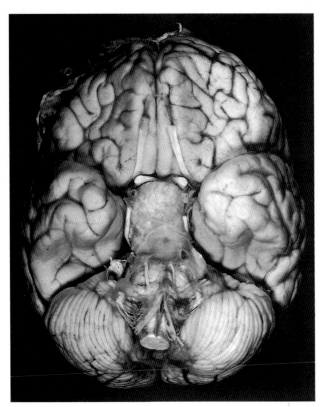

**FIGURE 9–92**   ADAMANTINOMATOUS CRANIOPHARYNGIOMA

This globoid craniopharyngioma compresses the optic chiasm and displaces cranial nerve III as well as the internal carotid and middle cerebral arteries. The 19-year-old woman's symptoms progressed over a period of 3 years through irregular menses, amenorrhea, headache, and eventually loss of vision.

"wet keratin," often undergoing calcification and apparent grossly as white flecks, are quite diagnostic (Fig. 9–99). Ossification of wet keratin may also be seen (Fig. 9–100).

**Immunohistochemical Features.** The lesions are immunoreactive for cytokeratins and EMA.

**Ultrastructural Features.** Ultrastructurally, both cohesive and loose-knit cells exhibit intermediate filament bundles (cytokeratin) and well-formed desmosomes, features of squamous differentiation.[17, 28, 48]

**Differential Diagnosis.** The demonstration of adamantinomatous epithelium or of wet keratin alone is diagnostic. Even in the absence of epithelium, a specimen of fibrous tissue derived from a calcified suprasellar mass accompanied by necrotic debris and cholesterol clefts provides a strong presumptive diagnosis of adamantinomatous craniopharyngiomas. The finding of only an attenuated layer of stratified squamous epithelium does not exclude the diagnosis but should prompt consideration of an epidermoid cyst. The latter are uniloculate, lined by a uniform layer of squamous epithelium resting upon a delicate fibrous capsule and filled with flaky, "dry keratin." In addition to orderly, diffuse, surface kera-

tinization, the epithelial cells lining epidermoid cysts feature keratohyalin granules. Furthermore, peripheral, picket fence–like cells are lacking. In those infrequent craniopharyngiomas wherein ordinary stratified squamous epithelium with surface maturation is a focal feature, thorough sampling is required to demonstrate adamantinomatous epithelium or wet keratin. The presence of calcification, machinery oil content, necrosis, and abundant fibrohistiocytic reaction generally serves to exclude epidermoid cyst.

Also in the differential is the *papillary craniopharyngioma* (see later), a tumor of adults, more often solid than cystic, and with a distinct tendency to involve the third ventricle. It is characterized by a pseudopapillary growth pattern and lacks adamantinomatous epithelium, as well as machinery oil content and "wet keratin" nodules. Degenerative fibrohistiocytic and xanthogranulomatous changes are far less frequent, and machinery oil content and calcification are lacking. Craniopharyngiomas with mixed adamantinomatous and papillary features are rare.

So-called *xanthogranuloma of the sellar region*[16] is also a candidate, particularly in the differential of an adamantinomatous tumor with advanced degenerative changes. Whether it is an entity or simply represents degenerative changes in a variety of sellar cysts is unsettled.

The infiltrative margins of an adamantinomatous craniopharyngioma provoke vigorous gliosis with abundant Rosenthal fiber formation in surrounding brain tissue. This exuberant reaction must not be mistaken for *pilocytic astrocytoma* (Fig. 9–101). Although gliosis is usually less cellular and lacks both microcysts and granular bodies, the distinction can be difficult.

**Treatment and Prognosis.** The natural history of adamantinomatous craniopharyngioma is unpredictable, but recurrence can be expected after incomplete resection. In two large series, the frequency of recurrence was substantial.[13, 49] Not surprisingly, recurrence is less likely after gross total resection (17%) than after subtotal removal, particularly without radiotherapy (58%).[49] Given the potential for operative damage to the hypothalamus, the extent to which craniopharyngiomas can, or should, be resected in toto is a subject of debate.[13, 15, 31, 49, 50] Recognizing the difficulties encountered in attempts at extirpation, partial resection, cyst drainage, and radiation therapy have all been used and credited with beneficial effects.[13, 50] There is general agreement that recurrent lesions become increasingly adherent to local structures and are, for practical purposes, unresectable. Operative implantation of tumor remote from the primary site is rarely seen.[6, 7, 24, 27, 38] The demonstration of receptors for estrogen, progesterone, and somatostatin in adamantinomatous tumors is of unknown clinical or therapeutic significance.[25, 47]

Despite reported differences in MIB-1 labeling indices between nonrecurring (3.4%) and recurrent tumors (13.2%),[35] some authors have found no clear prognostic relationship to such labeling indices.[12] Malignant transformation to squamous carcinoma has been described in only a single, previously irradiated case.[34]

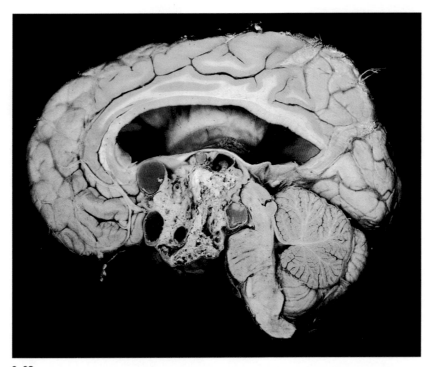

9–93

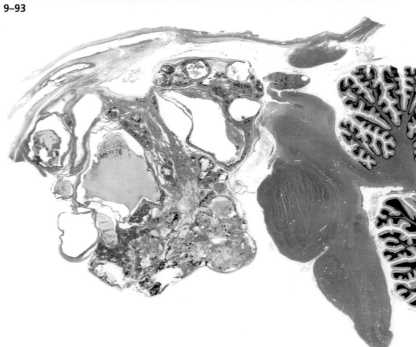

9–94

**FIGURES 9–93 AND 9–94**    ADAMANTINOMATOUS CRANIOPHARYNGIOMA

This multilobate, multicystic craniopharyngioma filled the third ventricle and produced hydrocephalus in an 11-year-old boy whose 3-year course included headaches and decreased visual acuity (Fig. 9–93). Suprasellar calcification was noted (see Fig. 9–90). The histologic section emphasizes nodular areas of cellularity interspersed among cysts, necrotic debris, and fibrous tissue (Fig. 9–94).

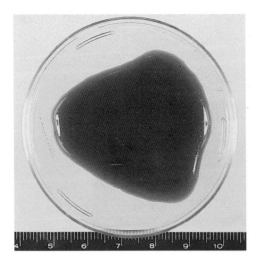

**FIGURE 9–95  CYST CONTENTS OF ADAMANTINOMATOUS CRANIOPHARYNGIOMA**

The presence of "machinery oil," glistening with droplets of cholesterol, is characteristic of adamantinomatous craniopharyngioma.

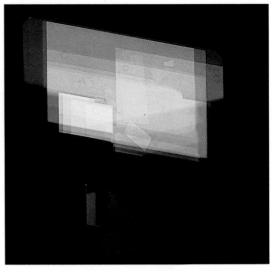

**FIGURE 9–96  CHOLESTEROL IN ADAMANTINOMATOUS CRANIOPHARYNGIOMA CONTENT**

The cholesterol crystals of a craniopharyngioma assume a distinctive layered, polygonal profile. Beginning as a diaphanous gray monolayer, opacity is imparted incrementally by lamination (unstained, polarized light, ×400).

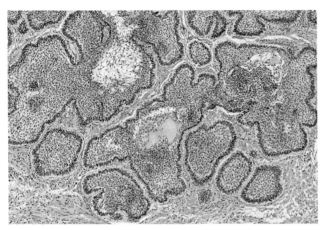

**FIGURE 9–97  ADAMANTINOMATOUS CRANIOPHARYNGIOMA**

The classical adamantinoma-like appearance of craniopharyngioma is unmistakable and diagnostic. The irregular interface with surrounding brain, seen here as macro- and microlobulation, complicates total tumor removal.

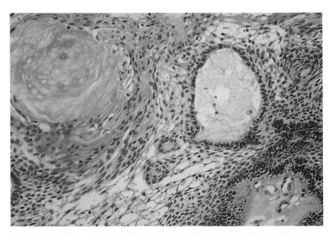

**FIGURE 9–98  ADAMANTINOMATOUS CRANIOPHARYNGIOMA**

In addition to palisaded epithelial cells, the lesion contains loosely cohesive squamous cells separated by intercellular fluid, a pattern termed stellate reticulum. Note also the presence of wet keratin.

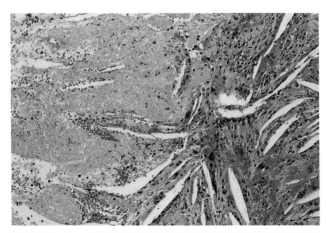

**FIGURE 9–99  ADAMANTINOMATOUS CRANIOPHARYNGIOMA**

Necrotic debris containing cholesterol clefts is a conspicuous feature of craniopharyngiomas and, even in the absence of epithelium, strongly suggests the diagnosis.

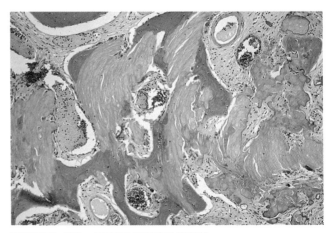

**FIGURE 9–100  ADAMANTINOMATOUS CRANIOPHARYNGIOMA**

Calcification may occur in association with epithelial cells, within keratin whorls, in amorphous debris, or within the stroma. In this example, ossification of wet keratin is a conspicuous feature.

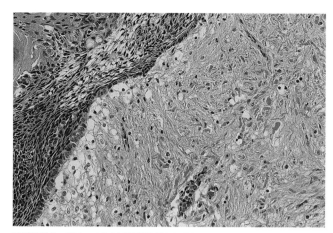

**FIGURE 9–101** ADAMANTINOMATOUS CRANIOPHARYNGIOMA

Craniopharyngiomas elicit vigorous gliosis with Rosenthal fiber formation, an appearance that closely mimics pilocytic astrocytoma.

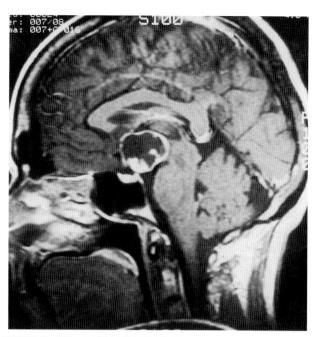

**FIGURE 9–102** PAPILLARY CRANIOPHARYNGIOMA

This unique variant of craniopharyngioma affects adults and often occupies the third ventricle. Although many lesions are solid, this example is cystic and demonstrates papillations similar to those illustrated in Figure 9–105.

## Papillary Craniopharyngioma

**Definition.** A very well differentiated, squamous, pseudopapillary neoplasm arising in the suprasellar region or third ventricle.

**General Comments.** In clinical, neuroradiologic, and histologic terms, this variant of craniopharyngioma differs from the adamantinomatous type.[11, 13, 18]

**Clinical Features.** Papillary craniopharyngiomas occur in adulthood with visual loss, signs of increased intracranial pressure, diminished mental acuity, and personality change. Radiographically, the sella is minimally or not at all affected because most tumors appear to arise within the third ventricle or the suprasellar space[27, 40] (Fig. 9–102). Unlike adamantinomatous craniopharyngioma, papillary tumors lack calcification. They vary from solid to cystic (Figs. 9–103 and 9–104; see Figs. 9–102 and 9–106). The unique concurrence of papillary craniopharyngioma and pineocytoma is probably coincidental.[23]

**Macroscopic Features.** Papillary craniopharyngiomas are solid or less often frankly cystic and feature conspicuous papillations (Figs. 9–105 and 9–106; see Fig. 9–104). Being well circumscribed, they lack the adhesive, ragged interface with adjacent brain that characterizes the adamantinomatous variant. The same is true of cholesterol-rich machinery oil content and calcification.

**Microscopic Features.** At the microscopic level, papillary craniopharyngiomas are formed of well-differentiated squamous epithelium and an anastomosing fibrovascular stroma (Fig. 9–107). Either naturally or artifactually, the epithelium separates along cracks and fissures to form crude pseudopapillae. Peripheral palisading of cells, stellate reticulin, and nodules of wet keratin—all features typical of the adamantinomatous

lesion—are lacking. Collagenous whorls often mimic keratin pearls, but the latter, as well as surface keratinization, are not a feature of papillary tumors. When present, ciliation and goblet cell formation are focal findings[11, 20, 32] (Fig. 9–108).

**Differential Diagnosis.** Although papillary craniopharyngiomas are highly distinctive, problems in differential diagnosis do arise. These center upon their distinction from the adamantinomatous variant, epidermoid cyst, and the occasional Rathke's cleft cyst with prominent squamous metaplasia. Although tumors with mixed adamantinomatous and papillary features do rarely occur, most craniopharyngiomas fall clearly into one group or the other.

Lastly, although the histogenesis of papillary craniopharyngioma is unclear, it may be linked to Rathke's cleft. This would explain why (1) some papillary craniopharyngiomas show focal ciliation of columnar epithelium and/or goblet cells (see Fig. 9–108)[11, 20, 32] and (2) occasional Rathke's cleft cysts feature conspicuous, bandlike squamous metaplasia beneath their mucinous or ciliated epithelial lining (see Fig. 9–115). In such cases, it is the lack of a solid component and the presence of extensive ciliation and/or mucin production that distinguish Rathke's cleft cyst. On occasion, however, squamous metaplasia is so marked that the distinction between Rathke's cleft cyst and papillary craniopharyngioma becomes blurred. Epithelial atrophy (see Fig. 9–113) as well as extensive xanthogranulomatous change (see Fig. 9–114) may also be seen in Rathke's cleft cyst.

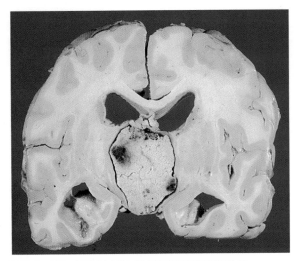

**FIGURE 9–103** PAPILLARY CRANIOPHARYNGIOMA

This large, solid example lies within the third ventricle. It occurred in a 61-year-old man who had undergone a prior unsuccessful surgery. He had experienced 5 years of progressive memory and visual disturbance as well as endocrine hypofunction. (Courtesy Dr. Ronald Kim, Long Beach, CA.)

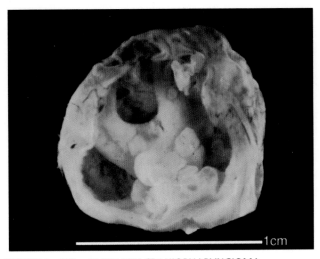

**FIGURE 9–106** PAPILLARY CRANIOPHARYNGIOMA

Papillary craniopharyngiomas are often solid, but some are cystic and show papillary ingrowth. Calcifications are typically absent. This lesion occurred in a 46-year-old woman with visual loss and headaches. A total excision was achieved.

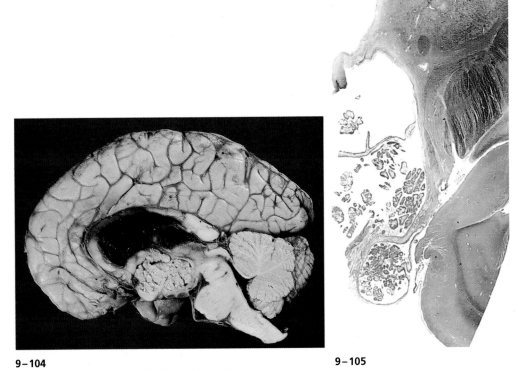

9–104                                             9–105

**FIGURES 9–104 AND 9–105** PAPILLARY CRANIOPHARYNGIOMA

A 31-year-old patient had experienced symptoms of hypopituitarism, headaches, and failing vision for 1 year. Intraventricular bleeding complicated shunt placement. The papillary architecture and third ventricular location of the tumor are readily apparent, both in the gross specimen (Fig. 9–104) and in a whole mount section (Fig. 9–105). In Figure 9–105, the medial temporal lobe is to the right of the illustration.

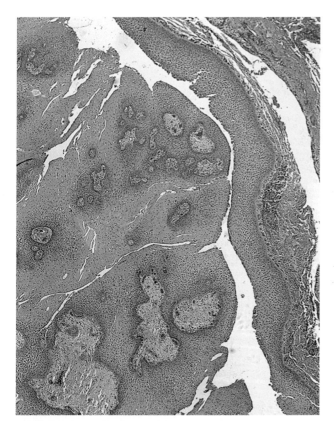

**FIGURE 9–107    PAPILLARY CRANIOPHARYNGIOMA**

At low magnification the basic lesion is a squamous neoplasm supported by fibrovascular cores. Note the absence of both an adamantinoma-like pattern and keratinizing nodules. At this magnification, the tumor shows dehiscence with resultant formation of pseudopapillae.

Unlike papillary craniopharyngiomas, epidermoid cysts lack papillations, show diffuse surface maturation with the formation of keratohyaline granules and anucleate squames, contain keratinous debris rather than fluid, and possess only a scant connective tissue capsule.

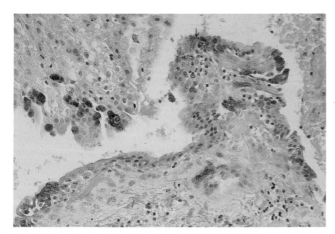

**FIGURE 9–108    PAPILLARY CRANIOPHARYNGIOMA**

Some squamous suprasellar neoplasms, otherwise identical to papillary craniopharyngioma, demonstrate mucus-producing columnar epithelium with squamous metaplasia (mucicarmine).

**Treatment and Prognosis.** Despite initial optimism based on a reported recurrence rate of only 4%,[11] subsequent series have suggested a prognosis for papillary craniopharyngioma that differs little from that of the adamantinomatous type.[13, 49]

# MISCELLANEOUS NEOPLASMS AND TUMOR-LIKE LESIONS

## Germ Cell Tumor

Germinoma, the most frequent of intracranial germ cell tumors, is identical to testicular and mediastinal seminoma and to ovarian dysgerminoma. It typically affects children, who first present with diabetes insipidus and only later with visual disturbance and/or hypopituitarism. Usually suprasellar in location, the soft gray tumor often adheres to the undersurface of the brain, where it is related to the optic chiasm and pituitary stalk. Primary intrasellar germinomas are exceptional.[3] Chapter 4 includes a detailed discussion of the pathobiology of this notably radiosensitive neoplasm. Only occasional germinomas evolve into more malignant variants of germ cell tumor.[1] Teratomas[2, 4] and various malignant germ cell tumors also affect the sellar region.

## Chordoma

The presumed origin of cranial chordoma from rostral remnants of the notochord places it in proximity to the sella turcica and prompts its consideration in the differential diagnosis of perisellar masses (see Chapter 1, pages 23 to 27). Only rare examples are entirely or largely intrasellar.[1–3] The distinction of so-called "chondroid chordoma" from chondrosarcoma of the skull base depends on demonstrating widespread cytokeratin and EMA staining in the former, not on S-100 protein reactivity. The latter, a regular feature of chondrosarcoma, is seen in fully half of chordomas.

## Postirradiation Neoplasia

The majority of postirradiation neoplasms of the sella and skull base are sarcomas,[1–4] including fibrosarcoma,[3, 4] osteosarcoma,[1] rhabdomyosarcoma,[2] and unclassifiable, poorly differentiated lesions. In most instances, the originally irradiated tumor was a pituitary adenoma[1, 3, 4] or retinoblastoma. In sarcomas associated with pituitary adenoma, the two elements are often intimately admixed. Radiation doses underlying the development of sarcomas generally exceed 20 Gy and the mean latency period is about 10 years. Postirradiation sarcomas are locally aggressive rather than metastasizing neoplasms. Nonetheless, postoperative survival is generally 1 year.

## Metastatic Neoplasms

Among tumors that secondarily involve the pituitary from adjacent osseous or dural deposits, metastatic carcinoma and hematopoietic neoplasms predominate. Most occur in the setting of disseminated disease. Symptoms include cranial nerve palsies (70%) and pituitary dysfunction (30%), most often of the posterior lobe (diabetes insipidus).

**Carcinoma.** Carcinomas of the breast and lung are the most common source of metastases to the sella.[1, 4] Such deposits are symptomatic in approximately one half of patients. Clinical expressions include diabetes insipidus, pituitary insufficiency, and retro-orbital pain. Median survival is approximately 6 months.[4] Local control minimally improves upon this figure.[4]

Secondary extension to the pituitary from osseous or capsular deposits is more frequent than are direct metastases to the gland. The latter affect mainly the posterior lobe, which has a direct arterial supply. In one series of metastatic carcinoma involving the anterior pituitary and simulating pituitary adenoma,[1] most were adenocarcinomas of mammary or renal origin.

Selective involvement of the hypothalamus, particularly of the median eminence, is an uncommon but characteristic metastatic pattern. In rare instances, a metastasis of a neuroendocrine carcinoma producing a hypothalamic hormone results in specific endocrinopathy by directly stimulating the pituitary.[2, 3]

**Hematopoietic Neoplasms.** Primary CNS lymphomas are increasing in frequency.[5] Unlike secondary lymphomas, which are typically meningeal based, most primary tumors involve deep parenchymal structures, particularly the basal ganglia and periventricular zones. Only a small proportion primarily affect the third ventricular region or hypothalamus. Most are diffuse B-cell lymphomas of large cell or immunoblastic type. Varying numbers of reactive T cells often contribute to the infiltrate. Endocrinopathy is a late occurrence and includes both diabetes insipidus and measurable hypothalamic-anterior pituitary dysfunction.

Leukemic involvement of the CNS is usually meningeal based and extensive. Acute and chronic lymphocytic leukemia is more frequent than the myelogenous variety. Diabetes insipidus may accompany sellar involvement, even during the preleukemic phase.[6]

## Other Neoplasms

The presence of neural tissue, meninges, bone, and nasal sinuses in the immediate vicinity of the sella turcica provides fertile soil for the development of various neoplasms and tumor-like lesions (see Figs. 9–1 and 9–2). Many are discussed elsewhere in this book. The spectrum includes chiasmal and hypothalamic astrocytomas (see Chapter 4), suprasellar meningioma with or without intrasellar extension,[16] primary intrasellar meningioma,[9] hemangiopericytoma,[12] plasmacytoma,[17] giant cell tumor of bone,[19] chondroma with or without Ollier's disease,[5, 13] osteolipoma,[7] schwannoma,[8, 18] lipoma,[6] angiolipoma,[11] hemangioblastoma in the setting of von Hippel–Lindau disease,[4] glomangioma,[1] paraganglioma,[2, 14, 20] malignant melanoma,[3, 15] and even salivary

gland tumors of the sellar region.[10] Granular cell tumor and pituicytoma of the sella, unusual forms of glioma, were discussed earlier.

## SELLAR REGION CYSTS

In addition to the two variants of craniopharyngioma already discussed, we recognize the separate identity of Rathke's cleft cyst, epidermoid cyst, mucocele, and pseudocyst of the pituitary. Strictly speaking, the arachnoid diverticulum underlying the primary empty sella syndrome is not a cyst but a secondary lesion related to either a structurally abnormal sellar diaphragm or to loss of intrasellar volume. As such, it is discussed separately (see later). Parasitic cysts are also dealt with separately. The nature of the often cystic xanthogranuloma of the sellar region remains unsettled (see later).

## Rathke's Cleft Cyst

**Definition.** A non-neoplastic cyst derived from glandular rests of Rathke's cleft in the region of the intermediate lobe.

**General Comments.** Rathke's cleft cysts of microscopic dimension are a common incidental finding at autopsy. Seen in 30% of normal pituitaries, fully 80% lie at the interface of the anterior and posterior lobes. The remainder are related to the pituitary stalk. Not surprisingly, such cysts also occur within the pharyngeal pituitary.

**Clinical Features.** On occasion, Rathke's cleft cysts are sufficiently large (1 cm or more) to produce endocrine or visual symptoms by compression of the pituitary gland, optic chiasm, or hypothalamus.[2, 6, 9, 13–15, 17] Endocrine effects include dysfunction of the gonadal, thyroid, and/or adrenal axes, growth retardation, and occasionally diabetes insipidus. Hyperprolactinemia related to "stalk section effect" is also common. Hydrocephalus is occasionally seen.

**Radiologic Features.** The cysts show variable signal characteristics but lack calcification. Like third ventricular colloid cysts, some show a high signal on T1-weighted MR images[5, 9] (Fig. 9–109), a feature highly suggestive of Rathke's cleft cyst.

**Macroscopic Features.** Although most examples are at least partly intrasellar, a minority are entirely suprasellar[1] (Figs. 9–110 and 9–111). One clinical and imaging study suggested that hemorrhage occasionally precipitates symptoms.[14] At surgery, the content of the thin-walled cyst varies from watery to viscid and from clear to opalescent.

**Histologic Features.** Although most cysts consist of a single layer of columnar, mucin-producing and/or ciliated cells (Fig. 9–112), some show variable degrees of pressure atrophy (Fig. 9–113) or xanthogranulomatous

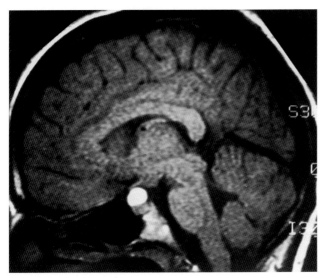

**FIGURE 9–109**  RATHKE'S CLEFT CYST

Because of their protein-rich contents, many Rathke's cleft cysts have high magnetic resonance signal intensity in the T1 mode. In the region of the sella turcica, a sharply demarcated, spherical lesion with this signal characteristic is strongly suggestive of this entity.

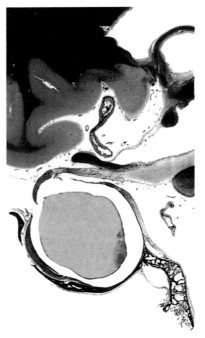

**FIGURE 9–111**  RATHKE'S CLEFT CYST

A 78-year-old man with hypopituitarism and a 6-year history of sellar enlargement died of gastrointestinal hemorrhage. Within the eroded expanded sella lies a thin-walled Rathke's cleft cyst, the mucinous contents of which have artifactually retracted from the epithelial wall. Because of compression, the adenohypophysis is reduced to a dark crescent in the anteroinferior floor of the sella.

reaction (Fig. 9–114). As in the similar colloid cyst of the third ventricle, the frequent presence of goblet cells suggests an endodermal derivation. Indeed, the immuno-histochemical and ultrastructural features of Rathke's cleft cyst are much the same as those of bronchial and enterogenous cysts.[10, 11, 18] Stromal amyloid is occasionally present.[3] In some cysts, proliferation of basal or reserve cells prompts extensive squamous metaplasia[6, 17] (Fig. 9–115). Given the high frequency of incidental pituitary adenomas in the normal pituitary gland, it is no surprise that occasional Rathke's cleft cysts are adenoma associated.[12, 16] Complex lesions in which two elements

occur in combination with squamous epithelium have been termed "transitional tumors."[4, 7] Their nature is poorly understood.

Aggressive resection of Rathke's cleft cysts can result in postoperative endocrine dysfunction, usually diabetes insipidus.[8, 16, 17] Even incomplete excision is curative.[8]

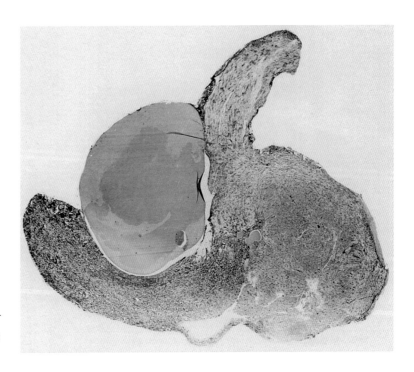

**FIGURE 9–110**  RATHKE'S CLEFT CYST

This asymptomatic Rathke's cleft cyst was an incidental autopsy finding. These cysts can not only extend into but also arise in the suprasellar region.

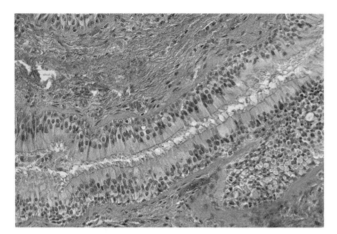

**FIGURE 9–112    RATHKE'S CLEFT CYST**

In a small lesion without pressure atrophy of the epithelium, the cells are tall and heavily ciliated. Some contain mucin.

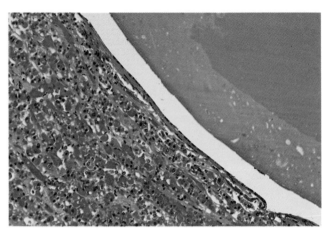

**FIGURE 9–113    RATHKE'S CLEFT CYST**

The epithelium may be low and atrophic.

## Miscellaneous Cysts

**Epidermoid Cyst.** These opalescent, unilocular, thin-walled cysts are lined by a uniform layer of keratinizing squamous cells and are filled with flaky, so-called "dry" keratin.[2] Morphologically, they are identical to epidermoid cysts occurring elsewhere and, in an adequate biopsy, are readily distinguished from craniopharyngiomas (see earlier). At least one convincing example of malignant transformation of an intrasellar epidermoid cyst has been documented.[5]

**Arachnoid Cyst.** Only infrequently do arachnoid cysts occur within the sella.[4] As expected, headache, visual symptoms, and anterior pituitary dysfunction may result. Their delicate walls consist of EMA-immunoreactive arachnoidal cells and a scant stroma.

**Mucocele.** Reactive in nature, these non-neoplastic, mucus-filled cysts are well known to occur in relation to nasal sinuses. For a full discussion, see Chapter 1 and Figures 1–31 and 1–32. Of examples affecting the sellar region, some represent a complication of transsphenoidal surgery[3] and others follow medical treatment of pituitary adenomas.[1]

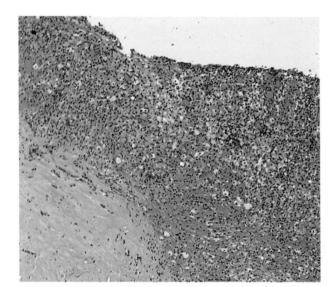

**FIGURE 9–114    RATHKE'S CLEFT CYST WITH XANTHOGRANULOMATOUS CHANGE**

Such lesions should not be mistaken for xanthogranulomatous reactions in some craniopharyngiomas and pituitary adenomas.

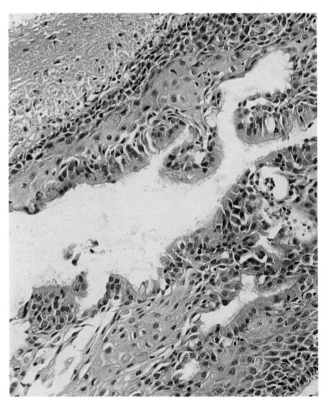

**FIGURE 9–115    RATHKE'S CLEFT CYST WITH SQUAMOUS METAPLASIA**

Extensive squamous metaplasia is noted in some Rathke's cleft cysts.

# INFLAMMATORY LESIONS

## Lymphocytic Hypophysitis

**Clinical Features.** Clinically, this inflammatory sellar mass typically occurs during late pregnancy or shortly after delivery with signs of pituitary insufficiency.[1, 2, 3, 5, 9] On occasion, it manifests as an isolated hormone deficiency.[7] Diabetes insipidus is infrequent.[3] Hyperprolactinemia, a common accompaniment, may be a reflection of tissue destruction or of "stalk section effect."[11, 14] Males are infrequently affected.[8, 12] In that pituitary enlargement can be significant and includes suprasellar extension, mass effects such as headache and visual disturbance may be seen.[1, 2, 3, 9, 11, 13]

**Radiologic Features.** Radiographically, the pituitary is symmetric and shows appreciable contrast enhancement[1, 2, 3, 7, 9, 11] (Fig. 9–116). Other chronic inflammatory lesions in the differential show a less striking female predilection, lack a temporal association with pregnancy, and differ in anatomic distribution as well as pathogenesis.[6]

**Macroscopic Features.** In contrast to pituitary adenoma, the main clinical differential, parenchyma affected by lymphocytic hypophysitis is firm.

**Microscopic Features.** Microscopically, the gland is overrun by lymphocytes as well as occasional plasma cells and histiocytes. Pituitary acini are often disrupted but clusters of adenohypophyseal cells are readily identified, even in advanced cases (Fig. 9–117). Lymphoid follicles with germinal centers are occasionally encountered. In contrast to giant cell granuloma (see later), granulomas and giant cells are lacking. Fibrosis eventually ensues and may become extensive.[10]

Lymphocytic hypophysitis clearly has an autoimmune basis, both cellular and humoral. This is affirmed by (1) the lymphocyte phenotype, which includes both T and B cells; (2) the presence in serum of antibodies directed toward either pituitary tissue or specific hormones, most often PRL[1, 3, 14] or ACTH; and (3) the concurrence of autoimmune infiltrates in other endocrine organs,[13] including thyroid, adrenal, or parathyroid. Rare examples of lymphocytic hypophysitis have been associated with systemic sarcoidosis[4] or retroperitoneal fibrosis.[13] Therapy consists of either a biopsy or a sparing surgical decompression followed by hormone replacement. Untreated lymphocytic hypophysitis may be fatal due to the effects of pituitary insufficiency.

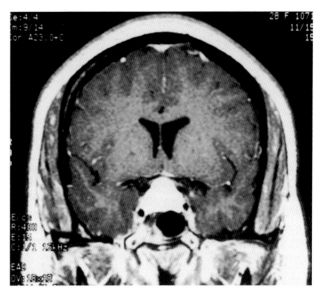

**FIGURE 9–116   LYMPHOCYTIC HYPOPHYSITIS**

This T1-weighted MR image with contrast enhancement shows marked symmetric enlargement of the pituitary with suprasellar extension. The patient was a 28-year-old female with postpartum visual loss.

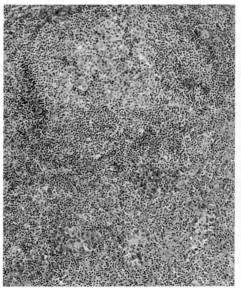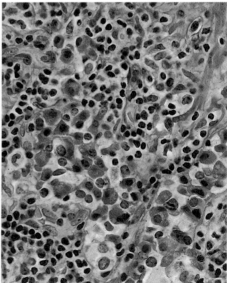

**FIGURE 9–117   LYMPHOCYTIC HYPOPHYSITIS**

The anterior lobe is overrun with a chronic inflammatory cell infiltrate (*left*), leaving trapped residual parenchyma (*right*).

## Giant Cell Granuloma

Also a cause of pituitary insufficiency, giant cell granuloma differs significantly from lymphocytic hypophysitis. Its predilection for females is less striking, and no real association with pregnancy has been noted.[2, 3, 4, 6, 7, 9] The clinical picture is one of anterior pituitary failure and occasionally diabetes insipidus. Because the gland may be enlarged during early-stage disease, the lesion mimics pituitary adenoma. Subsequently, it becomes shrunken and firm.

Histologically, the process involves the adenohypophysis and features noncaseating granulomatous inflammation. Extension into the posterior lobe or hypothalamus is rarely seen. The granulomas are well formed and consist in large part of giant cells with an occasional Schaumann body (Fig. 9–118). As a rule, lymphocytic infiltration is scant. With chronicity comes destruction of the gland and fibrosis. By definition, no organisms are identified with special stains or in culture. Experience with giant cell granuloma suggests that it is autoimmune in nature. Other endocrine organs, notably the thyroid, adrenals, or testes, may contain similar infiltrates. One reported example occurred in association with Crohn's disease.[1]

Giant cell granuloma appears to be a self-limited lesion, requiring only biopsy for confirmation of the diagnosis and perhaps decompression. Long-term hormone replacement therapy is often required. The principal differential diagnosis involves sarcoidosis, which, unlike giant cell granuloma, affects the posterior lobe and hypothalamus.[5, 8]

## Langerhans Cell Histiocytosis

To some extent, the CNS is involved in approximately 25% of cases of Langerhans histiocytosis.[1, 3, 5, 8] Only infre-

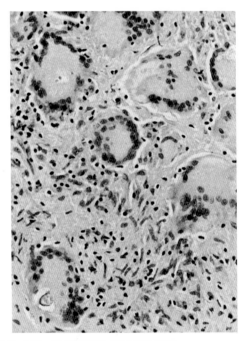

**FIGURE 9–118   GIANT CELL GRANULOMA**

Epithelioid and prominent multinucleated giant cells are characteristic of giant cell granuloma.

quently do signs of pituitary-hypothalamic axis involvement precede systemic manifestations.[8] Apparently clonal and perhaps neoplastic, Langerhans histiocytosis is discussed more fully on pages 146 to 148. Isolated involvement of the hypothalamus or pituitary is rare.[6, 7] The posterior lobe and the stalk are targeted, the result being hypothalamic dysfunction and diabetes insipidus with sparing of the anterior pituitary. The histiocytic infiltrate is variably CD68 and CD1A immunoreactive, whereas stains for lysozyme are negative.[4] Ultrastructurally, the finding of Birbeck granules is diagnostic.[2] Among histiocytoses affecting the CNS, Erdheim-Chester disease, a rare lesion affecting bone and brain, also enters into the differential. The same is true of Rosai-Dorfman disease. Both are discussed below.

## Xanthogranuloma of the Sellar Region and Pseudocyst

On occasion, a biopsy of a cystic, sellar region lesion yields only xanthomatous or xanthogranulomatous tissue composed of cholesterol clefts, macrophages, chronic inflammatory cells, necrotic debris, and hemosiderin deposits.[1, 2] It has been suggested that such lesions represent a distinct entity. Although neuroimaging and intraoperative features resemble those of craniopharyngioma, xanthogranulomas occur mainly in adolescents and young adults with longer preoperative symptoms, more severe endocrine deficits, and less in the way of visual disturbance. Furthermore, they seem to be mainly intrasellar, smaller in size, more easily resected, and associated with a more favorable outcome.[2] It is our opinion that, given the very nature of such chronic, degenerative lesions and the finding of squamous or adamantinomatous epithelium in some,[2] most are simply the end stage of one or several lesions, presumably craniopharyngioma or Rathke's cleft cyst.

On occasion, simple cysts unaccompanied by an epithelial lining are encountered within the pituitary gland. Such pseudocysts are considered to have originated from hemorrhage and necrosis in the anterior lobe or to be the residua of an adenoma that has undergone total apoplexy (see above).

## Rosai-Dorfman Disease

Although this well-known inflammatory disorder involves numerous organs, including the CNS,[1–4] only rare examples affect the sellar region.[3] The infiltrate consists of mononucleate or multinucleate (Touton-like), S-100 protein–immunoreactive giant cells and vacuolated histiocytes. Emperipolesis of lymphocytes, a typical feature, may be scant. The histiocytes of Rosai-Dorfman disease are CD1A and lysozyme immunonegative but are CD68 reactive.[2, 4] Ultrastructurally, Birbeck granules are lacking. Rosai-Dorfman disease is discussed in more detail in Chapter 2 on pages 96 to 97.

## Erdheim-Chester Disease

This rare disorder affects not only bone but the CNS as well.[1–5] The infiltrate includes often markedly vacuolated

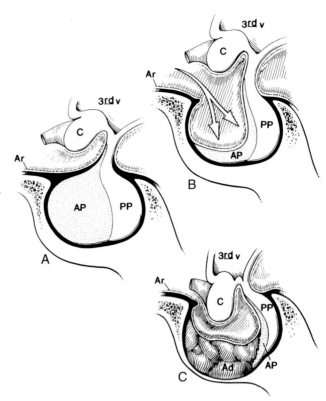

**FIGURE 9–119    EMPTY SELLA VARIANTS**

In contrast to the normal anatomy of the sella (*A*), the primary form of empty sella syndrome results from hypoplasia or absence of the sellar diaphragm, a situation that permits a pouch of arachnoid to come in contact with and compress the dorsal aspect of the pituitary (*B*). The secondary form of empty sella syndrome (*C*) occurs as a consequence of spontaneous infarction of a sellar neoplasm or of surgical or radiotherapeutic intervention. Ar, arachnoid; C, optic chiasm; 3rd v, third ventricle; AP, anterior pituitary; PP, posterior pituitary; Ad, adenoma.

mononucleate or multinucleate (Touton-like) cells, the latter having uniform round nuclei arranged in a peripheral ring. Eosinophils are scant. Immunostains show S-100 protein and/or CD68 staining, but not CD1A reactivity.[2, 4]

## Xanthoma Disseminatum

This rare condition has been found to involve the hypothalamus, pituitary, and dura.[1]

## INFECTIOUS LESIONS

### Abscess

Historically, the term pituitary abscess has been loosely applied to inflammatory masses as diverse as aseptic necrosis of a pituitary adenoma (pituitary apoplexy) and bacterial infection of either an adenoma[8] or the normal pituitary.[1] We limit use of the term to infectious lesions, the majority of which are simply pyogenic abscesses occurring in the setting of bacterial meningitis, sinusitis, sepsis, or immunosuppression.[2, 4, 5, 7, 8] Abscesses with a fungal etiology, usually aspergillosis, have also been described.[3, 9] There will always be cases in which the term abscess is applied to purulent-appearing lesions of

indeterminate etiology that lack evidence of an organism by either special stain or culture.[6]

## Miscellaneous Infections

Tuberculomas of the sellar region[2, 4] far outnumber such unusual lesions as cysticercosis[1] and echinococcosis.[3]

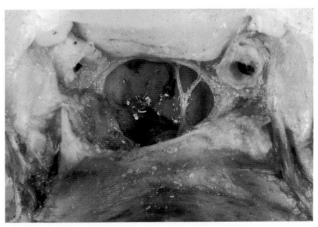

**FIGURE 9–120    EMPTY SELLA SYNDROME, PRIMARY TYPE**

An incompletely formed sellar diaphragm permits herniation of the arachnoid membrane into the sella.

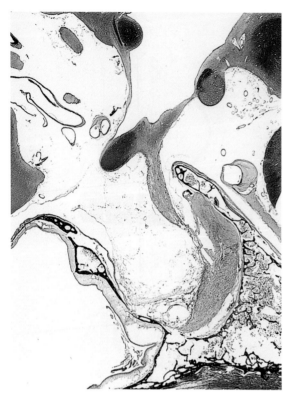

**FIGURE 9–121** EMPTY SELLA SYNDROME, PRIMARY TYPE

A pouch of arachnoid has entered the sella, causing displacement of, and traction on, the infundibulum as well as marked compression and atrophy of the gland. Comparison with Figure 9–1 demonstrates enlargement of the pituitary fossa and thinning of the sellar floor. The patient was a 72-year-old man with severe testicular and adrenocortical atrophy.

## MISCELLANEOUS NON-NEOPLASTIC PROCESSES

Occasionally occurring as sellar masses are cavernous angioma,[4,5] intravascular papillary endothelial hyperplasia,[4] extramedullary hematopoiesis,[1,2] and last but not least pseudotumor.[3]

## EMPTY SELLA SYNDROME

So-called empty sellas occur in two types. The primary form results from diverticular protrusion of an arachnoid pouch into the sella by way of an incompetent sellar diaphragm. In the secondary type, herniation of arachnoid follows loss of intrasellar volume related to infarction, radiation necrosis or atrophy, surgical resection of the pituitary gland, or involution of an adenoma (apoplexy)[1,2,4,5] (Fig. 9–119).

Primary empty sella syndrome may or may not be symptomatic and usually occurs in middle-age women. An association with hypertension and obesity has been noted.[1,2,4,5] Children are rarely affected.[3] Symptoms, if any, consist mainly of headaches. Endocrine hypofunction and hyperprolactinemia related to traction deformity of the pituitary stalk are uncommon. In rare instances, visual disturbance results from intrasellar prolapse of the chiasm. The long-term effect of pituitary

compression is posterior displacement of the gland, leaving only its flattened, crescent-shaped profile on the sellar floor (Figs. 9–120 and 9–121). In most cases, no surgical specimen is submitted. When one is available, it simply consists of normal-appearing arachnoid membrane with occasional aggregates of meningothelial cells.

## REFERENCES

### The Sellar Region and Normal Pituitary

1. Asa SL. Tumors of pituitary gland. In Atlas of Tumor Pathology. Fascicle 22. Ser 3. Washington, DC: Armed Forces Institute of Pathology, 1998, pp 1–214.
2. Horvath E, Kovacs K, Scheithauer BW, et al. Regional Neuropathology: The Pituitary and Hypothalamus. In Greenfield's Neuropathology. 5th ed. New York: Wiley Medical, 1997, pp 1007–1094.
3. Kovacs K, Horvath E. Tumors of the pituitary gland. In Atlas of Tumor Pathology. Fascicle 21. Ser 2. Washington, DC: Armed Forces Institute of Pathology, 1986.
4. Pernicone P, Scheithauer BW, Horvath E, et al. The pituitary and sellar region. In Sternberg S (ed). Histology for Pathologists. New York: Raven Press, 1992, pp 279–299.
5. Reeves WB, Bichat DG, Androli TE. The posterior pituitary and water metabolism. In Wilson JD, Foster DW, Kronenberg HN, et al (eds). Williams Textbook of Endocrinology. 9th ed. Philadelphia: WB Saunders, 1998, pp 341–387.
6. Scheithauer BW. The hypothalamus and neurohypophysis. In Kovacs K, Asa SL (eds). Functional Endocrine Pathology. 2nd ed. Malden, MA: Blackwell Science, 1998, pp 171–246.
7. Scheithauer BW, Horvath E, Kovacs K. Ultrastructure of the neurohypophysis. Microsc Res Tech 1992;20:177–186.
8. Scheithauer BW, Kovacs K, Horvath E. The adenohypophysis. In Lechago J, Gould VE (eds). Bloodworth's Pathology. 3rd ed. Baltimore: Williams & Wilkins, 1997, pp 85–152.
9. Scheithauer BW, Kovacs K, Young WF, et al. Neurohypophysis and hypothalamus. In Lechago J, Gould VE (eds). Bloodworth's Pathology. 3rd ed. Baltimore: Williams & Wilkins, 1997, pp 25–83.
10. Stefaneanu L, Kovacs K, Horvath E, et al. The adenohypophysis. In Stefaneanu L, Sasano H, Kovacs K (eds). Molecular and Cellular Pathology. London: Arnold Publishers, 2000, pp 75–117.
11. Thorner MO, Vance ML, Laws ER Jr, et al. The anterior pituitary. In Wilson JD, Foster DW, Kronenberg HN, et al (eds). Williams Textbook of Endocrinology. 9th ed. Philadelphia: WB Saunders, 1998, pp 249–340.

### Pituitary Neoplasia

1. Adelman LS, Post KD. Intraoperative frozen section techniques for pituitary adenomas. Am J Surg Pathol 1979;3:173–175.
2. Ahmed M, Rifai A, Al-Jurf M, et al. Classical pituitary apoplexy presentation and a follow-up of 13 patients. Horm Res 1989;31:125–132.
3. Anniko M, Tribukait B, Wersall J. DNA ploidy and cell phase in human pituitary tumors. Cancer 1984;53:1708–1713.
4. Asa SL. Tumors of pituitary gland. In Atlas of Tumor Pathology. Fascicle 22. Ser 3. Washington, DC: Armed Forces Institute of Pathology, 1998, pp 1–214.
5. Asa SL, Gerrie BM, Singer W, et al. Gonadotropin secretion in vitro by human pituitary null cell adenomas and oncocytomas. J Clin Endocrinol Metab 1986;62:1011–1019.
6. Asa SL, Kovacs K, Horvath E, et al. Sellar glomangioma. Ultrastruct Pathol 1984;7:49–54.
7. Asa SL, Scheithauer BW, Bilbao JM, et al. A case for hypothalamic acromegaly: a clinicopathological study of six patients with hypothalamic gangliocytomas producing growth hormone–releasing factor. J Clin Endocrinol Metab 1984;58:796–803.
8. Barrow DL, Tindall GT, Kovacs K, et al. Clinical and pathological effects of bromocriptine on prolactin-secreting and other pituitary tumors. J Neurosurg 1984;60:1–7.
9. Beauchesne P, Trouillas J, Barral F, et al. Gonadotropic pituitary carcinoma: case report. Neurosurgery 1995;37:810–816.
10. Berg KK, Scheithauer BW, Klee GG, et al. Alpha subunit in pituitary adenomas: a radioimmunoassay and immunohistochemical study. Adv Biosci 1988;69:397–411.

11. Bilbao JM, Horvath E, Kovacs K, et al. Intrasellar paraganglioma associated with hypopituitarism. Arch Pathol Lab Med 1978;102: 95–98.

12. Bilbao JM, Kovacs K, Horvath E, et al. Pituitary melanocorticotrophinoma with amyloid deposition. Can J Neurol Sci 1975;2: 199–202.

13. Bills DC, Meyer FB, Laws ER Jr, et al. A retrospective analysis of pituitary apoplexy. Neurosurgery 1993;33:602–609.

14. Black PM, Hsu DW, Klibanski A, et al. Hormone production in clinically nonfunctioning pituitary adenomas. J Neurosurg 1987; 66:244–250.

15. Boggild MD, Jenkinson S, Pistorello M, et al. Molecular genetic studies of sporadic pituitary tumors. J Clin Endocrinol Metab 1994;78:387–392.

16. Branch CL, Laws ER Jr. Metastatic tumors of the sella turcica masquerading as primary pituitary tumors. J Clin Endocrinol Metab 1987;65:469–474.

17. Calle-Rodrigue RD, Giannini C, Scheithauer BW, et al. Prolactinomas in male and female patients: a comparative clinicopathologic study. Mayo Clin Proc 1998;73:1046–1052.

18. Cardoso ER, Peterson EW. Pituitary apoplexy: a review. Neurosurgery 1984;14:363–373.

19. Colohan ART, Grady MS, Bonnin JM, et al. Ectopic pituitary gland simulating a suprasellar tumor. Neurosurgery 1986;20: 43–48.

20. Corenblum B, Sirek AMT, Horvath E, et al. Human mixed somatotrophic and lactotrophic pituitary adenomas. J Clin Endocrinol Metab 1976;42:857–863.

21. Costello RT. Subclinical adenoma of the pituitary gland. Am J Pathol 1936;12:205–215.

22. Cyrns VL, Alexander JM, Klibanski A, et al. The retinoblastoma gene in human pituitary tumors. J Clin Endocrinol Metab 1993;77:644–646.

23. Duello TM, Halmi NS. Immunocytochemistry of prolactin-producing human pituitary adenomas. Am J Anat 1980;158:463–469.

24. Ebersold M, Laws ER Jr, Scheithauer BW. Pituitary apoplexy treated by transsphenoidal surgery: a clinicopathologic and immunocytochemical study. J Neurosurg 1983;58:315–320.

25. Ebersold MJ, Quast LM, Laws ER Jr, et al. Long-term results in transsphenoidal removal of 100 clinically nonfunctioning immunocytochemically characterized pituitary adenomas. J Neurosurg 1986;64:713–719.

26. Egensperger R, Scheithauer BW, Horvath E, et al. Cushing's disease due to plurihormonal ACTH and gonadotropin-producing pituitary adenoma. Acta Neuropathol (Berl) 2001;102:398–403.

27. Fatourechi V, Gharib H, Scheithauer BW, et al. Pituitary thyrotropic adenoma associated with congenital hypothyroidism. Am J Med 1984;76:725–728.

28. Felix IA, Horvath E, Kovacs K. Massive Crooke's hyalinization in corticotroph cell adenomas of the human pituitary. Acta Neurochir (Wien) 1981;58:235–243.

29. Felix IA, Horvath E, Kovacs K, et al. Mammosomatotroph adenoma of the pituitary associated with gigantism and hyperprolactinemia: a morphologic study including immunoelectron microscopy. Acta Neuropathol (Berl) 1986;71:76–82.

30. Fitzgibbons PL, Appley AJ, Turner RR, et al. Flow cytometric analysis of pituitary tumors: correlation of nuclear antigen p105 and DNA content with clinical behavior. Cancer 1988;62: 1556–1560.

31. Flickinger JC, Nelson PB, Martinez AJ, et al. Radiotherapy of nonfunctional adenomas of the pituitary gland: results with long-term follow-up. Cancer 1989;63:2409–2414.

32. Gaffey TA, Scheithauer BW, DeBault LE, et al. Pituitary adenoma: a DNA flow cytometric study of 192 clinical pathologically characterized tumors. Endocrine Path (submitted).

33. Gaffey TA, Scheithauer BW, Lloyd RV, et al. Corticotroph cell carcinoma of the pituitary: a clinical pathologic study of four cases. J Neurosurg (submitted).

34. Gandour-Edwards R, Kapadia SB, Janacka IP, et al. Biologic markers of invasive pituitary adenomas involving the sphenoid sinus. Mod Pathol 1996;8:160–164.

35. Geddes JF, Jansen GH, Robinson SFD, et al. Gangliocytomas of the pituitary. Am J Surg Pathol 2000;24:607–613.

36. George D, Scheithauer BW, Kovacs K, et al. Crooke's cell adenoma of the pituitary: an aggressive variant. Am J Surg Pathol (submitted)

37. Gharib H, Carpenter PC, Scheithauer BW, et al. The spectrum of inappropriate pituitary thyrotropin secretion associated with hyperthyroidism. Mayo Clin Proc 1982;57:556–563.

38. Ghatak NR, Hirano A, Zimmerman HM. Intrasellar germinomas: a form of ectopic pinealoma. J Neurosurg 1969;31:670–675.

39. Girod C, Mazzuca M, Trouillas J, et al. Light microscopy, fine structure and immunohistochemistry studies of 278 pituitary adenomas. In Derome PJ, Jedynak CP, Peillon F (eds). Pituitary Adenomas: Biology, Pathophysiology, and Treatment. Paris: Esclepios Publishers, 1980, p 3.

40. Girod C, Trouillas J, Claustrat B. The human thyrotropic adenoma: pathologic diagnosis in five cases and critical review of the literature. Semin Diagn Pathol 1986;3:58–68.

41. Grigsby PW, Simpson JR, Fineberg B. Late regrowth of pituitary adenomas after irradiation and/or surgery: hazard function analysis. Cancer 1989;63:1308–1312.

42. Grisoli F, Vincentelli F, Rayband C, et al. Intrasellar meningioma. Surg Neurol 1983;20:36–41.

43. Hague K, Post KD, Morgello S. Absence of peritumoral Crooke's change is associated with recurrence in surgically treated Cushing's disease. Surg Neurol 2000;53:77–81.

44. Hampton TA, Scheithauer BW, Rojiani AM, et al. Salivary gland–like tumors of the sellar region. Am J Surg Pathol 1997;21: 421–434.

45. Hardy J. Transsphenoidal surgery of hypersecreting pituitary tumors. In Diagnosis and Treatment of Pituitary Tumors. International Congress Series No 303. Amsterdam: Excerpta Medica, 1973.

46. Heitz PU, Landolt AM, Zenklusen H-R, et al. Immunocytochemistry of pituitary tumors. J Histochem Cytochem 1987; 35:1005–1011.

47. Herman V, Drazin NZ, Gonsky R, et al. Molecular screening of pituitary adenomas for gene mutations and rearrangements. J Clin Endocrinol Metab 1993;77:50–55.

48. Hinton DR, Polk RK, Linse KD, et al. Characteristics of spherical amyloid protein from prolactin-producing pituitary adenoma. Acta Neuropathol 1997;93:43–49.

49. Hori A, Schmidt D, Rickels E. Pharyngeal pituitary development malformation tumorigenesis. Acta Neuropathol (Berl) 1999;98: 262–272.

50. Horvath E, Kovacs K. Gonadotrophic adenomas of the human pituitary: sex-related fine-structural dichotomy: histologic, immunocytochemical, and electron-microscopic study of 30 tumors. Am J Pathol 1984;117:429–440.

51. Horvath E, Kovacs K. Ultrastructural classification of pituitary adenomas. Can J Neurol Sci 1976;3:9–21.

52. Horvath E, Kovacs K, Killinger DW, et al. Silent corticotroph adenomas of the human pituitary gland: a histologic, immunocytologic, and ultrastructural study. Am J Pathol 1980;98: 617–638.

53. Horvath E, Kovacs K, Lloyd RV. Pars intermedia of the human pituitary revisited: morphologic aspects and frequency of hyperplasia of POMC-peptide immunoreactive cells. Endocrinol Pathol 1999;10:55.

54. Horvath E, Kovacs K, Scheithauer BW, et al. Pituitary adenoma with neuronal choristoma (PANCH): composite lesion or lineage infidelity. Ultrastruct Pathol 1994;18:565–574.

55. Horvath E, Kovacs K, Singer W, et al. Acidophilic stem cell adenoma of the human pituitary: clinical pathologic analysis of 15 cases. Cancer 1981;47:761–771.

56. Horvath E, Kovacs K, Singer W, et al. Acidophilic stem cell adenoma of the pituitary. Arch Pathol Lab Med 1977;101:594–599.

57. Horvath E, Kovacs K, Smyth H, et al. A novel type of pituitary adenoma: morphologic features and clinical correlations. J Clin Endocrinol Metab 1988;66:1111–1118.

58. Horvath E, Scheithauer BW, Kovacs K, et al. Pituitary adenomas producing growth hormone, prolactin, and one or more glycoprotein hormones: a histologic, immunohistochemical, and ultrastructural study of four surgically removed tumors. Ultrastruct Pathol 1983;5:171–183.

59. Horvath E, Scheithauer BW, Kovacs K, et al. Regional neuropathology: hypothalamus and pituitary. In Graham DI, Lantos PL (eds). Greenfield's Neuropathology. 6th ed. London: Arnold, 1997, pp 1007–1094.

60. Irofumi T, Herman V, Weiss M, et al. Purine-binding factor (nm23) gene expression in pituitary tumors: marker of adenoma invasiveness. J Clin Endocrinol Metab 1995;80:1733–1738.

61. Ironside JW, Royds JA, Jefferson AA, et al. Immunolocalization of cytokeratins in the normal and neoplastic human pituitary gland. J Neurol Neurosurg Psychiatry 1987;50:57–65.

62. Jacoby LB, Hedley-Whyte ET, Pulaski K, et al. Clonal origin of pituitary adenomas. J Neurosurg 1990;73:731–735.

63. Jefferson G: The invasive adenomas of the pituitary: In The Sherrington Lectures, III. Liverpool: University Press of Liverpool, 1955.

64. Kane LA, Leinung MG, Scheithauer BW, et al. Pituitary adenomas in childhood and adolescence. J Clin Endocrinol Metab 1994;79:1135–1140.

65. Karga HJ, Alexander JM, Hedley-Whyte ET, et al. Ras mutations in human pituitary tumors. J Clin Endocrinol Metab 1992;74:914–919.

66. Katz NS, Gregerman RI, Horvath E, et al. Thyrotroph cell adenoma of the human pituitary gland associated with primary hypothyroidism: clinical and morphological features. Acta Endocrinol (Copenh) 1980;95:41–48.

67. Kawamoto H, Kawamoto K, Mizoue T, et al. Matrix metalloproteinase-9 secretion by human pituitary adenomas detected by cell immunoblot analysis. Acta Neurochir (Wien) 1996;138:1142–1148.

68. Kawamoto H, Mizoue T, Arita K, et al. Expression of epithelial cadherin and cavernous sinus invasion in human pituitary adenomas. J Neurooncol 1997;34:105–109.

69. Kawamoto H, Vozumi I, Kawamoto K, et al. Type IV collagenase activity and cavernous sinus invasion in human pituitary adenomas. Acta Neurochir (Wien) 1996;138:390–395.

70. Kay S, Lees JK, Stout AP. Pituitary chromophobe tumors of the nasal cavity. Cancer 1950;3:695–704.

71. Kepes J. Transitional cell tumor of the pituitary gland developing from a Rathke's cleft cyst. Cancer 1978;41:337–343.

72. Kleinschmidt-DeMasters BK, Winston KR, Rubinstein D, et al. Ectopic pituitary adenoma of the third ventricle. Case report. J Neurosurg 1990;72:139–142.

73. Kontogeorgos G, Kovacs K, Horvath E, et al. Null cell adenomas, oncocytomas, and gonadotroph adenomas of the human pituitary: an immunocytochemical and ultrastructural analysis of 300 cases. Endocrinol Pathol 1993;4:20–27.

74. Kontogeorgos G, Scheithauer BW, Horvath E, et al. Double adenomas of the pituitary: a clinicopathological study of 11 tumors. Neurosurgery 1992;31:840–849.

75. Kovacs K, Asa SL, Horvath E, et al. Null cell adenomas of the pituitary: attempts to resolve their cytogenesis. In Lechago J, Kameya T (eds). Endocrine Pathology Update. Philadelphia: Field and Wood, 1990, pp 17–31.

76. Kovacs K, Horvath E. Pathology of growth hormone producing tumors of the human pituitary. Semin Diagn Pathol 1986;3: 18–33.

77. Kovacs K, Horvath E. Tumors of the pituitary gland. In Atlas of Tumor Pathology. Fascicle 21. Ser 2. Washington, DC: Armed Forces Institute of Pathology, 1986.

78. Kovacs K, Horvath E, Stefaneanu L, et al. Two cases of pituitary Crooke's cell adenoma without Cushing's disease: a histologic, immunocytochemical, electron microscopic and in situ hybridization study. Endocrinol Pathol 1999;10:65–72.

79. Kovacs K, Scheithauer BW, Horvath E, et al. The WHO classification of adenohypophysial neoplasms: a proposed five-tier scheme. Cancer 1996;78:502–510.

80. Kuratsu J-I, Matsukado Y, Miura M. Prolactinoma of pituitary with associated amyloid-like substances: case report. J Neurosurg 1983;59:1067–1070.

81. Lach B, Rippstein P, Benott BG, et al. Differentiating neuroblastoma of pituitary gland: neuroblastic transformation of epithelial adenoma cells. Case report. J Neurosurg 1996;85:953–960.

82. Landolt AM, Kleihues P, Heitz PU. Amyloid deposits in pituitary adenomas: differentiation of two types. Arch Pathol Lab Med 1987;111:453–458.

83. Landolt AM, Shibata T, Kleihues P. Growth rate of human pituitary adenomas. J Neurosurg 1987;67:803–806.

84. Laws ER Jr, Scheithauer BW, Carpenter S, et al. The pathogenesis of acromegaly: clinical and immunochemical analysis in 75 patients. J Neurosurg 1985;63:35–38.

85. Lees PD, Pickard JD, Chir M. Hyperprolactinemia, intrasellar pituitary tissue pressure, and the pituitary stalk compression syndrome. J Neurosurg 1987;67:192–196.

86. Leinung MC, Kane LA, Scheithauer BW, et al. Long-term treatment of Cushing's disease in childhood. J Clin Endocrinol Metab 1995;80:2475–2479.

87. Levy A, Lightman SL. Growth hormone–releasing hormone transcripts in human pituitary adenomas. J Clin Endocrinol Metab 1992;74:1474–1476.

88. Li JY, Racadot O, Kujas M, et al. Immunocytochemistry of four mixed pituitary adenomas and intrasellar gangliocytomas associated with different clinical syndromes: acromegaly, amenorrheagalactorrhea, Cushing's disease and isolated tumoral syndrome. Acta Neuropathol (Berl) 1989;77:320–328.

89. Lipper S, Isenberg HD, Kahn LB. Calcospherites in pituitary prolactinomas: a hypothesis for their formation. Arch Pathol Lab Med 1984;108:31–34.

90. Lloyd RV. Molecular biological analysis of pituitary disorders. In Lloyd RV (ed). Surgical Pathology of the Pituitary Gland. Philadelphia: WB Saunders, 1993, pp 85–93.

91. Lloyd RV, Chandler WF, Kovacs K, et al. Ectopic pituitary adenomas with normal anterior pituitary glands. Am J Surg Pathol 1986;10:546–552.

92. Lloyd RV, Chandler WF, McKeever PE, et al. The spectrum of ACTH-producing pituitary lesions. Am J Surg Pathol 1986;10: 618–626.

93. Lloyd RV, Gikas PW, Chandler WF. Prolactin and growth hormone–producing pituitary adenomas: an immunohistochemical and ultrastructural study. Am J Surg Pathol 1983;7:251–260.

94. Lloyd RV, Scheithauer BW, Kovacs K, et al. The immunophenotype of pituitary adenomas. Endocrinol Pathol 1996;7:145–150.

95. Lloyd RV, Wilson BS, Kovacs K, et al. Immunohistochemical localization of chromogranin in human hypophyses and pituitary adenomas. Arch Pathol Lab Med 1985;109:515–517.

96. Martinez AJ. The pathology of nonfunctional pituitary adenomas. Semin Diagn Pathol 1986;3:83–94.

97. Martinez AJ, Lee A, Moossy J, et al. Pituitary adenomas: clinicopathological and immunohistochemical study. Ann Neurol 1980;7: 24–36.

98. Martins AN, Hayes GJ, Kempe LG. Invasive pituitary adenomas. J Neurosurg 1965;22:268–276.

99. Masago A, Ueda Y, Kanai H, et al. Pituitary apoplexy after pituitary function test: a report of two cases and review of the literature. Surg Neurol 1995;43:158–165.

100. McComb DJ, Ryan N, Horvath E, et al. Subclinical adenomas of the human pituitary: new light on an old problem. Arch Pathol Lab Med 1983;107:488–491.

101. Mindermann T, Wilson CB. Pediatric pituitary adenomas. Neurosurgery 1995;36:259–269.

102. Mohr G, Hardy J. Hemorrhage, necrosis, and apoplexy in pituitary adenomas. Surg Neurol 1982;18:181–189.

103. Molinatti PA, Scheithauer BW, Randall RV, et al. Metastasis to pituitary adenoma. Arch Pathol Lab Med 1985;109:287–289.

104. Mori H, Mori S, Saitoh Y, et al. Effects of bromocriptine on prolactin-secreting pituitary adenomas. Cancer 1985;56:230–238.

105. Mori H, Mori S, Saitoh Y, et al. Growth hormone–producing pituitary adenoma with crystal-like amyloid immunohistochemically positive for growth hormone. Cancer 1985;55:96–102.

106. Mukai K. Pituitary adenomas: immunocytochemical study of 150 tumors with clinicopathologic correlation. Cancer 1983;52: 648–653.

107. Nakasu S, Nakasu Y, Kyoshima K, et al. Pituitary adenoma with multiple ciliated cysts: transitional cell tumor? Surg Neurol 1989; 31:41–48.

108. Nishio S, Mizuno J, Barrow DL, et al. Pituitary tumors composed of adenohypophysial adenoma and Rathke's cleft cyst elements: a clinicopathological study. Neurosurgery 1987;21:371–377.

109. Niwa J, Minase T, Mori M, et al. Immunohistochemical, electron microscopic, and morphometric studies of human prolactinomas after short-term bromocriptine treatment. Surg Neurol 1987;28: 339–374.

110. Palmer PE, Bogojavlensky S, Bhan AK, et al. Prolactinoma in wall of ovarian dermoid cyst with hyperprolactinemia. Obstet Gynecol 1990;75:540–543.

111. Parl FF, Cruz VE, Cobb CA, et al. Late recurrence of surgically removed prolactinomas. Cancer 1986;57:2422–2426.

112. Partington MD, Davis DH, Laws ER Jr, et al. Pituitary adenomas in childhood and adolescence: results of transsphenoidal surgery. J Neurosurg 1994;80:209–216.

113. Pernicone PJ, Scheithauer BW, Sebo PJ, et al. Pituitary carcinoma: a clinicopathologic study of 15 cases. Cancer 1997;79: 804–812.

114. Ramsay JA, Kovacs K, Scheithauer BW, et al. Metastatic carci-

noma to pituitary adenomas: a report of two cases. Exp Clin Endocrinol 1988;92:69–76.

115. Randall RV, Scheithauer BW, Laws ER Jr, et al. Pituitary adenomas associated with hyperprolactinemia: a clinical and immunohistochemical study of 97 patients operated on transsphenoidally. Mayo Clin Proc 1985;60:753–762.

116. Randall RV, Scheithauer BW, Laws ER Jr, et al. Pseudoprolactinomas. Trans Am Clin Climatol Assoc 1982;94:114–121.

117. Rhodes RH, Dusseau JJ, Boyd AS Jr, et al. Intrasellar neuraladenohypophyseal choristoma: a morphological and immunocytochemical study. J Neuropathol Exp Neurol 1982;41:267–280.

118. Riedel M, Noldus J, Saeger W, et al. Sellar lesions associated with isolated hyperprolactinaemia: morphological, immunocytochemical, hormonal and clinical results. Acta Endocrinol (Copenh) 1986;113:196–203.

119. Robert F. Electron microscopy of human pituitary tumors. In Tindall GT, Collins WF (eds). Clinical Management of Pituitary Disorders. New York: Raven Press, 1979, pp 113–131.

120. Robert F, Hardy J. Human corticotroph cell adenomas. Semin Diagn Pathol 1986;3:34–41.

121. Robert F, Pelletier G, Hardy J. Pituitary adenomas in Cushing's disease: histologic, ultrastructural, and immunocytochemical study. Arch Pathol Lab Med 1978;102:448–455.

122. Rock JP, Babu VR, Drumheller T, et al. Cytogenetic findings in pituitary adenoma: results of a pilot study. Surg Neurol 1993;40:224–229.

123. Saeki N, Sunami K, Sugaya Y, et al. MRI findings and clinical manifestations in Rathke's cleft cyst. Acta Neurochir (Wien) 1999;141:1055–1061.

124. Salassa RM, Kerns TP, Kernohan JW, et al. Pituitary tumors in patients with Cushing's syndrome. J Clin Endocrinol Metab 1959;19:1523.

125. Sano T, Kovacs K, Asa SL, et al. Immunoreactive luteinizing hormone in functioning corticotroph adenomas of the pituitary. Immunohistochemical and tissue culture studies of two cases. Virchows Arch [A] 1990;417:351–367.

126. Scheithauer BW, Horvath E, Kovacs K, et al. Plurihormonal pituitary adenomas. Semin Diagn Pathol 1986;3:69–82.

127. Scheithauer BW, Horvath E, Kovacs K, et al. Prolactin-producing adenoma and carcinoma with neuronal components—a metaplastic lesion. Pituitary 1999;1:197–206.

128. Scheithauer BW, Jaap AJ, Horvath E, et al. Clinically silent corticotroph tumors of the pituitary gland. Neurosurgery, 2000;47:723–729.

129. Scheithauer BW, Kovacs K, Horvath E, et al. Tumors of the adenohypophysis. In Solcia E, Kloppel G, Sobin LH (eds). Histologic Typing of Endocrine Tumors. The World Health Organization. Berlin: Springer, 2000, pp 15–29, 75–90.

130. Scheithauer BW, Kovacs K, Laws ER Jr, et al. Pathology of invasive pituitary tumors with special reference to functional classification. J Neurosurg 1986;65:733–744.

131. Scheithauer BW, Kovacs K, Randall RV, et al. Hypothalamic neuronal hamartoma and adenohypophyseal neuronal choristoma: their association with growth hormone adenoma of the pituitary gland. J Neuropathol Exp Neurol 1983;42:648–663.

132. Scheithauer BW, Kovacs K, Randall RV, et al. Pathology of excessive production of growth hormone. Clin Endocrinol 1986;15:655–681.

133. Scheithauer BW, Laws ER Jr, Kovacs K, et al. Pituitary adenomas of the multiple endocrine neoplasia type I syndrome. Semin Diagn Pathol 1987;4:205–211.

134. Scheithauer BW, Fereidooni F, Horvath E, et al. Pituitary carcinoma: A study of 11 cases. Ultrastruct Pathol (In press).

135. Schober R, Nelson D. Fine structure and origin of amyloid deposits in pituitary adenoma. Arch Pathol 1975;99:403–410.

136. Selman WR, Laws ER Jr, Scheithauer BW, et al. The occurrence of dural invasion in pituitary adenomas. J Neurosurg 1986;64:402–407.

137. Solero CL, Giombini S, Morello G. Suprasellar and olfactory meningiomas. Report on a series of 153 personal cases. Acta Neurochir (Wien) 1983;67:181–194.

138. Takahata T, Katayama Y, Tsubokawa T, et al. Ectopic pituitary adenoma occurring in the interpeduncular cistern. J Neurosurg 1995;83:1092–1094.

139. Thapar K, Kovacs K, Scheithauer BW, et al. Proliferative activity and invasiveness among pituitary adenomas and carcinomas: an analysis using the MIB-1 antibody. Neurosurgery 1996;38:99–107.

140. Thapar K, Kovacs K, Stefaneanu L, et al. Overexpression of the growth-hormone releasing hormone gene in acromegaly associated pituitary tumors: an event associated with neoplastic progression and aggressive behavior. Am J Pathol 1997;151:769–784.

141. Thapar K, Scheithauer BW, Kovacs K, et al. p53 expression in pituitary adenomas and carcinomas: correlation with invasive and tumor growth fractions. Neurosurgery 1996;38:765–777.

142. Thapar K, Yamata Y, Scheithauer BW, et al. Assessment of mitotic activity in pituitary adenomas and carcinomas. Endocrinol Pathol 1996;7:215–221.

143. Tindall GT, Kovacs K, Horvath E, et al. Human prolactin-producing adenomas and bromocriptine: a histological, immunocytochemical, ultrastructural, and morphologic study. J Clin Endocrinol Metab 1982;55:1178–1183.

144. Towfighi J, Salam MM, McLendon RE, et al. Ganglion cell–containing tumors of the pituitary gland. Arch Pathol Lab Med 1996;120:369–377.

145. Trouillas J, Girod C, Sassolas G, et al. The human gonadotrophic adenoma: pathologic diagnosis and hormonal correlations in 26 tumors. Semin Diagn Pathol 1986;3:42–57.

146. Urbanski SJ, Bilbao JM, Horvath E, et al. Intrasellar solitary plasmacytoma terminating in multiple myeloma: a report of a case including electron microscopical study. Surg Neurol 1980;14:233.

147. Velasco ME, Sindley SD, Roessmann V. Reticulin stain for frozen section diagnosis of pituitary adenomas. J Neurosurg 1977;46:548–550.

148. Wakai S, Fukushima T, Teramoto A, et al. Pituitary apoplexy: its incidence and clinical significance. J Neurosurg 1981;55:187–193.

149. Webster J, Peters JR, John R, et al. Pituitary stone: two cases of densely calcified thyrotrophin-secreting pituitary adenoma. Clin Endocrinol (Oxf) 1984;40:137–143.

150. Wilson CB, Tyrrell JB, Fitzgerald PA, et al. Neurosurgical aspects of Cushing's disease and Nelson's syndrome. In Tindall GT, Collins WF (eds). Clinical Management of Pituitary Disorders. New York: Raven Press, 1979, pp 229–238.

151. Wynne AG, Scheithauer BW, Young WF Jr, et al. Coexisting corticotroph and lactotroph adenomas: case report with reference to the relationship of corticotroph and prolactin excess. Neurosurgery 1992;30:919–23.

152. Young WF Jr, Scheithauer BW, Kovacs KT, et al. Gonadotroph adenoma of the pituitary gland: a clinicopathologic analysis of 100 cases. Mayo Clin Proc 1996;71:649–656.

153. Zambaziotis D, Kontogeorgos G, Kovacs K, et al. Intrasellar paraganglioma presenting as nonfunctioning pituitary adenoma. Arch Pathol Lab Med 1999;123:429–432.

154. Zimmerman D, Young WF Jr, Ebersold MJ, et al. Congenital gigantism due to growth hormone releasing hormone excess and pituitary hyperplasia with adenomatous transformation. J Clin Endocrinol Metab 1993;76:216–222.

## Pituitary Hyperplasia

1. Carey RM, Varma SK, Drake CR, et al. Ectopic secretion of corticotropin-releasing factor as a cause of Cushing's syndrome: a clinical, morphologic, and biochemical study. N Engl J Med 1984;311:13–20.

2. Horvath E, Kovacs K. Ultrastructural diagnosis of pituitary adenomas and hyperplasias. In Lloyd RV (ed). Surgical Pathology of the Pituitary Gland. Philadelphia, WB Saunders, 1993, pp 27, 52–84.

3. Horvath E, Kovacs K, Scheithauer BW. Pituitary hyperplasia. Pituitary 1999;1:169–180.

4. Horvath E, Kovacs K, Scheithauer BW. Surgical pathology of pituitary thyrotroph hyperplasia: an oxymoron? Endocrinol Pathol 1992;3(Suppl 1):514–515.

5. Horvath E, Scheithauer BW, Kovacs K, et al. Regional neuropathology: hypothalamus and pituitary. In Graham DI, Lantos PL (eds). Greenfield's Neuropathology. 6th ed. London: Arnold, 1997, pp 1007–1094.

6. Kovacs K, Stefaneanu L, Ezzat S, et al. Prolactin-producing pituitary adenoma in a male-to-female transsexual patient with protracted estrogen administration. A morphologic study. Arch Pathol Lab Med 1994;118:562–565.

7. Kovacs K, Stefaneanu L, Horvath E, et al. Pituitary corticotroph adenoma in a woman with long-standing Addison's disease: a

histologic, immunocytochemical, electron microscopic and in situ hybridization study. Endocrinol Pathol 1996;7:91–97.

8. Pioro E, Scheithauer BW, Laws ER, et al. Combined thyrotroph and lactotroph cell hyperplasia simulating prolactin-secreting pituitary "adenoma" in long-standing primary hypothyroidism. Surg Neurol 1988;29:218–226.

9. Saeger W, Ludecke DK. Pituitary hyperplasia: definition, light and electron microscopical structures and significance in surgical specimens. Virchows Arch [A] 1983;399:277–287.

10. Sano P, Kovacs K, Scheithauer BW, et al. Aging and human pituitary. Mayo Clin Proc 1993;68:971–977.

11. Sano T, Asa SL, Kovacs K. Growth hormone–releasing hormone–producing tumors: clinical, biochemical, and morphological manifestations. Endocr Rev 1988;9:357–373.

12. Scheithauer BW, Carpenter PC, Bloch B. Ectopic secretion of growth hormone releasing factor: report of a case of acromegaly with bronchial carcinoid tumor. Am J Med 1984;76:605–616.

13. Scheithauer BW, Kovacs K, Randall RV, et al. Hypothalamic neuronal hamartoma and adenohypophyseal neuronal choristoma: their association with growth hormone adenoma of the pituitary gland. J Neuropathol Exp Neurol 1983;42:648–663.

14. Scheithauer BW, Kovacs K, Randall RV, et al. Pituitary gland in hypothyroidism: histologic and immunocytologic study. Arch Pathol Lab Med 1985;109:499.

15. Scheithauer BW, Kovacs K, Randall RV. The pituitary in untreated Addison's disease: a histologic and immunocytologic study of 18 adenohypophyses. Arch Pathol Lab Med 1983;107: 484–487.

16. Scheithauer BW, Kovacs KT, Randall RV, et al. The effects of estrogen on the human pituitary: a clinicopathologic study. Mayo Clin Proc 1989;64:1077–1084.

17. Scheithauer BW, Sano T, Kovacs K, et al. The pituitary gland in pregnancy: a clinicopathologic and immunohistochemical study of 69 cases. Mayo Clin Proc 1990;65:461–474.

18. Stefaneanu L, Kovacs K, Lloyd R, et al. Pituitary lactotrophs and somatotrophs in pregnancy: a correlative in situ hybridization and immunocytochemical study. J Clin Endocrinol Metab 1992;62: 291–296.

19. Thorner MO, Perryman RL, Cronin MJ, et al. Somatotroph hyperplasia: successful treatment of acromegaly by removal of pancreatic islet tumor secreting a growth releasing factor. J Clin Invest 1982;70:965–977.

20. Wakabayashi I, Ihara T, Hattori M, et al. Presence of corticotroph-releasing factor–like immunoreactivity in human tumors. Cancer 1985;55:995–1000.

21. Young WF, Scheithauer BW, Gharib H, et al. Cushing's syndrome due to primary multinodular corticotroph hyperplasia. Mayo Clin Proc 1988;63:256–262.

22. Zimmerman D, Young WF Jr, Ebersold MJ, et al. Congenital gigantism due to growth hormone releasing hormone excess and pituitary hyperplasia with adenomatous transformation. J Clin Endocrinol Metab 1993;76:216–222.

## Pituicytoma and Granular Cell Tumor

1. Brat DJ, Scheithauer BW, Staugaitis SM, et al. Pituicytoma: a distinctive low grade glioma of the neurohypophysis. Am J Surg Pathol 2000;24:362–368.

2. Hurley TR, DiAngelo CM, Clasen RA, et al. Magnetic resonance imaging and pathological analysis of a pituicytoma: case report. Neurosurgery 1994;35:314–317.

3. Lafitte C, Aesch B, Henry-Lebras F, et al. Granular cell tumor of the pituitary stalk. J Neurosurg 1994;80:1103–1107.

4. Liwnicz BH, Liwnicz RG, Huff JS, et al. Giant granular cell tumor of the suprasellar area: immunocytochemical and electron microscopic studies. Neurosurgery 1984;15:246–251.

5. Luse SA, Kernohan JW. Granular-cell tumors of the stalk and posterior lobe of the pituitary gland. Cancer 1995;8:616–622.

6. Nishioka H, Li K, Llena JF, et al. Immunohistochemical study of granular cell tumors of the neurohypophysis. Virchows Arch [B] 1991;60:413–417.

7. Rossi ML, Bevan JS, Esiri MM, et al. Pituicytoma (pilocytic astrocytoma): case report. J Neurosurg 1987;67:768–672.

8. Schaller B, Kirsch E, Tolnay M, et al. Symptomatic granular cell tumor of the pituitary gland: case report and review of the literature. Neurosurgery 1998;42:166–171.

9. Scheithauer BW, Horvath E, Kovacs K. Ultrastructure of the neurohypophysis. Microsc Res Tech 1992;20:177–186.

10. Takei Y, Seyama S, Pearl GS, et al. Ultrastructural study of the human neurohypophysis. II. Cellular elements of neural parenchyma, the pituicytes. Cell Tissue Res 1980;205:273–287.

11. Vinores SA. Demonstration of glial fibrillary acidic (GFA) protein by electron immunocytochemistry in the granular cells of a choristoma of the neurohypophysis. Histochemistry 1991;96: 265–269.

## Craniopharyngioma

1. Adamson TE, Wiestler OD, Kleihues P, et al. Correlation of clinical and pathological features in surgically treated craniopharyngiomas. J Neurosurg 1990;73:12–17.

2. Akimura T, Kameda H, Abiko S, et al. Infrasellar craniopharyngioma. Neuroradiology 1989;31:180–183.

3. Altinors S, Senvall E, Erdogan A, et al. Craniopharyngioma of the cerebellopontine angle. J Neurosurg 1984;60:842–844.

4. Alvarez-Garijo JA, Froufe A, Taboada D, et al. Successful treatment of an odontogenic ossified craniopharyngioma: case report. J Neurosurg 1981;55:832–835.

5. Asa SL, Kovacs K, Bilbao JM. The pars tuberalis of the human pituitary: a histologic, immunohistochemical, ultrastructural and immunoelectron microscopic analysis. Virchows Arch [A] 1983;399:49–59.

6. Barloon TJ, Yuh WTC, Sato Y, et al. Frontal lobe implantation of craniopharyngioma by repeated needle aspirations. AJNR 1989;9: 406–407.

7. Baskin DS, Wilson CB. Surgical management of craniopharyngiomas: a review of 74 cases. J Neurosurg 1986;65:22–27.

8. Berstein ML, Buchino JJ. The histologic similarity between craniopharyngioma and odontogenic lesions: a reappraisal. Oral Surg 1983;56:502–511.

9. Boch AL, van Effenterre R, Kujas M. Craniopharyngioma in two consanguineous siblings: case report. Neurosurgery 1997;41: 1185–1187.

10. Cooper PR, Ransohoff J. Craniopharyngioma originating in the sphenoid bone: case report. J Neurosurg 1972;36:102–106.

11. Crotty TB, Scheithauer BW, Young WF Jr, et al. Papillary craniopharyngioma. A clinico-pathologic study of 48 cases. J Neurosurg 1995;83:206–214.

12. Dickey T, Raghaven R, Rushing E. MIB-1 (Ki-67) immunoreactivity as predictor of the risk of recurrence of craniopharyngioma produce pituitary hormones? Neurol Res 1999;58:567.

13. Duff JM, Meyer FB, Ilstrup DM, et al. The long-term outcome of surgically resected craniopharyngioma. Neurosurgery 2000;46(2):291–302.

14. Duff TA, Levine R. Intrachiasmatic craniopharyngioma: case report. J Neurosurg 1983;59:176–178.

15. Fischer EG, Welch K, Belli JA, et al. Treatment of craniopharyngioma in children: 1972–1981. J Neurosurg 1985;62:496–501.

16. Folkerth RD, Price DL Jr, Schwartz M, et al. Xanthomatous hypophysitis. Am J Surg Pathol 1998;22:736–741.

17. Ghatak NY, Hirano A, Zimmerman HM. Ultrastructure of a craniopharyngioma. Cancer 1971;27:1465–1475.

18. Giangaspero F, Burger PC, Osborne DR, et al. Suprasellar papillary squamous epithelioma ("papillary craniopharyngioma"). Am J Surg Pathol 1984;8:57–64.

19. Goldberg GM, Eshbaugh DE. Squamous cell nests of the pituitary gland as related to the origin of craniopharyngiomas: a study of their presence in the newborn and infants up to age four. Arch Pathol 1960;70:293–299.

20. Goodrich JT, Post KD, Duffy P. Ciliated craniopharyngioma. Surg Neurol 1985;24:105–111.

21. Gorlin RJ, Pindborg JJ, Redman RS, et al. The calcifying odontogenic cyst: a new entity and possible analogue of the cutaneous calcifying epithelioma of Malherbe. Cancer 1964;17:723–729.

22. Graziani N, Donnet A, Bugha TN, et al. Ectopic basisphenoidal craniopharyngioma: case report and review of the literature. Neurosurgery 1994;34:346–349.

23. Hazen S, Freidberg SR, Thomas C, et al. Multiple distinct intracranial tumors: association of pinealoma and craniopharyngioma: case report. Surg Neurol 1989;31:381–386.

24. Ho Lee J, Kim CY, Kim DG, et al. Postoperative ectopic seeding of craniopharyngioma. J Neurosurg 1999;90:796.

25. Honegger J, Renner C, Fahlbusch R, et al. Progesterone receptor gene expression in craniopharyngiomas and evidence for biological activity. Neurosurgery 1997;41:1359–1364.

26. Kalnins V, Rossi E. Odontogenic craniopharyngioma: a case report. Cancer 1965;18:899–906.

27. Lee JH, Kim C-Y, Kim DG, et al. Postoperative ectopic seeding of craniopharyngioma. J Neurosurg 1999;90:796.
28. Linden CN, Martinez CR, Gonzalvo AA, et al. Intrinsic third ventricle craniopharyngioma: CT and MR findings. J Comput Assist Tomogr 1989;13:362–368.
29. Liszczak T, Richardson EP Jr, Phillips JP, et al. Morphological, biochemical, ultrastructural, tissue culture and clinical observations of typical and aggressive craniopharyngiomas. Acta Neuropathol (Berl) 1978;43:191–203.
30. Luse SA, Kernohan JW. Squamous-cell nests of the pituitary gland. Cancer 1955;8:623–628.
31. Majlessi H, Shariat AS, Katirai A. Nasopharyngeal craniopharyngioma: case report. J Neurosurg 1978;49:119–120.
32. Matson DD, Crigler JF Jr. Management of craniopharyngioma in childhood. J Neurosurg 1969;30:377–390.
33. Matsushima T, Fukui M, Ohta M, et al. Ciliated and goblet cells in craniopharyngioma: light and electron microscopic study. Acta Neuropathol (Berl) 1980;50:199–205.
34. Nelson GA, Bastian FO, Schlitt M, et al. Malignant transformation in craniopharyngioma. Neurosurgery 1988;22:427–429.
35. Nishi T, Kuratsu JI, Takeshima H, et al. Prognostic significance of the MIB-1 labeling index for patient with craniopharyngioma. Int J Mol Med 1999;3;157–161.
36. Patrick BS, Smith RR, Bailey TO. Aseptic meningitis due to spontaneous rupture of craniopharyngioma cyst: case report. J Neurosurg 1974;41:387–390.
37. Pusey E, Kortman KE, Flannigan BD, et al. MR of craniopharyngiomas: tumor delineation and characterization. AJR 1987; 149:383–388.
38. Ragoowansi AT, Piepgras DG. Postoperative ectopic craniopharyngioma. Case report. J Neurosurg 1991;74:653–655.
39. Russell RWR, Pennybacker JB. Craniopharyngioma in the elderly. J Neurol Neurosurg Psychiatry 1961;24:1–13.
40. Sartoretti-Schefer S, Wichmann W, Aguzzi A, et al. MR differentiation of adamantinous and squamous-papillary craniopharyngiomas. AJNR 1997;18:77–87.
41. Satoh H, Uozumi T, Arita K, et al. Spontaneous rupture of craniopharyngioma cysts. A report of five cases and review of the literature. Surg Neurol 1993;40:414–419.
42. Seemayer TA, Blundell JS, Wiglesworth FW. Pituitary craniopharyngioma with tooth formation. Cancer 1972;29:423–430.
43. Solarski A, Panke ES, Panke TW. Craniopharyngioma in the pineal gland (Letter). Arch Pathol Lab Med 1978;102:490–491.
44. Sorva R, Jaaskinen J, Heiskanen O. Craniopharyngioma in children and adults: correlations between radiological and clinical manifestations. Acta Neurochir (Wien) 1987;89:3–9.
45. Szeifert GT, Pasztor E. Could craniopharyngiomas produce pituitary hormones? Neurol Res 1993;15:68–69.
46. Tachibana O, Yamashima T, Yamashita J, et al. Immunohistochemical expression of human chorionic gonadotropin and P-glycoprotein in human pituitary glands and craniopharyngiomas. J Neurosurg 1994;890:79–84.
47. Thapar K, Stefaneanu L, Kovacs K, et al. Estrogen receptor gene expression in craniopharyngiomas: an in situ hybridization study. Neurosurgery 1994;35:1012–1017.
48. Vilches J, Lopez A, Martinez MC, et al. Scanning and transmission electron microscopy of a craniopharyngioma: x-ray microanalytical study of the intratumoral mineralized deposits. Ultrastruct Pathol 1981;2:343–356.
49. Weiner HL, Wisoff JH, Rosenberg ME, et al. Craniopharyngiomas: a clinicopathological analysis of factors predictive of recurrence and functional outcome. Neurosurgery 1994;35: 1001–1011.
50. Wen B-C, Hussey DH, Staples J, et al. A comparison of the roles of surgery and radiation therapy in the management of craniopharyngiomas. J Radiat Oncol Biol Phys 1989;16:17–24.
51. Yamada H, Haratake J, Narasaki T, et al. Embryonal craniopharyngioma. Case report of the morphogenesis of a craniopharyngioma. Cancer 1995;75:2971–2977.

## Miscellaneous Neoplasms and Tumor-Like Lesions

### Germ Cell Tumor

1. Giuffre R, di Lorenzo N. Evolution of a primary intrasellar germinomatous teratoma into a choriocarcinoma. J Neurosurg 1975; 42:602–604.
2. Nishioka H, Ito H, Haraoka J, et al. Immature teratoma originat-
ing from the pituitary gland: case report. Neurosurgery 1999;44: 644–648.
3. Poon W, Ng HK, Wong K, et al. Primary intrasellar germinoma presenting with cavernous sinus syndrome. Surg Neurol 1988;30: 402–405.
4. Tobo M, Sumiyoshi A, Yamakawa Y. Sellar teratoma with melanotic progonoma: a case report. Acta Neuropathol (Berl) 1981;55:71–73.

### Chordoma

1. Leech RW, Scheithauer BW, Mitchell S. Chondroid chordoma presenting as cerebellar hemorrhage. Biomed Res (India) 1991; 2(1):127–133.
2. Mathews W, Wilson CB. Ectopic intrasellar chordoma: case report. J Neurosurg 1974;40:260–263.
3. Thodou E, Kontogeorgos G, Scheithauer BW, et al. Intrasellar chordoma mimicking pituitary adenoma. J Neurosurg 2000; 92:976–982.

### Postirradiation Neoplasia

1. Amine ARC, Sugar O. Suprasellar osteogenic sarcoma following radiation for pituitary adenoma: case report. J Neurosurg 1976; 44:88–91.
2. Jalalah S, Kovacs K, Horvath E, et al. Rhabdomyosarcoma in the region of the sella turcica. Acta Neurochir (Wien) 1987;88:142–146.
3. Pieterse S, Dinning TA, Blumbergs PC. Postirradiation sarcomatous transformation of a pituitary adenoma: a combined pituitary tumor: case report. J Neurosurg 1982;56:283–286.
4. Shi T, Farrell MA, Kaufmann JCE. Fibrosarcoma complicating irradiated pituitary adenoma. Surg Neurol 1984;22:277–283.

### Metastatic Neoplasms

1. Branch CL, Laws ER Jr. Metastatic tumors of the sella turcica masquerading as primary pituitary tumors. J Clin Endocrinol Metab 1987;65:469–474.
2. Carey RM, Varma SK, Drake CR, et al. Ectopic secretion of corticotropin-releasing factor as a cause of Cushing's syndrome: a clinical, morphologic, and biochemical study. N Engl J Med 1984;311:13–20.
3. Duchen LW. Metastatic carcinoma in the pituitary gland and hypothalamus. J Pathol Bacteriol 1966;91:347–355.
4. Morita A, Meyer FB, Laws ER. Symptomatic pituitary metastases. J Neurosurg 1998;89:69–70.
5. O'Neill BP, Tomlinson FH, Kurtin PJ, et al. Primary malignant non-Hodgkin's lymphoma of the brain: a clinicopathologic study of 89 cases. J Neuropathol Exp Neurol 1993;52:268.
6. Puolakka K, Korhonen T, Lahtinen R. Diabetes insipidus in preleukemic phase of acute myeloid leukemia in two patients with empty sella turcica. A report of two cases. Scand J Hematol 1984; 32:364–366.

### Other Neoplasms

1. Asa SL, Kovacs K, Horvath E, et al. Sellar glomangioma. Ultrastruct Pathol 1984;7:49–54.
2. Bilbao JM, Horvath E, Kovacs K, et al. Intrasellar paraganglioma associated with hypopituitarism. Arch Pathol Lab Med 1978;102: 95–98.
3. Copeland DD, Sink JD, Seigler HF. Primary intracranial melanoma presenting as a suprasellar tumor. Neurosurgery 1980; 6:542–545.
4. Dan NG, Smith DE. Pituitary hemangioblastoma in a patient with von Hippel–Lindau disease: case report. J Neurosurg 1975; 42:232–235.
5. De Divitiis E, Spaziante R, Cirillo S, et al. Primary sellar chondroma. Surg Neurol 1979;11:229–232.
6. Discepoli S. The lipoma of tuber cinereum. Tumor 1980;66: 123–130.
7. Friede RL. Osteolipomas of the tuber cinereum. Arch Pathol Lab Med 1977;101:369–372.
8. Goebel HH, Shimokawa K, Schaake T, et al. Schwannoma of the sellar region. Acta Neurochir (Wien) 1979;48:191–197.
9. Grisoli F, Vincentelli F, Rayband C, et al. Intrasellar meningioma. Surg Neurol 1983;20:36–41.
10. Hampton TA, Scheithauer BW, Rojiani AM, et al. Salivary gland–like tumors of the sellar region. Am J Surg Pathol 1997;21:424–434.
11. Lach B, Lesiuk H. Intracranial suprasellar angiolipoma: ultrastructural and immunohistochemical features. Neurosurgery 1994;34:163–167.

12. Mangiardi JR, Flamm ES, Cravioto H, et al. Hemangiopericytoma of the pituitary fossa: case report. Neurosurgery 1983; 13:58–61.
13. Pospiech J, Mehdorn HM, Reinhardt V, et al. Sellar chondroma in a case of Ollier's disease. Neurochirurgia (Stuttg) 1989;32: 30–35.
14. Scheithauer BW, Parameswaran A, Burdick B. Intrasellar paraganglioma: report of a case in a sibship of von Hippel–Lindau disease. Neurosurgery 1996;38:395–399.
15. Scholtz CL, Siu K. Melanoma of the pituitary: case report. J Neurosurg 1976;45:101–103.
16. Solero CL, Giombini S, Morello G. Suprasellar and olfactory meningiomas. Report on a series of 150 personal cases. Acta Neurochir (Wien) 1983;67:181–194.
17. Urbanski SJ, Bilbao JM, Horvath E, et al. Intrasellar solitary plasmacytoma terminating in multiple myeloma: a report of a case including electron microscopical study. Surg Neurol 1980;14:233.
18. Wilberger JE Jr. Primary intrasellar schwannoma: case report. Surg Neurol 1989;32:156–158.
19. Wolfe JT III, Scheithauer BW, Dahlin DC. Giant cell tumor of sphenoid bone: review of ten cases. J Neurosurg 1983;59: 322–327.
20. Zambaziotis D, Kontogeorgos G, Kovacs K, et al. Intrasellar paraganglioma presenting as nonfunctioning pituitary adenoma. Arch Pathol Lab Med 1999;123:429–432.

## Sellar Region Cysts

### Rathke's Cleft Cyst

1. Barrow DL, Spector RH, Takei Y, et al. Symptomatic Rathke's cyst located entirely in the suprasellar region: review of diagnosis, management, and pathogenesis. Neurosurgery 1985;16:766–772.
2. Baskin DS, Wilson CB. Transsphenoidal treatment of non-neoplastic intrasellar cysts. J Neurosurg 1984;60:8–13.
3. Concha S, Hamilton BPM, Millan JC, et al. Symptomatic Rathke's cleft cyst with amyloid stroma. J Neurol Neurosurg Psychiatry 1975;38:782–786.
4. Giuffre R, Gagliardi FM. Unusual hypophyseal tumour of Rathke's cleft origin. Neurochirurgia (Stuttg) 1968;11:81–89.
5. Inoue NY, Fukuda T, Shakudo M, et al. MR appearance of Rathke's cleft cysts. Neuroradiology 1988;30:155–159.
6. Iraci G, Giordano R, Gerosa M, et al. Ocular involvement in recurrent cyst of Rathke's cleft: case report. Ann Ophthalmol 1979;1:94–98.
7. Kepes JJ. Transitional cell tumor of the pituitary gland developing from a Rathke's cleft cyst. Cancer 1978;41:337–343.
8. Kleinschmidt-DeMasters BK, Lillehei KO, Stears JC. The pathologic, surgical, and MR spectrum of Rathke cleft cysts. Surg Neurol 1995;44:19–27.
9. Kucharczyk W, Peck WW, Kelly WM, et al. Rathke cleft cysts: CT, MR imaging, and pathologic features. Radiology 1987;165: 491–495.
10. Lach B, Scheithauer BW. Colloidal cyst of the third ventricle: a comparative ultrastructural study of neuraxis cysts and choroid plexus epithelium. Ultrastruct Pathol 1992;16:331–349.
11. Lach B, Scheithauer BW, Gregor A, et al. Colloid cyst of the third ventricle. A comparative immunohistochemical study of neuraxis cysts and choroid plexus epithelium. J Neurosurg 1993; 78:101–111.
12. Nishio S, Mizuno J, Barrow DL, et al. Pituitary tumors composed of adenohypophysial adenoma and Rathke's cleft cyst elements: a clinicopathological study. Neurosurgery 1987;21:371–377.
13. Roux FX, Constans JP, Monsaingeon V, et al. Symptomatic Rathke's cleft cysts; clinical and therapeutic data. Neurochirurgia (Stuttg) 1988;31:18–20.
14. Saeki N, Sunami K, Sugaya Y, et al. MRI findings and clinical manifestations in Rathke's cleft cyst. Acta Neurochir (Wien) 1999;41:1055–1061.
15. Steinberg GK, Koenig GH, Golden JB. Symptomatic Rathke's cleft cysts: report of two cases. J Neurosurg 1982;56:290–295.
16. Swanson SE, Chandler WF, Latack J, et al. Symptomatic Rathke's cleft cyst with pituitary adenoma: case report. Neurosurgery 1985;17:657–659.
17. Tomlinson FH, Scheithauer BW, Young WF Jr, et al. Rathke's cleft cyst—a clinicopathologic study of 31 cases (Abstract). Brain Pathology 1994;4:453.
18. Yoshida J, Kobayashi T, Kageyama N, et al. Symptomatic Rathke's cleft cyst: morphological study with light and electron microscopy and tissue culture. J Neurosurg 1977;47:451–458.

### Miscellaneous Cysts

1. Abe T, Ludecke. Mucocele-like formation leading to neurological symptoms in prolactin-secreting pituitary adenomas under dopamine agonist therapy. Surg Neurol 1999;52:274–279.
2. Boggan JE, Davis RL, Zorman G, et al. Intrasellar epidermoid cyst: case report. J Neurosurg 1983;58:411–415.
3. Hermon P, Lot G, Guichard JP, et al. Mucocele of the sphenoid sinus: a late complication of transsphenoidal pituitary surgery. Ann Otol Rhinol Laryngol 1998;107:765–768.
4. Meyer FB, Carpenter SM, Laws ER Jr. Intrasellar arachnoid cysts. Surg Neurol 1987;28:105–110.
5. Salyer D, Carter D. Squamous carcinoma arising in the pituitary gland. Cancer 1973;31:713–718.

## Inflammatory Lesions

### Lymphocytic Hypophysitis

1. Asa SL, Bilbao JM, Kovacs K, et al. Lymphocytic hypophysitis of pregnancy resulting in hypopituitarism: a distinct clinicopathologic entity. Ann Intern Med 1981;95:166–171.
2. Baskin DS, Townsend JJ, Wilson CB. Lymphocytic adenohypophysitis of pregnancy simulating a pituitary adenoma: a distinct pathological entity. J Neurosurg 1982;56:148–153.
3. Cosman F, Post KD, Holub DA, et al. Lymphocytic hypophysitis: report of 3 new cases and review of the literature. Medicine (Baltimore) 1989;68:240–256.
4. Hayashi H, Yamada K, Kuroki T, et al. Lymphocytic hypophysitis and pulmonary sarcoidosis. Report of a case. Am J Clin Pathol 1991;95:506–511.
5. Honnegger J, Fahlbusch R, Bornemann A, et al. Lymphocytic and granulomatous hypophysitis: experience with nine cases. Neurosurgery 1997;40:713–723.
6. Imura H, Nakao K, Shimatsu A, et al. Lymphocytic infundibuloneurohypophysitis as a cause of central diabetes insipidus. N Engl J Med 1993;329:683–689.
7. Jensen MD, Handwerger BS, Scheithauer BW, et al. Lymphocytic hypophysitis with isolated corticotropin deficiency. Ann Intern Med 1986;105:200–203.
8. Lee JH, Laws ER Jr, Guthrie BL, et al. Lymphocytic hypophysitis: occurrence in two men. Neurosurgery 1994;34:159–163.
9. Meichner RH, Riggio S, Manz HJ, et al. Lymphocytic adenohypophysitis causing pituitary mass. Neurology 1987;37:158–161.
10. Nishioka H, Ito H, Miki T, et al. A case of lymphocytic hypophysitis with massive fibrosis and the role of surgical intervention. Surg Neurol 1994;42:74–78.
11. Portocarrero CJ, Robinson AG, Taylor AL, et al. Lymphoid hypophysitis: an unusual cause of hyperprolactinemia and enlarged sella turcica. JAMA 1981;246:1811–1812.
12. Riedl M, Czech T, Slootweg J, et al. Lymphocytic hypophysitis presenting as a pituitary tumor in a 63-year-old man. Endocrinol Pathol 1995;6:159–166.
13. Sobrinho-Simoes M, Brandao A, Paiva ME, et al. Lymphoid hypophysitis in a patient with lymphoid thyroiditis, lymphoid adrenalitis, and idiopathic retroperitoneal fibrosis. Arch Pathol Lab Med 1985;109:230–233.
14. Wild RRA, Kepley M. Lymphocytic hypophysitis in a patient with amenorrhea and hyperprolactinemia: a case report. Reprod Med 1986;31:211–216.

### Giant Cell Granuloma

1. de Bruin WI, van't Verlaat JW, Graamans K, et al. Sellar granulomatous mass in a pregnant woman with active Crohn's disease. Neth J Med 1991;39:136–141.
2. Del Pozo JM, Roda JE, Montoya JG, et al. Intrasellar granuloma: a case report. J Neurosurg 1980;53:717–719.
3. Doniach I, Wright EA. Two cases of giant-cell granuloma of the pituitary gland. J Pathol Bacteriol 1951;63:69–79.
4. Hassoun P, Anayssi E, Salti I. A case of granulomatous hypophysitis with hypopituitarism and minimal pituitary enlargement. J Neurol Neurosurg Psychiatry 1985;48:949–951.
5. Lara-Caplan JI, Cuellar Olmedo L, Martinez Martin J, et al. Intrasellar mass with hypopituitarism as a manifestation of sarcoidosis. Case report. J Neurosurg 1990;73:283–286.
6. Miyamoto M, Sugawa H, Mori T, et al. A case of hypopituitarism due to granulomatous and lymphocytic adenohypophysitis with

minimal pituitary enlargement: a possible variant to lymphocytic adenohypophysitis. Endocrinol Jpn 1988;35:607–616.

7. Siqueira E, Tsung JS, Al-Kari MZ, et al. Case report: idiopathic giant cell granuloma of the hypophysis: an unusual cause of panhypopituitarism. Surg Neurol 1989;32:68–71.

8. Stern BJ, Krumholz A, John C, et al. Sarcoidosis and its neurological manifestations. Arch Neurol 1985;42:909–917.

9. Taylon C, Duff TA. Giant cell granuloma involving the pituitary gland: case report. J Neurosurg 1980;52:584–587.

### Langerhans' Histiocytosis

1. Bergmann M, Yuan Y, Bruck W, et al. Solitary Langerhans cell histiocytosis lesion of the parieto-occipital lobe. A case report and review of the literature. Clin Neurol Neurosurg 1997;99:50–55.

2. Erlandson RA. Diagnostic Transmission Electron Microscopy of Tumors: Clinical, Pathological, Immunohistochemical, and Cytogenetic Correlations: New York: Raven Press, 1994, pp 443–447.

3. Kepes JJ, Kepes M. Predominantly cerebral forms of histiocytosis X: A reappraisal of "Gagel's hypothalamic granuloma," "granuloma infiltrans of the hypothalamus" and "Ayala's disease" with a report of four cases. Acta Neuropathol (Berl) 1969;14:77–98.

4. Mazal PR, Hainfellner JA, Preiser J, et al. Langerhans cell histiocytosis of the hypothalamus: diagnostic value of immunohistochemistry. Clin Neuropathol 1996;15:87–91.

5. Montine TJ, Hollingshead SC, Ellis NG, et al. Solitary eosinophilic granuloma of the temporal lobe: a case report and long-term followup of previously reported cases. Clin Neuropathol 1994;13:225–228.

6. Nishio S, Mizuno J, Barrow DL, et al. Isolated histiocytosis X of the pituitary gland: case report. Neurosurgery 1987;21:718–721.

7. Ober KP, Alexander E Jr, Challa VR, et al. Histiocytosis X of the hypothalamus. Neurosurgery 1989;24:93–95.

8. Schmitt S, Wichmann W, Martin E, et al. Pituitary stalk thickening with diabetes insipidus preceding typical manifestations of Langerhans' cell histiocytosis in children. Eur J Pediatr 1993;152:399–401.

### Xanthogranuloma of Sellar Region

1. Folkerth RD, Price DL JR, Schwartz M, et al. Xanthomatous hypophysitis. Am J Surg Pathol 1998;22:736–741.

2. Paulus W, Honegger J, Keyvani K, et al. Xanthogranuloma of the sellar region: a clinicopathologic entity different from adamantinomatous craniopharyngioma. Acta Neuropathol (Berl) 1999;97:377–382.

### Rosai-Dorfman Disease

1. Foucar E, Rosai J, Dorfman R. Sinus histiocytosis with massive lymphadenopathy (Rosai-Dorfman disease): review of the entity. Semin Diagn Pathol 1990;7:19–73.

2. Jones RV, Colegial CH, Andriko JW. Extranodal sinus histiocytosis with massive lymphadenopathy (Rosai-Dorfman disease) of the central nervous system. J Neuropathol Exp Neurol 1997;56:613.

3. Kim M, Provias J, Bernstein M. Rosai-Dorfman disease mimicking multiple meningioma: case report. Neurosurgery 1995;36:1185–1187.

4. Resnick DK, Johnson BL, Lovely TJ. Rosai-Dorfman disease presenting with multiple orbital and intracranial masses. Acta Neuropathol (Berl) 1996;91:554–557.

### Erdheim-Chester Disease

1. Adle-Biassette H, Chetritt J, Bergemer-Fouquet AM, et al. Pathology of the central nervous system in Chester-Erdheim disease: report of three cases. J Neuropathol Exp Neurol 1997;56:1207–1216.

2. Babu R, Lansen T, Chadburn A, et al. Erdheim-Chester disease of the central nervous system. J Neurosurg 1997;86:888–892.

3. Evidente VG, Adler CH, Giannini C, et al. Erdheim-Chester disease with extensive intraaxial brain stem lesions presenting as a progressive cerebellar syndrome. Mov Disord 1998;13:576–581.

4. Oweity T, Scheithauer BW, Ching HS, et al. Multisystem Erdheim-Chester disease with massive hypothalamic-sellar involvement and hypopituitarism. Neurosurgery (in press).

5. Wright RA, Hermann RC, Parisi JE. Neurological manifestations of Erdheim-Chester disease. J Neurol Neurosurg Psychiatry 1999;66:72–75.

### Xanthoma Disseminatum

1. Hammond RR, Mackenzie IR. Xanthoma disseminatum with massive intracranial involvement. Clin Neuropathol 1995;14: 314–321.

## Infectious Lesions

### Abscess

1. Bjerre P, Riishede J, Lindholm J. Pituitary abscess. Acta Neurochir (Wien) 1983;68:187–193.

2. Domingue JN, Wilson CB. Pituitary abscesses: report of seven cases and review of the literature. J Neurosurg 1977;46:601–608.

3. Goldhammer Y, Smith JL, Yates BM. Mycotic intrasellar abscess. Trans Am Ophthalmol Soc 1974;72:66–78.

4. Leff RS, Martino RL, Pollock WJ, et al. Pituitary abscess after autologous bone marrow transplantation. Am J Hematol 1989;31: 62–64.

5. Lindholm J, Rasmussen P, Korsgaard O. Intrasellar or pituitary abscess. J Neurosurg 1973;38:616–619.

6. Lunardi P, Fraioli B, Ferrante L. Pituitary abscess: a case diagnosed preoperatively. Neurochirurgia (Stuttg) 1984;27:51–52.

7. Marks PV, Furneaux CE. Pituitary abscess following asymptomatic sphenoid sinusitis. J Laryngol Otol 1984;98:1151–1155.

8. Nelson PB, Haverkos H, Martinez AJ, et al. Abscess formation within pituitary tumors. Neurosurgery 1983;12:331–333.

9. Ramos-Gabatin A, Jordan RM. Primary pituitary aspergillosis responding to transsphenoidal surgery and combined therapy with amphotericin-B and 5-fluorocytosine: case report. J Neurosurg 1981;54:839–841.

### Miscellaneous Infections

1. Del Brutto OH, Guevara J, Sotelo J. Intrasellar cysticercosis. J Neurosurg 1988;69:58–60.

2. Delsedine M, Aguggia M, Cantello R, et al. Isolated hypophyseal tuberculoma: case report. Clin Neuropathol 1988;7: 311–313.

3. Osgen T, Bertan V, Kansu T, et al. Intrasellar hydatid cyst: case report. J Neurosurg 1984;60:647–648.

4. Ranjan A, Chandy MJ. Intrasellar tuberculoma. Br J Neurosurg 1994;8:179–185.

## Miscellaneous Non-Neoplastic Processes

1. Aarabi B, Haghshenas M, Rakeii V. Visual failure caused by suprasellar extramedullary hematopoiesis in beta thalassemia: case report. Neurosurgery 1998;42:922–926.

2. Badon SJ, Ansel J, Smith TW, et al. Diabetes insipidus caused by extramedullary hematopoiesis. Am J Clin Pathol 1985;38: 509–512.

3. Gartman JJ, Powers SK, Fortune M. Pseudotumor of the sellar and parasellar areas. Neurosurgery 1989;24:896–901.

4. Kristof RA, Van Roost D, Wolf HK, et al. Intravascular papillary endothelial hyperplasia of the sellar region. J Neurosurg 1997;86: 558–563.

5. Meyer FB, Lombardi D, Scheithauer B, et al. Extra-axial cavernous hemangiomas involving the dural sinuses. J Neurosurg 1990;73:187–192.

6. Sansone ME, Liwnicz BH, Mandybur TI. Giant pituitary cavernous hemangioma: case report. J Neurosurg 1980;53: 124–126.

## Empty Sella Syndrome

1. Gharib H, Frey HM, Laws ER Jr, et al. Coexistent primary empty sella syndrome and hyperprolactinemia: report of 11 cases. Arch Intern Med 1983;143:1383–1386.

2. Jaffer KA, Obbens EAMT, El Gammal TA. "Empty" sella: review of 76 cases. South Med J 1979;72:294–296.

3. Nass R, Engel M, Stoner E, et al. Empty sella syndrome in childhood. Pediatr Neurol 1986;2:224–229.

4. Neelon FA, Goree JA, Lebovitz HE. The primary empty sella: clinical and radiographic characteristics and endocrine function. Medicine (Baltimore) 1973;52:73–92.

5. Spaziante R, de Divitiis E, Stella L, et al. The empty sella. Surg Neurol 1981;16:418–426.`

# SPINE AND EPIDURAL SPACE

# 10

Neurologic function becomes extremely vulnerable as it funnels through the slender spinal cord and nerve roots. In this chapter we consider the primary and secondary lesions of the spine and epidural space that threaten the structural and functional integrity of this delicate extension of the nervous system (Figs. 10–1 and 10–2).

## CONGENITAL MALFORMATIONS (MENINGOCELE AND MENINGOMYELOCELE)

Spinal dysraphic states represent a morphologic continuum that ranges from the innocuous spina bifida occulta to gross, crippling deformities in which abnormal and exposed spinal cord tissue is elevated to, or rises above, the level of the skin. All occur most frequently in the lumbar area; cervical examples are uncommon.[10, 11] Thoracic lesions are often associated with neurofibromatosis type 1 (von Recklinghausen's disease).[4, 6] Most sizable lesions protrude in the posterior midline, whereas anterior and lateral examples[2, 13] are uncommon. Because the asymptomatic spina bifida does not usually require surgery, surgical specimens are derived from dysraphisms of intermediate severity.

As functional deficits are a direct expression of the anatomic abnormality, it is important to distinguish two categories of spinal dysraphic lesions: (1) those associated with malformation of the spinal cord and nerve roots and (2) the less common deformities confined to bone, soft tissue, and meninges. The former includes the meningomyelocele, myelocele, and so-called rachischisis. Although these three are usually depicted as distinct entities, they are a continuum of which only the meningomyelocele is likely to generate a surgical specimen (Figs. 10–3 and 10–4). Operative intervention for advanced, gaping lesions is largely reconstructive.[1]

The term meningocele is applied to the uncommon malformation that involves only bone, soft tissue, and meninges. Saccular in nature, it is noteworthy for its absence of abnormal neural tissue.

The translucent blue dome of the meningomyelocele transmits images of the enclosed spinal cord and nerve roots. The base is often girdled by skin (Figs. 10–5 and 10–6). The contents often include abnormal spinal cord, nerve roots, dorsal root ganglia, meninges, blood vessels, and hyalinized connective tissue (Figs. 10–7 to 10–10).

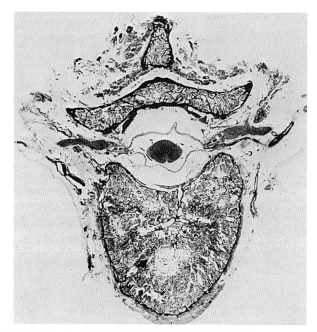

**FIGURE 10–1** ANATOMIC RELATIONS OF THE SPINE AND EPIDURAL SPACE

A horizontal section depicts the anatomic relations of the spine, epidural space, meninges, nerve roots, and spinal cord.

On rare occasion, striated muscle, islands of cartilage, or epidermal cysts[8, 9, 12] are included.

Microscopically, the surface of the sac may be covered by squamous epithelium or fibrous tissue, the former prone to ulceration and acute inflammation. The rare occurrence of carcinoma in association with a meningomyelocele is a medical curiosity.

It is unfortunate that the meningocele makes up such a small percentage of spinal dysraphic lesions because individuals with meningomyelocele have neuro-logic deficits referable to the local lesion and to the rostral malformative and obstructive lesions in the posterior fossa and upper spinal canal (Arnold-Chiari or Chiari II syndrome). In a meningocele or meningomyelocele, the leptomeninges immediately beneath the dermis typically have an alveolar rather than a membranous appearance (Fig. 10–11).[3, 15]

Of all the surgical specimens from congenital spinal lesions, a caudal tail is the most unusual.[14]

## INFLAMMATORY DISORDERS

### Tuberculosis

Disseminated osseous tuberculosis is particularly likely to affect the spine, with spinal cord compression a potential consequence of epidural granulomatous tissue and/or vertebral collapse.

Macroscopically, the tuberculous exudate forms a tenacious gray membrane or a mass lesion that replaces epidural fat and clings to the dura (Figs. 10–12 and 10–13). The character of the inflammatory response, with its epithelioid and giant cells, lymphocytes, and caseous necrosis, differs in no way from tuberculous reactions elsewhere (Fig. 10–14). Because there may be a paucity or absence of stainable organisms, culture is indicated.

Fortunately, chemotherapy usually arrests the course of the disease and prevents the marked angular kyphosis (gibbus) that characterizes end-stage spinal tuberculosis (Pott's disease)[1–5] (Fig. 10–15; see Figs. 10–12 and 10–13).

### Epidural Abscess

Suppurative infection of the epidural space may arise in continuity with a vertebral focus of disease or as a

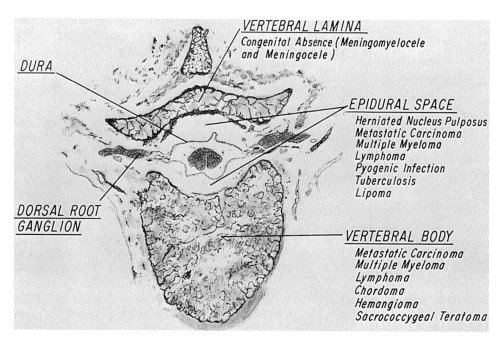

**FIGURE 10–2** TOPOGRAPHIC DISTRIBUTION OF LESIONS OF THE SPINE AND EPIDURAL SPACE

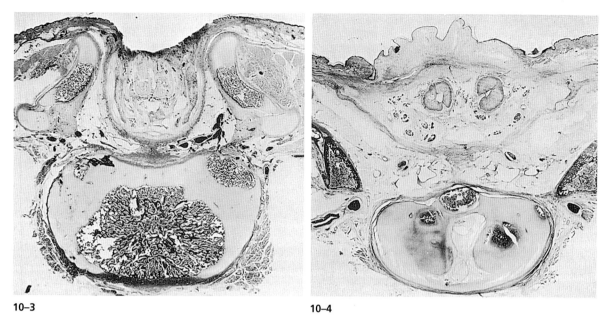

10–3                                                                  10–4

**FIGURES 10–3 AND 10–4**   SPINAL DYSRAPHIA

A defect common to the dysraphic states is absence of the posterior vertebral arches. Termed spina bifida, this defect may be (1) isolated and asymptomatic, (2) associated with herniation of meninges alone (meningocele), (3) accompanied by involvement of the nerve roots or spinal cord (meningomyelocele) (Fig. 10–3), or (4) associated with gross disturbances in the formation of the cord, such as reduplication (Fig. 10–4).

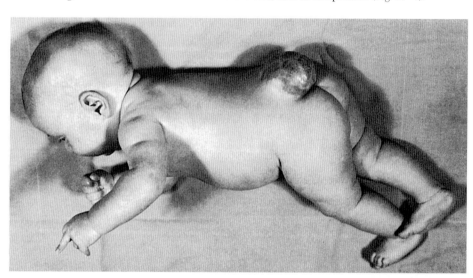

**FIGURE 10–5**
**MENINGOMYELOCELE**

This bulging, cystic lesion of the lumbosacral region features the typical collar of epidermis and translucent apex of meningomyelocele. At 2 months of age the infant's head size exceeded the 97th percentile; a ventriculoatrial shunt was placed. At 4 months the sacral lesion was excised. Fecal and urinary incontinence and lower extremity weakness attested to the participation of neural elements in the defect.

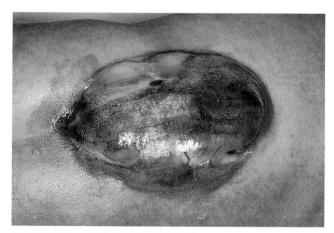

**FIGURE 10–6**   MENINGOMYELOCELE

The malformed spinal cord can be visualized through the lesion's translucent dome. (Courtesy of Dr. William E. Krauss, Rochester, MN.)

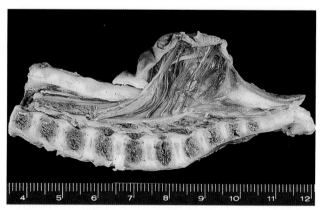

**FIGURE 10–7**   MENINGOMYELOCELE

This midsagittal section of the lumbosacral spine of a newborn with meningomyelocele reveals a defective spinal cord and the nerve roots. Note that the latter stretch across the rostral edge of the defect, enter the sac, and abruptly angle back to reenter the spinal canal and then exit through the dura. The patient also had a Chiari II (Arnold-Chiari) malformation.

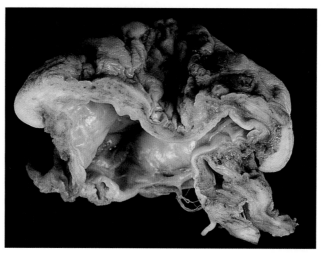

**10–8**

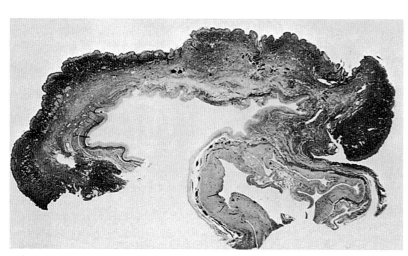

**10–9**

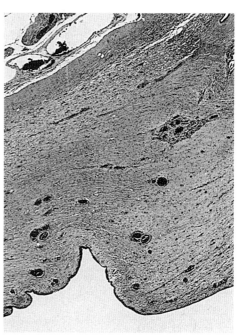

**10–10**

**FIGURES 10–8, 10–9, AND 10–10    MENINGOMYELOCELE**

This lesion was excised from the lumbosacral region of a 9-month-old male child in whom a ventriculoperitoneal shunt had been placed for the treatment of hydrocephalus. The lesion's cystic character is apparent in the bisected surgical specimen (Fig. 10–8) and in a whole mount histologic section (Fig. 10–9). The malformed tissue is formed of glia and neurons, lined by ependyma, and associated with nerve roots (Fig. 10–10).

hematogenous deposit from an extravertebral site such as skin or the genitourinary tract. Diabetes mellitus or intravenous recreational drug use explains some cases, but an extravertebral source or a predisposing factor is never forthcoming in others.[1–3] The inflammatory character of the lesion is often reflected in local tenderness, and its expansile quality is felt by signs and symptoms of nerve root or spinal cord compression. The thoracic region is most often affected. *Staphylococcus aureus* is the usual offending agent.[1–4]

Macroscopically, the suppuration of the acute lesion

affirms its infectious nature, whereas the proliferative component of chronic abscesses may simulate neoplasia. The proclivity for involvement of the dorsal aspect of the epidural space may be a consequence of the dura's adherence anteriorly to the posterior spinal ligament.

The duration of a bacterial process is chronicled histologically by the relative proportions of suppuration, granulation tissue, and collagen (Fig. 10–16). The predominant lymphocytic infiltrate in chronic lesions may simulate lymphoma.

## Other Inflammatory Disorders

Actinomycosis (Fig. 10–17),[3, 4] aspergillosis,[13, 19] blastomycosis,[3, 7] brucellosis,[17] coccidioidomycosis,[8] cryptococcosis,[9, 10] and echinococcosis[2, 15, 16, 20] represent rare "other" infections of the spine and epidural space. Amyloid deposits,[12, 14, 18] Langerhans cell histiocytosis,[1, 5, 11, 22] rheumatoid nodule,[6] and sarcoidosis[21] are additional inflammatory lesions of the spine.

## DEGENERATIVE AND REACTIVE PROCESSES

As summarized in Table 10–1 there are multiple degenerative and reactive lesions that impinge upon the spinal cord.

## Herniated Nucleus Pulposus

With age, a progressive series of structural and chemical alterations occur in the intervertebral disks that offset the normal balance between the restraining property of the anulus fibrosus and the expulsive force of the nucleus pulposus.[3, 4, 8] When the latter exceeds the former, nuclear material can extrude acutely through a defect in

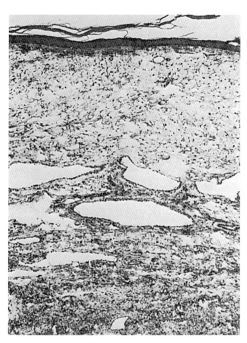

**FIGURE 10–11**   MENINGOCELE

The epidermis of this meningocele overlies vascularized areolar connective tissue devoid of neural elements. At operation, the nerve roots in the sac could be returned to the spinal canal.

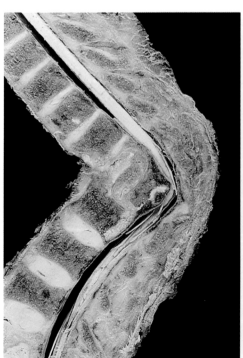
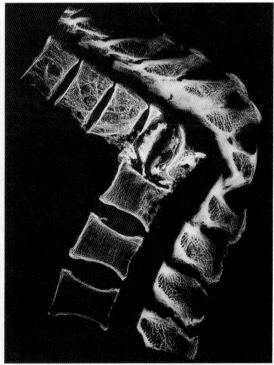

**FIGURES 10–12 AND 10–13**   TUBERCULOSIS

Vertebral collapse secondary to spinal tuberculosis produced the marked gibbus deformity characteristic of advanced Pott's disease. Caseous material marks the site of collapse. This tuberculous process in the cervical epidural space produced intermittent and ultimately fatal respiratory arrest in the 56-year-old man.

**TABLE 10–1**
**Degenerative and Reactive Lesions of the Spine Summarized**

Degenerative processes
   Herniated nucleus pulposus
   Synovial cyst
   Calcifying pseudoneoplasm of the neuraxis
   Amyloidosis
   Calcium pyrophosphate deposition
   Gouty tophus
   Hydroxyapatite crystal deposition
   Xanthoma and xanthogranuloma
Proliferative lesions
   Aneurysmal bone cyst
   Extramedullary hematopoiesis
   Fibrous dysplasia
   Langerhans cell histiocytosis
   Paget's disease
   Pigmented villonodular synovitis
Non-neoplastic vascular processes
   Arteriovenous malformation
   Cavernous angioma

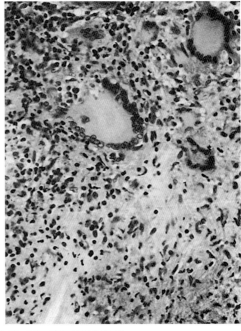

**FIGURE 10–14** TUBERCULOSIS

A 60-year-old man developed paraplegia, incontinence, and a sensory level at T5. Radiographs revealed destruction of the fifth and sixth thoracic vertebral bodies. Necrotic tissue encountered in the epidural space at surgery contained granulomatous inflammation with epithelioid cells, multinucleated giant cells, caseous necrosis, and acid-fast organisms.

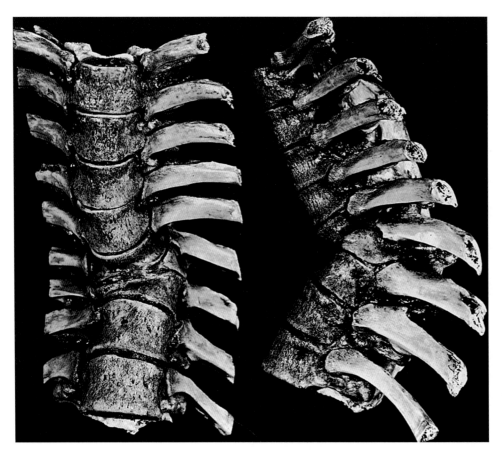

**FIGURE 10–15** TUBERCULOSIS

This severe angulation or gibbus was the sequel to destruction and collapse of vertebrae in a 28-year-old man with tuberculosis.

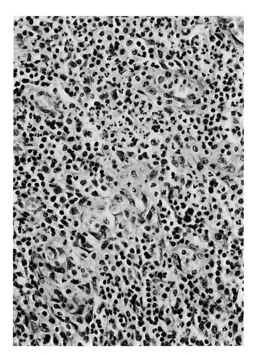

**FIGURE 10–16    PYOGENIC INFECTION**

An 18-year-old man developed severe midscapular pain followed on consecutive days by tingling and numbness in the legs, inability to void, and paraplegia. At laminectomy on the fourth day of his illness, purulent exudate was noted in the epidural space at the T5-7 level. The suppurative nature of the reaction is readily apparent. The presence of proliferating capillaries is consistent with a process of several days' duration.

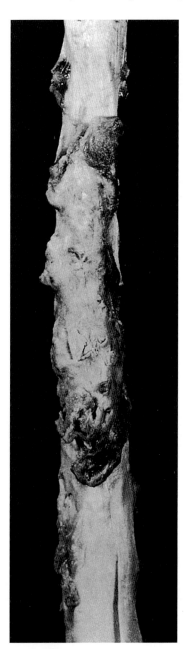

**FIGURE 10–17    ACTINOMYCOSIS**

This epidural actinomycotic abscess was present in a 23-year-old man with a 13-year history of cervical-facial induration associated with multiple fistulas.

the anulus and compress nerve roots or spinal cord. The incidence of symptomatic lumbar disk herniation exceeds the frequency of cervical herniations and greatly surpasses their occurrence at thoracic levels. In some cases, the herniated tissue loses continuity with the intervertebral space and becomes a sequestrum or free fragment. In most instances, however, there is prolapse but not detachment. Herniation in the midline, especially at thoracic levels, either elevates or penetrates the posterior longitudinal ligament, potentially with compression of the spinal cord (Fig. 10–18). More often, the protrusion is lateral, and the disk material is positioned to impinge upon a nerve root. Characteristically, the herniated nucleus compromises the spinal canal and displaces, but only rarely penetrates, the dura. The latter is an exceptional event that primarily occurs at the level of the L4-5 interspace.[1, 7, 9]

The histologic changes in the anulus fibrosus and nucleus pulposus are age related, and there is a fine line, if any, between these changes and the pathologic alterations observed in herniated disks. The anulus loses its lamellar architecture, develops fissures, and acquires both chondrocytes and blood vessels. Concomitantly, the nucleus undergoes gradual desiccation and fibrosis. Its chondrocytes become prominent and zones of necrosis, as well as cystic degeneration, make their appearance (Fig. 10–19). When seen in surgical specimens, these changes should not be confused with neoplasia. Although it is often assumed that the extruded tissue is an-

ulus fibrosus, histologic studies record the frequent presence of the hyaline cartilage from the endplate that covers the superior and inferior vertebral surfaces.[3] The normal anatomy of the intervertebral region and the degenerations that accrue with age have been subject to detailed study. Neovascularization of disk tissue was cited as a helpful diagnostic feature associated with prolapse[10] but was a common finding in nondetached tissues in another investigation.[3]

It comes as no surprise that a disparity exists between the clinical importance of the herniated nucleus pulposus and the lack of enthusiasm that attends its histopathologic examination. The pathologist quickly

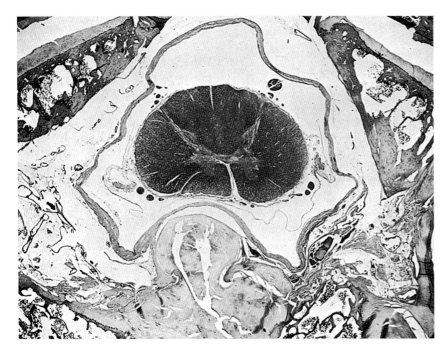

**FIGURE 10–18** HERNIATED NUCLEUS PULPOSUS

This central herniation of disk material was present in the thoracic spine of a 61-year-old man. The extruding nucleus traversed the anulus to protrude through a defect in the posterior spinal ligament, impinge upon the dura, and compress the spinal cord. Note resultant pallor of the anterior funiculi.

excludes the possibility of a metastatic neoplasm, labels the tissue "degenerative fibrocartilage," and perhaps regrets the rarity of such colorful disorders as ochronosis.[6]

In light of the marginal diagnostic reward, the need for histologic examination of routine disk specimens has been challenged,[2, 5] albeit not by all pathologists. We consider gross examination alone to be adequate; current guidelines do not mandate microscopic study.

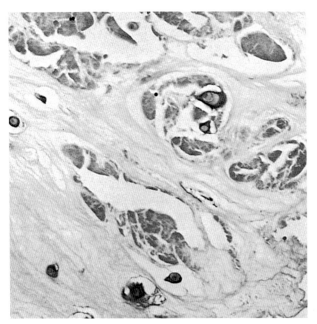

**FIGURE 10–19** HERNIATED NUCLEUS PULPOSUS

Cyst formation and chondrocyte prominence are common, age-related changes in the nucleus pulposus. Here they are evident in herniated disk material.

## Synovial Cyst

Synovial cysts are small, discrete, often pain-producing epidural masses related to the joints between vertebral facet joints (Fig. 10–20). Although thoracic and cervical examples appear from time to time,[1, 2] most arise in the lumbar area.[3–7] The encysted mucoid fluid conforms to that in synovial cysts at other sites.

Histologically, the largely fibrous wall contains elongated or more cuboidal synovial cells that align along the well-defined cavity but usually fall short of forming a continuous lamina that could be termed an epithelium (Fig. 10–21).

## Calcifying Pseudoneoplasm of the Neuraxis

As described also in Chapter 2 on pages 101 to 102, this is a distinctive, if difficult to describe, fibrocalcific reactive lesion of unknown pathogenesis. Intraspinally, the lesion is an expansile and somewhat destructive mass that can occur in patients of all ages and at all spinal levels (Fig. 10–22).[1, 2] Although it is usually extradural, occasional examples arise in the leptomeninges.[2] Histologically, the tissue is largely amorphous but at the same time is somewhat structured, with multinodular masses of fibrous connective tissue, peculiar granular debris, bone, and calcification (Fig. 10–23). Cells resembling epithelioid cells, with the same radial orientation seen in rheumatoid nodules, may frequent the periphery of the lobules in some cases (Fig. 10–24). Multinucleated cells mark some lesions.[1] Excision is curative.

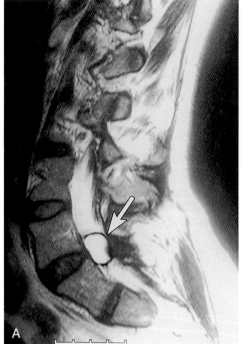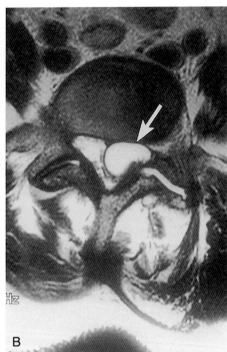

**FIGURE 10–20    SYNOVIAL CYST**

As seen in sagittal (A) and axial (B) T2-weighted MR images, the synovial cyst (arrows) is a bright discrete mass that here impinges on the dural sac. As is common, the lesion arises in the lumbar spine.

## Other Degenerative and Reactive Processes

Other degenerative and reactive processes include calcium pyrophosphate deposition,[10, 12, 15] extramedullary hematopoiesis,[2, 5] fibrous dysplasia,[11, 13] gouty tophus,[1, 6, 18] hydroxyapatite crystal deposition,[14] Paget's disease,[3, 17] pigmented villonodular synovitis,[4, 7, 8] and xanthoma and xanthogranuloma.[9, 16] Langerhans cell histiocytosis and amyloid deposits in the spine are described on pages 503, 504, and 522. Arteriovenous malformations are discussed on page 522.

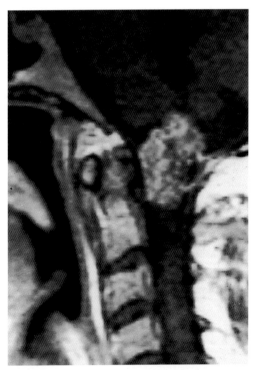

**FIGURE 10–22    CALCIFYING PSEUDONEOPLASM OF THE NEURAXIS**

Acute onset of arm pain prompted radiologic studies in this 39-year-old man. A destructive calcified epidural mass was found in the upper cervical region.

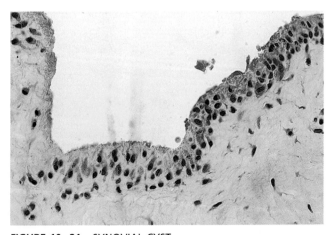

**FIGURE 10–21    SYNOVIAL CYST**

A discontinuous layer of epithelioid cells lines the mucin-containing cyst cavity.

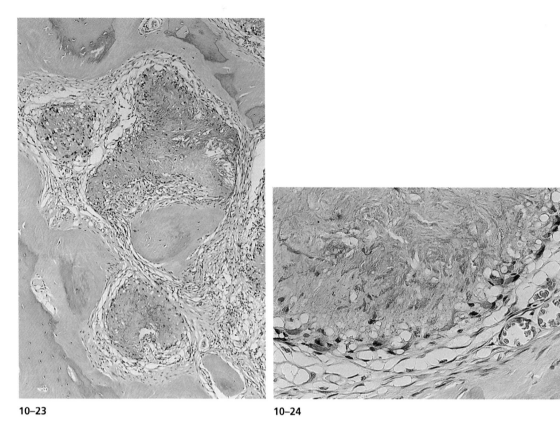

10–23                                          10–24

**FIGURES 10–23 AND 10–24**   CALCIFYING PSEUDONEOPLASM OF THE NEURAXIS

The lesion's lobular architecture and content of bone are apparent at low magnification (Fig. 10–23). The fibrillar quality of the amorphous material and the peripheral, incomplete rim of cuboidal cells are evident at high magnification (Fig. 10–24).

## NEOPLASMS AND OTHER TUMORS

As a region of the body with bone, soft tissues, lymphoid elements, peripheral nerve, and retroperitoneal and mediastinal components, all in close juxtaposition, it is not surprising that the spine and epidural space generates and accepts a diverse group of neoplasms and tumors. The principal lesions are recorded in Table 10–2.

## Chordoma

**Definition.**  A localized invasive and potentially metastasizing neoplasm presumptively derived from notochordal remnants.

**General Comments.**  Nearly all chordomas hug the midline along the axial skeleton. Clival examples constitute about 40% of all cases, with the remainder distributed unevenly along the vertebral axis. Cervical, thoracic, lumbar, and sacral segments are affected at ratios of 5:1:1:20, respectively.[2, 4, 17] Non-neoplastic notochordal tissue analogous to the clival "ecchordosis physaliphora" occurs as extraosseous nodules in the spinal canal,[10] as do somewhat larger, cord-compressive masses that seemingly represent neoplastic transforma-

tion of a notochordal rest.[12, 14] Intradural chordomas are most unusual.[15]

---

**TABLE 10–2**
**Spinal and Epidural Neoplasms and Selected Non-Neoplastic Masses Summarized**

| | |
|---|---|
| Amyloidoma | Hemangioma |
| Aneurysmal bone cyst | Hemangiopericytoma |
| Angiolipoma | Leiomyoma |
| Arteriovenous malformation | Leukemia |
| Carcinoid tumor | Lipoma |
| Cavernous angioma | Lipomatosis |
| Chondroblastoma | Lymphoma |
| Chondroma | Malignant fibrous histiocytoma |
| Chondromyxoid fibroma | Malignant hemangioendothelioma |
| Chondrosarcoma | Metastatic carcinoma |
| Chordoma | Multiple myeloma |
| Ependymoma | Neuroblastoma |
| Epithelioid hemangio- | Ossifying fibroma |
| endothelioma | Osteoblastoma |
| Ewing's sarcoma | Osteochondroma |
| Fibromatosis | Osteoid osteoma |
| Gangliocytoma | Osteosarcoma |
| Ganglioneuroblastoma | Plasmacytoma |
| Giant cell tumor | Sacrococcygeal teratoma |
| Giant sacral schwannoma | |

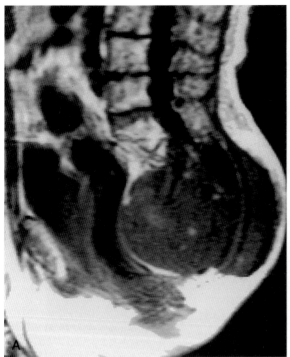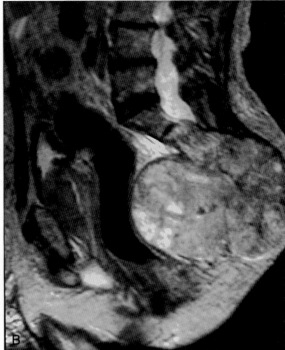

**FIGURE 10-25**    SACRAL CHORDOMA

As seen in a precontrast T1-weighted image (A) and a T2-weighted image (B), sacral chordomas are bone destructive and may undergo anterior extension into the pelvis.

**Clinical Features.** Pain is the generic symptom of chordoma at any level.[17] Anterior extension of sacral lesions adds rectal discomfort and dysfunction, whereas rostral lesions compress spinal roots and the spinal cord. In one case, a tumor's dissemination in the subarachnoid space followed penetration of the dura.[1]

**Radiologic Features.** Chordomas are characteristically lytic of bone, cast an anterior soft tissue shadow, and occasionally include calcification (Fig. 10–25).

**Macroscopic Features.** The lesion's destructive nature and lobular architecture are evident in specimens removed en bloc (Figs. 10–26 and 10–27), but most specimens consist only of semitranslucent tissue fragments.

**Microscopic Features.** The histologic features, including the classical lobularity and the presence of physaliphorous cells (Fig. 10–28), are discussed in detail in Chapter 1 on pages 23 to 27. Only rare spinal lesions have an anaplastic component.[6, 11, 16]

**Treatment and Prognosis.** Chordomas enlarge slowly, but inexorably, and permeate bone. The prognosis is related to the extent of resection. Total excision, a prerequisite for cure, is rarely attained,[8, 9] but radical resection is associated with a significantly longer time to recurrence than when only a subtotal removal is achieved.[17]

The median postoperative survival in one series was 6 years.[13] Infrequent metastases, more often in association with anaplastic lesions, target lung, bone, soft tissues, skin, and liver (Fig. 10–29).[3, 5, 7] The precise benefits of radiotherapy remain uncertain but appear to include delay of tumor recurrence.[17]

## Vertebral Hemangioma

As with their counterparts at other locations, vertebral hemangiomas are aggregates of thin-walled vessels with qualities more hamartomatous than neoplastic. As such, they are usually discovered incidentally during neuroradiologic or postmortem studies. Symptomatic examples occur with local pain and tenderness or with signs of nerve root or spinal cord compression.[1, 3, 4–7] As is the case for their cranial counterparts, the lesions have a distinctive neuroradiologic profile, being bright on both precontrast T1-weighted and T2-weighted images (Fig. 10–30). Seen best by computed tomography (CT), coarse bony trabeculae are characteristic.

At surgery, blood wells forth in artesian fashion from wormian vascular channels. The histologic appearance is less alarming, as only collapsed empty blood vessels remain (Fig. 10–31).[2] Hemangiomas are cured, or controlled, by either surgery or irradiation. Asymptomatic lesions rarely call for surgical attention.

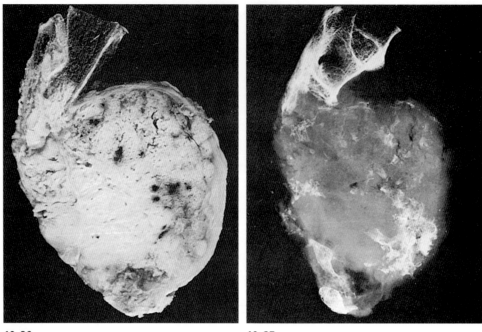

10–26                                    10–27

**FIGURES 10–26 AND 10–27**   SACRAL CHORDOMA

A 46-year-old man presented with coccygeal pain of several years' duration as well as a 1-year history of bowel, bladder, and sexual dysfunction. As seen in this gross sagittal section, the bulky and lobulated tumor destroys both the sacrum and coccyx and has undergone anterior pelvic extension.

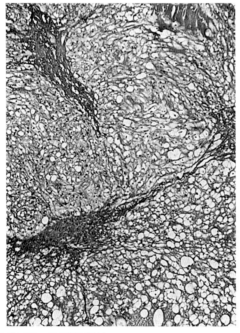

**FIGURE 10–28**   CHORDOMA

Histologically, the tumor features typical lobularity and is composed of vacuolated physaliphorous cells.

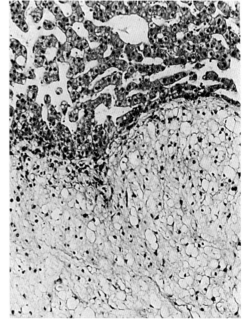

**FIGURE 10–29**   METASTATIC CHORDOMA

Three years after excision of a sacral chordoma, bowel and bladder obstruction necessitated a laparotomy. Two discrete hepatic metastases were encountered.

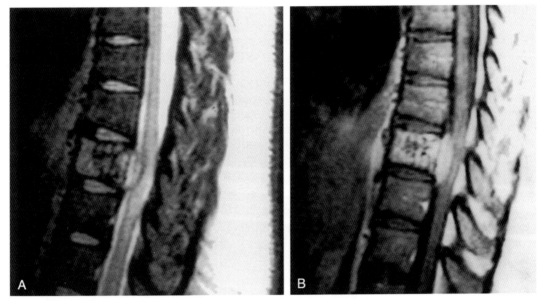

**FIGURE 10–30**   VERTEBRAL HEMANGIOMA

Typical of vertebral and calvarial hemangiomas is their bright signal on both T2-weighted (*A*) and precontrast T1-weighted images (*B*). The patient, a 29-year-old woman, presented with progressive myelopathy that had its onset as tingling in the feet. (Courtesy of Dr. Martin G. Pomper, Baltimore, MD.)

## Lipoma and Angiolipoma

As the spinal epidural space is filled with adipose tissue, it is not surprising that lipomas arise in this location or that some attain sufficient size to compress the spinal cord.[1, 3–6, 8] Most occur at the midthoracic level and affect women. A confident preoperative diagnosis can be established by fat suppression sequences that obliterate fat's intrinsically T1-bright magnetic resonance (MR) signal (see Fig. 10–29). The histologic appearance is so mundane that even the addition of a few blood vessels, as often occurs in spinal examples, is not enough to enhance their visual appeal. "Angiolipoma" is the glorified designation given to these hybrid lesions (Fig. 10–32).[2, 7]

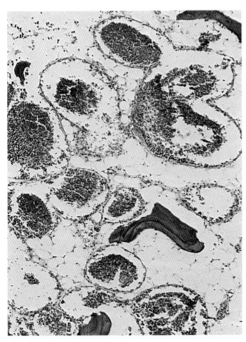

**FIGURE 10–31**   HEMANGIOMA

The typical vertebral hemangioma is composed of delicate serpiginous vascular channels.

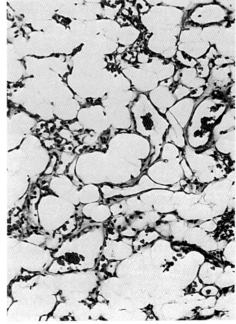

**FIGURE 10–32**   LIPOMA

Epidural lipomas may feature numerous, thin-walled blood vessels. The term angiolipoma is often applied to such lesions.

## Epidural Lipomatosis

As a focal form of adiposity, expansion of adipose tissue of the epidural space is a well-known, but uncommon, response to elevated levels of endogenous steroids (e.g., in Cushing's syndrome) or exogenous glucocorticoids.[2, 6, 7] This cloistered tissue also participates in exogenous obesity[1, 3, 5, 8] and appears to respond to local steroid injections.[4] Idiopathic expansion of epidural adipose tissue rarely occurs.[2] Because a reduction in steroid levels or a

curbing of caloric intake alleviates the problem, a surgical specimen is rarely forthcoming.

## Lymphoma and Leukemia

The generous vascularity of spinal bone marrow and its content of hematopoietic and systemic lymphoid cells readily explain the frequency with which vertebrae are involved in hematologic malignancies. Unlike the skull, with its intimate physical attachment to the dura, the

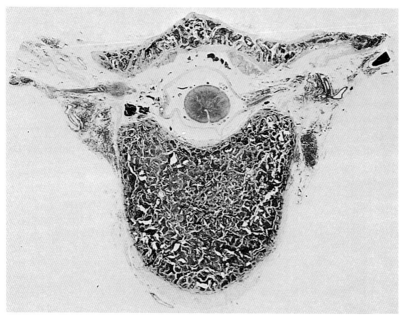

10–33

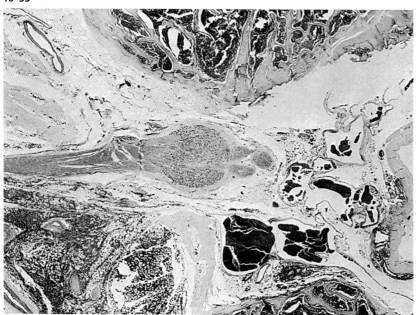

10–34

**FIGURES 10–33 AND 10–34    LYMPHOMA/LEUKEMIA**

Neoplastic cells replace the bone marrow, infiltrate paravertebral fat, and enter the spinal canal through the intervertebral foramina of this 42-year-old woman with acute lymphoblastic leukemia complicating a mixed lymphoma (Fig. 10–33). At higher magnification the dense infiltrate of neoplastic cells involves adipose tissue (*left*), passes inferior to the dorsal root ganglion, and adheres to the dura (*right*) (Fig. 10–34).

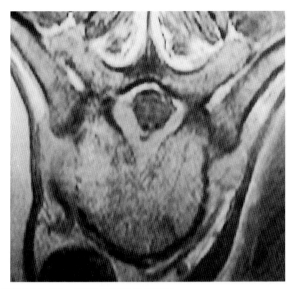

**FIGURE 10–35    HODGKIN'S DISEASE**

Hodgkin's disease can enter the spinal canal to compress the spinal cord, as occurred in this 26-year-old man.

spinal epidural space is a tissue compartment that offers little resistance to the expansion of neoplasms that penetrate the periosteum, spread through intervertebral foramina (Figs. 10–33 to 10–35), or embolize by way of vascular or lymphatic channels.

Although leukemic infiltrates may compress the spinal cord and produce functional deficits,[7, 9] lymphomatous involvement occurs with higher frequency and is of greater clinical consequence. Both entities affect adults most commonly and selectively target the midthoracic region. Signs and symptoms of spinal cord compression may be the initial presenting manifestation of the disease,[1–6, 8, 10, 11] but they are more often late events in the course of systemic lymphoma. Involvement of the epidural space occurs by direct extension from paraspinal sites, usually through intervertebral foramina. Metastatic carcinoma and myeloma more often spread directly from adjacent bone.

When the epidural compartment is unroofed at the time of surgery, the homogeneous, gray tumor is readily distinguished from the normal yellow and lobulated epidural fat (Figs. 10–36 and 10–37). The absence of

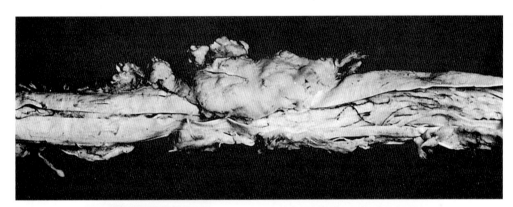

**10–36**

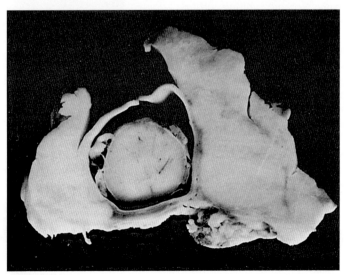

**10–37**

**FIGURES 10–36 AND 10–37    HODGKIN'S DISEASE**

A firm, white epidural mass literally strangles the thoracic spinal cord of this 32-year-old woman who developed hypoesthesias of the lower extremities during the terminal phase of a 7-year course of Hodgkin's disease.

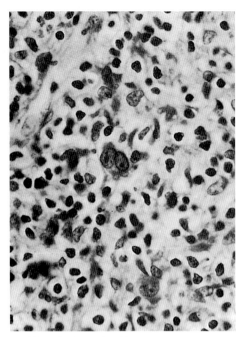

**FIGURE 10–38**    HODGKIN'S DISEASE

As at other sites, Hodgkin's disease of the spine and epidural space is characterized by Reed-Sternberg cells in association with variable numbers of lymphocytes and eosinophils as well as fibrous tissue and occasionally necrosis. This lesion of the mixed cellularity type was surgically removed from the thoracic epidural space of a 32-year-old man without previously recognized systemic disease.

the appropriate clinical setting, the disease is recognized radiologically. The tumor, or newly formed bone, diminishes or abolishes the T1-bright signal of the marrow's normal adipose tissue. Epidural infiltration usually follows lytic vertebral involvement that predisposes to pathologic fracture (Figs. 10–39 to 10–41). Common primary sites are lung, breast, and prostate.[2, 6, 7] Specific citations discuss spinal metastases from genitourinary tract, including prostate,[4, 10] lung,[5] breast,[3] and malignant melanoma.[8]

The reaction by the hosting bone is variable. Trabeculae are minimally affected in some cases but are destroyed in others. Of particular interest is the osteoblastic response that accompanies metastatic carcinomas of the prostate (Figs. 10–42 to 10–44).[9] Impingement of tumor upon sensory nerves, the basis of radicular pain, may occur as well (Fig. 10–45).

The appearance of the gross surgical specimen attests to the destructive character of most neoplastic lesions. Such specimens often have a fleshy consistency, zones of necrosis, and sequestered spicules of bone.

The ease with which the epithelial nature of metastatic carcinoma is recognized parallels its degree of differentiation (Fig. 10–46). Anaplastic examples may prompt consideration of lymphoma, myeloma, and peripheral primitive neuroectodermal tumor, issues discussed below on page 522.

appreciable lymphoid tissue in the normal epidural space obviates concern about reactive lymphoid hyperplasia. Relieved of this possibility, the differential diagnosis can focus on inflammatory and neoplastic conditions (Fig. 10–38). As previously noted, epidural inflammation is usually granulomatous or suppurative. These inflammatory entities are readily distinguished from leukemia or lymphoma. Notable among other neoplasms affecting the epidural space are multiple myeloma and metastatic carcinoma. On occasion, myeloma is sufficiently subtle in both tissue sections and smears as to be overlooked. Metastatic carcinoma, even when anaplastic, tends to grow as solid, often desmoplastic tissue, featuring foci of necrosis and, commonly, brisk mitotic activity. The epithelial nature of the lesion is clearly apparent in better differentiated examples.

## Metastatic Carcinoma

Surgical pathologists encounter metastatic carcinoma when acute spinal cord symptoms necessitate a diagnostic and decompressive laminectomy.[1] Such encounters have become less common because immediate steroid therapy and radiotherapy, rather than surgery, are often employed in the presence of known systemic disease. Local symptoms, usually pain, may be the initial manifestation; the thoracic spine is most often involved. In

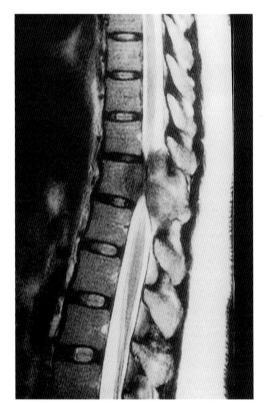

**FIGURE 10–39**    METASTATIC CARCINOMA

Metastatic deposit of follicular thyroid carcinoma compresses the spinal cord of a 35-year-old woman. (Courtesy of Dr. Elias Melhem, Baltimore, MD.)

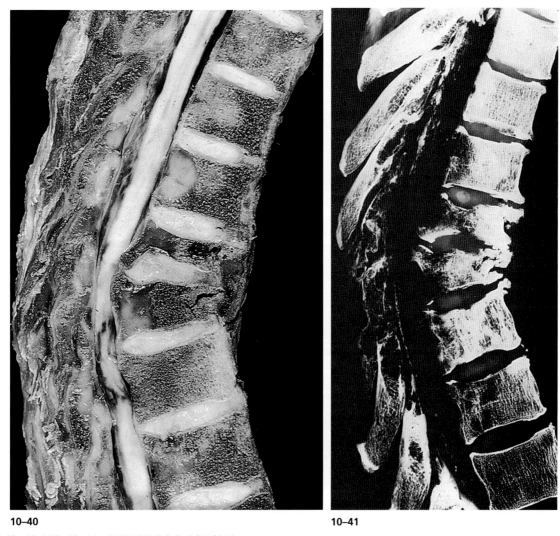

**10–40**                    **10–41**

**FIGURES 10–40 AND 10–41**   METASTATIC CARCINOMA

Three years after a right radical mastectomy, metastatic breast carcinoma produced vertebral collapse and paraparesis in a 55-year-old woman. The bisected spine discloses the typical fleshy character of metastatic cancer (Fig. 10–40). A radiograph emphasizes its destructiveness (Fig. 10–41).

## Multiple Myeloma and Plasmacytoma

Plasma cell neoplasia frequently affects the spine. Involvement of the epidural space is also a common event that is often precipitated by vertebral collapse (Figs. 10–47 to 10–50). The incidence is maximal during the fifth to the seventh decades, with preferential involvement of the thoracic segment. The collapsed vertebrae are readily seen by MR imaging (Fig. 10–47).[4, 8]

The grayish purple hue and the fleshy consistency of the neoplastic foci reflect the high cellularity. In patternless array, the tumor consists of obvious plasma cells, even in most anaplastic myelomas. Thus, cells with eccentric nuclei with "clock-face" chromatin, cytoplasmic basophilia, and a pale paranuclear Golgi zone are seen, if only focally. Binucleation may be conspicuous (Fig. 10–51). Kappa or lambda restriction establishes a clonal,

neoplastic process (Fig. 10–52). Although the utility of touch and smear preparations cannot be overstressed (Fig. 10–53), it must be admitted that plasma cells are sometimes more true to form in histologic sections than in cytologic preparations.

The diagnosis of "solitary" plasmacytoma of bone should be viewed with skepticism and entertained only after a thorough negative hematologic evaluation and, even then, characterized as a tentative diagnosis until confirmed by long-term follow-up. Unlike plasmacytomas in viscera, many spinal lesions evolve into multiple myeloma.[1–3, 5, 6] Occasional masses of amyloid and plasma cells may appear in the spine.[7] The neoplastic versus reactive nature of these remains in doubt.

Only a rare patient is cured of multiple myeloma despite aggressive therapy, such as high-dose chemotherapy with bone marrow transplantation.

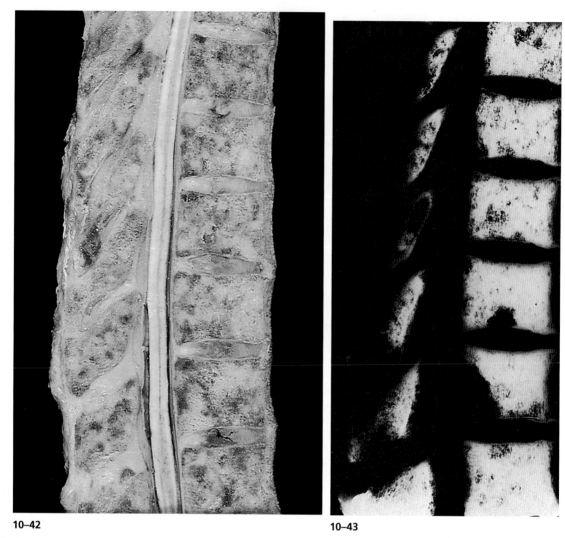

**10–42**

**10–43**

**FIGURES 10–42 AND 10–43** METASTATIC CARCINOMA

In contrast to the osteolysis seen in Figures 10–40 and 10–41, metastatic prostate cancer is usually osteoblastic. Nine years after apparently complete resection of the primary neoplasm, these lesions produced back pain in a 69-year-old patient.

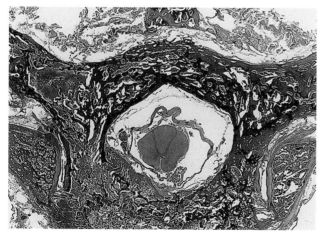

**FIGURE 10–44** METASTATIC CARCINOMA

Metastatic carcinoma of the prostate has resulted in a marked osteoblastic reaction in a thoracic vertebral body, its pedicles, and lamina. In addition, it has entered the epidural space to compress the spinal cord. The 53-year-old man had extensive bone metastases, including some to the skull.

## Neuroblastic and Neuronal Neoplasms

Neuroblastic and neuronal neoplasms, usually in children, occasionally appear as either primary lesions of the epidural space or secondary extensions of a paravertebral primary (Figs. 10–54 and 10–55).[1-6] Rare examples are hematogenous metastases. As fleshy, lobulated, and discrete masses, the lesions impinge upon the spinal cord and its nerve roots, producing signs and symptoms of cord compression as well as local and/or radicular pain. All levels of the spine are potential sites.

Microscopically, spinal neuroblastomas exhibit the expected neuroblasts, focal fibrillar background, patchy necrosis, and calcification. Ganglion cells enliven the ganglioneuroblastoma and, in association with Schwann cells, are the exclusive neuronal element in ganglioneuromas (Figs. 10–56 and 10–57).[7]

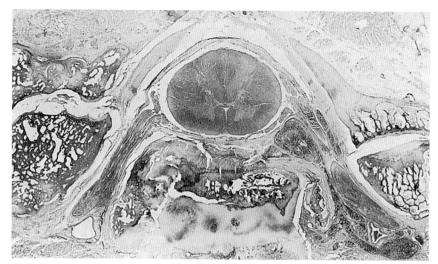

### FIGURE 10–45   METASTATIC CARCINOMA

A 45-year-old man with large cell undifferentiated carcinoma of the lung experienced progressive weakness of the right upper extremity. The responsible lesion was metastatic carcinoma, here seen as multiple dark lobules about a cervical nerve root on the right.

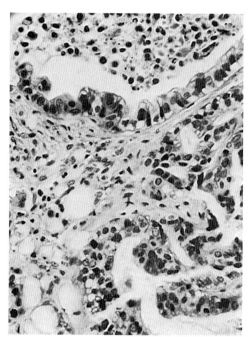

### FIGURE 10–46   METASTATIC CARCINOMA

The absence of epithelial structures in the epidural space simplifies the differential diagnosis of expansile lesions in this location. This gland-forming carcinoma that originated in the lung was surgically excised from the thoracic region in a 51-year-old man.

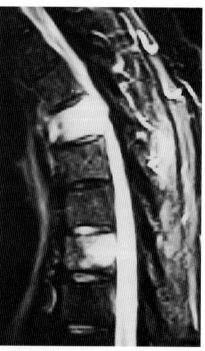

### FIGURE 10–47   MULTIPLE MYELOMA

The patient, a 43-year-old man, presented with back pain and signs of cord compression. Two collapsed vertebrae are readily evident.

### FIGURES 10–48 AND 10–49   MULTIPLE MYELOMA

Macroscopically (Fig. 10–48) and radiologically (Fig. 10–49), multiple myeloma is a markedly osteolytic lesion. Back pain brought this 73-year-old man to medical attention.

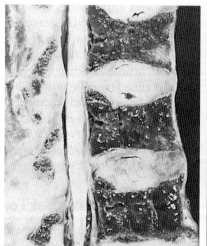

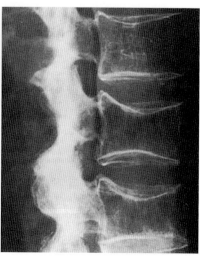

**10–48**

**10–49**

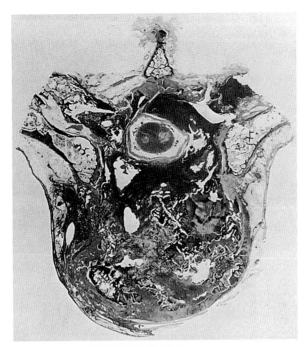

**FIGURE 10–50    MULTIPLE MYELOMA**

Involvement of the spine at the T9 level produced urinary retention and paresis in a 61-year-old man with multiple myeloma. This histologic cross section of the vertebra shows extensive bone involvement with obliteration of normal epidural tissues, massive encroachment upon the dura, and malacia of the spinal cord.

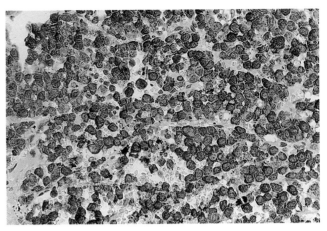

**FIGURE 10–52    MULTIPLE MYELOMA**

An immunohistochemical preparation for kappa-type immunoglobulin light chains establishes the monoclonality of the lesion seen in Figures 10–47 and 10–51.

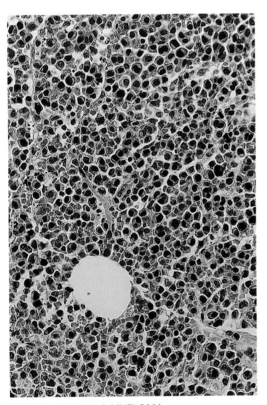

**FIGURE 10–51    MULTIPLE MYELOMA**

Plasma cells are identified by their rounded contours, eccentric nuclei with clock-face chromatin, sporadic binucleation, and dense basophilic cytoplasm. The presence of nuclear pleomorphism helps define these plasma cells as neoplastic.

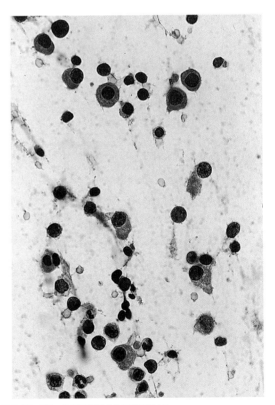

**FIGURE 10–53    MULTIPLE MYELOMA**

In providing cytologic details, touch preparations aid in the diagnosis of epidural neoplasms. Illustrated here are the classical features of plasma cells.

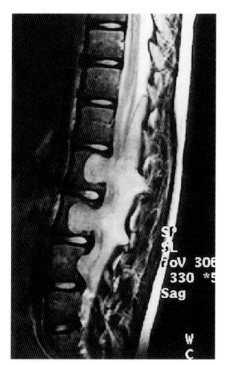

**FIGURE 10-54    GANGLIONEUROMA**

This large epidural mass compressed the spinal cord and eroded vertebral bodies in a 13-year-old.

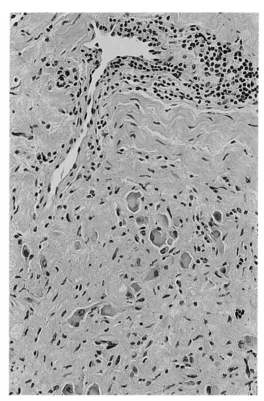

**FIGURE 10-56    GANGLIONEUROMA**

The lesion seen in Figure 10–54 contains scattered ganglion cells in a connective tissue matrix. Perivascular inflammatory cells, seen at the left, are a common feature of ganglion cell tumors.

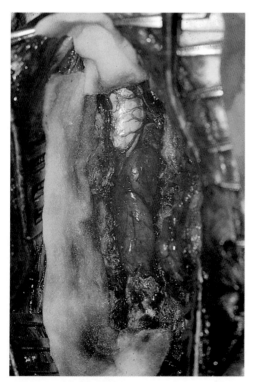

**FIGURE 10-55    GANGLIONEUROMA**

Spinal cord compression called attention to a thoracolumbar, paravertebral mass in a 2-year-old girl. At surgery, the discrete lobular lesion displaced the cord. An extraspinal component both entered the retroperitoneum and perirenal spaces and extended into paravertebral musculature. After a 5-year postoperative interval, the patient was free of recurrence.

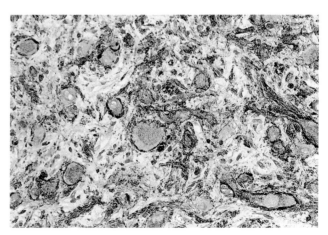

**FIGURE 10-57    GANGLIONEUROMA**

Granular "surface staining" for synaptophysin establishes the neuronal nature of the large cells seen in Figures 10–54 and 10–56.

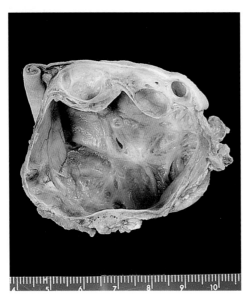

**FIGURE 10–58**    SACROCOCCYGEAL TERATOMA

A 4-day-old girl was born with a mass in the buttock. Of interest was a strong family history of twinning. The bisected orange-sized lesion included a large chamber with satellites of smaller cysts.

# Sacrococcygeal Teratoma

**Definition.** A usually well-differentiated germ cell neoplasm of the sacrum.

**General Comments.** Teratomatous growths in the sacrococcygeal region floridly express the proliferative and differentiating capacity of totipotential cells.

**Clinical Features.** Most of these uncommon lesions declare themselves during the neonatal period as a caudal deformity that can reach enormous proportions. Uncommonly, they appear later, in children and adults, when pain and mechanical interference with bowel, bladder, and sciatic nerve function herald their presence.[3, 4, 8–10, 12, 13, 15]

In accord with the sex distribution in patients with gonadal teratomas, but not for their counterparts in the pineal region, sacrococcygeal teratomas occur more often in females. Most originate in the coccygeal and presacral regions, from which sites they surface in the posterior midline or protrude laterally into a buttock. Alternatively or additionally, they may expand anteriorly and compress pelvic structures. Cleavage planes generally define tumor margins in the absence of infiltrative, malignant behavior. The latter is uncommon.

**Macroscopic Features.** Transection of the surgical specimen typically reveals a chaotic pattern of solid and cystic tissue (Fig. 10–58). The cysts vary in size, with their contents ranging from watery to mucinous or keratinous to sebaceous. The sebaceous material is often unpleasantly matted with hair. Solid regions may be strewn with calcium.

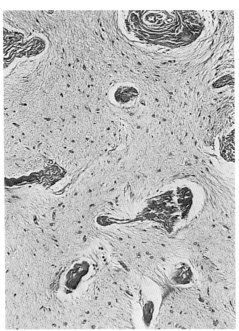

**10–59**

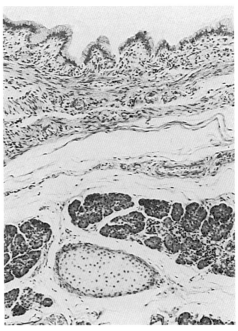

**10–60**

**FIGURES 10–59 AND 10–60**    SACROCOCCYGEAL TERATOMA

Neural elements frequently predominate in the sacrococcygeal teratoma (Fig. 10–59), and columnar epithelium, cartilage, and exocrine glands are often encountered (Fig. 10–60).

**Microscopic Features.** Histologic sections provide the gratification of multiple encounters with surprisingly well-differentiated tissues. Derivatives of all three germ layers may be represented and distributed in purposeless array.[4, 15] Ectodermal derivatives usually predominate, to form neuroectodermal, epidermoid, and dermoid structures. Neuroectoderm is represented by delicate, hypocellular, fibrillar tissue in which astroglia dominate but in which neurons of varying size, ependymal papillations, fronds of choroid plexus, and even pigmented choroidal epithelium are occasionally encountered (Fig. 10–59). Rosenthal's fibers may abound. Epidermoid and dermoid cysts complete the repertoire of ectodermal expression. Mesoderm contributes muscle, fibrous tissue, bone, and cartilage (Fig. 10–60); the latter should not be misinterpreted as the coccyx, an innocent bystander in the line of trespass. Embryonic endoderm may generate not only respiratory and intestinal epithelia but well-formed pancreas as well (see Fig. 10–60).

**Treatment and Prognosis.** The discrete nature of teratomas often permits gross total removal.[8, 13] The importance of removing the coccyx has been emphasized.[4, 11, 13]

Some teratomas contain more primitive tissues. The presence of immature, as opposed to malignant, elements is not a poor prognostic factor.[14] A grading system similar to that applied to ovarian teratomas has been advocated.[4] A small number of tumors are overtly malignant owing to their content of other germ cell components, which include embryonal carcinoma[2, 3, 15] and yolk sac tumor.[3, 4, 8, 13] A Wilms tumor element has also been reported.[16] In one series, the production of alpha-fetoprotein was positively correlated with the presence of yolk sac components.[8] Malignant behavior, as expressed as local invasion and distant metastases, is largely reserved for lesions detected after the neonatal period.[5-9] Although incompletely resected or undetected lesions may remain stable for decades, rare examples undergo late malignant transformation.[1, 11]

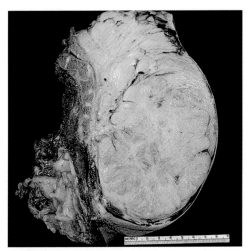

**FIGURE 10–61**   SACRAL EPENDYMOMA

Massive ependymomas of the myxopapillary type can arise in perisacral soft tissues. This example originated in postsacral soft tissues of an obese adult male who noted discomfort on sitting.

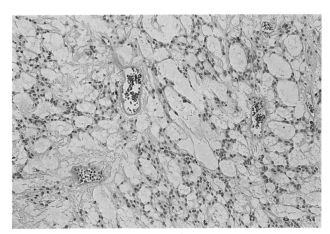

**FIGURE 10–62**   SACRAL EPENDYMOMA

Sacral ependymomas typically show features of myxopapillary ependymoma of the filum terminale but are often somewhat more epithelial in appearance.

## Sacral Ependymoma

Ependymomas occasionally occur primarily in the sacrum or parasacral soft tissues without an associated intradural mass (Figs. 10–61 and 10–62). Immunohistochemistry for glial fibrillary acidic protein (GFAP) can be used to confirm the glial nature of these sometimes pleomorphic, and diagnostically confusing, myxopapillary lesions. These unusual and potentially aggressive neoplasms are discussed in the section on ependymomas in

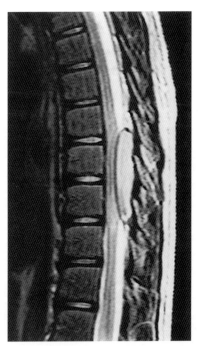

**FIGURE 10–63**   PERIPHERAL PRIMITIVE NEUROECTODERMAL TUMOR/EWING'S SARCOMA

Signs and symptoms of spinal cord compression called attention to this epidural mass in a 1-year-old girl.

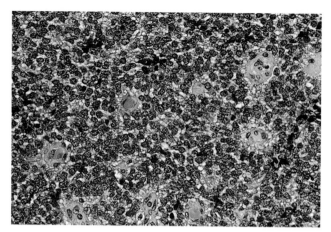

**FIGURE 10–64** PERIPHERAL PRIMITIVE NEUROECTODERMAL TUMOR/EWING'S SARCOMA

Sheets of uniform small cells without conspicuous anaplasia are typical of peripheral primitive neuroectodermal tumor.

Chapter 11 on page 565. Ectopic ependymal tissue in the sacrum is the logical source of these lesions.

## Miscellaneous Neoplasms and Non-Neoplastic Tumors

A partial list of spinal lesions that come to neurosurgical attention includes epidural amyloidoma,[9] aneurysmal bone cyst,[3, 5, 11, 14, 19, 29, 32, 35, 39, 40, 47] arteriovenous malformation, carcinoid tumor,[55] chondroblastoma,[63] chondroma,[26, 38, 61] chondromyxoid fibroma,[51] chondrosarcoma,[6, 7, 12, 22, 64] mesenchymal chondrosarcoma,[16] epithelioid hemangioendothelioma,[20] peripheral primitive euroectodermal tumor or Ewing's sarcoma (Figs. 10–63 to 10–65),[5, 54, 57] fibromatosis,[36, 37] and giant cell tumor.[5, 10, 13, 15, 41]

Still others include hamartoma,[44] intraosseous schwannoma,[8] parachordoma,[62] giant sacral schwannoma[2, 17, 49, 53, 60] hemangiopericytoma,[23, 45] leiomyoma,[33, 58] malignant fibrous histiocytoma,[59] malignant hemangioen-

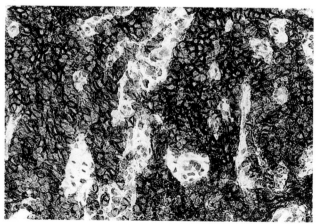

**FIGURE 10–65** PERIPHERAL PRIMITIVE NEUROECTODERMAL TUMOR/EWING'S SARCOMA

The lesions are immunoreactive with the O13 antibody to the Mic-2 gene product.

dothelioma,[30] ossifying fibroma,[48] osteoma,[52] osteoblastoma,[5, 21, 27, 31, 34, 43, 56] osteochondroma,[4, 5, 25, 28, 46, 50] osteoid osteoma,[1, 5, 34] and osteosarcoma.[5, 18, 24, 42]

## REFERENCES

### Congenital Malformations (Meningocele and Meningomyelocele)

1. Akar Z. Myelomeningocele. Surg Neurol 1995;43:113–118.
2. Barami K, Pereira J, Canady AI. Anterolateral lumbar lipomyelomeningocele: case report and review of the literature. Neurosurgery 1997;41:1421–1424.
3. Chadduck WM, Uthman EO. Squamous cell carcinoma and meningomyelocele. Neurosurgery 1984;14:601–603.
4. Dolynchuk KN, Teskey J, West M. Intrathoracic meningocele associated with neurofibromatosis: case report. Neurosurgery 1990;27:485–487.
5. Dyck P, Wilson CB. Anterior sacral meningocele: case report. J Neurosurg 1980;53:548–552.
6. Erkulvrawatr S, El Gammal T, Hawkins J, et al. Intrathoracic meningoceles and neurofibromatosis. Arch Neurol 1979;36:557–559.
7. Ivamoto HS, Wallman LJ. Anterior sacral meningocele. Arch Neurol 1974;31:345–346.
8. Leibowitz E, Barton W, Sadighi P, et al. Anterior sacral meningocele contiguous with a pelvic hamartoma. J Neurosurg 1984;61:188–190.
9. Mitgang RN. Teratoma occurring within a myelomeningocele: case report. J Neurosurg 1972;37:448–451.
10. Nishino A, Shirane R, So K, et al. Cervical myelocystocele with Chiari II malformation: magnetic resonance imaging and surgical treatment. Surg Neurol 1998;49:269–273.
11. Pang D, Dias MS. Cervical myelomeningoceles. Neurosurgery 1993;33:363–373.
12. Quigley MR, Schinco F, Brown JT. Anterior sacral meningocele with an unusual presentation: case report. J Neurosurg 1984;61:790–792.
13. Sogani KC, Kalani BP. Paravertebral lumbar meningomyelocele: report of two cases. J Neurosurg 1972;37:746–748.
14. Spiegelmann R, Schinder E, Mintz M, et al. The human tail: a benign stigma: case report. J Neurosurg 1985;63:461–462.
15. Thorp RH. Case reports and technical notes; carcinoma associated with myelomeningocele: case report. J Neurosurg 1967;27:446–448.

### Tuberculosis

1. Martin NS. Pott's paraplegia. J Bone Joint Surg Br 1971;53:596–608.
2. Moon M-S. Spine update. Tuberculosis of the spine. Controversies and a new challenge. Spine 1997;22:1791–1797.
3. Nussbaum ES, Rockswold GL, Bergman TA, et al. Spinal tuberculosis: a diagnostic and management challenge. J Neurosurg 1995;83:243–247.
4. Rezai AR, Lee M, Cooper PR, et al. Modern management of spinal tuberculosis. Neurosurgery 1995;36:87–98.
5. Shanley DJ. Tuberculosis of the spine: imaging features. AJR 1995;164:659–664.

### Epidural Abscess

1. Curling OD Jr, Gower DJ, McWhorter JM. Changing concepts in spinal epidural abscess: a report of 29 cases. Neurosurgery 1990;27:185–192.
2. Hlavin ML, Kaminski HJ, Ross JS, et al. Spinal epidural abscess: a ten-year perspective: experimental and clinical studies. Neurosurgery 1990;27:177–184.
3. Khanna RK, Malik GM, Rock JP, et al. Spinal epidural abscess: evaluation of factors influencing outcome. Neurosurgery 1996;39:958–964.
4. Nussbaum ES, Rigamonti D, Standiford H, et al. Spinal epidural abscess: a report of 40 cases and review. Surg Neurol 1992;38:225–231.

## Other Inflammatory Disorders

1. Acciarri N, Paganini M, Fonda C, et al. Langerhans cell histiocytosis of the spine causing cord compression: case report. Neurosurgery 1992;31:965–968.
2. Apt WL, Fierro JL, Calderón C, et al. Vertebral hydatid disease. Clinical experience with 27 cases. J Neurosurg 1976;44:72–76.
3. Baylin GJ, Wear JM. Blastomycosis and actinomycosis of the spine. Am J Roentgenol Radium Ther Nucl Med 1953;69: 395–398.
4. Brown JR. Human actinomycosis. A study of 181 subjects. Hum Pathol 1973;4:319–330.
5. Dickinson LD, Farhat SM. Eosinophilic granuloma of the cervical spine. A case report and review of the literature. Surg Neurol 1991;35:57–63.
6. Friedman H. Intraspinal rheumatoid nodule causing nerve root compression. Case report. J Neurosurg 1970;32:689–691.
7. Greenwood RC, Voris HC. Systemic blastomycosis with spinal cord involvement. Case report. J Neurosurg 1950;7:450–454.
8. Ingham SD. Coccidioidal granuloma of the spine with compression of the spinal cord. Bull Los Angeles Neurol Soc 1936;1:41–45.
9. Lara R. Extradural toruloma in the lumbo-sacral region. Surg Neurol 1975;3:211–213.
10. Litvinoff J, Nelson M. Extradural lumbar cryptococcosis. Case report. J Neurosurg 1978;49:921–923.
11. Maggi G, de Sanctis N, Aliberti F, et al. Eosinophilic granuloma of C4 causing spinal cord compression. Childs Nerv Syst 1996;12:630–632.
12. Marcelli C, Pérennou D, Cyteval C, et al. Amyloidosis-related cauda equina compression in long-term hemodialysis patients. Three case reports. Spine 1996;21:381–385.
13. Mawk JR, Erickson DL, Chou SN, et al. *Aspergillus* infections of the lumbar disc space. Report of three cases. J Neurosurg 1983;58:270–274.
14. Mullins KJ, Meyers SP, Kazee AM, et al. Primary solitary amyloidosis of the spine: a case report and review of the literature. Surg Neurol 1997;48:405–408.
15. Pandey M, Chaudhari MP. Primary hydatid cyst of sacral spinal canal: case report. Neurosurgery 1997;40:407–409.
16. Tekkök I, Benli K. Primary spinal extradural hydatid disease: report of a case with magnetic resonance characteristics and pathological correlation. Neurosurgery 1993;33:320–323.
17. Tekkök IH, Berker M, özcan OE, et al. Brucellosis of the spine. Neurosurgery 1993;33:838–844.
18. Villarejo F, Diaz CP, Perla C, et al. Spinal cord compression by amyloid deposits. Spine 1994;19:1178–1181.
19. Wagner DK, Varkey B, Sheth NK, et al. Epidural abscess, vertebral destruction, and paraplegia caused by extending infection from an aspergilloma. Am J Med 1985;78:518–522.
20. Wani MA, Taheri SA, Babu ML, et al. Primary spinal extradural hydatid cyst. Neurosurgery 1989;24:631–632.
21. Weissman MN, Lange R, Kelley C, et al. Intraspinal epidural sarcoidosis: case report. Neurosurgery 1996;39:179–181.
22. Yeom J-S, Lee C-K, Shin HY, et al. Langerhans' cell histiocytosis of the spine. Spine 1999;24:1740–1749.

## Herniated Nucleus Pulposus

1. Blikra G. Intradural herniated lumbar disc. J Neurosurg 1969;31:676–679.
2. Boutin P, Hogshead H. Surgical pathology of the intervertebral disc. Is routine examination necessary? Spine 1992;17: 1236–1238.
3. Brock M, Patt S, Mayer H-M. The form and structure of the extruded disc. Spine 1992;17:1457–14561.
4. Coventry MB, Ghormley RK, Kernohan JW. The intervertebral disc: its microscopic anatomy and pathology. Part II. Changes in the intervertebral disc concomitant with age. J Bone Joint Surg 1945;27:233–247.
5. Daftari TK, Levine J, Fischgrund JS, et al. Is pathology examination of disc specimens necessary after routine anterior cervical discectomy and fusion? Spine 1996;21:2156–2159.
6. Feild JR, Higley GB Sr, DeSaussure RL Jr. Ochronosis with ruptured lumbar disc. Case report. J Neurosurg 1963;20:348–351.
7. Hodge CJ, Binet EF, Kieffer SA. Intradural herniation of lumbar intervertebral discs. Spine 1978;3:346–350.
8. Markolf KL, Morris JM. The structural components of the intervertebral disc. A study of their contributions to the ability of the disc to withstand compressive forces. J Bone Joint Surg Am 1974;56:675–687.
9. Smith RV. Intradural disc rupture. Report of two cases. J Neurosurg 1981;55:117–120.
10. Weidner N, Rice DT. Intervertebral disk material: criteria for determining probable prolapse. Hum Pathol 1988;19:406–410.

## Synovial Cyst

1. Fransen P, Pizzolato GP, Otten P, et al. Synovial cyst and degeneration of the transverse ligament: an unusual cause of high cervical myelopathy. Case report. J Neurosurg 1997;86:1027–1030.
2. Goffin J, Wilms G, Plets C, et al. Synovial cyst at the C1-C2 junction. Neurosurgery 1992;30:914–916.
3. Howington JU, Connolly ES, Voorhies RM. Intraspinal synovial cysts: 10-year experience at the Ochsner Clinic. J Neurosurg 1999;91:193–199.
4. Hsu KY, Zucherman JF, Shea WJ, et al. Lumbar intraspinal synovial and ganglion cysts (facet cysts). Ten-year experience in evaluation and treatment. Spine 1995;20:80–89.
5. Munz M, Tampieri D, Robitaille Y, et al. Spinal synovial cyst: case report using magnetic resonance imaging. Surg Neurol 1990;34:431–434.
6. Silbergleit R, Gebarski SS, Brunberg JA, et al. Lumbar synovial cysts: correlation of myelographic, CT, MR, and pathologic findings. AJNR 1990;11:777–779.
7. Yarde WL, Arnold PM, Kepes JJ, et al. Synovial cysts of the lumbar spine: diagnosis, surgical management, and pathogenesis. Report of eight cases. Surg Neurol 1995;43:459–465.

## Calcifying Pseudoneoplasm of the Neuraxis

1. Bertoni F, Unni K, Dahlin DC, et al. Calcifying pseudoneoplasms of the neural axis. J Neurosurg 1990;72:42–48.
2. Qian J, Rubio A, Powers JM, et al. Fibro-osseous lesions of the central nervous system. Report of four cases and literature review. Am J Surg Pathol 1999;23:1270–1275.

## Other Degenerative and Reactive Processes

1. Bonaldi VM, Duong H, Starr MR, et al. Tophaceous gout of the lumbar spine mimicking an epidural abscess: MR features. AJNR 1996;17:1949–1952.
2. Buetow PC, Perry JJ, Geyer CA. Gd-DTPA enhancement in CNS extramedullary hematopoiesis. AJNR 1990;11:411–412.
3. Cartlidge NEF, McCollum JPK, Ayyar RAD. Spinal cord compression in Paget's disease. J Neurol Neurosurg Psychiatry 1972;35:825–828.
4. Clark LJP, McCormick PW, Domenico DR, et al. Pigmented villonodular synovitis of the spine. Case report. J Neurosurg 1993;79:456–459.
5. Dibbern DA Jr, Loevner LA, Lieberman AP, et al. MR of thoracic cord compression caused by epidural extramedullary hematopoiesis in myelodysplastic syndrome. AJNR 1997;18: 363–366.
6. Duprez TP, Malghem J, Vande Berg BC, et al. Gout in the cervical spine: MR pattern mimicking diskovertebral infection. AJNR 1996;17:151–153.
7. Gezen F, Akay KM, Aksu AY, et al. Spinal pigmented villonodular synovitis. A case report. Spine 1996;21:642–645.
8. Giannini C, Scheithauer BW, Wender DE, et al. Pigmented villonodular synovitis of the spine: a clinical, radiological, and morphological study of 12 cases. J Neurosurg 1996;84:592–597.
9. Kim D-S, Kim T-S, Choi J-U. Intradural extramedullary xanthoma of the spine: a rare lesion arising from the dura mater of the spine: case report. Neurosurgery 1996;39:182–185.
10. Kuzma BB, Goodman JM, Renkens KL. Cervical myelopathy secondary to calcium pyrophosphate crystal deposition in the alar ligament. Surg Neurol 1997;47:498–499.
11. Montoya G, Evarts CM, Dohn DF. Polyostotic fibrous dysplasia and spinal cord compression: case report. J Neurosurg 1968;29: 102–105.
12. Muthukumar N, Karuppaswamy U, Sankarasubbu B. Calcium pyrophosphate dihydrate deposition disease causing thoracic cord compression: case report. Neurosurgery 2000;46:222–225.

13. Nabarro MN, Giblin PE. Monostotic fibrous dysplasia of the thoracic spine. Spine 1994;19:463–465.
14. Scully RE (ed). Case records of the Massachusetts General Hospital. Case 37-1991. N Engl J Med 1991;325:794–799.
15. Shaffrey CI, Munoz EL, Sutton CL, et al. Tumoral calcium pyrophosphate dihydrate deposition disease mimicking a cervical spine neoplasm: case report. Neurosurgery 1995;37:335–339.
16. Shimosawa S, Tohyama K, Shibayama M, et al. Spinal xanthogranuloma in a child: case report. Surg Neurol 1993;39: 138–142.
17. Teng P, Gross SW, Newman CM. Compression of spinal cord by osteitis deformans (Paget's disease), giant-cell tumor and polyostotic fibrous dysplasia (Albright's syndrome) of vertebrae: a report of four cases. J Neurosurg 1951;8:482–493.
18. Wald SL, McLennan JE, Carroll RM, et al. Extradural spinal involvement by gout. Case report. J Neurosurg 1979;50:236–239.

## Chordoma

1. Aleksic S, Budzilovich GN, Nirmel K, et al. Subarachnoid dissemination of thoracic chordoma. Arch Neurol 1979;36:652–654.
2. Bjornsson J, Wold LE, Ebersold MJ, et al. Chordoma of the mobile spine. A clinicopathologic analysis of 40 patients. Cancer 1993;71:735–740.
3. Chambers PW, Schwinn CP. Chordoma. A clinicopathologic study of metastasis. Am J Clin Pathol 1979;72:765–776.
4. D'Haen B, De Jaegere T, Goffin J, et al. Case report. Chordoma of the lower cervical spine. Clin Neurol Neurosurg 1995;97: 245–248.
5. Hall WA, Clark HB. Sacrococcygeal chordoma metastatic to the brain with review of the literature. J Neurooncol 1995;25: 155–159.
6. Hruban RH, May M, Marcover RC, et al. Lumbo-sacral chordoma with high-grade malignant cartilaginous and spindle cell components. Am J Surg Pathol 1990;14:384–389.
7. Jenkins CNJ, Colquhoun IR. Case report: symptomatic metastasis from a sacrococcygeal chordoma. Clin Radiol 1995;50:416–417.
8. Klekamp J, Samii M. Spinal chordomas--results of treatment over a 17-year period. Acta Neurochir (Wien) 1996;138:514–519.
9. Ozaki T, Hillmann A, Winkelmann W. Surgical treatment of sacrococcygeal chordoma. J Surg Oncol 1997;64:274–279.
10. Rengachary SS, Grotte DA, Swanson PE. Extradural ecchordosis physaliphora of the thoracic spine: case report. Neurosurgery 1997;41:1198–1202.
11. Rone R, Ramzy I, Duncan D. Anaplastic sacrococcygeal chordoma. Fine needle aspiration cytologic findings and embryologic considerations. Acta Cytol 1986;30:183–188.
12. Sebag G, Dubois J, Beniaminovitz A, et al. Extraosseous spinal chordoma: radiographic appearance. AJNR 1993;14:205–207.
13. Sundaresan N, Galicich JH, Chu FCH, et al. Spinal chordomas. J Neurosurg 1979;50:312–319.
14. Tomlinson FH, Scheithauer BW, Miller GM, et al. Extraosseous spinal chordoma. Case report. J Neurosurg 1991;75:980–984.
15. Vaz RM, Pereira JC, Ramos U, et al. Intradural cervical chordoma without bone involvement. Case report. J Neurosurg 1995;82:650–653.
16. Wichmann AP, Latz DM. [The transformation of a cervical chordoma into an anaplastic tumor. A case report and review of the literature.]. Strahlenther Onkol 1993;169:121–125.
17. York JE, Kaczaraj A, Abi-Said D, et al. Sacral chordoma: 40-year experience at a major cancer center. Neurosurgery 1999;44:74–79.

## Vertebral Hemangioma

1. Bremnes RM, Hauge HN, Sagsveen R. Radiotherapy in the treatment of symptomatic vertebral hemangiomas: technical case report. Neurosurgery 1996;39:1054–1058.
2. Dorfman HD, Steiner GC, Jaffe HL. Vascular tumors of bone. Hum Pathol 1971;2:349–376.
3. Fox MW, Onofrio BM. The natural history and management of symptomatic and asymptomatic vertebral hemangiomas. J Neurosurg 1993;78:36–45.
4. Graziani N, Bouillot P, Figarella-Branger D, et al. Cavernous angiomas and arteriovenous malformations of the spinal epidural space: report of 11 cases. Neurosurgery 1994;35:856–864.
5. Harrington JF Jr, Khan A, Grunnet M. Spinal epidural cavernous angioma presenting as a lumbar radiculopathy with analysis of magnetic resonance imaging characteristics: case report. Neurosurgery 1995;36:581–584.
6. Harrison MJ, Eisenberg MB, Ullman JS, et al. Symptomatic cavernous malformations affecting the spine and spinal cord. Neurosurgery 1995;37:195–205.
7. Nguyen JP, Djindjian M, Gaston A, et al. Vertebral hemangiomas presenting with neurologic symptoms. Surg Neurol 1987;27:391–397.

## Lipoma and Angiolipoma

1. Anson JA, Cybulski GR, Reyes M. Spinal extradural angiolipoma: a report of two cases and review of the literature. Surg Neurol 1990;34:173–178.
2. Labram EK, El-Shunnar K, Hilton DA, et al. Revisited: spinal angiolipoma—three additional cases. Br J Neurosurg 1999;13: 25–29.
3. Mascalchi M, Arnetoli G, Dal Pozzo G, et al. Spinal epidural angiolipoma: MR findings. AJNR 1991;12:744–745.
4. Pagni CA, Canavero S. Spinal epidural angiolipoma: rare or unreported? Neurosurgery 1992;31:758–764.
5. Preul MC, Leblanc R, Tampieri D, et al. Spinal angiolipomas. Report of three cases. J Neurosurg 1993;78:280–286.
6. Provenzale JA, McLendon RE. Spinal angiolipomas: MR features. AJNR 1996;17:713–719.
7. Turgut M. Spinal angiolipomas: report of a case and review of the cases published since the discovery of the tumour in 1890. Br J Neurosurg 1999;13:30–40.
8. Yamashita K, Fuji T, Nakai T, et al. Extradural spinal angiolipoma: report of a case studied with MRI. Surg Neurol 1993;39:49–52.

## Epidural Lipomatosis

1. Beges C, Rousselin B, Chevrot A, et al. Epidural lipomatosis. Interest of magnetic resonance imaging in a weight-reduction treated case. Spine 1994;19:251–254.
2. Haddad S, Hitchon PW, Godersky JC. Idiopathic and glucocorticoid-induced spinal epidural lipomatosis. J Neurosurg 1991; 74:38–42.
3. Kumar K, Nath RK, Nair CPV, et al. Symptomatic epidural lipomatosis secondary to obesity. Case report. J Neurosurg 1996; 85:348–350.
4. McCullen GM, Spurling GR, Webster JS. Epidural lipomatosis complicating lumbar steroid injections. J Spinal Disord 1999; 12:526–529.
5. Robertson SC, Traynelis VC, Follett KA, et al. Idiopathic spinal epidural lipomatosis. Neurosurgery 1997;41:68–75.
6. Roy-Camille R, Mazel CH, Husson JL, et al. Symptomatic spinal epidural lipomatosis induced by a long-term steroid treatment. Review of the literature and report of two additional cases. Spine 1991;16:1365–1371.
7. Sandberg DI, Lavyne MH. Symptomatic spinal epidural lipomatosis after local epidural corticosteroid injections: case report. Neurosurgery 1999;45:162–165.
8. Van Rooij WJJ, Borstlap ACW, Canta LR, et al. Lumbar epidural lipomatosis causing neurogenic claudication in two obese patients. Case report. Clin Neurol Neurosurg 1994;96:181–184.

## Lymphoma and Leukemia

1. Di Marco A, Campostrini F, Garusi GF. Non-Hodgkin lymphomas presenting with spinal epidural involvement. Acta Oncol 1989;28:485–488.
2. Eeles RA, O'Brien P, Horwich A, et al. Non-Hodgkin's lymphoma presenting with extradural spinal cord compression: functional outcome and survival. Br J Cancer 1991;63:126–129.
3. Epelbaum R, Haim N, Ben-Shahar M, et al. Non-Hodgkin's lymphoma presenting with spinal epidural involvement. Cancer 1986;58:2120–2124.
4. Grant JW, Kaech D, Jones DB. Spinal cord compression as the first presentation of lymphoma—a review of 15 cases. Histopathology 1986;10:1191–1202.
5. Higgins SA, Peschel RE. Hodgkin's disease with spinal cord compression. A case report and a review of the literature. Cancer 1995;75:94–98.
6. Lyons MK, O'Neill BP, Marsh R, et al. Primary spinal epidural non-Hodgkin's lymphoma: report of eight patients and review of the literature. Neurosurgery 1992;30:675–680.
7. Michalevicz R, Burstein A, Razon N, et al. Spinal epidural compression in chronic lymphocytic leukemia. Cancer 1989;64: 1961–1964.

8. Mohammed WA, Doshi R. Spinal epidural malignant lymphoma presenting with spinal cord compression. Clin Neuropathol 1995;14:237–240.
9. Mostafvi H, Lennarson PJ, Traynelis VC. Granulocytic sarcoma of the spine. Neurosurgery 2000;46:78–84.
10. Perry JR, Deodhare SS, Bilbao JM, et al. The significance of spinal cord compression as the initial manifestation of lymphoma. Neurosurgery 1993;32:157–162.
11. Salvati M, Cervoni L, Artico M, et al. Primary spinal epidural non-Hodgkin's lymphomas: a clinical study. Surg Neurol 1996;46: 339–344.

## Metastatic Carcinoma

1. Chamberlain MC, Kormanik PA. Epidural spinal cord compression: a single institution's retrospective experience. Neurooncology 1999;1:120–123.
2. Constans JP, De Divitiis E, Donzelli R, et al. Spinal metastases with neurological manifestations. Review of 600 cases. J Neurosurg 1983;59:111–118.
3. Landreneau FE, Landreneau RJ, Keenan RJ, et al. Diagnosis and management of spinal metastases from breast cancer. J Neurooncol 1995;23:121–134.
4. Liskow A, Chang CH, DeSanctis P, et al. Epidural cord compression in association with genitourinary neoplasms. Cancer 1986;58: 949–954.
5. Pedersen AG, Bach F, Melgaard B. Frequency, diagnosis, and prognosis of spinal cord compression in small cell bronchogenic carcinoma. A review of 817 consecutive patients. Cancer 1985;55: 1818–1822.
6. Sioutos PJ, Arbit E, Meshulam CF, et al. Spinal metastases from solid tumors. Analysis of factors affecting survival. Cancer 1995;76:1453–1459.
7. Sørensen PS, Børgesen SE, Rohde K, et al. Metastatic epidural spinal cord compression. Results of treatment and survival. Cancer 1990;65:1502–1508.
8. Spiegel DA, Sampson JH, Richardson WJ, et al. Metastatic melanoma to the spine. Demographics, risk factors, and prognosis in 114 patients. Spine 1995;20:2141–2146.
9. Yamaguchi T, Tamai K, Yamato M, et al. Intertrabecular pattern of tumors metastatic to bone. Cancer 1996;78:1388–94.
10. Zelefsky MJ, Scher HI, Krol G, et al. Spinal epidural tumor in patients with prostate cancer. Clinical and radiographic predictors of response to radiation therapy. Cancer 1992;70:2319–2325.

## Multiple Myeloma and Plasmacytoma

1. Cervoni L, Celli P, Salvati M, et al. Solitary plasmacytoma of the spine: relationship of IGM to tumour progression and recurrence. Acta Neurochir (Wien) 1995;135:122–125.
2. Delauche-Cavallier MC, Laredo JD, Wybier M, et al. Solitary plasmacytoma of the spine. Long-term clinical course. Cancer 1988;61:1707–1714.
3. Holland J, Trenkner DA, Wasserman TH, et al. Plasmacytoma. Treatment results and conversion to myeloma. Cancer 1992;69: 1513–1517.
4. Lecouvet FE, Vande Berg BC, Maldague BE, et al. Vertebral compression fractures in multiple myeloma. Part I. Distribution and appearance at MR imaging. Radiology 1997;204:195–199.
5. Loftus CM, Michelsen CB, Rapoport F, et al. Management of plasmacytomas of the spine. Neurosurgery 1983;13:30–36.
6. McLain RF, Weinstein JN. Solitary plasmacytomas of the spine: a review of 84 cases. J Spinal Disord 1989;2:69–74.
7. Mullins KJ, Meyers SP, Kazee AM, et al. Primary solitary amyloidosis of the spine: a case report and review of the literature. Surg Neurol 1997;48:405–408.
8. Rahmouni A, Divine M, Mathieu D, et al. Detection of multiple myeloma involving the spine: efficacy of fat-suppression and contrast-enhanced MR imaging. AJR 1993;160:1049–1052.

## Neuroblastic and Neuronal Neoplasms

1. Balakrishnan V, Rice MS, Simpson DA. Spinal neuroblastomas. Diagnosis, treatment, and prognosis. J Neurosurg 1974;40: 631–638.
2. Hayes FA, Green AA, O'Connor DM. Chemotherapeutic management of epidural neuroblastoma. Med Pediatr Oncol 1989;17:6–8.
3. Holgersen LO, Santulli TV, Schullinger JN, et al. Neuroblastoma

with intraspinal (dumbbell) extension. J Pediatr Surg 1983;18: 406–411.
4. Massad M, Haddad F, Slim M, et al. Spinal cord compression in neuroblastoma. Surg Neurol 1985;23:567–572.
5. Mutluer S, Ersahin Y, Binatli ö, et al. Dumbbell ganglioneuromas in childhood. Childs Nerv Syst 1993;9:182–184.
6. Punt J, Pritchard J, Pincott JR, et al. Neuroblastoma: a review of 21 cases presenting with spinal cord compression. Cancer 1980;45:3095–3101.
7. Scoville WB, Polcyn JL, Dunsmore RH. Spinal ganglioneuroma. End results and differential diagnosis. J Neuropathol Exp Neurol 1956;15:85–92.

## Sacrococcygeal Teratoma and Sacral Ependymoma

1. Chen KTK. Squamous cell carcinoma arising in sacrococcygeal teratoma (Letter). Arch Pathol Lab Med 1980;104:336.
2. Chretien PB, Milam JD, Foote FW, et al. Embryonal adenocarcinomas (a type of malignant teratoma) of the sacrococcygeal region. Clinical and pathologic aspects of 21 cases. Cancer 1970;26: 522–535.
3. Conklin J, Abell MR. Germ cell neoplasms of sacrococcygeal region. Cancer 1967;20:2105–2117.
4. Dehner LP. Gonadal and extragonadal germ cell neoplasms of sacrococcygeal region. Hum Pathol 1983;14:493–511.
5. Dewan PA, Davidson PM, Campbell PE, et al. Sacrococcygeal teratoma: has chemotherapy improved survival? J Pediatr Surg 1987;22:274–277.
6. Donnellan WA, Swenson O. Benign and malignant sacrococcygeal teratomas. Surgery 1968;64:834–846.
7. Ein SH, Mancer K, Adeyemi SD. Malignant sacrococcygeal teratoma—endodermal sinus, yolk sac tumor—in infants and children: a 32-year review. J Pediatr Surg 1985;20:473–477.
8. Gonzalez-Crussi F, Winkler RF, Mirkin DL. Sacrococcygeal teratoma in infants and children. Relationship of histology and prognosis in 40 cases. Arch Pathol Lab Med 1978;102:420–425.
9. Grosfeld JL, Ballantine TVN, Lowe D, et al. Benign and malignant teratomas in children: analysis of 85 patients. Surgery 1976;80:297–305.
10. Hickey RC, Layton JM. Sacrococcygeal teratoma: emphasis on the biological history and early therapy. Cancer 1954;7: 1031–1043.
11. Lahdenne P, Heikinheimo M, Nikkanen V, et al. Neonatal benign sacrococcygeal teratoma may recur in adulthood and give rise to malignancy. Cancer 1993;72:3727–3731.
12. Miles RM, Stewart GS Jr. Sacrococcygeal teratomas in adults. Ann Surg 1974;179:676–683.
13. Tapper D, Lark EE. Teratomas in infancy and childhood: a 54-year experience at the Children's Hospital Medical Center. Ann Surg 1983;198:398–410.
14. Valdiserri RO, Yunis EJ. Sacrococcygeal teratomas: a review of 68 cases. Cancer 1981;48:217–221.
15. Waldhausen JA, Kilman JW, Vellios F, et al. Sacrococcygeal teratoma. Surgery 1963;54:933–949.
16. Ward SP, Dehner LP. Sacrococcygeal teratoma with nephroblastoma (Wilms' tumor): a variant of extragonadal teratoma in childhood. A histologic and ultrastructural study. Cancer 1974;33: 1355–1363.

## Miscellaneous Neoplasms and Non-Neoplastic Tumors

1. Abe E, Sato K, Okada K, et al. Selective en bloc resection of osteoid osteoma of the superior articular process of the sacral spine. Spine 1993;18:2336–2339.
2. Abernathey CD, Onofrio BM, Scheithauer B, et al. Surgical management of giant sacral schwannomas. J Neurosurg 1986;65: 286–295.
3. Ameli NO, Abbassioun K, Saleh H, et al. Aneurysmal bone cysts of the spine. Report of 17 cases. J Neurosurg 1985;63:685–690.
4. Arasil E, Erdem A, Yüceer N. Osteochondroma of the upper cervical spine. A case report. Spine 1996;21:516–8.
5. Beer SJ, Menezes AH. Primary tumors of the spine in children. Natural history, management, and long-term follow-up. Spine 1997;22:649–659.
6. Blaylack RL, Kempe LG. Chondrosarcoma of the cervical spine: case report. J Neurosurg 1976;44:500–503.
7. Camins MB, Duncan AW, Smith J, et al. Chondrosarcoma of the spine. Spine 1978;3:202–209.

8. Chang C-J, Huang J-S, Wang Y-C, et al. Intraosseous schwannoma of the fourth lumbar vertebra: case report. Neurosurgery 1998;43:1219–1222.

9. Cloft HJ, Quint DJ, Markert JM, et al. Primary osseous amyloidoma causing spinal cord compression. AJNR 1995;16:1152–1154.

10. Cohen DM, Dahlin DC, MacCarty CS. Vertebral giant-cell tumor and variants. Cancer 1964;17:461–472.

11. Cory DA, Fritsch SA, Cohen M, et al. Aneurysmal bone cysts: imaging findings and embolotherapy. AJR 1989;153:369–373.

12. Crowell RM, Wepsic JG. Thoracic cord compression due to chondrosarcoma in two cousins with hereditary multiple exostoses: report of two cases. J Neurosurg 1972;36:86–89.

13. Dahlin DC. Giant-cell tumor of vertebrae above the sacrum: a review of 31 cases. Cancer 1977;39:1350–1356.

14. De Cristofaro R, Biagini R, Boriani S, et al. Selective arterial embolization in the treatment of aneurysmal bone cyst and angioma of bone. Skeletal Radiol 1992;21:523–527.

15. Di Lorenz N, Spallone A, Nolletti A, et al. Giant cell tumors of the spine: a clinical study of six cases, with the emphasis on the radiologic features, treatment, and follow-up. Neurosurgery 1980;6:29–34.

16. Di Lorenzo N, Palatinsky E, Artico M, et al. Dural mesenchymal chondrosarcoma of the lumbar spine: case report. Surg Neurol 1989;31:470–472.

17. Dominguez J, Lobato RD, Ramos A, et al. Giant intrasacral schwannomas: report of six cases. Acta Neurochir (Wien) 1997;139:954–959.

18. Dowdle JA Jr, Winter RB, Dehner LP. Postirradiation: osteosarcoma of the cervical spine in childhood: a case report. J Bone Joint Surg 1977;59:969–971.

19. Dysart SH, Swengel RM, Van Dam BE. Aneurysmal bone cyst of a thoracic vertebra. Treatment by selective arterial embolization and excision. Spine 1992;17:846–848.

20. Ellis TS, Schwartz A, Starr JK, et al. Epithelioid hemangioendothelioma of the lumbar vertebral column: case report and review of literature. Neurosurgery 1996;38:402–407.

21. Epstein N, Benjamin V, Pinto R, et al. Benign osteoblastoma of a thoracic vertebra: case report. J Neurosurg 1980;53:710–713.

22. Evans HL, Ayala AG, Romsdahl MM. Prognostic factors in chondrosarcoma of bone: a clinicopathologic analysis with emphasis on histologic grading. Cancer 1977;40:813–818.

23. Fathie K. Hemangiopericytoma of the thoracic spine: case report. J Neurosurg 1970;32:371–374.

24. Fielding JW, Fietti VG, Hughes JEO, et al. Primary osteogenic sarcoma of the cervical spine. J Bone Joint Surg 1976;58:892–894.

25. Fiumara E, Scarabino T, Guglielmi G, et al. Osteochondroma of the L-5 vertebra: a rare cause of sciatic pain: case report. J Neurosurg 1999;91:219–222.

26. Gaetani P, Tancioni F, Merlo P, et al. Spinal chondroma of the lumbar tract: case report. Surg Neurol 1996;46:534–539.

27. Gelberman RH, Olson CO. Benign osteoblastoma of the atlas: a case report. J Bone Joint Surg 1974;56:808–810.

28. George B, Atallah A, Laurian C, et al. Cervical osteochondroma (C2 level) with vertebral artery occlusion and second cervical nerve root irritation. Surg Neurol 1989;31:459–464.

29. Gladden ML Jr, Gillingham BL, Hennrikus W, et al. Aneurysmal bone cyst of the first cervical vertebrae in a child treated with percutaneous intralesional injection of calcitonin and methylprednisolone. A case report. Spine 2000;25:527–530.

30. Glenn JN, Reckling FW, Mantz FA. Malignant hemangioendothelioma in a lumbar vertebra: a rare tumor in an unusual location. J Bone Joint Surg 1974;56:1279–1282.

31. Griffin JB. Benign osteoblastoma of the thoracic spine: case report with fifteen-year follow-up. J Bone Joint Surg 1978;60:833–835.

32. Gupta VK, Gupta SK, Khosla VK, et al. Aneurysmal bone cysts of the spine. Surg Neurol 1994;42:428–432.

33. Hekster REM, Lambooy N, van Hall EV, et al. Hormone-dependent spinal leiomyoma. Surg Neurol 1994;41:330–333.

34. Janin Y, Epstein JA, Carras R, et al. Osteoid osteomas and osteoblastomas of the spine. Neurosurgery 1981;8:31–8.

35. Koci TM, Mehringer CM, Yamagata N, et al. Aneurysmal bone cyst of the thoracic spine: evolution after particulate embolization. AJNR 1995;16:857–860.

36. Kriss TC, Warf BC. Cervical paraspinous desmoid tumor in a child: case report. Neurosurgery 1994;35:956–959.

37. Lidov MW, Stollman AL, Wolfe D, et al. Fibromatosis involving the epidural space. AJNR 1995;16:885–888.

38. Lozes G, Fawaz A, Perper H, et al. Chondroma of the cervical spine: case report. J Neurosurg 1987;66:128–130.

39. Martinez V, Sissons HA. Aneurysmal bone cyst. A review of 123 cases including primary lesions and those secondary to other bone pathology. Cancer 1988;61:2291–2304.

40. McArthur RA, Fisher RG. Aneurysmal bone cyst involving the vertebral column: a case report. J Neurosurg 1966;24:772–776.

41. Meyers SP, Yaw K, Devaney K. Giant cell tumor of the thoracic spine: MR appearance. AJNR 1994;15:962–964.

42. Mnaymneh W, Brown M, Tejada F, et al. Primary osteogenic sarcoma of the second cervical vertebra: case report. J Bone Joint Surg 1979;61:460–462.

43. Mori Y, Takayasu M, Saito K, et al. Benign osteoblastoma of the odontoid process of the axis: a case report. Surg Neurol 1998;49:274–277.

44. Morris GF, Murphy K, Rorke LB, et al. Spinal hamartomas: a distinct clinical entity. J Neurosurg 1998;88:954–961.

45. Muraszko KM, Antunes JL, Hilal SK, et al. Hemangiopericytomas of the spine. Neurosurgery 1982;10:473–479.

46. O'Connor GA, Roberts TS. Spinal cord compression by an osteochondroma in a patient with multiple osteochondromatosis. Case report. J Neurosurg 1984;60:420–423.

47. Ohry A, Lipschitz M, Shemesh Y, et al. Disappearance of quadriparesis due to a huge cervicothoracic aneurysmal bone cyst. Surg Neurol 1988;29:307–310.

48. Ohyama T, Ohara S, Momma F, et al. Ossifying fibroma of the thoracolumbar spine: a case report and review of the literature. Surg Neurol 1992;37:231–235.

49. Ortolan EG, Sola CA, Gruenberg MF, et al. Giant sacral schwannoma. A case report. Spine 1996;21:522–526.

50. Quirini GE, Meyer JR, Herman M, et al. Osteochondroma of the thoracic spine: an unusual cause of spinal cord compression. AJNR 1996;17:961–964.

51. Ramani PS. Chondromyxoid fibroma: a rare cause of spinal cord compression: case report. J Neurosurg 1974;40:107–109.

52. Rengachary SS, Sanan A. Ivory osteoma of the cervical spine: case report. Neurosurgery 1998;42:182–185.

53. Salvant JB Jr, Young HF. Giant intrasacral schwannoma: an unusual cause of lumbosacral radiculopathy. Surg Neurol 1994;41:411–412.

54. Scheithauer BW, Egbert BM. Ewing's sarcoma of the spinal epidural space: report of two cases. J Neurol Neurosurg Psychiatry 1978;11:1031–1035.

55. Schnee CL, Hurst RW, Curtis MT, et al. Carcinoid tumor of the sacrum: case report. Neurosurgery 1994;35:1163–1167.

56. Shikata J, Yamamuro T, Iida H, et al. Benign osteoblastoma of the cervical vertebra. Surg Neurol 1987;27:381–385.

57. Spaziante R, de Divitiis E, Giamundo A, et al. Ewing's sarcoma arising primarily in the spinal epidural space: fifth case report. Neurosurgery 1983;12:337–341.

58. Steel TR, Pell MF, Turner JJ, et al. Spinal epidural leiomyoma occurring in an HIV-infected man. Case report. J Neurosurg 1993;79:442–445.

59. Teddy PJ, Esiri MM. Malignant fibrous histiocytoma producing spinal cord compression. J Neurol Neurosurg Psychiatry 1979;42:838–842.

60. Turk PS, Peters N, Libbey NP, et al. Diagnosis and management of giant intrasacral schwannoma. Cancer 1992;70:2650–2657.

61. Waga S, Tochia H, Sakakura M. Chondroma of the spine in a newborn infant: case report. Neurosurgery 1979;4:181–182.

62. Wiebe BM, Jensen K, Laursen H. Parachordoma of the sacrococcygeal region—a neuroepithelial tumor. Clin Neuropathol 1995;14:343–346.

63. Wisniewski M, Toker C, Anderson PJ. Chondroblastoma of the cervical spine: case report. J Neurosurg 1973;38:763–766.

64. Yorke JE, Berk RH, Fuller GN, et al. Chondrosarcoma of the spine: 1954 to 1997. J Neurosurg 1999;90:73–78.

# SPINAL MENINGES, SPINAL NERVE ROOTS, AND SPINAL CORD

# 11

As emphasized throughout this text, anatomic considerations greatly facilitate the study of surgical specimens from the nervous system and its coverings. This is particularly true within the close confines of the spinal intradural compartment, where the anatomic position of a lesion guides one's thoughts logically through a differential diagnosis (Figs. 11–1 and 11–2).

## SPINAL MENINGES

## Neoplasms

### Meningioma

**General Comments.** Meningiomas constitute one fourth to one third of all primary intraspinal tumors. Aside from the rare examples that appear to be radiation

527

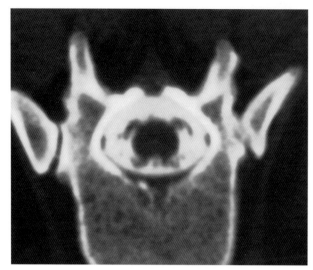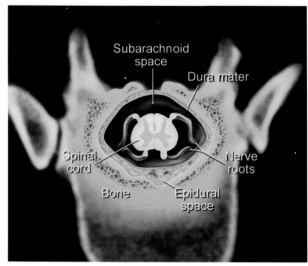

**FIGURE 11–1**   NORMAL ANATOMY OF THE SPINE, MENINGES, NERVE ROOTS, AND SPINAL CORD

A normal CT myelogram illustrates the multiple, often juxtaposed, structures and anatomic compartments in the spine.

induced[16] or those that arise in genetically mispro-grammed individuals with neurofibromatosis type 2 (NF2), the etiology of spinal meningiomas is unknown. Multiplicity is common in NF2 but is also observed in rare families in which a specific genetic defect has not been identified.[3]

**Clinical Features.** Like their intracranial counterparts, meningiomas occur primarily after the fourth decade.[1, 5, 14] Whereas intracranial meningiomas show a consistent 3:2 predilection for females, this ratio is even higher among intraspinal examples. For several series of the latter, a ratio of 4:1 has been reported.[12, 14, 17]

Meningiomas arise primarily in the thoracic region. The cervical region is affected less often, the lumbar area only rarely, and the sacral region almost never.[1, 5, 14] The predilection of the distinctive clear cell variant for the lumbar region is discussed on page 59.

Spinal meningiomas originate from meningothelial cells making up arachnoid villi in the proximity of dorsal root ganglia.[8] This concentration of precursor cells ex-plains the high incidence of meningiomas adjacent to spinal nerve roots, with occasional examples mimicking schwannoma.[13]

Most meningiomas remain within the intradural space, although a few penetrate the dura or exit through a root sleeve to reach the adipose tissue of the epidural compartment.[2] Only rarely does a lesion continue its in-filtration into regional soft tissue and bone.[7] Rare menin-giomas appear to arise primarily in the epidural com-partment[4, 10, 14] or the skin.[19] Only rarely are spinal meningiomas intramedullary.[18]

Given the spatial limitations of the spinal canal, meningiomas generally become symptomatic earlier in their evolution than do their intracranial counterparts. They are also less likely to become entangled in nonre-sectable structures, and rarely do they invade nearby bone. The latter occurrence is largely restricted to

meningiomas that arise primarily in the epidural space.[14] Only uncommonly do meningiomas appear to arise pri-marily in the epidural compartment.[4, 10, 14] These appear to be more common in children.[2, 4, 7, 11, 15]

**Radiologic Features.** A dural base, contrast enhance-ment, and "dural tails" are classical features (Fig. 11–3). Densely calcified lesions are dark in T2-weighted mag-netic resonance (MR) images.

**Macroscopic Features.** Most spinal meningiomas are globoid (Figs. 11–4 and 11–5), but a few exceptions as-sume a carpet-like, en plaque configuration. Reflecting the variable proportions of neoplastic cells, collagen, and psammoma bodies, meningiomas range in consistency from soft to firm to even gravelly. Whereas thoracic meningiomas are usually situated laterally, cervical exam-ples are more likely to be anterior.[14] Most meningiomas remain within the intradural space, although a few pene-trate the dura or exit through root sleeves to reach the adipose tissue of the epidural compartment.[2] Only rarely does a lesion continue its infiltration into regional soft tissue and bone.[2]

**Microscopic Features.** Although they span the same histologic spectrum as the intracranial meningiomas dis-cussed in Chapter 2, highly calcified psammomatous le-sions are overrepresented (Fig. 11–6). An unusual menin-gioma, the clear cell variant, favors the lumbar region—a level rarely visited by other subtypes (Fig. 11–7).[9, 20] The histopathology of meningiomas is discussed in detail on pages 52 to 63. Atypical and malignant meningiomas are rare in the spinal meninges.

**Differential Diagnosis.** If elongated meningothelial cells and collagen are abundant (Fig. 11–8), the differ-ential diagnosis of the spinal meningioma usually focuses on *schwannoma*. Features that exclude the latter include

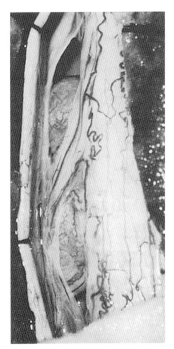

**FIGURE 11–4   MENINGIOMA**

Intraspinal meningiomas are discrete masses usually situated laterally near a nerve root. This thoracic lesion produced numbness and weakness in the legs of a 60-year-old woman. (From Burger PC, Vogel FS. Frozen section interpretation in surgical neuropathology. II. Intraspinal lesions. Am J Surg Pathol 1978;2:81.)

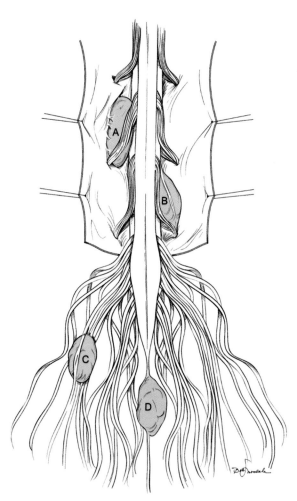

**FIGURE 11–2   TOPOGRAPHIC DISTRIBUTION OF COMMON NEOPLASMS OF THE SPINAL MENINGES, NERVE ROOTS, AND SPINAL CORD**

Dura-based lesions are usually meningiomas or the uncommon solitary fibrous tumors and hemangiopericytomas (A). With the exception of the rare clear cell subtype, meningiomas are rare at this low level. Discrete neoplasms of the nerve roots (B and C) are usually schwannomas, but in the cauda equina (C) they may also be paragangliomas or myxopapillary ependymomas. Hemangioblastomas can arise from nerve roots, especially in von Hippel–Lindau disease. The conus medullaris filum terminale (D) is host to ependymoma, usually myxopapillary, and paraganglioma.

whorls and psammomatous calcifications. With the exception of the rare melanotic psammomatous variant, schwannomas are not calcified. The immunohistochemical distinctions between meningiomas and schwannomas are discussed in Chapter 2 on page 70. In brief, meningiomas are reactive for epithelial membrane antigen and show little positivity for S-100 protein. They lack immunoreactivity for collagen type IV, laminin, Leu 7, and glial fibrillary acidic protein (GFAP). Schwannomas have pericellular reticulin; meningiomas do not.

**FIGURE 11–3   MENINGIOMA**

Meningiomas are discrete extra-axial lesions that displace rather than infiltrate spinal cord parenchyma. In this T1-weighted magnetic resonance image, the tumor shows characteristic dense enhancement after injection of contrast material. (Courtesy of Dr. John T. Curnes, Greensboro, NC.)

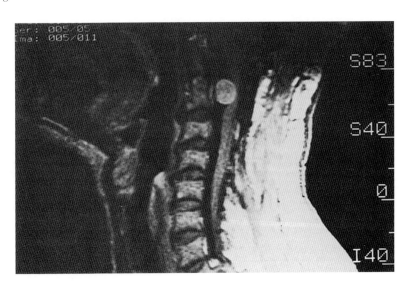

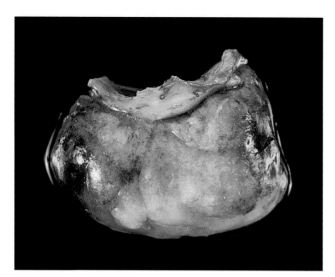

**FIGURE 11–5**  MENINGIOMA

Meningiomas are nodular, discrete, spherical neoplasms with a firm dural attachment.

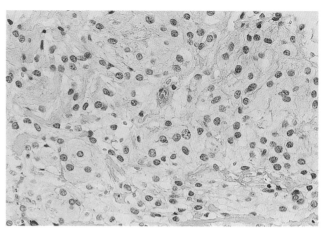

**FIGURE 11–7**  CLEAR CELL MENINGIOMA

Clear cell meningiomas are overrepresented in meninges of the cauda equina region. Classical features of meningiomas, such as whorls and psammoma bodies, are rarely seen in this uncommon variant. Ill-defined whorls are seen here.

A cellular lesion without psammoma bodies raises the issue of *hemangiopericytoma*. This differential is discussed in Chapter 2 on page 69.

An entity newly described in the spinal canal, *solitary fibrous tumor*, deserves consideration because its less cellular portions may exhibit cellular polarity and collagen contents similar to those of fibrous meningioma. Cellular areas may resemble hemangiopericytoma. Solitary fibrous tumors are discussed on pages 71 to 73 and 534.

**Diagnostic Checklist**

- Is this "fibrous meningioma" not really a schwannoma?
- Have solitary fibrous tumor and hemangiopericytoma been excluded?

**Treatment and Prognosis.** Almost all spinal meningiomas are amenable to total excision. Although they may recur when incompletely resected,[6, 12, 14] a surgical specimen of a recurrent spinal meningioma is most unusual.

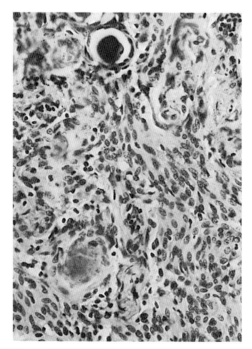

**FIGURE 11–6**  MENINGIOMA

Whorls and psammoma bodies characterize most spinal meningiomas.

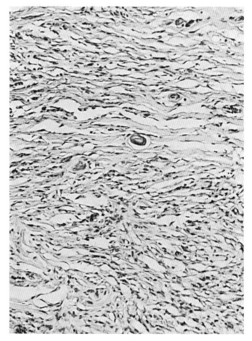

**FIGURE 11–8**  MENINGIOMA

Elongated cells and abundant collagen are features of fibrous meningiomas. The presence of psammoma bodies helps distinguish this lesion from both schwannoma and solitary fibrous tumor.

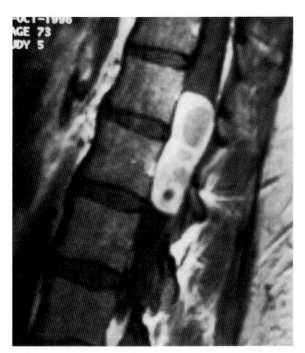

**FIGURE 11–9**   HEMANGIOPERICYTOMA

As illustrated in this T12-L1 mass in a 28-year-old woman, meningeal hemangiopericytomas are discrete, intradural-extramedullary, and contrast enhancing.

## Hemangiopericytoma

Intraspinal hemangiopericytomas are less common than their intracranial counterparts but are otherwise identi-cal in their clinicopathologic features.[1-4] The latter include onset during adulthood, intradural-extramedullary position (Fig. 11–9), macroscopic circumscription, lobularity (Fig. 11–10), a distinctive histologic appearance (Fig. 11–11), local aggressiveness, frequent recurrences, and propensity for late distant metastasis.[2, 4] The differential diagnosis between hemangiopericytoma and meningioma is discussed in Chapter 2 on pages 69 and 81. Solitary fibrous tumor, another differential contender, is discussed on pages 72, 73, and 534.

### Melanocytic Neoplasms

The rare intraspinal neoplasms derived from meningeal melanocytes (Figs. 11–12 and 11–13) range, through difficult-to-grade transitional forms, from low-grade melanocytomas to incontrovertibly malignant melanomas.[1-11] Melanocytic tumors are discussed in greater detail on pages 73 and 85 in Chapter 2. Whereas many melanocytomas are cured by surgery, most melanomas are refractory to irradiation or chemotherapy and recur locally and/or widely seed the neuraxis.[1] The differential diagnosis between melanocytic lesions and melanotic schwannomas is discussed on page 75.

### Tumors of Adipose Tissue

**Definition.** Neoplastic or malformative masses of mature adipose tissue.

**General Comments.** Lipomatous masses of yellow fat are an infrequent cause of spinal cord and nerve root

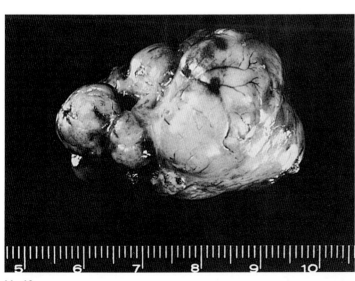

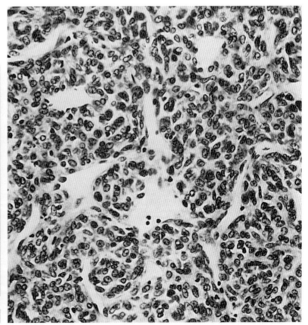

**11–10**                                              **11–11**

**FIGURES 11–10 AND 11–11**   HEMANGIOPERICYTOMA

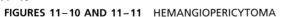

Intradural hemangiopericytomas are discrete, lobulated masses grossly deceptively similar to meningiomas. This cervical lesion occurred in a 43-year-old woman. The discovery of a clavicular metastasis 1 year later underscored the malignant nature of this neoplasm. Figure 11–1 illustrates the basic histologic appearance of the hemangiopericytoma.

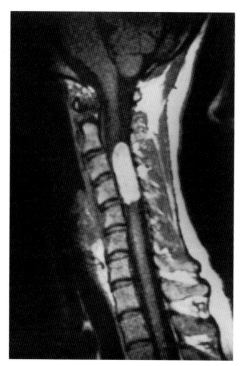

**FIGURE 11–12    RECURRENT MELANOCYTIC NEOPLASM**

Primary meningeal melanocytic tumors usually occur as discrete, contrast-enhancing, intradural-extramedullary masses. This lesion produced signs of spinal cord compression in a 20-year-old woman. A sizable recurrence was detected 20 months after the initial, incomplete, resection. The initial lesion was a melanocytoma. The recurrence was a well-differentiated melanoma.

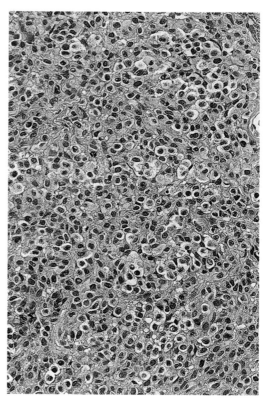

**FIGURE 11–13    MALIGNANT MELANOMA**

Slight cellular atypia, prominent nucleoli, and scattered mitotic figures characterized the recurrent melanoma shown in Figure 11–12.

compression. Some are asymptomatic incidental findings, whereas others are bona fide tumors requiring surgical decompression. Patients of all ages are affected. Although encountered throughout the intradural space, isolated lipomas favor the cervical and upper thoracic regions.[1, 2, 4, 5, 7, 11] In the lower spinal canal, "lipomas" are more often malformative in nature and are generally associated with spina bifida, meningocele, dermal sinus, or

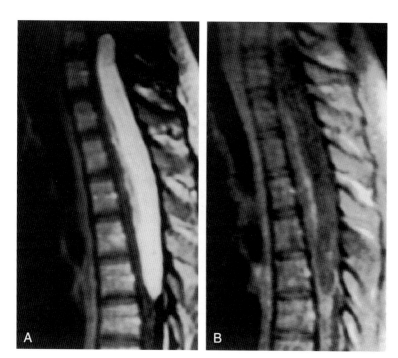

**FIGURE 11–14    LIPOMA**

Preoperatively, intradural lipomas are readily identified by their intrinsic bright signal in precontrast T1-weighted images (A) and their "disappearance" on "fat suppression" sequences (B). The patient, a 19-year-old woman with a C6 mass, complained of neck pain and weakness in the legs.

a subcutaneous adipose tissue mass.[6, 8, 10, 12, 13, 15] The terms lipomeningocele and leptomyelolipoma are often applied to such embryologic misadventures. Yet another form of lipoma is the fatty tissue associated with the tethered cord syndrome, as discussed on pages 544 to 545.

**Radiologic Features.** Fat is readily visualized on computed tomography and MR imaging. The latter, when images with and without fat suppression can be compared, permits the radiologist to identify the lesions with confidence (Fig. 11–14).

**Macroscopic Features.** The bright yellow lesions are often adherent to the spinal cord and may burrow superficially into its substance (Fig. 11–15). This intimacy with neural tissue may extend to the nerve roots that course through the lobulated yellow mass.

**Microscopic Features.** The bulk of a lipomatous lesion is lost into the alcohols and xylenes of the histology laboratory, sparing for microsections only the familiar chicken wire pattern of mature adipose tissue (Figs. 11–16 and 11–17). Skeletal or smooth muscle, neuroglia, and fibrous tissue are casual components in some lumbosacral lipomas with developmental origins.[9, 15] Although they are unresectable because of encasement of nerve roots and intimate attachment to the spinal cord, significant long-term improvement can follow incomplete excision.[1, 5, 12]

The hibernoma is a "sleeper" in the intradural space.[3, 14]

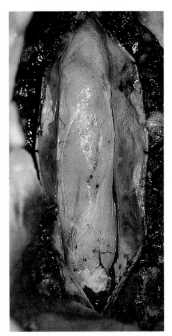

**FIGURE 11–15    LIPOMA**

Intraoperatively, the color of lipomas makes their basic nature unmistakable. (Courtesy of Dr. Wiliam E. Krauss, Rochester, MN.)

## Other Primary Meningeal Tumors

**Mesenchymal Chondrosarcoma.** Rarely does this distinctive tumor make an intraspinal appearance, and then

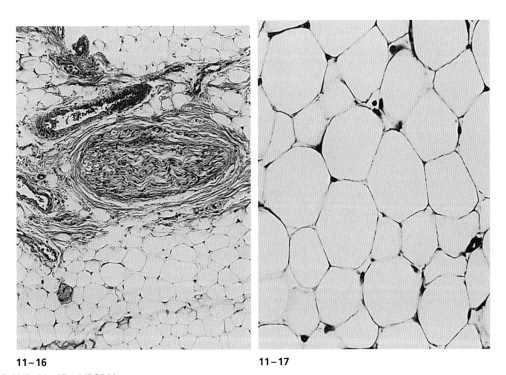

11–16                         11–17

**FIGURES 11–16 AND 11–17    LIPOMA**

Histologic sections emphasize the composition of adult adipose tissue and its intimacy with nerve roots.

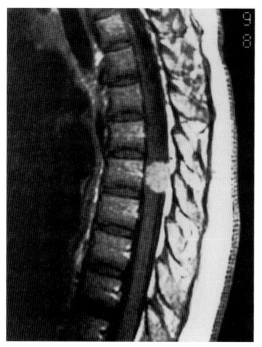

**FIGURE 11–18  MESENCHYMAL CHONDROSARCOMA**

Intraspinal mesenchymal chondrosarcomas usually occur as a dura-based, meningioma-like mass. As is typical, the patient was young, 12 years old, and presented with paraplegia and urinary retention.

it does so typically as a dura-based mass (Figs. 11–18 and 11–19). Although patients of all ages are affected, children and young adults are most often targeted.[8, 11–13] The entity is discussed on pages 84 to 85 of Chapter 2.

**Solitary Fibrous Tumor.** As an offender of the nervous system, solitary fibrous tumor is a recently described entity.[3] Most occur intracranially, but the spinal

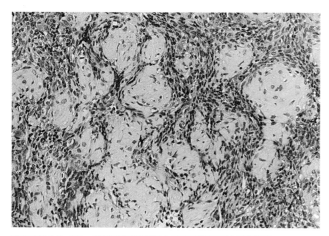

**FIGURE 11–19    MESENCHYMAL CHONDROSARCOMA**

The biphasic, densely cellular, and cartilaginous composition is typical of this neoplasm at any site.

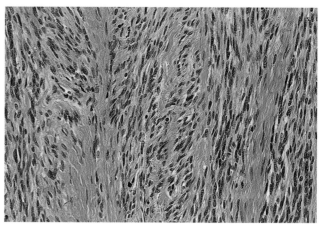

**FIGURE 11–20    SOLITARY FIBROUS TUMOR**

Histologically, solitary fibrous tumors closely resemble fibrous meningioma. The lesion was immunoreactive for CD34 and BCL-2.

region is not off limits. Irrespective of location, solitary fibrous tumors occur as dura-based, meningioma-like masses (Fig. 11–20).[1–3, 9, 14] The pathologic features and the differential diagnosis with fibrous meningioma and emangiopericytoma are discussed on page 72.

**Leiomyosarcoma.** As is discussed in Chapter 2 on page 84, malignant smooth muscle tumors affecting the central nervous system (CNS) can arise in immunocompromised patients. Intraspinal examples have been reported.[4, 7]

**Meningeal Gliomatosis.** Diffuse gliomas in the meninges are, in most instances, seedings from a primary glioma of the brain or spinal cord. In rare instances, no primary is found and the process is assumed to have arisen primarily within the leptomeninges.[5, 6, 10]

### Metastatic Carcinoma and Lymphoma

Gravity and the free flow of the cerebrospinal fluid within the craniospinal subarachnoid space aid and abet the dissemination of carcinomas in the leptomeninges (Figs. 11–21 and 11–22). The provenance of such cells is variable, but most are carcinomas metastatic from lung, stomach, or breast. Although spinal involvement is often overshadowed by intracranial disease, the clinical features of some cases are predominantly or exclusively spinal.[1, 4–8] Focal, discrete extramedullary masses may occur with or without evidence of diffuse leptomeningeal disease.[2] Although the milieu differs, the pathologic aspects of intracranial and intraspinal metastases are interchangeable. The greater number of intraspinal nerve roots puts them at high risk of involvement. These may become heavily infiltrated by malignant cells (Figs. 11–23 and 11–24). Unusually diffuse and multicentric lymphomatous involvement of brain and peripheral nerves is termed neurolymphomatosis.[3]

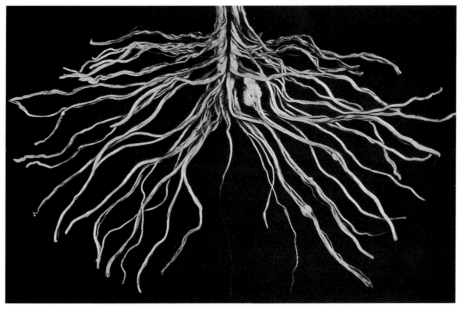

11–21

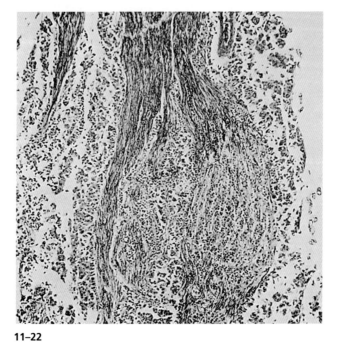

11–22

**FIGURES 11–21 AND 11–22**   METASTATIC CARCINOMA

Multiple implants of lung carcinoma metastatic to the cauda equina of a 58-year-old man resemble the nitrogen-fixing nodules on the roots of a legume (Fig. 11–21). The implant situated in the 5 o'clock position is illustrated in the histologic section in Figure 11–22, where the poorly differentiated epithelial cells have permeated fascicles to splay and destroy nerve fibers.

### Seeding of Primary Intracranial Neoplasms

Any primary brain tumor that reaches the ventricular system or the subarachnoid space is free to disseminate throughout the cerebrospinal fluid pathways. Medulloblastoma and supratentorial small cell embryonal tumors (primitive neuroectodermal tumors or PNETs), germ cell tumors, and high-grade gliomas are most likely to exploit this opportunity.[1, 3, 6, 7] Uncommonly, histologically benign lesions such as pilocytic astrocytoma may do likewise.[2, 4, 5] Secondary lesions of the spinal meninges usually occur in

the setting of a known primary. Hence, they are often diagnosed by radiologic and/or cytologic means. Only a small proportion come to surgical attention.

## Cystic Lesions

An understanding of the origin and character of cystic lesions within the spinal canal is facilitated by an approach based on anatomic localization. The epidural

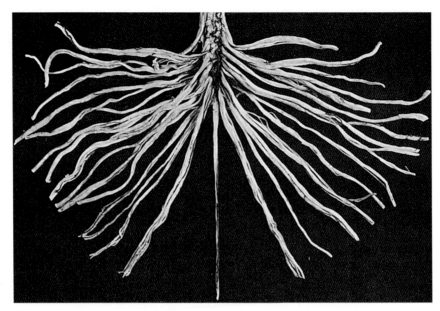

11–23

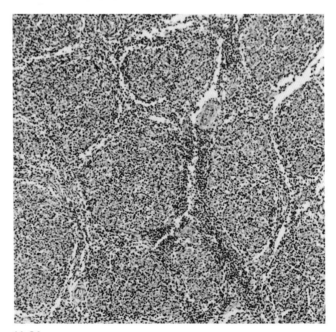

11–24

**FIGURES 11–23 AND 11–24    LEUKEMIA**

In contrast to the usually nodular carcinomatous metastases in the cauda equina, there is diffuse enlargement of all roots in this 32-year-old man with acute myelomonocytic leukemia. Malignant cells had been identified during cytologic examination of cerebrospinal fluid. The root enlargement is made more apparent by comparison with uninvolved roots of Figure 11–21 and is readily appreciated in the histologic section of Figure 11–24.

compartment has its epidural meningeal cyst, and the intradural chamber houses arachnoidal, ependymal, epidermoid, dermoid, and enterogenous cysts. The perineurial sleeve spawns Tarlov cysts that encompass the dorsal root and its ganglion (Fig. 11–25).

### Epidural Meningeal Cyst

More a diverticulum than a cyst, this lesion usually retains some communication with the subarachnoid space through a slender pedicle from the dura.[5, 10, 15, 40, 47] Although individual lesions lack this connection, it is assumed that a communication once existed, an inference supported by the report of one noncommunicating cyst that contained myelographic contrast material introduced 23 years earlier.[24] Such cysts are most often situated in the posterior midline (Figs. 11–26 and 11–27). Histologically, they are bilayered and consist of a thick dura-like layer of collagen as well as an inner, less constant membrane of arachnoid (Fig. 11–28).

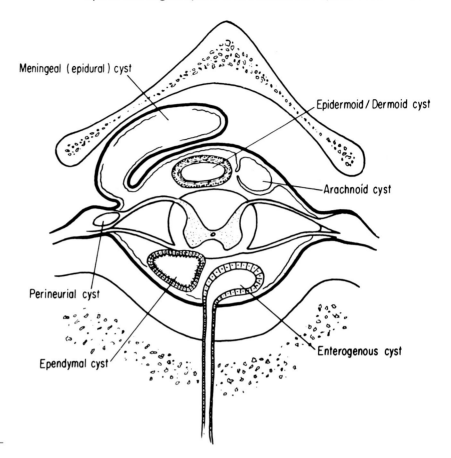

**FIGURE 11–25**  CYSTIC LESIONS OF THE MENINGEAL SPACES AND NERVE ROOTS

## Arachnoid Cyst

The spinal arachnoid cyst is more a diverticulum than a cyst.[1, 9, 13, 19, 45] Multiple lesions are common. As with intracranial arachnoid cysts, their origin is obscure and has been variably attributed to trauma, hemorrhage, inflammation, or genetic influences. Histologically, they are formed of delicate connective tissue with a covering of meningothelial cells.

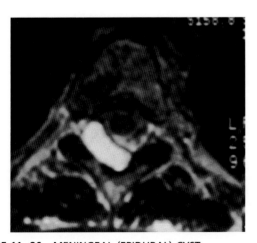

**FIGURE 11–26**  MENINGEAL (EPIDURAL) CYST

As in this 61-year-old woman with low back pain, epidural cysts are typically bright on T2-weighted MR images and displace the spinal cord anteriorly.

## Ependymal Cyst

In the intradural space, true cysts composed of simple cuboidal to columnar ciliated epithelium have been designated ependymal cysts.[14, 20] It remains to be seen whether these are truly ependymal rather than neurenteric.

## Epidermoid and Dermoid Cysts

Most of these lesions are presumed to arise from embryologically displaced tissues. This hypothesis is supported by their frequent association with spina bifida and an occasional connection with skin via a dermal sinus.[3, 28, 43] There is circumstantial evidence that yet other "epidermoids" arise from cutaneous cells that have been displaced into the intradural space by a lumbar puncture needle.[7, 27] Both epidermoid[7, 22, 27] and dermoid[2, 8] cysts are most frequent in the lumbosacral region. The majority are extramedullary, but an occasional example lies partly embedded within the spinal cord.[22] A rare example is entirely intramedullary.[42] Although discrete, the cysts may be adherent to the cord or be inextricably bound to spinal nerve roots. Both the thin-walled epidermoid cyst and the better encapsulated dermoid lesion project a glistening white or cream-colored appearance that reflects their contents of either flaky keratin or greasy sebaceous material (Fig. 11–29). Keratinizing squamous epithelium lines both lesions, but the wall of dermoid cysts contains sebaceous glands and hair

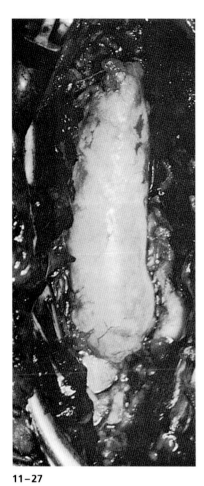

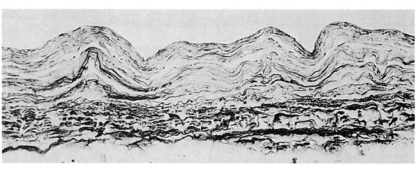

11-28

11-27

**FIGURES 11-27 AND 11-28   MENINGEAL (EPIDURAL) CYST**

Weakness and paresthesias in the legs of a 46-year-old man drew attention to this typically smooth, cylindrical meningeal cyst positioned in the epidural space overlying the thoracic cord (Fig. 11-27). Characteristically, the thick-walled lesion resembles dura and is attached at the exit of a nerve root (T9). A histologic section demonstrates its composition of fibrous connective tissue resembling dura (Fig. 11-28). (Courtesy of Dr. Guy L. Odom, Durham, NC.)

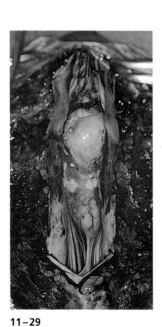

11-29                  11-30

**FIGURES 11-29 AND 11-30   DERMOID CYST**

Characteristically, the dermoid is a "pearly" cyst. Here it is entangled in the cauda equina of an 8-year-old girl presenting with urinary retention and saddle hypoesthesia (Fig. 11-29). Well-differentiated squamous epithelium lines the cyst and is accompanied by hair follicles and sebaceous glands lying within its fibrous wall (Fig. 11-30). (Courtesy of Dr. Guy L. Odom, Durham, NC.)

follicles (Fig. 11–30). Cyst contents can contaminate and irritate the subarachnoid space if a capsular rent liberates the contents.[44]

### Neurenteric and Bronchogenic Cysts

Uncommon intradural cysts presumably arise from displaced remnants of the developing gastrointestinal tract and from the respiratory system. They are termed neurenteric[6, 11, 12, 21, 25, 31, 32, 39] and bronchogenic cysts, respectively.[50] Descriptions of "teratomatous" cysts occasionally appear in the literature, but the distinction from cysts of endodermal origin is unclear because simple columnar epithelium is common to both.[18, 38, 41] Endodermal lesions, particularly neurenteric cysts, occur along the entire spinal axis, usually ventral to the spinal cord. Dorsally situated examples are exceptional.[26]

It is perhaps not surprising, given their malformative nature, that endodermal cysts may be associated with enterogenous cysts of the mediastinum or with duplications of the gastrointestinal tract. Not only are malformations of the vertebral bodies common, but the cysts may communicate with the abdomen or thorax through a defect in the vertebral column. As a consequence of the caudad movement of the vertebrae relative to that of the spinal cord during embryologic development, bone defects may be several segments lower than the cyst. A midline defect in the skin of the back is a rare signal lesion.[32]

Macroscopically, the lesion is an opalescent, smooth-surfaced mass (Fig. 11–31).

Microscopically, the most elementary lesion has a well-differentiated columnar epithelium with or without cilia and mucus globules (Fig. 11–32). This rests upon a periodic acid–Schiff (PAS)–positive basement membrane. Rare, more intriguing lesions have a well-formed gastric mucosa,[23] transitional epithelium,[30] intestine-like muscularis, serous and mucous glands, and cartilage-containing facsimiles of bronchi.[21, 50] These cysts react

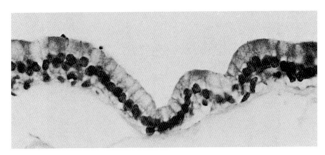

**FIGURE 11–32**    ENTEROGENOUS CYST

Weakness and numbness of the right arm prompted myelography in a 52-year-old woman. An intradural extramedullary lesion at the C2-3 level was approached surgically and excised as a translucent cyst. The uniform layer of mucus-secreting columnar cells is characteristic of enterogenous cyst. Although it did not communicate with gastrointestinal structures, there were bony abnormalities of the spine anterior to the cyst.

with antibodies to cytokeratins, epithelial membrane antigen, and carcinoembryonic antigen.[49] Electron microscopy reveals the expected features of well-differentiated columnar epithelium seated on a uniform basal lamina. Apical junctional complexes bind adjacent cells.[16, 17, 29, 33, 34, 37]

### Perineurial (Tarlov) Cysts

Perineurial or Tarlov cysts occur in the sacral region and are usually bilateral. Presumably, they evolve through degenerative changes that create a cleavage between the epineurium and perineurium of exiting nerve roots or dorsal root ganglion.[4, 35, 36, 46, 48] Although the differential diagnosis includes synovial cyst, the distinction is generally self-evident, as judged from the anatomic site of the lesion. Although symptomatic relief may be sought through surgical decompression or cyst drainage, only rarely does this lesion become a surgical specimen. Collagenous tissue and nerve fascicles are seen.

## Inflammatory Lesions

Many of the inflammatory lesions discussed in Chapter 3 may be encountered in the spinal meninges as well. They are often identified by analysis of cerebrospinal fluid rather than by the tissue specimens discussed in this book.

### Sarcoidosis

Sarcoidosis is an exception because it occurs as a mass or as a diffuse contrast-enhancing leptomeningeal process (Fig. 11–33).[2–5, 8, 9] The principal histopathologic features, granulomas, are familiar to pathologists (Fig. 11–34).

### Hypertrophic Pachymeningitis

The term hypertrophic pachymeningitis is descriptive of fibrous thickening of the dura associated with a chronic inflammatory infiltrate. The disorder may represent a

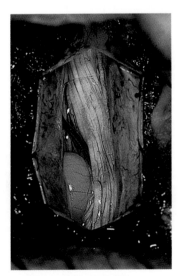

**FIGURE 11–31**    ENTEROGENOUS CYST

The smooth-surfaced mucus-filled cyst compresses the spinal cord. (Courtesy of Dr. William E. Krauss, Rochester, MN.)

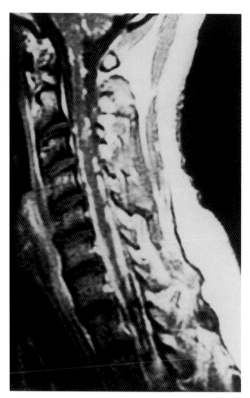

**FIGURE 11–33**    SARCOIDOSIS

Extensive meningeal contrast enhancement is typical of meningeal sarcoidosis.

single entity or a pathologic process with many causations. When nerve roots are involved, the lesion is painful; impingement upon the spinal cord may produce sensorimotor deficits. The cervical region is most often affected.[1, 6, 7]

## Arachnoid Plaques

Dorsally situated, wafer-like arachnoid plaques are common incidental postmortem findings within the arach-

noid membrane of the thoracolumbar spinal cord. At surgery the white, scalloped, brittle lesions are little more than a nuisance because they obscure the surgeon's view of the real medullary lesion at hand. Only a rare example is symptomatic.[1-3] Histologically, the hyaline lesions are sufficiently lamellated to resemble bone, but they are rarely calcified.

## SPINAL NERVE ROOTS

## Primary Neoplasms

### Schwannoma and Melanocytic Schwannoma

**Definition.** Neoplasms derived from the nerve sheath.

**General Comments.** The abrupt transition from the central to the peripheral nervous system occurs in the spinal roots within 1 or 2 mm of the pial surface. Distal to this point, Schwann's cells replace oligodendrocytes as the myelinating element. The family of neoplasms attributed to Schwann's cells includes the siblings schwannoma and neurofibroma, although the histogenesis of the latter is unclear as discussed in Chapter 12. By far the most common member of the duo is the schwannoma in its solitary sporadic form (Fig. 11–35). The same, but multifocal, neoplasm arises in the setting of

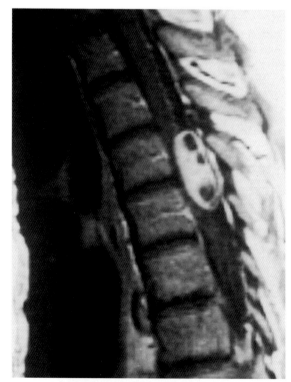

**FIGURE 11–35**    SCHWANNOMA

Schwannomas are discrete, intradural-extramedullary, contrast-enhancing masses. This example occurred in a 52-year-old man with a 2-year history of subcostal pain and progressive leg weakness. Note the presence of intratumoral cysts, a common feature of sizable schwannomas at any site.

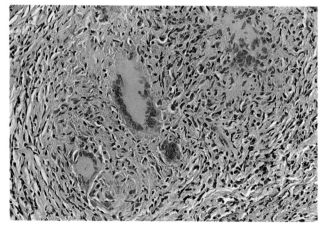

**FIGURE 11–34**    SARCOIDOSIS

A biopsy of the lesions shown in Figure 11–33 showed discrete, noncaseating granulomas typical of sarcoidosis.

NF2,[10] and multiple schwannomas occasionally appear independent of a dysgenetic syndrome.[6, 13] As a rule, nerve root neurofibromas have a genetic basis in NF1.

**Clinical Features.** Schwannomas may originate from nerve roots at all spinal levels, from the cervicomedullary junction to the cauda equina.[21] The incidence curve peaks during the fifth and sixth decades. Like their intracranial counterparts, the tumors favor sensory nerves, dorsal roots predominantly.

Symptoms commonly attributed to schwannomas include radiating pain in the distribution of an affected root and weakness caused by spinal cord compression.[21] Many of the multiple nerve root schwannomas in patients with NF2 are asymptomatic for long periods.[8]

**Radiologic Features.** Although most spinal schwannomas are entirely intradural, some pass through the intervertebral foramen to form a dumbbell- or hourglass-shaped mass. Only a small number penetrate the dura and directly enter the extradural space. The expansive nature of many schwannomas is manifest radiographically as widening of an intervertebral foramen, a feature analogous to the common expansion of the internal auditory meatus produced by vestibular schwannomas. Osseous destruction, usually compressive rather than invasive in nature, is common with the large tumors that affect the sacrum.

Schwannomas are predictably contrast enhancing; cysts are a common feature of large lesions (Fig. 11–35).[22] Although schwannomas can burrow into the cord, rarely are they entirely intramedullary, as discussed on page 571.

Highly melanotic schwannomas have characteristic imaging features, that is, brightness in precontrast T1-weighted images and darkness in T2-weighted images.

**Macroscopic Features.** Schwannomas of spinal nerve roots are soft, glistening, discrete, lobulated, and sometimes cystic (Fig. 11–36). Smaller lesions are often only

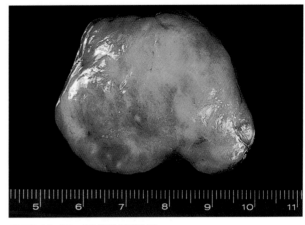

**FIGURE 11–37   SCHWANNOMA**

Extensive xanthomatous change lends yellowness to some schwannomas.

appended to the nerve of origin, whereas large neoplasms stretch and splay the root beyond recognition across the surface of the mass. Internally, some schwannomas are yellow (Fig. 11–37), as are two other intraspinal tumors, hemangioblastoma and lipoma. Melanotic schwannomas are variably pigmented (Fig. 11–38).

**Microscopic Features.** Spinal schwannomas do not differ histologically from those that arise elsewhere (Fig. 11–39) except that Verocay bodies are perhaps more common in spinal lesions than in their vestibular counterpart.

The *cellular schwannoma* is a variant that may cause diagnostic confusion because it is often monomorphic and often contains scattered mitoses (Fig. 11–40).[5, 7, 19] In concept, the diagnosis rests on finding several features of typical schwannoma including a thick collagenous capsule, hyaline vessels, Verocay bodies, cytologic uniformity, and lack of cytologic malignancy despite occasional degenerative atypia. In practice, this may be difficult in a small, nonrepresentative specimen. Cellular schwannomas are discussed in detail in Chapter 12 on pages 599 to 601.

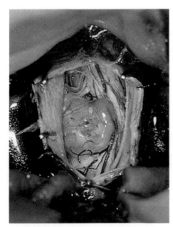

**FIGURE 11–36   SCHWANNOMA**

The root of origin is splayed across the discrete, intradural-extramedullary mass. (Courtesy of Dr. William E. Krauss, Rochester, MN.)

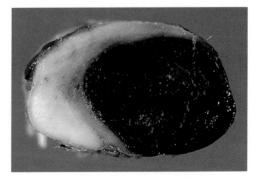

**FIGURE 11–38   MELANOTIC SCHWANNOMA**

Rare schwannomas are intensely melanotic. (Courtesy of Dr. Arnulf H. Koeppen, Albany, NY.)

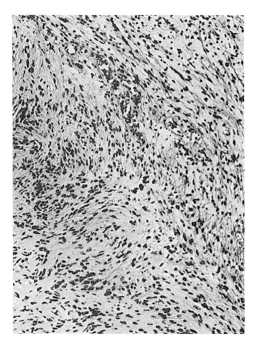

**FIGURE 11–39** SCHWANNOMA

Spinal schwannomas share the histologic features of schwannomas occurring at other sites. In this lesion, compacted spindle cells (*left*) abut areas of lower cellularity and looser texture, the Antoni A and B tissues, respectively.

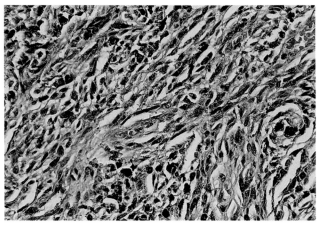

**FIGURE 11–41** MELANOTIC SCHWANNOMA

Fascicular architecture is a common feature in melanocytic lesions.

On rare occasion, the surgeon uncovers a sinister black tumor that macroscopically and microscopically mimics a melanoma (Fig. 11–38). Termed melanotic schwannomas, such tumors are usually discrete and extramedullary like conventional schwannomas,[2, 9, 11, 12, 14] but a few appear to arise directly within the substance of the cord.[15] Most are composed of spindle cells, but epithelioid forms are occasionally seen. Melanin is present in variable quantities within tumor cells, scattered free in the stroma, or aggregated in melanophages (Fig. 11–41).

Pericellular reticulin staining is prominent as it is in all schwannomas. Melanotic schwannomas are S-100 and HMB-45 positive but, unlike melanoma, show pericellular type IV collagen or laminin staining (Fig. 11–42).

Ultrastructurally, the cells are surrounded by basal lamina, burdened with melanosomes, and driven to varying degrees of maturation.[12, 14, 16] An uncommon variant, the psammomatous melanotic schwannoma, features not only melanin but also psammoma bodies and is part of a recognized complex discussed in Chapter 12 on pages 601 to 602.[4]

**Differential Diagnosis.** Above the level of the cauda equina, the differential diagnosis of an extramedullary schwannoma embraces *meningioma*, a tumor often situated laterally adjacent to the nerve root exit zone. As a rule, meningiomas can be distinguished readily by their firm attachment to dura, hemispheric shape, and often gritty texture. Histologically, the diagnostic whorls and

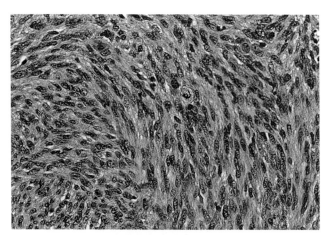

**FIGURE 11–40** CELLULAR SCHWANNOMA

High cellularity and scattered mitoses should not be taken as evidence of a malignancy in schwannomas. Compact, somewhat fascicular architecture (Antoni A tissue) markedly predominates or is the exclusive pattern in cellular schwannomas.

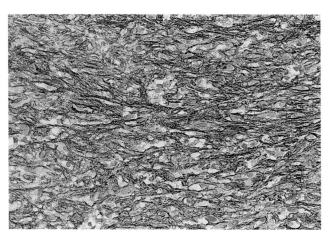

**FIGURE 11–42** SCHWANNOMA

Pericellular immunoreactivity for collagen type IV is characteristic of schwannomas.

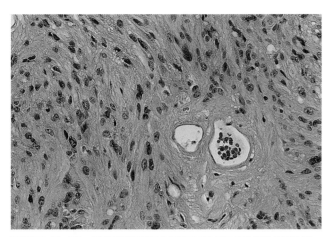

**FIGURE 11–43**    EPENDYMOMA RESEMBLING SCHWANNOMA

Some ependymomas resemble schwannoma, as here where the tumor has a fascicular architecture, low cellularity, and only inconspicuous perivascular pseudorosettes.

psammoma bodies are often prominent. Contrastingly, schwannomas are uniformly S-100 protein immunoreactive, whereas only a minority of meningiomas, particularly fibrous tumors, are positive and then usually only minimally.[24]

At the level of the cauda equina, the differential diagnosis expands to include *paraganglioma* and *ependymoma*. Between these two additions, only the ependymoma, usually one of the tanycytic variety, may sufficiently resemble a schwannoma to generate concern (Fig. 11–43). Immunoreactivity for GFAP (Fig. 11–44) and lack of reticulin staining readily identify the ependymoma.

*Solitary fibrous tumor*, an unusual dura-based lesion, may also resemble a schwannoma (see Fig. 11–20).[3] Only lately described in the CNS, it is discussed on pages 71 to 73 and 534.

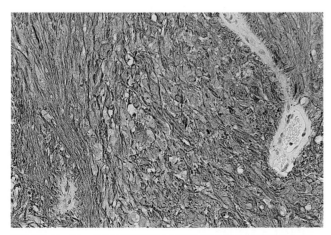

**FIGURE 11–44**    EPENDYMOMA RESEMBLING SCHWANNOMA

Positivity of cellular processes for GFAP helps establish the diagnosis of ependymoma, but caution is in order because fully half of schwannomas are also reactive for this antigen. Reticulin or collagen IV stains can be used to show widespread intercellular staining in schwannomas (see Fig. 11–42.)

The presence of scattered mitoses in a cellular schwannoma raises concern about the possibility of a *malignant peripheral nerve sheath tumor (MPNST)*. Admittedly, the latter is rare in the intradural compartment.[20] Unlike MPNST, cellular schwannomas are uniformly reactive for S-100 protein, type IV collagen, and laminin stains for basement membranes.

Distinguishing melanocytic schwannomas from *melanocytoma*, a well-differentiated melanocytic lesion, rests largely on the lesion's appearance in the standard histologic sections. Whereas the melanocytic schwannoma exhibits at least some unmistakable features of conventional schwannoma, most melanocytomas are composed of plump, polygonal cells organized in nests. Chromatin is open, and nucleoli are often prominent. A uniform pericellular pattern of reticulin staining favors the diagnosis of schwannoma. This differential diagnosis is also discussed on pages 75, 601 to 602.

### Diagnostic Checklist

- Is this "schwannoma" not really a tanycytic ependymoma?
- Is this seemingly malignant neoplasm not really just a cellular schwannoma?
- Has solitary fibrous tumor been excluded?

**Treatment and Prognosis.** Almost all intraspinal schwannomas lend themselves to total excision. Incompletely removed examples can regrow,[10] but many do not regain sufficient size to become symptomatic.[21] Cellular schwannomas have never been reported to metastasize.[20] The prognosis for patients with a cellular schwannoma is also favorable, but experience indicates a significantly higher frequency of recurrence for this schwannoma variant.[5] In one series of cellular schannomas, there were 8 recurrences among 29 cases.[5] As previously noted, giant sacral schwannomas, conventional or cellular, may destroy bone.[1]

Although local recurrence and even metastasis have been noted after incomplete resection of melanotic schwannomas, benign-appearing examples generally behave in a manner similar to conventional, nonpigmented schwannomas. Some melanotic schwannomas that exhibit malignant behavior show prominent nucleoli, mitoses, necrosis, and invasive growth.

### *Neurofibroma*

Involvement of spinal nerve roots by neurofibroma is decidedly uncommon outside the setting of NF1[10, 17] Although often multiple (Figs. 11–45 and 11–46), such syndrome-associated tumors may be asymptomatic. The cervical region is usually affected.[20] Macroscopically, the tumor produces diffuse expansion of intradural and extradural portions of the root, with the tumor's mucinous matrix contributing softness, translucency, and a glistening appearance (Fig. 11–47; see Fig. 11–46). Neoplastic cells permeate the nerve root and separate axis cylinders (Figs. 11–48 and 11–49). Unlike schwannomas, plexiform neurofibromas are gelatinous and solid. Because they are also intrinsic to the nerve of origin, they are more likely to extend into both intradural and extradural

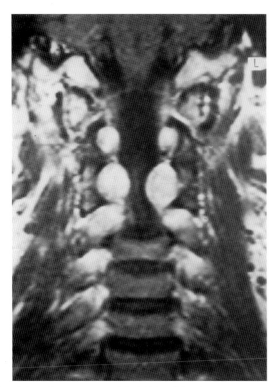

**FIGURE 11–45**   MULTIPLE NEUROFIBROMAS IN NEUROFIBROMATOSIS 1

Multiple contrast-enhancing neurofibromas overrun nerve roots in this 18-year-old patient with neurofibromatosis 1. Multiple decompressions had been required to retard progressive quadriparesis.

compartments. Although the lesions are usually histologically benign, their location and multiplicity create a complex medical problem that cannot be solved surgically.[18] Overall, life expectancy of such patients with nerve root neurofibromas is shortened.[20] Chapter 12 (pages 606 and 636) discusses the microscopic features of neurofibromas and the lesion's potential for malignant degeneration. The latter has appeared in the cauda equina.[23]

### Other Primary Neoplasms of Spinal Nerve Roots

Paragangliomas and ependymomas arising in nerve roots (see Fig. 11–2) are discussed on pages 567 and 561 respectively. Hemangioblastomas, especially in the setting of von Hippel–Lindau disease, may also arise in a nerve root, as discussed on page 565. A spinal nerve root is a most unusual venue for an adrenal adenoma.[1]

## Secondary Neoplasms (Carcinoma, Leukemia, and Lymphoma)

As they traverse the subarachnoid space, spinal nerve roots are bathed in cerebrospinal fluid and are thus exposed to vagrant tumor cells seeking a point of attachment. The leptomeningeal dissemination of epithelial

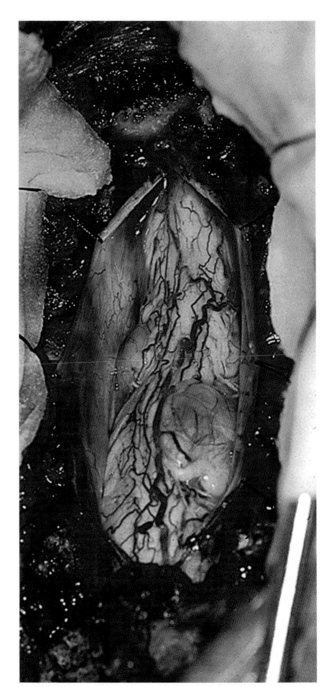

**FIGURE 11–46**   MULTIPLE NEUROFIBROMAS IN NEUROFIBROMATOSIS 1

The relationship of the lesions to nerve roots is apparent at the time of surgery. (Courtesy of Dr. William E. Krauss, Rochester, MN.)

and hematopoietic neoplasms is discussed on pages 534 to 535.

## SPINAL CORD

### Congenital Malformations

Congenital malformations of the spinal cord can be categorized as the glaring externally evident dysraphisms and

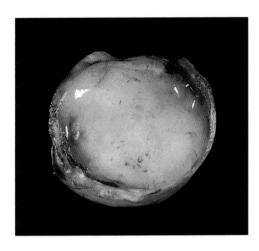

**FIGURE 11–47    NEUROFIBROMA**

A 64-year-old woman with multiple cutaneous neurofibromas and an intrathoracic neurofibroma developed progressive paraparesis. Attached to the left C1 nerve root was this typically solid, fusiform, and glistening plexiform neurofibroma.

the internal changes, if any, that accompany spina bifida occulta. Among the former are meningomyelocele and diastematomyelia, as discussed in Chapter 10 on pages 499 to 500. Aberrations associated with spina bifida occulta include lipomatous lesions such as lipomeningocele and tethered cord.

Generically, the term *tethered cord* denotes any abnormal anchoring of the spinal cord in the lumbosacral region. It is usually seen in children but occasionally occurs in adults.[3, 6] Tethering can be a sequela of surgical repair of dysraphic states.[5] An association with müllerian neoplasms has been reported.[8, 11] In a more restricted sense, tethered cord denotes congenital low placement of the conus medullaris without other malformative lesions[2, 4, 9, 10, 12, 13] (Fig. 11–50). Relief from resulting neurologic and urologic symptoms is sought by transection of the taut filum with the intent of releasing tension on the caudally drawn conus. The conus is not, however, invariably low lying.[14, 15] Surgical specimens, if any, consist solely of a segment of filum terminale, identifiable by its central core of ependymocytes, surrounded by fibroadipose tissue (Fig. 11–51). Skeletal muscle is seen in some cases.[1] Adipose tissue is occasionally encountered in the fila of normal patients and is not, of itself, abnormal.[7]

## Inflammatory Disorders

### Demyelinating Disease and Transverse Myelopathy (Myelitis)

The misinterpretation of a *demyelinating disease* for a neoplasm is an error with potentially serious consequences. The chance of this diagnostic misadventure can be minimized by always entertaining the possibility of this common disorder when examining spinal cord le-

sions, especially those from youthful adults (Fig. 11–52). Vigilance is required because such specimens are often minute, the zone of demarcation between the lesion and the normal parenchyma is often unsampled, and the clinical possibility of a demyelinating disease is frequently not transmitted to the pathologist. Thus, routinely, all cord lesions should be carefully evaluated for the principal hallmark of demyelinating disease, namely the presence of macrophages.[18] Immunohistochemical markers, such as HAM-56 and KP-1, should be used liberally. The pitfalls in the diagnosis of demyelinating diseases are discussed in Chapter 3 on pages 113 to 119.

*Transverse myelopathy* or *myelitis* is a vaguely defined entity that, like demyelinating disease, compromises the cord's conductivity of impulses. Sudden loss of motor and sensory functions and sphincter dysfunctions are typical presenting symptoms. Unlike demyelinating disease, transverse myelitis is more likely to affect the entire cross section of the cord and to extend over multiple segments. It is also more likely to produce a tumefaction.[4, 7, 17] Although the etiology is usually unresolved, some cases are postinfectious,[7, 12] others are associated with systemic lupus erythematosus,[7, 8, 10, 11, 14] and still others are seemingly ischemic in origin because symptoms may be related to the distribution of the anterior spinal artery.[7] No explanation is forthcoming in other cases.[3] Some cases are, in light of subsequent events, the initial manifestation of multiple sclerosis.[15]

Transverse myelopathy is a disorder without pathognomonic abnormalities. Some cases arise in the setting of lupus erythematosus.[5] Macrophages and sometimes a chronic inflammatory infiltrate are typical features. The similarity to demyelinating disease is therefore obvious, and a distinction between the two conditions cannot always be drawn. Devic's disease, a demyelinating process, is intermediate between the two. In association with similar lesions in the optic pathways, the latter disorder produces a myelopathy more destructive and extensive than that of the classical demyelinating diseases.[1, 16] Although the principal role of the pathologist is to avoid labeling tissue from transverse myelopathy as a neoplasm, clinicians are often left in a quandary as to the appropriate treatment of a process responsible for what may be a devastating neurologic deficit.

A noninflammatory myelopathy as a late effect of radiation is occasionally encountered in surgical and autopsy specimens.[2, 6, 9, 13]

### Other Inflammatory Disorders

Inflammatory lesions of spinal cord parenchyma are submitted uncommonly as surgical specimens. The references provide citations regarding pyogenic abscess,[2, 5, 12, 20, 30, 33, 34, 37] tuberculosis (Figs. 11–53 and 1–54),[1, 10, 15, 19, 22, 31] brucellosis,[3] coccidioidomycosis,[30] cryptococcosis,[6, 21, 29] cysticercosis,[7, 9, 17, 25, 28, 40] ecchinococcosis,[21] schistosomiasis,[4, 23, 35, 36, 39] granulomatous angiitis,[13, 42] toxoplasmosis,[32] Langerhans cell histiocytosis,[16] Rosai-Dorfman disease,[27] and paraneoplastic

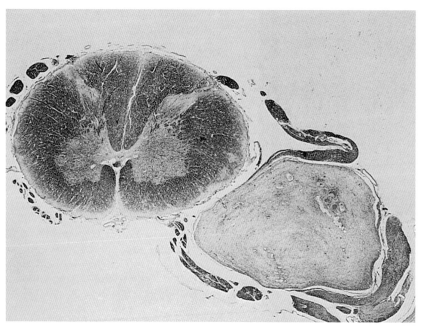

**11–48**

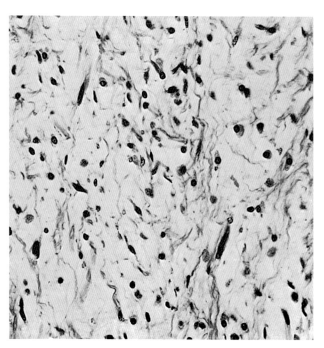

**11–49**

**FIGURES 11–48 AND 11–49**   NEUROFIBROMA

This neurofibroma (Fig. 11–48) occurred in the setting of neurofibromatosis type 1 in the patient pictured in Figure 12–79. The wavy spindle cells, which lie loosely and haphazardly distributed in a pale matrix, serve to distinguish this lesion from schwannoma (Fig. 11–49). Neurofibromas of spinal nerve roots are far less common than schwannomas.

disease.[14] Like tuberculosis, sarcoidosis may affect the meninges, spinal cord, or both.[8, 11, 18, 24, 26, 38, 41]

## Vascular Malformations

The literature surrounding the classification of spinal vascular malformations is as ensnarling as the lesions

themselves. Practicality dictates the consideration of two principal categories.

### Cavernous Angioma

One entity, composed of thick-walled, hyaline vessels, has been variously labeled cavernous angioma,[3, 4, 6–8, 11, 12, 15, 18] more simply as a vascular malformation,[10] or even more

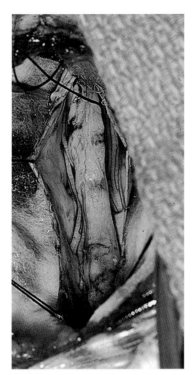

**FIGURE 11–50   TETHERED CORD**

This conus medullaris is inferiorly displaced and the filum terminale is thickened with fibroadipose tissue. The latter is markedly larger than adjacent nerve roots. (Courtesy of Dr. W. Jerry Oakes, Durham, NC.)

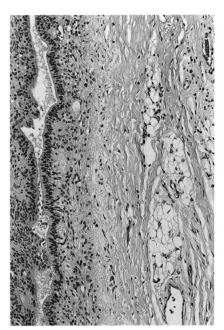

**FIGURE 11–51   TETHERED CORD**

Adipose tissue thickens the filum terminale in patients with tethered cord syndrome. Note remnants of the normal central canal in the center of the filum (at left center).

noncommittally as a vascular lesion.[14] It is possible that these are not all the same entity, but they do share certain clinicopathologic features; among them are (1) the development of insidious neurologic symptoms, (2) an angiographically occult mass that can simulate a glioma, and (3) a re-

luctance to sudden hemorrhage. MR scans hint at its vascular nature by disclosing a hemosiderin-rich rim in some cases (Fig. 11–55). Macroscopically, it shares the discreteness and composition of closely packed vessels of cavernous malformations at any site (Fig. 11–56).

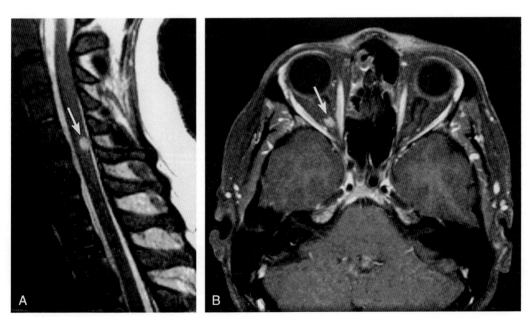

**FIGURE 11–52   DEMYELINATING DISEASE (DEVIC'S DISEASE)**

Coincident lesions in the spinal cord (A) and visual pathways (B) characterize this variant of demyelinating disease. (Courtesy of Dr. Martin G. Pomper, Baltimore, MD.)

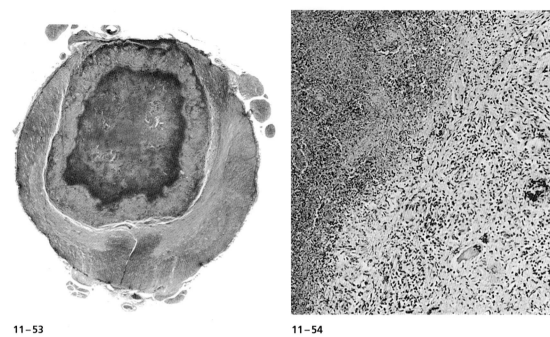

11–53                                                    11–54

**FIGURES 11–53 AND 11–54**   TUBERCULOMA

Although tuberculoma is an unusual lesion in the spinal cord, the appearance of this example is typical, with its central core of caseous necrosis and peripheral rim of firm, viable tissue. Surprisingly, this 39-year-old man manifested only minor sensory disturbances in the legs during terminal stages of his disseminated disease (Fig. 11–53). The histologic appearance is also characteristic, with caseous necrosis, a margin of epithelioid cells, a sprinkling of multinucleated giant cells, and an outer rim of lymphocytes (Fig. 11–54).

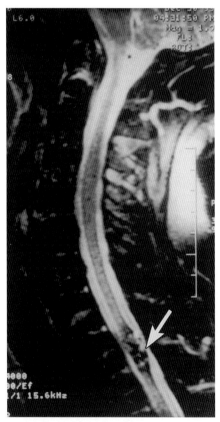

**FIGURE 11–55**   CAVERNOUS ANGIOMA

Left chest numbness and left lower extremity weakness called attention to this discrete, T1-2 intramedullary lesion (*arrow*) in a 40-year-old man. As is typical of "cavernomas," the T2-weighted image discloses the dark signal of hemosiderin.

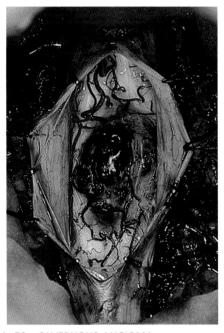

**FIGURE 11–56**   CAVERNOUS ANGIOMA

Exposed at surgery, the lesion is a dark, botryoid mass of closely opposed vessels. (Courtesy of Dr. William E. Krauss, Rochester, MN.)

Histologically, the hyalinized, often thrombosed, and sometimes recanalized vessels form compact conglomerates or lie individually in the gliotic cord parenchyma (Fig. 11–57).[10, 14] Because gliosis may be impressive and Rosenthal fibers abundant, an erroneous diagnosis of glioma may be entertained.

### Arteriovenous Malformation

The arteriovenous malformation consists of large, serpentine vessels that throw their coils about the cord and exiting nerve roots (Fig. 11–58). Most vessels lie on the dorsal surface of the cord and consist largely of veins, some arterialized. Smaller numbers of hyalinized vessels, somewhat resembling those of cavernous angioma, lie within cord parenchyma (Figs. 11–59 and 11–60). Symptoms are attributed to pressure or ischemia and only rarely to hemorrhage. In light of their arteriographic, macroscopic, and microscopic features, these complex lesions are similar to intracranial arteriovenous malformation as described in Chapter 7 on pages 405 to 407.[1, 5, 13] As a rule, the conspicuous large vessels encountered by the surgeon are not the shunting "nidus" but only the secondarily enlarged feeding or draining vessels. The actual point of shunting may be intradural, extradural, or occasionally within the substance of the dura itself.[1, 9, 16] The effect of hemodynamic back pressure upon spinal cord parenchyma is allegedly the basis of the observed myelopathy in some cases.[2, 17]

## Neoplasms

### Astrocytic Neoplasms

As in the brain, astrocytic neoplasms can be divided into the infiltrative, diffuse or fibrillary astrocytomas, of varying grade, and discrete lesions, that is, pilocytic astrocytoma (Fig. 11–61 and Table 11–1).

Although a precise correlation between histologic tumor type, radiographic images, and intraoperative appearance remains to be established, astrocytomas of the spinal

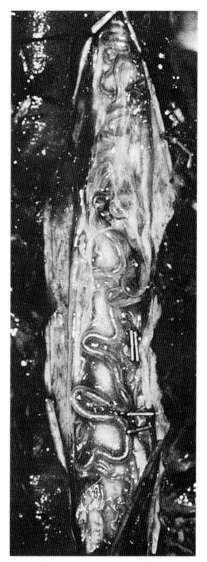

**FIGURE 11–58    ARTERIOVENOUS MALFORMATION**

This vascular malformation meanders over the dorsal surface of the thoracic spinal cord of a 55-year-old man with lower extremity sensorimotor deficits. (Courtesy of Dr. Guy L. Odom, Durham, NC.)

cord can thus be divided into two clinicopathologically distinct groups; one is the diffuse or diffusely infiltrative astrocytoma and the other is the better circumscribed pilocytic astrocytoma, discussed on pages 555 to 557. This

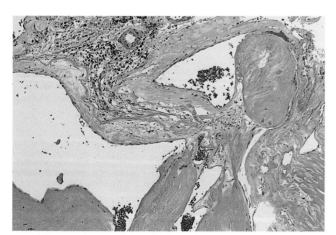

**FIGURE 11–57    CAVERNOUS ANGIOMA**

Malformed vessels abut hemosiderin-stained parenchyma in the lesion seen in Figure 11–55.

**TABLE 11–1**
**Spinal Cord Neoplasms by Architectural Features**

Discrete, contrast enhancing, with or without a cyst (syrinx)
   Ependymoma
   Pilocytic astrocytoma
   Hemangioblastoma
   Paraganglioma
   Intramedullary schwannoma
Ill defined, contrast enhancing
   Grade IV astrocytoma (glioblastoma multiforme)
Ill defined, nonenhancing
   Grade II or III (anaplastic) fibrillary astrocytoma

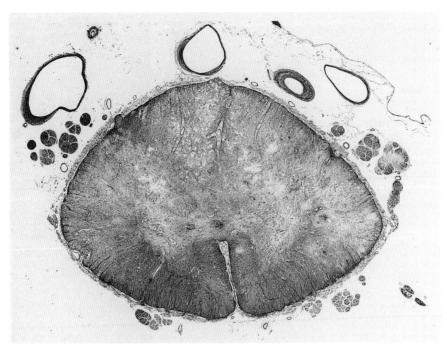

**11–59**

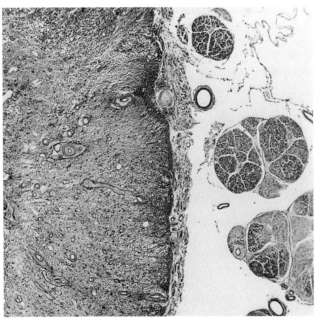

**11–60**

**FIGURES 11–59 AND 11–60** VASCULAR MALFORMATION

Redundant meningeal blood vessels of this spinal cord vascular malformation are abnormally large and are variously composed of smooth muscle and fibrous tissue (Fig. 11–59). Typically, the underlying cord contains a plethora of small hyalinized vessels and shows ischemic effects, including loss of myelin and gliosis (Fig. 11–60).

dichotomy is not always apparent in published series, which often combine the two tumors under the imprecise term "low-grade astrocytoma." When applied to a given lesion, the latter designation can have serious consequence for the patient because the two tumor types differ in their growth pattern, biologic behavior, optimal therapy, and prognosis. Every effort should be made to distinguish pilocytic and diffuse astrocytomas.[12]

The diagnosis of a spinal astrocytic neoplasm can be extremely challenging, with the difficulty exacerbated by the small size of the specimen and mechanical as well as frozen section artifacts. In this situation, the specialities of neurosurgery, radiology, and pathology must converge to assess the lesion accurately and fully.

## Diffuse (Infiltrative) Astrocytomas

**Definition.** Infiltrative astrocytomas that range from grade II to IV.

**General Comments.** These rather uncommon lesions occur in both children and adults. A small percentage arise in association with neurofibromatosis; prior radiotherapy is implicated in the genesis of a rare example.[5] Most are "spontaneous."

**Clinical Features.** Pain, motor deficits, sensory disturbances, and abnormalities of sphincter function are the common symptoms. An insidious onset with gradual progression characterizes the better differentiated lesions. A more acute onset typifies anaplastic lesions (e.g., glioblastoma).

**Radiologic Features.** MR imaging reveals an ill-defined, expansile process that extends over several segments (Figs. 11–61 and 11–62). Although one or more cysts are not uncommon, extensive syrinx formation is more often associated with discrete intramedullary neoplasms such as pilocytic astrocytoma, ependymoma, and hemangioblastoma. Typically, there is no well-circumscribed mass in grade II examples. An irregular zone of contrast enhancement characterizes grade IV (glioblastoma) examples (Fig. 11–63). See Table 11–1 for a summary of intramedullary neoplasms by architectural features.

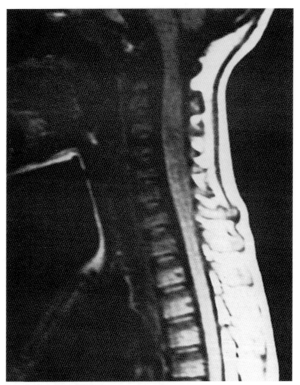

**FIGURE 11–62    ASTROCYTOMA**

Diffuse astrocytomas produce fusiform, nonenhancing widening of the cord. The patient was a 9-year-old girl with arm weakness and shoulder pain.

**Macroscopic Features.** The lesions produce a fusiform enlargement without sharply defined borders (Fig. 11–64). Neoplastic cells permeate the parenchyma and often impart a faint yellow color. Tumor consistency varies in relation to the degree of cellularity. It is therefore firm in hypocellular regions where the parenchyma

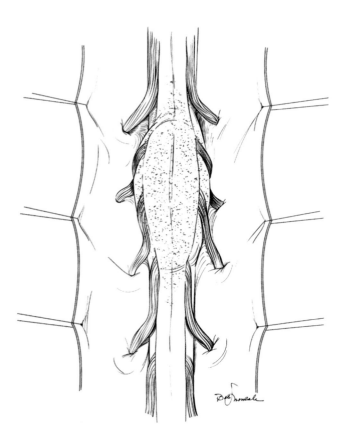

**FIGURE 11–61    INFILTRATIVE GLIOMAS OF THE SPINAL CORD**

A minority of spinal cord gliomas "diffusely" infiltrate the spinal cord without clearly defined borders. With the exception of a rare oligodendroglioma, these neoplasms are "diffuse astrocytomas" of grades II to IV.

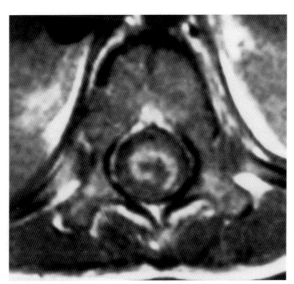

**FIGURE 11–63    GLIOBLASTOMA MULTIFORME**

Glioblastomas in the spinal cord are usually contrast enhancing and can show the same "ring" or "rim" conformation seen in the brain. The 3-year-old patient died 5 months after surgery.

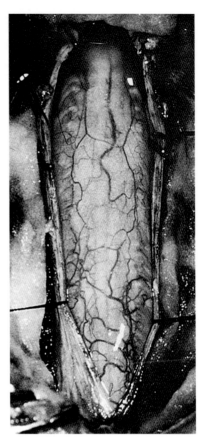

**FIGURE 11–64** ASTROCYTOMA

As depicted in Figure 11–1 and shown in this operative photograph of a cervical spinal cord example, grade II astrocytomas produce a fusiform enlargement of the cord without the formation of a defined mass. The 12-year-old patient presented with weakness and wasting of the upper extremities.

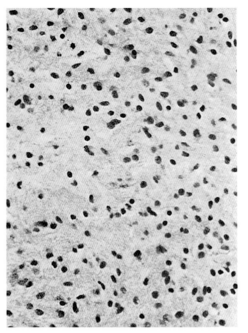

**FIGURE 11–65** DIFFUSE ASTROCYTOMA

Well-differentiated diffuse astrocytomas consist of uniform randomly distributed mature-appearing glia with minimal variation in nuclear size and shape.

cord is among the most difficult in the surgical pathology of the CNS. Consideration must always be given to the possibility that the lesion represents gliosis or a tumor other than an astrocytoma. Demyelinating disease must receive consideration as well.

is largely intact, soft in regions of hypercellularity, and gelatinous or grumous in areas of degeneration or necrosis. In addition to the intrinsic cysts, some tumors have a non-neoplastic syrinx at their rostral or caudal extremities.

**Microscopic Features.** In contrast to infiltrative astrocytomas of the brain, those arising in spinal cord are more often well differentiated (grade II) (Fig. 11–65). Nonetheless, tumors of grades III (Fig. 11–66) and IV (glioblastoma) (Figs. 11–67 and 11–68) also occur. The cells of the grade II lesions vary from case to case. In some, cytoplasm is scant and the cells' atypical nuclei appear naked in a background of intact gray or white matter. In others, the cytoplasm is more conspicuous and the cells are either fibrillary or gemistocytic. As anaplasia appears, the cells become increasingly pleomorphic and closely packed. Anaplastic (grade III) astrocytomas feature atypia in addition to mitotic activity, whereas microvascular proliferation and necrosis complete the description of glioblastoma multiforme.

**Differential Diagnosis.** The diagnosis of the well-differentiated (grade II) diffuse astrocytoma of the spinal

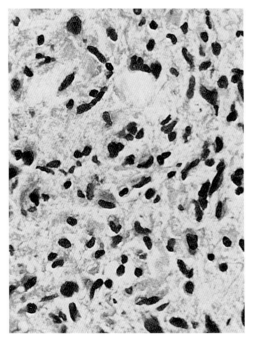

**FIGURE 11–66** ANAPLASTIC ASTROCYTOMA

Only a few spinal cord astrocytomas are as pleomorphic as this example.

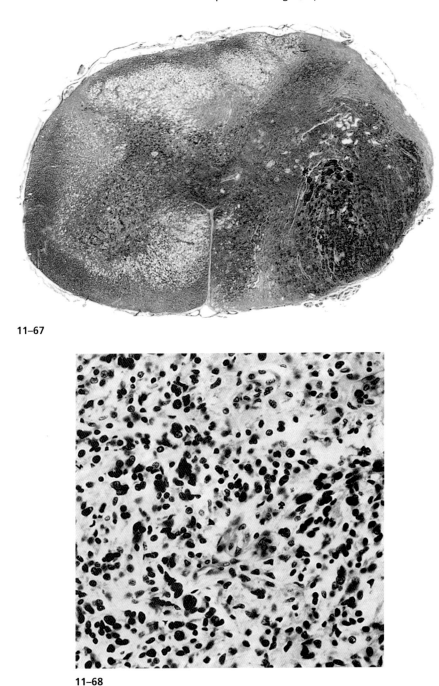

11–67

11–68

**FIGURES 11–67 AND 11–68**    GLIOBLASTOMA MULTIFORME

The spectrum of astrocytic neoplasms of the spinal cord includes glioblastoma multiforme. The cervical spinal cord is overrun by small anaplastic glial cells. Note the glomeruloid vascular proliferation.

The issue of *gliosis versus glioma*, a recurrent theme in the diagnosis of astrocytoma at any site in the CNS, is especially relevant in the spinal cord. Here, as in the brain, gliosis is a morphologically heterogeneous process in which two principal types can be identified—diffuse and piloid.

*Fibrillary gliosis* is more a process of hypertrophy than of hyperplasia. The cells assume a gemistocytic appearance with glassy cytoplasm and distinctive radiating and tapering processes (Fig. 11–69). With resolution or removal of the exciting stimulus, the cytoplasm of such cells reverts to its more normal resting state (Figs. 11–70 and 11–71). Subacute gliosis accompanies *demyelinating disease* or other processes and may be mixed with or surround any primary or metastatic neoplasm. In any case, one should not be too taken with the cytologic features of subacute gliosis and infer the presence of an astrocytoma on the basis of scattered cells with reactive atypical nuclei and prominent pink cytoplasm (see Fig. 11–69). The issue of whether a specimen represents gliosis or tumor

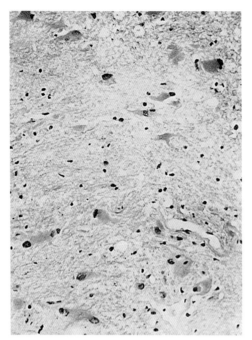

**FIGURE 11–69    REACTIVE GLIOSIS**

Astrocytes with prominent eosinophilic cytoplasmic processes characterize reactive gliosis of the "fibrillary" type. An intramedullary schwannoma was the inciting lesion.

rests in part upon cellularity. Without a clear-cut increase, twofold or more, the diagnosis of astrocytoma should be made with great caution. In reactive lesions, subacute gliosis can divert attention from evidence of the lesion's true nature, i.e., a macrophage-rich process. Again, the density of the astrocytes becomes critical. It is generally the prominence (hypertrophy) of astrocytes that is increased in reactive lesions, not their number. The differential diagnosis of astrocytoma and demyelinating disease is discussed in Chapter 3 on page 118.

The second type of gliosis, chronic *piloid gliosis*, is created by prominent, often elongated cells, often accompanied by Rosenthal fibers. This glial response is common in the spinal cord, as it is in hypothalamus and cerebellum. At microscopic and even macroscopic levels, this reactive process may resemble pilocytic astrocytoma, as discussed on pages 213 and 557. Pilocytic gliosis is particularly prominent around such chronic discrete intramedullary tumors as ependymoma (see Figs. 11–77 and 11–78) and hemangioblastoma.

Once the differential of glioma versus gliosis has been resolved, one must distinguish diffuse astrocytoma from other intramedullary neoplasms, including *pilocytic astrocytoma, ependymoma,* and *hemangioblastoma.* It is worth a reminder, however, that ependymomas with a highly fibrillar background and hemangioblastoma as seen in frozen section can resemble

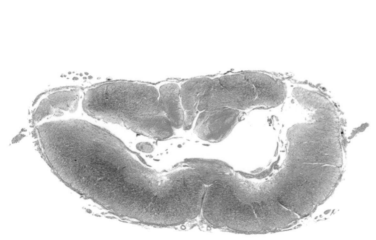

**11–70**

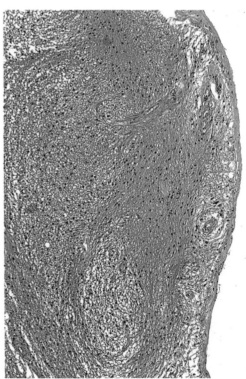

**11–71**

**FIGURES 11–70 AND 11–71    SYRINGOMYELIA WITH REACTIVE GLIOSIS**

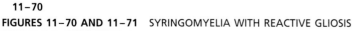

A syrinx often induces intense gliosis, here apparent in the posterior columns just above the syrinx (Fig. 11–70). Histologically, these reactive cells often exhibit cytologic and architectural features similar to those of well-differentiated fibrillary astrocytoma (Fig. 11–71).

fibrillary astrocytoma (see Fig. 11–106). Table 11–1 summarizes architectural features of spinal cord tumors.

If the differential diagnosis of low-grade diffuse astrocytoma is difficult in permanent sections, a frozen section diagnosis can be even more challenging. The pathologist must be aware of the consequences of such a diagnosis and should proceed with the greatest caution. To avoid creating a needless neurologic defect in the presence of a presumably unresectable lesion, most surgeons terminate the operation upon receiving a frozen section diagnosis of fibrillary astrocytoma. All available clinical and radiographic information should be considered while freezing as little of the specimen as possible. The radiographic images become especially important. For example, a neuroimaging finding of a solid, contrast-enhancing nodule with an accompanying cyst or syrinx is evidence that the lesion is probably not a fibrillary or diffuse astrocytoma. One should carefully reconsider before assigning this diagnosis of a low-grade diffuse astrocytoma in the presence of such an image. Unless tissue was set aside for permanent sections, no additional specimen will be submitted and all final permanent sections will be compromised by freezing artifacts.

The often repetitive biopsy–frozen section–report to the operating room sequence can be trying for both surgeon and pathologist when it appears that no specific diagnosis is forthcoming, and that further sampling risks a postoperative neurologic deficit. At this juncture, a dialogue is critical in order to make the most of the remaining tissue. Unless there is some unusual compelling reason for an additional frozen section, we are careful to save a portion by forgoing a repeated frozen section that is likely to be nondiagnostic. Before terminating the procedure, the surgeon deserves a clearly expressed opinion about the certainty of the preliminary diagnosis and must be informed if it seems likely that a definite diagnosis may not be possible on the basis of permanent sections.

### Diagnostic Checklist

- Is the "diffuse astrocytoma" really not just gliosis as part of a reactive condition?
- Is this "astrocytoma" or "anaplastic astrocytoma" seen in a frozen section not really hemangioblastoma?
- Is this "astrocytoma" not really a tanycytic ependymoma?

**Treatment and Prognosis.** Regrettably, there are few clinical studies wherein a clear distinction is made between diffuse and pilocytic astrocytomas of the spinal cord. One large study found both 5- and 10-year survival rates for all patients with diffuse astrocytoma to be 15%.[12] Another study, of children, found a significant difference in survival between patients with low-grade astrocytomas (pilocytic and grade II astrocytomas combined) and those with grade III and grade IV tumors.[3] Patients with pilocytic lesions appeared to do better than those with grade II astrocytomas. Patients with grade III and IV lesions all succumbed within 2½ years of diagnosis,[12] and similarly poor survival has been reported by others.[11] Local recurrence and cerebrospinal fluid spread

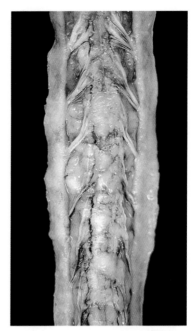

**FIGURE 11–72    SPINAL GLIOBLASTOMA WITH CEREBROSPINAL FLUID DISSEMINATION**

Malignant astrocytomas of the spinal cord are prone to dissemination in the subarachnoid space. (Courtesy of Dr. Caterina Giannini, Rochester, MN.)

are typical terminal events in association with high-grade lesions (Fig. 11–72).[2-4, 6, 18] Lacking a clear differentiation between pilocytic and diffuse tumors, most studies are difficult to interpret with respect to prognosis and the need for adjuvant therapy.[1, 3, 7-10, 13, 15, 17]

### Pilocytic Astrocytoma

**Definition.** A generally well-circumscribed, often cystic, astrocytoma composed of variable proportions of loose and compact tissue.

**General Comments.** The relative frequency of pilocytic versus diffuse astrocytoma is unclear. In one study of 12 astrocytomas of the spinal cord in children, 4 were pilocytic.[16] In another series of 73 pediatric spinal cord astrocytomas, there were 28 pilocytic neoplasms, 21 grade II tumors, 21 grade III neoplasms, and 3 glioblastomas.[3] In a larger series of 79 patients, mostly adults, 54% were found to be pilocytic, 32% diffuse, and 14% not classifiable as either.[12]

**Clinical Features.** Both children and adults are affected, with presenting signs and symptoms common to intramedullary tumors, that is, weakness, sensory deficits, and pain.[12, 14, 16]

**Radiologic Features.** Radiographic findings in pilocytic astrocytomas of spinal cord have yet to be described completely. In our experience, these tumors are discrete, frequently cyst associated, and typically contrast enhancing (Fig. 11–73).[16] As summarized in Table 11–1, this

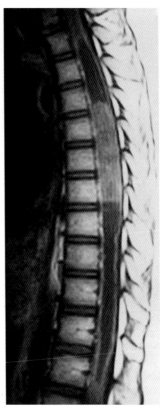

**FIGURE 11–73**   PILOCYTIC ASTROCYTOMA

In contrast to the diffuse astrocytomas, pilocytic lesions are well circumscribed and enhance with gadolinium. As in this 11-year-old girl, a large cyst often accompanies the lesion.

architecture is shared with other discrete intramedullary tumors such as ependymoma and hemangioblastoma (see. Figs. 11–79 and 11–102). A syrinx may extend from either end of the lesion. The term holocord astrocytoma is applied to remarkable examples wherein the entire spinal cord is affected. Descriptively, in light of their

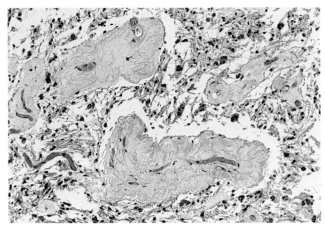

**FIGURE 11–75**   PILOCYTIC ASTROCYTOMA

A compact, noninfiltrative growth pattern and hyalinized vessels are typical of pilocytic astrocytomas. The cytologic "atypia" is considered degenerative in nature and should not be interpreted as evidence of malignancy.

silhouettes, long thin pilocytic astrocytomas are sometimes labeled pencil gliomas.[14] The other discrete intramedullary neoplasms are given in Table 11–1.

**Microscopic Features.** Pilocytic astrocytomas of the spinal cord may feature the full spectrum of patterns exhibited by optic, hypothalamic, and cerebellar examples (Figs. 11–75 and 11–76). The features by which pilocytic astrocytomas may simulate high-grade diffuse astrocytomas are discussed in detail in the section on pilocytic astrocytomas in Chapter 4 on pages 209 to 210. Suffice it to say that degenerative nuclear atypia may be conspicuous and suggest a grade III lesion. The same is true of the rare mitotic figures. The finding of hyalinized vessels, a common feature of pilocytic astrocytoma, is helpful evidence of the tumor's chronicity and low grade.

**Differential Diagnosis.** The process of differential diagnosis as applied to spinal pilocytic astrocytomas differs

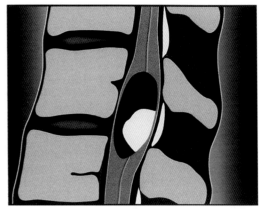

**FIGURE 11–74**   INTRAMEDULLARY TUMOR WITH SYRINX

A discrete contrast-enhancing mass, here with an associated cyst, is typical of pilocytic astrocytoma, ependymoma, and hemangioblastoma. (From Passe TJ, Beauchamp NJ, Burger PC. Neuroimaging in the identification of low-grade and nonneoplastic CNS lesions. The Neurologist 1999;5:293–299.)

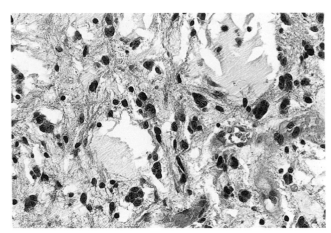

**FIGURE 11–76**   PILOCYTIC ASTROCYTOMA

Microcysts are common in pilocytic astrocytomas.

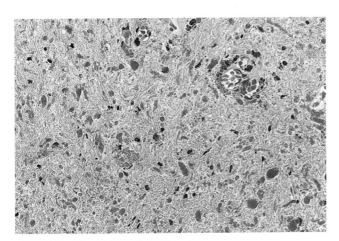

**FIGURE 11–77    PILOID GLIOSIS**

This abundance of Rosenthal fibers in such a highly fibrillar background is more consistent with piloid gliosis than with pilocytic astrocytoma.

somewhat from that employed in the assessment of well-differentiated diffuse astrocytomas. In the latter instance, it is the very determination of abnormality that can be the greatest challenge. In the case of pilocytic astrocytoma, the tissue is obviously abnormal and the principal concern is to decide whether it is chronic *piloid gliosis* or a neoplasm.

Macroscopic and radiographic characteristics weigh heavily in the process of differential diagnoses. A focal solid enlargement speaks strongly in favor of pilocytic astrocytoma, whereas an ill-defined expansion extending over several spinal segments is most consistent with a *diffuse astrocytoma*. A syrinx is a more likely associate of the pilocytic lesion but may also accompany other discrete lesions such as *ependymoma* and *hemangioblastoma*. Syringomyelia, an idiopathic, non-neoplastic lesion, is another consideration. In a *wall of a syrinx*, either with or without an associated neoplasm, there can be little cellular pleomorphism, with small nuclei residing in a fibrillary, process-rich matrix (see Figs. 11–70 and 11–71). In other cases there is a flagrant pilocytic response with elongated process-containing cells that can be misinterpreted readily as pilocytic astrocytoma (Figs. 11–77 and 11–78). Such gliosis is generally solid without microcystic change. Scattered Rosenthal fibers are commonly present. On the other hand, subacute gliosis featuring gemistocytic astrocytes is seen in active, evolving processes such as demyelinating disease. To complicate matters, pilocytic astrocytomas can have their own reactive cyst wall with Rosenthal fibers.

**Treatment and Prognosis.** There is little information about the prognosis for patients with pilocytic astrocytomas of the spinal cord, but the expected favorable nature of the lesion was confirmed in one study in which both the 5- and 10-year survival rates were 81%.[12] Similar results were noted in another investigation.[3] These figures match those associated with supratentorial pilocytic tumors.

## Ependymomas

**Definition.** Variably fibrillar and epithelial neoplasms derived from the ependyma.

**General Comments.** Ependymomas, the most common gliomas of the spinal cord, can be divided into (1) the classical cellular lesion and its variants and (2) the myxopapillary lesion. The former share histologic features with intracranial ependymomas, whereas the myxopapillary lesions are histologically distinctive and largely restricted to the conus medullaris and filum terminale.

### Cellular Ependymoma

**Clinical Features.** The incidence curve peaks during the fourth and fifth decades and flattens symmetrically toward the extremes of life. Spinal ependymomas of the classical, or cellular, type can be multifocal in the setting of NF2.[11] Most spinal cord ependymomas are intramedullary, but occasional examples, although intradural, arise outside the spinal cord.[10, 16, 28]

**Radiologic Features.** Ependymomas are discrete, contrast-enhancing masses (Figs. 11–79 and 11–80 and Table 11–1). They may have dark, hemosiderin-rich regions evident in T2-weighted images.[9] An associated peritumoral cyst is not uncommon.

**Macroscopic Features.** Primary intramedullary ependymomas usually remain within the substance of the spinal cord as a discrete mass. At surgery, affected segments are fusiformly enlarged. Upon incision of the cord, the discrete character and central location (Fig. 11–81) of the tumor quickly become apparent. Ependymomas are usually solid but can be cystic.

The intramedullary ependymoma is, overall, well circumscribed, but the pathologist may hear from the surgeon at some point during the operation that the lesion merges somewhat with the parenchymal tissue.

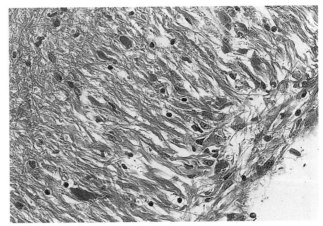

**FIGURE 11–78    PILOID GLIOSIS**

This zone of reactive gliosis surrounding an ependymoma illustrates the similarity between long-standing gliosis of this type and pilocytic astrocytoma.

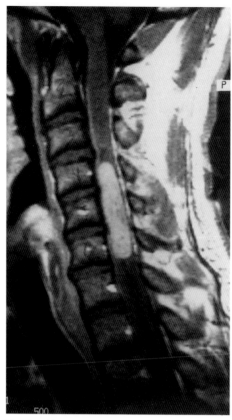

**FIGURE 11–79** EPENDYMOMA

Most spinal ependymomas are discrete, contrast enhancing, and intramedullary. This example occurred in a 37-year-old man with back pain.

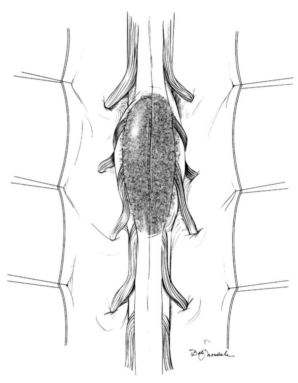

**FIGURE 11–80** DISCRETE INTRAMEDULLARY TUMOR

Solid, largely noninfiltrating tumors include ependymoma, pilocytic astrocytoma, hemangioblastoma, and rarer lesions such as schwannoma. Ependymomas are the most common.

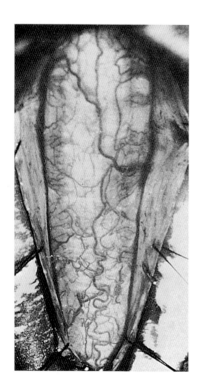
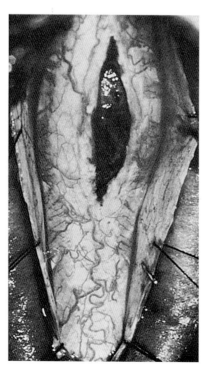

**FIGURE 11–81** EPENDYMOMA

Intramedullary ependymomas segmentally expand the cord. In this case, opening of the enlarged segment relieved the intrinsic pressure and delivered a discrete, fleshy neoplasm through the lips of the incision. The cervical lesion expressed itself first as weakness while playing tennis and then as diminished arm strength in a 53-year-old physician. (Courtesy of Dr. Guy L. Odom, Durham, NC.)

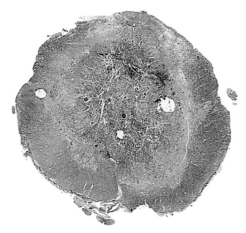

**FIGURE 11–83**    EPENDYMOMA

As seen in a whole mount section, spinal ependymomas are discrete masses.

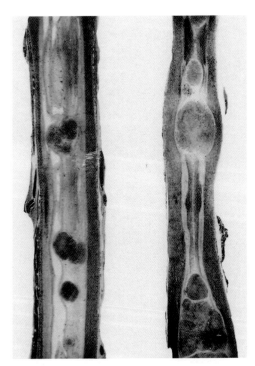

**FIGURE 11–82**    MULTIPLE EPENDYMOMAS IN NEUROFIBROMATOSIS 2

The origin of spinal cord ependymomas from the region of the central canal is apparent in these multiple lesions.

Although ill-defined borders are more characteristic of fibrillary astrocytomas than ependymomas, some macroscopic merging with the spinal cord parenchyma is in no way inconsistent with ependymoma.

**Microscopic Features.** Spinal ependymomas are discrete masses (Figs. 11–82 and 11–83). Most consist of cellular sheets interrupted by perivascular anuclear zones or pseudorosettes (Fig. 11–84). Less often, true rosettes, canals, or simple epithelial surfaces appear. Occasionally, even perivascular pseudorosettes are inconspicuous and the diagnosis of ependymoma may not come to mind. Nodules of collagenized tissue and foamy macrophages are sometimes present.[26]

There are two uncommon variants of spinal ependymoma related to the cellular type just described: (1) the tanycytic variety[4] and (2) the subependymoma.[2,8,13,18,21] The former is a poorly defined entity that is a paucicellular or moderately cellular, vaguely fascicular lesion with inconspicuous pseudorosettes that are best appreciated at low magnification (Fig. 11–85). It is not surprising that these tumors are often misinterpreted as schwannoma or pilocytic astrocytoma, particularly in frozen sections.

The spinal subependymoma is identical to its intracranial counterpart discussed on pages 250 to 254 of Chapter 4. Nodular in architecture, its typically uniform nuclei cluster within delicate, often circumferential skeins of fibril-rich processes (Fig. 11–86). Pure subependymomas are rare in the spinal cord.[8, 18, 21]

Dense stromal collagenization may rarely be found in ependymomas.[23]

High-grade ependymomas with high cellularity, increased cytologic atypia, numerous mitoses, and microvascular proliferation are uncommon in the spinal cord.

**Features in Frozen Sections.** The diagnosis of spinal ependymomas in a frozen section can be stressful because cytologic features of the ependymoma often simulate those of astrocytoma (Fig. 11–87). The correct identification of an ependymoma during the surgical

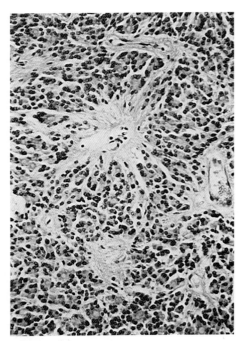

**FIGURE 11–84**    EPENDYMOMA

Ependymomas of the spinal cord share all of the histologic features of their intracranial counterparts. Note prominent perivascular anucleate zones and clustering of cells in small rosettes.

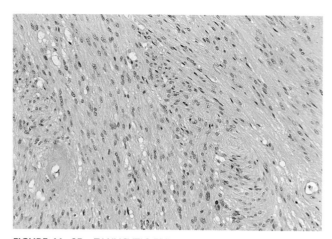

**FIGURE 11–85** TANYCYTIC EPENDYMOMA

The uncommon variant of ependymoma is composed of elongated cells and may resemble astrocytoma, particularly the pilocytic variety. Distinguishing features are its sharp circumscription, nuclear characteristics with distinct micronucleoli, and the finding of subtle perivascular pseudorosettes.

procedure is crucial because diagnosis of fibrillary astrocytoma prompts termination of the procedure and, at least temporarily, precludes the chance of a curative total excision.

**Cytologic Features.** Smears can complement the frozen sections as they highlight the small, dark, oval ependymal nuclei as well the cells' attachment to vessels by tapered processes (Fig. 11–88).

**Differential Diagnosis.** The differential diagnosis of spinal cord ependymomas should begin with a review of the operative description and the neuroimaging characteristics. Almost by definition, ependymomas are discrete and contrast enhancing. They share this feature, however, with other spinal neoplasms, including hemangioblastoma, pilocytic astrocytoma, schwannoma, and

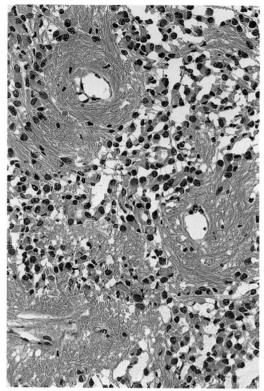

**FIGURE 11–87** EPENDYMOMA

The cells of ependymoma often appear "gemistocytic" in frozen section preparations. The lesion was, however, radiologically and macroscopically discrete and noninfiltrative. It also contains perivascular pseudorosettes.

paraganglioma (Table 11–1). It is also critical to be certain that the tissue obtained at biopsy represents the substance of the neoplasm and not merely tissue from either the cyst wall or the spinal cord parenchyma directly surrounding the lesion. These regions consist of compacted piloid astrocytes, often with Rosenthal fibers.

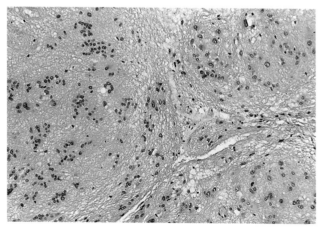

**FIGURE 11–86** SUBEPENDYMOMA

Clustered nuclei and a highly fibrillar background are the essential features of this tumor.

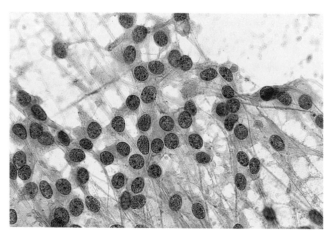

**FIGURE 11–88** EPENDYMOMA

A smear preparation shows the uniform nuclei, distinct micronucleoli, and cytoplasmic processes typical of ependymoma.

This appearance closely simulates that of *pilocytic astrocytoma*, a lesion that can have its own Rosenthal fiber–containing cyst wall. In some instances, the distinction is virtually impossible (see Figs. 11–77 and 11–78). Awareness that a lesion is cystic should generate a "prove it to me" attitude on the part of the pathologist, requiring verification that the tissue is not simply a portion of a cyst wall.

*Diffuse astrocytoma*, although not a discrete lesion when low grade, enters into the differential at the microscopic level because some ependymomas are highly fibrillar. This feature of fibrillarity is exaggerated in frozen sections of ependymomas, wherein fibril-rich processes and gemistocytic cytologic features are exaggerated (see Fig. 11–87). This is doubly true of the tanycytic variant, a lesion that is easily confused with an astrocytoma even in permanent sections. As previously noted, perivascular pseudorosettes, the principal distinguishing feature of the ependymoma, may be inconspicuous or, rarely, lacking. Their presence, even when vague, can be emphasized by their GFAP positivity. Perhaps most important, the ependymoma's characteristic solid, noninfiltrative growth pattern serves to distinguish it from infiltrating diffuse astrocytomas. Thus, while appearing astrocytic because of prominent fibrillarity, ependymomas are composed solely of neoplastic tissue. The absence of "overrun" spinal cord parenchyma interspersed among the tumor cells is an important negative feature.

*Hemangioblastoma* shares the discreteness and frequency of cysts comparable to ependymomas. Distinctively, however, hemangioblastomas possess lipidized stromal cells set into extensive reticulin-rich vascular stroma. Foci of extramedullary erythropoiesis help confirm the diagnosis in a minority of cases.

**Treatment and Prognosis.** As discrete masses, spinal ependymomas can often be removed in toto.[7] Recurrence is unusual.

### Myxopapillary Ependymoma

**Clinical Features.** This distinctive lesion usually occurs in adults[19, 22, 24] and rarely in children. Neurologic symptoms include either sphincter disturbances or deficits related to compression or involvement of the conus medullaris or sacral nerve roots. Myxopapillary ependymomas also occasionally arise intracranially, and at this site they may be difficult to distinguish from mucin-rich pilocytic astrocytomas.[12]

Neoplasms with an identical myxopapillary architecture can arise extradurally in the presacral or postsacral regions,[1, 27, 31] presumably from congenital ependymal cell rests that themselves closely resemble the tumor[20] (see Figs. 10–61 and 10–62). These "ectopic" ependymomas are discussed in Chapter 10 on pages 521 to 522.

**Radiologic Features.** Lying low in the lumbar region, the masses are discrete and contrast enhancing (Fig. 11–89). The abundant mucin that characterizes these lesions can be visualized radiologically as hyperintensity or whiteness on nonenhanced T1-weighted MR images.[9]

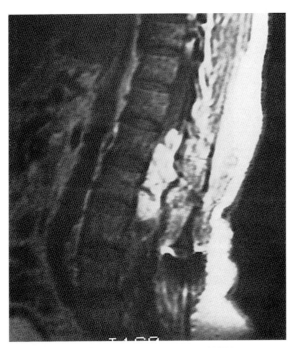

**FIGURE 11–89**    MYXOPAPILLARY EPENDYMOMA

Typical myxopapillary ependymomas are lobulated, discrete masses arising from the filum terminale with or without involvement of the conus medullaris. (Courtesy of Dr. John T. Curnes, Greensboro, NC.)

**Macroscopic Features.** The myxopapillary ependymoma is a well-defined, soft, saccular mass that may secondarily adhere to the nerve roots of the cauda equina or extend cephalad to involve the conus medullaris (Figs. 11–90 and 11–91).[5, 17, 22] Uncommonly, they appear to arise from a nerve root.

**Microscopic Features.** Primarily because of their distribution of stromal mucin, myxopapillary ependymomas are distinctive overall, but they vary considerably in cytologic appearance from case to case. They are variably papillary, epithelial, or fibrillar (Figs. 11–92 and 11–93). Characteristically, mucin is abundant and often located within the walls of the vessels (Fig. 11–94; see Fig. 11–93) and, less commonly, as a diffuse deposition (Fig. 11–95). The cells of the classical lesion appear epithelial, as they are seated upon vessels. Gland-like spaces and arrays reminiscent of papillae are created, but true papillations are uncommon.

So-called balloons are interesting structural features in myxopapillary lesions. These structures are small, round, eosinophilic formations that stain with PAS, alcian blue, Masson's trichrome, and in reticulin preparations (Figs. 11–96 and 11–97). At the ultrastructural level, they consist of collagen-rich stroma surrounded by tumor cell processes that rest on basal laminae.[24]

A variety of other patterns in caudal ependymomas overlap histologically with the classical myxopapillary lesion but are neither distinctly epithelial nor papillary. These are discussed in the following section on differential diagnosis.

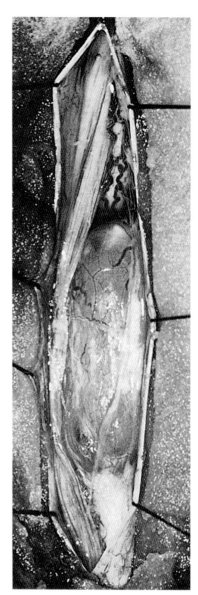

**FIGURE 11–90** MYXOPAPILLARY EPENDYMOMA

Many ependymomas are sausage-shaped masses. Unlike schwannoma with its nerve root attachment and thicker capsule, myxopapillary ependymomas are quite vascular and delicately invested, as are paragangliomas at this site. This lesion occurred in an 11-year-old boy with back pain and weakness of the left leg. (Courtesy of Dr. Richard S. Kramer, Durham, NC.)

Solid architecture, cellular pleomorphism, and considerable degenerative nuclear atypia characterize a distinctive ependymoma variant referred to as the giant cell type (Fig. 11–98).[32] This lesion occurs mainly in the cauda equina region. Mitoses are rare and, as in the classical lesions,[19] the MIB-1 or Ki-67 labeling index is low.[32] Experience with the giant cell variant is limited, but with short-term follow-up reported examples have not recurred.[32] Anaplastic forms of myxopapillary ependymoma are not recognized.

**Immunohistochemical Features.** Myxopapillary lesions are immunoreactive for GFAP (Fig. 11–99) and

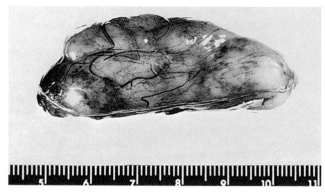

**FIGURE 11–91** MYXOPAPILLARY EPENDYMOMA

The discrete character of ependymomas of the filum terminale is emphasized by this surgical specimen from a 30-year-old woman with back and leg pain.

S-100 protein. The processes of the perivascular tumor cells are most strongly positive, and the more epithelial elements are less likely to react.[19, 24] Stains for collagen IV may highlight perivascular basal lamina.

**Cytologic Features.** The perivascular mucin (Fig. 11–100) and the processes reaching to vessels are readily apparent.

**Ultrastructural Features.** Myxopapillary ependymomas resemble conventional ependymomas but feature an abundance of basal laminae.[24, 25] Microtubular aggregates

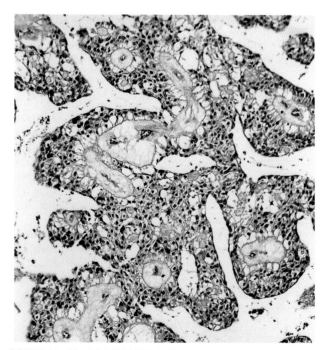

**FIGURE 11–92** MYXOPAPILLARY EPENDYMOMA

Some lesions are prominently papillary. Note the characteristic collar of mucinous material that surrounds blood vessels within the core of the papillae.

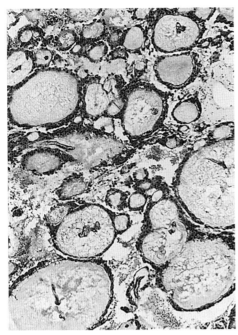

**FIGURE 11–93**    MYXOPAPILLARY EPENDYMOMA

The distinctive morphology of myxopapillary ependymoma of the filum terminale is created by collars of epithelial cells that surround mucin about a central blood vessel.

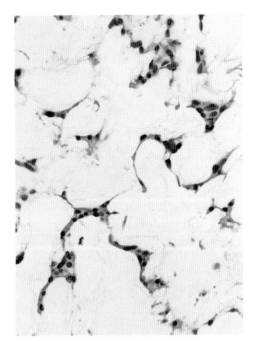

**FIGURE 11–95**    MYXOPAPILLARY EPENDYMOMA

Some tumors are particularly mucin rich.

within rough endoplasmic reticulum, a feature of no known significance, have been described.[6, 25]

**Differential Diagnosis.** This centers primarily upon the two other discrete intradural lesions that frequent this region: (1) schwannoma and (2) paraganglioma (Fig. 11–101). In regard to *schwannoma*, the precise site of origin is, in concept, helpful because ependymomas usually arise in the filum terminale, whereas schwannomas originate from nerve roots. At surgery, however, the precise localization is not always clear. As a result, the

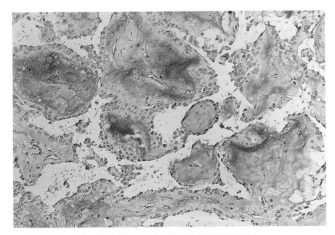

**FIGURE 11–94**    MYXOPAPILLARY EPENDYMOMA

Staining with alcian blue can highlight the stroma and its content of mucopolysaccharide.

pathologist is often presented with "tumor of the cauda equina region" that contains elements of the CNS (conus medullaris and filum terminale) and also the peripheral nervous system (spinal nerve roots). In most instances, the distinctive histologic appearance of ependymal lesions quickly resolves the issue. Nonetheless, one occasionally encounters a paucicellular ependymoma with a fascicular architecture simulating schwannoma (see Fig. 11–43). Such ependymomas usually feature uniform nuclei with delicate nucleoli and ependymal pseudorosettes, albeit subtle. They lack nuclear-cytoplasmic inclusions as well as Antoni A and B tissue. Ependymomas have a delicate rather than densely collagenous capsule. The presence of pericellular reticulin assuredly identifies the schwannoma, as does extensive immunoreactivity for type IV collagen or laminin (see Fig. 11–42). Both tumors are S-100 protein immunoreactive, although schwannomas are more so. The opposite is true of GFAP staining (see Fig. 11–44).

*Paraganglioma* also enters into the differential diagnosis of myxopapillary ependymoma. Although situated in the caudal dural sac, it more often arises from nerve roots than does the ependymoma. Focally, the cells of a paraganglioma are oriented about blood vessels to form papillary structures (see Fig. 11–101). Generally, however, the two lesions bear little resemblance. The finding of a Zellballen pattern, or ganglion cells, confirms the diagnosis of paraganglioma, as does staining for chromogranin. The distinction is discussed in more detail on page 569.

The mucinous matrix and an occasional "strung out" pattern of tumor cells in myxopapillary formations may simulate *chordoma*. Mucin distribution in the noto-

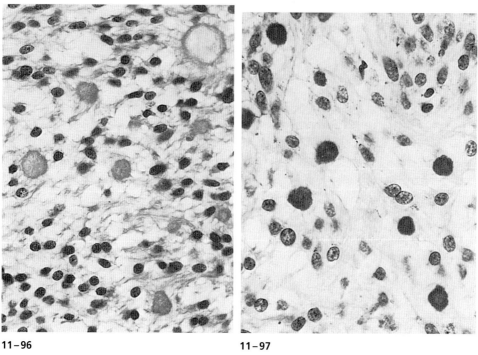

11–96                                          11–97

**FIGURES 11–96 AND 11–97**    MYXOPAPILLARY EPENDYMOMA

"Balloons," a feature of some but not all myxopapillary ependymomas, are distinctive spherical structures consisting of stromal collagen fibrils (Fig. 11–96). To a varying extent, they stain positively in trichrome, reticulin, alcian blue, and PAS (Fig. 11–97, PAS).

chordal lesion is diffuse and tends not to be confined in perivascular spaces. Chordomas are strongly reactive for low-molecular-weight keratin as well as epithelial membrane antigen. They lack GFAP staining. Only rarely are they intradural. The classical extradural chordoma and the rare extradural ependymoma do share a mucinous background and cells with epithelial features.

**Treatment and Prognosis.** Myxopapillary ependymomas are often lifted cleanly from the operative bed. Others are dissected piecemeal but nevertheless in toto.

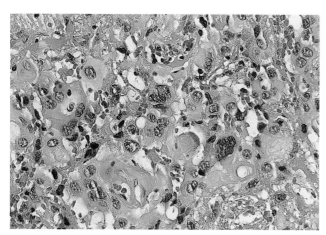

**FIGURE 11–98**    "GIANT CELL" EPENDYMOMA

This uncommon pleomorphic variant of ependymoma occurs primarily in the filum terminale.

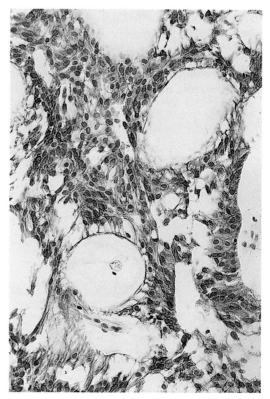

**FIGURE 11–99**    MYXOPAPILLARY EPENDYMOMA

Myxopapillary ependymomas are often strongly GFAP positive.

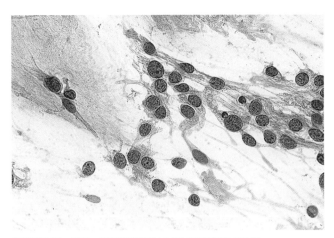

**FIGURE 11–100    MYXOPAPILLARY EPENDYMOMA**

A mucoid matrix and cells showing nuclear uniformity and process formation are well seen in smear preparations.

The chance of recurrence is low in either setting. Nonetheless, a small percentage recur locally and have the potential to disseminate in the spinal subarachnoid space.[24, 30] Radiotherapy for myxopapillary ependymomas is generally reserved for subtotally removed examples.[19, 22, 24] Some authors recommend radiation therapy for tumors removed totally but in a piecemeal fashion.[29] However, there is no consensus on this issue.

The locally invasive qualities of ectopic, extradural myxopapillary ependymomas are expressed by infiltration of soft tissue and destruction of sacral bone. The stage is then set for late recurrence and distant metastasis.[3, 14, 15]

## Oligodendroglioma

In one large historical series of 301 primary intramedullary tumors of the spinal cord, 8 (3%) were considered oligodendrogliomas.[8] Modern methods might show some of these lesions to be clear cell ependymomas or neurocytic tumors. The rarity of case reports in the modern literature attests to the low incidence of spinal oligodendrogliomas.[1–8]

## Ganglion Cell Tumors

Although rare, ganglion cell tumors are recognized entities in the spinal cord.[1–8]

## Hemangioblastoma

**Clinical Features.** Like their cerebellar counterpart, spinal hemangioblastomas occur primarily in adults (third to fifth decades), preferentially affect men,[1, 9] and show an occasional association with additional features of von Hippel–Lindau disease.[2, 4–6] Their morphology is also identical; the tumors are discrete, highly vascular, and often lipid rich. Despite the vascularity, spontaneous hemorrhage is uncommon.[10]

**Radiologic Features.** The neoplasm itself is discrete and contrast enhancing (Fig. 11–102 and Table 11–1).

Many have associated cysts, syringes, above or below the mass. Although the spinal cord proper is the usual site, the neoplasm can arise on a nerve root, especially in von Hippel–Lindau syndrome, or on the filum terminale.[7]

**Macroscopic Features.** The tumors abut the leptomeninges. The high vascularity of the lesion is reflected in compensatory enlargement of leptomeningeal vessels that may be sufficiently prominent to simulate a vascular malformation (Fig. 11–103).[3] Depending on the degree of lipidization, the tumors have a distinctive red-yellow variegation on cut section (Fig. 11–104). Most spinal hemangioblastomas are intramedullary, but some appear to arise in a nerve root.[2, 8] The posterior half of the cord and the dorsal roots are affected more often than are comparable ventral structures.[1]

**Microscopic Features.** The homology between the spinal and cerebellar hemangioblastoma extends to the microscopic level, where varying proportions of feeder vessels and capillaries enmesh stromal cells in a pervasive reticular network (Fig. 11–105). The histopathology of the hemangioblastoma is discussed in greater detail in Chapter 4, pages 329 and 336.

**Differential Diagnosis.** The diagnosis is usually self-evident when the entity is considered. Without this awareness, however, the tumor's cellularity and nuclear pleomophism make astrocytoma too strong a candidate, especially at the time of frozen section (Fig. 11–106).

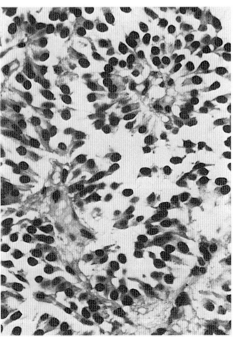

**FIGURE 11–101    INTRASPINAL PARAGANGLIOMA SIMULATING MYXOPAPILLARY EPENDYMOMA**

The apparent fibrillarity and artifactual papillae of this intraspinal paraganglioma mimic myxopapillary ependymoma. The mucoid matrix characteristic of myxopapillary ependymoma is lacking.

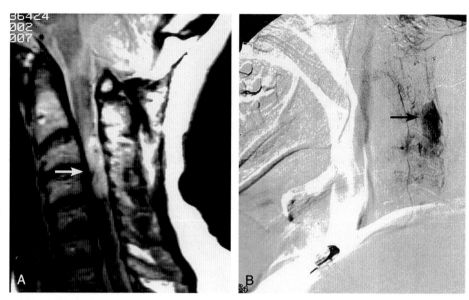

**FIGURE 11–102** HEMANGIOBLASTOMA

Hemangioblastomas are discrete contrast-enhancing masses (A). The high vascularity is apparent here in the vertebral angiogram (B). The patient with von Hippel–Lindau disease had been operated upon previously for a cerebellar hemangioblastoma. (Courtesy of Dr. Martin G. Pomper, Baltimore, MD.)

The cellular crowding and the occasional nuclear pleomorphism accentuated by the freezing process can create the impression of even a grade III (anaplastic) astrocytoma. At this juncture, review of radiologic studies, particularly MR imaging, is particularly valuable. Aware of these findings, the pathologist will be disposed to consider the diagnosis and be better prepared to deal with specimens taken from the cyst wall before the nodule is encountered. The latter can be quite small relative to the overall dimensions of the cyst. Although not specific,

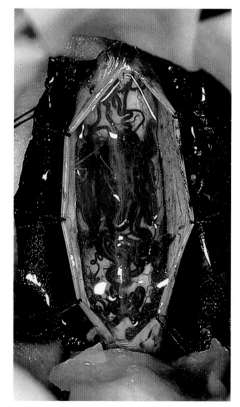

**FIGURE 11–103** HEMANGIOBLASTOMA

The profusion of feeding and draining vessels can misrepresent the lesion as a vascular malformation. (Courtesy of Dr. Wiliam E. Krauss, Rochester, MN.)

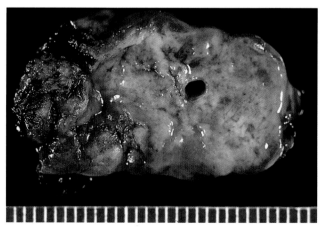

**FIGURE 11–104** HEMANGIOBLASTOMA

As in the case of hemangioblastomas occurring at other sites, most spinal hemangioblastomas are distinctively variegated, ranging from red to yellow.

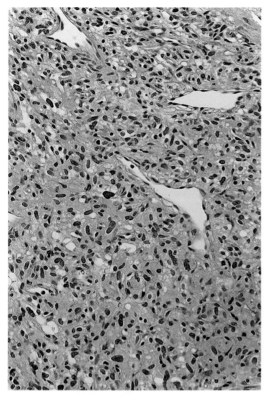

**FIGURE 11–105    HEMANGIOBLASTOMA**

Vacuolated interstitial or "stromal" cells are always present, but vary in prominence and degree of lipidization.

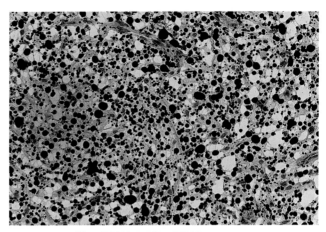

**FIGURE 11–107    HEMANGIOBLASTOMA**

The fat in the cytoplasmic vacuoles of the hemangioblastoma's stromal cells, illustrated in Figures 11–105 and 11–106, is best seen with fat stains such as oil red O.

a positive fat stain on the frozen tissue helps confirm the diagnosis (Fig. 11–107).

**Treatment and Prognosis.** The discrete nature of the spinal lesion often permits curative excision.[1, 9] The role of radiation therapy for residual neoplasm has not been fully defined.

### Paraganglioma

**Definition.** A neuroendocrine neoplasm similar to paragangliomas in other body sites.

**Clinical Features.** Paragangliomas are uncommon neoplasms in the cauda equina region. Most occur in adults. Delicately encapsulated, soft, and vascular, they usually arise from the filum terminale, less often from a nerve root[2, 3, 6] (Fig. 11–108; see Fig. 11–2).

**Radiologic Features.** Paragangliomas are discrete and contrast enhancing (see Table 11–1).[5]

**Microscopic Features.** Histologically, most paragangliomas display the characteristic Zellballen architecture (Figs. 11–109 and 11–110). In addition, neuroendocrine or carcinoid tumor-like patterns are commonly observed. Ganglion cells occur in close to 50% of lesions[2, 3] (Fig. 11–111). Such large neurons may lie in clusters, often in a fibrillar Schwann cell–rich stroma, or may be found as they appear to emerge in transition from chief cells.

**Features in Frozen Sections.** The discrete, noninfiltrative nature of the lesion is well seen. Although not as evident as in permanent sections, a lobular architecture is apparent (Fig. 11–112)

**Cytologic Features.** The distinctive nuclei of chief cells with a "salt-and-pepper," chromatin pattern are fea-

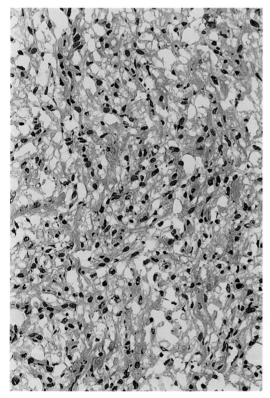

**FIGURE 11–106    HEMANGIOBLASTOMA**

In frozen sections, hemangioblastomas often resemble astrocytomas. Nevertheless, the vacuolated appearance of lipid-containing stromal cells is often evident.

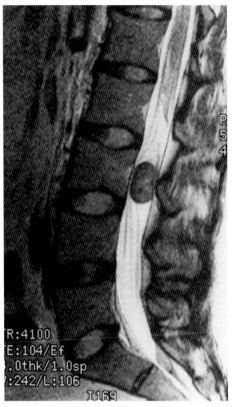

**FIGURE 11–108    PARAGANGLIOMA**

The dark, discrete lesion stands out in relief against the white CSF in this T2-weighted MR image.

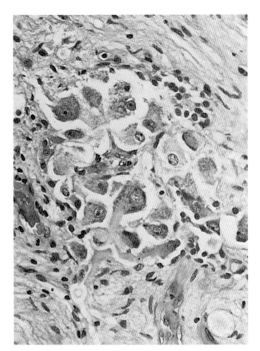

**FIGURE 11–111    PARAGANGLIOMA**

Aggregates of ganglion cells may enrich a Schwann cell matrix.

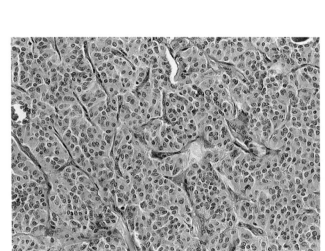

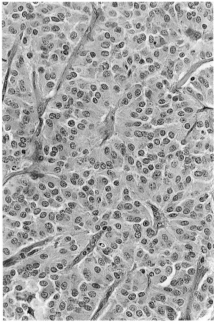

11–109                                            11–110

**FIGURES 11–109 AND 11–110    PARAGANGLIOMA**

The lobules of paraganglioma cells, termed "Zellballen," and the epithelial quality of their constituent cells are apparent at both low (Fig. 11–109) and high (Fig. 11–110) magnification.

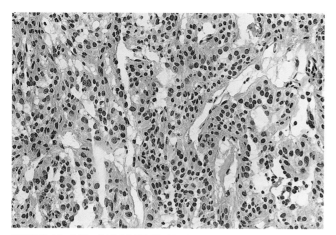

**FIGURE 11–112**   PARAGANGLIOMA

Although partially obscured by frozen section artifact, the typical lobular architecture of paraganglioma is still evident.

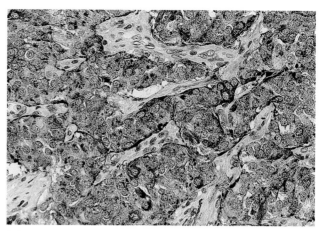

**FIGURE 11–114**   PARAGANGLIOMA

The cells are immunoreactive for chromogranin.

tures that are well seen in cytologic preparations (Fig. 11–113).

**Immunohistochemical Features.** Chief cells are reactive for chromogranin (Fig. 11–114) and synaptophysin. Variable reactivity for neurotransmitter substances such as somatostatin, serotonin, and leu-enkephalin is com-

monly manifest.[2, 3] Delicate sustentacular cells, often perilobular and perivascular in distribution, are S-100 (Fig. 11–115) and often GFAP reactive.

**Ultrastructural Features.** Electron-dense sustentacular cells surround lobules and embrace clusters of chief cells (Fig. 11–116). They lack granules and contain occasional intermediate filaments. Dense-core granules can be visualized in chief cells (Fig. 11–117).[1, 3]

**Differential Diagnosis.** The diagnosis of the paraganglioma in the cauda equina rests largely on an awareness of the entity. Although it may resemble *myxopapillary ependymoma* superficially, the paraganglioma lacks mucin within the walls of blood vessels, is not a fibrillary lesion, and is not diffusely GFAP positive.

**Treatment and Prognosis.** Gross total excision and cure are possible in almost all instances.[2, 3] Recurrence

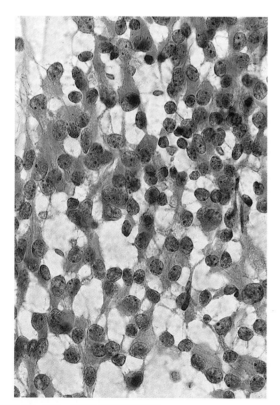

**FIGURE 11–113**   PARAGANGLIOMA

In a smear preparation, nuclear roundness, "salt-and-pepper" chromatin, and regimentation of cells help distinguish paraganglioma from myxopapillary ependymoma. In contrast to the latter, paragangliomas lack long cell processes.

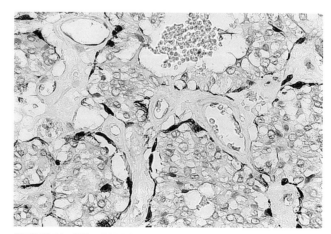

**FIGURE 11–115**   PARAGANGLIOMA

S-100–positive sustentacular cells surround lobules of chief cells.

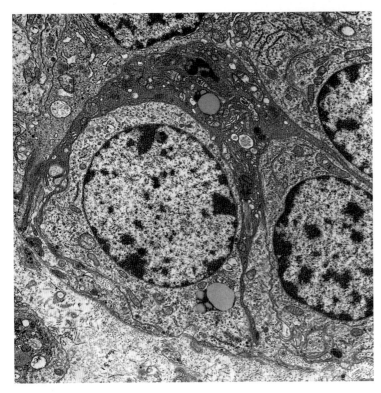

**FIGURE 11–116** PARAGANGLIOMA

Sustentacular cells are electron dense, often contain some intermediate filaments, and lack neurosecretory granules. One such cell is seen here cornered by four chief cells.

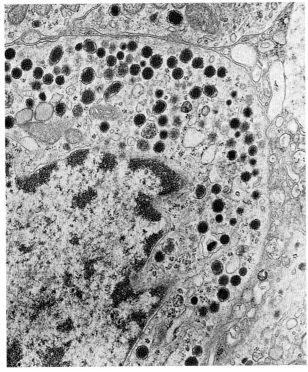

**FIGURE 11–117** PARAGANGLIOMA

Dense-core granules, even when present in small numbers, are diagnostically important in the identification of paragangliomas.

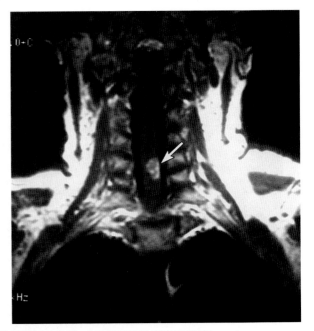

**FIGURE 11–118** METASTATIC CARCINOMA

A large pulmonary carcinoma (*arrow*) was the source of this metastasis to the spinal cord, as seen in a contrast-enhanced image.

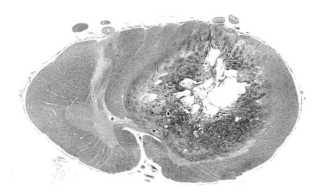

**FIGURE 11–119**   METASTATIC CARCINOMA

As in the brain, metastases to the spinal cord are usually localized to the gray matter. The primary was in the lung.

is limited virtually to cases in which only biopsies are performed or tumors are subtotally resected.[3] Metastasis to the CNS parenchyma is exceedingly uncommon.[4]

### Intramedullary Schwannoma

Small perivascular bundles of peripheral nerves normally occur within the spinal cord and logically are the source of intramedullary schwannomas.[3, 5] Short of a capsule, these rare lesions share the macroscopic and microscopic features of schwannomas that occur classically on intraspinal nerve roots.[2, 4, 6] Rare examples are melanotic.[1, 7]

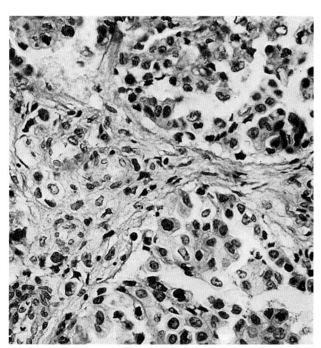

**FIGURE 11–120**   METASTATIC CARCINOMA

This uncommon example of carcinoma metastatic to the spinal cord is clearly alien tissue because of its anaplasia, epithelial appearance, and collagenous stroma. This lesion was removed from the conus medullaris of a 48-year-old man with a pulmonary primary.

### Metastatic Neoplasms

Uncommon as surgical specimens, intramedullary metastases need little comment other than a reminder that they may appear in biopsy material, usually in the setting of a known, already metastasizing cancer (Fig. 11–118).[1, 2, 4] Not surprisingly, the lung is the most common source. Anatomically, the lesion typically resides in an anterior or ventral gray horn,[2, 3] with symptoms reflecting this unilaterality (Figs. 11–119 and 11–120).[4]

### Other Intramedullary Neoplasms

There is an assortment of neoplasms that only rarely affect the spinal cord directly. Its members include germinoma,[8, 15, 22] atypical teratoid or rhabdoid tumor,[20] hamartoma,[1, 19] lipoma,[2, 13, 18] lymphomatoid granulomatosis,[6] meningioma,[21] neurocytoma,[23, 24] pleomorphic xanthoastrocytoma,[7] primary CNS lymphoma,[5, 10, 11, 14] primitive neuroectodermal tumor,[3,9] and teratoma.[4, 12, 16, 17]

## REFERENCES

**Meningioma**

1. Brown MH. Intraspinal meningiomas: a clinical and pathologic study. Arch Neurol Psychiatry 1942;47:271–292.
2. Calogero JA, Moossy J. Extradural spinal meningiomas: report of four cases. J Neurosurg 1972;37:442–447.
3. Chaparro MJ, Young RF, Smith M, et al. Multiple spinal meningiomas: a case of 47 distinct lesions in the absence of neurofibromatosis or identified chromosomal abnormality. Neurosurgery 1993;32:298–302.
4. Chen H-J, Lui C-C, Chen L. Spinal epidural meningioma in a child. Childs Nerv Syst 1992;8:465–467.
5. Cushing H, Eisenhardt L. Meningiomas—Their Classification, Regional Behavior, Life History, and Surgical End Results. Springfield, IL: Charles C Thomas, 1938.
6. Feiring EH, Barron K. Late recurrence of spinal-cord meningioma. J Neurosurg 1962;19:652–6.
7. Fournier D, Mercier P, Pouplard F, et al. Invasive character of an intradural spinal meningioma in early childhood. Childs Nerv Syst 1993;9:28–32.
8. Hassin GB. Villi (pacchionian bodies) of the spinal arachnoid. Arch Neurol Psychiatry 1930;23:65–78.
9. Holtzman RNN, Jormark SC. Nondural-based lumbar clear cell meningioma; case report. J Neurosurg 1996;84:264–266.
10. Ibrahim AW, Satti MB, Ibrahim EM. Extraspinal meningioma: case report. J Neurosurg 1986;64:328–303.
11. Kaya U, Özden B, Turantan I, et al. Spinal epidural meningioma in childhood: a case report. Neurosurgery 1982;10:746–747.
12. Klekamp J, Samii M. Surgical results for spinal meningiomas. Surg Neurol 1999;52:552–562.
13. Kumar S, Kaza RC, Maitra TK, et al. Extradural spinal meningioma arising from a nerve root. J Neurosurg 1980;52:728–729.
14. Levy W Jr, Bay J, Dohn D. Spinal cord meningioma. J Neurosurg 1982;57:804–812.
15. Motomochi M, Makita Y, Nabeshima S, et al. Spinal epidural meningioma in childhood. Surg Neurol 1980;13:5–7.
16. Patronas NJ, Brown F, Duda EE. Multiple meningiomas in the spinal canal. Surg Neurol 1980;13:78–80.
17. Roux F-X, Nataf F, Pinaudeau M, et al. Intraspinal meningiomas: review of 54 cases with discussion of poor prognosis factors and modern therapeutic management. Surg Neurol 1996;46:458–464.
18. Salvati M, Artico M, Lunardi P, et al. Intramedullary meningioma: case report and review of the literature. Surg Neurol 1992;37:42–45.
19. Zaaroor M, Borovich B, Bassan L, et al. Primary cutaneous extravertebral meningioma. J Neurosurg 1984;60:1097–1098.

20. Zorludemir S, Scheithauer BW, Hirose T, et al. Clear cell meningioma: a clinicopathologic study of a potentially aggressive variant of meningioma. Am J Surg Pathol 1995;19:493–505.

**Hemangiopericytoma**

1. Guthrie B, Ebersold M, Scheithauer B, et al. Meningeal hemangiopericytoma: histopathological features, treatment, and long-term follow-up of 44 cases. Neurosurgery 1989;25:514–522.
2. Harris DJ, Fornasier VL, Livingston KE. Hemangiopericytoma of the spinal cord: report of three cases. J Neurosurg 1978;49:914–920.
3. Mena H, Ribas JL, Pezeshkpour GH, et al. Hemangiopericytoma of the central nervous system: a review of 94 cases. Hum Pathol 1991;22:84–91.
4. Osborne DR, Dubois P, Drayer B, et al. Primary intracranial meningeal and spinal hemangiopericytoma: radiologic manifestations. Am J Neuroradiol 1981;2:69–74.

**Melanocytic Neoplasms**

1. Brat D, Giannini C, Scheithauer BW, et al. Primary melanocytic neoplasms of the central nervous system. Am J Surg Pathol 1999;23:745–754.
2. Clarke DB, Leblanc R, Bertrand G, et al. Meningeal melanocytoma. Report of a case and a historical comparison. J Neurosurg 1998;88:116–121.
3. Clifford JH, McClintock HG, Lubchenco AE. Primary spinal cord melanoma: case report. J Neurosurg 1968;29:410–413.
4. Czarnecki EJ, Silbergleit R, Gutierrez J. MR of spinal meningeal melanocytoma. AJNR 1997;18:180–182.
5. Hirano A, Carton CA. Primary malignant melanoma of the spinal cord. J Neurosurg 1960;17:935–944.
6. Kiel FW, Starr LB, Hansen JL. Primary melanoma of the spinal cord. J Neurosurg 1961;18:616–629.
7. Lach B, Russell N, Benoit B, et al. Cellular blue nevus ("melanocytoma") of the spinal meninges: electron microscopic and immunohistochemical features. Neurosurgery 1988;22:773–780.
8. Litofsky NS, Zee C-S, Breeze RE, et al. Meningeal melanocytoma: diagnostic criteria for a rare lesion. Neurosurgery 1992;31:945–948.
9. O'Brien TF, Moran M, Miller JH, et al. Meningeal melanocytoma. Arch Pathol Lab Med 1995;119:542–546.
10. Steinberg JM, Gillespie JJ, MacKay B, et al. Meningeal melanocytoma with invasion of the thoracic spinal cord. J Neurosurg 1978;48:818–824.
11. Tatagiba M, Böker D-K, Brandis A, et al. Meningeal melanocytoma of the C8 nerve root: case report. Neurosurgery 1992;31:958–961.

**Tumors of Apidose Tissue**

1. Ammerman BJ, Henry JM, De Girolami U, et al. Intradural lipomas of the spinal cord: a clinicopathologic correlation. J Neurosurg 1976;44:331–336.
2. Caram PC, Scarcella G, Carton CA. Intradural lipomas of the spinal cord: with particular emphasis on the "intramedullary" lipomas. J Neurosurg 1957;14:28–42.
3. Chitoku S, Kawai S, Watabe Y, et al. Intradural spinal hibernoma: case report. Surg Neurol 1998;49:509–513.
4. Drapkin AJ. High cervical intradural lipoma. J Neurosurg 1974;41:699–704.
5. Ehni G, Love JG. Intraspinal lipomas: report of cases, review of the literature, and clinical and pathologic study. Arch Neurol Psychiary 1945;53:1–28.
6. Endoh M, Iwasaki Y, Koyanagi I, et al. Spontaneous shrinkage of lumbosacral lipoma in conjunction with a general decrease in body fat: case report. Neurosurgery 1998;43:150–151; discussion 1–2.
7. Giuffre R. Intradural spinal lipomas: review of the literature (99 cases) and report of an additional case. Acta Neurochir (wien) 1966;14:69–95.
8. Harrison MJ, Mitnick RJ, Rosenblum BR, et al. Leptomyelolipoma: analysis of 20 cases. J Neurosurg 1990;72:360–367.
9. Knierim DS, Wacker M, Peckham N, et al. Lumbosacral intramedullary myolipoma: case report. J Neurosurg 1987;66:457–459.
10. Lassman LP, James CCM. Lumbosacral lipomas: critical survey of 26 cases submitted to laminectomy. J Neurol Neurosurg Psychiatry 1967;30:174–181.

11. Maggi G, Alberti F, Colucci MR, et al. Spinal entramedullary angiolipoma. Childs Nerv Syst 1996;12:346–349.
12. McLone DG, Naidich TP. Laser resection of fifty spinal lipomas. Neurosurgery 1986;18:611–615.
13. Pierre-Kahn A, Lacombe J, Pichon J, et al. Interspinal lipomas with spina bifida: prognosis and treatment in 73 cases. J Neurosurg 1986;65:756–761.
14. Shuangshoti S, Menakanit W. Intraspinal hibernoma. Br J Surg 1974;61:580–582.
15. Walsh JW, Markesbery WR. Histologic features of congenital lipomas of the lower spinal canal. J Neurosurg 1980;52:564–569.

**Other Primary Meningeal Tumors**

1. Alston SR, Francel PC, Jane JA Jr. Solitary fibrous tumor of the spinal cord. Am J Surg Pathol 1997;21:477–483.
2. Brunori A, Cerasoli S, Donati R, et al. Solitary fibrous tumor of the meninges: two new cases and review of the literature. Surg Neurol 1999;51:636–640.
3. Carneiro SS, Scheithauer BW, Nascimento AG, et al. Solitary fibrous tumor of the meninges: a lesion distinct from fibrous meningioma. Am J Clin Pathol 1996;106:217–224.
4. De Vries J, Scheremet R, Altmannsberger M, et al. Primary leiomyosarcoma of the spinal leptomeninges. J Neurooncol 1994;18:25–31.
5. Heye N, Iglesias JR, Tönsen K, et al. Primary leptomeningeal gliomatosis with predominant involvement of the spinal cord. Acta Neurochir (wien) 1990;102:145–148.
6. Kalyan-Raman UP, Cancilla PA, Case MJ. Solitary, primary malignant astrocytoma of the spinal leptomeninges. J Neuropathol Exp Neurol 1983;42:517–521.
7. Kidooka M, Okada T, Takayama S, et al. Primary leiomyosarcoma of the spinal dura mater. Neuroradiology 1991;33:173–174.
8. Lee S-T, Lui T-N, Tsai M-D. Primary intraspinal dura mesenchymal chondrosarcoma. Surg Neurol 1989;31:54–57.
9. Malek AM, Weller SJ, Price DL Jr, et al. Solitary fibrous tumor presenting as a symptomatic intraspinal mass: case report. Neurosurgery 1997;40:844–847.
10. Ramsay DA, Goshko V, Nag S. Primary spinal leptomeningeal astrocytoma. Acta Neuropathol (Berl) 1990;80:338–341.
11. Ranjan A, Chacko G, Joseph T, et al. Intraspinal mesenchymal chondrosarcoma. J Neurosurg 1994;80:928–930.
12. Rushing EJ, Mena H, Smirniotopoulos JG. Mesenchymal chondrosarcoma of the cauda equina. Clin Neuropathol 1995;14:150–153.
13. Scheithauer BW, Rubinstein LJ. Meningeal mesenchymal chondrosarcoma. Cancer 1978;42:2744–2752.
14. Vorster SJ, Prayson RA, Lee JH. Solitary fibrous tumor of the thoracic spine. Case report and review of the literature. J Neurosurg 2000;92:217–202.

**Metastatic Carcinoma and Lymphoma**

1. Chamberlain MC. Comparative spine imaging in leptomeningeal metastases. J Neurooncol 1995;23:233–238.
2. Chow TSF, McCutcheon IE. The surgical treatment of metastatic spinal tumors within the intradural extramedullary compartment. J Neurosurg 1996;85:225–230.
3. Diaz-Arrastia R, Younger DS, Hair L, et al. Neurolymphomatosis: a clinicopathologic syndrome re-emerges. Neurology 1992;42:1136–1141.
4. Gonzalez-Vitale JC, Garcia-Bunuel R. Meningeal carcinomatosis. Cancer 1976;37:2906–2911.
5. Griffin JW, Thompson RW, Mitchinson MJ. Lymphomatous leptomeningitis. Am J Med 1971;51:200–208.
6. Little JR, Dale AJD, Okazaki H. Meningeal carcinomatosis: clinical manifestations. Arch Neurol 1974;30:138–143.
7. Olson ME, Chernik NL, Posner JB. Infiltration of the leptomeninges by systemic cancer: a clinical and pathologic study. Arch Neurol 1974;30:122–137.
8. Parsons M. The spinal form of carcinomatous meningitis. Am J Med 1972;41:509–519.

**Seeding of Primary Intracranial Neoplasms**

1. Bryan P. CSF seeding of intracranial tumors: a study of 96 cases. Clin Radiol 1974;25:355–360.
2. Carins H, Russell DS. Intracranial and spinal metastases in gliomas of the brain. Brain 1931;54:377–420.

3. Grabb PA, Albright AL, Pang D. Dissemination of supratentorial malignant gliomas via the cerebrospinal fluid in children. Neurosurgery 1992;30:64–71.
4. Pollack IF, Hurtt M, Pang D, et al. Dissemination of low grade intracranial astrocytomas in children. Cancer 1994;73:2869–2878.
5. Polmeter FE, Kernohan JW. Meningeal gliomatosis: a study of forty-two cases. Arch Neurol Psychiatry 1947;57:593–616.
6. Schwaninger M, Patt S, Henningsen P, et al. Spinal canal metastases: a late complication of glioblastoma. J Neuroncol 1992;12:93–98.
7. Vertosick FT Jr, Selker RG. Brain stem and spinal metastases of supratentorial glioblastoma multiforme: a clinical series. Neurosurgery 1990;27:516–522.

## Cystic Lesions (All)

1. Aarabi B, Pasternack G, Hurko O, et al. Familial intradural arachnoid cysts. J Neurosurg 1979;50:826–829.
2. Bailey IC. Dermoid tumors of the spinal cord. J Neurosurg 1970;33:676–681.
3. Barkovich AJ, Edwards MSB, Cogen PH. MR evaluation of spinal dermal sinus tracts in children. AJNR 1991;12:123–129.
4. Bartels RHMA, Van Overbeeke JJ. Lumbar cerebrospinal fluid drainage for symptomatic sacral nerve root cysts: an adjuvant diagnostic procedure and/or alternative treatment? Technical case report. Neurosurgery 1997;40:861–865.
5. Bergland RM. Congenital intraspinal extradural cyst: report of three cases in one family. J Neurosurg 1968;28:495–499.
6. Birch BD, McCormick PC. High cervical split cord malformation and neurenteric cyst associated with congenital mirror movements: case report. Neurosurgery 1996;38:813–816.
7. Boyd HR. Iatrogenic intraspinal epidermoid: report of a case. J Neurosurg 1966;24:105–107.
8. Cavazzani P, Ruelle A, Michelozzi G, et al. Spinal dermoid cysts originating in intracranial fat drops causing obstructive hydrocephalus: case reports. Surg Neurol 1995;43:466–470.
9. Chen H-J, Chen L. Traumatic interdural arachnoid cyst in the upper cervical spine. J Neurosurg 1996;85:351–353.
10. Cloward RB, Bucy PC. Spinal extradural cyst and kyphosis dorsalis juvenilis. Surg Neurol 1993;39:469–473.
11. Devkota UP, Lam JMK, Ng H-K, et al. An anterior intradural neurenteric cyst of the cervical spine: complete excision through the central corpectomy approach–case report. Neurosurgery 1994;35:1150–1154.
12. Dorsey JF, Tabrisky J. Intraspinal and mediastinal foregut cyst compressing the spinal cord. Neurosurgery 1966;24:562–567.
13. Fujimura M, Tominaga T, Koshu K, et al. Cine-mode magnetic resonance imaging of a thoracic intradural arachnoid cyst: case report. Surg Neurol 1996;45:533–536.
14. Gainer JV Jr, Chou SM, Nugent GR, et al. Ependymal cyst of the thoracic spinal cord. J Neurol Neurosurg Psychiatry 1974;37:974–977.
15. Hamburger CH, Büttner A, Weiss S. Dural cysts in the cervical region. J Neurosurg 1998;89:310–313.
16. Hirano A, Ghatak NR, Wisoff HS, et al. An epithelial cyst of the spinal cord. An electron microscopic study. Acta Neuropathol (Berl) 1971;18:214–223.
17. Ho L, Tiel R. Intraspinal bronchogenic cyst: ultrastructural study of the lining epithelium. Acta Neuropathol (Berl) 1989;78:513–520.
18. Hoefnagel D, Benirschke K, Duarte J. Teratomatous cysts within the vertebral canal: observation on the occurrence of sex chromatin. J Neurol Neurosurg Psychiatry 1962;25:159–164.
19. Hoffmann GT. Cervical arachnoidal cyst. Report of a 6-year old negro male with recovery from quadriplegia. J Neurosurg 1960;17:327–303.
20. Iwahashi H, Kawai S, Watabe Y, et al. Spinal intramedullary ependymal cyst: a case report. Surg Neurol 1999;52:357–361.
21. Kim C-Y, Wang K-C, Choe G, et al. Neurenteric cyst: its various presentations. Childs Nerv Syst 1999;15:333–341.
22. King AB. Intramedullary epidermoid tumor of the spinal cord. J Neurosurg 1957;14:353–357.
23. Knight G, Griffiths T, Williams I. Gastrocystoma of the spinal cord. Br J Surg 1955;42:635–638.
24. Lake PA, Minckler J, Scanlan RL. Spinal epidural cyst: theories of pathogenesis. J Neurosurg 1974;40:774–778.
25. LeDoux MS, Faye-Petersen OM, Aronin PA, et al. Lumbosacral neurenteric cyst in an infant. J Neurosurg 1993;78:821–825.
26. MacDonald RL, Schwartz ML, Lewis AJ. Neurenteric cyst located dorsal to the cervical spine: case report. Neurosurgery 1991;28:583–588.
27. Manno NJ, Uihlein A, Kernohan JW. Intraspinal epidermoids. J Neurosurg 1962;19:754–765.
28. Matson DD, Jerva MJ. Recurrent meningitis associated with congenital lumbo-sacral dermal sinus tract. J Neurosurg 1966;25:288–297.
29. Matsushima T, Fukui M, Egami H. Epithelial cells in a so-called intraspinal neurenteric cyst: a light and electron microscopic study. Surg Neurol 1985;24:656–660.
30. Mendel E, Lese GB, Gonzalez-Gomez I, et al. Isolated lumbosacral neurenteric cyst with partial sacral agenesis: case report. Neurosurgery 1994;35:1159–1163.
31. Menezes AH, Ryken TC. Craniocervical intradural neurenteric cysts. Pediatr Neurosurg 1995;22:88–95.
32. Millis RR, Holmas AE. Enterogenous cyst of the spinal cord with associated intestinal reduplication, vertebral anomalies, and a dorsal dermal sinus. J Neurosurg 1973;38:73–77.
33. Morita Y, Kinoshita K, Wakisaka S, et al. Claws of cilia: further observation of ciliated epithelium in neurenteric cyst. Virchows Arch [A] 1991;418:263–265.
34. Morita Y, Kinoshita K, Wakisaka S, et al. Fine surface structure of an intraspinal neurenteric cyst: a scanning and transmission electron microscopy study. Neurosurgery 1990;27:829–833.
35. Nathan H, Rosner S. Multiple meningeal diverticula and cysts associated with duplications of the sheaths of spinal nerve posterior roots. J Neurosurg 1977;47:68–72.
36. Paulsen RD, Call GA, Murtagh FR. Prevalence and percutaneous drainage of cysts of the sacral nerve root sheath (Tarlov cysts). AJNR 1994;15:293–297.
37. Prasad VSSV, Reddy DR, Murty JMK. Cervico-thoracic neurenteric cyst: clinicoradiological correlation with embryogenesis. Childs Nerv Syst 1996;12:48–51.
38. Rewcastle NB, Francoeur J. Teratomatous cysts of the spinal canal: with "sex chromatin" studies. Arch Neurol 1964;11:91–99.
39. Rhaney K, Barclay GPT. Enterogenous cysts and cogential diverticula of the alimentary canal with abnormalities of the vertebral column and spinal cord. J Pathol Bacteriol 1959;77:457–471.
40. Rohrer DC, Burchiel KJ, Gruber DP. Intraspinal extradural meningeal cyst demonstrating ball-valve mechanism of formation. J Neurosurg 1993;78:122–125.
41. Rosenbaum TJ, Soule EH, Onofrio BM. Teratomatous cyst of the spinal canal. J Neurosurg 1978;49:292–297.
42. Roux A, Mercier C, Larbrisseau A, et al. Intramedullary epidermoid cysts of the spinal cord. Case report. J Neurosurg 1992;76:528–533.
43. Sakai K, Sakamoto K, Kobayashi N, et al. Dermoid cyst within an upper thoracic meningocele. Surg Neurol 1996;45:287–292.
44. Scearce TA, Shaw C-M, Bronstein AD, et al. Intraventricular fat from a ruptured sacral dermoid cyst: clinical, radiographic, and pathologic correlation: case report. J Neurosurg 1993;78:666–668.
45. Shimizu H, Tominaga T, Takahashi A, et al. Cine magnetic resonance imaging of spinal intradural arachnoid cysts. Neurosurgery 1997;41:95–100.
46. Tarlov IM. Spinal perineurial and meningeal cysts. J Neurol Neusurg Psychiatry 1970;33:833–843.
47. Uemura K, Yoshizawa T, Matsumura A, et al. Spinal extradural meningeal cyst: case report. J Neurosurg 1996;85:354–356.
48. Van de Kelft E, Van Vyve M. Chronic perineal pain related to sacral meningeal cysts. Neurosurgery 1991;29:223–226.
49. Whiting DM, Chou SM, Lanzieri CF, et al. Cervical neurenteric cyst associated with Klippel-Feil syndrome: a case report and review of the literature. Clin Neuropathol 1991;10:285–290.
50. Yamashita J, Maloney AFJ, Harris P. Intradural spinal bronchiogenic cyst. J Neurosurg 1973;39:240–245.

## Inflammatory Lesions

1. Ashkenzai E, Constantini S, Pappo S, et al. Hypertrophic spinal pachymeningitis: report of two cases and review of the literature. Neurosurgery 1991;28:730–732.
2. Day AL, Sypert GW. Spinal cord sarcoidosis. Ann Neurol 1977;1:79–85.
3. Graf M, Wakhloo A, Schmidtke K, et al. Sarcoidosis of the spinal cord and medulla oblongata. A pathological and neuroradiological case report. Clin Neuropathol 1994;13:19–25.

4. Jallo GI, Zagzag D, Lee M, et al. Intraspinal sarcoidosis: diagnosis and management. Surg Neurol 1997;48:514–521.
5. Lin S-K, Wu T, Wai Y-Y. Case report; intramedullary spinal tuberculomas during treatment of tuberculous meningitis. Clin Neurol Neurosurgery 1994;96:71–78.
6. Mikawa Y, Watanabe R, Hino Y, et al. Hypertrophic spinal pachymeningitis. Spine 1994;19:620–625.
7. Rosenfeld JV, Kaye AH, Davis S, et al. Pacymeningitis cervicalis hypertrophica: case report. J Neurosurg 1987;66:137–139.
8. Scully RE (ed). Weekly clinicopathological exercises; case 8-1998. Case record of the Massachusetts General Hospital. N Engl J Med 1998;338:747–754.
9. Terunuma H, Konno H, Iizuka H, et al. Sarcoidosis presenting as progressive myelopathy. Clin Neuropathol 1998;7:77–80.

**Arachnoid Plaques**

1. McCulloch GAJ. Arachnoid calcification producing spinal cord compression. J Neurol Neurosurg Psychiatry 1975;38:1059–1062.
2. Nagpal RD, Gokhale SD, Parikh VR. Ossification of spinal arachnoid with unrelated syringomyelia: case report. J Neurosurg 1975;42:222–225.
3. Nizzoli V, Testa C. A case of calcification in the spinal arachnoid giving rise to spinal cord compression. J Neurol Sci 1968;7:381–384.

**Schwannoma, Melanocytic Schwannoma, and Neurofibroma**

1. Abernathy CD, Onofrio BM, Scheithauer, B, et al. Surgical management of giant sacral schwannomas. J Neurosurg 1986;65:286–295.
2. Bagchi AK, Sarkar SK, Chakraborti DP, et al. Melanotic spinal schwannoma. Surg Neurol 1975;3:79–81.
3. Carneiro SS, Scheithauer BW, Nascimento AG, et al. Solitary fibrous tumor of the meninges: a lesion distinct from fibrous meningioma. A clinicopathologic and immunohistochemical study. Am J Clin Pathol 1996;106:217–224.
4. Carney JA. Psmmomatous melanotic schwannoma. A distinctive, heritable tumor with special associations, including cardiac myxoma and the Cushing syndrome. Am J Surg Pathol 1990;14:206–222.
5. Casadei GP, Scheithauer BW, Hirose T, et al. Cellular schwannoma. A clinicopathologic, DNA flow cytometric, and proliferation marker study of 70 patients. Cancer 1995;75:1109–1119.
6. Daras M, Koppel BS, Heise CW, et al. Multiple spinal intradural schwannomas in the absence of von Recklinghausen's disease. Spine 1993;18:2556–2559.
7. Deruaz JP, Janzer RC, Costa J. Cellular schwannomas of the intracranial and intraspinal compartment: morphological and immunological characteristics compared with classical benign schwannomas. J Neuropathol Exp Neurol 1993;52:114–118.
8. Egelhoff JC, Bates DJ, Ross JS, et al. Spinal MR findings in neurofibromatosis types 1 and 2. AJNR 1992;13:1071–1077.
9. Killeen RM, Davy CL, Bauserman SC. Melanocytic schwannoma. Cancer 1988;62:174–183.
10. Kleamp J, Samii M. Surgery of spinal nerve sheath tumors with special reference to neurofibromatosis. Neurosurgery 1998;42:279–290.
11. Limas C, Tio FO. Meningeal melanocytoma ("melanotic meningioma"). Its melanocytic origin as revealed by electron microscopy. Cancer 1972;30:1286–1294.
12. Lowman RM, LiVolsi VA. Pigmented (melanotic) schwannomas of the spinal canal. Cancer 1980;46:391–397.
13. MacCollin M, Woodfin W, Kronn D, et al. Schwannomatosis: a clinical and pathologic study. Neurology 1996;46:1072–1079.
14. Mandybur TI. Melanotic nerve sheath tumors. J Neurosurg 1974;41:187–192.
15. Marchese MJ, McDonald JV. Intramedullary melanotic schwannoma of the cervical spinal cord. Surg Neurol 1990;33:353–355.
16. Mennemeyer RP, Hallman KO, Hammar SP, et al. Melanotic schwannoma: clinical and ultrastructural studies of three cases with evidence of intracellular melanin synthesis. Am J Surg Pathol 1979;3:3–10.
17. Nadkarni TD, Rekate HL, Coons SW. Plexiform neurofibroma of the cauda equina. Case report. J Neurosurg 1999;91:112–115.
18. Pollack IF, Colak A, Fitz C, et al. Surgical management of spinal cord compression from plexiform neurofibromas in patients with neurofibromatosis 1. Neurosurgery 1998;43:248–256.

19. Seppälä MT, Halti MJJ. Spinal malignant nerve-sheath tumor or cellular schwannoma? A striking difference in prognosis. J Neurosurg 1993;79:528–532.
20. Seppälä MT, Haltia MJJ, Sankila RJ, et al. Long-term outcome after removal of spinal neurofibroma. J Neurosurg 1995;82:572–577.
21. Seppälä MT, Haltia MJJ, Sankila RJ, et al. Long-term outcome after removal of spinal schwannoma: a clinicopathological study of 187 cases. J Neurosurg 1995;83:621–626.
22. Shiono T, Yoshikawa K, Iwasaki N. Huge lumbar spinal cystic neurinomas with unusual MR findings. AJNR 1995;16:881–882.
23. Thomeer RT, Bots GT, Van Dulken H, et al. Neurofibrosarcoma of the cauda equina: case report. J Neurosurg 1981;54:409–411.
24. Winek RR, Scheithauer BW, Wick MR. Meningioma, meningeal hemangiopericytoma (angioblastic meningioma), peripheral hemangiopericytoma, and acoustic schwannoma. A comparative immunohistochemical study. Am J Surg Pathol 1989;13:251–261.

**Other Primary Neoplasms of Spinal Nerve Roots**

1. Mitchell A, Scheithauer BW, Sasano H, et al. Symptomatic intradural adrenal adenoma of the spinal nerve root: report of two cases. Neurosurgery 1993;32:658–661; discussion 61–62.

**Congenital Malformations**

1. Brown PG, Shaver EG. Myolipoma in a tethered cord. Case report and review of the literature. J Neurosurg 2000;92:214–216.
2. Gokay H, Barlas O, Hepgul KT, et al. Tethered cord in the adult mimicking the lumbar disc syndrome: report of two cases. Surg Neurol 1993;39:440–442.
3. Gupta SK, Khosla VK, Sharma BS, et al. Tethered cord syndrome in adults. Surg Neurol 1999;52:362–370.
4. Hall WA, Albright AL, Brunberg JA. Diagnosis of tethered cords by magnetic resonance imaging. Surg Neurol 1988;30:60–64.
5. Inoue HK, Kobayashi S, Ohbayashi K, et al. Treatment and prevention of tethered and retethered spinal cord using a Gore-Tex surgical membrane. J Neurosurg 1994;80:689–693.
6. Iskandar BJ, Fulmer BB, Hadley MN, et al. Congenital tethered spinal cord syndrome in adults. J Neurosurg 1998;88:958–961.
7. McLendon RE, Oakes WJ, Heinz ER, et al. Adipose tissue in the filum terminale: a computed tomographic finding that may indicate tethering of the spinal cord. Neurosurgery 1988;22:873–876.
8. Molleston MC, Roth KA, Wippold FJ II, et al. Tethered cord syndrome from a choristoma of müllerian origin. J Neurosurg 1991;74:497–500.
9. Pang D, Wilberger JE Jr. Tethered cord syndrome in adults. J Neurosurg 1982;57:32–47.
10. Raghavan N, Barkovich AJ, Edwards M, et al. MR imaging in the tethered spinal cord syndrome. AJR 1989;152:843–862.
11. Rougier A, Vital C, Caillaud P. Uterus-like mass of the conus medullaris with associated tethered cord. Neurosurgery 1993;33:328–331.
12. Scully RE (ed). Case records of the Massachusetts General Hospital: case 47-1992. N Engl J Med 1992;327:1581–1588.
13. Simon RH, Donaldson JO, Ramsby GR. Tethered spinal cord in adult siblings. Neurosurgery 1981;8:241–244.
14. Warder DE, Oakes WJ. Tethered cord syndrome and the conus in a normal position. Neurosurgery 1993;33:374–378.
15. Warder DE, Oakes WJ. Tethered cord syndrome: the low-lying and normally positioned conus. Neurosurgery 1994;34:597–600.

**Demyelinating Disease and Transverse Myelopathy (Myelitis)**

1. Baudoin D, Gambarelli D, Gayraud D, et al. Devic's neuromyelitis optica: a clinicopathological review of the literature in connection with a case showing fatal dysautonomia. Clin Neuropathol 1998;17:175–183.
2. Berlit P, Schwechheimer K. Neuropathological findings in radiation myelopathy of the lumbosacral cord. Eur Neurol 1987;27:29–34.
3. Campi A, Filippi M, Comi G, et al. Acute transverse myelopathy: spinal and cranial MR study with clinical follow-up. AJNR 1995;16:115–123.
4. Choi KH, Leeks, Chung SO, et al. Idiopathic transverse myelitis: MR characteristics. AJNR 1996;17:1151–1160.
5. Deodhar AA, Hochenedel T, Bennett RM. Longitudinal involvement of the spinal cord in a patient with lupus related transverse myelitis. J Rheumatol 1999;26:446–449.

6. Itabashi HH, Bebin J, DeJong RN. Postirradiation cervical myelopathy. Report of two cases. Neurology 1957;7:844–852.
7. Jeffery DR, Mandler RN, Davis LE. Transverse myelitis: retrospective analysis of 33 cases, with differentiation of cases associated with multiple sclerosis and parainfectious events. Arch Neurol 1993;50:532–535.
8. Kuzma BB, Goodman JM. Spinal cord swelling and brain lesions in lupus myelitis. Surg Neurol 1997;48:200–202.
9. Phuphanich S, Jacobs M, Murtagh FR, et al. MRI of spinal cord radiation necrosis simulating recurrent cervical cord astrocytoma and syringomyelia. Surg Neurol 1996;45:362–365.
10. Provenzale J, Bouldin TW. Lupus-related myelopathy: report of three cases and review of the literature. J Neurol Neurosurg Psychiatry 1992;55:830–835.
11. Provenzale JM, Barboriak DP, Gaensler EHL, et al. Lupus-related myelitis: serial MR findings. AJNR 1994;15:1911–1917.
12. Rosenfeld J, Taylor CL, Atlas SW. Myelitis following chickenpox: a case report. Neurology 1993;43:1834–1836.
13. Schultheiss TE, Stephens LC, Maor MH. Analysis of the histopathology of radiation myelopathy. Int J Radiat Oncol Biol Phys 1988;14:27–32.
14. Simeon-Aznar CP, Tolosa-Vilella C, Cuenca-Luque R, et al. Transverse myelitis in systemic lupus erythematosus: two cases with magnetic resonance imaging. Br J Rheumatol 1992;31:555–558.
15. Simnad VI, Pisani DE, Rose JW. Multiple sclerosis presenting as transverse myelopathy: clinical and MRI features. Neurology 1997;48:65–73.
16. Tartaglino LM, Friedman DP, Flanders AE, et al. Multiple sclerosis in the spinal cord: MR appearance and correlation with clinical parameters. Radiology 1995;195:725–732.
17. Tartaglino LM, Heiman-Patterson T, Friedman DP, et al. MR imaging in a case of postvaccination myelitis. AJNR 1995;16:581–582.
18. Zagzag D, Miller DC, Kleinman GM, et al. Demyelinating disease versus tumor in surgical neuropathology. Am J Surg Pathol 1993;17:537–545.

## Other Inflammatory Disorders

1. Arseni C, Samitca DC-T. Intraspinal tuberculous granuloma. Brain 1960;83:285–292.
2. Bartels RHMA, Gonera EG, Van der Spek JAN, et al. Intramedullary spinal cord abscess. A case report. Spine 1995;20:1199–1204.
3. Bingöl A, Yücemen N, Meco O. Medically treated intraspinal "Brucella" granuloma. Surg Neurol 1999;52:570–576.
4. Budzilovich GN, Most H, Feigin I. Pathogenesis and latency of spinal cord schistosomiasis. Arch Pathol 1964;77:383–388.
5. Byrne RW, Von Roenn KA, Whisler WW. Intramedullary abscess: a report of two cases and a review of the literature. Neurosurgery 1994;35:321–326.
6. Carton CA, Mount LA. Neurosurgical aspects of cryptococcosis. J Neurosurg 1951;8:143–156.
7. Castillo M, Quencer RM, Post MJD. MR of intramedullary spinal cysticercosis. AJNR 1988;9:393–395.
8. Chitoku S, Kawai S, Watabe Y, et al. Multiple intramedullary spinal sarcoidosis: case report. Surg Neurol 1997;48:522–526.
9. Corral I, Quereda C, Moreno A, et al. Intramedullary cysticercosis cured with drug treatment. A case report. Spine 1996;21:2284–2287.
10. Dastur DK, Wadia NH. Spinal meningitides with radiculomyelopathy: part 2. Pathology and pathogenesis. J Neurol Sci 1969;8:261–297.
11. Day AL, Sypert GW. Spinal cord sarcoidosis. Ann Neurol 1977;1:79–85.
12. Erlich JH, Rosenfeld JV, Fuller A, et al. Acute intramedullary spinal cord abscess: case report. Surg Neurol 1992;38:287–290.
13. Giovanni MA, Eskin TA, Mukherji SK, et al. Granulomatous angiitis of the spinal cord: a case report. Neurosurgery 1994;34:540–543.
14. Glantz MJ, Biran H, Myers ME, et al. The radiographic diagnosis and treatment of paraneoplastic central nervous system disease. Cancer 1994;73:168–175.
15. Graf M, Wakhloo A, Schimidtke K, et al. Sarcoidosis of the spinal cord and medulla oblongata. A pathological and neuroradiological case report. Clin Neuropathol 1994;13:19–25.

16. Hamilton B, Connolly ES, Mitchell WT Jr. Isolated intramedullary histiocytosis-X of the cervical spinal cord. Case report. J Neurosurg 1995;83:716–718.
17. Holtzman RNN, Hughes JEO, Sachdev RK, et al. Intramedullary cysticercosis. Surg Neurol 1986;26:187–191.
18. Jallo GI, Zagzag D, Lee M, et al. Intraspinal sarcoidosis: diagnosis and management. Surg Neurol 1997;48:514–521.
19. Jenkins RB. Intradural spinal tuberculoma with genitourinary symptoms. Arch Neurol 1963;8:539–543.
20. Koppel BS, Daras M, Duffy KR. Intramedullary spinal cord abscess. Neurosurgery 1990;26:145–146.
21. Ley A Jr, Marti A. Intramedullary hydatid cyst. Case report. J Neurosurg 1970;33:457–459.
22. Lin S-K, Wu T, Wai Y-Y. Intramedullary spinal tuberculomas during treatment of tuberculous meningitis. Clin Neurol Neurosurg 1994;96:71–78.
23. Liu LX. Spinal and cerebral schistosomiasis. Semin Neurol 1993;13:189–199.
24. Martin CA, Murali R, Trasi SS. Spinal cord sarcoidosis. Case report. J Neurosurg 1984;61:981–982.
25. Mohanty A, Venkatrama SK, Das S, et al. Spinal intramedullary cysticercosis. Neurosurgery 1997;40:82–78.
26. Nagai H, Ohtsubo K, Shimada H. Sarcoidosis of the spinal cord. Report of an autopsy case and review of the literature. Acta Pathol Jpn 1985;35:1007–1022.
27. Osenbach RK. Isolated extranodal sinus histiocytosis presenting as an intramedullary spinal cord tumor with paraplegia. J Neurosurg 1996;85:692–696.
28. Queiroz LDS, Filho AP, Callegaro D, et al. Intramedullary cysticercosis. Case report, literature review and comments on pathogenesis. J Neurol Sci 1975;26:61–70.
29. Ramamurthi B, Anguli VC. Intramedullary cryptococcic granuloma of the spinal cord. J Neurosurg 1954;11:622–624.
30. Rand CW. Coccidioidal granuloma. Report of two cases simulating tumor of the spinal cord. Arch Neurol Psychiatry 1930;23:502–511.
31. Ratkliff JK, Connolly ES. Intramedullary tuberculoma of the spinal cord. Case report and review of the literature. J Neurosurg 1999;90:125–128.
32. Resnick DK, Comey CH, Welch WC, et al. Isolated toxoplasmosis of the thoracic spinal cord in a patient with acquired immunodeficiency syndrome. Case report. J Neurosurg 1995;82:493–496.
33. Rifaat M, El-Shafei I, Samra K, et al. Intramedullary spinal abscess following spinal puncture. Case report. J Neurosurg 1973;38:366–367.
34. Rogg JM, Benzil DL, Haas RL, et al. Intramedullary abscess, an unusual manifestation of a dermal sinus. AJNR 1993;14:1393–1395.
35. Scully RE (ed). Case records of the Massassachusetts General Hospital: case 47-1996. N Engl J Med 1996;334:382–389.
36. Selwa LM, Brunberg JA, Mandell SH, et al. Spinal cord schistosomiasis: a pediatric case mimicking intrinsic cord neoplasm. Neurology 1991;41:755–757.
37. Tacconi L, Arulampalam T, Johnston FG, et al. Intramedullary spinal cord abscess: case report. Neurosurgery 1995;37:817–819.
38. Terunuma H, Konno H, Iizuka H, et al. Sarcoidosis presenting as progressive myelopathy. Clin Neuropathol 1988;7:77–80.
39. Ueki K, Parisi JE, Onofrio BM. Schistosoma mansoni infection involving the spinal cord. J Neurosurg 1995;82:1065–1067.
40. Venkataramana NK, Jain VK, Das BS, et al. Intramedullary cysticercosis. Clin Neurol Neurosurg 1989;91:337–341.
41. Vighetto A, Fischer G, Collet P et al. Intramedullary sarcoidosis of the cervical spinal cord. J Neurol Neurosurg Psychaiatry 1985;48:477–479.
42. Yoong MF, Blumbergs PC, North JB. Primary (granulomatous) angiitis of the central nervous system with multiple aneurysms of spinal arteries. J Neurosurg 1993;79:603–607.

## Vascular Malformations

1. Bao Y-H, Ling F. Classification and therapeutic modalities of spinal vascular malformations in 80 patients. Neurosurgery 1997;40:75–81.
2. Bret P, Salzmann M, Bascoulergue Y, et al. Dural arteriovenous fistula of the posterior fossa draining into the spinal medullary veins—an unusual cause of myelopathy: case report. Neurosurgery 1994;35:965–969.

3. Canavero S, Pagni CA, Duca S, et al. Spinal intramedullary cavernous angiomas: a literature metaanalysis. Surg Neurol 1994;41:381–388.
4. Cantore G, Delfini R, Cervoni L, et al. Intramedullary cavernous angiomas of the spinal cord: report of six cases. Surg Neurol 1995;43:448–452.
5. Connolly ES Jr, Zubay GP, McCormick PC, et al. The posterior approach to a series of glomus (type II) intramedullary spinal cord arteriovenous malformations. Neurosurgery 1998;42:774–786.
6. Cristante L, Herrmann H-D. Radical excision of intramedullary cavernous angiomas. Neurosurgery 1998;43:424–431.
7. Furuya K, Sasaki T, Suzuki I, et al. Intramedullary angiographically occult vascular malformations of the spinal cord. Neurosurgery 1996;39:1123–1132.
8. Harrison MJ, Eisenberg MB, Ullman JS, et al. Symptomatic cavernous malformations affecting the spine and spinal cord. Neurosurgery 1995;37:195–205.
9. Lee TT, Gromelski EB, Bowen BC, et al. Diagnostic and surgical management of spinal dural arteriovenous fistulas. Neurosurgery 1998;43:242–247.
10. Montine TJ, O'Keane JC, Eskin TA, et al. Vascular malformations presenting as spinal cord neoplasms: case report. Neurosurgery 1995;36:194–198.
11. Ogilvy CS, Louis DN, Ojemann RG. Intramedullary cavernous angiomas of the spinal cord: clinical presentation, pathological features, and surgical management. Neurosurgery 1992;31:219–280.
12. Pagni CA, Canavero S, Forni M. Report of a cavernoma of the cauda equina and review of the literature. Surg Neurol 1990;33:124–131.
13. Rosenblum B, Oldfield EH, Doppman JL, et al. Spinal arteriovenous malformations: a comparison of dural arteriovenous fistulas and intradural AVM's in 81 patients. J Neurosurg 1987;67:795–802.
14. Schwartz TH, Chang Y, Stein BM. Unusual intramedullary vascular lesion: report of two cases. Neurosurgery 1997;40:1295–1301.
15. Sharma R, Rout D, Radhakrishnan VV. Intradural spinal cavernomas. Br J Neurosurg 1992;6:351–356.
16. Symon L, Kuyama H, Kendall B. Dural arteriovenous malformations of the spine: clinical features and surgical results in 55 cases. J Neurosurg 1984;60:238–247.
17. Versari PP, D'Aliberti G, Talamonti G, et al. Progressive myelopathy caused by intracranial dural arteriovenous fistula: report of two cases and review of the literature. Neurosurgery 1993;33:914–918.
18. Vishteh AG, Sankhla S, Anson JA, et al. Surgical resection of intramedullary spinal cord cavernous malformations: delayed complications, long-term outcomes, and association with cryptic venous malformations. Neurosurgery 1997;41:1094–1101.

### Astrocytic Neoplasms

1. Alvisi C, Cerisoli M, Giulioni M. Intramedullary spinal gliomas: long-term results of surgical treatments. Acta Neurochir (Wien) 1984;70:169–179.
2. Andrews AA, Enriques L, Renaudin J, et al. Spinal intramedullary glioblastoma with intracranial seeding. Arch Neurol 1978;35:244–245.
3. Boufett E, Pierre-Kahn A, Marchal JC, et al. Prognostic factors in pediatric spinal cord astrocytoma. Cancer 1998;83:2391–2399.
4. Ciappetta P, Salvati M, Capoccia G, et al. Spinal glioblastomas: report of seven cases and review of the literature. Neurosurgery 1991;28:302–306.
5. Clifton MD, Ammromin GD, Perry MC, et al. Spinal cord glioma following irradiation for Hodgkin's disease. Cancer 1980;45:2051–2055.
6. Cohen AR, Wisoff JH, Allen JC, et al. Malignant astrocytomas of the spinal cord. J Neurosurg 1989;70:50–54.
7. Cristante L, herrmann H-D. Surgical management of intramedullary spinal cord tumors: functional outcome and sources of morbidity. Neurosurgery 1994;35:69–76.
8. Epstein F, Epstein N. Surgical treatment of spinal cord astrocytomas of childhood. J Neurosurg 1982;57:685–689.
9. Epstein FJ, Farmer J-P, Freed D. Adult intramedullary astrocytomas of the spinal cord. J Neurosurg 1992;77:355–359.
10. Guidetti B, Mercuri S, Vagnozzi R. Long-term results of the surgical treatment of 129 intramedullary spinal gliomas. J Neurosurg 1981;54:323–330.
11. Jyothirmayi R, Madhavan J, Nair MK et al. Conservative surgery and radiotherapy in the treatment of spinal cord astrocytoma. J Neurooncol 1997;33:205–211.
12. Minehan KJ, Shaw EG, Scheithauer BW, et al. Spinal cord astrocytoma: pathological and treatment considerations. J Neurosurg 1995;83:590–595.
13. O'Sullivan C, Jenkin RD, Doherty MA, et al. Spinal cord tumors in children: long-term results of combined surgical and radiation treatment. J Neurosurg 1994;81:507–512.
14. Rauhut F, Reinhardt V, Budach V, et al. Intramedullary pilocytic astrocytomas—a clinical and morphological study after combined surgical and photon or neutron therapy. Neurosurg Rev 1989;12:309–313.
15. Reimer R, Onofrio BM. Astrocytomas of the spinal cord in children and adolescents. J Neurosurg 1985;63:669–675.
16. Rossitch E Jr, Zeidman SM, Burger PC, et al. Clinical and pathological analysis of spinal cord astrocytomas in children. Neurosurgery 1990;27:193–196.
17. Sandler HM, Papadopoulos SM, Thornton AF Jr, et al. Spinal cord astrocytomas: results of therapy. Neurosurgery 1992;30:490–493.
18. Tijssen CC, Sluzewski M. Spinal astrocytoma with intracranial metastases. J Neurooncol 1994;18:49–52.

### Ependymomas

1. Anderson MS. Myxopapillary ependymomas presenting in the soft tissue over the sacrococcygeal region. Cancer 1966;19:585–590.
2. Bardella L, Artico M, Nucci F. Intramedullary subependymoma of the cervical spinal cord. Surg Neurol 1988;29:326–329.
3. Davis C, Barnard RO. Malignant behavior of myxopapillary ependymoma. J Neurosurg 1985;62:925–929.
4. Friede RL, Pollak A. The cytogenetic basis for classifying ependymomas. J Neuropathol Exp Neurol 1978;37:103–118.
5. Gagliardi FM, Cervoni L, Domenicucci M, et al. Ependymomas of the filum terminale in childhood: report of four cases and review of the literature. Childs Nerv Syst 1993;9:3–6.
6. Ho K-L. Microtubular aggregates within rough endoplasmic reticulum in myxopapillary ependymoma of the filum terminale. Arch Pathol Lab Med 1990;114:956–960.
7. Hoshimaru M, Koyama T, Hashimoto N, et al. Results of microsurgical treatment for intramedullary spinal cord ependymomas: analysis of 36 cases. Neurosurgery 1999;44:264–269.
8. Jallo GI, Zagzag D, Epstein F. Intramedullary subependymoma of the spinal cord. Neurosurgery 1996;38:251–257.
9. Kahan H, Sklar EML, Post MJD, et al. MR characteristics of histopathologic subtypes of spinal ependymoma. AJNR 1996;17:143–150.
10. Katoh S, Ikata T, Inoue A, et al. Intradural extramedullary ependymoma. A case report. Spine 1995;20:2036–2038.
11. Lee M, Rezai AR, Freed D, et al. Intramedullary spinal cord tumors in neurofibromatosis. Neurosurgery 1996;38:32–37.
12. Maruyama R, Koga K, Nakahara T, et al. Cerebral myxopapillary ependymoma. Hum Pathol 1992;23:960–962.
13. Matsumura A, Hori A, Spoerri O. Spinal subependymoma presenting as an extramedullary tumor: case report. Neurosurgery 1988;23:115–117.
14. Mavroudis C, Townsend JJ, Wilson CB. A metastasizing ependymoma of the cauda equina. J Neurosurg 1977;47:771–775.
15. Morantz RA, Kepes JJ. Extraspinal ependymomas: report of three cases. J Neurosurg 1979;51:383–391.
16. Moser FG, Tuvia J, LaSalla P, et al. Ependymoma of the spinal nerve root: case report. Neurosurgery 1992;31:962–964.
17. O'Sullivan C, Jenkin RD, Doherty MA, et al. Spinal cord tumors in children: long-term results of combined surgical and radiation treatment. J Neurosurg 1994;81:507–512.
18. Pagni CA, Canavero S, Giordana MT, et al. Spinal intramedullary subependymomas: case report and review of the literature. Neurosurgery 1992;30:115–117.
19. Prayson RA. Myxopapillary ependymomas: a clincopathologic study of 14 cases including MIB-1 and p53 immunoreactivity. Mod Pathol 1997;10:304–310.
20. Pulitzer DR, Martin PC, Collins PC, et al. Subcutaneous sacrococcygeal ("myxopapillary") ependymal rests. Am J Surg Pathol 1988;12:672–677.
21. Salvati M, Raco A, Artico M, et al. Subependymoma of the spinal cord: case report and review of the literature. Neurosurg Rev 1992;15:65–69.

22. Schweitzer JS, Batzdorf U. Ependymoma of the cauda equina region: diagnosis, treatment, and outcome in 15 patients. Neurosurgery 1992;30:202–207.
23. Soeur M, Monseu G, Ketelbant P, et al. Intramedullary ependymoma producing collagen: a clinical and patholgical study. Acta Neuropathol 1979;47:159–160.
24. Sonneland PRL, Scheithauer BW, Onofrio BM. Myxopapillary ependymoma: a clinicopathologic and immunocytochemical study of 77 cases. Cancer 1985;56:883–893.
25. Specht CS, Smith TW, DeGirolami U, et al. Myxopapillary ependymoma of the filum terminale: a light and electron microscopic study. Cancer 1986;58:310–317.
26. Takahashi H, Goto J, Emura I, et al. Lipidized (foamy) tumor cells in a spinal cord ependymoma with collagenous metaplasia. Acta Neuropathol (Berl) 1998;95:421–425.
27. Vagaiwala MR, Robinson JS, Galicich JH, et al. Metastasizing extradural ependymoma of the sacrococcygeal region: case report and review of literature. Cancer 1979;44:326–333.
28. Wagle WA, Jaufman B, Mincy JE. Intradural extramedullary ependymoma: MR-pathologic correlation. J Compnt Assist Tomogr 1988;12:705–707.
29. Wen B-C, Hussey DH, Hitchon PW, et al. The role of radiation therapy in the management of ependymomas of the spinal cord. Int J Radiat Oncol Biol Phys 1991;20:781–786.
30. Woesler B, Moskopp D, Kuchelmeister K, et al. Intracranial metastasis of a spinal myxopapillary ependymoma. A case report. Neurosurg Rev 1998;21:62–65.
31. Wolff M, Santiago H, Duby MM. Delayed distant metastasis from a subcutaneous sacrococcygeal ependymoma. Cancer 1972;30:1046–1067.
32. Zec N, De Girolami U, Schofield DE, et al. Giant cell ependymoma of the filum terminale: a report of two cases. Am J Surg Pathol 1996;20:1091–1101.

### Oligodendroglioma

1. Alvisi C, Cerisoli M, Giulioni M. Intramedullary spinal gliomas: long-term results of surgical treatments. Acta Neurochir (Wien) 1984;70:169–179.
2. Cristante L, Herrmann H-D. Surgical management of intramedullary spinal cord tumors: functional outcome and sources of morbidity. Neurosurgery 1994;35:69–76.
3. Eneström S, Gröntoft O. Oligodendroglioma of the spinal cord: report of one case. Acta Pathol Microbiol Scand 1957;40:396–400.
4. Garcia JH, Lemmi H. Ultrastructure of oligodendroglioma of the spinal cord. Am J Clin Pathol 1970;54:757–765.
5. Gilmer-Hill HS, Ellis WG, Imbesi SG, et al. Spinal oligodendroglioma with gliomatosis in a child. Case report. J Neurosurg 2000;92:109–113.
6. O'Brien CP, Lehrer HZ, Harkin JC. Extensive oligodendrogliomas of the spinal cord with associated bone changes. Neurology 1968;18:887–890.
7. Russell JR, Bucy PC. Oligodendroglioma of the spinal cord. J Neurosurg 1949;6:433–437.
8. Slooff JL, Kernohan JW, MacCarty CS. Primary Intramedullary Tumors of the Spinal Cord and Filum Terminale. Philadelphia: WB Saunders, 1964.

### Ganglion Cell Tumors

1. Azzarelli B, Luerssen TG, Wolfe TM. Intramedullary secretory gangliocytoma. Acta Neuropathol (Berl) 1991;82:402–407.
2. Hamburger C, Buttner A, Weis S. Ganglioglioma of the spinal cord: report of two rare cases and review of the literature. Neurosurgery 1997;41:1410–1416.
3. Miller G, Towfighi J, Page RB. Spinal cord ganglioglioma presenting as hydrocephalus. J Neuroncol 1990;9:147–152.
4. Ng THK, Fung CF, Goh W, et al. Ganglioneuroma of the spinal cord. Surg Neurol 1991;35:147–151.
5. Park SH, Chi JG, Cho BK, et al. Spinal cord ganglioglioma in childhood. Pathol Res Pract 1993;189:189–196.
6. Russo CP, Katz DS, Corona RJ Jr, et al. Gangliocytoma of the cervicothoracic spinal cord. AJNR 1995;16:889–891.
7. Sibilla L, Martelli A, Farina L, et al. Ganglioneuroblastoma of the spinal cord. AJNR 1995;16:875–877.
8. Wald U, Levy PJ, Rappaport ZH, et al. Conus ganglioglioma in a 2.5-year-old-boy. Case report. J Neurosurg 1985;62:142–144.

### Hemangioblastoma

1. Browne TR, Adams RD, Roberson GH. Hemangioblastoma of the spinal cord: review and report of five cases. Arch Neurol 1976;33:435–414.
2. Ismail SM, Cole G. Von Hippel–Lindau syndrome with microscopic hemangioblastomas of the spinal nerve roots. J Neurosurg 1984;60:1279–1281.
3. Krishnan KR, Smith WT. Intramedullary hemangioblastoma of the spinal cord associated with pial varicosities simulating intradural angioma. J Neurol Neurosurg Psychiatry 1961;24:350–352.
4. Mock A, Levi A, Drake JM. Spinal hemangioblastoma, syrinx, and hydrocephalus in a two-year-old child. Neurosurgery 1990;27:799–802.
5. Neumann HPH, Eggert HR, Weigel K, et al. Hemangioblastomas of the central nervous system. A 10 year study with special reference to von Hippel–Lindau syndrome. J Neurosurg 1989;70:24–30.
6. Rojiani AM, Elliott K, Dorovini-Zis K. Extensive replacement of spinal cord and brainstem by hemangioblastoma in a case of von Hippel–Lindau disease. Clin Neuropathol 1991;10:297–302.
7. Tibbs RE Jr, Harkey HL, Raila FA. Hemangioblastoma of the filum terminale: case report. Neurosurgery 1999;44:221–223.
8. Wisoff HS, Suzuki Y, Llena JF, et al. Extramedullary hemangioblastoma of the spinal cord: case report. J Neurosurg 1978;48:461–464.
9. Xu Q-W, Bao W-M, Mao R-L, et al. Magnetic resonance imaging and microsurgical treatment of intramedullary hemangioblastoma of the spinal cord. Neurosurgery 1994;35:671–676.
10. Yu JS, Short P, Schumacher J, Chapman PH, et al. Intramedullary hemorrhage in spinal cord hemangioblastoma: report of two cases. J Neurosurg 1994;81:937–940.

### Paraganglioma

1. Hirose T, Sano, Mori K, et al. Paraganglioma of the cauda equina: an ultrastructural and immunohistochemical study of two cases. Ultrastruct Pathol 1988;12:235–243.
2. Moran CA, Rush W, Mena H. Primary spinal paragangliomas: a clinicopathological and immunohistochemical study of 30 cases. Histopathology 1997;31:167–173.
3. Sonneland PRL, Scheithauer BW, LeChago J, et al. Paraganglioma of the cauda equina region. Clinicopathologic study of 31 cases with special reference to immunocytology and ultrastructure. Cancer 1986;58:1720–1735.
4. Strommer KN, Brandner S, Sarioglu AC, et al. Symptomatic cerebellar metastasis and late local recurrence of a cauda equina paraganglioma. J Neurosurg 1995;83:166–169.
5. Sundgren P, Annertz M, Englund E, et al. Paragangliomas of the spinal canal. Neuroradiology 1999;41:788–794.
6. Toyota B, Barr HWK, Ramsay D. Hemodynamic activity associated with a paraganglioma of the cauda equina. J Neurosurg 1993;79:451–455.

### Intramedullary Schwannoma

1. Acciarri N, Padovani R, Riccioni L. Intramedullary melanotic schwannoma. Report of a case and review of the literature. Br J Neurosurg 1999;13:322–325.
2. Gorman PH, Rigamonti D, Joslyn JN. Intramedullary and extramedullary schwannoma of the cervical spinal cord—case report. Surg Neurol 1989;32:459–462.
3. Koeppen AH, Ordinario AT, Barron KD. Aberrant intramedullary peripheral nerve fibers. Arch Neurol 1968;18:567–573.
4. Melanica JL, Pimentel JC, Conceição I, et al. Intramedullary neuroma of the cervical spinal cord: case report. Neurosurgery 1996;39:594–598.
5. Riggs HE, Clary WU. A case of intramedullary sheath cell tumor of the spinal cord: consideration of vascular nerves as a source of origin. J Neuropathol Exp Neurol 1957;16:332–336.
6. Ross DA, Edwards MSB, Wilson CB. Intramedullary neurilemomas of the spinal cord: report of two cases and review of the literature. Neurosurgery 1986;19:458–464.
7. Solomon RA, Handler MS, Sedelli RV, et al. Intramedullary melanotic schwannoma of the cervicomedullary junction. Neurosurgery 1987;20:36–38.

### Metastatic Neoplasms

1. Connolly ES Jr, Winfree McCormick PC, et al. Intramedullary spinal cord metastasis: report of three cases and review of the literature. Surg Neurol 1996;46:329–338.

2. Costigan DA, Winkelman MD. Intramedullary spinal cord metastasis. A clinicopathological study of 13 cases. J Neurosurg 1985;62:227–233.
3. Hashizume Y, Hirano A. Intramedullary spinal cord metastasis: pathologic findings in five autopsy cases. Acta Neuropathol (Berl) 1983;61:214–218.
4. Schiff D, O'Neill BP. Intramedullary spinal cord metastases: clinical features and treatment outcome. Neurology 1996;47:906–912.

## Other Intramedullary Neoplasms

1. Brownlee RE, Clark AW, Sevick RJ, et al. Symptomatic hamartoma of the spinal cord associated with neurofibromatosis type 1: case report. J Neurosurg 1998;88:1099–1103.
2. Caram PC, Scarcella G, Carton CA. Intradural lipomas of the spinal cord: with particular emphasis on the "intramedullary" lipomas. J Neurosurg 1974;41:699–704.
3. Deme S, Ang L-C, Skaf G, et al. Primary intramedullary primitive neuroectodermal tumor of the spinal cord: report and review of the literature. Neurosurgery 1997;41:1417–1420.
4. Harrington ES, Kell JF Jr. Intraspinal teratoma, with report of a case. J Neuropathol Exp Neurol 1955;14:214–221.
5. Hautzer NW, Aiyesimoju A, Robitaille Y. "Primary" spinal intramedullary lymphomas: a review. Ann Neurol 1983;14:62–66.
6. Herderscheê D, Troost D, de Visser M, et al. Lymphomatoid granulomatosis: clinical and histopathological report of a patient presenting with spinal cord involvement. J Neurol 1998;235:432–434.
7. Herpers MJHM, Freling G, Beuls EAM. Pleomorphic xanthoastrocytoma in the spinal cord. Case report. J Neurosurg 1994;80:564–569.
8. Itoh Y, Mineura K, Sasajima H, et al. Intramedullary spinal cord germinoma: case report and review of the literature. Neurosurgery 1996;38:187–191.
9. Kepes JJ, Belton K, Roessmann U, et al. Primitive neuroectodermal tumors of the cauda equina in adults with no detectable primary intracranial neoplasm—three case studies. Clin Neuropathol 1985;4:1–11.
10. Klein P, Zientek G, VandenBerg SR, et al. Primary CNS lymphoma: lymphomatous meningitis presenting as a cauda equina lesion in an AIDS patient. Can J Neurol Sci 1990;17:329–331.
11. Knopp EA, Chynn KY, Hughes J. Primary lymphoma of the cauda equina: myelographic, CT myelographic, and MR appearance. AJNR 1994;15:1187–1189.
12. Koen JL, McLendon RE, George TM. Intradural spinal teratoma: evidence for a dysembryogenic origin. Report of four cases. J Neurosurg 1998;89:844–851.
13. Maggi G, Aliberti F, Colucci MR, et al. Spinal intramedullary angiolipoma. Childs Nerv Syst 1996;12:346–349.
14. McDonald AC, Nicoll JAR, Rampling R. Intramedullary non-Hodgkin's lymphoma of the spinal cord: a case report and literature review. J Neurooncol 1995;23:257–263.
15. Miyauchi A, Matsumoto K, Kohmura E, et al. Primary intramedullary spinal cord germinoma. Case report. J Neurosurg 1996;84:1060–1061.
16. Nicoletti GF, Passanisi M, Platania N, et al. Intramedullary spinal cystic teratoma of the conus medullaris with caudal exophytic development: case report. Surg Neurol 1994;41:106–111.
17. Poeze M, Herpers MJHM, Tjandra B, et al. Intramedullary spinal teratoma presenting with urinary retention: case report and review of the literature. Neurosurgery 1999;45:379–385.
18. Razack N, Jimenez OF, Aldana P, et al. Intramedullary holocord lipoma in an athlete: case report. Neurosurgery 1998;42:394–397.
19. Riley K, Palmer CA, Oser AB, et al. Spinal cord hamartoma: case report. Neurosurgery 1999;44:1125–1128.
20. Rosemberg S, Menezes Y, Sousa MR, et al. Primary malignant rhabdoid tumor of the spinal dura. Clin Neuropathol 1994;13:221–224.
21. Salvati M, Artico M, Lunardi P, et al. Intramedullary meningioma: case report and review of the literature. Surg Neurol 1992;37:42–45.
22. Slagel DD, Goeken JA, Platz CA, et al. Primary germinoma of the spinal cord: a case report with 28-year follow-up and review of the literature. Acta Neuropathol (Berl) 1995;90:657–659.
23. Stephan CL, Kepes JJ, Arnold P, et al. Neurocytoma of the cauda equina. Case report. J Neurosurg 1999;90:247–251.
24. Tatter SB; Borges LF, Louis DN. Central neurocytomas of the cervical spinal cord. Report of two cases. J Neurosurg 1994;81:288–293.

# THE PERIPHERAL NERVOUS SYSTEM

# 12

Tumors and tumor-like lesions of the peripheral nervous system are generally classified as soft tissue processes, but most differ significantly from neoplasms in that category, given their neuroepithelial nature, histologic diversity, origin in a distinct anatomic compartment, and frequent association with genetic disorders. The spectrum includes not only tumors but also hamartomas; hyperplasias; reactive processes, including "true neuromas"; and inflammatory or infectious lesions simulating neoplasia. The diagnosis and classification of nerve sheath lesions require correlation of clinical and surgical data, as well as attention to histochemical and immunocytologic features. Application of these methods permits the virtual "dissection" of peripheral nerve lesions. Although largely supplanted by immunocytochemistry, electron microscopy still plays a diagnostic role.

Applying modern investigative methods to large clinicopathologic studies has advanced our understanding of the nature and behavior of long-recognized as well as new entities. Our discussion here focuses solely on lesions encountered in the setting of surgical neuropathology. Because medical disorders of nerve are beyond the scope of this work, the reader is referred to an authoritative text on the subject.[1]

## SPECIMEN ASSESSMENT

Tumors of peripheral nerve usually present either as clinically and grossly apparent tumors of the nerve proper or as soft tissue tumors of inapparent type secondarily involving nerve. In either case, a meaningful approach to the assessment of these lesions includes (1) photographically recording their gross appearance before dissection; (2) obtaining three-dimensional measurements and describing their gross appearance in terms of configuration, demarcation, texture, color, and precise relation to a nerve; and (3) sectioning the specimen along the axis of the nerve. Alternatively, when its configuration is cylindric, for example in intraneural perineurioma or plexiform neurofibroma, multiple cross sections may be more revealing than longitudinal sections. Cut surfaces should be promptly photographed to avoid changes in color resulting from exposure to air. Sampling is also of importance, particularly with grossly heterogeneous lesions. We recommend one section per centimeter of a lesion's greatest dimension. Circumferential as well as proximal and distal margins must be carefully sampled. Specimen inking is encouraged. In addition to optimal fixation for light microscopy, setting aside fixed tissue for electron microscopy is important. Although 3% glutaraldehyde or Trump's solution (4% glutaraldehyde and 4% formaldehyde) is optimal, fixation in ordinary 10% buffered formalin will suffice. In selected instances, quick freezing of samples in liquid nitrogen for molecular genetic study, or obtaining fresh tissue for cytogenetic, tissue culture, or flow cytometric study may also be useful.

## NORMAL ANATOMY

### Macroscopic Features

The anatomy of the peripheral nervous system is complex (Fig. 12–1) and includes not only multiple distinct compartments (intradural-extradural, intraspinal-extraspinal) and nerve segments (roots, trunks, branches, ganglia) but also a variety of cell types. Of the latter, some are limited to nervous tissue (Schwann and perineurial cells, neurons), whereas others are common to soft tissue (adipose, fibroblastic, and endothelial cells). Thus, a few words regarding the organization and anatomy of the system are in order.

As a rule, neurons giving rise to motor nerve fibers lie within the central nervous system, either in brain stem nuclei or in anterior horns of the spinal cord. In contrast, neurons from which sensory nerve fibers originate lie within either cranial nerve or spinal dorsal root ganglia. Portions of motor and sensory nerve fibers situated in the brain or spinal cord are myelinated by oligodendrocytes. In contrast, their distal, intraneural portions are ensheathed by Schwann cells. Whereas cranial nerves are sensory, motor, or mixed in function, peripheral nerves are predominantly of mixed type and contain autonomic nerve fibers as well. Anterior (motor) and posterior (sensory) spinal nerve roots exit the cord separately. Unlike spinal nerves, cranial nerves originate from the brain at irregular intervals and do not form dorsal and ventral roots. Instead, efferent and afferent fibers exit and enter brain at the same site.

Within the subarachnoid space, cranial and spinal nerve root sheaths acquire an arachnoidal element that

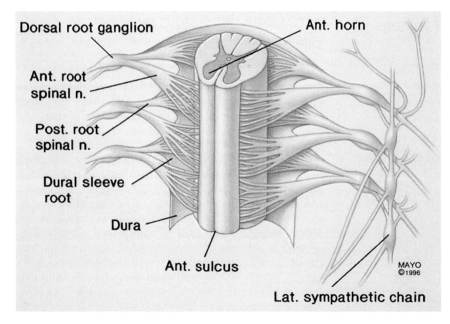

**FIGURE 12–1   NORMAL NERVE**

Schematic illustration of the sensorimotor and autonomic nerves, as well as their ganglia, relative to the spinal cord and meninges.

becomes confluent with the perineurium of peripheral nerve. Nerve roots also become surrounded by a dural sheath that exits the central nervous system through cranial or intervertebral foramina. Upon exiting, roots give rise to spinal nerve trunks that divide into dorsal and ventral rami. The latter fuse to form major plexuses, such as the brachial, lumbar, and sacral. Thus, nerve plexuses receive fibers from multiple cord segments. Eventually, motor nerve fibers terminate on muscle endplates, whereas sensory fibers end in specialized sensory structures.

Autonomic nerves are of either sympathetic or parasympathetic type and innervate primarily viscera and blood vessels. Sympathetic preganglionic fibers arise from the intermediolateral gray columns of the thoracic and lumbar spinal cord, exit in unmyelinated form via anterior nerve roots, and terminate on neurons of sympathetic ganglia lying in the paravertebral region. In contrast, parasympathetic preganglionic fibers are craniosacral in origin. The ganglia in which they terminate lie near or within innervated structures. A schematic representation of the relationship of sensorimotor and autonomic nerves and ganglia to the spinal cord and meninges is illustrated in Figure 12–1.

## Microscopic Features

Peripheral nerve is divided into three basic elements: epineurium, perineurium, and endoneurium (Figs. 12–2 and 12–3). Each has unique morphologic characteristics. Thus an understanding of the pathology of nerves is aided by familiarity with their anatomy, as well as histochemical and immunocytologic staining reactions. Table 12–1 provides an overview.

In the immediate surroundings of a peripheral nerve, fibrous tissue condenses to form an often distinct layer encircling the nerve and filling the interstices between fascicles (Fig. 12–4). Termed epineurium, this layer is no different in structure, function, or reaction to injury from

mesenchymal tissue at other sites. Around large nerves, it is relatively abundant and contains arteries, veins, and lymphatics. In contrast, small, single-fascicle nerves possess little more than a scant rim of adipose tissue. The periphery of the nerve proper begins with the perineurium, a compact layer of concentrically arranged polygonal and flattened cells that sharply delimits peripheral and autonomic nerve fascicles as well as ganglia (Fig. 12–5). Its thickness is directly related to fascicle size. Although perineurial cells are functionally distinctive and neuroepithelial in nature, they are often erroneously termed perineurial "fibroblasts" or "epithelial" cells. Emphasizing the individuality of perineurium is its immunoreactivity for epithelial membrane antigen (EMA) (Fig. 12–6) and lack of staining for S-100 protein. By contrast, Schwann cells are S-100 protein positive and not EMA reactive.[2, 7] Basement membrane normally surrounds both these cell types and is immunoreactive for both collagen IV and laminin. Ultrastructural studies demonstrate pericellular basement membrane, a structural feature of perineurial and Schwann cells, but not of fibroblasts.[4] Other distinctive features of perineurial cells include abundant micropinocytotic vesicles, electron-dense cytoplasm, and numerous tight junctions. The last accounts for the diffusion barrier characteristics of perineurium,[1, 9] which maintains the physiologic milieu of the endoneurium. At the terminations of nerves, perineurium contributes to the architecture of various specialized motor and sensory structures, such as pacinian and Meissner's corpuscles.[3, 10]

Surrounded by the perineurium, the endoneurial space contains axons, Schwann cells and their myelin sheaths, fibroblasts, macrophages, mast cells, blood vessels, and a collagenous, albumin-rich matrix (Figs. 12–3 and 12–7). Particularly when associated with myelin sheaths, Schwann cells are readily recognized on both hematoxylin and eosin (H&E) and Luxol fast blue–periodic acid-Schiff (PAS) stains (Figs. 12–7 and 12–8). Their nuclei are round or crescentic in cross section and are bluntly elongated in longitudinal

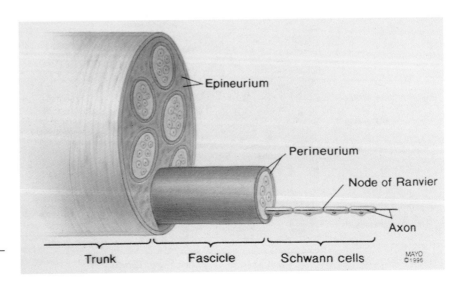

**FIGURE 12–2    NORMAL NERVE**

Schematic illustration of the basic architecture of a normal nerve.

**TABLE 12–1**
**Histologic and Immunohistochemical Techniques for Peripheral Nerve**

| Stain | Feature Demonstrated |
| --- | --- |
| **General stains** | |
| Hematoxylin and eosin | Detection of large, well-myelinated axons and Schwann and perineurial cells |
| Reticulin | Basement membrane–surrounding Schwann cells in normal nerve are barely evident, but are more readily demonstrated in nerve sheath tumors |
| Masson trichrome | Fibrosis; myelin, red |
| Alcian blue | Glycosaminoglycans, blue |
| Toluidine blue | Mast cells, metachromatic; general stain for semithin plastic sections |
| Congo red | Amyloid |
| **Stains for myelin** | |
| Luxol fast blue | Myelin, blue; can be combined with silver stains for axons |
| Periodic acid–Schiff | Degenerating myelin and macrophages; perineurium |
| Osmium | Myelin, black |
| **Stains for axons** | |
| Bodian, Bielschowsky, or Palmgren (silver stains) | Axons, black |
| **Immunocytochemistry** | |
| S-100 protein | Schwann cells, normal and neoplastic |
| Leu-7 (CD56) | Schwann cells, normal and neoplastic |
| Glial fibrillary acidic protein | Some Schwann cells and Schwann cell tumors |
| Myelin basic protein | Myelin |
| Epithelial membrane antigen | Perineurial cells |
| Synaptophysin | Axons, neurons |
| Neurofilament protein | Axons, neurons |
| Collagen IV, laminin | Basement membrane |

profile. A periaxonal spiral of tightly wound Schwann cell cytoplasm is the substance of myelin (Fig. 12–9).[1, 9] Early in its formation, incorporation of axons—the initial step in myelin wrapping—begins with pincer-like encirclement of an axon segment. This is followed by approximation and fusion of the Schwann cell plasma membrane,[2, 9] the result being a focus of "double membrane" termed the mesaxon. Subsequent winding of the Schwann cell membrane results in the formation of a sheath that varies in thickness. In contrast, unmyelinated fibers, typically multiple, lie individually encased within simple cuffs of Schwann cell cytoplasm that do not undergo spiral lamination and myelin formation (see Fig. 12–9).

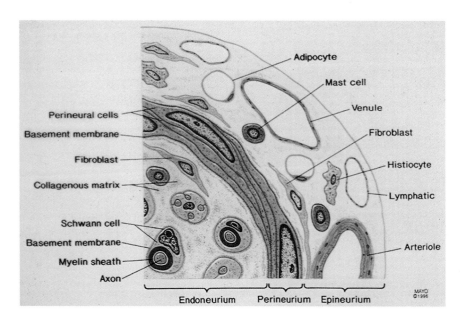

**FIGURE 12–3  NORMAL NERVE**

Schematic illustration of the essential elements of epineurium, perineurium, and endoneurium.

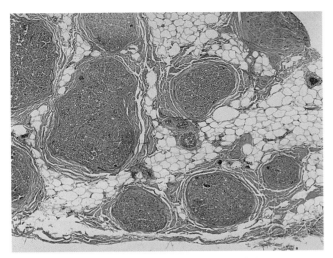

**FIGURE 12-4    NORMAL NERVE—CROSS SECTION**

Multiple fascicles are seen embedded in fibrofatty epineurial tissue.

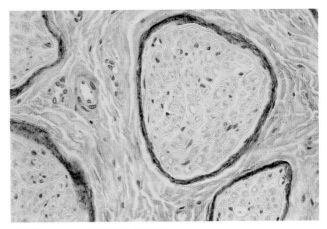

**FIGURE 12-6    NORMAL NERVE**

The perineurium is immunoreactive for epithelial membrane antigen.

Whether myelin-producing or not, Schwann cells encompass axons of all sizes. In histologic section, the Masson trichrome stain vividly contrasts the red color of myelin against the green endoneurial collagen. More myelin specific is the Luxol fast blue method. When combined with silver impregnations for axons, such as the Bodian or Bielschowsky stains, one can simultaneously visualize myelin and encircled neuronal processes (see Fig. 12–8). Viewed on cross section, the myelin sheaths appear as thick-walled cylinders, often with prominent, artifactual radial fractures. In longitudinal sections, the sheath is also fractured, producing an artifactual herringbone pattern not seen in central nervous system tissues. Nodes of Ranvier are difficult to visualize in paraffin-embedded material but are readily seen in semithin plastic sections and in "tease" preparations that isolate single fibers. Therein, myelinated axons appear as chains of elongated sausages, the nodes producing peri-

odic constrictions between the "links." Each link represents the myelin wrap of a single Schwann cell. Myelinated axons vary in size but are larger than those that are unmyelinated. Both the thickness of the myelin layer and the internodal distances are proportional to axon diameters. Myelin consists largely of lipids (75%) and, to a lesser extent, of proteins. Among the latter are $P_o$, a glycoprotein and the principal protein of peripheral myelin, as well as myelin-associated glycoprotein, a product solely of myelin-forming Schwann cells.

Axons are classified according to their diameter, which is directly related to conduction velocity. Most nerves contain both large, myelinated fibers and small, unmyelinated fibers. Only sizable myelinated axons are visible by light microscopy; unmyelinated axons are not. On Masson trichrome stain, axons in cross section have a red, dot-like profile. In longitudinal perspective, only slender filaments are evident. The same is true on H&E

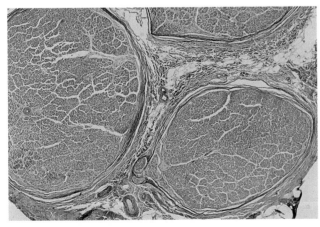

**FIGURE 12-5    NORMAL NERVE**

Varied Luxol fast blue–periodic acid-Schiff (PAS) stain showing three fascicles each surrounded by PAS-positive perineurium. The endoneurium contains nerve fibers surrounded by a blue myelin sheath.

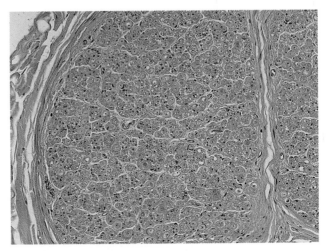

**FIGURE 12-7    NORMAL NERVE**

H&E stained section demonstrates a fascicle surrounded by perineurium and containing numerous nerve fibers. Myelinated axons appear as dots, each surrounded by a myelin cuff. Note the perineurial septa.

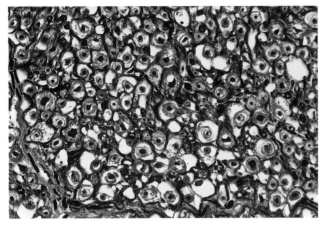

**FIGURE 12-8   NORMAL DORSAL NERVE ROOT**

Luxol fast blue–periodic acid-Schiff–Bielschowsky stain showing a content of heavily myelinated nerve fibers.

stain and neurofilament protein immunostain, in which even large fibers frequently enter and exit the plane of section and appear more like ribbons than cylinders (Fig. 12–10 *A, B*). It is for this reason that cross sections of nerve are more informative. Axonal number and range of size are best seen in toluidine blue–stained Epon-embedded sections. The relationship of Schwann cells to axons is readily apparent on S-100 protein immunostain (Fig. 12–10*C*).

Whereas endoneurial fibroblasts are difficult to distinguish from Schwann cells in paraffin-embedded material, semithin plastic sections show them to possess distinctive, elongated, bipolar processes and to be randomly disposed within endoneurial collagen. At the ultrastructural level, fibroblasts are devoid of pericellular basal lamina, and endoneurial collagen is readily evident as fibrils with characteristic periodicity (see Fig. 12–3). The capacity for collagen formation, so freely attributed to fibroblasts, belongs to Schwann cells as well. The

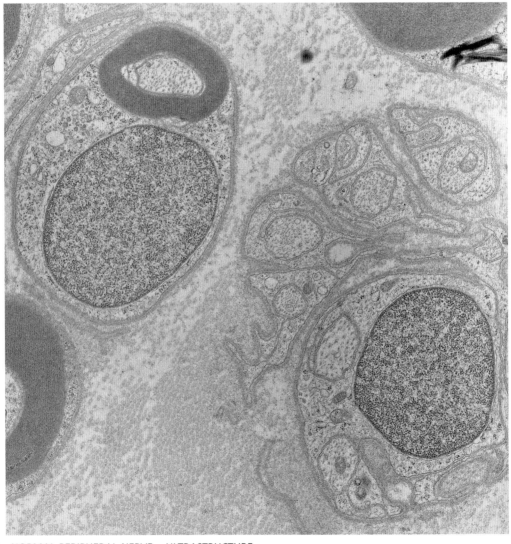

**FIGURE 12-9   NORMAL PERIPHERAL NERVE—ULTRASTRUCTURE**

This cross section of a normal sural nerve shows the relation of one Schwann cell to a myelinated axon (*upper left*) and the relation of another to unmyelinated axons (*lower right*). The basal lamina, which distinguishes Schwann cells from fibroblasts, traces the outline of the cells ($\times$ 15,000).

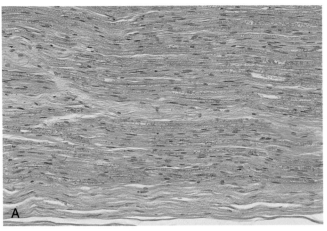

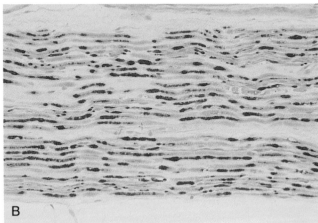

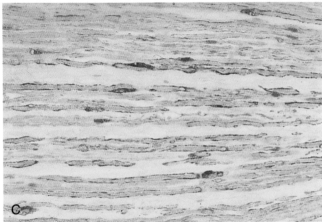

**FIGURE 12–10** NORMAL PERIPHERAL NERVE—
LONGITUDINAL SECTION

On H&E stained section (*A*), barely discernible axons are seen as
delicate threads obscured by myelin. Axons are demonstrated on
neurofilament protein immunostain (*B*). Schwann cells and their
nuclei (*C*) are S-100 protein immunoreactive.

contribution of endoneurial blood vessels to the "blood-
nerve barrier" is due to both lack of endothelial fenes-
trations and the presence of tight junctions.[1, 9] Endoneurium has no lymphatics.

Dorsal root (sensory) and autonomic ganglia are
highly specialized structures consisting of large neurons,
perineuronal satellite cells (modified Schwann cells),
and axons (Fig. 12–11 *A* to *C*). Sensory ganglia differ in
that they possess a dural sheath, are greater in size,
have larger ganglion cells with more centrally situated
nuclei, and exhibit axonal myelination.

For a more in-depth discussion of the structure and
function of peripheral nerve, the reader is directed to
authoritative texts on the subject.[5, 8]

## REACTIVE LESIONS

Among the non-neoplastic lesions discussed, some
clinically mimic neoplasms. Of these, the only "true
neuromas"—that is, processes composed of both axons
and nerve sheath elements—are traumatic neuroma
and localized hypertrophic neuropathy. The term can
also be applied to mucosal neuromas and palisaded encapsulated neuromas of skin. Both are beyond the scope
of this chapter. Also discussed are lesions that are more
degenerative in nature, including interdigital neuritis
(Morton's neuroma) and nerve cysts or "ganglia."

## Traumatic Neuroma

**Definition.** A non-neoplastic, disorganized proliferation
of axons and accompanying Schwann and perineural
cells, all in a collagenous stroma and occurring at the
site of partial or complete nerve transection.

**General Comments.** Both proliferative and reparative
changes follow partial or complete transection of a
nerve. These include growth of new axons from the
proximal stump and cellular alterations preparatory to
reinnervation in the distal segment.[2] When orderly, the
result is a reconstituted nerve. Frequently, however, the
process is unsuccessful, and a tender, painful nodule
arises at the site of injury. Traumatic neuromas are not
limited to readily traumatized, superficially situated
nerves. Also affected are visceral sites of previous
surgery, such as the gallbladder,[3] in which the neuromas
are rarely polypoid,[7] and bile ducts.[6] Examples occurring
in mastectomy scars may show granular cell change.[5]
Most traumatic neuromas become symptomatic months
to years after surgery. Only rare visceral lesions are
unassociated with prior surgery.[4] Autoamputation of a
supernumerary digit in utero may also be followed by
traumatic neuroma formation.[8]

**Macroscopic Features.** At sites of complete transection and nerve retraction, traumatic neuromas present as

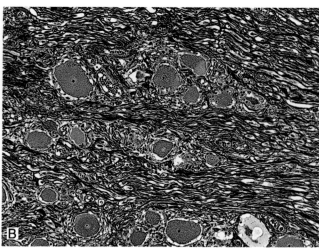

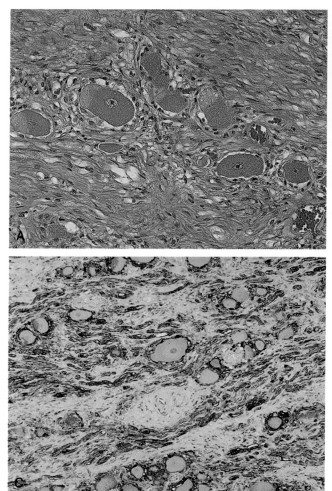

**FIGURE 12–11   NORMAL DORSAL ROOT GANGLION**

Ganglion cells (A) lie clustered and separated by bundles of myelinated nerve fibers. The nerve fibers are heavily myelinated (blue) (B). Ganglion cells with their centrally situated nuclei are surrounded by S-100 protein–immunopositive satellite cells (C).

firm, demarcated but nonencapsulated, bulbous masses arising at the proximal stump (Fig. 12–12). On cut section they appear pale and gray. When occurring in an incompletely transected nerve, the lesion may assume a fusiform contour (Fig. 12–13A). On longitudinal section, the proximal nerve segment splays and disappears into the lesion (Fig. 12–14A). Injury to a nerve plexus may result in the formation of multiple neuromas. Most traumatic neuromas are 1 to 2 cm in size; only a rare example approaches 5 cm.

**Microscopic Features.** Given their cellular makeup, which includes the full spectrum of nerve components, and the tendency to form abortive fascicles, traumatic neuromas represent the consummate "true neuroma." The key feature of traumatic neuromas is their haphazard arrangement of bundles of regenerating nerve fibers (i.e., axons) ensheathed by Schwann cells (Figs. 12–13B and 12–14A). In more organized examples, the bundles resemble microfascicles, some with a delicate investment of perineurium (Fig. 12–14B). Myelination varies but is generally scant. An occasional lesion features granular cell change.[5] As previously stated, traumatic neuromas are nonencapsulated. Peripherally, they merge with fibrocollagenous tissue, and some even extend into adipose tissue or nearby skeletal muscle. Chronic inflamma-

tion and a foreign body giant cell reaction are occasionally seen at the site of prior trauma.

**Immunohistochemical Features.** Axons, their ensheathing Schwann cells, and the perineurial cells that often surround microfascicles show neurofilament protein, S-100 protein, and EMA immunoreactivity, respectively.

**Ultrastructural Features.** Early-phase lesions often contain axons that are unmyelinated, whereas the Schwann cells in older lesions frequently show varying degrees of myelin formation. When present, microfascicles are surrounded by well-differentiated perineurial cells. The specific fine structural features of these various elements were discussed earlier in the Normal Anatomy section.

**Differential Diagnosis.** Generally, the diagnosis of traumatic neuroma poses no problem. *Schwannoma* and *intraneural neurofibroma* are readily distinguished by encapsulation, cellular monomorphism, and characteristic tissue patterns (Antoni A and B tissue) on the one hand, and by mucin-rich stroma, sparse content of axons, and the uniform perineurial layer delimiting fascicles on the other.

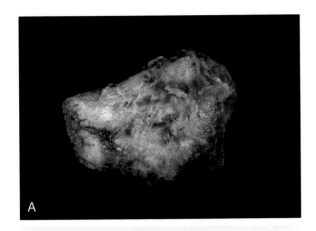

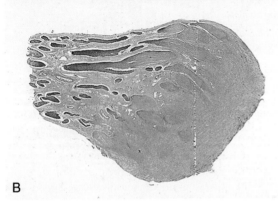

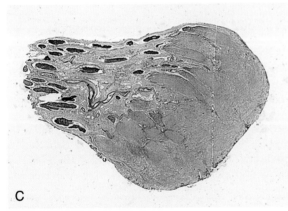

**FIGURE 12–12** TRAUMATIC NEUROMA

The club-shaped proximal stump (*A*) transected from the remainder of the nerve (*left*) forms a firm, bulbous mass. On H&E stain (*B*), longitudinally oriented eosinophilic nerve fibers are seen to disappear along sprouted axons of the neuroma. The collagen content of the neuroma is readily apparent on trichrome stain (*C*).

**Treatment and Prognosis.** The formation of a traumatic neuroma can be avoided if, at the time of nerve injury, the ends of the traumatized nerves are optimally approximated to promote reinnervation. Graft replacement is also an option. Resection of traumatic neuromas is curative, but at the time of excision the proximal nerve stump should be embedded in normal soft tissue to avoid recurrence. In a patient with a prior malignancy, surgery may be required to distinguish visceral traumatic neuromas from recurrent neoplasm.[1]

# Localized Interdigital Neuritis (Morton's Neuroma)

**Definition.** A localized, degenerative process characterized by nerve fiber loss and fibrosis, typically involving a plantar digital nerve.

**Clinical and Radiologic Features.** Localized interdigital neuritis typically affects the foot and is attributed to chronic, repetitive trauma, or to effects of ischemia.[3, 4] In most cases the condition is unilateral and affects adult women. Worsened by exercise and relieved by rest, it is attributed to ill-fitting shoes. Symptoms consist of severe paroxysmal pain between the third and fourth toes. Point tenderness is also noted on compression of the interspace. A similar lesion may affect the hands, usually of men with chronic occupational trauma.

**Macroscopic Features.** Localized interdigital neuritis consists of a firm, fusiform enlargement of the fourth plantar digital nerve at its bifurcation (Fig. 12–15). On its surface, the nerve sheath may be adherent to the intermetatarsal bursa and the nearby digital artery. Most lesions measure approximately 1 cm and resemble a traumatic neuroma or neurofibroma.

**Microscopic Features.** The degenerative nature of localized interdigital neuritis is readily apparent, all compartments of the nerve being involved. Basic architectural features of the nerve are retained, but fibrosis of epineurium and hyalinization of vessels, sometimes thrombosed, are conspicuous features (Fig. 12–16*A, B*). Mucinous degeneration is common (see Fig. 12–16*A*), even in early lesions. In chronic stage lesions, axons and myelin are often markedly decreased (Fig. 12–16*C*). Other late findings are laminated collagenous nodules within endoneurium (Fig. 12–16*D*) and elastic tissue deposition in interfascicular tissue. Inflammation is insignificant.

**Immunohistochemical and Ultrastructural Features.** Neurofilament protein and S-100 protein immunostains show a reduction in axons and Schwann cells, respectively. Electron microscopy reveals collagen deposition, most notably in endoneurium; multilayering of basal membrane about vessels; and degenerative changes in nerve fibers.[2]

**Differential Diagnosis.** Traumatic neuromas must be distinguished from true neoplasms of the nerve sheath. The former consists of an overgrowth of axons and Schwann cells, which stands in stark contrast to the atrophy and striking fibrosis that characterize localized interdigital neuritis. *Neurofibromas* are proliferative in nature and consist in large part of Schwann cells and fibroblasts that separate axons and enlarge nerve fascicles. *Schwannomas* are also proliferative, consist entirely of Schwann cells, feature distinctive Antoni A and B patterns, and primarily displace rather than incorporate nerve fibers.

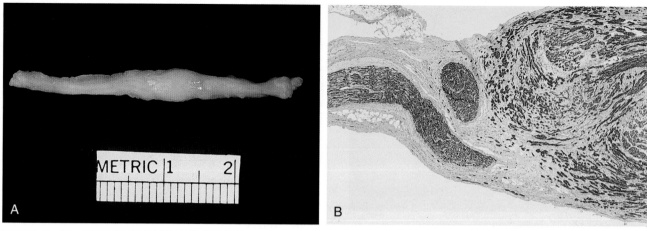

**FIGURE 12–13    INCOMPLETELY TRANSECTED NERVE WITH TRAUMATIC NEUROMA**

On gross examination (A), the neuroma appears as a nodular fibrous mass in continuity with viable proximal nerve fibers and atrophic distal fibers. On neurofilament protein immunostain (B), two sizable proximal fascicles are seen to give rise to individual and less well-formed bundles of regenerating axons.

**Treatment and Prognosis.** Aside from palliation by a change in shoe style or steroid or anesthetic injection, resection remains the only therapeutic option.[1, 5] Failure of neurectomy in 10% of cases is usually due to subsequent formation of a traumatic neuroma.[6]

## Localized Hypertrophic Neuropathy

**Definition.** A rare, sporadic lesion characterized grossly by segmental hypertrophy of a peripheral nerve and microscopically by "onion bulb" hyperplasia of Schwann cells. It differs from intraneural perineurioma, a distinctive lesion composed of perineurial cells engaged in pseudo–onion bulb formation.

**General Comments and Clinical Features.** Localized hypertrophic neuropathy is a reactive rather than a neoplastic process. Unlike hypertrophic sensorimotor neuropathies, for example, Dejerine-Sottas and Charcot-Marie-Tooth diseases, it has no genetic basis. Instead, it is thought to result from repeated episodes of demyelination and remyelination. Only a few cases of localized hypertrophic neuropathy have been described.[1–3, 6] All occurred in adults, none of whom showed evidence of neurofibromatosis.

**Macroscopic Features.** Localized hypertrophic neuropathy is a focal lesion. In only one instance did the process involve two nerves.[6] Either cranial[1, 2] or spinal nerves are affected.[3, 6] Both cranial nerve examples involved a trigeminal nerve. The nerves appear fusiform and feature enlarged fascicles. Lesion length varies from 2 to 15 cm.[6]

**Microscopic Features.** Histologically the onion bulbs consist of whorls of cytologically normal Schwann cells surrounding myelinated axons (Fig. 12–17A). The fascicles also contain a hypocellular, mucopolysaccharide-

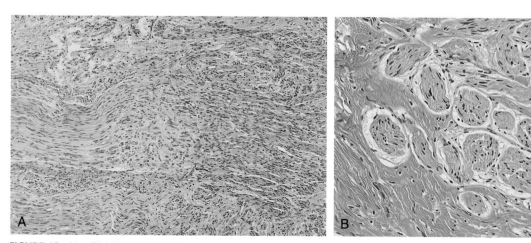

**FIGURE 12–14    TRAUMATIC NEUROMA**

H&E stained section (A) shows the transition between a proximal fascicle (left) and disordered, regenerated axons constituting the neuroma (right). In contrast, a long-standing neuroma (B) shows the well-formed microfascicles in a collagenous stroma.

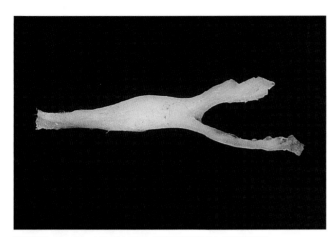

**FIGURE 12–15** LOCALIZED INTERDIGITAL NEURITIS (MORTON'S NEUROMA)

The lesion is a firm, pale gray, fusiform expansion of the digital plantar nerve.

rich, collagen-containing matrix (Fig. 12–17A). Alcian blue–positive matrix is abundant and separates the onion bulbs. Axons and myelin are readily demonstrated on special stains (see Table 12–1).

**Immunohistochemical and Ultrastructural Features.** The onion bulbs and their central Schwann sheaths stain strongly for S-100 protein (Fig. 12–17B). Their single central axon is neurofilament protein positive. EMA reactivity is limited to perineurium. Ultrastructurally the onion bulbs consist of multiple layers of normal-appearing Schwann cells encircling myelinated axons. The essential features of Schwann cells were discussed earlier under Normal Anatomy.

**Differential Diagnosis.** Localized hypertrophic neuropathy should not be confused with *intraneural perineurioma*, a tumor of perineurial cells that affects major nerves[4] but is strongly immunoreactive for epithelial membrane protein; S-100 protein reactivity is limited to normal Schwann sheaths. Intraneural perineurioma is discussed in detail later on pages 612 to 614. Also in the differential diagnosis are *Charcot-Marie-Tooth disease*, *Dejerine-Sottas disease*, and *chronic inflammatory demyelinating polyneuropathy*.[5] All are easily distinguished from localized hypertrophic neuropathy by clinical criteria.

**Treatment and Prognosis.** Localized hypertrophic neuropathy is an indolent process. Not all examples are

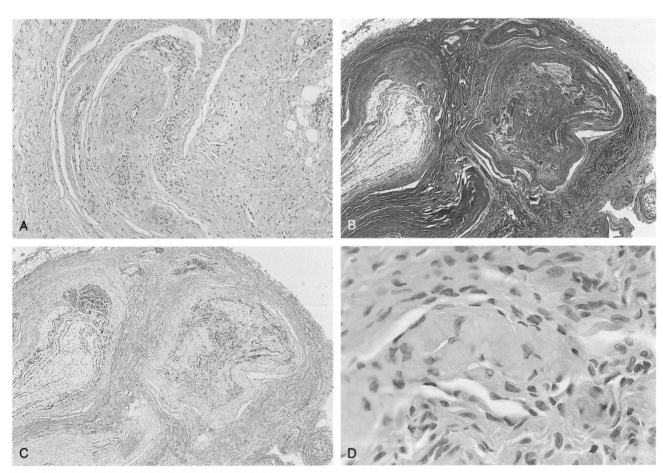

**FIGURE 12–16** LOCALIZED INTERDIGITAL NEURITIS

Low-power micrograph (A) shows a fascicle of the digital nerve exhibiting endo-, peri-, and epineurial fibrosis. The change is most apparent on trichrome stain (B). Nerve fiber loss within two fascicles is marked on this immunostain for neurofilament protein (C). Intraneural collagenous nodules are a characteristic feature of this lesion (D).

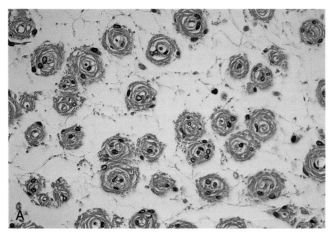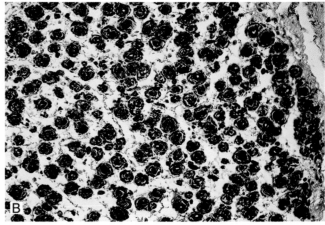

**FIGURE 12–17**    LOCALIZED HYPERTROPHIC NEUROPATHY

Individually distributed in a mucinous matrix (A), the onion bulbs are composed of S-100 protein–immunoreactive Schwann cells (B).

tumefactive.[2] Given the lack of specific therapy, biopsy confirmation is usually followed by supportive observation.

## Nerve Cyst or "Ganglion"

**Definition.** A mucin-filled cystic, longitudinal expansion of nerve caused by intraepineurial intrusion of mucinous fluid originating from a nearby joint.

**General Comments.** Nerve cysts or "ganglia" are reactive/degenerative in nature and etiologically related to mechanical stress.[12] Favored nerves include the peroneal at the level of the tibiofibular joint, the ulnar nerve at the level of the wrist[2, 5] or elbow, the median nerve,[4] posterior interosseous nerve,[3] and the radial nerve. Peroneal examples have been particularly well characterized. Careful dissection and injection studies of peroneal intraneural ganglia have shown that most arise by extension from the tibiofibular joint and travel along the articular branch of that nerve.[11] Rare nerve cysts, involving the suprascapular, tibial, and sural nerves, have also been described. Rare examples purportedly arise in nearby bone.[1, 6] Only a small minority of cysts remote from joints appear to arise de novo in epineurial tissue.

**Clinical Features.** Nerve cysts affect primarily males.[9] Their age range is very broad and most occur in adults. Sensorimotor symptoms result from nerve compression. A tender, fluctuant mass may be evident on physical examination. Tinel's sign, that is, paresthesia following percussion, is often elicited. Electromyography discloses a conduction disturbance. Ultrasonography and MRI imaging confirm the diagnosis.

**Macroscopic Features.** The gross characteristics of nerve cysts vary. The majority are small and measure but a few centimeters. Large examples (10 cm or more) are less common. When the cyst is solitary and large, it may simply displace aggregated fascicles of the nerve. In other cases, multiple small cystic spaces irregularly disfigure its course (Fig. 12–18A). Contiguity of what

appear to be multiple cysts may be difficult to confirm, even by injection studies. When ruptured, the cysts drain a clear fluid that varies in consistency from liquid as joint fluid to decidedly viscid.

**Microscopic Features.** Histologically, cross sections of the nerve show a single well-formed lumen and/or multiple small lumens within the epineurium. Chronic ganglia possess fibrous walls, whereas those of short duration are often smaller, delicate, and surrounded by loose textured, mucin-containing connective tissue. Those showing multiple lumina (Fig. 12–18B) appear to arise from multidirectional intrusion of fluid along routes of least resistance. Such cysts were once thought to originate in epineurium, but current evidence indicates that they too have their origin from joint space.[11] In summary, nerve sheath cysts are composed entirely of fibrocollagenous tissue and mucin. None possess an epithelial lining. Spindle cells in their walls are fibroblastic or myofibroblastic in nature.

**Immunohistochemical and Ultrastructural Features.** Nerve cysts feature vimentin and perhaps actin immunoreactivity, but lack staining for S-100 protein and epithelial membrane antigen. Ultrastructurally, the cyst walls contain conventional fibroblasts and myofibroblasts.[9]

**Differential Diagnosis.** The differential diagnosis of nerve sheath cysts includes markedly cystic examples of *schwannoma*. Ganglia are hypocellular, lack a biphasic (Antoni A and B) patterns, and are composed of fibroblasts rather than sinuous, S-100 protein immunoreactive Schwann cells.

**Treatment and Prognosis.** The conventional treatment of nerve cysts is surgical. Simple drainage, marsupialization, and subtotal excision have all been utilized. Whereas simple drainage is often followed by cyst recurrence, excision may result in significant nerve deficit.[6] Most operated patients experience excellent pain relief but only some restoration of nerve function.[10] The

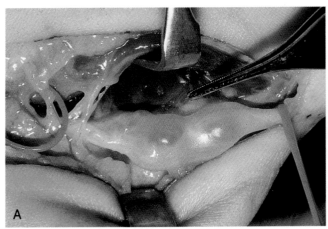
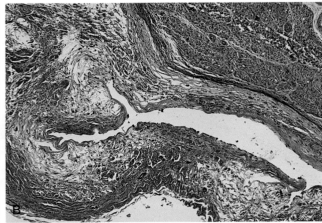

**FIGURE 12–18    NERVE CYST OR "GANGLION"**

This cyst of the median nerve is complex and exhibits multiple interconnected spaces filled with viscid fluid (*A*). Yet another example of a nerve cyst affecting the peroneal nerve is seen on trichrome stain to reside in epineurium (*B*). Note the displaced nerve fascicle (*upper right*).

overall rate of nerve cyst recurrence is underestimated but has been said to be as low as 7% and as high as 23%.[7, 8]

## INFLAMMATORY AND INFECTIOUS LESIONS SIMULATING TUMOR

### Inflammatory Pseudotumor of Nerve

Also termed "plasma cell granuloma" and "inflammatory myofibroblastic tumor," these idiopathic lesions are localized tumefactions composed of chronic inflammatory and reactive mesenchymal cells. The various synonyms reflect the heterogeneous nature of the process. The clinical presentation of inflammatory pseudotumor may mimic malignancy. Identical lesions affect lung, lymph node, brain, and orbit, as well as soft tissue sites. Reports of inflammatory pseudotumor involving nerves are few.[1, 3–6] Affected nerves include the facial, greater auricular, and sciatic. Grossly they appear fusiform or nodular in configuration. By definition, the infiltrate is limited to epineurium. Careful dissection may permit their separation from nerve (Fig. 12–19*A*).

Inflammatory pseudotumors vary considerably in composition, ranging from patchy lymphoplasmacellular inflammation with fibrous reaction (Fig. 12–19*B*) to nodular lymphoid hyperplasia and even uni- to multinucleate histiocyte infiltrates. Immunohistochemistry shows the lymphocytes to be polyclonal and mainly of T-cell type. Tumors composed primarily of histiocytes are strongly immunoreactive for CD68, but they lack both CD1A and S-100 protein reactivity, thereby excluding Langerhans' histiocytosis and Rosai-Dorfman disease.

The differential diagnosis depends largely on the predominant inflammatory response but includes *lymphoma* and *infection*. The benign cytology and mixed immunophenotype of the infiltrate exclude the former. By definition, microorganisms are lacking, and cultures

are negative. Neither tumefactive Langerhans' histiocytosis nor Rosai-Dorfman disease have been reported as primary within nerve. Lastly, nonspecific inflammation and benign fibroproliferative lesions, such as fibromatosis, may also affect nerve, particularly in the head and neck region.[2, 7–9] The treatment of choice is biopsy and nerve-sparing microsurgical resection. Only one reported lesion has recurred.[1]

### Sarcoidosis

Characterized by noncaseating granulomatous inflammation, this idiopathic systemic disorder affects the nervous system in approximately 5% of cases.[1] In many instances the peripheral nervous system is involved, mainly the facial nerve.[3] Patients vary in age from adolescents to the elderly; most are female, and many are black. Only in a small minority of cases is nerve involvement tumefactive. Mono- or polyneuropathy may be seen, and nerve roots can be affected. Among spinal nerves, the peroneal, median, radial, and phrenic nerves, as well as the cauda equina nerve roots, are most often involved.[2] All nerve compartments, including epineurium, perineurium, and endoneurium, may contain noncaseating granulomas. By definition, microorganisms are lacking, and cultures are negative. Nerve injury may be due to compression or to accompanying lymphocytic angiitis. The principal differential diagnosis includes fungal and mycobacterial infection. Clinical, radiographic, and laboratory features generally establish the diagnosis. Not surprisingly, the prognosis of patients with sarcoidosis of peripheral nerve is more favorable than of those with central nervous system involvement.

### Leprosy

Caused by *Mycobacterium leprae* infection, this chronic disease is the most common treatable cause of peripheral neuropathy worldwide. It occurs not only in the tropics

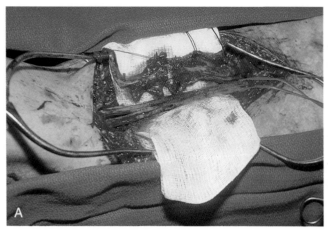
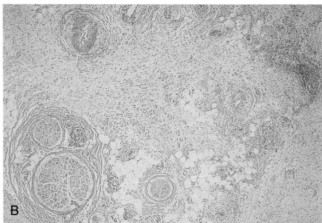

**FIGURE 12–19**    INFLAMMATORY PSEUDOTUMOR OF NERVE

This operative photograph (A) of a reported case[6] shows the intact normal sciatic nerve to be surrounded by a layer of fibroinflammatory epineurial tissue dissected free of the nerve. The lesion (B) consists of a cytologically benign lymphocyte and plasma cell infiltrate within epineurium. Note the trapped normal nerve fascicles (*lower left*).

but in temperate zones as well. The pathology of nerve involvement has been well documented.[2] Superficially situated nerves are particularly affected. Only a minority of people are susceptible to infection, children more so than adults. Of its two major forms—lepromatous and tuberculoid leprosy—the latter more often produces nerve enlargement (Fig. 12–20A). Microscopically the lesions consist of epithelioid granulomas only rarely associated with caseation (Fig. 12–20B). Lymphocytic infiltrates often accompany the epithelioid histiocytes. Destruction of nerve fibers is extensive. On Fite stain organisms are rarely evident within histiocytes and Langhans-type giant cells. A particularly intense response to the bacilli results in the formation of a mass—a so-called "cold abscess." For a discussion of the differential diagnosis of leprosy, the reader is referred to an authoritative text.[1] Specific antimicrobial therapy is curative.

# HAMARTOMA AND CHORISTOMA

## Lipofibromatous Hamartoma

**Definition.** A benign overgrowth of epineurial adipose and fibrous tissue, with or without associated macrodactyly, usually involving the upper extremity.

**Clinical Features.** This very uncommon, sporadically occurring overgrowth of epineurial fibroadipose tissue results in compression neuropathy.[1, 6, 11, 12] In the upper extremity, most but not all lesions occur in the distal arm and hand.[5, 10] The lower extremity may also be affected. A large percentage of lipofibromatous hamartomas are present at birth. "True macrodactyly," enlargement of bones in addition to soft tissue, typifies some cases. No association with neurofibromatosis

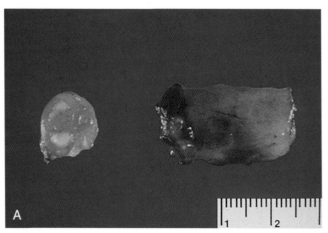
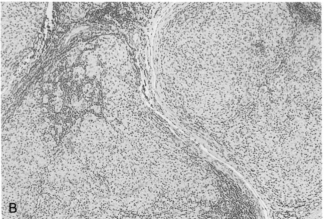

**FIGURE 12–20**    TUBERCULOID LEPROSY

Occasionally this variant of leprosy causes marked enlargement of a peripheral nerve (A). Microscopically, the fascicles contain numerous noncaseating granulomas (B) but are largely devoid of bacilli.

1 (NF1) has been reported, but one example reportedly arose in the setting of Klippel-Trénaunay-Weber syndrome.[1] Symptoms consist of sensorimotor deficits. Not surprisingly, median nerve lesions may present as carpal tunnel syndrome.

**Macroscopic Features.** Lipofibromatous hamartomas are yellow-gray, often sausage-shaped masses of fat containing one or more centrally situated nerves (Fig. 12–21A). In some instances the lesion follows not only the course of the main nerve but its branches as well.

**Microscopic Features.** The epineurium of the affected nerve is expanded by mature adipose tissue (Fig. 12–21B). As a result of chronic compression, entrapped nerves often demonstrate axon and myelin loss, as well as concentric layers of perineurial cells around nerve fibers. The latter somewhat resemble pseudo–onion bulbs of intraneural perineurioma and have been studied ultrastructurally.[13] Microfascicle formation may also be seen. Long-standing lesions also feature intraneural collagen deposition.

**Differential Diagnosis.** Various adipose lesions enter into the differential diagnosis, including *soft tissue lipoma*. The distinction is readily made at surgery, because such lesions are composed entirely of adipose tissue, are delicately encapsulated, and lack an intimate association with nerve. The occasional lobular lipoma of the epineurium lacks tubular ensheathment of nerve. Because cranial nerves are devoid of epineurium, so-called lipomas of cranial nerve roots are more complex developmental lesions.[3, 4, 7, 8] Of these, some contain additional tissue elements, including muscle. Such lesions are discussed in the next section, Neuromuscular Choristoma.

**Treatment and Prognosis.** Excision, although curative, often results in functional deficits.[2, 9] Intraneural dissection[13] or decompression alone may be more beneficial.

## Neuromuscular Choristoma

**Definition.** Also termed neuromuscular hamartoma, this non-neoplastic mass lesion consists of mature skeletal muscle and peripheral nerves, the myocytes being intimately associated with nerve fibers and encompassed by perineurium.

**General Comments.** The nature of this rare lesion is unsettled, but parallels have been drawn to muscle-containing "lipomas" of the lumbar sac,[3] the capacity of neuroectoderm to undergo mesenchymal differentiation ("ectomesenchyme"),[7] and the occurrence of skeletal muscle heterotopias within normal laryngeal nerves.[11] In any event, the lesion is non-neoplastic.

**Clinical Features.** Sporadic in occurrence, neuromuscular choristomas are rare; only a small number have been reported.[4, 8] An occasional example is congenital, but most present in childhood or adolescence. There is no sex predilection. Some lesions produce neurologic symptoms, whereas others present with only mass effects. Involvement of major nerve trunks is the rule, but small nerves may be affected.[2] Cranial nerve examples[12] and multiple lesions[2, 9] are infrequent. The same is true of associated malformations, such as intradural lipoma and skeletal anomalies.[3, 9]

**Macroscopic Features.** Nodular, firm, and often brown in color, most neuromuscular choristomas are globular masses; only a minority somewhat retain the shape of the nerve. Nearly all have been associated with a sizable if not a major nerve, branches of which enter and exit the mass and insinuate themselves within the lesion. On cut surface, nodules of neuromuscular tissue are often separated by fibrous septae. Electrical stimulation of the lesion results in its contraction.

**Microscopic Features.** Neuromuscular choristomas consist of disordered, well-differentiated skeletal muscle

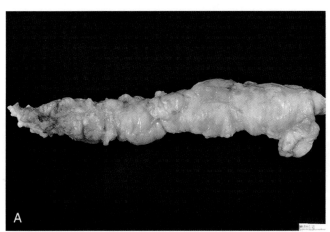
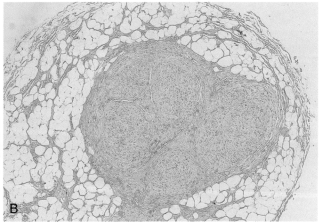

**FIGURE 12–21    LIPOFIBROMATOUS HAMARTOMA OF NERVE**

This massive, sausage-shaped expansion of epineurium (*A*) has encased the distal median and digital nerves at the level of the wrist and thumb. Note the transected, residual nerve stump (*left*). On cross section (*B*), such nerves lie embedded in fibroadipose tissue.

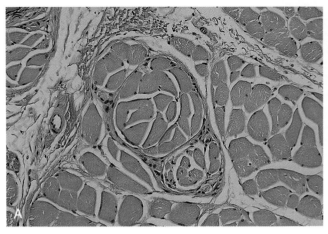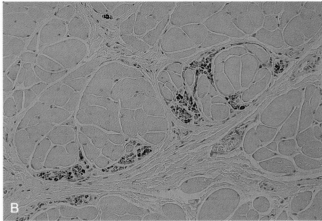

**FIGURE 12–22** NEUROMUSCULAR CHORISTOMA

Note nodules of skeletal muscle intimately admixed with bundles of nerve fibers of varying size (A). The latter are best seen on neurofilament protein immunostain (B).

bundles and individual fibers that are haphazardly distributed among myelinated nerves. A careful search often shows at least grouped or individual myocytes lying in endoneurium among individual nerve fibers rather than simply between fascicles (Fig. 12–22A). One unique example featured not only skeletal but also smooth muscle.[10] As a rule, muscle bundles predominate, particularly at the center of the lesion. Histochemical stains for axons (Bodian, Bielschowsky's) and myelin (Luxol fast blue) are useful in highlighting the neural component.

**Immunohistochemical and Ultrastructural Features.** The neural component of neuromuscular choristoma is particularly well seen on immunostains for neurofilament protein (Fig. 12–22B) and S-100 protein. As expected, the muscular component is immunoreactive for the full spectrum of skeletal muscle markers. Only a single reported example of neuromuscular choristoma has been studied ultrastructurally.[10]

**Differential Diagnosis.** Both *peripheral nerve sheath tumors with myoid differentiation* and rhabdomyoma enter into the differential diagnosis. Only a single example of neurofibroma with rhabdomyomatous components, a so-called "benign triton tumor," has been reported.[6] The patternless, loose-textured, mucin-rich stroma of *neurofibroma* tissue is alien to neuromuscular choristoma. Conversely, normal-appearing nerve fascicles and highly organized muscle are not seen in neurofibroma of this unusual type. Unlike neuromuscular choristoma, *malignant peripheral nerve sheath tumor (MPNST) with rhabdomyosarcomatous components (malignant triton tumor)* is an NF1-associated, cytologically malignant, spindle cell neoplasm. It contains only a minor myoid component. Although the central, muscle-rich component of neuromuscular choristoma may simulate *rhabdomyoma,* the latter consists entirely of muscle and lacks a neural component. *Cranial nerve lipoma,* an often muscle-containing lipomatous lesion of cranial nerve roots and ganglia, may be confused with

neuromuscular choristoma. The finding of a definite adipose component and lack of the intimate "muscle-in-nerve" element aids in the distinction. Last, a *fibromatosis (desmoid tumor)* component may either initially overshadow or postoperatively overrun the underlying neuromuscular choristoma.[1, 8]

**Treatment and Prognosis.** Neuromuscular choristomas are benign and are cured by simple resection. An occasional example spontaneously regresses.[5] Thus the approach should be conservative and nerve sparing. In some instances, a concurrent or postoperative fibromatosis necessitates an amputation.[8]

# BENIGN PERIPHERAL NERVE SHEATH TUMORS

In addition to variants of schwannoma and neurofibroma, the clinicopathologic features of which are well known, two perineurioma variants have come to be recognized. These and other lesions in the expanding spectrum of benign peripheral nerve sheath tumors are the subject of this section.

## Schwannoma Variants

### Conventional Schwannoma

**Definition.** A benign, encapsulated nerve sheath tumor composed entirely of Schwann cells.

**General Comments.** Because Schwann cells are a universal constituent of peripheral nerve, schwannomas are encountered at a variety of sites and include intracranial, intraspinal, and extraspinal examples. Even parenchymal tumors have been described.[6] Intracranial tumors are discussed in Chapter 4, and intraspinal lesions in Chapter 11. Extraspinal schwannomas may arise from motor, sensory, or autonomic nerves and are usually encountered as solitary lesions in adults. Multiple schwannomas have an association with neurofibromatosis 2 (NF2) as well as with schwannomatosis, a recently characterized condition.[28, 29] Radiation therapy seemingly induces some schwannomas.[36]

In addition to conventional schwannomas, three other morphologic variants are worthy of note.[11, 35] These are cellular schwannoma, a tumor often mistaken for MPNST; plexiform schwannoma, which usually involves dermal and subcutaneous tissue; and melanotic schwannoma, a subset of which is associated with Carney's complex.[4, 5] Each is discussed in turn.

**Macroscopic Features.** Although incipient schwannomas arise as local proliferations within a nerve fascicle (Fig. 12–23A, B), most symptomatic tumors have acquired sufficient size to deflect the parent nerve over the surface of the tumor (Fig. 12–23C, D). The nerve may become so attenuated as to preclude detection. Most schwannomas, mucosal examples excepted,[17] are

well-encapsulated, firm, globular to multinodular (Fig. 12–24A) masses lying eccentric to their parent nerve. In contrast, intraneural neurofibromas are delicately invested, soft, often fusiform enlargements of the affected nerve. In the early phase, schwannomas are solid and tan on cut surface (Fig. 12–24B). In contrast, long-standing lesions are often large, partly cystic and hemorrhagic, and yellow due to xanthomatous degeneration (Fig. 12–24C). Marked cystic change may also be seen (Fig. 12–24D). Intradural schwannomas (Fig. 12–25A) or paraspinal tumors showing intraspinal extension through a foramen (Fig. 12–25B) may compress the spinal cord. Mucosal schwannomas are rare and are unencapsulated (Fig. 12–26).

**Microscopic Features.** Typical schwannomas are encapsulated tumors (Fig. 12–27A) featuring hyalinized vessels (Fig. 12–27B). The majority exhibit two distinct histologic patterns referred to as Antoni A and B (Fig. 12–28A, B). The former consists of elongated, tightly

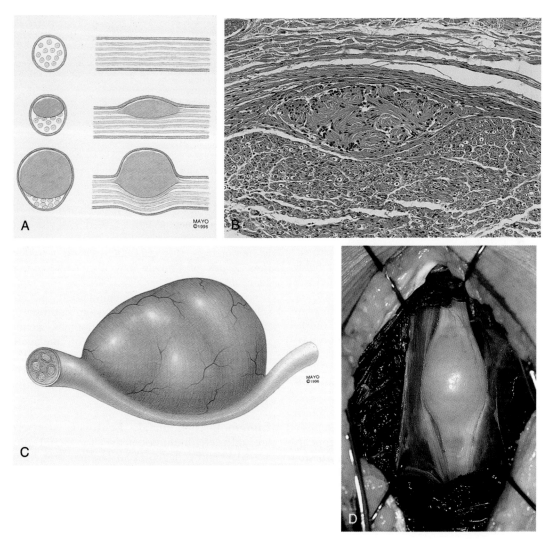

**FIGURE 12–23    SCHWANNOMA**

Schematic illustration (A) and micrograph (B) of the relationship of a growing schwannoma to its parent nerve. Another schematic illustration (C) and an operative photograph (D) show the eccentric growth of the tumor relative to the nerve. The protruding belly of the tumor lies atop the remainder of the nerve (C, D).

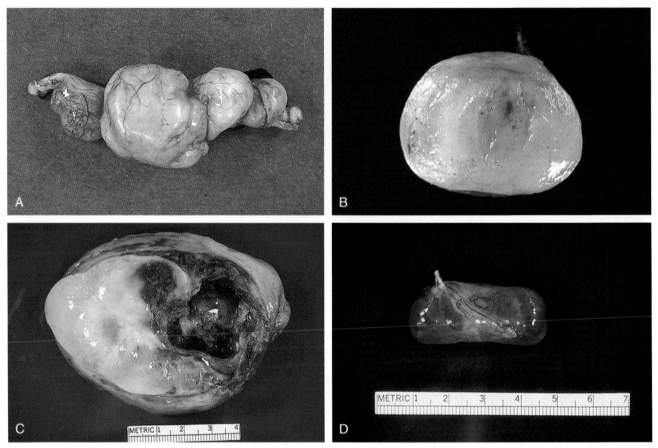

**FIGURE 12–24    SCHWANNOMA**

Externally and on cut section, the gross appearance of schwannomas varies, with some tumors being multinodular (A). On cut section, they may be solid and yellow-tan in color (B), necrotic and hemorrhagic with cystic change (C), or thin walled and almost entirely cystic (D).

compacted cells with fusiform and tapered nuclei (Fig. 12–28A). Palisades created by alignment of nuclei alternating with cytoplasm-rich, anucleate zones (Verocay bodies; Fig. 12–28C) produce a staggered pattern, which is either regimented over several low-power fields or jumbled in distribution (Fig. 12–28D). The anucleate zones are often fibrillar appearing and consist of elongated cytoplasmic processes (Fig. 12–28C). In contrast, Antoni B tissue consists of an unstructured meshwork of loosely disposed cells with rounded, hyperchromatic nuclei and short, disordered processes (Fig. 12–28B). Foamy histiocytes may be abundant. The histochemical and ultrastructural features of Antoni B tissue suggest it results from a degenerative process.[37] Pyknotic Schwann cell nuclei are particularly common in Antoni B tissue, wherein they superficially resemble lymphocytes (Fig. 12–28B). In addition to the appearances described, occasional schwannomas show microcytics in which the "lining cells" appear pseudoepithelial (Fig. 12–28E). Such cytologic and histologic variation in schwannomas makes smear preparations of marginal utility (Fig. 12–28F). Less common patterns include neurofibroma-like tissue, whorl formation, epithelioid features, and mucinous change (Fig. 12–29).

Degenerative changes are a common feature of schwannomas. So-called "ancient schwannomas" contain cells with large, bizarre, hyperchromatic nuclei (Fig.

12–30A).[3, 9] Such degenerative changes are of no prognostic significance. When marked, vascular sclerosis may result in ischemic, infarct-like necrosis (Fig. 12–30B) or in hemorrhage (Fig. 12–30C) with hemosiderin deposition. Zones of fibrosis may also be encountered (Fig. 12–30D).

Although pigment accumulation in conventional schwannoma is due to cytoplasmic lipofuscin accumulation, some peripheral schwannomas contain "true" melanin.[15, 25] Of these, one form of "melanotic schwannoma" is psammomatous and associated with an inherited multisystem disorder (Carney's complex).[4] These special variants are discussed later under the heading Melanotic Schwannoma.

**Immunohistochemical Features.** All schwannomas are diffusely immunoreactive for S-100 protein (Fig. 12–31A) and collagen IV or laminin (Fig. 12–31B). The latter highlights pericellular basal lamina, as do reticulin stains (Fig. 12–31C). Leu-7 and occasionally myelin basic protein staining is also observed.[22] In contrast, neurofibromas show less uniform S-100 protein reactivity, a reflection of their variable content of Schwann cells, fibroblasts, and perineurial-like cells. Vimentin immunoreactivity is observed in virtually all forms of peripheral nerve sheath tumor. Although it attests to "immunoviability" of the tissue sample, vimentin staining

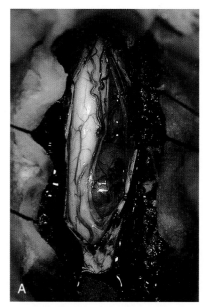 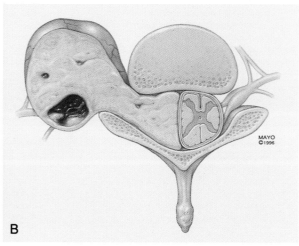

**FIGURE 12–25   SCHWANNOMA AND THE SPINAL CORD**

Intradural examples (*A*), as well as paraspinous tumors with intraspinal extension (*B*), can displace the spinal cord.

is of little diagnostic use, being present in nearly all soft tissue tumors.[16] Bona fide positivity for glial fibrillary acidic protein (GFAP) is observed in approximately half of schwannomas (Fig. 12–31*D*),[22, 24, 30] a factor of importance in the assessment of CNS lesions, particularly of the cerebellopontine angle wherein exophytic gliomas are also encountered.

**Ultrastructural Features.** At the ultrastructural level, schwannoma cells exhibit intertwining processes and two diagnostically helpful features, pericellular basement membranes enveloping individual cells and intercellular "long-spacing" collagen (Fig. 12–32).[10, 12, 33, 37]

**Molecular and Cytogenetic Features.** In a recent chromosome banding study, clonal abnormalities were

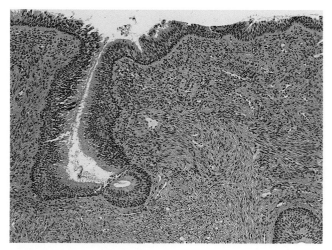

**FIGURE 12–26   SCHWANNOMA**

Mucosal tumors, such as this nasal example, lack a capsule. Note its abutment with the epithelial layer.

seen in half or more of benign nerve sheath tumors.[31] Karyotypic abnormalities in schwannomas were independent of their site of origin and included loss of chromosome 22q material, loss of a sex chromosome, and trisomy 7. In contrast, neurofibromas only infrequently showed karyotypic abnormalities.

**Differential Diagnosis.** Schwannomas must be distinguished from *neurofibromas*, of the localized intraneural type. A number of clinicopathologic features aid the process (Tables 12–2 and 12–3). As previously noted, most schwannomas present as discrete masses, eccentric to the parent nerve, surrounded by a collagenous capsule, and prone to cyst formation as well as xanthomatous change. In contrast, *localized intraneural neurofibromas* produce fusiform symmetric expansion of the nerve, are delicately encapsulated, have a mucoid texture, and are translucent on cut section. In schwannomas, remaining fascicles of the parent nerve are peripherally displaced, and reside mainly on the tumor surface. Only occasional nerve fibers of the affected fascicle lie within the tumor. In neurofibromas, nerve fibers tend to be dispersed throughout or centrally concentrated. Widely separated axons are often difficult to identify, particularly in large tumors and ones cut in cross section. We find it convenient to use either Masson trichrome or Luxol fast blue stains to highlight their myelin sheaths. Simpler yet is the use of immunostains for neurofilament protein. Unlike schwannomas, which consist entirely of Schwann cells, neurofibromas are loose textured and consist of disordered and dispersed Schwann cells, perineurial-like cells, and fibroblasts. This admixture is reflected in nonuniform immunoreactivity for S-100 protein. Occasional schwannomas display somewhat indeterminate features, including both typical Antoni A tissue and a looser, myxoid, slightly fascicular pattern resembling neurofibroma (see Fig. 12–29*A*).

**TABLE 12–2**
**Clinicopathologic Comparison of Schwannoma and Neurofibroma**

| Schwannoma | Neurofibroma* |
|---|---|
| Non–NF1 associated/occasional NF2 or schwannomatosis associated | NF1 associated/non–NF2 associated |
| Frequently affects extremities | Frequently involves the trunk |
| Usually solitary | Frequently solitary |
| Nerve often identified | Nerve infrequently identified |
| Eccentric to nerve | Incorporates nerve |
| Globular or plexiform | Fusiform, globular, plexiform, or diffuse |
| Encapsulated | Delicately surrounded by perineurium and epineurium (solitary and plexiform neurofibroma); no capsule (diffuse neurofibroma) |
| Nonmucoid, soft to firm | Mucoid and firm |
| Tan to yellow, opaque | Gray-tan, opalescent |
| High cellularity | Low to moderate cellularity |
| Biphasic Antoni A and B patterns | Uniphasic pattern with gradual changes in cellularity |
| Scant or no stromal mucin | Mucin-rich matrix |
| Axons often absent | Axons often present |
| Palisading and Verocay bodies | Wagner-Meissner or rarely pacinian-like corpuscles; no palisading |
| Composed of Schwann cells | Composed of Schwann cells, perineurial-like cells, fibroblasts, and transitional cells |
| Mast cells infrequent | Mast cells frequent |
| Malignant transformation extremely rare | Malignant transformation rare (2% of patients with NF1) |

*Exclusive of plexiform neurofibroma.
NF, neurofibromatosis.

Most such lesions are straightforward schwannomas, as evidenced by a thick fibrous capsule, hyalinized vasculature, hemosiderin deposits, absence of dispersed axons, and paucity of mucopolysaccharides. Neurofibromas containing Schwann cell nodules of varying size may also be encountered (see later). Such "mixed" patterns are well recognized, especially in the setting of NF1.

Considerable nuclear pleomorphism, often accompanied by tumor hyalinization and decreased cellularity, may be seen in long-standing or in large tumors (see Fig. 12–30A).[3, 9] Such "degenerative nuclear atypia" is not indicative of malignancy; proliferative activity is lacking. Just the same, taken out of context or viewed under high magnification, the considerable cellularity of Antoni A and B regions of some schwannomas may prompt an erroneous diagnosis of *MPNST*. This mistake is especially frequent with "cellular schwannoma" (Figs. 12–33 and 12–34A, B),[7, 14, 39, 40] a monomorphous, spindle cell tumor simulating MPNST and discussed later.

Lastly, the plexiform variant of schwannoma must be distinguished from *plexiform neurofibroma*[21, 23] (see later), a typically more extensive, deeply situated lesion

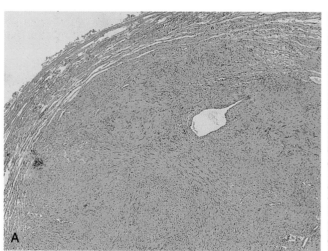
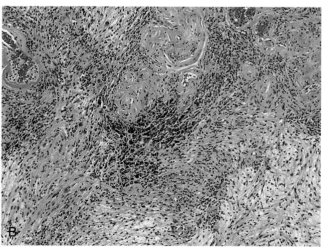

**FIGURE 12–27**   SCHWANNOMA

Key morphologic features include a distinct collagenous capsule (A) and vascular hyalinization (B).

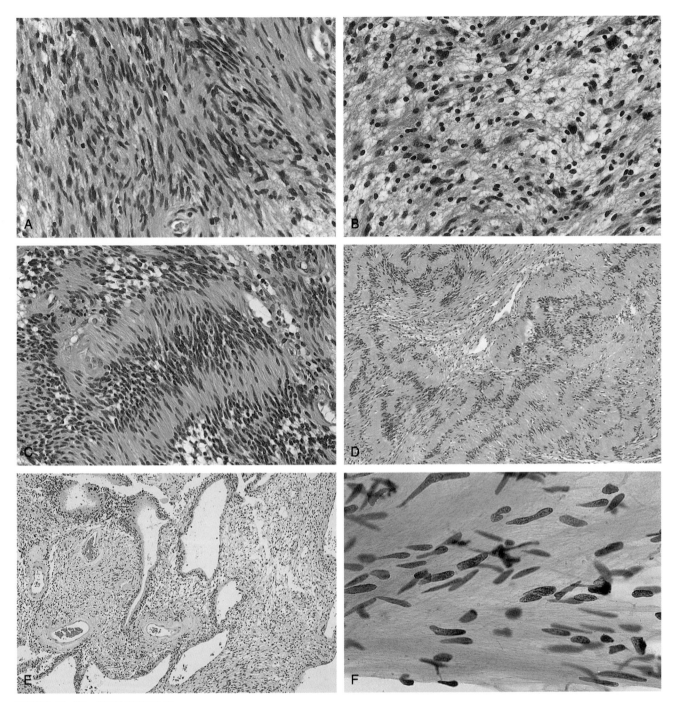

**FIGURE 12–28**    SCHWANNOMA

Typical tumors feature a biphasic histologic pattern that includes compact tissue (*A*) consisting of spindle cells with elongated nuclei (Antoni A pattern) and loose-textured tissue (Antoni B pattern) consisting of jumbled multipolar cells with round nuclei (*B*). So-called Verocay bodies (*C*) consist of staggered, alternating arrangements of nuclei and cytoplasmic processes in Antoni A tissue. Such arrangements can be orderly (*D, lower right*) or not (*D, upper left*). Formation of microcysts with pseudoepithelial linings (*E*) is relatively common. This morphologic variation in schwannomas confounds the interpretation of smear preparations, as does the tissue's reluctance to form a thin smear (*F*). The long, tapered nucleus are, nevertheless, distinctive.

strongly associated with NF1. The latter is fully discussed on pages 608 to 611.

**Treatment and Prognosis.** Despite their potential for regrowth following incomplete excision, schwannomas are benign and only rarely become malignant.[2, 32, 34, 35, 42, 43] Bone remodeling due to chronic compressive growth often affects spinal foramina. Significant bone destruction

is uncommon[7, 20] but may be seen in so-called "giant sacral schwannomas".[1]

## Cellular Schwannoma

**Definition.** A hypercellular schwannoma composed largely or exclusively of Antoni A tissue, devoid of telltale Verocay bodies, and exhibiting variable mitotic activity.

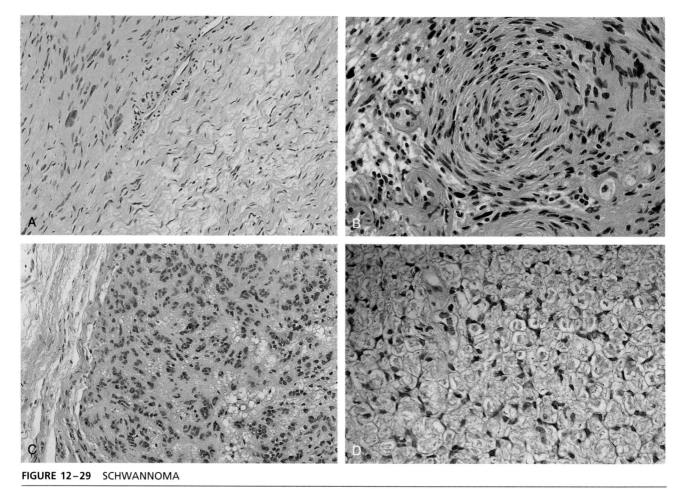

**FIGURE 12–29    SCHWANNOMA**

Pattern variations include loose-textured tissue resembling neurofibroma (*A, lower right*), whorl formation (*B*), tight clustering of epithelioid tumor cells (*C*), and mucinous change (*D*).

**General Comments.** Cellular schwannomas are now well characterized.[7, 27, 35, 39, 40] This common variant of schwannoma is mistaken for MPNST in about 10% of cases.[7] Nearly all examples are solitary; an NF1 association is unusual.[7] Only 5% occur in childhood.[7] Most are situated in the paravertebral regions of the pelvis, retroperitoneum, and mediastinum or in the intraspinal space.[27, 39, 40] Among the latter, fully one third are "dumbbell tumors" often associated with bone erosion. Distal peripheral nerves are uncommonly involved. Only a minority arise in cranial nerves, usually the fifth or eighth.[7, 20] The head and neck region may also be affected. As a rule, cellular schwannomas are slow growing.

**Macroscopic Features.** Cellular schwannomas are encapsulated, expansile masses resembling conventional schwannomas. Ranging from 1 to 20 cm in size, only one third to one half are nerve associated.[7, 39] In most instances, the tumors are globular. Their cut surface appears homogeneously tan without apparent necrosis, cyst formation, or xanthomatous change (Fig. 12–33A). An occasional example is grossly plexiform (Fig. 12–33B).[41] Cellular schwannomas are more often bone destructive than are conventional schwannomas.[7, 20]

**Microscopic Features.** The presence of basic schwannoma features, such as a thick capsule, vascular hyalinization, and schwannian cytology (Fig. 12–34A, B) generally confirms the diagnosis, as do classic immunotypic and ultrastructure fractures (see later). Subcapsular chronic inflammation and patchy histiocyte infiltrates are ancillary features (Fig. 12–34A, C). Although not required for the diagnosis, mitoses in small number are usually present (Fig. 12–34B); brisk mitotic activity is uncommon. In one series,[7] MIB-1 labeling indices varied considerably; median values in nonrecurring and recurring tumors were similar (6% and 8%, respectively). Fully two thirds of tumors were diploid, and the remainder were either tetraploid or aneuploid. Immunoreactivity for p53 was seen in approximately 50% of cases, but at low levels. The occasional finding of degenerative nuclear atypia or of focal, nonpalisading necrosis may cause confusion with MPNST. This misdiagnosis occurred in 10% of cases in one large series.[7]

**Immunohistochemical and Ultrastructural Features.** Cellular schwannomas exhibit the same immunophenotype (Fig. 12–35) and fine structural features (see Fig. 12–32) as conventional schwannomas.[7, 40]

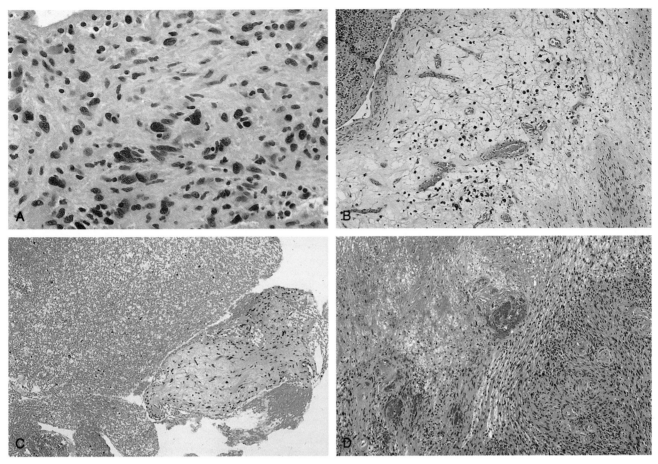

**FIGURE 12–30    SCHWANNOMA**

Degenerative changes include nuclear hyperchromasia and pleomorphism (*A*), widespread stromal hyalinization (*B*), necrosis due to vascular thrombosis (*C*), and hemorrhage, in which the finding of aspirated tumor fragments may secure the diagnosis (*D*).

**Differential Diagnosis.** The distinction of cellular schwannoma from *conventional schwannoma* and, more importantly, from *MPNST* is summarized in Table 12–3. The distinction of cellular schwannoma from *leiomyoma* (smooth muscle actin-positive) and from *meningioma* or *soft tissue perineurioma* (both EMA-positive) generally poses no problem.

**Treatment and Prognosis** Cellular schwannomas are benign. Nonetheless, tumors that are centrally situated (intracranial, intraspinal, and sacral) are quite prone to recur (30% to 40%) following incomplete resection.[7] To date, no cellular schwannoma has transformed to MPNST, metastasized, or behaved in a clinically malignant manner.

### Plexiform Schwannoma

This form of schwannoma exhibits a plexiform or multinodular pattern of growth.[35, 41] Although the parent nerve is not always evident, the lesion does involve superficially situated dermal and or subcutaneous nerves (Fig. 12–36*A*, *B*).[21, 23, 35] Most plexiform schwannomas arise in an extremity or in the head and neck region; cranial nerves are usually spared. Deeply situated tumors[38] and visceral examples[8, 18] are uncommon.

Histologically, the proliferation of Schwann cells clearly lies within nerves (Fig. 12–36*C*). This is confirmed by the finding of residual axons and perineurium on neurofilament protein and EMA stain, respectively. Most plexiform schwannomas are sporadic, but some occur in the setting of schwannomatosis,[14, 21] a recently described condition.[28, 29] Only a rare example arises in association with NF1[21, 23] or NF2.[19] A small proportion of plexiform schwannomas recur if incompletely excised.[21, 23, 35]

### Melanotic Schwannoma

Schwannomas that contain true (melanosome-associated) melanin are rare.[15, 25, 35] Their peak incidence is somewhat earlier than that of conventional schwannomas. Unlike the latter, their degree of encapsulation varies. Most affect spinal nerves, but an association with sympathetic ganglia is relatively frequent. Melanotic schwannomas consist in varying proportion of epithelioid to spindle cells (Fig. 12–37*A*, *B*). Thus, they resemble melanoma. Degenerative nuclear changes are commonly seen (Fig. 12–37*C*). At the immunohistochemical and ultrastructural (Fig. 12–38) levels, the tumors exhibit a mixed phenotype with features of both Schwann cells and melanocytes. For example, they show immunoreactivity for markers of both schwannoma (S-100 protein, collagen IV, laminin) and melanoma (HMB45,

**TABLE 12–3**
**Conventional Schwannoma, Cellular Schwannoma, and Malignant Peripheral Nerve Sheath Tumor (MPNST):
Differential Diagnosis**

| Findings | Conventional Schwannoma | Cellular Schwannoma | MPNST |
|---|---|---|---|
| **Gross** | Usually globoid, encapsulated tumor with abundant homogeneous light tan tissue; may be cystic or hemorrhagic and show yellow patches. No gross necrosis. | Usually globoid, encapsulated tumor, firmer than classic schwannoma, and homogeneously tan. Occasional patches of yellow, but no gross necrosis. | Fusiform or globoid, pseudoencapsulated (infiltrative of surrounding tissues), firm, cream-tan, usually grossly necrotic tumor. |
| **Microscopic** | Antoni A and B areas with Verocay bodies; commonly find hyalinized and thick-walled blood vessels and lipid-laden histiocytes. Mitotic figures infrequent. Rarely see malignant transformation. | Mainly hypercellular Antoni A tissue. Cells are arranged in fascicles or whorls and may show marked hyperchromasia and nuclear pleomorphism. Notable are lymphoid deposits in capsule or perivascular area. Commonly find thick-walled blood vessels and collections of lipid-laden histiocytes. Rare foci of necrosis. Mitoses not uncommon but usually number no more than 4/10 HPF. | Markedly hypercellular, fasciculated, spindle cell tumor generally consisting of a uniform size and pronounced hyperchromasia. Geographic necrosis and mitotic counts in excess of 4/10 HPF are common. Epithelioid cells predominate in about 5% of tumors, and 15% show heterologous glandular or sarcomatous elements. |
| **Immunohisto-chemical** | Diffuse and strong expression of S-100 protein. | Diffuse and strong expression of S-100 protein. | S-100 protein expression in scattered cells of 50–70% of cases. |
| **Electron microscopy** | Well-differentiated cells with long, often interlacing cytoplasmic processes coated by basement membrane on their free surfaces. Intercellular, long-spacing collagen common. | Similar to classic schwannoma. Increased cellularity. More nuclear atypia and occasional residual arrays of long, basement membrane–coated cytoplasmic processes. Long-spacing collagen less common. | Poorly differentiated cells with more pleomorphic nuclei, thick cytoplasmic processes, and sometimes patchy basement membrane. Long-spacing collagen rarely seen. |
| **Clinical behavior** | May cause bone erosion and can recur if incompletely excised. Thus far 5 reported examples with malignant transformation that followed a malignant clinical course. | May cause bone erosion and recur if incompletely excised. Thus far no clinically malignant examples. | Has a proclivity to invade and destroy nearby soft tissue, recur locally, and metastasize distantly (usually to lung). About 90% are high-grade lesions. |

HPF, high-power field.

melan A, tyrosine hydroxylase). Ultrastructurally, they exhibit pericellular or perilobular basal lamina formation as well as variably pigmented melanosomes.

Melanotic schwannomas occur in two forms: nonpsammomatous tumors[15] and ones containing psammoma bodies (see Fig. 12–37D).[5] The majority of nonpsammomatous tumors involve spinal nerves, whereas psammomatous lesions often affect viscera as well (gastrointestinal tract, heart). In either case, cranial nerves may also be involved. Approximately half of patients with psammomatous schwannomas have Carney's complex,[4] an autosomal disorder caused by a mutation of the PKA holoenzyme[26] and variously featuring facial lentigines, cardiac or cutaneous myxomas, endocrine hyperfunction (Cushing's syndrome due to multinodular adrenal cortical hyperplasia or acromegaly due to pituitary adenoma), and calcifying Sertoli cell tumors.[4]

Approximately 10% of melanotic schwannomas are malignant.[25] Such tumors typically feature invasion rather than circumscription (Fig. 12–39A), show areas of necrosis (Fig. 12–39B), and exhibit cytologic malignancy as evidenced by violaceous macronucleoli and brisk mitotic activity (Fig. 12–39C), including abnormal mitoses.

# Neurofibroma

**Definition.** Neurofibromas are benign peripheral nerve sheath tumors of diffuse, localized intraneural, plexiform, or massive type consisting of Schwann cells, perineurial-like cells, fibroblasts, and cells with intermediate features. Many, but not all, are associated with a recognizable nerve. As a result, residual axons, myelinated or unmyelinated, are frequently found.

**General Comments.** The recognition of neurofibroma and its distinction from schwannoma is important. In both clinical and pathologic terms, these two principal peripheral nerve sheath tumors differ significantly (see Table 12–2). Recognition of the highly varied gross and microscopic features of these lesions is clinically relevant, because some neurofibromas are associated with NF1 or have a propensity to transform to MPNST.[6]

The fundamental nature of neurofibromas is coming into focus. Both the multiplicity of lesions in NF1 and their cellular heterogeneity suggest a hyperplastic nature. However, X chromosome inactivation studies showing monoclonality,[30] recent genetic studies showing only

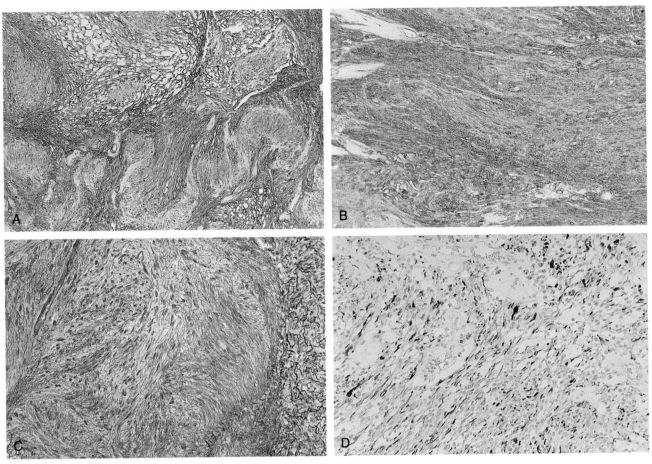

**FIGURE 12–31    SCHWANNOMA**

The immunoprofile includes widespread S-100 protein reactivity (A), stronger in Antoni A than in Antoni B; collagen IV staining (B), a reflection of the pericellular basement membrane so conspicuous on reticulin stain (C); and positivity for glial fibrillary acidic protein (D), a common feature of schwannoma and neurofibroma.

the Schwann cell element to have an NF1 deletion,[23] and the well-known tendency of some neurofibromas to transform to MPNST[28] all support a neoplastic nature. With respect to tumorigenesis, all NF1 patients possess one nonfunctional NF1 gene as a germline mutation. Evidently, neurofibromas are initiated by a second, somatic mutation.[16] Non–NF1-associated neurofibromas also occur as a result of alterations in the NF1 gene. MPNSTs that arise in transformation from neurofibromas apparently reflect the additional loss or mutation of one or more tumor suppressor genes.

Neurofibromas are a key feature of NF1, but most are sporadic lesions. Only a rare example occurs in the setting of NF2. Despite their common cellular makeup, several forms of neurofibroma have been described. Their clinical presentation and gross appearances differ considerably and include (1) cutaneous neurofibromas of both localized and diffuse type, (2) intraneural neurofibroma of localized or plexiform type, (3) massive soft tissue tumors often composed of both diffuse and plexiform elements, and (4) visceral neurofibromas. Although morphologic overlap is seen, the clinicopathologic characteristics of these lesions differ. Their gross appearance reflects their individual manners of growth

and spread. For example, cutaneous lesions presumably arise in minute nerves before diffusely infiltrating dermal and subcutaneous tissues. Intraneural neurofibromas originate in sizable nerves and undergo endoneurial spread with resultant fusiform enlargement of the affected fascicle. Involvement of multiple fascicles and their branches is the basis of plexiform neurofibromas, with their "bag of worms" configuration. Plexiform tumors often exhibit an element of diffuse soft tissue infiltration as well. Conversely, when adequately sampled, massive soft tissue neurofibromas often feature a minor plexiform component. In addition to the finding of numerous cutaneous neurofibromas, both plexiform and massive soft tissue tumors are manifestations of NF1. These variants of neurofibroma, which differ in nosologic terms from those historically applied,[12] are discussed below.

## Cutaneous Neurofibroma: Localized and Diffuse

**Clinical Features.** Unlike intraneural neurofibromas in deeper soft tissues, cutaneous neurofibromas are largely extraneural proliferations. Presumably originating from

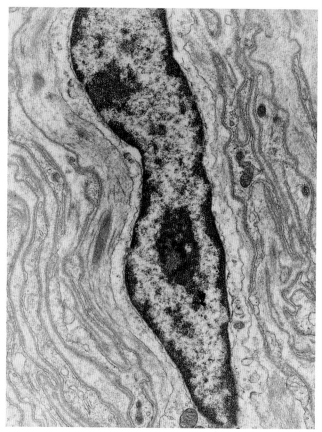

**FIGURE 12–32   SCHWANNOMA**

Ultrastructural features include cells with long cytoplasmic processes enshrouded by basement membrane. Interstitial long-spacing collagen, or "Luse bodies" (not shown), is also a common feature (× 16,000).

small peripheral nerves in dermis or subcutaneous tissue, most elevate the skin as soft, hemispheric to pedunculated lesions (localized cutaneous neurofibroma) (Fig. 12–40A), with no particular distribution. They are painless and freely movable and range in size up to 2 cm. The vast majority of localized cutaneous neurofibromas

are solitary and sporadic, occurring in patients 20 to 30 years of age.[28] When multiple, they are a cardinal feature of NF1 and are evident at puberty. In later life, NF1-associated tumors may be innumerable.

In contrast, diffuse cutaneous neurofibromas are relatively uncommon. They form plaque-like, cutaneous and subcutaneous lesions (Fig. 12–40B), often affecting the head and neck region of children or young adults. An association with NF1 is seen in approximately 10% of cases.

**Macroscopic Features.** Often polypoid (Fig. 12–40A), localized cutaneous neurofibromas may be overlain by a café au lait spot. On cut section they are relatively circumscribed but not encapsulated. Most are gray-tan in color and lack degenerative changes.

Although distinguishing localized from diffuse cutaneous neurofibromas is usually easy, mixed patterns are occasionally seen. The term "diffuse" is applied to large, plaque-like lesions (Fig. 12–40B). Ill defined and yellow-white on cut section, with a texture more adipose-rich than that of localized cutaneous neurofibromas, they consist of diffusely infiltrated, thickened dermal and subcutaneous tissue (Fig. 12–40B). Diffuse tumors more often entrap than displace cutaneous adnexa (Fig. 12–40C). Spread along subcutaneous connective tissue septa is a common feature (Fig. 12–40B). Some tumors exhibit a plexiform element as well.

**Microscopic   Features.** Microscopically, cutaneous neurofibromas may or may not be separated from overlying epidermis by a grenz zone (Fig. 12–40C). Deep portions are typically less defined. Particularly in diffuse lesions, the patternless proliferation overgrows dermal blood vessels, nerves, and adnexa (Fig. 12–40C). The twisted and angulated nuclei of the neurofibroma cells are set in a delicate to dense matrix of wavy collagen that often obscures cell processes (Fig. 12–40D). As a rule, the neural nature of cutaneous neurofibromas is readily apparent. This is particularly true of diffuse tumors in which fascicles of wavy Schwann cells are seen,

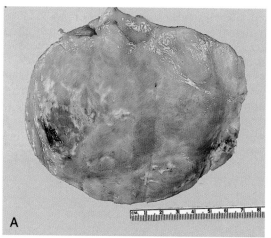
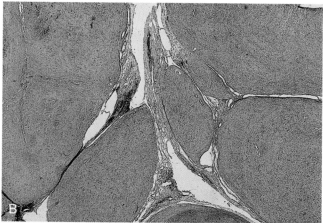

**FIGURE 12–33   CELLULAR SCHWANNOMA**

Globular (A) or occasionally plexiform in configuration (B), cellular schwannomas are often solid and fleshy. The focus of necrosis (A) is the site of a prior biopsy.

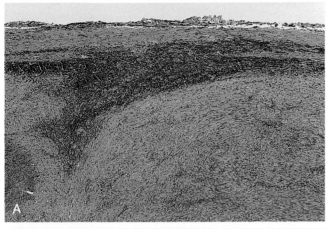

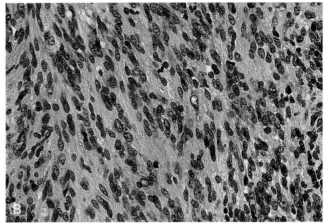

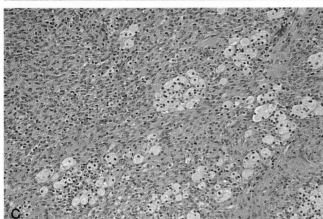

**FIGURE 12–34**   CELLULAR SCHWANNOMA

Characteristic histologic features include a substantial capsule with subcapsular chronic inflammation (*A*), increased cellularity with low-level mitotic activity (*B*), and often patchy histiocytic infiltrates (*C*).

or when cell arrangements superficially resemble tactile end organs, more often Meissner's than pacinian corpuscles.[31] The rare finding of melanin in neurofibroma cells underscores their neural crest derivation.[8, 21]

**Immunohistochemical and Ultrastructural Features.** The majority of cells in cutaneous neurofibromas

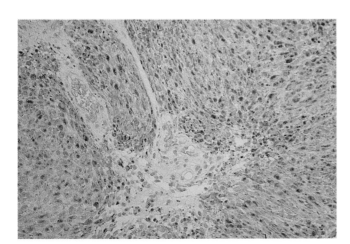

**FIGURE 12–35**   CELLULAR SCHWANNOMA

As in conventional schwannoma and in contrast to malignant peripheral nerve sheath tumor, S-100 protein immunoreactivity is uniform.

are S-100 protein immunoreactive (Fig. 12–41*A*). Attempts to find their parent nerve or nerves by applying neurofilament protein immunostains usually highlight only scattered axons. Ultrastructurally, it is the well-differentiated Schwann cells that encompass collagen bundles (Fig. 12–41*B*).

**Treatment and Prognosis.** The superficial location of localized and diffuse cutaneous neurofibromas usually permits their complete excision. Recurrence, even after partial removal, is rare. Malignant transformation is also rare.

### Localized Intraneural Neurofibroma

**Definition.** A proliferation of neurofibromatous tissue within a single nerve fascicle of varying size that typically results in a fusiform mass.

**General Comments.** Unlike the infiltrative, cutaneous forms of neurofibroma, intraneural tumors are far less common and arise in larger, more deeply situated nerves. Their larger size, more frequent association with NF1, and potential for malignant transformation makes them of greater clinical significance.

**Clinical Features.** Whereas superficially situated neurofibromas of the localized intraneural type are palpable and asymptomatic, deep tumors often present with pain or dysesthesia in the distribution of the nerve. A small

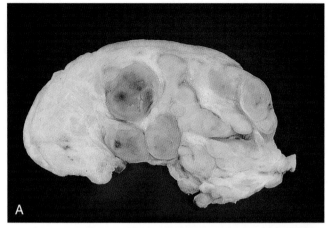

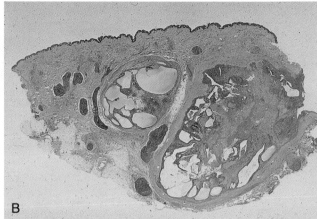

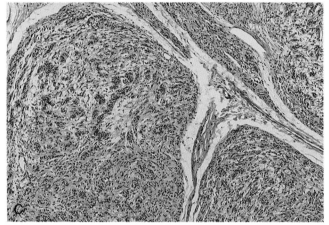

**FIGURE 12–36**   PLEXIFORM SCHWANNOMA

This exceptionally large example (*A*) clearly shows plexiform profiles of massively enlarged subcutaneous nerves. A smaller subcutaneous tumor (*B*) is multicystic. At higher magnification (*C*), the profiles are seen to be composed entirely of Schwann cells; axons are inconspicuous.

number are incidental radiographic findings. When these tumors are viewed in cross section, MRI scans often exhibit a characteristic "target sign."[1] Although intraneural neurofibromas occur at a variety of sites, including viscera, most arise in large nerves related to the cervical, brachial, or lumbosacral plexuses. Multiple intraneural neurofibromas of spinal nerve roots are usually associated with NF1 (see Fig. 12–78*D*). In contrast, solitary intraneural neurofibromas only infrequently show this association. Spinal nerve root lesions may be both intra- and extraspinal ("dumbbell tumors").

**Macroscopic Features.** The gross appearance of localized intraneural neurofibromas is typically that of a fusiform intraneural mass (Fig. 12–42). On cut section they vary in texture and color, ranging from gelatinous to fibrous and translucent to opaque tan, depending on their collagen content (Fig. 12–43). Neurofibromas may overrun either dorsal root (Fig. 12–44) or sympathetic ganglia.

**Microscopic Features.** Localized intraneural neurofibromas are characterized by a chaotic array of wavy Schwann cells bundled or dispersed in a mucopolysaccharide matrix containing variable amounts of collagen (see Fig. 12–43*B, D*). As the parent nerve merges with the bulk of a localized intraneural neurofibroma, its fibers splay and become widely separated within the matrix and among neoplastic cells.

Neurofibromas containing large, often bizarre, hyperchromatic cells with smudgy chromatin are termed "atypical neurofibromas" (Fig. 12–45). Such cells are nonproliferative and of no prognostic significance.

So-called "cellular neurofibromas" are hypercellular, feature somewhat enlarged nuclei, and show increased proliferative activity and p53 expression (Fig. 12–46).[11, 28] Such tumors are incompletely understood but appear to represent precursors of MPNST. The precise cutoff between these lesions is subjective,[28] but criteria are addressed in the section on MPNST (see below).

**Immunohistochemical Features.** Neurofibromas are reactive for vimentin, S-100 protein, and, in most cases, Leu-7.[10, 13, 14, 20, 28, 32] Staining for S-100 protein is always present, but highlights only a portion of the cells. Immunoelectron microscopy shows S-100 protein to reside in cells with schwannian features, not in perineurial-like or fibroblastic cells.[13] Reactivity of Schwann cells for GFAP is also commonly seen.[14, 15, 18] Tactile corpuscle-like structures are also S-100 protein reactive.[28] EMA staining is rarely seen in perineurial-like cells,[22] but it reliably labels perineurium surrounding the tumor. Collagen IV reactivity labels both Schwann and perineurial-like cells.[3] Minor CD34 reactivity is seen in cells of indeterminate type.[33] As a rule, axons are demonstrable on neurofilament protein stain, but their density is inversely proportional to tumor size.

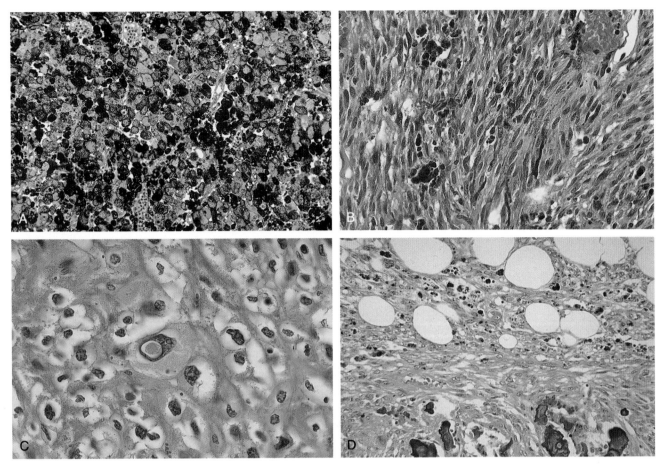

**FIGURE 12–37    MELANOTIC SCHWANNOMA**

Histologic features vary considerably, ranging from epithelioid (A) to spindle cells (B). Degenerative nuclear changes, such as pleomorphism, hyperchromasia, and cytoplasmic nuclear inclusions, are common (C). Tumors associated with Carney's complex (D) feature psammoma bodies and often adipose-like cells.

**Ultrastructural Features.** Attention has focused on the often dominant Schwann components of neurofibromas,[5, 13] but characteristic perineurial-like cells as well as fibroblasts are also present.[7, 28] Schwann cells may be

intimately associated with axons, but they also show a tendency to wrap about collagen bundles. Unlike Schwann cells, perineurial-like cells feature incomplete basal laminae, unbranched processes, and prominent pinocytotic vesicles.[7] Fibroblasts show abundance of rough endoplasmic reticulum and lack basal laminae.

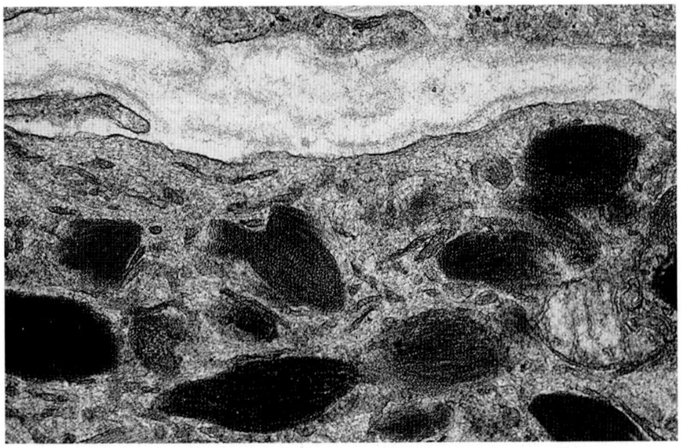

**Molecular and Cytogenetic Features.** A recent chromosome banding study of benign nerve sheath tumors and MPNSTs showed that neurofibromas exhibit clonal karyotypic abnormalities less often than do schwannomas or MPNSTs.[19]

**Differential Diagnosis.** The principal differential diagnosis is *schwannoma*. The distinguishing features of localized intraneural neurofibroma and schwannoma are summarized in Table 12–2. Ganglioneuromas, which contain numerous Schwann cells arrayed in bundles, also mimic neurofibromas. Neurofibromas can overrun sensory and autonomic ganglia, thus trapping normal ganglia and surrounding satellite cells. Ganglioneuromas differ from such neurofibromas in several ways, including (1) the neoplastic nature of the neurons, evidenced by their disarray, pleomorphism, binucleation, cytoplasmic vacuolation, and fewer accompanying satellite cells; (2)

**FIGURE 12–38    MELANOTIC SCHWANNOMA**

At the ultrastructural level, the cells exhibit cytoplasmic melanosomes and surface basal lamina ($\times$ 38,900).

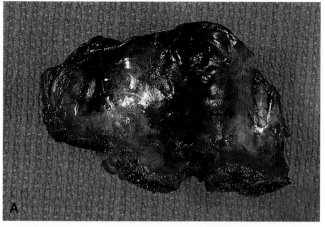

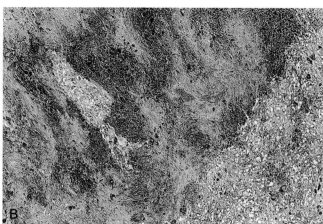

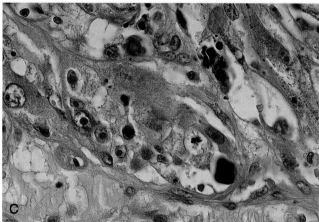

**FIGURE 12–39**    MALIGNANT MELANOTIC SCHWANNOMA

In addition to invasion of soft tissue (A) or bone, these tumors often feature necrosis (B), brisk mitotic activity, and violaceous macronucleoli (C).

the high content of axons present throughout their substance, even in areas remote from ganglion cells; and (3) the fact that the axons of overrun dorsal root ganglia are myelinated, whereas those of ganglioneuromas are not.

### Plexiform Neurofibroma

**Definition.** Neurofibromatous involvement of multiple fascicles of a nerve and often of its branches.

**General Comments.** With infrequent exception,[17] plexiform neurofibromas are pathognomonic of NF1 and involve the same nerves as do localized intraneural neurofibromas. Plexiform elements are common in large neurofibromas of the diffuse cutaneous type and in massive soft tissue neurofibromas. Most visceral and mesenteric tumors are of the plexiform type.

**Macroscopic Features.** Resembling a "bag of worms" or a braided rope composed of distended fascicles, the appearance of these tumors varies, depending on the configuration of the parent nerve. Some branch; others do not. Those prone to branch come to resemble worm-like, complex tangles of gelatinous fascicles (Fig. 12–47). These are readily evident on MRI scan (Fig. 12–48). In contrast, relatively nonbranching nerves, such as the sciatic, resemble a thick rope, some reaching hawser proportions (Figs. 12–47C and 12–65 B, C). The fascicular makeup of such brawny nerves is accentuated

as fascicles bulge from the freshly cut surface. These vary from gelatinous to firm and are often semitranslucent. The color and texture of the lesion are indicators of its relative mucin and collagen content. Affected nerves may be of sensorimotor or autonomic type.

**Microscopic Features.** Plexiform neurofibromas consist of mucin-rich expansions of fascicles in which cellularity and collagen content vary. With few exceptions, their essential histologic features are the same as those of localized intraneural neurofibroma. Since the diameter of affected nerves is generally smaller, axons are not as dispersed. Instead, they tend to be centrally concentrated within the core of the affected fascicles (Fig. 12–49A to C). In addition, structures resembling Meissner's and pacinian corpuscles may be a prominent architectural feature of plexiform tumors, particularly in their commonly occurring extraneural components.[29, 31] As previously noted, the ratio of cells to stromal mucin and collagen varies considerably. Like localized intraneural neurofibromas, plexiform tumors may also feature a "shredded carrot" pattern of collagen deposition.

Plexiform neurofibromas are particularly prone to malignant transformation. Hypercellularity, nuclear enlargement, and mitotic activity are worrisome features, but a diagnosis of MPNST should be made with caution. The subject of MPNST arising in neurofibroma is discussed in detail later. Because it can be a focal change, careful specimen sampling is imperative. As in schwan-

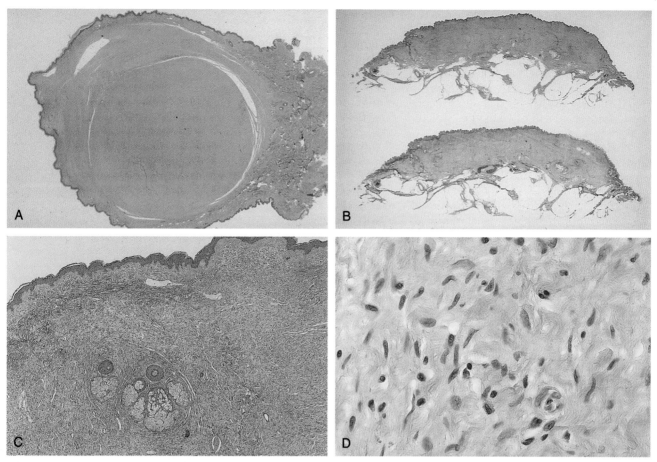

**FIGURE 12–40    CUTANEOUS NEUROFIBROMA**

Whether localized and pedunculated (A) or diffuse (B), cutaneous neurofibromas are generally unassociated with a recognizable nerve. Particularly in diffuse lesions, cutaneous adnexa are often trapped (C), and the proliferation extends into subcutaneous connective tissue septa (B). At higher magnification, the typical cytologic features of neurofibroma cells in their variably collagenous stroma are readily evident (D).

nomas, the simple finding of scattered large cells with pleomorphic nuclei and smudgy hyperchromasia is of no importance. Such tumors are termed "atypical neurofibromas."[28] Their nuclear changes are considered "degenerative" in nature and not indicative of malignancy. Of

greater significance is distinguishing a "cellular neurofibroma" element in plexiform tumors from early MPNST, a subject discussed earlier under Localized Intraneural Neurofibroma and later under Conventional Malignant Peripheral Nerve Sheath Tumor.

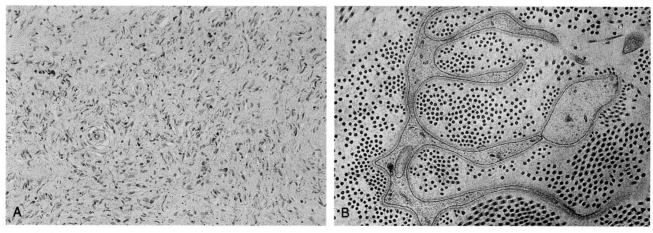

**FIGURE 12–41    DIFFUSE CUTANEOUS NEUROFIBROMA**

Immunopositivity for S-100 protein is evident in many, but not all, cells (A). The processes of a Schwann cell are seen to envelop stromal collagen fibers (B). Note the continuous basal lamina on the cell surface (× 26,400).

### Immunohistochemical and Ultrastructural Features.
The basic characteristics of plexiform neurofibromas are the same as those of localized intraneural neurofibromas (Fig. 12–49A to C).[14] Immunoreactivity for S-100 protein is seen in many but not all cells (Fig. 12–49D). When present, tactile corpuscle-like structures are also S-100 protein reactive.[28] The ultrastructural features of plexiform tumors and of tactile-like structures have been well studied.[7, 30]

**Differential Diagnosis.** Few lesions enter into consideration; most affect skin and superficial soft tissue. *Plexiform schwannomas* differ in (1) their uniform composition of Schwann cells, (2) the presence of occasional Verocay bodies, (3) the relative lack of stromal mucin, (4) the lack of a diffuse extraneural component, (5) the large size of their cells, and (6) uniform S-100 protein immunopositivity. *Plexiform fibrohistiocytic tumors* (1) show a female predilection; (2) are small and firm in texture and do not appear like a "bag of worms"; (3) lack an underlying nerve association; (4) consist of myofibroblasts, epithelioid, and giant cells; and (5) show HHF35 and KP-1 immunoreactivity rather than S-100 protein staining.

**Treatment and Prognosis.** Plexiform neurofibromas are approached surgically due to their mass effects.

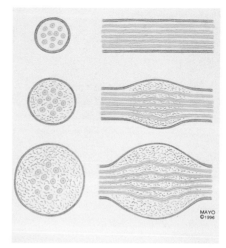

**FIGURE 12–42**    LOCALIZED INTRANEURAL NEUROFIBROMA

The configuration of the normal nerve is altered by an interstitial accumulation of neurofibroma cells and varying quantities of stromal mucin. The result is fusiform expansion of the nerve and dispersion of axons.

Encountering worm-like nerves coursing within fascial planes, the surgeon may be tempted to follow each of their repetitively dividing branches, to the neurologic

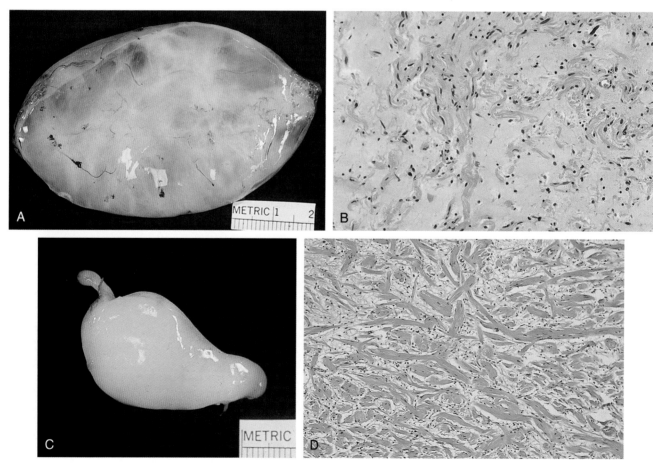

**FIGURE 12–43**    LOCALIZED INTRANEURAL NEUROFIBROMA

The tumors vary in consistency from translucent (*A*) and hypocellular (*B*) to tan in color and opaque (*C*) due to accumulation of collagen (*D*). The latter often takes the form of a "shredded carrots" appearance.

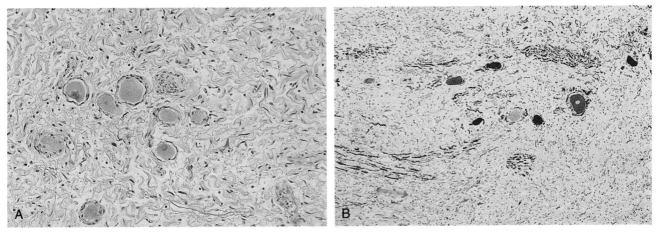

**FIGURE 12–44**  LOCALIZED INTRANEURAL NEUROFIBROMA WITH DORSAL ROOT GANGLION INVOLVEMENT

Note the uniform size and cytologic characteristics of these trapped dorsal root ganglion cells accompanied by numerous satellite cells (A). The underlying anatomy of the ganglion is best seen on neurofilament protein immunostains (B) in which fascicles of axons are seen to traverse the structure.

detriment of the patient. Fully 5% to 10% of plexiform neurofibromas undergo malignant transformation (see Fig. 12–65B). Patients whose tumors transform are usually older and are more prone to experience a recurrence than are those whose tumors remain benign.[17]

### Massive Soft Tissue Neurofibroma

Once termed "elephantiasis neuromatosa" when presenting in its extreme form, this uncommon variant of neurofibroma occurs only in NF1. It produces marked enlargement of either a region, often the shoulder or pelvic girdle (Fig. 12–50A), or a single limb, as in "localized gigantism."[26, 27] Pendulous or cape-like folds of neurofibromatous tissue are a common feature (see Fig. 12–77B). Soft tissue infiltration is widespread and includes muscle (Fig. 12–50B). A plexiform component is frequent, as is

the finding of structures resembling Meissner's or pacinian corpuscles (Fig. 12–50B, C).[29, 31] Pigmented Schwann cells are occasionally seen and may be abundant.[2, 8, 21] Malignant transformation is very uncommon.

### Visceral Neurofibroma

This category consists of solitary or multiple, sporadic or NF1-associated neurofibromas of localized or plexiform type. Viscera affected include the gastrointestinal tract (Fig. 12–51A, B), which may also feature ganglioneuromatosis (Fig. 12–51C), the liver, and the genitourinary tract (Fig. 12–51D).[4] Cardiac or laryngeal examples are rare.[24, 25] In some cases the process is limited to viscera; whether this is a situation analogous to "segmental neurofibromatosis" affecting other sites or the result of a selective trophic effect is unclear.[9]

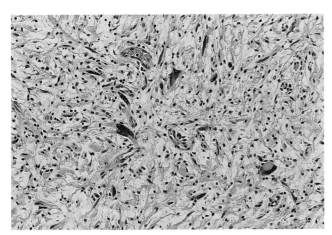

**FIGURE 12–45**  ATYPICAL NEUROFIBROMA

The finding of bizarre hyperchromatic Schwann cells in an otherwise cytologically atypical neurofibroma is of no clinical significance. Such cells are degenerative in nature and show little or no proliferative activity.

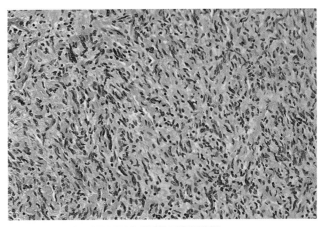

**FIGURE 12–46**  CELLULAR NEUROFIBROMA

This lesion is characterized by hypercellularity, mild nuclear enlargement, and often occasional mitotic figures. These features differ quantitatively from those of low-grade malignant peripheral nerve sheath tumor (see Fig. 12–67A).

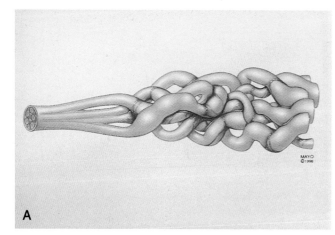

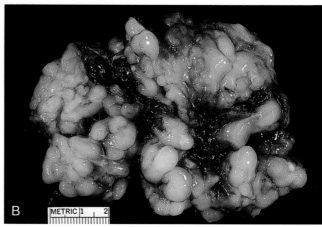

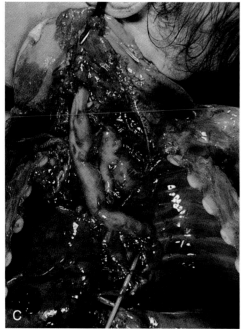

**FIGURE 12–47** PLEXIFORM NEUROFIBROMA

A schematic diagram (*A*) shows the multiple fascicles of the parent nerve (transected at left) giving way to the entwined and markedly enlarged fascicles constituting the tumor. A surgical specimen (*B*) underscores the architectural complexity of the tumor. A mediastinal example (*C*) occurring in a 9-month-old girl massively enlarged the cervical plexus and proved fatal owing to laryngeal compression.

# Perineurioma

Perineurial or perineurial-like cells contribute to the formation of a variety of nerve sheath lesions, both reactive (traumatic neuroma, interdigital neuroma) and neoplastic (perineurioma, neurofibroma, rare MPNSTs). Two benign nerve sheath tumors, one intraneural and the other located in soft tissue, are composed entirely of perineurial cells.[17] Both exhibit abnormalities of chromosome 22 and are discussed below.[5, 8]

## *Intraneural Perineurioma*

**Definition.** An intraneural neoplasm composed exclusively of perineurial cells and characterized by pseudo–onion bulb formation.

**General Comments.** Once considered reactive in nature,[9, 17] intraneural perineuriomas were only recently characterized as neoplasms.[5] Formerly, they were designated "localized hypertrophic neuropathy," but that term is now reserved for an unrelated process—a localized, nonhereditary Schwann cell proliferation featuring true onion bulb formation (see Localized Hypertrophic Neuropathy).

**Clinical Features.** Intraneural perineuriomas typically present in adolescents and young adults. A history of trauma is uncommon.[4, 14] No sex predilection is noted. Motor symptoms are more frequent than sensory disturbances.[5] Denervation is evident on electromyography and may result in muscle atrophy. Although the affected nerve is occasionally palpable, the lesion is best visualized as segmental nerve enlargement on MRI scan. Spinal nerves are far more often involved than are cranial nerves.[12]

**Macroscopic Features.** This distinctive form of perineurioma produces a several-fold, cylindric enlargement of the nerve. Individual fascicles appear coarse and firm (Fig. 12–52). Most intraneural perineuriomas measure between 2 and 10 cm in length. Much larger examples are rare.[5] Involvement of more than a single nerve root is also exceptional.[5] Intraneural perineuriomas do not feature plexiform growth.

**Microscopic Features.** The histologic features of intraneural perineurioma are best seen on cross section of a fascicle of the nerve. The key feature is pseudo–onion bulb formation. Fascicles may be only partially affected (Fig. 12–53A).[18] Pseudo–onion bulbs consist of multilayer cuffs of perineurial cells surrounding single or several nerve fibers (Fig. 12–53B, C). Particularly large whorls may contain numerous fibers. Occasional whorls even surround capillaries (Fig. 12–53B). The number of perineurial cell layers varies but may be five or more. Little cytologic atypia is seen. As a rule, nuclei are elongated, chromatin is delicate, and mitoses are absent or rare. Bodian or Bielschowsky stains for axons, as well as the Luxol fast blue–PAS stain for myelin, show the central nerve fibers to advantage. In long-standing lesions, nerve fibers may be few or nearly absent due to the chronic compressive effects of collagen deposition (Fig. 12–54).

**Immunohistochemical Features.** EMA immunoreactivity is the key feature of pseudo–onion bulbs

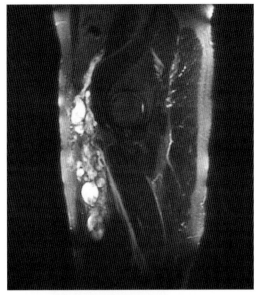

**FIGURE 12–48** PLEXIFORM NEUROFIBROMA

The radiographic features of this neoplasm, as seen on a magnetic resonance imaging scan with contrast, reflect its worm-like, multinodular architecture.

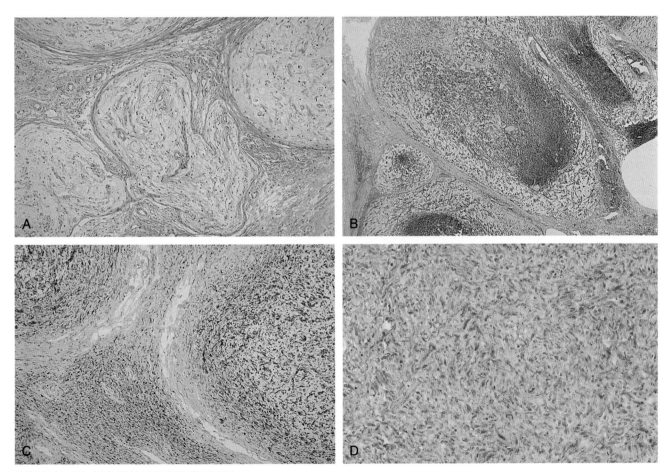

**FIGURE 12–49** PLEXIFORM NEUROFIBROMA

Note the expansion of multiple nerve fascicles by neurofibroma cells and an accompanying mucin-rich matrix. The nerve fibers within these fascicles are variously aggregated and dispersed (A). Aggregated residual nerve fibers are best seen on neurofilament protein immunostain (B). An S-100 protein immunopreparation shows reactivity of neurofibroma cells not only within the two fascicles but also in the often present epineurial and diffuse soft tissue component accompanying these lesions (C). As in localized intraneural neurofibroma, only the Schwann cell element is S-100 protein immunoreactive (D). Perineurial-like and fibroblastic cells lack staining.

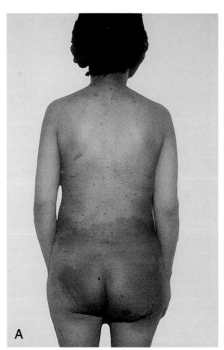

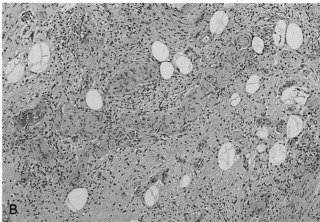

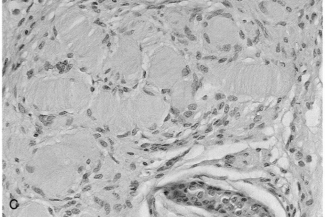

**FIGURE 12–50** MASSIVE SOFT TISSUE NEUROFIBROMA

Note asymmetric enlargement of the right buttock by a very diffuse soft tissue neurofibroma (*A*). The lesion is overlain by widespread cutaneous pigmentation. Microsections demonstrate neurofibroma cells percolating throughout adipose tissue. Pseudo-meissnerian corpuscles are also seen, being a common feature of this tumor type (*B, C*).

(Fig. 12–55*A*).[3, 5] Neurofilament protein and S-100 protein immunostaining is limited to axons and Schwann cells, respectively (Fig. 12–55*B, C*). MIB-1 labeling indices are generally low, ranging from 5% to 15%.[5] p53 protein immunoreactivity may also be expressed,[17] but its significance is uncertain.

**Ultrastructural Features.** The cells engaged in pseudo–onion bulb formation are disposed in multiple layers around myelinated or unmyelinated axons and their accompanying Schwann cells (Fig. 12–56). Perineurial cells possess thin processes whose surfaces exhibit pinocytotic vesicles and often discontinuous basement membrane.

**Differential Diagnosis.** Due to the superficial resemblance of pseudo–onion bulbs to the true onion bulbs that characterize *hereditary sensorimotor neuropathies* (Dejerine-Sottas disease, Charcot-Marie-Tooth disease), these entities are drawn into the differential diagnosis. The distinction is made largely on clinical grounds, because both disorders are hereditary and generalized. Also in the differential diagnosis is *localized hypertrophic neuropathy* (see earlier), a more globular lesion composed of less crowded, true onion bulbs.[1] The latter are composed of S-100 protein–immunoreactive Schwann cells. Last, although *neurofibromas* occasionally feature whorled structures superficially resembling the pseudo–onion bulbs of perineuriomas, these are composed of Schwann

cells and are S-100 protein rather than EMA immunoreactive.

**Treatment and Prognosis.** Intraneural perineuriomas are benign. Although resection, if deemed necessary, is curative, a more conservative approach is generally taken. Even if only partly functional, affected nerves should be preserved. Therefore, only a single fascicle should be biopsied to establish the diagnosis before excision and nerve graft placement is undertaken. Intraneural perineuriomas are not known to recur.

### Soft Tissue Perineurioma

**Definition.** A soft tissue tumor consisting of well-differentiated perineurial cells.

**General Comments.** Once termed "storiform perineurial fibroma,"[15] the perineurial nature of this soft tissue tumor is now well established.[8, 11, 12, 19] Its immunohistochemical and ultrastructural features permit a definitive diagnosis. As in intraneural perineuriomas, at least partial deletion of chromosome 22 is a frequent finding.[7]

**Clinical Features.** Soft tissue perineuriomas occur over a broad range of patient ages and generally affect subcutaneous tissues. The leg is a favored site,[16, 17, 19] and the hands are often affected.[6] Visceral perineuri-

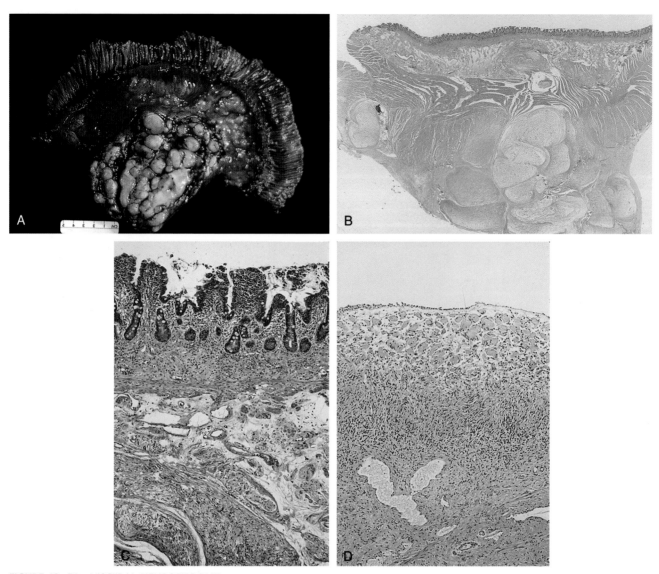

**FIGURE 12–51    VISCERAL NEUROFIBROMA**

Neurofibromas also affect deep viscera, including small bowel and mesentery (A). Another example is shown in transverse section exhibiting an underlying mesenteric plexiform component (B). Ganglioneuromatosis (C) may also be a feature. Involvement of the urinary bladder (D) is rare. This example featured numerous pseudo-meissnerian corpuscles.

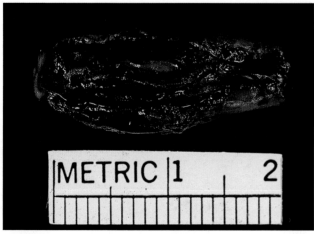

**FIGURE 12–52    INTRANEURAL PERINEURIOMA**

Grossly, the affected fascicles appear enlarged and coarse.

omas are rare.[17, 20] One example arose in the nose and maxillary sinus.[8] To date, only a single intracranial example has been described—a tumor of the choroid plexus.[7] No association has been reported with either form of neurofibromatosis. Soft tissue perineuriomas are benign. So-called perineurial MPNSTs are discussed later.

**Macroscopic Features.** With rare exception,[10] soft tissue perineuriomas are unassociated with a nerve. They are discrete but unencapsulated, nodular, or ovoid in configuration, and range in size from 1.5 to 2 cm. On cut surface, most soft tissue perineuriomas are white to tan and rubbery (Fig. 12–57A). An occasional large tumor shows regressive changes akin to those of schwannoma, including myxoid degeneration, extensive collagen deposition, dystrophic calcification, and even osseous metaplasia.[2, 17]

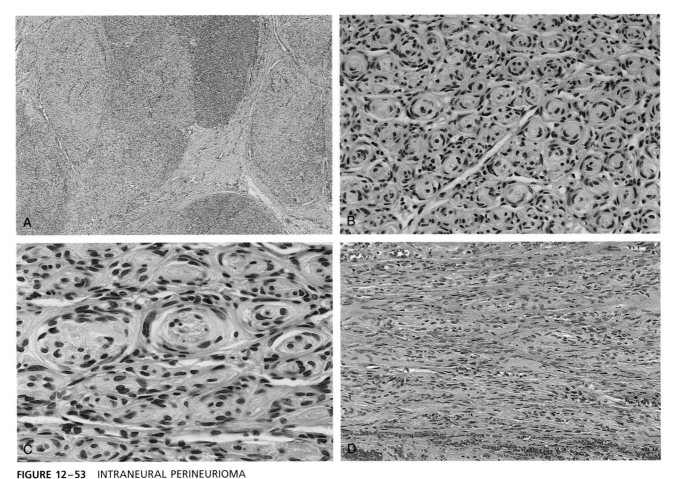

**FIGURE 12–53** INTRANEURAL PERINEURIOMA

On this cross section of an affected nerve, fascicle involvement is seen to vary (*A*). The telltale pseudo–onion bulbs not only wrap around nerve fibers but also encircle occasional capillaries (*B*). Some larger pseudo–onion bulbs surround numerous nerve fibers (*C*). Longitudinal sections show a characteristic "ropey" appearance of the thickly ensheathed nerve fibers (*D*).

**Microscopic Features.** Histologically, the capsules of soft tissue perineuriomas are thin compared with those of schwannomas. The histologic pattern varies considerably and includes bundles of spindle cells, storiform arrangements, interweaving fascicles, and loose whorls (Fig. 12–57B).[17] Crack-like separation of cell bundles is also a common feature. The same is true of dissection and encirclement of collagen bundles (Fig. 12–57C). Most soft tissue perineuriomas are collagen rich, but those arising in the hands are often markedly sclerotic.[6] The cytologic features of soft tissue perineurioma cells include variation in nuclear shape, ranging from elongated and curved to often twisted and disk shaped (Fig. 12–57D). Cell processes are typically long and very slender. Nuclear atypia rarely consists of more than hyperchromasia. Marked degenerative atypia, as occurs in ancient schwannomas and atypical neurofibromas, is rarely seen.[2, 17] Mitoses are few or absent, and necrosis is lacking. Psammoma bodies are occasionally seen in small numbers.[19]

**Immunohistochemical Features.** Analogous to intraneural perineuriomas (see earlier), the key feature of soft tissue perineuriomas is their EMA immunoreactivity.[3] This and the lack of S-100 protein staining clearly distinguish perineurial from Schwann cell neoplasms. Nonetheless, they share some features—namely, pericellular staining for laminin and type IV collagen, a reflection of the presence of basal lamina. Reactivity for CD34 may also be seen. Stains for myoid markers are negative.

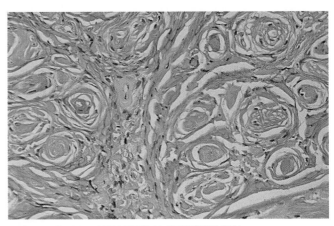

**FIGURE 12–54** INTRANEURAL PERINEURIOMA

Advanced hyalinization may be seen in long-standing lesions. Note marked loss of nerve fibers on Luxol fast blue–periodic acid-Schiff stain.

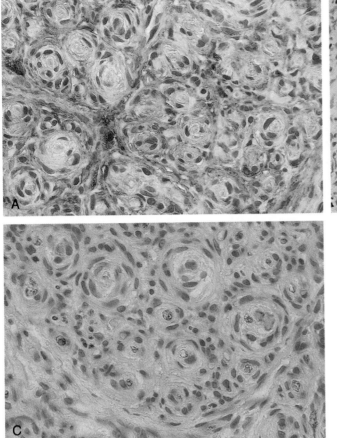

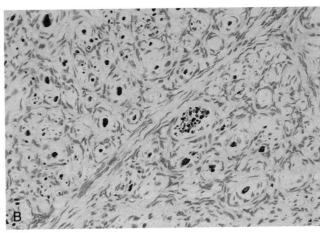

**FIGURE 12–55   INTRANEURAL PERINEURIOMA**

The immunoprofile includes epithelial membrane antigen staining of perineurial cells constituting the pseudo–onion bulbs (*A*), neurofilament protein reactivity of single or grouped axons (*B*), and S-100 protein positivity of accompanying Schwann sheaths (*C*).

**Ultrastructural Features.** Soft tissue perineuriomas consist of ultrastructurally normal perineurial cells in variably dense collagenous stroma.[8, 12, 13] Diagnostic features include long, thin cytoplasmic processes; relatively sparse organelles and intermediate filaments; surface pinocytotic vesicles; discontinuous basement membranes; and rudimentary intercellular junctions. Cell processes frequently dissect among and encircle collagen.[8, 12, 13]

**Differential Diagnosis.** Lesions to be distinguished include mainly benign and low-grade malignant spindle cell tumors with a collagenous stroma. Immunohistochemistry is most informative, but electron microscopy plays an ancillary role. Processes to be considered include *dermatofibrosarcoma protuberans* and *solitary fibrous tumor* (both are more strongly CD34 positive), *myoepithelioma* (cytokeratin and actin positive), *fibroma*, *low-grade fibrosarcoma*, and *fibromyxoid sarcoma*.[8] Fibrous lesions lack EMA and collagen IV reactivity. With the exception of *schwannoma*, all lesions mentioned lack pericellular basal lamina.

**Treatment and Prognosis.** The optimal treatment of soft tissue perineurioma is gross total excision. None has recurred or metastasized. Thus, the prognosis is excellent, even when lesions are subtotally resected.

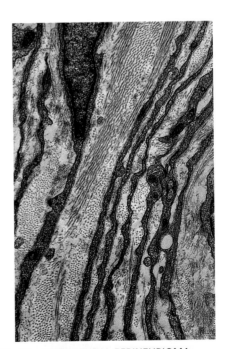

**FIGURE 12–56   INTRANEURAL PERINEURIOMA**

Ultrastructurally, the lesion consists mainly of perineurial cells circumferentially enwrapping nerve fibers. Their very thin cell processes feature conspicuous pinocytotic vesicles and often incomplete surface basal lamina (×18,500).

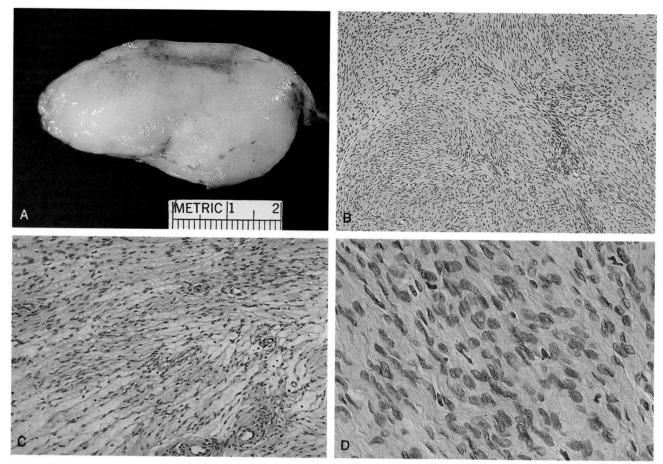

**FIGURE 12–57** SOFT TISSUE PERINEURIOMA

Unassociated with nerve, these benign soft tissue tumors are discrete and delicately encapsulated (*A*). Architecturally solid, such tumors lack the mucin-rich texture of neurofibroma and the yellow hue of the lipid deposition that typifies schwannomas. Their vague fascicles and whorls consist of cells with elongated processes (*B*) that often dissect between and surround bundles and nodules of collagen (*C*). The nuclear configuration of these tumors varies from spindle or plump to wavy or twisted (*D*).

## Granular Cell Tumor

**Definition.** A histologically benign tumor of probable Schwann cell derivation, composed of large, granular cells rich in secondary lysosomes.

**General Comments.** Much speculation has surrounded the histogenesis of these tumors.[10, 17, 19, 20] Once termed "granular cell myoblastoma" and thought to be myogenic in nature, granular cell tumors are now known to be neural in derivation. Both cranial[5] and spinal nerves[22] may be affected. Other indicators of their neurogenic nature include their immunophenotype (see below) and ultrastructure, which include schwannian attributes,[1, 4, 5, 9, 10, 16, 17] and the occasional finding of granular cell change in schwannomas and neurofibromas.[22] Malignant granular cell tumors are rare and may be indistinguishable from the benign variant at the histologic level. An unrelated form of granular cell tumor, arising from infundibular glia, is discussed in Chapter 9.

**Clinical Features.** Granular cell tumors occur at all ages, but their frequency peaks somewhat in mid to later life. Most occur in females, and blacks are preferentially affected.[21, 22, 28] Up to 10% are multiple.[3, 15, 24] The great majority occur in skin and subcutaneous tissue, particularly of the head and neck. Fully 25% arise in the tongue[2, 13] and oral cavity.[29] Mammary lesions, most of which are subcutaneous rather than parenchymal, represent 5% to 15%.[7] Visceral tumors affect mainly the respiratory tract, particularly the larynx.[21] Approximately 5% involve the gastrointestinal tract, usually the esophagus,[11] biliary tree,[27] large bowel,[3, 23] or perianal region.

**Macroscopic Features.** Granular cell tumors occurring at non-neural sites tend to form rather circumscribed, nodular lesions measuring less than 3 cm in maximal dimension. Most are superficially situated and reside in dermal and subcutaneous tissue (Fig. 12–58A). Of these, only a minority extend into muscle. Those affecting nerve are usually extraneural in location but may also involve perineurium (Fig. 12–58B). Occasional dermal examples show a plexiform pattern of nerve involvement (Fig. 12–58C).[14, 22] Visceral examples are rare and reside mainly in lamina propria and the submucosal region (Fig. 12–58D).[3, 11, 23]

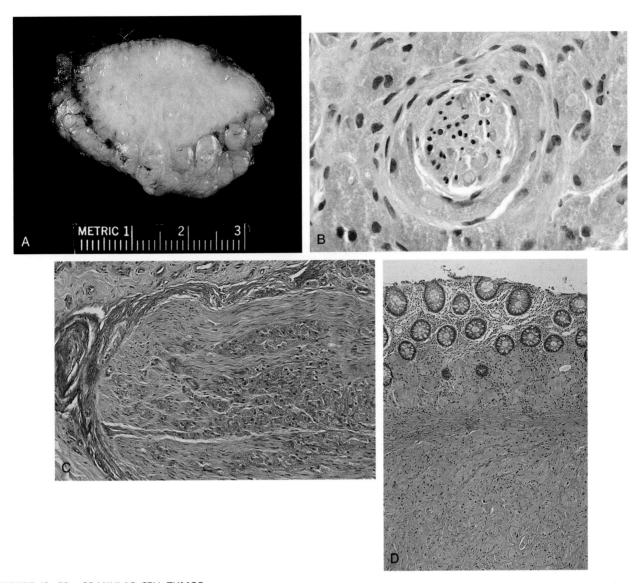

**FIGURE 12–58**   GRANULAR CELL TUMOR

Granular cell tumors, as in this skin and subcutaneous tissue lesion (A), appear circumscribed yet as not encapsulated. Affected nerves in such tumors often show perineurial involvement (B). Endoneurial plexiform-like growth is less common (C). Lack of a capsule is a conspicuous feature in visceral examples such as this colonic example (D).

**Microscopic Features.** The cells comprising granular cell tumor grow in sheet-like, nested, lobular or ribbon patterns (Fig. 12–59A). Their stroma varies, but occasional examples are markedly collagenous. Limited infiltration of soft tissue is frequently seen. The cytologic features of the tumor cells are distinctive (Fig. 12–59A). Monotonous in quality, they range in configuration from polyhedral to elongated, with small, somewhat hyperchromatic nuclei containing minute nucleoli. Degenerative nuclear atypia may be seen. Cytoplasm is relatively abundant and granular owing to its high content of lysosomes. Eosinophilic globules, some surrounded by a halo, may also be conspicuous. Both granules and globules are PAS positive and diastase resistant (Fig. 12–59B). Multinucleation, nuclear pleomorphism, conspicuous nucleoli, mitotic figures, and necrosis are uncommon features but, when present, are suggestive of malignancy. Refractile eosinophilic lysosomes termed

"angulate bodies" are often seen within stromal histiocytes (Fig. 12–59C).

**Immunohistochemical Features.** The immunophenotype of granular cell tumors is distinctive but not entirely specific. It includes reactivity for S-100 protein (see Fig. 12–59D),[1, 4] the macrophage markers $\alpha_1$-antichymotrypsin[26] and CD68,[9, 12] neuron-specific enolase,[9] and vimentin. Only a minority show Leu-7 reactivity.[16] Staining for the myelin-associated proteins P0 and P2 has been reported.[18] Whereas some authors have found myelin basic protein reactivity in a substantial proportion of lesions,[16] others have not.[6] Stains for collagen IV or laminin often show circumscription of cell lobules.[22]

**Ultrastructural Features.** The cytoplasmic granularity noted at the light microscopic level is due to the presence of innumerable pleomorphic lysosomes. These include

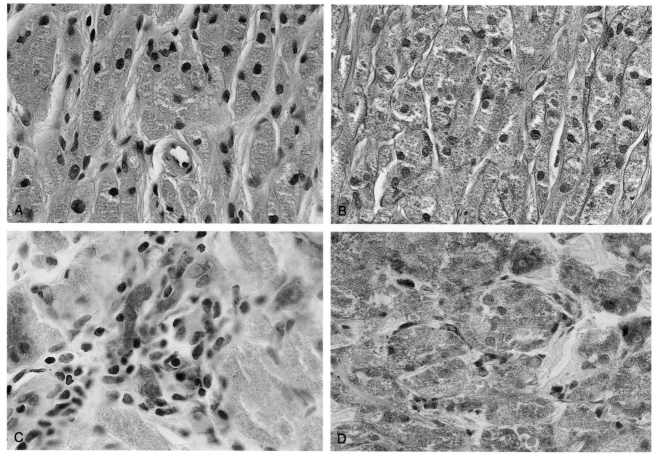

**FIGURE 12–59** GRANULAR CELL TUMOR

The neoplastic cells are polygonal to elongated in configuration and feature coarsely granular cytoplasm on H&E stain (*A*). The granules are strongly positive for periodic acid-Schiff (PAS) (*B*). Non-neoplastic, interstitial histiocytes frequently contain elongated, PAS-positive lysosomes ("angulate bodies") (*C*). Uniform cytoplasmic positivity for S-100 protein is the rule (*D*).

autophagosomes, residual bodies, multivesicular bodies, and material resembling ceroid lipofuscin.[1, 4, 10, 17, 20, 24] Angulate bodies within stromal histiocytes consist of membrane-bound, parallel arrays of microtubules and scant, dense lipid bodies.[8, 24, 25]

**Differential Diagnosis.** This discussion is limited to the differential diagnosis of granular cell tumor affecting nerve. Whereas *schwannoma* and *neurofibroma* occasionally contain granular cells, these are never widespread, despite the expression of CD8 immunoreactivity in schwannomas.[12] The distinction of granular cell tumor from *granular cell leiomyoma* may require either immunostaining for muscle markers, such as HHF35 and smooth muscle actin, or the performance of electron microscopy.

Of greatest importance is the distinction between benign and *malignant granular cell tumors*. This is often difficult at the light microscopic level. Some lesions, however, do show cellular pleomorphism, marked hyperchromasia, mitotic activity, and focal necrosis—features lacking in benign granular cell tumors. Malignant granular cell tumors are often large. A discussion of malignant granular cell tumors is found on pages 632 to 633.

**Treatment and Prognosis.** Local excision with negative margins is curative. Recurrence rates are less than 10% when margins appear free of involvement and are reportedly 20% to 50% following incomplete excision.[2]

# Ganglioneuroma

**Definition.** A benign tumor composed of mature autonomic ganglion cells, occasional satellite or "capsular" cells, and abundant unmyelinated axons with accompanying Schwann cells.

**General Comments.** The histogenesis of ganglioneuromas remains in question. No doubt they originate in neuroblasts, but whether these are normal in nature and mature apace with development or pass through a "neuroblastoma" phase remains unclear. Because some neuroblastomas undergo neuronal maturation spontaneously or after therapy,[8, 26] it is conceivable that ganglioneuromas also represent fully differentiated neuroblastomas. Admittedly, differences in the distributions of the two tumors argue against this notion.

**Clinical Features.** Ganglioneuromas usually occur at sites of autonomic ganglia, notably sympathetic ganglia of the mediastinum, retroperitoneum, and pelvis. The adrenal medulla is also a favored site. Head and neck lesions have been reported at the skull base, in the parapharyngeal region, or in cranial nerve ganglia.[10] In addition, visceral examples[29] arise from parasympathetic ganglia and occur in localized as well as diffuse form. Localized gastrointestinal lesions are rare and sporadic in occurrence,[4, 18, 23, 33, 35] whereas diffuse lesions occur in the setting of multiple endocrine neoplasia type IIb. Ganglioneuromas have also been documented in the choroid of the eye,[32] posterior cranial fossa,[13] and spinal intradural space.[16]

Occasional ganglioneuromas are endocrinologically functional. Best known are tumors that produce vasoactive intestinal polypeptide (VIP) with resultant "watery diarrhea syndrome" (Verner-Morrison syndrome).[20, 31] Hypertension,[21] virilization,[1] and myasthenia gravis[22] have also been reported. In some cases, low levels of catecholamine metabolites (vanilmandelic acid and homovanillic acid) are found.[17] The association of ganglioneuroma with NF1 is well known but rare. Occasionally ganglioneuromas are familial but unassociated with a syndrome.[24]

**Radiologic Features.** Ganglioneuromas appear as single, sharply defined masses that, on computed tomography scans, may show minor amorphous calcification. Contrast enhancement and cyst formation are best seen on MRI scans.

**Macroscopic Features.** Sizable, circumscribed, and variable in shape (Fig. 12–60A), most ganglioneuromas measure less than 15 cm. Truly gigantic examples have nevertheless been reported. Many are solid, but cyst formation is common. On cut section ganglioneuromas appear homogeneous, tan, and often translucent (Fig. 12–60A). Few show grossly evident calcification. Most tumors possess a thin pseudocapsule (Fig. 12–60B), which may be focally incomplete. The result is an irregular interface with adjacent soft tissue (Fig. 12–60C). Centrally situated tumors often surround important anatomic structures. Both features may complicate resection. Ganglioneuromas are rarely multiple, but one example reportedly involved an entire segment of the sympathetic chain.[28] Rare lesions arise in the organ of Zuckerkandl.[34] Occasional ganglioneuromas originate in other lesions, such as pheochromocytomas.[7, 15]

**Microscopic Features.** The essential features of ganglioneuroma include ganglion cells, their long axons with accompanying Schwann sheaths, and occasional perineurial satellite cells. By definition, neuroblasts are lacking. The distribution of ganglion cells varies from widely scattered (see Fig. 12–60B, C) to clustered (Fig. 12–61A). Generous sampling of large tumors is imperative, because whole fields may be devoid of ganglion cells, thus mimicking

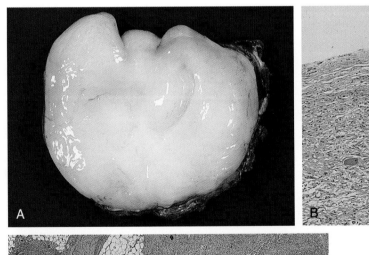
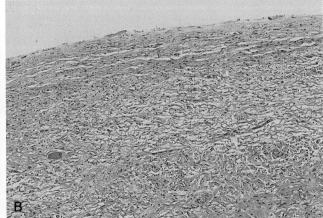
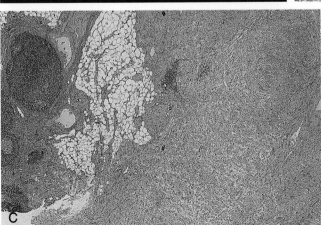

**FIGURE 12–60    GANGLIONEUROMA**

Globular to somewhat irregular in contour (A), ganglioneuromas vary from delicately encapsulated (B) to somewhat infiltrative of surrounding tissue (C). Because the ganglion cells can be dispersed or localized, entire fields may mimic neurofibroma (B, C).

neurofibroma (Fig. 12–60B, C). The cytoplasm of the ganglion cell is abundant eosinophilic to amphophilic, and contains single to multiple vesicular nuclei, each with a prominent nucleolus. Nissl substance varies from inconspicuous to prominent. Distinguishing neoplastic from normal ganglion cells is the tendency of the former toward pleomorphism, multinucleation, vacuolation, and the presence of pale, spherical cytoplasmic inclusions, some of which resemble Lewy bodies. Grimelius' stains frequently show argyrophilia. Perineuronal satellite cells, with their typically flattened nuclei, vary in number (Fig. 12–61A, B). The axons are abundant and are either aligned in bundles or separated in more loose textured fashion. Their small diameter is readily evident on Bodian and Bielschowsky's silver impregnations. Peanut agglutinin, a marker of advanced neuronal differentiation, also labels these cells and their processes.[11] Although Schwann cells ensheathing the axons are numerous, myelination is absent on Luxol fast blue stain (Fig. 12–61C).

Degenerative changes are frequent and include the accumulation of pigmented lysosomes ("neuromelanin")[9] within ganglion cells,[9] stromal collagen deposition or mucin accumulation, vascular hyalinization with frequent evidence of prior hemorrhage, cystic change, patchy coarse calcifications, and lymphocytic inflammation that should not be mistaken for the presence of neuroblasts.

Rare "composite ganglioneuroma-pheochromocytomas" do occur. Although the two components are often separate and distinct,[2, 7, 34] an occasional tumor clearly shows gradual transition of pheochromocytoma to ganglioneuroma.[6]

**Immunohistochemical Features.** The ganglion cells and axons of ganglioneuroma are strongly immunoreactive for synaptophysin, neurofilament protein (Fig. 12–62A), tubulin, and neuron-specific enolase.[3, 25] The Schwann sheaths are positive for S-100 protein (Fig. 12–62B) and occasionally for myelin basic protein[30] or GFAP. Staining for laminin and collagen IV highlights basal cell lamina surrounding Schwann cells. Of the various hormones produced by ganglioneuromas, VIP is most often found, even in cases unassociated with Verner-Morrison syndrome (Fig. 12–62C).

**Ultrastructural Features.** The ganglion cells of ganglioneuroma possess sizable, typically round to oval nuclei with prominent nucleoli, abundant cytoplasm with well-developed endoplasmic reticulum, prominent Golgi complexes, numerous pleomorphic lysosomes, and scattered 90 to 130 nm neurosecretory granules. Intermediate filaments (neurofilament) are best seen in axonal processes. Axonal terminations contain secretory granules and clear vesicles. Tubular inclusions[19] and others resembling Pick bodies[5] have also been reported. Like conventional Schwann cells, the satellite cells that surround neoplastic ganglion cells exhibit surface basal lamina. The stroma often contains collagen, both normal and the long-spacing type ("Luse bodies").

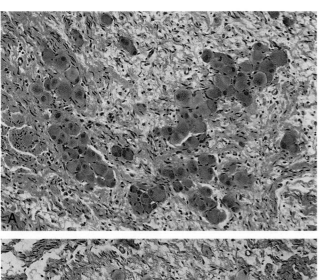

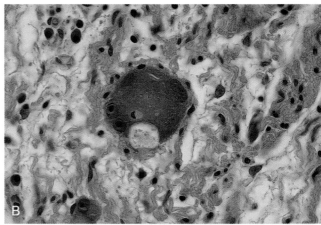

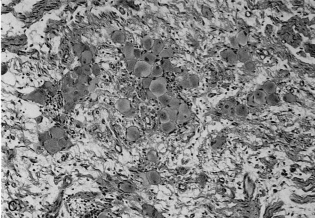

**FIGURE 12–61   GANGLIONEUROMA**

The neoplastic ganglion cells often lie clustered, their cell bodies molded to one another (A). Bi- or multinucleation (A, B) is commonly seen. The same is true of cytoplasmic vacuolation (B). Myelin is lacking on Luxol fast blue–periodic acid-Schiff stain (C).

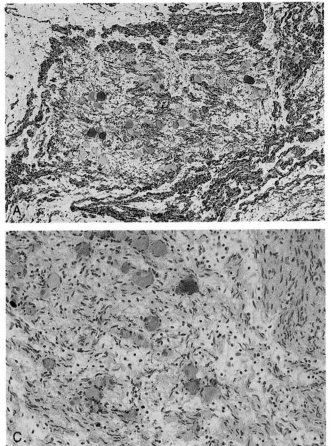

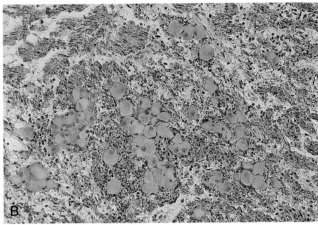

**FIGURE 12–62**   GANGLIONEUROMA

The immunophenotype of the tumor is predictable and includes sheaves of neurofilament protein–positive axons (*A*), S-100 protein–reactive Schwann cells (*B*), and neuronal cell bodies often containing neurotransmitter substances—in this case, vasoactive intestinal polypeptide (*C*) in a patient without Verner-Morrison syndrome.

**Differential Diagnosis.** Principal lesions in the differential diagnosis include *neurofibroma* and *schwannoma*, neither of which features constituent ganglion cells or an abundance of nerve fibers. Because both tumors may overrun dorsal root or sympathetic ganglia, the finding of ganglion cells within their substance may prompt consideration of ganglioneuroma. However, regular distribution of ganglion cells, even in overrun ganglia, lack of dysmorphic neurons, and the presence of myelin in affected dorsal root ganglia aid in the distinction. Unlike ganglioneuromas, neurofibromas typically show extensive stromal mucin accumulation. In contrast, schwannomas are distinguished by their thick capsules, hyaline vessels, Antoni A and B patterns, and Verocay bodies. Composite *ganglioneuroma-pheochromocytoma* also enters into the differential diagnosis but is readily eliminated by adequate tissue sampling. The same is true of *ganglioneuroblastoma*, particularly the stroma-rich type.[27] Here again, adequate sampling reveals only mature ganglion cells. The finding of small neurons lacking vesicular nuclei with prominent nucleoli and possessing little cytoplasm should prompt a search for neuroblasts. Distinguishing the latter from lymphocytes is accomplished by immunostaining for neuronal (synaptophysin, neuron-specific enolase) or hematopoietic (leukocyte common antigen, CD3) markers. *Immature ganglioneuroma*, a relatively uncommon lesion, is characterized by a broad range of neuronal maturation, rare or absent neuroblasts, and abundant axons unassociated with Schwann cells (Fig. 12–63). Lastly, ganglioneuroma components may be seen in so-called *ectomesenchymoma*,[12] *gangliorhabdomyosarcoma*,[14] and rare examples of ganglioneuroma that have undergone transformation to MPNST (see the discussion of MPNST ex-schwannoma, below).

**Treatment and Prognosis.** Ganglioneuromas are benign and characteristically produce mass effects rather than endocrinopathy. Resection is curative.

The rare finding of ganglioneuromatous tissue in regional lymph nodes or at other sites suggests maturation of a prior neuroblastoma metastasis. In such cases, the prognosis is excellent.

## PRIMARY MALIGNANT TUMORS OF NERVE

Although a variety of cells are native to nerve sheath and epineurium, this chapter focuses largely on malignant neoplasms derived from Schwann cells. In comparison, perineurial MPNSTs are rare, as are malignant granular cell tumors and primitive neuroectodermal tumor (PNET) of nerve. Each is discussed in the following sections. Table 12–4 lists other tumors and tumor-like lesions of nerve not discussed in this chapter.

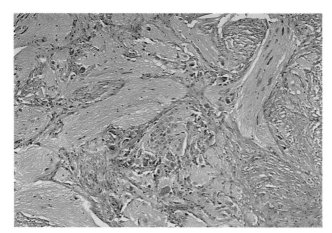

**FIGURE 12-63**   IMMATURE GANGLIONEUROMA

Unlike conventional ganglioneuromas, the processes of these uncommon tumors lack significant ensheathing by Schwann cells. Careful scrutiny may reveal occasional neuroblasts, but neuronal maturation is the rule.

## Conventional Malignant Peripheral Nerve Sheath Tumor

**Definition.** A malignant tumor showing variable Schwannian or, less frequently, perineurial or an element of fibroblastic differentiation. Mesenchymal tumors of epineurial soft tissue and endothelial cells are not included in this designation.

**General Comments.** MPNSTs are uncommon, accounting for approximately 5% of malignant soft tissue tumors.[10, 31, 62] Their recognition is greatly aided by any of the following: (1) origin in nerve, (2) derivation from neurofibroma,[7, 23, 52] or (3) occurrence in the setting of NF1.[18] MPNSTs unassociated with nerve pose a greater diagnostic challenge, requiring immunohistochemical or ultrastructural verification of their neural nature. Most MPNSTs are derived from neurofibroma or originate in a normal peripheral nerve.[7, 23, 52] Although the majority show some features of Schwann cell differentiation, many tumors are frankly anaplastic. Occasional MPNSTs show some fibroblastic or perineurial features.[19-21, 26, 52] Thus the encompassing designation "malignant peripheral nerve sheath tumor" is more appropriate than either "neurofibrosarcoma" or "neurogenic sarcoma." The term "malignant schwannoma" is particularly misleading, in that most MPNSTs bear no resemblance to schwannoma. Furthermore MPNST ex-schwannoma is exquisitely rare,[68] as are MPNSTs arising from Schwann cell components of ganglioneuroma or ganglioneuroblastoma[49] or from the sustentacular cells of pheochromocytoma.[39, 41, 51]

**Clinical Features.** As a rule, MPNSTs occur in young to middle-aged adults. Only about 15% occur in childhood.[8, 35] A majority are NF1 associated,[7, 23] in which case they generally affect younger individuals. Approximately 5% of patients with NF1 have been said to develop MPNSTs,[7, 29] although the best documented study sets the figure at somewhat under 2%.[54] Multiple MPNSTs are rare and appear to occur only in the setting

**TABLE 12-4**
**Miscellaneous Tumors and Tumor-Like Lesions of Nerve**

Reactive lesions
 Pacinian neuroma
 Endometriosis
Hyperplastic lesions
 Palisaded encapsulated neuroma
  Mucosal neuroma
  Mucosal neuromatosis
  Intestinal ganglioneuromatosis of multiple endocrine
   neoplasia IIB
Benign neurogenic tumors
 Nerve sheath myxoma
 Neurothekeoma
Benign and malignant non-neurogenic tumors and tumor-like
 lesions
 Adrenal adenoma of nerve root
 Ectopic meningioma
 Paraganglioma of nerve root
 Lipoma
 Rhabdomyoma
 Vascular tumors
  Hemangioma
  Angiomatosis of nerve
  Glomangioma
 Hemangiopericytoma
 Lymphoma—primary

of NF1.[27, 29] Approximately 10% to 20% of MPNSTs arise at a site of prior irradiation,[9, 12, 23] the mean latency being 15 years.[7]

Most MPNSTs involve sizable spinal nerves. Of these, the sciatic is most often affected.[7, 61] Neuroimaging characteristics (irregular margins and lack of homogeneity on MRI scans) often, but not invariably, distinguish MPNSTs from benign nerve sheath tumors (Fig. 12-64). Cranial nerve MPNSTs are very uncommon; most affect either the trigeminal[1, 69] or acoustic nerves.[17, 33, 42] With few exceptions, such tumors arise de novo rather than in transition from schwannoma. Only single examples of intracerebral[55] and intraventricular[58] MPNST have been reported. Visceral examples are also rare and typically occur in association with NF1.[13, 14, 30]

**Macroscopic Features.** MPNSTs vary in their appearance, as modified by the presence or absence of a precursor lesion. Those arising within nerve are more often fusiform than globular in configuration (Fig. 12-65A). MPNSTs originating in plexiform neurofibromas may be grossly obvious (Fig. 12-65B, C) or a microscopic finding. Therefore, thorough sampling is required. Tumors arising in soft tissue and grossly unassociated with nerve, pose a greater diagnostic challenge (Fig. 12-65D) because they require ancillary studies to demonstrate nerve sheath differentiation. The pseudocapsules of such tumors consist of infiltrated soft tissue (Fig. 12-65E).

Most MPNSTs exceed 5 cm in size and are surrounded by a pseudocapsule consisting of involved surrounding tissue (Fig. 12-65D). Their cut surface is firm, gray or tan, and often mottled by zones of hemorrhage or necrosis (Fig. 12-65A, C). It is of note that low- to intermediate-grade MPNSTs may lack

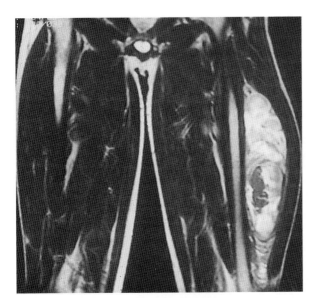

**FIGURE 12–64**  MALIGNANT PERIPHERAL NERVE SHEATH TUMOR

On neuroimaging, this large tumor shows irregularity of outline, an indicator of invasion, and heterogeneous enhancement, a reflection of necrosis or variation of tumor grade.

degenerative changes and thus resemble benign nerve sheath tumors.

Careful sampling of MPNSTs is important. It serves to identify an associated nerve or neurofibroma, reveals the presence of heterologous elements, and determines histologic grade. One section per centimeter of greatest tumor dimension is suggested. For tumors arising in sizable nerves, sampling along their length permits assessment of the extent of intraneural spread (Fig. 12–66A). Intraoperatively, this is of obvious importance for the determination of negative proximal and distal margins. Such spread is particularly important in paraspinous lesions, which often show proximal extension (Fig. 12–66B).[27]

**Microscopic Features.** MPNSTs exhibit greater histologic variation than any soft tissue tumor. Their neural nature may not be apparent on routine H&E stain. Diagnostically helpful features include the identification of an involved nerve or ganglion or of an underlying neurofibroma of the localized or plexiform type (Fig. 12–67A). Most tumors are highly cellular and consist of mitotically active spindle cells with hyperchromatic nuclei and eosinophilic cytoplasm. In "neural-appearing" tumors, nuclei are often tapered and exhibit a wavy contour (Fig. 12–67B). Reflecting the morphologic variation of MPNSTs, their constituent cells often resemble those of synovial sarcoma (Fig. 12–67C), fibrosarcoma (herringbone pattern; Fig. 12–67D), malignant fibrous histiocytoma (pleomorphic cells, storiform pattern; Fig. 12–67E), or a monotonous, undifferentiated tumor (Fig. 12–67F). Tumors that feature epithelial-like cells (epithelioid MPNST) mimic carcinoma or melanoma (see below). In addition, heterologous tumors feature frankly epithelial (glandular, squamous, neuroendocrine elements) or

mesenchymal (rhabdomyoblasts, cartilage, bone) disfferentiation (see later).

As a rule, MPNSTs are high grade, cellular tumors exhibiting brisk mitotic activity and necrosis. The latter is often geographic in nature and associated with palisading (Fig. 12–68).[23, 52] Only about 15% are low-grade tumors showing less cellularity, fewer hyperchromatic cells and mitotic figures, lack of necrosis, and occasionally transition from neurofibroma.[7] The very existence of low-grade MPNSTs requires their distinction from neurofibromas. This is not easy, and no correlative morphologic-prognostic studies have addressed the issue. We believe that the distinction of low-grade MPNST from "cellular neurofibroma" rests on several findings, including cell crowding, nuclear enlargement (at least three times the size of ordinary neurofibroma nuclei), and hyperchromasia.[52] In the absence of these findings, low-level mitotic activity must not be overinterpreted as indicative of malignancy. As noted earlier, hypercellular neurofibromas with occasional mitoses ("cellular neurofibromas") and neurofibromas with degenerative nuclear atypia ("atypical neurofibromas") should not be mistaken for MPNSTs.

**Immunohistochemical Features.** Although a useful marker of peripheral nerve sheath tumor, S-100 protein is nonspecific. Fully 30% to 65% of MPNSTs are reactive.[4, 18, 25, 62] Low-grade tumors may show relatively widespread staining (see Fig. 12–68), but high-grade tumors, which constitute the majority of MPNSTs, often show only individual, scattered or clustered immunoreactive cells. Leu-7 staining is also variable and a reflection of schwannian differentiation.[25, 57, 63] The same is true of the basement membrane components collagen IV and laminin[3, 45] and of GFAP. High-grade MPNSTs are typically immunonegative for GFAP, but an occasional low-grade example shows limited reactivity.[15, 25] Staining for EMA in other than "glandular MPNSTs" is rare and suggests perineurial differentiation.[19, 21] Because vimentin is found in virtually all soft tissue tumors, we use it to confirm the immunoviability of a specimen. In the identification of MPNSTs, we, like others,[57, 63] advocate an immunobattery approach that relies heavily on antisera to S-100 protein and Leu-7.

**Ultrastructural Features.** Although benign peripheral nerve sheath tumors consist of well-differentiated cells of schwannian or perineurial type, most MPNSTs exhibit few specific features. Indeed, many appear undifferentiated. The remainder offer only suggestions of schwannian differentiation, notably inconspicuous processes, poorly formed cell junctions, and scant surface basement membrane. Only low-grade MPNSTs show obvious schwannian features in the form of conspicuous, entwined processes joined by rudimentary junctions and coated by basal lamina.[6, 11, 18–20, 59] Occasional cytoplasmic filaments and microtubules are nonspecific findings. Only rare MPNSTs show features of perineurial differentiation,[19–21] including remarkably thin cytoplasmic processes with surface pinocytotic vesicles, discontinuous basement membrane, and primitive junctions. Occasional tumors appear fibroblastic, showing an abundance of rough endoplasmic reticulum.

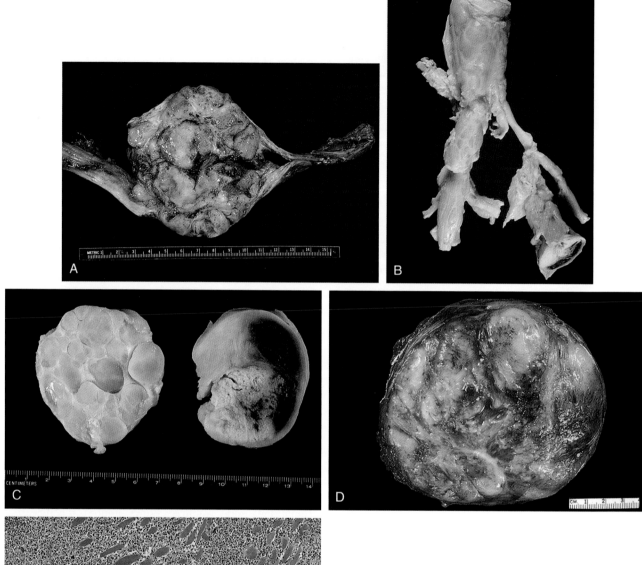

**FIGURE 12–65**  MALIGNANT PERIPHERAL NERVE SHEATH TUMOR

This nerve-associated tumor (*A*), bivalved to show its cut surface, features zones of necrosis. Fully half of malignant peripheral nerve sheath tumors (MPNSTs) arise in neurofibromas of either the localized intraneural or the plexiform type. The latter may be particularly impressive, as in this sciatic and tibial nerve example in a 30-year-old (*B*), in which cross sections show variation from massive fascicle expansion to total replacement of anatomic landmarks (*C*). Tumors unassociated with a recognizable nerve (*D*) pose a diagnostic challenge, requiring the application of ancillary methods, such as immunohistochemistry and ultrastructural study, to confirm their neural nature. The pseudocapsules of MPNSTs are composed of infiltrated peritumoral soft tissue (*E*).

**Molecular and Cytogenetic Features.** To date, no consistent cytogenetic changes have been observed in MPNSTs.[24, 37, 38, 48] Triploidy is common,[24, 37] as is loss of the NF1 locus (band 17q11) and of the band containing the tumor suppressor gene p53 (17p13).

The development of MPNST appears to be a multistep process initiated by mutation of one or both copies of the NF1 gene. A subsequent event would be the loss of one or both copies of a tumor suppressor gene, likely p53. Loss or deletion of 17p in nearly all MPNSTs and the occurrence of point mutations in exon 4 of the p53 gene in many cases supports this notion.[36] Also in accord is the frequent demonstration of strong p53 protein immunoreactivity.[16] In a recent study of plexiform neurofibromas undergoing transition to MPNST, 13% of the benign neurofibroma compo-

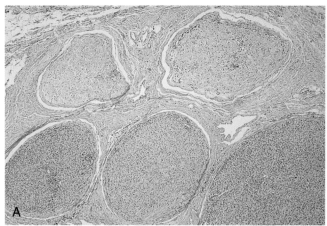

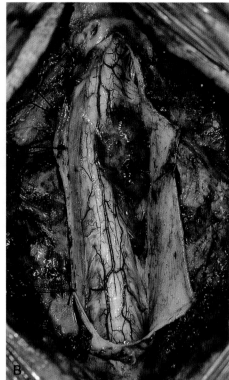

**FIGURE 12–66**    MALIGNANT PERIPHERAL NERVE SHEATH TUMOR

Intraneural extension is common in nerve-based tumors (A). Assessment of nerve margins is therefore important. Proximal intraneural extension, particularly from paraspinous tumors, can reach the intradural compartment and compress the spinal cord (B).

nent showed p53 staining, compared with 80% of the MPNST component.[32]

According to a recent chromosome banding study,[37] MPNSTs all exhibit clonal abnormalities; the karyotype is complex, with numerous structural and numerical changes. Loss of chromosome 21 was seen in only 1 of 20 cases studied. No differences were noted between sporadic and NF1-associated tumors. Although triploid and tetraploid clones were more frequent in high-grade tumors, no overall prognostic correlations were found. Karyotyping does, however, discriminate between benign and malignant nerve sheath tumors.

A recent comparative genomic hybridization study found gains in chromosomes 7, 8q, 15q, and 17q to be characteristic of MPNSTs but not of benign nerve sheath tumors.[53]

**Differential Diagnosis.** Principal lesions entering into the differential of MPNST are presented in Table 12–5, which summarizes their immunoprofile and points of distinction from schwannoma, perineurioma, fibrosarcoma, leiomyosarcoma, synovial sarcoma, and epithelioid sarcoma. Among these, several deserve special mention. Because some MPNSTs exhibit a herringbone pattern, *fibrosarcoma* is mimicked. However, fibrosarcomas lack immunoreactivity for S-100 protein and Leu-7 and are ultrastructurally devoid of surface basement membrane. Instead, they show far greater development of rough endoplasmic reticulum. *Leiomyosarcomas* differ in cytologic terms, being composed of cells with blunt-ended nuclei or abundant eosinophilic cytoplasm in which fibrils are evident on trichrome and phosphotungstic acid–hematoxylin stains. Occasional leiomyosarcomas are S-100

protein immunoreactive, but they also stain for muscle markers, such as desmin and muscle-specific actin (HHF35). *Monophasic synovial sarcoma* also differs in cytologic terms, being composed of closely packed spindle cells with nuclei that are plumper than those of conventional MPNST. They also feature irregularly distributed, dense bands of collagen and occasional calcifications. Approximately half of *synovial sarcomas* show cytokeratin or EMA staining.[46] As in leiomyosarcoma, occasional synovial sarcomas show S-100 protein staining. At the ultrastructural level, synovial sarcomas often feature greater numbers of intercellular junctions, occasional lumens containing microvilli, and scant intercellular spaces. The cytogenetics and molecular genetics of synovial sarcomas also differ significantly from those of MPNSTs.[47, 66]

**Treatment and Prognosis.** Surgery, particularly wide, en bloc resection, is the treatment of choice for MPNST that involves soft tissue.[23] Postoperative radiation leads to a significant reduction in local recurrence.[64] Postoperative radiation (60 Gy), as well as brachytherapy and intraoperative electron irradiation, also significantly improve survival.[64] To date, chemotherapy has proved ineffective in the treatment of MPNST.

The overall prognosis of patients with MPNST is similar to that in other high-grade sarcomas. Two large studies with long-term follow-up reported a tumor-related mortality of approximately 65%.[7, 23] Overall 5- and 10-year survival rates range from 34% to 52% and from 23% to 34%, respectively.[7, 23, 64]

A number of factors negatively influence survival. These include central location of the tumor,[7, 27] lesion size greater than 5 cm[7] or 10 cm,[23] extent of resection,[27, 64]

**TABLE 12–5**
**Immunohistochemistry in the Differential Diagnosis of Malignant Peripheral Nerve Sheath Tumor (MPNST)**

| | Schwann-oma | Peri-neurioma | MPNST | Fibrosar-coma/MFH | Leiomyo-sarcoma | Synovial Sarcoma | Epithelioid Sarcoma |
|---|---|---|---|---|---|---|---|
| Vimentin | + | + | + | +/+ | + | + | + |
| Cytokeratin | − | − | − (Glandular +) | − | Occasional | (Bi- and monophasic +) | + |
| Desmin | − | − | (Triton +) | +/− | + | − | |
| Glial fibrillary acidic protein | 20% | − | Rare | − | − | − | − |
| Muscle-specific actin (HHF35) | − | − | − (Triton +) | − | + | − | − |
| HMB-45 | (Melanotic +) | − | − | − | − | − | − |
| S-100 protein | >95% | − | 50% | − | Occasional | Occasional | − |
| Leu-7 | 50–60% | − | 30–40% | − | 10–20% | 25–40% | − |
| Myelin basic protein | 50% | − | 10% | − | − | − | − |
| Epithelial membrane antigen | − | + | (Glandular differentiation) | − | − | (Bi- and monophasic +) | + |
| Carcinoembryonic antigen | − | − | " | − | − | Glands +/− | − |
| Chromogranin | − | − | " | − | − | − | − |
| Factor VIII | − | − | (Angiosarcoma differentiation) | − | − | − | − |
| CD34 | − | +/− | " | − | Occasional | − | + |
| CD68 (KP-1) | + | +/− | +/− | −/+ | − | − | − |
| Laminin and collagen IV | + | + | 25–30% | − | + | 10% | 10% |

MFH, malignant fibrous histiocytoma.

p53 immunoreactivity,[16] tumor recurrence,[23] and metastasis.[64] The significance of NF1 association is unsettled; some series find it to be a negative prognostic indicator,[7] whereas others report no prognostic significance.[23, 27, 56] The meaningfulness of histologic subtype, tumor grade, DNA ploidy, and proliferation indices remains unsettled.

## Malignant Peripheral Nerve Sheath Tumor Variants

**Epithelioid MPNST.** This distinctive tumor represents less than 5% of MPNSTs and is composed largely or entirely of malignant epithelioid cells.[52] The finding of only focal, cytologically malignant epithelioid cell change in a schwannoma may represent a precursor lesion.[34] Epithelioid MPNSTs frequently affect the legs, arms, and inguinal regions. Prognostically, they differ with respect to superficial versus deep location.[5, 28] A nerve origin is noted in approximately half of cases. No association with NF1 has been reported. Histologically, these tumors simulate large cell carcinoma and amelanotic melanoma (Fig. 12–69A, B). Unlike the conventional MPNSTs, nearly 80% of epithelioid tumors express diffuse, strong S-100 protein immunoreactivity (Fig. 12–69C). Furthering the mimicry of carcinoma, an occasional example shows cytokeratin or EMA immunostaining.[2] Pericellular basal lamina is commonly present, as evidenced by membrane pattern staining for collagen IV and laminin. Electron microscopy plays a role in the diagnosis of this rare tumor.[60] The treatment of epithelioid MPNST is the same as that of conventional MPNST. Deeply situated tumors are associated with a higher mortality.[5, 28]

**MPNST with Divergent Differentiation.** Only rare nerve sheath tumors show divergent differentiation. Nearly all are malignant. The spectrum includes tumors with skeletal muscle ("triton tumor"), bone, or cartilage differentiation (Fig. 12–70A to C),[65, 67] those with an angiosarcomatous element,[50] and ones with true epithelium.[65, 66] Termed "glandular MPNST," the last type usually features mucin-producing epithelium (Fig. 12–70D), but squamous and even neuroendocrine components may be seen. With few exceptions,[43] the epithelial elements are benign appearing. Occasional tumors show both mesenchymal and epithelial differentiation ("pluridirectional MPNST").[4, 52, 66] Collectively, tumors with divergent differentiation show a frequent association with NF1 and have a poorer prognosis, than conventional MPNST. For detailed discussions of these variants, the reader is referred to a comprehensive text.[52]

**MPNST with Perineurial Differentiation.** This subset of MPNSTs is not fully understood. Too few cases have been reported.[19–22, 52] The tumors (1) can be low or high grade; (2) feature whorls and often storiform arrangements of cells with elongated, sometimes collagen-encompassing processes; (3) exhibit EMA instead of S-100 protein immunoreactivity; (4) show variable ultrastructural features of perineurial differentiation; and (5) vary in biologic behavior based on grade.[21] Although transition from low to high grade has been documented,[26] transformation of benign perineurioma to perineurial MPNST has not.[26]

**MPNST Arising in Other Nervous System Tumors.** Rare examples of MPNST arise in transition from schwan-

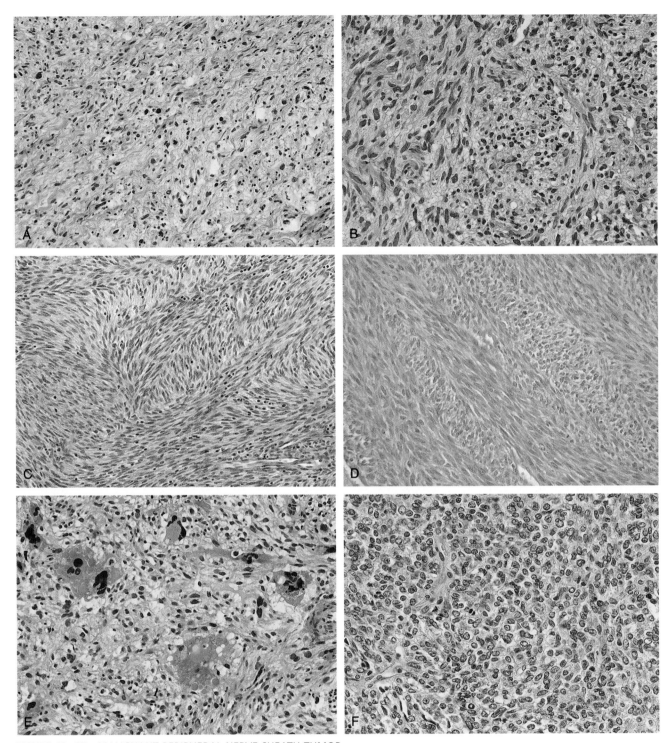

**FIGURE 12–67**   MALIGNANT PERIPHERAL NERVE SHEATH TUMOR

Histologic variation characterizes this tumor group. It ranges from low-grade lesions (*A, B*) arising in neurofibromas (*A*) and showing increased cellularity, nuclear size, and mitotic figures to high-grade tumors (*B*). Of the latter, some exhibit schwannoma- or synovial sarcoma-like features (*B, C*), whereas others feature fibrosarcoma-like herringbone arrangements of spindle cells (*D*), conspicuous giant cells that suggest malignant fibrous histiocytoma (*E*), or crowded cells without specific differentiation (*F*).

noma, ganglioneuroma or ganglioneuroblastoma,[44] and pheochromocytoma.[39, 41, 51] The clinicopathologic features of each of these tumors has recently been summarized.[52]

MPNST ex-schwannoma is particularly worthy of mention.[40, 52, 68] Its morphology differs from that of cel-lular schwannoma and conventional MPNST. Most cases feature the emergence of a malignant epithelioid or a small, round cell component (Fig. 12–71) within a conventional schwannoma. The behavior of MPNST ex-schwannoma is that of conventional MPNST.

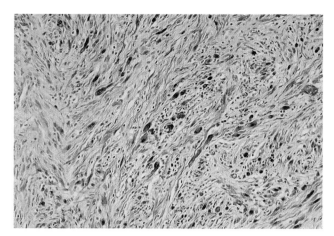

**FIGURE 12–68**   MALIGNANT PERIPHERAL NERVE SHEATH TUMOR

Although nearly half of these tumors lack immunohistochemical markers of nerve sheath, and most of the remainder show little staining, low-grade lesions may be quite immunoreactive. This grade 2 tumor shows conspicuous S-100 protein positivity.

## Primitive Neuroectodermal Tumor of Nerve

Since the initial description of a PNET of the ulnar nerve,[12] only a few additional examples have been published.[2, 3, 7, 9–11, 13] The term "peripheral neuroepithe-lioma" has also been applied. To date, all such tumors have occurred in adults, none in association with NF1. Most such tumors involve sizable nerves of the extremities. The designation PNET is limited to tumors composed entirely of "primitive" neuroectodermal cells and should not be applied to rare examples of conventional MPNST that demonstrate PNET elements.[4, 5]

**Microscopic Features.** PNETs are highly malignant tumors presumably derived from the neural crest. Histologically, they have been designated "small blue cell" tumors because they consist of monotonous, poorly differentiated round cells disposed in a sheet or lobular pattern. Many, but not all, feature a fibrillar background. Nuclei are small, and cytoplasm is scant. Homer Wright rosettes, a feature of neuroblastic differentiation, may be seen (Fig. 12–72A), but ganglion cells are generally not. Flexner-Wintersteiner rosettes or canals of the type seen in medulloepithelioma are also a rarity.

**Immunohistochemical, Ultrastructural, and Cytogenetic Features.** PNETs are far more often immunoreactive for neuron-specific enolase, CD99 (Fig. 12–72B), and synaptophysin than for neurofilament protein.

Ultrastructurally, they consist of rounded cells with occasional short, neuritic processes containing microtubules, scant cytoplasm with few organelles, and rare dense-core granules.

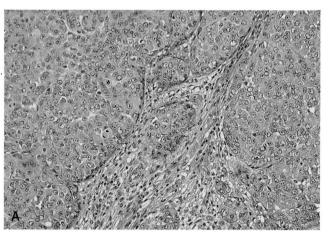

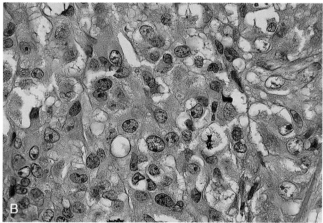

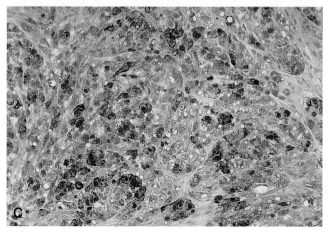

**FIGURE 12–69**   MALIGNANT PERIPHERAL NERVE SHEATH TUMOR

The subset of "malignant epithelioid schwannoma" often mimics carcinoma (A). This tumor's large cells, with open chromatin, prominent nucleoli, and abundant cytoplasm (B), are strongly S-100 protein immunoreactive (C).

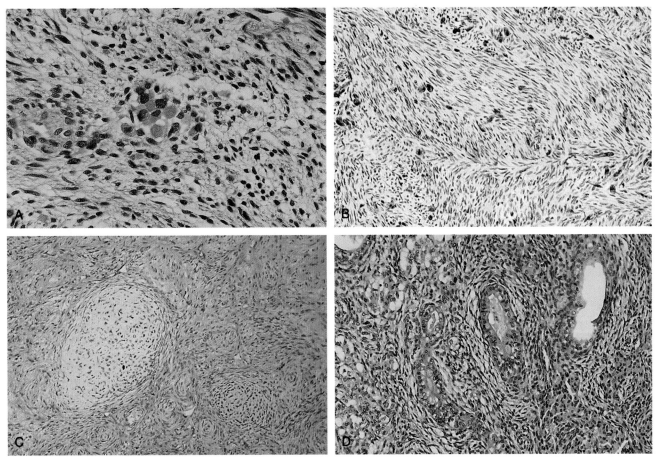

**FIGURE 12–70    MALIGNANT PERIPHERAL NERVE SHEATH TUMOR**

Divergent differentiation is seen in approximately 10% of these tumors. Those termed "Triton tumors" feature skeletal muscle differentiation (*A*), as evidenced by desmin immunoreactivity (*B*). Cartilaginous differentiation is less frequently seen (*C*). "Malignant glandular schwannomas" (*D*) are rare and exhibit well-differentiated, columnar, mucin-producing epithelium. Squamous or neuroendocrine epithelium may also be seen.

Although most soft tissue PNETs show a reciprocal translocation of chromosomes 11 and 22 (q21:q12),[14] no nerve-based PNETs have been cytogenetically studied to date.

Some small cell tumors of peripheral nerve included among PNETs lack specific immunohistochemical or molecular markers.[1]

**Differential Diagnosis.** Unlike *neuroblastomas*, the principal differential diagnosis, peripheral PNETs occur in patients older than 10 years; affect soft tissue or bone; are cholinergic rather than adrenergic in character; lack metabolite excretion; stain for CD99; are far more often immunoreactive for vimentin, and rarely exhibit immunoreactivity for neurofilament protein; ultrastructurally show relatively scant neuronal differentiation (neurites and secretory granules); feature different chromosomal abnormalities, namely, translocation 11:22 rather than del 1(q-), homogeneously stained regions, and double minutes; exhibit *c-myc* rather than *n-myc* oncogene expression; and are associated with lower survival frequencies in the setting of both local (50% versus 80%) and disseminated (10% versus 20%) disease. *Poorly differentiated synovial sarcoma* also enters into the differential diagnosis. Given their varied im-

munophenotype, which includes reactivity for PNET and nerve sheath–associated antigens,[6] cytogenetic or molecular genetic confirmation of the synovial sarcoma–associated translocation (X;18) may be necessary.

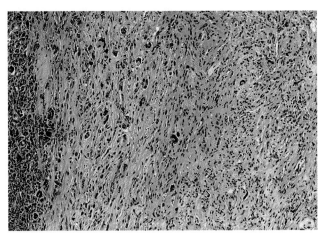

**FIGURE 12–71    MALIGNANT PERIPHERAL NERVE SHEATH TUMOR EX-SCHWANNOMA**

This rare form of malignant peripheral nerve sheath tumor originates in a preexisting schwannoma. The malignant component is typically small cell or epithelioid in cytology.

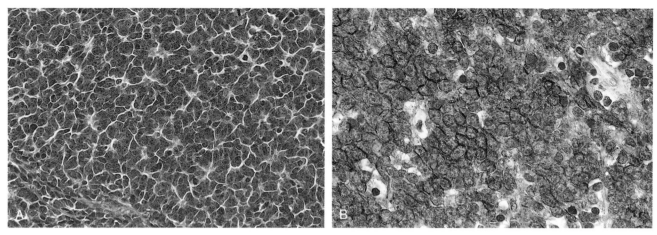

**FIGURE 12–72**   PRIMITIVE NEUROECTODERMAL TUMOR

These tumors, which are rarely primary in nerve, consist of small cells often featuring Homer Wright–type rosettes (A) and show immunoreactivity for CD99 (B).

**Treatment and Prognosis.** As a tumor group, PNETs exhibit locally aggressive behavior and are prone to undergo disseminated spread to lung, bone, and lymph nodes.[8] Their survival relative to stage was noted above in a comparison with neuroblastoma.

## Malignant Granular Cell Tumor

**Definition.** The malignant counterpart of conventional granular cell tumor. The lesion is composed of granular, S-100 protein–immunoreactive cells containing numerous secondary lysosomes.

**General Comments.** Although at one time the existence of malignant granular cell tumor was questioned,[7] they have now been well characterized.[3–5, 9, 12] Diagnostic criteria rightly include histologic malignancy (see below), but some tumors undergo metastasis despite benign histology.

**Clinical Features.** Malignant granular cell tumors occur in adults and affect primarily the trunk and extremities, particularly the thighs. At least two reported examples have originated in large nerves.[13, 15]

**Macroscopic Features.** Whether relatively circumscribed or infiltrative, most malignant granular cell tumors are sizable (5 to 15 cm). As previously noted, a nerve association is rare. On cut section, necrosis may be grossly apparent.

**Microscopic Features.** Malignant granular cell tumors form sheets or irregular lobules of polygonal to somewhat spindled cells with strongly PAS-positive and diastase-resistant granules and globules. PAS-positive angulate bodies are also seen within accompanying macrophages. Although some tumors appear histologically benign, those with malignant features express at least three of the following: hypercellularity, pleomorphism, prominent spindling of neoplastic cells, high nu-

clear cytoplasmic ratio, nucleolar prominence, brisk mitotic activity, and frequent necrosis (Fig. 12–73).[4] Clinically malignant but histologically benign granular cell tumors cannot be diagnosed with confidence at the H&E level.[6] Nonetheless, finding several low-power fields featuring enlarged, pleomorphic, vesicular or hyperchromatic nuclei, as well as prominent nucleoli, suggests probable malignancy. Simply the presence of an occasional mitotic figure is insufficient for the diagnosis. The same is true of limited infiltration of soft tissue. On the other hand, destructive growth and lymphatic or vascular invasion warrant a malignant designation.

**Immunohistochemical Features.** Malignant granular cell tumors are vimentin, S-100 protein, and neuron-specific enolase immunoreactive.[1, 3, 10, 11] The significance of occasional carcinoembryonic antigen staining is unresolved. Although benign granular cell tumors are CD68 positive,[8] not all malignant examples stain for this antigen. Collagen IV reactivity outlines occasional lobules. In one series, half of histologically malignant

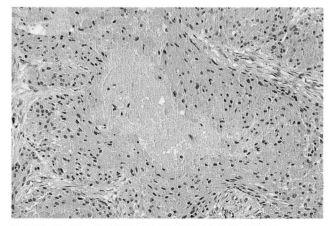

**FIGURE 12–73**   MALIGNANT GRANULAR CELL TUMOR

These rare tumors feature cytologic atypia, mitotic activity, and often necrosis.

granular cell tumors showed MIB-1 labeling indices of 10% to 50%[4]; nearly 70% showed extensive p53 staining as well.

**Ultrastructural Features.** Electron microscopy does not distinguish benign from malignant granular cell tumors, but pleomorphic nuclei and multiple coarse nucleoli are in keeping with the latter. Innumerable cytoplasmic lysosomes and the occasional finding of basal lamina surrounding cell clusters are common in both benign and malignant lesions. Specialized junctions are lacking. Angulate bodies (lysosomes) are also seen in interstitial histiocytes.[2, 14]

**Differential Diagnosis.** The major differential diagnosis is *benign granular cell tumor*. Their comparative features were previously discussed in this section. *Granular cell leiomyosarcoma* is distinguishable on immunostains by its reactivity for myoid markers (smooth muscle actin, muscle common actin [HHF35], desmin). The distinction of malignant granular cell tumor from *alveolar soft part sarcoma* is generally easy, given its organoid and alveolar growth pattern; the presence of PAS-positive, needle-like cytoplasmic crystalloids; and lack of S-100

protein staining. The crystalloids of alveolar soft part sarcoma are distinctive, appearing rhomboid at the ultrastructural level.

**Treatment and Prognosis.** The treatment of choice of malignant granular cell tumor is wide, en bloc excision. Neither radiation nor chemotherapy is beneficial. In most instances, metastases develop within 2 years of the initial resection. One large series assessing the prognostic significance of a variety of clinicopathologic parameters found that only advanced patient age and MIB-1 labeling indices greater than 10% adversely affected survival.

## METASTATIC NEOPLASMS

Carcinoma, sarcoma, neurotropic melanoma, and leukemia-lymphoma are well-known to secondarily affect nerves, either by direct extension or metastasis. The incidence of nerve involvement varies. Some lesions simply compress or encase the nerve, whereas others infiltrate epineurium, perineurium, or endoneurium. In most instances the involved nerves are small.

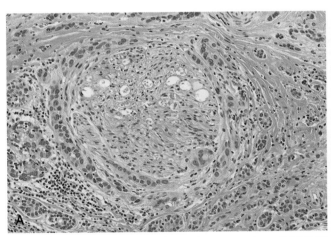

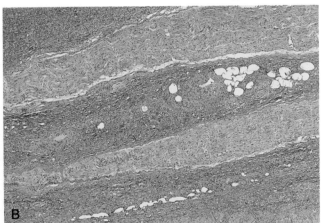

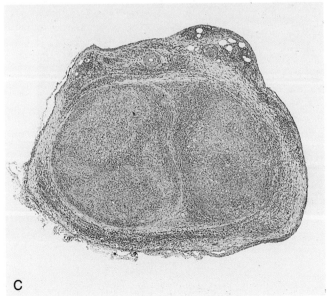

**FIGURE 12–74** SECONDARY TUMORS OF NERVE

Of non-neural tumors involving nerve, carcinomas are most frequent. Adenoid cystic carcinoma (*A*) is particularly prone to perineurial space involvement. Sarcomas more often affect the epineurium, as shown in an example of angiosarcoma separating nerve fascicles (*B*).
Hematopoietic tumors, such as this example of a T-cell lymphoma (*C*), often involve the endoneurial space.

## Carcinoma

The anatomic compartment most often involved by secondary tumors is the "perineurial space," a potential rather than physiologic space that permits the spread of infiltrative tumors within nerve. Among neoplasms using this route, carcinomas are most common, specifically adenocarcinoma of the prostate, adenoid cystic carcinoma of salivary glands (Fig. 12–74A, see also Fig. 1–83), squamous carcinoma of the head and neck region,[2, 8] and ductal carcinoma of the breast. Significant proximal spread within this space is of clinical importance, because it brings the tumor within reach of the central nervous system and facilitates so-called meningeal carcinomatosis. Although carcinomas and sarcomas may involve the perivascular sleeves of arteries that traverse the perineurium and enter the endoneurium, lymphoma-leukemia cells do so more readily. Endoneurium is infrequently involved by carcinoma, but this is not the case for sensory ganglia. The latter are rendered susceptible to invasion due to their lack of a blood-ganglion barrier.

It is important to note that benign epithelial proliferations occasionally gain access to perineurium or endoneurium. These include mammary fibrocystic change,[14] prostatic hypertrophy,[4] benign gallbladder lesions,[5] and vasitis nodosa.[18] Intraneural inclusions of normal tissue, such as prostate[4] and pancreas,[7] may also be encountered. Affected nerves are generally small.

## Sarcoma

Secondary involvement of nerve by sarcomas is well recognized.[3] Among such tumors, nearly half affect peripheral nerve by simple displacement, adherence, or encasement. Invasion of sizable nerves is less frequent and is generally associated with high-grade tumors that destroy epineurium (see Fig. 12–74B) and infiltrate perineurium. In any case, actual involvement of endoneurium is infrequent. As with carcinomas, extension within the perineurial space may be appreciable.

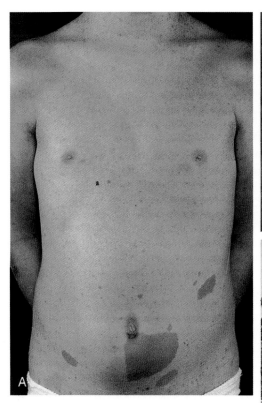

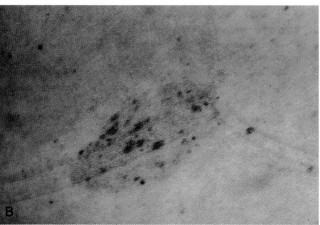

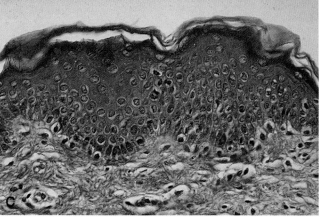

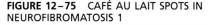

**FIGURE 12–75**    CAFÉ AU LAIT SPOTS IN NEUROFIBROMATOSIS 1

The multiple lesions in this case (A) vary in size and are demarcated from surrounding skin. Note the dermatomal distribution of the largest lesion. Among the earliest features of neurofibromatosis 1, café au lait spots enlarge slowly in early life and become increasingly pigmented over time. Freckling of intertriginous skin (B) is also a common finding. In both instances, pigmentation (C) is due to an increase in melanosomes within phagolysosomes, not of melanocytes.

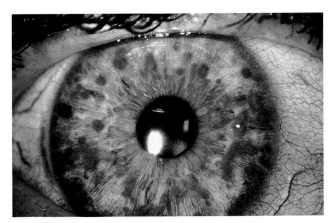

**FIGURE 12-76**    LISCH NODULE IN NEUROFIBROMATOSIS 1

This characteristic, circumferential lesion of the iris affects the vast majority of neurofibromatosis 1 patients. The elevated brown nodules on the iris readily distinguished from iris nevi, which are flat and involve only a segment of the iris.

## Neurotropic Melanoma

Among melanomas, it is the desmoplastic variant that often exhibits neurotropism, invading and extending along peripheral nerves.[1, 12, 15] Most desmoplastic melanomas arise in sun-exposed skin of the head and neck region in elderly male patients. Histologically, they often lack an intraepidermal component and appear "neuroid" owing to their tendency to form nerve-like bundles.[16] Being highly malignant, they are prone to frequent recurrence and metastasis.[10] Many, but not all, are immunoreactive for S-100 protein.[10, 17] Curiously, most are negative for the melanocytic marker HMB-45.[10] Ultrastructurally, the neoplastic cells of desmoplastic melanoma have abundant rough endoplasmic reticulum, a fibroblastic feature, intermediate filaments, scant melanosomes, cytoplasmic processes, focal basement membranes, and rudimentary cell junctions.[9]

## Lymphoma-Leukemia

Hematopoietic tumors affect nerve roots, ganglia, and cranial peripheral nerves. Although the process may be widespread, its distribution is often nonuniform. Infiltrates typically involve the subperineurial zone and endoneurium (see Fig. 12-74C). In most cases, involvement of the nerve occurs in the setting of systemic disease. On occasion, non-Hodgkin's lymphomas are primary within and limited to nerve.[13]

## Miscellaneous Secondary Neoplasms

PNETs of soft tissue may secondarily affect nerve, thus making a bona fide diagnosis of peripheral PNET difficult.

Carcinomas rarely metastasize to a nerve sheath tumor, most often to a schwannoma.[6, 11]

## NEUROFIBROMATOSIS

Neurofibromatosis is the most frequent of the phakomatoses, a group of disorders that also includes

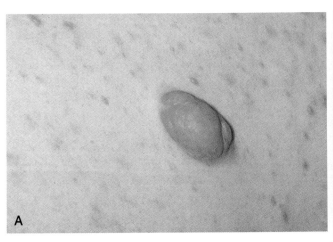
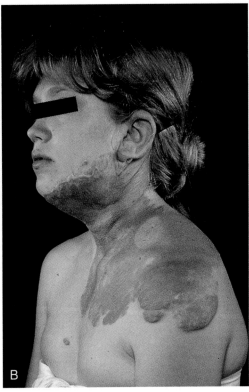

**FIGURE 12-77**    CUTANEOUS NEUROFIBROMAS IN NEUROFIBROMATOSIS 1

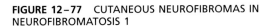

Note the single, dominant, localized neurofibroma (A) in a field of minute lesions. A large, diffuse, cutaneous neurofibroma (B) with an underlying plexiform component forms a cape-like tumor, accompanied by diffuse cutaneous pigmentation.

**TABLE 12–6**
**Comparative Features of Neurofibromatosis 1 and 2**

| | NF1 (Peripheral Form; von Recklinghausen's Disease) | NF2 (Central Form) |
|---|---|---|
| Incidence | 1/3000 | 1/40,000 |
| Prevalence | 60/100,000 | 0.01/100,000 |
| Inheritance | Autosomal dominant | Autosomal dominant |
| Sporadic recurrence | 50% | 50% |
| Chromosome location | 17q11.2 | 22q12 |
| Encoded protein | Neurofibromin | Merlin (schwannomin) |
| Café au lait spots | Often multiple and large | Small, rarely more than 6 |
|   One or more |   About 90% of patients |   40% of patients |
|   Six or more |   At least 70% of patients | |
| Cutaneous neurofibromas | Most patients | Rare |
| Cutaneous schwannomas | Not associated | 70% |
| Multiple Lisch nodules | Very common | Not associated |
| Cataracts | Not associated | 60–80% |
| Skeletal malformations | Common | Not associated |
| Astrocytomas (optic, cerebellar, cerebral) | Moderate incidence | Infrequent |
| Pheochromocytoma | Occasionally seen | Not associated |
| Malignant peripheral nerve sheath tumor | Approximately 2% | Not seen |
| Intellectual impairment | Associated | Not associated |
| Vestibular schwannoma | Not associated | Most cases (usually bilateral) |
| Meningioma | Uncommon | Common |
| Spinal cord ependymoma | Not associated | Common |
| Meningioangiomatosis | Not associated | Occasional |
| Schwannosis | Not associated | Common |
| Glial hamartomas | Occasional | Very common |
| Syringomyelia | Not associated | Associated |
| Posterior subcapsular cataracts | Not associated | Common |
| Ganglioneuroma | Occasional | Not associated |
| Gastrointestinal autonomic nerve tumor | Occasional | Not associated |
| Paraganglioma, including duodenal gangliocytic variant | Occasional | Not associated |
| Foregut carcinoid tumor, including duodenal calcifying somatostatinoma | Occasional | Not associated |
| Juvenile xanthogranuloma | Occasional | Not associated |
| Rhabdomyosarcoma | Occasional | Not associated |
| Juvenile leukemia | Occasional | Not associated |

tuberous sclerosis, neurocutaneous melanosis, Sturge-Weber syndrome, and two lesser-known conditions—hypomelanosis of Ito and incontinentia pigmenti. All but Sturge-Weber syndrome are heritable, the pattern being autosomal dominant. The spectrum of lesions encountered in neurofibromatosis is diverse and includes hyperplasia, hypoplasia, hamartoma, and benign as well as malignant neoplasms. The majority are neuroectodermal or mesenchymal processes. All races are affected. There is no sex predilection.

Neurofibromatosis is not a single disease but a group of genetic disorders. At least eight variants have been described.[17] The two principal forms, NF1 and NF2, are distinctive and exhibit only minimal clinical overlap (Table 12–6). Both have their basis in genetic alterations of a tumor suppressor gene that impart a 10-fold increase in the risk of malignancy.

## Neurofibromatosis 1

Also termed "peripheral neurofibromatosis" and "von Recklinghausen's disease," NF1 is the most common form of neurofibromatosis. Ostensibly, the affected gene, which resides near that of the nerve growth factor receptor,[22] modulates cell proliferation and differentiation.[5, 26]

Only half of cases are familial. Although penetrance is high, expression is variable.[17–19] Thus only a minority of patients are significantly affected. Criteria for the clinical diagnosis of NF1 are summarized in Table 12–7. As indicated, no single criterion is pathognomonic of the condition. Café au lait spots are the earliest expression of the

**TABLE 12–7**
**Diagnostic Criteria for Neurofibromatosis 1 (NF1)**

The patient should have two or more of the following:
1. Six or more café au lait spots:
    1.5 cm or larger in postpubertal individuals
    0.5 cm or larger in prepubertal individuals
2. Two or more neurofibromas of any type, or one or more plexiform neurofibromas
3. Freckling in the axilla or groin
4. Optic glioma (tumor of the optic pathway)
5. Two or more Lisch nodules (benign iris hamartomas)
6. A distinctive bony lesion:
    Dysplasia of the sphenoid bone
    Dysplasia or thinning of the long bone cortex
7. A first-degree relative with NF1

From Gutmann DH, Aylsworth A, Carey JC, et al. The diagnostic evaluation and multidisciplinary management of neurofibromatosis 1 and neurofibromatosis 2. JAMA 1997; 278:51–57.

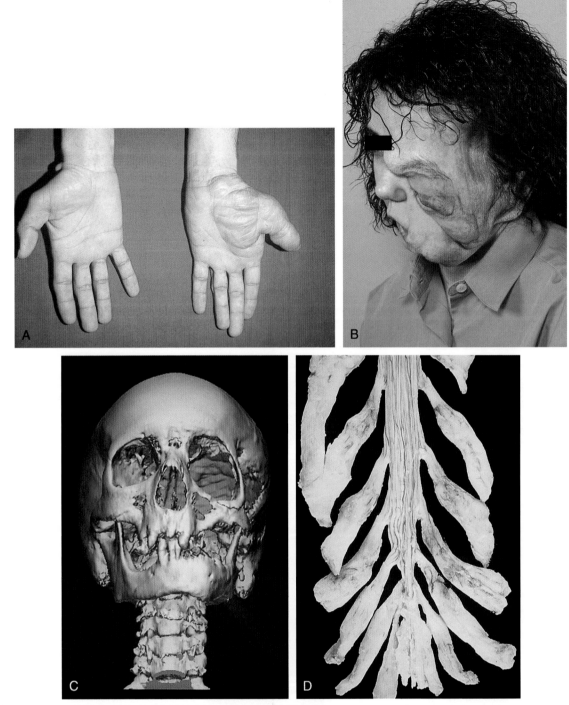

**FIGURE 12–78**    PLEXIFORM NEUROFIBROMA IN NEUROFIBROMATOSIS 1

This lesion (*A*) presents as a protuberant, bag-like enlargement of one thenar eminence. Another example, a disfiguring tumor of the left face associated with osseous dysplasia, consists of plexiform neurofibroma with accompanying diffuse soft tissue extension (*B*). The corresponding computer reconstruction shows the typical orbital asymmetry (*C*). Plexiform neurofibromas may also involve the intradural components of multiple spinal nerve roots (*D*).

disease (Fig. 12–75*A*). Most become apparent in childhood, but occasional examples are congenital. Pigmentation or "freckling" of intertriginous skin (Fig. 12–75*B*) is also of diagnostic importance. Both these pigmentary lesions are due to an excess of melanin in "macromelanosomes" (melanosome-containing phagolysosomes) (Fig. 12–75*C*), not to an increase in melanocytes. Café

au lait spots may be seen in unrelated disorders, such as McCune-Albright syndrome, and occur in small number in normal individuals. A distinctive ocular abnormality of NF1, Lisch nodules of the iris, consists of macroscopic aggregates of pigmented cells (Fig. 12–76).

Neurofibromas are also a key feature of NF1. Their clinicopathologic spectrum was discussed earlier on pages

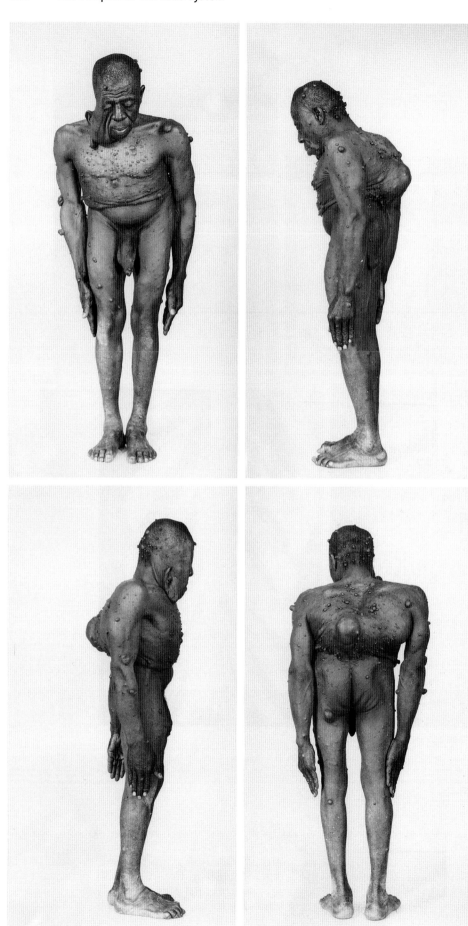

**FIGURE 12–79** ADVANCED NEUROFIBROMATOSIS 1

This statue-like figure of a 57-year-old man portrays the full spectrum of external manifestations of neurofibromatosis 1, including cutaneous neurofibromas, café au lait spots, "elephantiasis neuromatosa," and kyphoscoliosis.

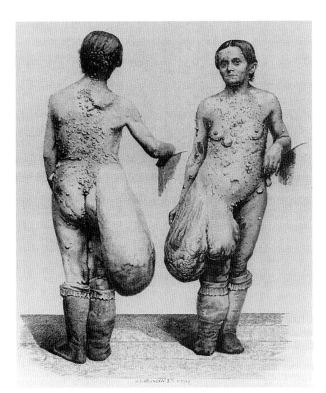

**FIGURE 12–80**   MASSIVE SOFT TISSUE NEUROFIBROMA IN NEUROFIBROMATOSIS 1

As depicted by Virchow's *Krankhafte Geschwulste* in 1856, the patient shows obvious cutaneous neurofibromas, occasional café au lait spots, and massive "elephantiasis neuromatosa." Note the typical facies, characterized by a broad, rectangular forehead.

602 to 611. Despite cellular heterogeneity at the light and electron microscopic levels, one recent genetic study suggested that only their Schwann cell component expresses the telltale genetic abnormality of the disorder.[15] Neurofibromas are presumed to be monoclonal processes[23] arising as the result of a second, somatic mutation in patients already having one nonfunctional NF1

gene. The occurrence of malignant transformation in a neurofibroma is attributable to loss or mutation of yet another tumor suppressor gene, for example, p53.[6, 14] Most neurofibromas make their appearance at about the time of puberty. All four morphologic variants occur in NF1— namely, localized and diffuse cutaneous neurofibromas (Fig. 12–77), localized intraneural tumors, plexiform neurofibromas (Fig. 12–78), and massive soft tissue examples (Figs. 12–79 and 12–80). Of these, plexiform and massive soft tissue lesions are virtually pathognomonic of the disease. The same is true of numerous cutaneous neurofibromas. On occasion, however, a small, often cutaneous plexiform neurofibroma is unassociated with other stigmata or a family history of NF1. Such lesions may be due to a local somatic mutation.[18] This also appears to be the basis of so-called segmental neurofibromatosis, a condition in which neurofibromas are limited to an anatomic region.[16, 20] Such patients do not genetically transmit the defect.

Whether sporadic or NF1 associated, so-called visceral neurofibromatosis is a rare condition. Lesions may be solitary or multiple, localized or plexiform. External manifestations of the disease may be few. As previously noted, various organs are affected, especially the upper gastrointestinal tract (esophagus, stomach, small bowel). Urinary bladder involvement is rare.[1] Other NF1-associated visceral lesions include ganglioneuromatosis, gastrointestinal stromal tumors,[9, 10] and various neuroendocrine neoplasms. Multiple intestinal neurofibromas may also result from translocation of chromosomes 12 and 14.[25] Visceral MPNSTs are rare and usually NF1 associated.[3, 4, 11]

Although a detailed discussion of NF1-associated central nervous system lesions is beyond the scope of this chapter, astrocytomas of the pilocytic or diffuse fibrillary type are commonly encountered in surgical pathology practice and deserve mention. In NF1, pilocytic tumors often involve the optic nerve, classically in a bilateral fashion. The cerebellum, thalamus, brain stem, and cerebrum are also favored sites. Most pilocytic tumors present early in childhood or adolescence. Of the

---

**TABLE 12–8**
**Diagnostic Criteria for Neurofibromatosis 2 (NF2)**

Individuals with the following clinical features should have confirmed (definite) NF2:
Bilateral or vestibular schwannoma (VS)
  or
Family history of NF2 (first-degree family relative)
  Plus
  1. Unilateral VS <30 years or
  2. Any two of the following: meningioma, glioma schwannoma, juvenile posterior subscapular lenticular opacities or juvenile cortical cataract
Individuals with the following clinical features should be evaluated for NF (presumptive or probable NF2):
  Unilateral VS <30 years plus at least one of the following: meningioma, glioma, schwannoma, juvenile posterior subscapular lenticular opacities, or juvenile cortical cataract
  Multiple meningiomas (two or more) plus unilateral VS <30 years or one of the following: glioma, schwannoma, juvenile posterior subscapular lenticular opacities, or juvenile cortical cataract

From Gutmann MD, Aylsworth A, Carey JC, et al. The diagnostic evaluation and multidisciplinary management of neurofibromatosis 1 and neurofibromatosis 2. JAMA 1997;278:51–57.

diffuse astrocytomas occurring in NF1, fully half are malignant. Neuroglial hamartomas of the brain and retina also occur in NF1. Aside from tumors of the nervous system, a variety of other neoplasms may be seen in NF1(see Table 12–6).

## Neurofibromatosis 2

Localized to an abnormality on chromosome 22,[8, 21] NF2 or "central neurofibromatosis" is also inherited in an autosomal dominant manner and with high penetrance.[27] The condition is far less common than NF1 and is heterogeneous in its presentation.[2] Most patients present in the second or third decade, and fully half represent new mutations. Strict diagnostic criteria have been formulated (Table 12–8). From a neurologic point of view, the disease is more devastating than NF1. The clinicopathologic features of the two conditions are compared in Table 12–6. Classic features of NF2 include bilateral eighth nerve schwannoma, as well as multiple ependymomas and meningiomas. Meningioangiomatosis is also NF2 associated.[7] A genetically related disorder termed "schwannomatosis" has recently been characterized and consists of multiple schwannomas of spinal and less often cranial nerves. Some are plexiform. Eighth nerve involvement is not a feature.[12, 13] An NF2 neuropathy has also been described.[24]

## APPENDIX: DIFFERENTIAL DIAGNOSIS OF TUMORS AND TUMOR-LIKE LESIONS OF NERVE

| Lesion | Differential |
|---|---|
| 1. Tumor-like lesions | |
|   a. Reactive lesions | |
|     (1) Traumatic neuroma | Neurofibroma, palisaded encapsulated neuroma, mucosal neuroma |
|     (2) Plantar (Morton's) neuroma | Traumatic neuroma |
|     (3) Pacinian neuroma | Nerve sheath myxoma |
|     (4) Nerve cyst | Nerve sheath myxoma, cystic schwannoma |
|     (5) Inflammatory pseudotumor | Infection, lymphoma |
|   b. Inflammatory and infectious lesions | |
|   c. Hyperplastic lesions | |
|     (1) Palisaded encapsulated neuroma (PEN) | Plexiform schwannoma, leiomyoma |
|     (2) Mucosal neuromatosis, ganglioneuroma/ganglioneuromatosis | Traumatic neuroma, PEN, ganglioneuroma(tosis) |
|     (3) Localized hypertrophic neuropathy | Intraneural perineurioma |
|   d. Hamartomas | |
|     (1) Fibrolipomatous hamartoma | Lipoma |
|     (2) Neuromuscular choristoma | Rhabdomyoma, benign and malignant "triton tumor" |
| 2. Benign tumors | |
|   a. Schwannoma (neurilemoma) | Neurofibroma, leiomyoma, palisaded myofibroblastoma, PEN |
|     (1) Cellular schwannoma | Malignant peripheral nerve sheath tumor (MPNST), fibrosarcoma, leiomyosarcoma |
|     (2) Plexiform schwannoma | Plexiform neurofibroma, plexiform fibrohistiocytic tumor |
|     (3) Melanotic schwannoma | Melanoma, pigmented dermatofibrosarcoma protuberans, melanotic neurofibroma |
|   b. Neurofibroma | |
|     (1) Diffuse (cutaneous) | Dermatofibroma, dermatofibrosarcoma protuberans, mucinosis, myxoid fibrous histiocytoma, spindle cell lipoma |
|     (2) Localized | Schwannoma, myxoma, ganglioneuroma |
|     (3) Plexiform | Plexiform schwannoma |
|     (4) Divergent differentiation (glandular, rhabdomyomatous pigmented, etc.) | |
|   c. Perineurioma | Localized hypertrophic neuropathy |
|   d. Nerve sheath myxoma and neurothekeoma | Myxoid neurofibroma and schwannoma, soft tissue myxoma, mucinosis, myxoma, myxoid malignant fibrous histiocytoma |
|   e. Granular cell tumor | Malignant granular cell tumor, granular epithelioid leiomyoma, hibernoma, rhabdomyoma, paraganglioma, alveolar soft part sarcoma |
|   f. Ganglioneuroma | Schwannoma, neurofibroma |
|   g. Miscellaneous lesions | |
|     (1) Paraganglioma (cauda equina) | Ependymoma (filum terminale) |
|     (2) Lipoma | Lipofibromatous hamartoma |
|     (3) Hemangioma | Angiomatosis |
|     (4) Hemangioblastoma | Metastatic renal cell carcinoma |
|     (5) Adrenal adenoma | Metastatic renal cell carcinoma, granular cell tumor |
|     (6) Angiomatosis of nerve | Hemangioma |

3. Malignant tumors
  a. MPNST

    (1) MPNST variants
      (a) Epithelioid MPNST
      (b) MPNST with divergent (mesenchymal/
          epithelial) differentiation
      (c) Schwannoma with malignant transformation

      (d) MPNST arising from ganglioneuroma
          or ganglioneuroblastoma
      (e) Malignant perineurioma
  b. Malignant tumors of possible peripheral nerve origin
    (1) Primitive neuroectodermal tumor
      (peripheral neuroepithelioma)
    (2) Malignant granular cell tumor

  c. Secondary neoplasms

Cellular neurofibroma, cellular schwannoma, fibrosarcoma, leiomyosarcoma, monophasic synovial sarcoma, neurotropic melanoma, clear cell sarcoma

Melanoma, carcinoma, rhabdoid tumor, clear cell sarcoma
Synovial sarcoma, rhabdomyosarcoma, osteo- and chondrosarcoma, carcinoma
Cellular schwannoma, metastatic carcinoma, primitive neuroectodermal tumor

Conventional MPNST

Small cell carcinoma/sarcoma, lymphoma

Granular cell tumor, granular variant of leiomyosarcoma, alveolar soft part sarcoma, rhabdoid tumor
Carcinoma, sarcoma, neurotropic melanoma, meningioma

# REFERENCES

## Introduction
1. Dyck PJ, Thomas PK (eds). Peripheral Neuropathy. Philadelphia: WB Saunders, 1993.

## Normal Anatomy
1. Angevine JB. The nervous tissue. In Bloom W, Fawcett DW, (eds). A Textbook of Histology. New York: Chapman and Hall, 1994, pp 309–364.
2. Ariza A, Bilbao JM, Rosai J. Immunohistochemical detection of epithelial membrane antigen in normal perineurial cells and perineuriomas. Am J Surg Pathol 1988;12:678–683.
3. Bell J, Bolanowski S, Holmes MH. The structure and function of pacinian corpuscles—a review. Prog Neurobiol 1994;42:79–128.
4. Erlandson RA, Woodruff JM. Peripheral nerve sheath tumors: an electron microscopic study of 43 cases. Cancer 1982;49:273–287.
5. Gardner E, Bunge RP. Gross anatomy of the peripheral nervous system. In Dyck PJ, Thomas PK (eds). Peripheral Neuropathy. 3rd ed. Philadelphia: WB Saunders, 1993, pp 8–27.
6. Nathaniel EJH, Pease DC. Collagen and basement membrane formation by Schwann cells during nerve regeneration. J Ultrastruct Res 1963;9:550–560.
7. Perentes E, Nakagawa Y, Ross G, et al. Expression of epithelial membrane antigen in perineurial cells and their derivatives: an immunohistochemical study with multiple markers. Acta Neuropathol (Berl) 1987;75:160–165.
8. Scheithauer BW, Woodruf JW, Erlandson RA. The normal peripheral nervous system. In Rosai J, Sobin LH (eds). Atlas of Tumor Pathology: Tumors of the Peripheral Nervous System. Series 3. Washington, DC: Armed Forces Institute of Pathology, 2000, pp. 7–27.
9. Thomas PK, Berthold CH, Ochoa J. Microscopic anatomy of the peripheral nervous system. In Dyck PJ, Thomas PK (eds). Peripheral Neuropathy. Philadelphia: WB Saunders, 1993, pp 28–92.
10. Vega JA, Haro JJ, Del Valle ME. Immunohistochemistry of human cutaneous Meissner and pacinian corpuscles. Microsc Res Tech 1996;34:351–361.

## Traumatic Neuroma
1. Das Gupta TW, Brasfield RD. Amputation neuromas in cancer patients. N Y State J Med 1969;69:2129–2132.
2. Dyck PJ, Giannini C, Lais A. Pathologic alterations of nerves. In Dyck PJ, Thomas PK (eds). Peripheral Neuropathy. 3rd ed. Philadelphia: WB Saunders, 1993, pp 514–596.
3. Elhag AM, Al Awadi NZ. Amputation neuroma of the gallbladder. Histopathology 1992;21:586–587.
4. Matsuoka J, Tanaka N, Kojima K, et al. A case of traumatic neuroma of the gallbladder in the absence of previous surgery and cholelithiasis. Acta Med Okayama 1996;50:273–277.

5. Rosso R, Scelsi M. Granular cell traumatic neuroma—a lesion occurring in mastectomy scars. Arch Pathol Lab Med 2000;124:709–711.
6. Rush BF Jr, Stefaniwsky AB, Sasso A, et al. Neuroma of the common bile duct. J Surg Oncol 1988;39:17–21.
7. Sano T, Hirose T, Kagawa N, et al. Polypoid traumatic neuroma of the gallbladder. Arch Pathol Lab Med 1985;109:574–576.
8. Shapiro L, Juhlin E, Brownstein MH. Rudimentary polydactyly: an amputation neuroma. Arch Dermatol 1973;108:223–225.

## Localized Interdigital Neuritis (Morton's Neuroma)
1. Bennett GL, Graham CE, Mauldin DM. Morton's interdigital neuroma: a comprehensive treatment protocol. J Foot Ankle Surg 1995;16:760–763.
2. Lassmann G, Lassmann H, Stockinger L. Morton's metatarsalgia: light and electron microscopic observations and their relation to entrapment neuropathies. Virchows Arch A 1976;370:307–321.
3. Reed RJ, Bliss BO. Morton's neuroma: regressive and productive intermetatarsal elastofibrosis. Arch Pathol 1973;95:123–129.
4. Scotti TM. The lesion of Morton's metatarsalgia (Morton's toe). Arch Pathol 1957;63:91–102.
5. Wu KK. Morton's interdigital neuroma: a clinical review of its etiology, treatment, and results. J Foot Ankle Surg 1996;25:112–119.
6. Young G, Lindsey J. Etiology of symptomatic recurrent interdigital neuromas. J Am Podiatr Med Assoc 1993;83:255–258.

## Localized Hypertrophic Neuropathy
1. Baskin DS, Townsend JJ, Wilson CB. Isolated hypertrophic interstitial neuropathy of the trigeminal nerve associated with trigeminal neuralgia. J Neurosurg 1981;55:987–990.
2. Chang Y, Horoupian DS, Jordan J, Steinberg G. Localized hypertrophic mononeuropathy of the trigeminal nerve. Arch Pathol Lab Med 1993;117:170–176.
3. Chow SM. Role of macrophages in onion-bulb formation in localized hypertrophic mononeuritis (LHN). Clin Neuropathol 1991;10:112–121.
4. Emory TS, Scheithauer BW, Hirose T, et al. Intraneural perineurioma: a clonal neoplasm associated with abnormalities of chromosome 22. Am J Clin Pathol 1995;103:696–704.
5. Suarez GA, Giannini C, Bosch EP, et al. Immune brachial plexus neuropathy: suggestive evidence for an inflammatory immune pathogenesis. Neurology 1996;26:559–561.
6. Yassini PR, Sauter K, Schochet SS, et al. A localized hypertrophic mononeuropathy involving spinal roots and associated with sacral meningocele. J Neurosurg 1993;79:774–778.

## Nerve Cyst or "Ganglion"
1. Donahue F, Turkel DH, Mnaymneh W, Mnaymneh LG. Intraosseous ganglion cyst associated with neuropathy. Skeletal Radiol 1996;25:675–678.

2. Gurdjian ES, Larsen RD, Linder DW. Intraneural cyst of peroneal and ulnar nerves: report of two cases. J Neurosurg 1965; 23:76–78.

3. Hashizume H, Nishida K, Nanba Y, et al. Intraneural ganglion of the posterior interosseous nerve with lateral elbow pain. J Hand Surg 1995;20:649–651.

4. Jaradeh S, Sanger JR, Maas EF. Isolated sensory impairment of the thumb due to an intraneural ganglion cyst in the median nerve. J Hand Surg 1995;20:475–478.

5. Jenkins SA. Solitary tumors of peripheral nerve trunks. J Bone Joint Surg 1952;34:401–411.

6. Nucci F, Artico M, Santoro A, et al. Intraneural synovial cyst of the peroneal nerve: report of two cases and review of the literature. Neurosurgery 1990;26:339–344.

7. Orf G. Intraneurale ganglienzysten. Schweiz Arch Neurol Neurochir Psychiatr 1972;110:55–67.

8. Robert R, Resche F, Lajat Y, et al. Kyste synovial intraneural du sciatique poplite externe. A propos d'un cas. Neurochirurgie 1980;26:135–143.

9. Scherman BM, Bilbao JM, Hudson AR, Briggs RT. Intraneural ganglion: a case report with electron microscopic observations. Neurosurgery 1981;8:487–490.

10. Sotelo D, Frankel VH. Intraneural ganglion of the peroneal nerve: a cause of peripheral neuropathy. Bull Hosp Joint Dis Orthop Inst 1982;42:230–235.

11. Spinner RJ, Atkinson JLD, Kline DG, Tiel RL. Peroneal intraneural ganglia. The importance of the articular branch: A unifying theory (abstract). Clin Anat 14: 464, 2001.

12. Weller RO, Cervos-Navarro J. Pathology of Peripheral Nerves. London: Butterworth, 1977, pp 153–154.

### Inflammatory Pseudotumor of Nerve

1. Beer TW, Carr NJ, Weller RO. Inflammatory pseudotumor of peripheral nerve (Letter). Am J Surg Pathol 1998;2:1035–1036.

2. Fanous MM, Margo CE, Hamed LM. Chronic idiopathic inflammation of the retropharyngeal space presenting with sequential abducens palsies. J Clin Neuroophthalmol 1992;12:154–157.

3. George DH, Scheithauer BW, Hilton DL, et al. Juvenile xanthogranuloma of peripheral nerve: a case report. Am J Surg Pathol 2001;25:521–526.

4. Keen M, Conley J, McBride T, et al. Pseudotumor of the pterygomaxillary space presenting as anesthesia of the mandibular nerve. Laryngoscope 1986;96:560–563.

5. Scheithauer BW, Woodruff JM, Erlandson RA. Inflammatory and infectious lesions simulating tumors of nerve. In Rosai J, Sobin LH (eds). Atlas of Tumor Pathology: Tumors of the Peripheral Nervous System. Series 3. Washington, DC: Armed Forces Institute of Pathology, 2000, pp 57–67.

6. Weiland TL, Scheithauer BW, Rock MG, Sargent JM. Inflammatory pseudotumor of nerve. Am J Surg Pathol 1996;20:1212–1218.

7. Wiseman JB, Arriaga MA, Houston GD, Boyd EM. Facial paralysis and inflammatory pseudotumor of the facial nerve in a child. Otolaryngol Head Neck Surg 1995;113:826–828.

8. Wold LE, Weiland LH. Tumefactive fibro-inflammatory lesions of the head and neck. Am J Surg Pathol 1983;7:477–482.

9. Yanagihara N, Segoe M, Gyo K, Ueda N. Inflammatory pseudotumor of the facial nerve as a cause of recurrent facial palsy: case report. Am J Otol 1991;12:199–202.

### Sarcoidosis

1. Delaney P. Neurologic manifestations of sarcoidosis: review of the literature with a report of 23 cases. Ann Intern Med 1977;87:336–345.

2. Scheithauer BW, Woodruff JM, Erlandson RA. Inflammatory and infectious lesions simulating tumors of nerve. In Rosai J, Sobin LH (eds). Atlas of Tumor Pathology: Tumors of the Peripheral Nervous System. Series 3. Washington, DC: Armed Forces Institute of Pathology, 2000, pp 57–67.

3. Silverstein A, Feuer MM, Stiltzbach LE. Neurologic sarcoidosis: study of 18 cases. Arch Neurol 1965;12:1–11.

### Leprosy

1. Sabin TD, Swift TR, Jacobson RR. Leprosy. In Dyck PJ, Thomas PK (eds). Peripheral Neuropathy. 3rd ed. Philadelphia: WB Saunders, 1993, pp 1354–1379.

2. Scheithauer BW, Woodruff JM, Erlandson RA. Inflammatory and infectious lesions simulating tumors of nerve. In Rosai J, Sobin LH (eds). Atlas of Tumor Pathology: Tumors of the Peripheral Nervous System. Series 3. Washington, DC: Armed Forces Institute of Pathology, 2000, pp 57–67.

### Lipofibromatous Hamartoma

1. Amadio PC, Reiman HM, Dobyns JH. Lipofibromatous hamartoma of nerve. J Hand Surg 1988;13A:67–75.

2. Bergman FO, Blom SE, Stenström SJ. Radical excision of a fibrofatty proliferation of the median nerve, with no neurological loss of symptoms. Plast Reconr Surg 1970;46:375–380.

3. Christensen WN, Long DM, Epstein JI. Cerebellopontine angle lipoma. Hum Pathol 1986;17:739–743.

4. Fukui M, Tanaka A, Kitamura K, Okudera T. Lipoma of the cerebellopontine angle: case report. J Neurosurg 1977;46:544–547.

5. Gouldesbrough DR, Kinny SJ. Lipofibromatous hamartoma of the ulnar nerve at the elbow: brief report. J Bone Joint Surg 1989;71:331–332.

6. Guthikonda M, Rengachary SS, Balko MG, van Loveren H. Lipofibromatous hamartoma of the median nerve: case report with magnetic resonance imaging correlation. Neurosurgery 1994; 35:127–132.

7. Mattern WC, Blattner RE, Werth J, et al. Eighth nerve lipoma: case report. J Neurosurg 1980;53:397–400.

8. Olson JE, Glasscock ME III, Britton BH: Lipomas of the internal auditory canal. Arch Otolaryngol 1978;104:431–436.

9. Paletta FX, Senay LC Jr. Lipofibromatous hamartoma of median nerve and ulnar nerve: surgical treatment. Plast Reconstr Surg 1981;68:915–921.

10. Price AJ, Compson JP, Calonje E. Fibrolipomatous hamartoma of nerve arising in the brachial plexus. J Hand Surg 1995;1:16–18.

11. Scheithauer BW, Woodruff JM, Erlandson RA. Hamartoma and choristoma. In Rosai J, Sobin LH (eds). Atlas of Tumor Pathology: Tumors of the Peripheral Nervous System. Series 3. Washington, DC: Armed Forces Institute of Pathology, 2000, pp 95–104.

12. Silverman TA, Enzinger FM. Fibrolipomatous hamartoma of nerve: a clinicopathologic analysis of 26 cases. Am J Surg Pathol 1985;9:7–14.

13. Terzis JK, Daniel RK, Williams HB, Spencer PS. Benign fatty tumors of the peripheral nerves. Ann Plast Surg 1978;1:193–216.

### Neuromuscular Choristoma

1. Boman F, Palan C, Floquet A, et al. Neuromuscular hamartoma. Ann Pathol 1991;11:36–41.

2. Bonneau R, Brochu P. Neuromuscular choristoma: a clinicopathologic study of two cases. Am J Surg Pathol 1983;7:521–528.

3. Chapon F, Hubert P, Mandard JC, et al. Spinal lipoma associated with a neuromuscular hamartoma: report of one case. Ann Pathol 1991;11:345–348.

4. Kusuzaki K, Emoto K, Murata H, et al. Nerve contact with muscle component in neuromuscular hamartoma. Anticancer Res 2000;20:3807–3811.

5. Louhimo I, Rapola J. Intraneural muscular hamartoma: a report of two cases in small children. J Pediatr Surg 1972;7:696–699.

6. Markel SF, Enzinger FM. Neuromuscular hamartoma—a benign "triton tumor" composed of mature neural and striated muscle elements. Cancer 1982;49:140–144.

7. Masson P. Tumeurs Humaines. Paris: Librairie Maloine, 1956, pp 973–975.

8. Mitchell A, Scheithauer BW, Ostertag H, et al. Neuromuscular choristoma. Am J Clin Pathol 1995;103:460–465.

9. Orlandi E. A case of rhabdomyoma of the sciatic nerve. Arch Sci Med 1895;19:113–37.

10. Van Dorpe JV, Sciot R, De Vos R, et al. Neuromuscular choristoma (hamartoma) with smooth and striated muscle component: case report with immunohistochemical and ultrastructural analysis. Am J Surg Pathol 1997;9:1090–1095.

11. Zak FG, Lawson W. An anatomic curiosity: intraneural striated muscle fibers in the human larynx. J Laryngol Otol 1975;89:199–201.

12. Zwick DL, Livingston K, Clapp L, et al. Intracranial trigeminal nerve rhabdomyoma/choristoma in a child: a case report and discussion of possible histogenesis. Hum Pathol 1989;20:390–392.

## Schwannoma Variants

1. Abernathy CD, Onofrio BM, Scheithauer BW, et al. Surgical management of giant sacral schwannomas. J Neurosurg 1986;65:286–295.
2. Akimoto J, Ito H, Kudo M. Primary intracranial malignant schwannoma of trigeminal nerve: a case report with review of the literature. Acta Neurochir (Wien) 2000;142:591–595.
3. Argenyi ZB, Balogh K, Abraham AA. Degenerative (ancient) changes in benign cutaneous schwannoma—a light-microscopic, histochemical and immunohistochemical study. J Cutan Pathol 1993;20:148–153.
4. Carney JA, Gordon H, Carpenter PC, et al. The complex of myxomas, spotty pigmentation, and endocrine overactivity. Medicine (Baltimore) 1985;64:270–283.
5. Carney JA. Psammomatous melanotic schwannoma: a distinctive, heritable tumor with special associations, including cardiac myxoma and the Cushing syndrome. Am J Surg Pathol 1990;14:206–222.
6. Casadei GP, Komori T, Scheithauer BW, et al. Intracranial parenchymal schwannoma. J Neurosurg 1993;79:217–222.
7. Casadei GP, Scheithauer BW, Hirose T, et al. Cellular schwannoma: a clinicopathologic, DNA flow cytometric, and proliferation marker study of 70 patients. Cancer 1995;75:1109–1119.
8. Cokelaere K, Sciot R, Geboes K. Esophageal plexiform schwannoma. Int J Surg Pathol 2000;8:353–357.
9. Dahl I. Ancient neurilemmoma (schwannoma). Acta Pathol Microbiol Scand 1977;85:812–818.
10. Dickersin GR. The electron microscopic spectrum of nerve sheath tumors. Ultrastruct Pathol 1987;11:103–146.
11. Enzinger FM, Weiss SW. Benign tumors of peripheral nerves. In Soft Tissue Tumors. 3rd ed. St. Louis: CV Mosby, 1995, pp 829–843.
12. Erlandson RA, Woodruff JM. Peripheral nerve sheath tumors: an electron microscopic study of 43 cases. Cancer 1982;49:273–287.
13. Ferry JA, Dickersin GR. Pseudoglandular schwannoma. Am J Clin Pathol 1988;89:546–552.
14. Fletcher CDM, Davies SE, McKee PH. Cellular schwannoma: a distinct pseudosarcomatous entity. Histopathology 1987;11:21–35.
15. Font RL, Truong LD. Melanotic schwannoma of soft tissues: electron-microscopic observations and review of literature. Am J Surg Pathol 1984;8:129–138.
16. Gould VE, Moll R, Moll I, et al. The intermediate filament complement of the spectrum of nerve sheath neoplasms. Lab Invest 1986;55:463–474.
17. Hasegawa SL, Mentzel T, Fletcher CDM. Schwannomas of the sinonasal tract and nasopharynx. Mod Pathol 1997;10:777–784.
18. Hirose T, Scheithauer BW, Sano T. Giant plexiform schwannomas: report of two cases with soft tissue and visceral involvement. Mod Pathol 1997;11:1075–1081.
19. Ishida T, Kuroda M, Motoi T, et al. Phenotypic diversity of neurofibromatosis 2: association with plexiform schwannoma. Histopathology 1998;32:264–270.
20. Ishii N, Sawamura Y, Tada M, Abe H. Acoustic cellular schwannoma invading the petrous bone: case report. Neurosurgery 1996;38:576–578.
21. Iwashita T, Enjoji M. Plexiform neurilemoma: a clinicopathological and immunohistochemical analysis of 23 tumours from 20 patients. Virchows Arch A 1987;411:305–309.
22. Johnson MD, Glick AD, Davis BW. Immunohistochemical evaluation of Leu-7, myelin basic-protein, S100-protein, glial-fibrillary acidic-protein, and LN3 immunoreactivity in nerve sheath tumors and sarcomas. Arch Pathol Lab Med 1988;112:155–160.
23. Kao GF, Laskin WB, Olsen TG. Solitary cutaneous plexiform neurilemmoma (schwannoma): a clinicopathologic, immunohistochemical, and ultrastructural study of 11 cases. Mod Pathol 1989;2:22–26.
24. Kawahara E, Oda Y, Ooi A, et al. Expression of glial fibrillary acidic protein (GFAP) in peripheral nerve sheath tumors. Am J Surg Pathol 1988;12:115–120.
25. Killeen RM, Davy GL, Bauserman SC. Melanocytic schwannoma. Cancer 1988;62:174–183.
26. Kirschner LS, Sandrini F, Monbo J, et al. Genetic heterogeneity and spectrum of mutations of the PRKAR1A gene in patients with Carney complex. Hum Mol Genet 2000;9:3037–3046.
27. Lodding P, Kindblom LG, Angervall L, Stenman G. Cellular schwannoma: a clinicopathologic study of 29 cases. Virchows Arch Pathol Anat Histopathol 1990;416:237–248.
28. MacCollin M, Ramesh V, Jacoby LB, et al. Mutational analysis of patients with neurofibromatosis 2. Am J Hum Genet 1994;55:314–320.
29. MacCollin M, Woodfin W, Kronn D, Short MP. Schwannomatosis: a clinical and pathologic study. Neurology 1996;36:1072–1079.
30. Memoli VA, Brown EF, Gould VE. Glial fibrillary acidic protein (GFAP) immunoreactivity in peripheral nerve sheath tumors. Ultrastruct Pathol 1984;7:269–275.
31. Mertens F, Dal Cin P, De Wever I, et al. Cytogenetic characterization of peripheral nerve sheath tumors: a report of the CHAMP study group. J Pathol 2000;190:31–38.
32. Mikami Y, Hidaka T, Akisada T, et al. Malignant peripheral nerve sheath tumor arising in benign ancient schwannoma: a case report with an immunohistochemical study. Pathol Int 2000;50:156–161.
33. Ramsey HJ. Fibrous long-spacing collagen in tumors of the nervous system. J Neuropathol Exp Neurol 1965;24:40–48.
34. Robey SS, deMent SH, Eaton KK, Aoun H. Malignant epithelioid peripheral nerve sheath tumor arising in a benign schwannoma. Surg Neurol 1987;28:441–446.
35. Scheithauer BW, Woodruf JW, Erlandson RA. Schwannoma. In Rosai J, Sobin LH (eds). Atlas of Tumor Pathology: Tumors of the Peripheral Nervous System. Series 3. Washington, DC: Armed Forces Institute of Pathology, 2000, pp 105–176.
36. Shore-Freedman E, Abrahams C, Recant W, Schneider AB. Neurilemomas and salivary gland tumors of the head and neck following childhood irradiation. Cancer 1983;51:2159–2163.
37. Sian CS, Ryan SF. The ultrastructure of neurilemoma with emphasis on Antoni B tissue. Hum Pathol 1981;12:145–160.
38. Tomita K, Mori K, Miyajima Y, Nakashima T. Plexiform schwannoma of the neck extending deeply to the mediastinum. Acta Otolaryngol 1998;539:106–109.
39. White W, Shiu MH, Rosenblum M, Woodruff JM. Cellular schwannoma: a clinicopathologic study of 52 cases. Cancer 1990;66:1266–1275.
40. Woodruff JM, Godwin TA, Erlandson RA, et al. Cellular schwannoma: a variety of schwannoma sometimes mistaken for a malignant tumor. Am J Surg Pathol 1981;5:733–744.
41. Woodruff JM, Marshall ML, Godwin TA, et al. Plexiform (multinodular) schwannoma: a tumor simulating the plexiform neurofibroma. Am J Surg Pathol 1983;7:691–697.
42. Woodruff JM, Selig AM, Crowley K, Allen PW. Schwannoma (neurilemoma) with malignant transformation a rare, distinctive peripheral-nerve tumor. Am J Surg Pathol 1994;18:882–895.
43. Yousem SA, Colby TV, Urich H. Malignant epithelioid schwannoma arising in a benign schwannoma: a case report. Cancer 1985;55:2799–2803.

## Neurofibroma

1. Bhargava R, Parham DM, Lasater OE, et al. MR imaging differentiation of benign and malignant peripheral nerve sheath tumors: use of the target sign. Pediatr Radiol 1997;27:124–129.
2. Bird CC, Willis RA. The histogenesis of pigmented neurofibromas. J Pathol 1969;97:631–637.
3. Chanoki M, Ishii M, Fukai K, et al. Immunohistochemical localization to type I, III, IV, V, and IV collagens and laminin in neurofibroma and neurofibrosarcoma. Am J Dermatol 1991;13:365–373.
4. Cheng L, Scheithauer BW, Leibovich BC, et al. Neurofibroma of the urinary bladder. Cancer 1999;86:505–513.
5. Dickersin GR. The electron microscopic spectrum of nerve sheath tumors. Ultrastruct Pathol 1987;11:103–146.
6. Enzinger FM, Weiss SW. Soft Tissue Tumors. 2nd ed. St. Louis: CV Mosby, 1988, p 725.
7. Erlandson RA, Woodruff JM. Peripheral nerve sheath tumors: an electron microscopic study of 43 cases. Cancer 1982;49:273–287.
8. Fetsch JF, Michal M, Miettinen M. Pigmented (melanotic) neurofibroma: a clinicopathologic and immunohistochemical analysis of 19 lesions from 17 patients. Am J Surg Pathol 2000;24:331–343.
9. Fuller CE, Williams GT. Gastrointestinal manifestations of type 1 neurofibromatosis (von Recklinghausen's disease). Histopathology 1991;19:1–11.
10. Gould VE, Moll R, Moll I, et al. The intermediate filament complement of the spectrum of nerve sheath neoplasms. Lab Invest 1986;55:463–474.

11. Halling KC, Scheithauer BW, Halling AC, et al. p53 Expression in neurofibroma and malignant peripheral nerve sheath tumor: an immunohistochemical study of sporadic and NF-1 associated tumors. Am J Clin Pathol 1996;106:282–288.

12. Harkin JC, Reed RJ. Tumors of the Peripheral Nervous System. Washington, DC: Armed Forces Institute of Pathology, 1969, p 51.

13. Hirose T, Sano T, Hizawa K. Ultrastructural localization of S-100 protein in neurofibroma. Acta Neuropathol (Berl) 1986;69:103–110.

14. Johnson MD, Glick AD, Davis BW. Immunohistochemical evaluation of Leu-7, myelin basic-protein, S100-protein, glial-fibrillary acidic-protein, and LN3 immunoreactivity in nerve sheath tumors and sarcomas. Arch Pathol Lab Med 1988;112:155–160.

15. Kawahara E, Oda Y, Ooi A, et al. Expression of glial fibrillary acidic protein (GFAP) in peripheral nerve sheath tumors: a comparative study of immunoreactivity of GFAP, vimentin, S-100 protein, and neurofilament in 38 schwannomas and 18 neurofibromas. Am J Surg Pathol 1988;12:115–120.

16. Kluwe L, Friedrich RE, Mautner VF. Allelic loss of the NF1 gene in NF1-associated plexiform neurofibromas. Cancer Genet Cytogenet 1999;113:65–69.

17. McCarron KF, Goldblum JR. Plexiform neurofibroma with and without associated malignant peripheral nerve sheath tumor: a clinicopathologic and immunohistochemical analysis of 54 cases. Mod Pathol 1998;11:612–617.

18. Memoli VA, Brown EF, Gould VE. Glial fibrillary acidic protein (GFAP) immunoreactivity in peripheral nerve sheath tumors. Ultrastruct Pathol 1984;7:269–275.

19. Mertens F, Dal Cin P, De Wever I, et al. Cytogenetic characterization of peripheral nerve sheath tumours: a report of the CHAMP study group. J Pathol 2000;190:31–38.

20. Nakajima T, Watanabe S, Sato Y, et al. An immunoperoxidase study of S-100 protein distribution in normal and neoplastic tissues. Am J Surg Pathol 1982;6:715–727.

21. Payan MJ, Gambarelli D, Keller P, et al. Melanotic neurofibroma: a case report with ultrastructural study. Acta Neuropathol (Berl) 1986;69:148–152.

22. Perentes E, Nakagawa Y, Ross GW, et al. Expression of epithelial membrane antigen in perineurial cells and their derivatives: an immunohistochemical study with multiple markers. Acta Neuropathol (Berl) 1987;75:160–165.

23. Perry A, Roth KA, Banerjee R, et al. NF1 deletions in S-100 protein–positive and negative cells of sporadic and neurofibromatosis 1 (NF1)–associated plexiform neurofibromas and MPNSTs. Am J Pathol 2001;25:57–61.

24. Pleasure J, Geller SA. Neurofibromatosis in infancy presenting with congenital stridor. Am J Dis Child 1967;113:390–393.

25. Pung S, Hirsch EF. Plexiform neurofibromatosis of the heart and neck. Arch Pathol 1955;59:341–346.

26. Rawlings CE III, Wilkins RH, Cook WA, Burger PC. Segmental neurofibromatosis. Neurosurgery 1987;20:946–949.

27. Roth RR, Martines R, James WD. Segmental neurofibromatosis. Arch Dermatol 1987;123:917–920.

28. Scheithauer BW, Woodruff JW, Erlandson RA. Neurofibroma. In Rosai J, Sobin LH (eds): Atlas of Tumor Pathology: Tumors of the Peripheral Nervous System. Series 3. Washington, DC: Armed Forces Institute of Pathology, 2000, pp 177–218.

29. Schochet SS Jr, Barret DAH. Neurofibroma with aberrant tactile corpuscles. Acta Neuropathol (Berl) 1974;28:161–165.

30. Skuse GR, Kosciolek BA, Rowley PT. The neurofibroma in von Recklinghausen neurofibromatosis has a unicellular origin. Am J Hum Genet 1991;49:600–607.

31. Smith TW, Bhawan J. Tactile-like structures in neurofibromas: an ultrastructural study. Acta Neuropathol (Berl) 1980;50:233–236.

32. Weiss SW, Langloss JM, Enzinger FM. Value of S-100 protein in the diagnosis of soft tissue tumors with particular reference to benign and malignant Schwann cell tumors. Lab Invest 1983; 49:299–308.

33. Weiss SW, Nickoloff BJ. CD-34 is expressed by a distinctive cell population in peripheral nerve, nerve sheath tumors, and related lesions. Am J Surg Pathol 1993;17:1039–1045.

## Perineurioma

1. Anthony DC, Ward WA, McAlister JA, Scheithauer BW. Ultrastructural comparison of perineurioma ("localized hypertrophic neuropathy") and hereditary and hypertrophic neuropathy. J Neuropathol Exp Neurol 1990;49:296.

2. Aoki T, Hisaoka M, Hashimoto H, et al. Giant degenerative perineurial cell tumor. Skeletal Radiol 1996;25:757–761.

3. Ariza A, Bilbao JM, Rosai J. Immunohistochemical detection of epithelial membrane antigen in normal perineurial cells and perineurioma. Am J Surg Pathol 1988;12:678–683.

4. Bilbao JM, Khoury NJS, Hudson AR, Briggs SJ. Perineurioma (localized hypertrophic neuropathy). Arch Pathol Lab Med 1984;108:557–560.

5. Emory TS, Scheithauer BW, Hirose T, et al. Intraneural perineurioma: a clonal neoplasm associated with abnormalities of chromosome 22. Am J Clin Pathol 1995;103:696–704.

6. Fetch JF, Miettinen M. Sclerosing perineurioma. Am J Surg Pathol 1997;21:1433–1442.

7. Giannini C, Scheithauer BW, Cosgrove T, et al. Intraventricular perineurioma—case report. Neurosurgery 1998;43:1478–1481.

8. Giannini C, Scheithauer BW, Jenkins RB, et al. Soft tissue perineurioma: evidence for an abnormality of chromosome 22, criteria for diagnosis, and review of the literature. Am J Surg Pathol 1997;21:164–173.

9. Johnson PC, Kline DG. Localized hypertrophic neuropathy: possible focal perineurial barrier defect. Acta Neuropathol (Berl) 1989;77:514–518.

10. Landini G, Kitano M. Meningioma of the mandible. Cancer 1992;69:2917–2920.

11. Lazarus SS, Trombetta LD. Ultrastructural identification of a benign perineurial cell tumor. Cancer 1978;41:1823–1829.

12. Li D, Schauble B, Moll C, Fisch U. Intratemporal facial nerve perineurioma. Laryngoscope 1996;106:328–333.

13. Ohno T, Park P, Akai M, et al. Ultrastructural study of perineurioma. Ultrastruct Pathol 1988;12:495–504.

14. Peckham NH, O'Boynick PL, Meneses A, Kepes JJ. Hypertrophic mononeuropathy: a report of two cases and review of the literature. Arch Pathol Lab Med 1982;106:534–537.

15. Reed RJ, Harkin JC. Supplement to Tumors of the Peripheral Nervous System. Series 2. Fascicle 3 (Supplement). Washington, DC: Armed Forces Institute of Pathology, 1983, pp S15–S16.

16. Robson A, Calonje E. Perineurioma: a clinico-pathological analysis of eleven cases. J Pathol 2000;190:69A.

17. Scheithauer BW, Woodruff JM, Erlandson RA. Miscellaneous benign neurogenic tumors. In Rosai J, Sobin LH (eds): Atlas of Tumor Pathology: Tumors of the Peripheral Nervous System. Series 3. Washington, DC: Armed Forces Institute of Pathology, 2000, pp 219–282.

18. Stanton C, Perentes E, Phillips L, VandenBerg SR. The immunohistochemical demonstration of early perineurial change in the development of localized hypertrophic neuropathy. Hum Pathol 1988;19:1455–1457.

19. Tsang WY, Chan JK, Chow LT, Tse CC. Perineurioma: an uncommon soft tissue neoplasm distinct from localized hypertrophic neuropathy and neurofibroma. Am J Surg Pathol 1992;16: 756–763.

20. Val-Bernal JF, Hernando M, Garijo MF, Villa P. Renal perineurioma in childhood. Gen Diagn Pathol 1997;143:75–81.

## Granular Cell Tumor

1. Abenoza P, Sibley RK. Granular cell myoma and schwannoma: fine structural and immunohistochemical study. Ultrastruct Pathol 1987;11:19–28.

2. Alessi DM, Zimmerman MC. Granular cell tumors of the head and neck. Laryngoscope 1988;98:810–814.

3. Bodic O, Couderc JP, Guilliere P. Tumeur á cellules granulluses colique plurifocale. Ann Pathol 1992;12:130–134.

4. Buley ID, Gatter KC, Kelly PM, et al. Granular cell tumors revisited: an immunohistochemical and ultrastructural study. Histopathology 1988;12:263–274.

5. Carvalho GA, Lindeke A, Tatagiba M, et al. Cranial granular-cell tumor of the trigeminal nerve: case report. J Neurosurg 1994;81:795–798.

6. Clark HB, Minesky JJ, Agrawal D, Agrawal HC. Myelin basic protein and P2 protein are not immunohistochemical markers for Schwann cell neoplasms: a comparative study using antisera to S-100, P2, and myelin basic proteins. Am J Pathol 1985;121:96–101.

7. DeMay RM, Kay S. Granular cell tumor of the breast. Pathol Annu 1984;19:121–148.

8. Dingemans KP, Mooi WJ, van den Bergh Weeman MA. Angulate lysosomes. Ultrastruct Pathol 1983;5:113–122.

9. Filie AC, Lage JM, Azumi N. Immunoreactivity of S-100 protein, alpha-1 antitrypsin, and CD68 in adult and congenital granular cell tumors. Mod Pathol 1996;9:888–892.

10. Fisher ER, Wechsler H. Granular cell myoblastoma—a misnomer: electron microscopic and histochemical evidence concerning its Schwann cell derivation and nature (granular cell schwannoma). Cancer 1962;15:936–954.

11. Goldblum JR, Rice TW, Zuccaro G, Richter JE. Granular cell tumors of the esophagus: a clinical and pathologic study of 13 cases. Ann Thorac Surg 1996;62:860–865.

12. Kurtin PJ, Bonin DM. Immunohistochemical demonstration of the lysosome associated glycoprotein CD 68 (KP-1) in granular cell tumors and schwannomas. Hum Pathol 1994;25:1172–1178.

13. Lack EE, Worsham GF, Callihan MD, et al. Granular cell tumor: a clinicopathologic study of 110 patients. J Surg Oncol 1980;13:301–316.

14. Lee J, Bhawan J, Wax F, Farber J. Plexiform granular cell tumor: a report of two cases. Am J Dermatopathol 1994;16:537–541.

15. Martin RW, Nelder KH, Boyd AS, Coates PW. Multiple cutaneous granular cell tumors and neurofibromatosis in childhood. Arch Dermatol 1990;126:1051–1056.

16. Mazur MT, Shultz JJ, Myers JL. Granular cell tumor: immunohistochemical analysis of 21 benign tumors and one malignant tumor. Arch Pathol Lab Med 1990;114:692–696.

17. Miettinen M, Lehtonen E, Lehtola H, et al. Histogenesis of granular cell tumour—an immunohistochemical and ultrastructural study. J Pathol 1984;142:221–229.

18. Mukai M. Immunohistochemical localization of S-100 protein and peripheral nerve myelin proteins (P2 protein, P0 protein) in granular cell tumors. Am J Pathol 1983;112:139–146.

19. Ordonez NG, Mackay B. Granular cell tumor: a review of the pathology and histogenesis. Ultrastruct Pathol 1999;23:207–222.

20. Ordonez NG. Granular cell tumor: a review and update. Adv Anat Pathol 1999;6:186–203.

21. Peterson LJ. Granular cell tumor: review of the literature and report of a case. Oral Surg Oral Med Oral Pathol 1974;37:728–735.

22. Scheithauer BW, Woodruff JM, Erlandson RA. Miscellaneous benign neurogenic tumors. In Rosai J, Sobin LH (eds). Atlas of Tumor Pathology: Tumors of the Peripheral Nervous System. Series 3. Washington, DC: Armed Forces Institute of Pathology, 2000, pp 219–282.

23. Seo IS, Azarelli B, Warner TF, et al. Multiple visceral and cutaneous granular cell tumors: ultrastructural and immunocytochemical evidence of Schwann cell origin. Cancer 1984;53:2104–2110.

24. Shintaku M, Sasaki M. Angulate body cell: an immunohistochemical and ultrastructural study. Brain Tumor Pathol 1992;9:41–47.

25. Sobel HJ, Marquet E. Granular cells and granular cell lesions. Pathol Ann 1974;9:43–79.

26. Soini Y, Miettinen M. Widespread immunoreactivity for alpha-1-antichymotrypsin in different types of tumors. Am J Clin Pathol 1988;90:131–136.

27. te Boekhorst DS, Gerhards MF, van Gulik TM, Gouman DJ. Granular cell tumor at the hepatic duct confluence with mimicking Klatskin tumor—a report of two cases and degenerative arthritis review of the literature. Digest Surg 2000;17:299–303.

28. Vance SF III, Hudson RP Jr. Granular cell myoblastoma: clinicopathologic study of forty-two patients. Am J Clin Pathol 1969;33:208–211.

29. Wright BA, Jackson D. Neural tumors of the oral cavity, a review of the spectrum of benign and malignant oral tumors of the oral cavity and jaw. Oral Surg Oral Med Oral Pathol 1980;49:509–522.

### Ganglioneuroma

1. Aguirre P, Scully RE. Testosterone-secreting adrenal ganglioneuroma containing Leydig cells. Am J Surg Pathol 1983;7:699–705.

2. Balázs M. Mixed pheochromocytoma-ganglioneuroma producing catecholamines and various neuropeptides. Acta Med Scand 1988;224:403–408.

3. Becker H, Wirnsberger G, Ziervogel K, Hofler H. Immunohistochemical markers in ganglioneuroblastomas. Acta Histochem Suppl 1990;38:107–114.

4. Beer TW. Solitary ganglioneuroma of the rectum: report of two cases. J Clin Pathol 1992;45:353–355.

5. Bender BL, Ghatak NR. Light and electron microscopic observations on a ganglioneuroma. Acta Neuropathol (Berl) 1978;42:7–10.

6. Brady S, Lechan RM, Schwaitzberg SD, et al. Composite pheochromocytoma/ganglioneuroma of the adrenal gland associated with multiple endocrine neoplasia 2A: case report with immunohistochemical analysis. Am J Surg Pathol 1997;21:102–108.

7. Chetty R, Duhig JD. Bilateral pheochromocytoma-ganglioneuroma of the adrenal in type 1 neurofibromatosis. Am J Surg Pathol 1993;17:837–841.

8. Garvin JH Jr, Lack EE, Berenberg W, Frantz CN. Ganglioneuroma presenting with differentiated skeletal metastases: report of a case. Cancer 1984;54:357–360.

9. Graham DG. On the origin and significance of neuromelanin. Arch Pathol Lab Med 1979;103:359–362.

10. Johnson DC, Teleg M, Eberle RC. Simultaneous occurrence of a ganglioneuroma and a neurilemmoma of the vagus nerve: a case report. Otolaryngol Head Neck Surg 1981;89:75–76.

11. Kahn HJ, Baumal R, Thorner PS, Chan H. Binding of peanut agglutinin to neuroblastoms and ganglioneuromas: a marker for differentiation of neuroblasts into ganglion cells. Pediatr Pathol 1988;8:83–93.

12. Karcioglu Z, Someren A, Mathes SJ. Ectomesenchymoma: a malignant tumor of migratory neural crest (ectomesenchyme) remnants showing ganglionic, schwannian, melanocytic, and rhabdomyoblastic differentiation. Cancer 1977;39:2486–2496.

13. Keefe JF, Kobrine AI, Kempe LG. Primary ganglioneuroma of the posterior cranial fossa: case report. Mil Med 1976;141:115–116.

14. Kodet R, Kasthuri N, Marsden HB, et al. Gangliorhabdomyosarcoma: a histopathologic and immunohistochemical study of three cases. Histopathology 1986;10:181–193.

15. Lam KY, Lo CY. Composite pheochromocytoma-ganglioneuroma of the adrenal gland: an uncommon entity with distinctive clinicopathologic features. Endocr Pathol 1999;10:343–352.

16. Levy DI, Bucci MN, Weatherbee L, Chandler EF. Intradural extramedullary ganglioneuroma: case report and review of the literature. Surg Neurol 1992;37:216–218.

17. Lucas K, Gula MJ, Knisely AS, et al. Catecholamine metabolites in ganglioneuroma. Med Pediatr Oncol 1994;22:240–243.

18. Markaki S, Edwards C. Intrapulmonary ganglioneuroma: a case report. Arch Anat Cytol Pathol 1987;35:183–184.

19. Matsuda M, Nagashima K. Cytoplasmic tubular inclusion in ganglioneuroma. Acta Neuropathol (Berl) 1984;64:81–84.

20. Mendelsohn G, Eggleston JC, Olson JL, et al. Vasoactive intestinal peptide and its relationship to ganglion cell differentiation in neuroblastic tumors. Lab Invest 1979;41:144–149.

21. Moore PJ, Biggs PJ. Compound adrenal medullary tumor. South Med J 1995;88:475–478.

22. Nagashima F, Hayashi J, Araki Y, et al. Silent mixed ganglioneuroma/pheochromocytoma which produces vasoactive intestinal polypeptide. Int Med 1993;32:63–66.

23. Nassiri M, Ghazi C, Stivers JR, Nadji M. Ganglioneuroma of the prostate: a novel finding in neurofibromatosis. Arch Pathol Lab Med 1994;118:938–939.

24. Robertson CM, Tyrrell JC, Pritchard J. Familial neural crest tumours. Eur J Pediatr 1991;150:789–792.

25. Sasaki A, Ogawa A, Nakazato Y, et al. Distribution of neurofilament protein and neuron-specific enolase in peripheral neuronal tumors. Virchows Arch Pathol Anat 1985;407:33–41.

26. Scheithauer BW, Woodruff JW, Erlandson RA. Miscellaneous benign neurogenic tumors. In Rosai J, Sobin LH (eds). Atlas of Tumor Pathology: Tumors of the Peripheral Nervous System. Series 3. Washington, DC: Armed Forces Institute of Pathology, 2000, pp 259–277.

27. Shimada H, Chatten J, Newton WA Jr, et al. Histopathologic prognostic factors in neuroblastic tumors: definition of subtypes of ganglioneuroblastoma and an age-linked classification of neuroblastomas. J Natl Cancer Inst 1984;73:405–416.

28. Shotton JC, Milton CM, Allen JP. Multiple ganglioneuroma of the neck. J Laryngol Otol 1992;106:277–278.

29. Stout AP. Ganglioneuroma of the sympathetic nervous system. Surg Gynecol Obstet 1947;84:101–110.

30. Trojanowski JQ, Molenaar WM, Baker DL, et al. Neural and neuroendocrine phenotype of neuroblastomas, ganglioneuroblastomas, ganglioneuromas and mature versus embryonic human adrenal medullary cells. Prog Clin Biol Res 1991;366:335–341.

31. Trump DL, Livingston JN, Baylin SB. Watery diarrhea syndrome in an adult with ganglioneuroma-pheochromocytoma:

identification of vasoactive intestinal peptide, calcitonin, and catecholamines and assessment of their biologic activity. Cancer 1977; 40:1526–1532.

32. Wogg JJ, Albert DM, Craft J, et al. Choroidal ganglioneuroma in neurofibromatosis. Graefes Arch Clin Exp Ophthalmol 1983; 220:25–31.

33. Wyman HE, Chappell BS, Jones WR Jr. Ganglioneuroma of bladder: report of case. J Urol 1950;63:526–532.

34. Yoshimi N, Tanaka T, Hara A, et al. Extra-adrenal pheochromocytoma-ganglioneuroma: a case report. Pathol Res Pract 1992; 188:1098–1100.

35. Zarabi M, LaBach JP. Ganglioneuroma causing acute appendicitis. Hum Pathol 1982;13:1143–1146.

## Malignant Peripheral Nerve Sheath Tumors

1. Akimoto J, Ito H, Kudo M. Primary intracranial malignant schwannoma of trigeminal nerve: a case report with review of the literature. Acta Neurochir (Wien) 2000;142:591–595.

2. Axiotis CA, Merino MJ, Tsokos M, Yang JJ. Epithelioid malignant peripheral nerve sheath tumor with squamous differentiation: a light microscopic, ultrastructural, and immunohistochemical study. Surg Pathol 1990;3:301–308.

3. Chanoki M, Ishii M, Fukai K, et al. Immunohistochemical localization of type I, II, III, IV, V, and VI collagens and laminin in neurofibroma and neurofibrosarcoma. Am J Dermatol 1991;13: 365–373.

4. Daimaru Y, Hashimoto H, Enjoji M. Malignant peripheral nerve sheath tumors (malignant schwannomas): an immunohistochemical study of 29 cases. Am J Surg Pathol 1985;9:434–444.

5. DiCarlo EF, Woodruff JM, Bansal M, Erlandson RA. The purely epithelioid malignant peripheral nerve sheath tumor. Am J Surg Pathol 1986;10:478–490.

6. Dickersin GR. The electron microscopic spectrum of nerve sheath tumors. Ultrastruct Pathol 1987;11:103–146.

7. Ducatman BS, Scheithauer BW, Piepgras DG, et al. Malignant peripheral nerve sheath tumor: a clinicopathologic study of 120 cases. Cancer 1986;57:2006–2021.

8. Ducatman BS, Scheithauer BW, Piepgras DG, Reiman HM. Malignant peripheral nerve sheath tumors in childhood. J Neurooncol 1984;2:241–248.

9. Ducatman BS, Scheithauer BW. Post-irradiation neurofibrosarcoma. Cancer 1983;51:1028–1033.

10. Enzinger FM, Weiss SW. Malignant tumors of the peripheral nerves. In Soft Tissue Tumors. 3rd ed. St. Louis: CV Mosby, 1995, pp 889–928.

11. Erlandson RA, Woodruff JM. Peripheral nerve sheath tumors: an electron microscopic study of 43 cases. Cancer 1982;49:273–287.

12. Foley KM, Woodruff JM, Ellis FT, Posner J. Radiation induced malignant and atypical PNST. Ann Neurol 1980;7:311–318.

13. Gennatas CS, Exarhakos G, Kondi-Pafiti A, et al. Malignant schwannoma of the stomach in a patient with neurofibromatosis. Eur J Surg Oncol 1988;14:251–254.

14. Ghrist TD. Gastrointestinal involvement in neurofibromatosis. Arch Intern Med 1963;112:357–362.

15. Gray MH, Rosenberg AE, Dickersin GR, Bhan AK. Glial fibrillary acidic protein and keratin expression by benign and malignant nerve sheath tumors. Hum Pathol 1989;20:1089–1096.

16. Halling KC, Scheithauer BW, Halling AC, et al. p53 Expression in neurofibroma and malignant peripheral nerve sheath tumor: an immunohistochemical study of sporadic NF-1 associated tumors. Am J Clin Pathol 1996;106:282–288.

17. Han DH, Kim DG, Chi JG, et al. Malignant triton tumor of the acoustic nerve: case report. J Neurosurg 1992;76:874–877.

18. Herrera GA, Pinto de Moraes H. Neurogenic sarcoma in patients with neurofibromatosis (von Recklinghausen's disease): light, electron microscopy, and immunohistochemistry study. Virchows Arch A 1984;403:361–376.

19. Hirose T, Hasegawa T, Kudo E. Malignant peripheral nerve sheath tumors: an immunohistochemical study in relation to ultrastructural features. Hum Pathol 1992;23:865–870.

20. Hirose T, Sano T, Hizawa K. Heterogeneity of malignant schwannomas. Ultrastruct Pathol 1988;12:107–116.

21. Hirose T, Scheithauer BW, Sano T. Perineurial malignant peripheral nerve sheath tumor: a clinicopathologic, immunohistochemical and ultrastructural study of seven cases. Am J Surg Pathol 1998;22:1368–1373.

22. Hirose T, Sumitomo M, Kudo E, et al. Malignant peripheral nerve sheath tumor (MPNST) showing perineurial cell differentiation. Am J Surg Pathol 1989;13:613–620.

23. Hruban RH, Shiu MH, Senie RT, Woodruff JM. Malignant peripheral nerve sheath tumors of the buttock and lower extremity: a study of 43 cases. Cancer 1990;66:1253–1265.

24. Jhanwar SC, Chen Q, Li FP, et al. Cytogenetic analysis of soft tissue sarcomas: recurrent chromosome abnormalities in malignant peripheral nerve sheath tumors (MPNST). Cancer Genet Cytogenet 1994;78:138–144.

25. Johnson TL, Lee MW, Meis JM, et al. Immunohistochemical characterization of malignant peripheral nerve sheath tumors. Surg Pathol 1991;4:121–135.

26. Karaki S, Mochida J, Lee YH, et al. Low-grade malignant perineurioma of the paravertebral column, transforming into a high-grade malignancy. Pathol Int 1999;49:820–825.

27. Kourea HP, Bilsky MH, Leung DH, et al. Subdiaphragmatic and intrathoracic paraspinal malignant peripheral nerve sheath tumor: a clinicopathologic study of 25 patients and 26 tumors. Am J Cancer 1998;82:2191–2203.

28. Laskin WB, Weiss SW, Brathauer GL. Epithelioid variant of malignant peripheral nerve sheath tumor (malignant epithelioid schwannoma). Am J Surg Pathol 1991;15:1136–1145.

29. Leslie MD, Cheung KY. Malignant transformation of neurofibromas at multiple sites in a case of neurofibromatosis. Postgrad Med J 1987;63:131–133.

30. Levy D, Khatib R. Intestinal neurofibromatosis with malignant degeneration: report of a case. Dis Colon Rectum 1960;3:140–144.

31. Lewis JJ, Brennan MR. Soft tissue sarcomas. Curr Probl Surg 1996;33:817–872.

32. McCarron KF, Goldblum JR. Plexiform neurofibroma with and without associated malignant peripheral nerve sheath tumor: a clinicopathologic and immunohistochemical analysis of 54 cases (Abstract). Mod Pathol 1997;10:11A.

33. McLean CA, Laidlaw JD, Brownbill DS, Gonzales MF. Recurrence of acoustic neurilemmoma as a malignant spindle-cell neoplasm: case report. J Neurosurg 1990;73:946–950.

34. McMenamin ME, Fletcher CDM. Expanding the spectrum of malignant change in schwannomas—epithelioid malignant change, epithelioid malignant peripheral nerve sheath tumor, and epithelioid angiosarcoma: a study of 17 cases. Am J Surg Pathol 2001;25:13–25.

35. Meis JM, Enzinger FM, Martz KL, Neal JA. Malignant peripheral nerve sheath tumors (malignant schwannomas) in children. Am J Surg Pathol 1992;16:694–707.

36. Menon AG, Anderson KM, Riccardi VM, et al. Chromosome 17p depletions and p53 gene mutations associated with the formation of malignant neurofibrosarcoma in von Recklinghausen neurofibromatosis. Proc Natl Acad Sci 1990;87:5435–5439.

37. Mertens F, Dal Cin P, De Wever I, et al. Cytogenetic characterization of peripheral nerve sheath tumours: a report of the CHAMP study group. J Pathol 2000;190:31–38.

38. Mertens F, Rydholm A, Bauer HF, et al. Cytogenetic findings in malignant peripheral nerve sheath tumors. Int J Cancer 1995;61: 793–798.

39. Miettinen M, Saari A. Pheochromocytoma combined with malignant schwannoma: unusual neoplasm of the adrenal medulla. Ultrastruct Pathol 1988;12:513–527.

40. Mikami Y, Hidaka T, Akisada T, et al. Malignant peripheral nerve sheath tumor arising in benign ancient schwannoma: a case report with an immunohistochemical study. Pathol Int 2000;50:156–161.

41. Min KW, Clemens A, Bell J, Dick H. Malignant peripheral nerve sheath tumor and pheochromocytoma: a composite tumor of the adrenal. Arch Pathol Lab Med 1988;112:266–270.

42. Mrak RE, Flanigan S, Collins CL. Malignant acoustic schwannoma. Arch Pathol Lab Med 1994;118:557–561.

43. Nagasaka T, Lai R, Sone M, et al. Glandular malignant peripheral nerve sheath tumor—an unusual case showing histologically malignant glands. Arch Pathol Lab Med 2000;124:1364–1368.

44. Navarro O, Nunez-Santos E, Daneman A, et al. Malignant peripheral nerve-sheath tumor arising in a previously irradiated neuroblastoma: report of 2 cases and a review of the literature. Pediatr Radiol 2000;30:176–180.

45. Ogawa K, Oguchi M, Yamabe H, et al. Distribution of collagen type IV in soft tissue tumors: an immunohistochemical study. Cancer 1986;58:269–277.

46. Ordonez NG, Mahfouz SM, Mackay B. Synovial sarcoma: an immunohistochemical and ultrastructural study. Hum Pathol 1990; 21:733–749.
47. Ramalingam P, Hoschar A, Barr F, et al. A clinical, morphologic and molecular genetic analysis of 33 cases of malignant peripheral nerve sheath tumor (MPNST). Mod Pathol 2001;14:81.
48. Riccardi VM, Elder DW. Multiple cytogenetic aberrations in neurofibrosarcomas complicating neurofibromatosis. Cancer Genet Cytogenet 1986;23:199–209.
49. Ricci A Jr, Parham DW, Woodruff JM, et al. Malignant peripheral nerve sheath tumors arising from ganglioneuromas. Am J Surg Pathol 1984;8:19–29.
50. Ruckert RI, Fleige B, Rogalla P, Woodruff JM. Schwannoma with angiosarcoma—report of a case and comparison with other types of nerve tumors with angiosarcoma. Cancer 2000;89:1577–1585.
51. Sakaguchi N, Sano K, Makoto I, et al. A case of von Recklinghausen's disease with bilateral pheochromocytoma—malignant peripheral nerve sheath tumors of the adrenal and gastrointestinal autonomic nerve tumors. Am J Surg Pathol 1996; 20:889–897.
52. Scheithauer BW, Woodruf JW, Erlandson RA. Primary malignant tumors of peripheral nerve. In Rosai J, Sobin LH (eds). Atlas of Tumor Pathology: Tumors of the Peripheral Nervous System. Series 3. Washington, DC: Armed Forces Institute of Pathology, 2000, pp 303–372.
53. Schmidt H, Taubert H, Meye A, et al. Gains in chromosomes 7, 8q, 15q and 17q are characteristic changes in malignant but not in benign peripheral nerve sheath tumors from patients with Recklinghausen's disease. Cancer Lett 2000;155:181–190.
54. Sorenson SA, Mulvihill JJ, Nielsen A. Long-term follow-up of von Recklinghausen neurofibromatosis: survival and malignant neoplasms. N Engl J Med 1986;314:1010–1015.
55. Stefanko SZ, Vuzevski VD, Maas AI, Van Vroonhoven CC. Intracerebral malignant schwannoma. Acta Neuropathol (Berl) 1986;71:321–325.
56. Storm FK, Eilber FR, Mirra J, Morton DL. Neurofibrosarcoma. Cancer 1980;45:126–129.
57. Swanson PE, Scheithauer BW, Wick MR. Peripheral nerve sheath neoplasms: clinicopathologic and immunochemical observations. In Rosen PP, Fechner RE (eds). Pathology Annual. Stanford, CT: Appleton and Lange, 1995, pp 1–82.
58. Takahashi Y, Sugita Y, Abe T, et al. Intraventricular malignant triton tumor. Acta Neurochir (Wien) 2000;142:473–476.
59. Taxy JB, Battifora H, Trujillo Y, Dorfman HD. Electron microscopy in the diagnosis of malignant schwannoma. Cancer 1981;48:1381–1391.
60. Taxy JB, Battifora H. Epithelioid schwannoma: diagnosis by electron microscopy. Ultrastruct Pathol 1981;2:19–24.
61. Thomas J, Piepgras DG, Scheithauer BW, et al. Neurogenic tumors of the sciatic nerve: a clinicopathologic study of 35 cases. Mayo Clin Proc 1983;58:640–647.
62. Weiss SW, Langloss JM, Enzinger FM. Value of S-100 protein in the diagnosis of soft tissue tumors with particular reference to benign and malignant Schwann cell tumors. Lab Invest 1983; 49:299–308.
63. Wick MR, Swanson PE, Scheithauer BW, Manivel JC. Malignant peripheral nerve sheath tumor: an immunohistochemical study of 62 cases. Am J Clin Pathol 1987;87:425–433.
64. Wong WM, Hirose T, Scheithauer BW, et al. Malignant peripheral nerve sheath tumor: analysis of treatment outcome. Int J Radiat Oncol Biol Phys 1998;42:351–360.
65. Woodruff JM, Chernik N, Smith M, et al. Peripheral nerve tumors with rhabdomyosarcomatous differentiation (malignant "triton" tumors). Cancer 1973;32:426–439.
66. Woodruff JM, Christensen WN. Glandular peripheral nerve sheath tumors. Cancer 1993;72:3618–3628.
67. Woodruff JM, Perino G. Non–germ cell or teratomatous malignant tumors showing additional rhabdomyoblastic differentiation, with emphasis on the malignant triton tumor. Semin Diagn Surg Pathol 1994;11:69–81.
68. Woodruff JM, Selig AM, Crowley K, Allen PW. Schwannoma (neurilemoma) with malignant transformation a rare, distinctive peripheral-nerve tumor. Am J Surg Pathol 1994;18:882–895.
69. Yamashiro S, Nagashiro S, Mimata C, et al. Malignant trigeminal schwannoma associated with xeroderma pigmentosum—case report. Neurol Med Chir (Tokyo) 1994;34:817–820.

**Primitive Neuroectodermal Tumor of Nerve**

1. Abe S, Imamura T, Park P, et al. Small round-cell type of malignant peripheral nerve sheath tumor. Mod Pathol 1998;11: 747–753.
2. Akeyson EW, McCutcheon IE, Pershouse MA, et al. Primitive neuroectodermal tumor of the median nerve—case report with cytogenetic analysis. J Neurosurg 1996;85:163–169.
3. Bolen JW, Thorning D. Peripheral neuroepithelioma: a light and electron microscopic study. Cancer 1980;46:2456–2462.
4. DiCarlo EF, Woodruff JM, Bansal M, Erlandson RA. The purely epithelioid malignant peripheral nerve sheath tumor. Am J Surg Pathol 1986;10:478–490.
5. Enzinger FM. Case twelve. In Proceedings of Forty-ninth Annual Anatomic Pathology Slide Seminar of the American Society of Clinical Pathologists. Chicago: ASCP, 1983, pp 90–96.
6. Folpe AL, Schmidt RA, Chapman D, Gown AM. Poorly differentiated synovial sarcoma—immunohistochemical distinction from primitive neuroectodermal tumors and high-grade malignant peripheral nerve sheath tumors. Am J Surg Pathol 1998;22: 673–682.
7. Harper PG, Pringle J, Souhami RL. Neuroepithelioma—a rare malignant peripheral nerve tumor of primitive origin: report of two new cases and a review of the literature. Cancer 1981;48: 2282–2287.
8. Marina NM, Etcubanas E, Parham DM, et al. Peripheral primitive neuroectodermal tumor (peripheral neuroepithelioma) in children: a review of the St. Jude's experience and controversies in diagnosis and management. Cancer 1989;64:1952–1960.
9. Nesbit KA, Vidone RA. Primitive neuroectodermal tumor (neuroblastoma) arising in sciatic nerve of a child. Cancer 1976;37: 1562–1570.
10. Scheithauer BW, Woodruf JW, Erlandson RA. Primary malignant tumors of peripheral nerve. In Rosai J, Sobin LH (eds). Atlas of Tumor Pathology: Tumors of the Peripheral Nervous System. Series 3. Washington, DC: Armed Forces Institute of Pathology, 2000, pp 303–372.
11. Stout AP, Murray MR. Neuroepithelioma of the radial nerve with a study of its behaviour in vitro. Rev Can de Biol 1942;1: 651–659.
12. Stout AP. A tumor of the ulnar nerve. Proc N Y Pathol Soc 1918; 18:2–11.
13. Stout AP. Tumors of the peripheral nerve system. In Atlas of Tumor Pathology. Series 1. Fascicle 6. Washington, DC: Armed Forces Institute of Pathology, 1949.
14. Whang-Peng J, Triche TJ, Knutset T, et al. Cytogenetic characterization of selected small round cell tumor of childhood. Cancer Genet Cytogenet 1986;21:185–208.

**Malignant Granular Cell Tumor**

1. Buley ID, Gatter KC, Kelly PMA, et al. Granular cell tumours revisited: an immunohistological and ultrastructural study. Histopathology 1988;12:263–274.
2. Dingemans KP, Mooi WJ, van den Bergh Weeman MA. Angulate lysosomes. Ultrastruct Pathol 1983;5:113–122.
3. Enzinger FM, Weiss SW. Soft Tissue Tumors. 2nd ed. St. Louis: CV Mosby, 1988, p 757.
4. Fanburg-Smith JC, Meis-Kindblom JM, Fante R, Kindblom LG. Malignant granular cell tumor of soft tissue: diagnostic criteria and clinicopathologic correlation. Am J Surg Pathol 1998;22: 779–794.
5. Gamboa LG. Malignant granular cell myoblastoma. Arch Pathol 1955;60:663–668.
6. Geisinger KR, Kawamoto EH, Marshall RB, et al. Aspiration exfoliative cytology including ultrastructure of a malignant granular-cell tumor. Acta Cytol 1985;29:593–597.
7. Harkin JC, Reed RJ. Atlas of Tumor Pathology. Series 2. Fascicle 3. Washington, DC: Armed Forces Institute of Pathology, 1969, p 156.
8. Kurtin PJ, Bonin DM. Immunohistochemical demonstration of the lysosome associated glycoprotein CD 68 (KP-1) in granular cell tumors and schwannomas. Hum Pathol 1994;25:1172–1178.
9. MacKenzie DH. Malignant granular cell myoblastoma. J Clin Pathol 1967;20:739–742.
10. Mazur MT, Shultz JJ, Myers JL. Granular cell tumor: immunohistochemical analysis of 21 benign tumors and one malignant tumor. Arch Pathol Lab Med 1990;114:692–696.

11. Miettinen M, Lehtonen E, Lehtola H, et al. Histogenesis of granular cell tumour—an immunohistochemical and ultrastructural study. J Pathol 1984;142:221–229.

12. Scheithauer BW, Woodruf JW, Erlandson RA. Primary malignant tumors of peripheral nerve. In Rosai J, Sobin LH (eds). Atlas of Tumor Pathology: Tumors of the Peripheral Nervous System. Series 3. Washington, DC: Armed Forces Institute of Pathology, 2000, pp 303–372.

13. Shimamura K, Osamura RY, Ueyama Y, et al. Malignant granular cell tumor of the right sciatic nerve. Cancer 1984;53:524–529.

14. Shintaku M, Sasaki M. Angulate body cell: an immunohistochemical and ultrastructural study. Brain Tumor Pathol 1992;9:41–47.

15. Usui M, Ishii S, Yamawaki S, et al. Malignant granular cell tumor of the radial nerve: an autopsy observation with electron microscopic and tissue culture studies. Cancer 1977;39:1547–1555.

## Metastatic Neoplasms

1. Ackerman AB, Godomski J. Neurotrophic malignant melanoma and other neurotrophic neoplasms in the skin. Am J Dermatopathol 1984;6:63–80.

2. Ballantyne AJ, McCarten AB, Ibanez ML. The extension of cancer of the head and neck through peripheral nerves. Am J Surg 1963;106:651–667.

3. Barber JR, Coventry MB, McDonald JR. Spread of soft tissue sarcoma of extremities along peripheral nerve trunks. J Bone Joint Surg 1957;39:534–540.

4. Carstens PH. Perineurial glands in normal and hyperplastic prostates. J Urol 1980;123:686–688.

5. Cavazza A, Asioli S, Martella EM, et al. Neural infiltration in benign gallbladder lesions: description of a case. Pathologica 1998;90:42–45.

6. Chambers PW, Davis RL, Buck FS. Metastases to primary intracranial meningiomas and neurilemomas. Arch Pathol Lab Med 1980;104:350–354.

7. Costa J. Benign epithelial inclusions in pancreatic nerves (Letter). Am J Clin Pathol 1977;67:306–307.

8. Dodd GD, Dolan PA, Ballantyne AJ, et al. The dissemination of tumors of the head and neck via the cranial nerves. Radiol Clin North Am 1970;8:445–461.

9. From L, Hanna W, Kahn HJ, et al. Origin of the desmoplasia in desmoplastic malignant melanoma. Hum Pathol 1983;14:1072–1080.

10. Longacre TA, Egbert BM, Rouse RV. Desmoplastic and spindle cell malignant melanoma: an immunohistochemical study. Am J Surg Pathol 1996;20:1489–1500.

11. Ni K, Dehner LP. Schwannoma with metastatic carcinoma of the breast: an unconventional form of glandular peripheral nerve sheath tumor. Hum Pathol 1995;26:457–459.

12. Reed RJ, Leonard DD. Neurotropic melanoma: a variant of desmoplastic melanoma. Am J Surg Pathol 1979;3:301–311.

13. Roncaroli F, Poppi M, Riccioni L, Frank F. Primary non-Hodgkin's lymphoma of the sciatic nerve followed by localization in the central nervous system: case report and review of the literature. Neurosurgery 1997;40:618–622.

14. Taylor HB, Norris JH. Epithelial invasion of nerves in benign diseases of the breast. Cancer 1967;20:2245–2249.

15. Warner TF, Ford CN, Hafez GR. Neurotropic melanoma of the face invading the maxillary nerve. J Cutan Pathol 1985;12:520–527.

16. Warner TF, Hafez GR, Finch RE, Brandenberg JH. Schwann cell features in neurotropic melanoma. J Cutan Pathol 1981;8:177–187.

17. Warner TF, Lloyd RC, Hafez GR, Angevine JM. Immunocytochemistry of neurotropic melanoma. Cancer 1984;53:254–257.

18. Zimmerman KG, Johnson PC, Paplanus SH. Nerve invasion by benign proliferating ductules in vasitis nodosa. Cancer 1983;51:2066–2069.

## Neurofibromatosis

1. Cheng L, Scheithauer BW, Leibovich BC, et al. Neurofibroma of the urinary bladder. Cancer 1999;86:505–513.

2. Eldridge R, Parry DM, Kaiser-Kupfer MI. Clinical heterogeneity and natural history based on 39 individuals in 9 families and 16 sporadic cases. Proceedings of the Eighth International Congress on Human Genetics. Am J Hum Genet 1991;49:133.

3. Gennatas CS, Exarhakos G, Kondi-Pafiti A, et al. Malignant

schwannoma of the stomach in a patient with neurofibromatosis. Eur J Surg Oncol 1988;14:261–264.

4. Ghrist TD. Gastrointestinal involvement in neurofibromatosis. Arch Intern Med 1963;112:357–362.

5. Gutmann DH, Collins FS. Neurofibromatosis type 1: beyond positional cloning. Arch Neurol 1993;50:1185–1193.

6. Halling KC, Scheithauer BW, Halling AC, et al. p53 Expression in neurofibroma and malignant peripheral nerve sheath tumor: an immunohistochemical study of sporadic and NF-1 associated tumors. Am J Clin Pathol 1996;106:282–288.

7. Halper J, Scheithauer BW, Okazaki H, Laws ER Jr. Meningo-angiomatosis: a report of six cases with special reference to the occurrence of neurofibrillary tangles. J Neuropathol Exp Neurol 1986;45:426–446.

8. Kanter WR, Eldridge R, Fabricant R, et al. Central neurofibromatosis with bilateral acoustic neuroma: genetic, clinical and biochemical distinctions from peripheral neurofibromatosis. Neurology 1980;30:851–859.

9. Kindblom LG, Remotti HE, Aldenborg F, Meis-Kindblom JM. Gastrointestinal pacemaker cell tumor (GIPACT): gastrointestinal stromal tumors show phenotypic characteristics of the interstitial cells of Cajal. Am J Pathol 1998;152:1259–1269.

10. Lauwers GY, Erlandson RA, Casper ES, et al. Gastrointestinal autonomic nerve tumors: a clinicopathological, immunohistochemical, and ultrastructural study of 12 cases. Am J Surg Pathol 1993;17:887–897.

11. Levy D, Khatib R. Intestinal neurofibromatosis with malignant degeneration: report of a case. Dis Colon Rectum 1960;3:140–144.

12. MacCollin M, Ramesh V, Jacoby LB, et al. Mutational analysis of patients with neurofibromatosis 2. Am J Hum Genet 1994;55:314–320.

13. MacCollin M, Woodfin W, Kronn D, Short MP. Schwannomatosis: a clinical and pathologic study. Neurology 1996;46:1072–1079.

14. Menon AG, Anderson KM, Riccardi VM, et al. Chromosome 17p deletions and p53 gene mutations associated with the formation of malignant neurofibrosarcoma in von Recklinghausen neurofibromatosis. Proc Natl Acad Sci 1990;87:5435–5439.

15. Perry A, Roth KA, Banerjee R, et al. NF1 deletions in S-100 protein–positive and negative cells of sporadic and neurofibromatosis 1 (NF1)–associated plexiform neurofibromas and MPNSTs. Am J Pathol 2001;25:57–61.

16. Rawlings CE III, Wilkins RH, Cook WA, Burger PC. Segmental neurofibromatosis. Neurosurgery 1987;20:946–949.

17. Riccardi VM, Lewis RA. Penetrance of von Recklinghausen neurofibromatosis: a distinction between predecessors and descendants. Am J Hum Genet 1988;24:284–289.

18. Riccardi VM. Neurofibromatosis: Phenotype, Natural History, and Pathogenesis. 2nd ed. Baltimore: Johns Hopkins University Press, 1992.

19. Riccardi VM. Neurofibromatosis: clinical heterogeneity. Curr Probl Cancer 1982;71:1–34.

20. Roth RR, Martines R, James WD. Segmental neurofibromatosis. Arch Dermatol 1987;123:917–920.

21. Rouleau GA, Wertelecki W, Haines JL, et al. Genetic linkage of bilateral acoustic neurofibromatosis to a DNA marker on chromosome 22. Nature 1987;329:246–248.

22. Seizinger BR, Rouleau GA, Ozelius LJ, et al. Genetic linkage of von Recklinghausen neurofibromatosis to the nerve growth factor receptor gene. Cell 1987;49:589–594.

23. Skuse GR, Kosciolek BA, Rowley PT. The neurofibroma in von Recklinghausen neurofibromatosis has a unicellular origin. Am J Hum Genet 1991;49:600–607.

24. Thomas PK, King RH, Chiang TR, et al. Neurofibromatosis neuropathy. Muscle Nerve 1990;13:93–101.

25. Verhest A, Heimann R, Verschraegen J, et al. Hereditary intestinal neurofibromatosis. II. Translocation between chromosomes 12 and 14. Neurofibromatosis 1988;1:33–36.

26. von Deimling A, Krone W, Menon AG. Neurofibromatosis type 1: pathology, clinical features and molecular genetics. Brain Pathol 1995;5:153–162.

27. Wertelecki W, Rouleau GA, Superneau DW, et al. Neurofibromatosis 2: clinical and DNA linkage studies of a large kindred. N Engl J Med 1988;319:278–283.

# INDEX

Note: **Boldface** type refers to main discussion. Page numbers followed by the letter f refer to figures; those followed by the letter t refer to tables.

**649**

ISBN 0-443-06506-3